Heart Disease in Women

Susan Wilansky, M.D.

Attending Cardiologist
Southern California Kaiser Permanente
Medical Group
Orange County, California

James T. Willerson, M.D.

Medical Director
Texas Heart Institute
Chief of Cardiology
St. Luke's Episcopal Hospital
Edward Randall III Chair in Internal Medicine
The University of Texas–Houston Medical School
Alkek-Williams Distinguished Professor
President
The University of Texas Health Science Center at Houston
Houston, Texas

CHURCHILL LIVINGSTONE
An Imprint of Elsevier Science
New York Edinburgh London Philadelphia

CHURCHILL LIVINGSTONE
An Imprint of Elsevier Science

The Curtis Center
Independence Square West
Philadelphia, Pennsylvania 19106

Library of Congress Cataloging-in-Publication Data

Heart disease in women / [editors]. Susan Wilansky, James T. Willerson.—1st ed.

p. cm.

ISBN 0–443–07900–5

1. Heart disease in women. I. Wilansky, Susan. II. Willerson, James T. III. Title.

RC682 .H3835 2002 616.1′2′0082—dc21

DNLM/DLC 2001017366

Acquisitions Editor: Emily Barrosse
Project Manager: Natalie Ware

HEART DISEASE IN WOMEN ISBN 0–443–07900–5

Printed in the United States of America.

Last digit is the print number: 9 8 7 6 5 4 3 2 1

DEDICATION

*We dedicate this book to our families,
our students, and our patients.*

CONTRIBUTORS

EZZAT I. ABOULEISH, M.D.
Professor Emeritus, The University of Texas–Houston Medical School; Anesthesiologist, Memorial Hermann Hospital, Houston, Texas
Chapter 26—Management of Valvular Heart Disease

REETA ACHARI, M.D.
Neurologist, Memorial Hermann Hospital; St. Luke's Episcopal Hospital; The Institute for Rehabilitation & Research, Houston, Texas
Chapter 22—Cerebrovascular Disease

KAROLINA ADAM, M.D.
Clinical Assistant Professor, Department of Obstetrics and Gynecology, Baylor College of Medicine, Houston, Texas
Chapter 26—Management of Valvular Heart Disease

CARINA M. ALFARO-FRANCO, M.D., F.A.C.C.
Assistant Clinical Professor of Medicine, Upstate Medical University; Attending Physician, St. Joseph's Hospital Health Center, Syracuse, New York
Chapter 9—Invasive Diagnostic Testing

JAMES K. ALEXANDER, M.D.
Professor of Medicine (Cardiology), Baylor College of Medicine; Staff Physician, Houston Veterans Administration Hospital, Houston, Texas
Chapter 6—Behavioral Barriers to Health; Chapter 33—Pulmonary Emboli

H. VERNON ANDERSON, M.D.
Professor of Medicine, The University of Texas–Houston Medical School, Houston, Texas
Chapter 3—Coronary Artery Disease: Overview; Chapter 5—Coronary Artery Disease: Risk Factors; Chapter 9—Invasive Diagnostic Testing

PAOLO ANGELINI, M.D.
Clinical Professor of Internal Medicine, Baylor College of Medicine; Senior Cardiologist, Texas Heart Institute and St. Luke's Episcopal Hospital, Houston, Texas
Chapter 11—Coronary Artery Disease: Therapy

FRANK C. ARNETT, M.D.
Professor and Chairman, Department of Internal Medicine, The University of Texas–Houston Medical School, The University of Texas Health Science Center at Houston; Chief, Medical Service, Memorial Hermann Hospital, Houston, Texas
Chapter 41—Collagen Vascular Disease: Pathophysiology, Clinical Recognition, Diagnosis, and Management

EDDY BARASCH, M.D.
Associate Professor of Medicine, The University of Texas–Houston Medical School; Director, Echocardiography Laboratory, Memorial Hermann Hospital, Houston, Texas
Chapter 8—Noninvasive Diagnostic Testing

MICHAEL A. BELFORT, M.B.B.CH., M.R.C.O.G., M.D., F.R.C.S., F.A.C.O.G.
Professor of Obstetrics and Gynecology, University of Utah Medical School, Salt Lake City; Director, Department of Maternal Fetal Medicine, Utah Valley Regional Medical Center, Provo, Utah
Chapter 27—Pregnancy: Hypertension; Chapter 28—Peripartum Cardiomyopathy

L. MAXIMILIAN BUJA, M.D.
Dean of the Medical School and Professor of Pathology and Laboratory Medicine, The University of Texas–Houston Medical School; Member of the Board of Directors and Staff Physician, Memorial Hermann Hospital System, Houston; Chief of Cardiovascular Pathology, Texas Heart Institute at St. Luke's Episcopal Hospital, Houston, Texas
Chapter 1—Cardiovascular System in Women: Anatomy; Chapter 4—Coronary Artery Disease: Anatomy, Overview

ALLEN P. BURKE, M.D.
Adjunct Professor of Pathology, Georgetown University; Associate Chair, Cardiovascular Pathology; Armed Forces Institute of Pathology, Washington, D.C.
Chapter 4—Coronary Artery Disease: Anatomy

JANICE L. B. BYRNE, M.D.
Associate Professor, Department of Obstetrics and Gynecology, University of Utah, Salt Lake City, Utah
Chapter 5—Coronary Artery Disease: Risk Factors

AGUSTIN CASTELLANOS, M.D.
Professor of Medicine, University of Miami School of Medicine; Director, Clinical Electrophysiology, University of Miami/Jackson Memorial Medical Center, Miami, Florida
Chapter 38—Sudden Cardiac Death

GRACE L. CHUA, M.D., F.A.C.C., F.R.C.P.C.
Staff Cardiologist, York Central Hospital, Toronto, Ontario, Canada
Chapter 18—Hypertrophic Cardiomyopathy

JACK M. COLMAN, M.D., F.R.C.P.C.
Assistant Professor of Medicine, University of Toronto; Attending Cardiologist, University of Toronto Congenital Cardiac Centre for Adults, Toronto General Hospital/ University Health Network and Mount Sinai Hospital, Toronto, Ontario, Canada
Chapter 24—Congenital Heart Disease: Pathophysiology, Clinical Recognition, Diagnosis, and Management

DENTON A. COOLEY, M.D.
President and Surgeon-in-Chief, Texas Heart Institute at St. Luke's Episcopal Hospital; Clinical Professor of Surgery, The University of Texas–Houston Medical School, Houston, Texas
Chapter 20—Aortic Diseases and Aortic Dissection

GERALD S. CYPRUS, M.D.
Professor of Medicine, Baylor College of Medicine; Associate Chief of Medicine, The Methodist Hospital; Medical Director, Baylor Internal Medicine Consultants, Houston, Texas
Chapter 2—Cardiovascular System in Women: Physiology; Chapter 32—Deep Vein Thrombosis

JAMIE DOUCET, M.D.
Cardiologist, Colorado Cardiovascular Center, Boulder, Colorado
Chapter 11—Coronary Artery Disease: Therapy

ANNE HAMILTON DOUGHERTY, M.D.
Professor of Medicine, The University of Texas–Houston Medical School; Attending Cardiologist, Memorial Hermann Hospital, Houston, Texas
Chapter 2—Cardiovascular System in Women: Physiology

KATHRYN DOUGHERTY, C.R.I.T., R.C.U.T.
Peripheral Vascular Research Assistant, St. Luke's Episcopal Hospital, Houston, Texas
Chapter 21—Peripheral Vascular Disease

ANDREW FARB, M.D.
Assistant Professor of Medicine and Pathology, Georgetown University; Staff Cardiovascular Pathologist, Armed Forces Institute of Pathology, Washington, D.C.
Chapter 4—Coronary Artery Disease: Anatomy

JOHN A. FARMER, M.D.
Associate Professor of Medicine, Baylor College of Medicine; Chief, Section of Cardiology, Ben Taub General Hospital, Houston, Texas
Chapter 5—Coronary Artery Disease: Risk Factors

O. H. FRAZIER, M.D.
Professor of Surgery, The University of Texas–Houston Medical School; Clinical Associate Professor of Surgery, Department of Thoracic Surgery, The University of Texas M.D. Anderson Cancer Center; Clinical Professor, Department of Surgery, Baylor College of Medicine; Chief of the Cardiopulmonary Transplant Service and Co-Director of the Cardiovascular Research Laboratories, Texas Heart Institute and St. Luke's Episcopal Hospital, Houston, Texas
Chapter 11—Coronary Artery Disease: Therapy; Chapter 16—Dilated Cardiomyopathy

HERBERT L. FRED, M.D.
Professor of Medicine, The University of Texas Health Science Center at Houston; Clinical Director, Department of Internal Medicine, Lyndon B. Johnson General Hospital, Houston, Texas
Chapter 33—Pulmonary Emboli

ADAANI E. FROST, M.D.
Professor of Medicine, Baylor College of Medicine; Medical Director, Lung Transplantation, The Methodist Hospital and St. Luke's Episcopal Hospital, Houston, Texas
Chapter 31—Primary Pulmonary Hypertension and Pregnancy; Chapter 40—Pulmonary Hypertension: Pathophysiology, Clinical Recognition, Diagnosis, and Management

JANE M. GERACI, M.D., M.P.H.
Assistant Professor of Medicine, Department of General Internal Medicine, Ambulatory Treatment & Emergency Care, Division of Internal Medicine, The University of Texas M.D. Anderson Cancer Center, Houston, Texas
Chapter 10—Coronary Artery Disease: Clinical Consequences

LARRY C. GILSTRAP III, M.D.
Professor and Chairman, Division of Maternal-Fetal Medicine, The University of Texas–Houston Medical School, Houston, Texas
Chapter 26—Management of Valvular Heart Disease; Chapter 27—Pregnancy: Hypertension

ANTONIO M. GOTTO, JR., M.D., D.PHIL.
The Stephen and Suzanne Weiss Dean, Professor of Medicine, Cornell University, Joan and Sanford I. Weill Medical College, New York, New York
Chapter 5—Coronary Artery Disease: Risk Factors

K. LANCE GOULD, M.D.
Martin Bucksbaum Distinguished University Chair, Professor and Director, Weatherhead P.E.T. Center for Preventing and Reversing Atherosclerosis, The University of Texas–Houston Medical School, Houston, Texas
Chapter 8—Noninvasive Diagnostic Testing

STEPHANIE GROSZ, M.D.
Associate Professor of Medicine, University of South Alabama; Clinical Electrophysiologist, Providence Hospital, Mobile Infirmary, Springhill Medical Center, and University of South Alabama Medical Center, Mobile, Alabama
Chapter 39—Neurally Mediated Syncopal Syndromes

RAMESH HARIHARAN, M.D., M.R.C.P. (UK)
Cardiology Fellow, Baylor College of Medicine; Cardiology Fellow, Texas Heart Institute and St. Luke's Episcopal Hospital, Houston, Texas
Chapter 33—Pulmonary Emboli

LOUISE HARRIS, M.B., F.R.C.P.C.
Associate Professor, Department of Medicine, University of Toronto; Clinical Electrophysiologist, Toronto General Hospital, Toronto, Ontario, Canada
Chapter 29—Arrhythmias in Pregnancy

MARIA C. HENDERSON-EVERHARDUS, B.S.N., R.N., C.V.N., R.V.T.
Manager, Peripheral Vascular Laboratory; Chair, Vascular Nursing Education, St. Luke's Episcopal Hospital, Houston, Texas
Chapter 21—Peripheral Vascular Disease

LISA M. HOLLIER, M.D., M.P.H.
Assistant Professor, Division of Maternal-Fetal Medicine, The University of Texas–Houston Medical School, Houston, Texas
Chapter 26—Management of Valvular Heart Disease

MOHAMMAD HADI KADIVAR, M.D.
Research Assistant, Baylor College of Medicine; Research Assistant, St. Luke's Episcopal Hospital, Houston, Texas
Chapter 36—Ventricular Tachycardia

BRIAN KIRSHON, M.D.
Houston Perinatal Associates, Houston, Texas
Chapter 26—Management of Valvular Heart Disease

ZVONIMIR KRAJCER, M.D.
Clinical Professor of Medicine, Baylor College of Medicine and The University of Texas Health Science Center at Houston; Director, Peripheral Vascular Intervention, Texas Heart Institute and St. Luke's Episcopal Hospital, Houston, Texas
Chapter 21—Peripheral Vascular Disease

JOHN C. LaROSA, M.D.
President, SUNY Downstate Medical Center, Brooklyn, New York
Chapter 11—Coronary Artery Disease: Therapy

VICTOR R. LAVIS, M.D.
Professor, Internal Medicine (Endocrinology), The University of Texas–Houston Medical School; Attending Physician, Internal Medicine (Endocrinology), Memorial Hermann Hospital, Houston, Texas
Chapter 2—Cardiovascular System in Women: Physiology

MARCY LIM, M.D.
Cardiologist, Cardiovascular Association, Memorial Hermann Hospital, Houston; Northeast Medical Center Hospital, Humble; Kingwood Hospital, Kingwood, Texas
Chapter 8—Noninvasive Diagnostic Testing

JAMES J. LIVESAY, M.D.
Associate Surgeon, Texas Heart Institute and St. Luke's Episcopal Hospital; Clinical Associate Professor of Surgery, The University of Texas–Houston Medical School, Houston, Texas
Chapter 22—Cerebrovascular Disease

BEVERLY H. LORELL, M.D.
Professor of Medicine, Harvard Medical School; Director, Program in Heart Failure; Director, Hemodynamic Research Laboratory, Beth Israel Deaconess Medical Center, Boston, Massachusetts
Chapter 17—Congestive Heart Failure

MAUREEN LOWERY, M.D.
Associate Professor of Medicine and Medical Director, Cardiovascular Outpatient Center and Non-Invasive Diagnostic Laboratories, University of Miami School of Medicine, Jackson Memorial Hospital, Miami, Florida
Chapter 38—Sudden Cardiac Death

SUSANNA MAK, M.D., F.R.C.P.C.
Clinical Research Fellow, Mount Sinai Hospital, University of Toronto, Toronto, Ontario, Canada
Chapter 29—Arrhythmias in Pregnancy

DANIEL B. MARK, M.D., M.P.H.
Professor of Medicine, Duke University Medical Center; Director, Outcomes Research and Assessment Group, Duke Clinical Research Institute, Durham, North Carolina
Chapter 7—Coronary Artery Disease: Clinical Recognition: Risk Assessment Screening

EDWARD K. MASSIN, M.D.
Clinical Professor of Internal Medicine (Cardiology), The University of Texas–Houston Medical School; Clinical Professor of Medicine, Baylor College of Medicine, Houston, Texas
Chapter 16—Dilated Cardiomyopathy

ALI MASSUMI, M.D.
Clinical Professor of Medicine, Baylor College of Medicine; Director, Center for Cardiac Arrhythmias and Electrophysiology, Texas Heart Institute and St. Luke's Episcopal Hospital, Houston, Texas
Chapter 35—Supraventricular Tachycardia; Chapter 36—Ventricular Tachycardia; Chapter 39—Neurally Mediated Syncopal Syndromes

A. IAIN McGHIE, M.D.
Clinical Assistant Professor of Medicine, University of Missouri at Kansas City; Consulting Cardiologist, Mid-America Heart Institute, St. Luke's Hospital of Kansas City, Kansas City, Missouri
Chapter 8—Noninvasive Diagnostic Testing

JUDITH K. MICKELSON, M.D.
Professor of Clinical Medicine, Department of Internal Medicine (Cardiology), University of Cincinnati; University Hospital, University of Cincinnati Medical Center, Cincinnati, Ohio
Chapter 10—Coronary Artery Disease: Clinical Consequences

DIANNA M. MILEWICZ, M.D., Ph.D.
Professor and Director, Division of Medical Genetics; Vice-Chair, Department of Internal Medicine, The University of Texas–Houston Medical School, Houston, Texas
Chapter 20—Aortic Diseases and Aortic Dissection

SUSAN D. MUELLER, M.D.
Network Medical Director, Aetna Inc., Houston, Texas
Chapter 23—Pregnancy, Hemodynamic Alterations, and the Cardiovascular System; Chapter 30—Drugs and Pregnancy

ROBERT J. MYERBURG, M.D.
Director, Division of Cardiology, University of Miami School of Medicine, Miami, Florida
Chapter 38—Sudden Cardiac Death

TIMOTHY J. MYERS, B.S.
Manager, Clinical Research and Regulatory Affairs, Cardiovascular Surgery Research Laboratory, Texas Heart Institute at St. Luke's Episcopal Hospital, Houston, Texas
Chapter 16—Dilated Cardiomyopathy

SHAHLA NADER, M.D.
Professor, Departments of Obstetrics and Gynecology and Internal Medicine (Endocrinology), The University of Texas–Houston Medical School; Attending Physician, Memorial Hermann Hospital, Houston, Texas
Chapter 2—Cardiovascular System in Women: Physiology

SHERIF F. NAGUEH, M.D.
Assistant Professor of Medicine, Baylor College of Medicine; Assistant Professor of Medicine, The Methodist Hospital, Houston, Texas
Chapter 12—Aortic Valve Disease

NANCY A. NUSSMEIER, M.D.
Clinical Associate Professor of Anesthesiology, The University of Texas–Houston Medical School; Director of Cardiovascular Anesthesia Research and Staff Cardiovascular Anesthesiologist, Texas Heart Institute and St. Luke's Episcopal Hospital, Houston, Texas
Chapter 11—Coronary Artery Disease: Therapy

PHILIP R. ORLANDER, M.D.
Professor of Medicine and Director, Endocrinology, The University of Texas–Houston Medical School; Chief, Endocrinology & Metabolism, Memorial Hermann Hospital, Lyndon B. Johnson General Hospital, Houston, Texas
Chapter 5—Coronary Artery Disease: Risk Factors

VINCENZO PASCERI, M.D., Ph.D.
Cardiology Fellow, Texas Heart Institute and St. Luke's Episcopal Hospital, Houston, Texas
Chapter 32—Deep Vein Thrombosis

ERIC D. PETERSON, M.D., M.P.H.
Associate Professor of Medicine, Division of Cardiology; Director, Cardiovascular Outcomes Research and Quality, Duke University Medical Center, Durham, North Carolina
Chapter 7—Coronary Artery Disease: Clinical Recognition: Risk Assessment Screening

CHARLES POLLICK, M.B.Ch.B.
Medical Director, Non-Invasive Cardiology, Good Samaritan Hospital, Los Angeles, California
Chapter 13—Mitral Valve Disease

HARRY RAKOWSKI, M.D., F.R.C.P.C., F.A.C.C.
Professor of Medicine, University of Toronto, Toronto, Ontario, Canada
Chapter 18—Hypertrophic Cardiomyopathy

SUSAN M. RAMIN, M.D.
Associate Professor, Director, Division of Maternal-Fetal Medicine, The University of Texas–Houston Medical School, Houston, Texas
Chapter 27—Pregnancy: Hypertension

PRISCILLA RAY, M.D.
Clinical Professor, Department of Psychiatry, Baylor College of Medicine; Active Staff, St. Luke's Episcopal Hospital; Active Staff, The Methodist Hospital, Houston, Texas
Chapter 10—Coronary Artery Disease: Clinical Consequences

GEORGE J. REUL, Jr., M.D.
Clinical Professor, Department of Surgery, Division of Thoracic and Cardiac Surgery, The University of Texas–Houston Medical School; Clinical Professor, Department of Surgery, Baylor College of Medicine; Associate Chief of Surgery and Director, Peripheral Vascular Laboratory, Texas Heart Institute and St. Luke's Episcopal Hospital, Houston, Texas
Chapter 21—Peripheral Vascular Disease

CARLOS RIZO-PATRON, M.D.
Assistant Professor of Medicine, Section of Cardiology, Baylor College of Medicine, Houston; Assistant Clinical Professor of Medicine, Texas Tech University School of Medicine, Lubbock, Texas
Chapter 37—Heart Block

ROXANN ROKEY, MD, F.A.C.C., F.A.C.P.
Professor of Medicine, University of Wisconsin, Madison, Wisconsin; Director, Adult Congenital Heart Disease, Co-Director, Echocardiography, Department of Cardiology, Marshfield Clinic, Marshfield, Wisconsin
Chapter 28—Peripartum Cardiomyopathy

HAZIM J. SAFI, M.D.
Professor of Surgery and Chairman, Department of Cardiothoracic and Vascular Surgery, The University of Texas–Houston Medical School; Memorial Hermann Hospital, Houston, Texas
Chapter 20—Aortic Diseases and Aortic Dissection

GARETH SEAWARD, M.B.B.Ch., F.R.C.S.C.
Assistant Professor, Department of Obstetrics and Gynecology, University of Toronto; Specialist, Maternal-Fetal Medicine, Director, Labor and Delivery Unit, Mount Sinai Hospital, Toronto, Ontario, Canada
Chapter 24—Congenital Heart Disease: Pathophysiology, Clinical Recognition, Diagnosis, and Management

MATHEW SERMER, M.D., F.R.C.S.C.
Associate Professor, Obstetrics and Gynecology, University of Toronto; Head of Obstetrics and Maternal-Fetal Medicine, Mount Sinai Hospital, Toronto, Ontario, Canada
Chapter 24—Congenital Heart Disease: Pathophysiology, Clinical Recognition, Diagnosis, and Management

RALPH SHABETAI, M.D., F.A.C.P., F.A.C.C.
Professor of Medicine Emeritus, University of California at San Diego; Attending Physician, University of California at San Diego Medical Center, San Diego; Attending Physician, Veterans Administration Health Care System, La Jolla, California
Chapter 34—Pericardial Disease: Pathophysiology, Clinical Recognition, Diagnosis, and Management

LESLEE J. SHAW, Ph.D.
Duke University, Durham, North Carolina; Director, Outcomes Research, Atlanta Cardiovascular Research Institute, Atlanta, Georgia
Chapter 7—Coronary Artery Disease: Clinical Recognition: Risk Assessment Screening

SAMUEL C. SIU, M.D., S.M.
Associate Professor of Medicine, University of Toronto; Research Director, University of Toronto Congenital Cardiac Centre for Adults, Toronto General Hospital; Director of Echocardiography, University Health Network and Mount Sinai Hospital, Toronto, Ontario, Canada
Chapter 24—Congenital Heart Disease: Pathophysiology, Clinical Recognition, Diagnosis, and Management

RICHARD W. SMALLING, M.D., Ph.D.
Professor of Medicine, Jay Brent Sterling Professor of Cardiovascular Medicine, The University of Texas–Houston Medical School; Director, Catheterization Laboratories, Memorial Hermann Hospital, Houston, Texas
Chapter 9—Invasive Diagnostic Testing

RAYMOND F. STAINBACK, M.D.
Clinical Assistant Professor of Medicine, Baylor College of Medicine; Medical Director, Adult Echocardiography Laboratory, Texas Heart Institute and St. Luke's Episcopal Hospital, Houston, Texas
Chapter 14—Tricuspid and Pulmonary Valve Disease

LYNNE W. STEVENSON, M.D.
Associate Professor of Medicine, Harvard Medical School; Director, Cardiomyopathy and Heart Failure Service, Brigham and Women's Hospital, Boston, Massachusetts
Chapter 17—Congestive Heart Failure

NEIL E. STRICKMAN, M.D.
Associate Professor of Medicine, Baylor College of Medicine; Interventionalist, Director, Peripheral Vascular Disease Section, Texas Heart Institute and St. Luke's Episcopal Hospital, Houston, Texas
Chapter 21—Peripheral Vascular Disease

THOMAS J. TAKACH, M.D.
Cardiovascular Surgery Fellow, Texas Heart Institute and St. Luke's Episcopal Hospital, Houston, Texas
Chapter 21—Peripheral Vascular Disease; Chapter 22—Cerebrovascular Disease

KARA THOMPSON, M.D.
Consultant, Texas Cardiovascular Consultants, Austin, Texas
Chapter 3—Coronary Artery Disease: Overview

MARGARET O. UTHMAN, M.D.
Associate Professor of Pathology and Laboratory Medicine, Vice Chair for Education, Department of Pathology and Laboratory Medicine, and Assistant Dean for Educational Programs, The University of Texas–Houston Medical School; Director, Hematology Laboratory, Memorial Hermann Hospital, Houston, Texas
Chapter 1—Cardiovascular System in Women: Anatomy; Chapter 4—Coronary Artery Disease: Anatomy

J. HAJO VAN BOCKEL, M.D.
Professor of Surgery, Leiden University; Chief of Vascular Surgery, Leiden University Medical Center, Leiden, The Netherlands
Chapter 21—Peripheral Vascular Disease

WILLIAM K. VAUGHN, Ph.D.
Vice President, Biostatistics and Epidemiology, Texas Heart Institute at St. Luke's Episcopal Hospital, Houston, Texas
Chapter 5—Coronary Artery Disease: Risk Factors

CARLOS VILLAR-CORDOVA, M.D.
Cardiovascular Senior Fellow, Department of Neurology, The University of Texas–Houston Medical School, Houston, Texas
Chapter 22—Cerebrovascular Disease

ROLLO P. VILLAREAL, M.D.
Cardiology Fellow, Texas Heart Institute and St. Luke's Episcopal Hospital, Houston, Texas
Chapter 8—Noninvasive Diagnostic Testing; Chapter 35—Supraventricular Tachycardia

RENU VIRMANI, M.D.
Clinical Professor, Department of Pathology, Georgetown University, Washington, D.C.; Clinical Research Professor, Department of Pathology, Vanderbilt University, Nashville, Tennessee; Chair, Department of Cardiovascular Pathology, Armed Forces Institute of Pathology, Washington, D.C.
Chapter 4—Coronary Artery Disease: Anatomy

E. DOUGLAS WIGLE, M.D.
Professor of Medicine, University of Toronto; Staff Cardiologist, Toronto General Hospital, Toronto, Ontario, Canada
Chapter 18—Hypertrophic Cardiomyopathy

SUSAN WILANSKY, M.D.
Attending Cardiologist, Southern California Kaiser Permanente Medical Group, Orange County, California
Chapter 6—Behavioral Barriers to Health; Chapter 11—Coronary Artery Disease: Therapy; Chapter 19—Pathophysiology, Clinical Recognition, Therapy, and Prevention of Hypertension; Chapter 25—Valvular Heart Disease: Pathophysiology, Clinical Recognition, Diagnosis, and Management

JAMES T. WILLERSON, M.D.
Medical Director, Texas Heart Institute; Chief of Cardiology, St. Luke's Episcopal Hospital; Edward Randall III Chair in Internal Medicine, The University of Texas–Houston Medical School; Alkek-Williams Distinguished Professor and President, The University of Texas Health Science Center at Houston, Houston, Texas
Chapter 4—Coronary Artery Disease: Anatomy
Chapter 8—Noninvasive Diagnostic Testing; Chapter 11—Coronary Artery Disease: Therapy; Chapter 20—Aortic Diseases and Aortic Dissection; Chapter 23—Pregnancy, Hemodynamic Alterations, and the Cardiovascular System; Chapter 30—Drugs and Pregnancy; Chapter 32—Deep Vein Thrombosis; Chapter 34—Pericardial Disease: Pathophysiology, Clinical Recognition, Diagnosis, and Management; Chapter 41—Collagen Vascular Disease: Pathophysiology, Clinical Recognition, Diagnosis, and Management

JAMES M. WILSON, M.D.
Clinical Assistant Professor, Baylor College of Medicine; Assistant Chief of Cardiology, Co-Associate Director of Cardiology Education, Texas Heart Institute and St. Luke's Episcopal Hospital, Houston, Texas
Chapter 21—Peripheral Vascular Disease

ANDREA G. WITLIN, D.O.
Assistant Professor, The University of Texas Medical Branch, Galveston, Texas
Chapter 27—Hypertension

ANNA WOO, M.D., F.R.C.P.C.
Assistant Professor of Medicine, University of Toronto; Staff Cardiologist, Toronto General Hospital, Toronto, Ontario, Canada
Chapter 18—Hypertrophic Cardiomyopathy

AMY L. WOODRUFF, M.D.
Cardiology Fellow, Texas Heart Institute and St. Luke's Episcopal Hospital, Houston, Texas
Chapter 35—Supraventricular Tachycardia

FRANK M. YATSU, M.D.
Professor, Department of Neurology, The University of Texas–Houston Medical School, Houston, Texas
Chapter 22—Cerebrovascular Disease

BARRY JAMES ZELUFF, M.D.
Clinical Professor of Medicine, The E. L. Wagner, M.D., Volunteer Faculty Chair of Internal Medicine, Baylor College of Medicine, Houston, Texas
Chapter 15—Infective Endocarditis

WILLIAM A. ZOGHBI, M.D.
Professor of Medicine, Baylor College of Medicine; Director, Echocardiographic Research Laboratories, The Methodist Hospital, Houston, Texas
Chapter 12—Aortic Valve Disease

PREFACE

Heart disease in women is an important topic. Many persons believe that it has received inadequate attention from physicians and even from women themselves. Some women maintain that serious attention to heart and vascular diseases has focused primarily on men, because heart attacks generally occur earlier in men, leading to relatively early disability and sometimes death.

However, just as it is in men, heart disease is also the major cause of death and disability in women. Heart attacks in the postmenopausal years, and heart muscle (cardiomyopathies) and valvular heart diseases in the premenopausal years, are very serious problems for women. Some forms of heart disease may even be more difficult to recognize and treat in women than in men. Therefore, one cannot arbitrarily assume that what applies to men also applies to women, especially with regard to the different forms of treatment.

For these reasons, we have produced this textbook, *Heart Disease in Women,* which discusses a wide range of important issues related to women and heart disease. In some areas, the medical community's knowledge is incomplete and needs to be enhanced. We are committed to furthering the search for new knowledge and to publishing periodic updates of this text. By drawing on the wisdom of some of today's leading specialists, this book provides us with a solid foundation upon which to build.

We would like to express our sincere appreciation to the contributors, without whose time, effort, and expertise our text would not exist. We owe special thanks to Marianne Mallia, Virginia Fairchild, Christina Chambers, Jude Richard, and Jackie McCollum at the Texas Heart Institute, who edited and managed the project through its final stages. Finally, we are most appreciative of the continued cooperation and encouragement of our publisher, W.B. Saunders, and especially of the help we received there from Natalie Ware, production manager, and Carol DiBerardino, manuscript editor.

James T. Willerson, M.D.
Susan Wilansky, M.D.

NOTICE

CONTENTS

SECTION VIII
PREGNANCY

SECTION IX
VASCULAR DISEASE

SECTION X
PERICARDIAL DISEASE

SECTION XI
ARRHYTHMIAS

SECTION XII
PULMONARY HYPERTENSION

SECTION XIII
COLLAGEN VASCULAR DISEASE

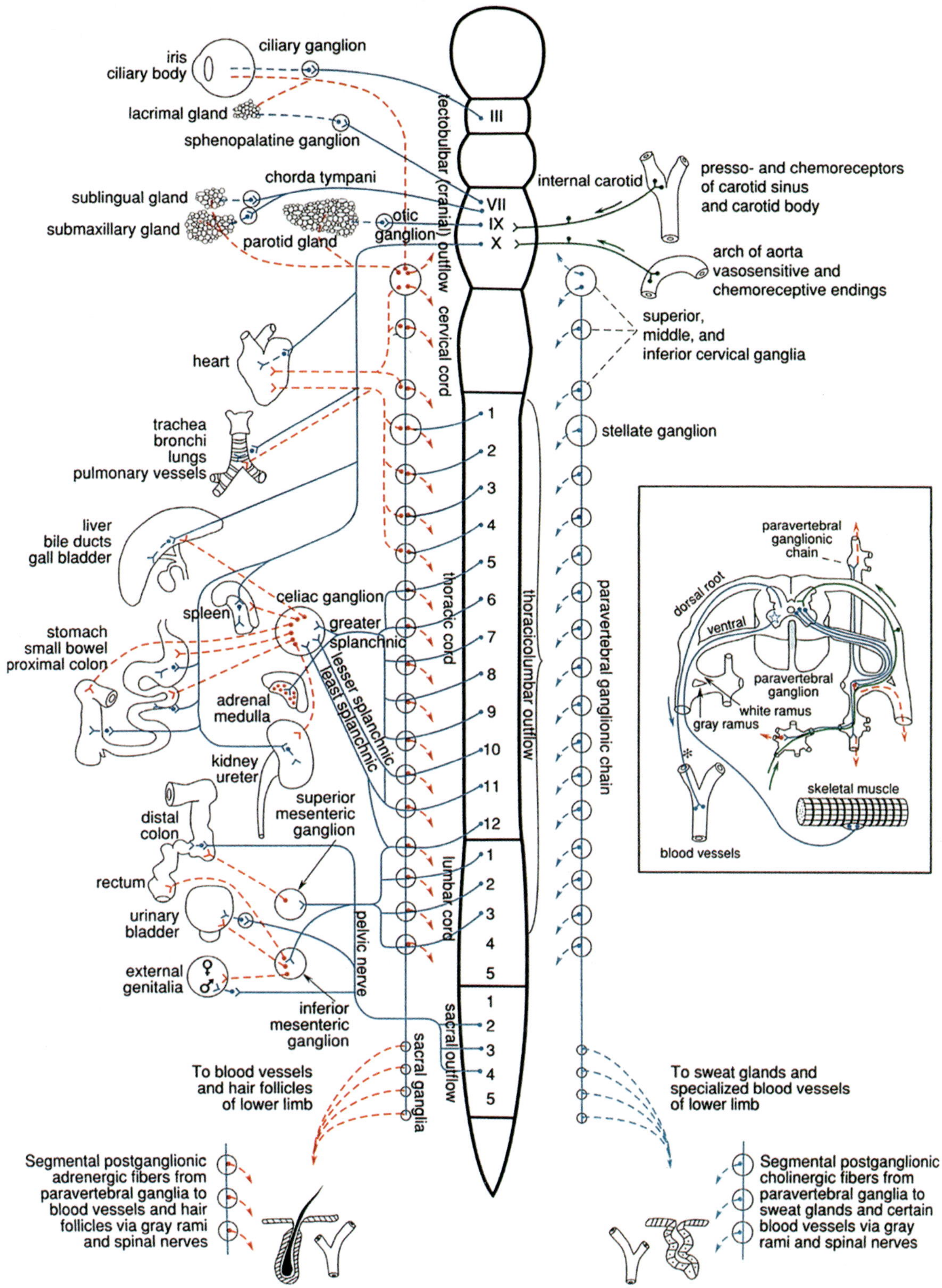

COLOR PLATE 2–1. Diagram of the autonomic nerves and effector organs. Blue = cholinergic; red = adrenergic; green = visceral afferent; solid lines = preganglionic; broken lines = postganglionic. The insert demonstrates the finer details of the ramification of adrenergic fibers at a typical segment of the spinal cord, the path of visceral afferent nerves, the cholinergic nature of somatic motor nerves to skeletal muscle, and the presumably cholinergic nature of vasodilator fibers in the dorsal roots of the spinal nerves. (From Lefkowitz RJ, Hoffman BB, Taylor P: Neurotransmission: the autonomic and somatic motor nervous systems. In Hardman JG, et al (eds): Goodman and Gilman's The Pharmacological Basis of Therapeutics, 9th ed. McGraw-Hill, New York, 1996, p 105.)

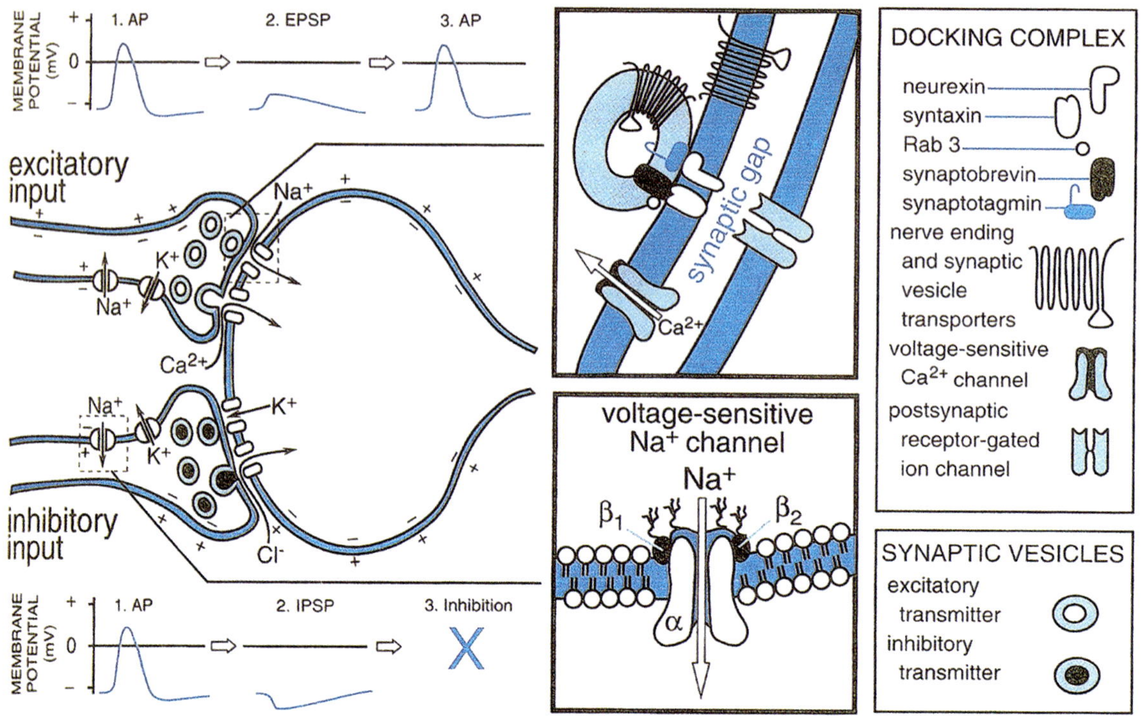

COLOR PLATE 2–2. Neurotransmission. The nerve action potential (AP) arrives at the presynaptic terminal, initiating release of an excitatory or inhibitory neurotransmitter from synaptic vesicles into the intercellular cleft by exocytosis. The neurotransmitter then diffuses across the cleft and stimulates receptors on the postsynaptic cell membrane. An excitatory transmitter produces a localized depolarization, the excitatory postsynaptic potential (EPSP), by increasing permeability to cation. An inhibitory transmitter results in selective increase in permeability to K^+ or Cl^-, resulting in a localized hyperpolarization, the inhibitory postsynaptic potential (IPSP). The summation of collective EPSP and IPSP determines whether or not a full AP results. (From Lefkowitz RJ, Hoffman BB, Taylor P: Neurotransmission: the autonomic and somatic motor nervous systems. In Hardman JG, et al (eds): Goodman and Gilman's The Pharmacological Basis of Therapeutics, 9th ed. McGraw-Hill, New York, 1996, p 105.)

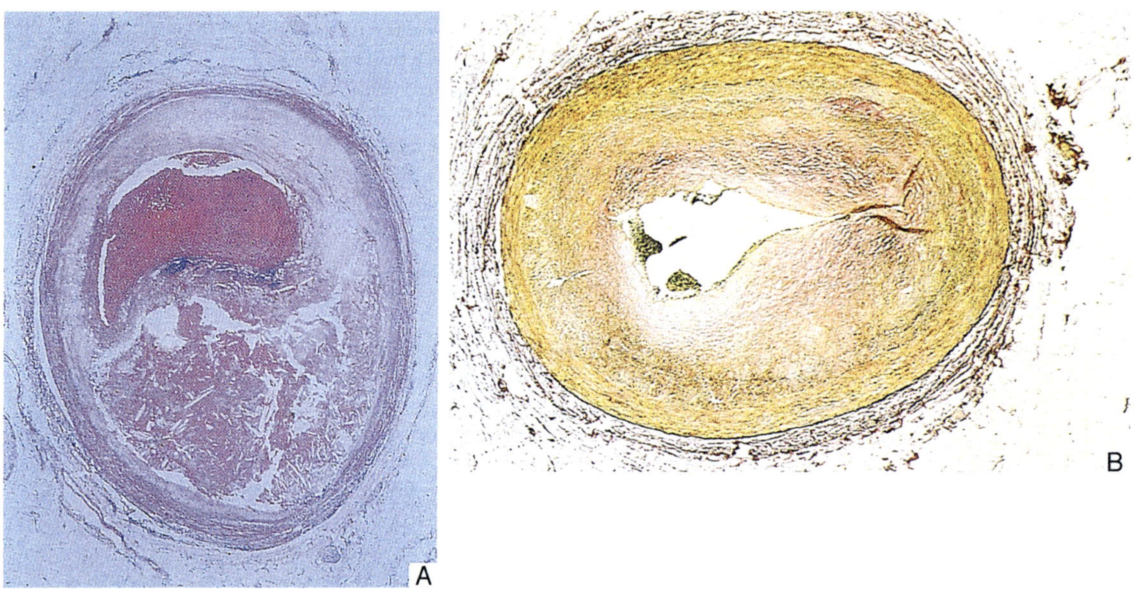

COLOR PLATE 4–1. *A*, A typical atherosclerotic plaque in which plaque has ruptured, leading to the development of coronary artery thrombosis. Such a patient may or may not have had angina at effort before the plaque rupture and thrombosis, and may have abruptly developed severe chest pain and a myocardial infarction (MI) with plaque rupture and coronary artery thrombosis. *B*, The neointimal proliferation occurring with restenosis after coronary artery angioplasty, leading to coronary artery luminal diameter narrowing and the need for an additional revascularization procedure. Patients who develop coronary heart disease after cardiac transplantation also demonstrate this same alteration in their coronary arteries (i.e., neointimal proliferation). Native atheromas have substantial fibroproliferative alterations as well. (*A*, From Becker AE, Anderson RH: Cardiac Pathology, Gower Medical, London, 1988. *B*, From Hurst JW, Anderson RH, Becker AE, et al: Atlas of the Heart. Gower Medical, New York, 1988, p 63 with permission.)

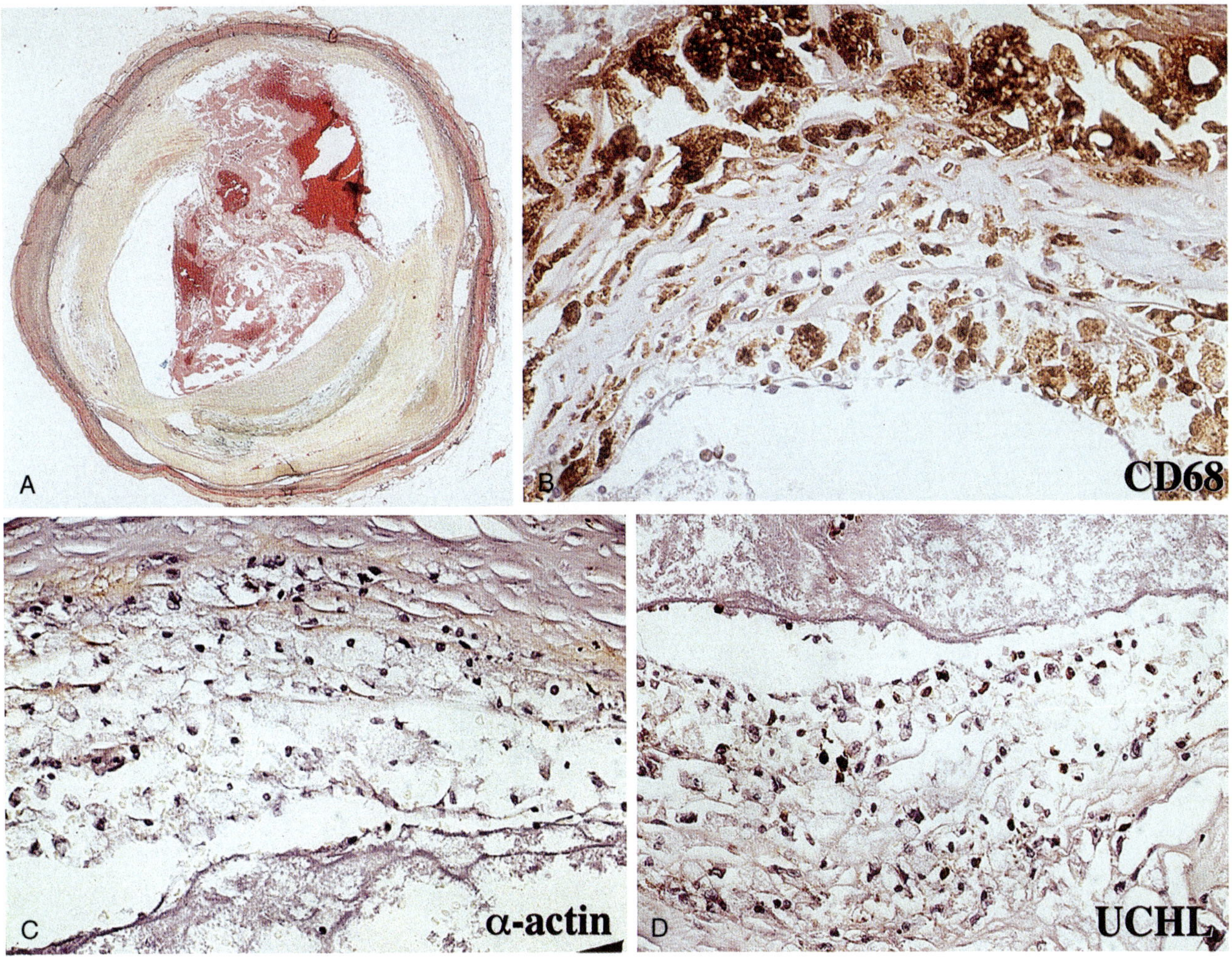

COLOR PLATE 4–2. Acute plaque rupture. Movat pentachrome stain *(A)* demonstrates a thin fibrous cap *(center)*, hemorrhage into lipid core *(top)*, and luminal thrombus *(bottom)*. The fibrous cap is thinned centrally and does not appear intact. An immunohistochemical stain for CD 68 to identify macrophages (*B*, brown staining) shows an abundance of macrophages within the region of the fibrous cap. There are relatively few smooth muscle cells as demonstrated by an antibody against smooth muscle (alpha) actin *(C)*. Similarly, there is little or no brown staining when an antibody against surface marker for T cells (UCHL, *D*) is applied. Acute plaque ruptures are very infrequent as a cause of thrombosis in premenopausal women; however, they account for a significant proportion of coronary thrombus in postmenopausal women. *B*, The morphology of plaque rupture shows the thin fibrous cap, large number of inflammatory cells beneath or on the surface of the plaque, and an adjacent lipid core.

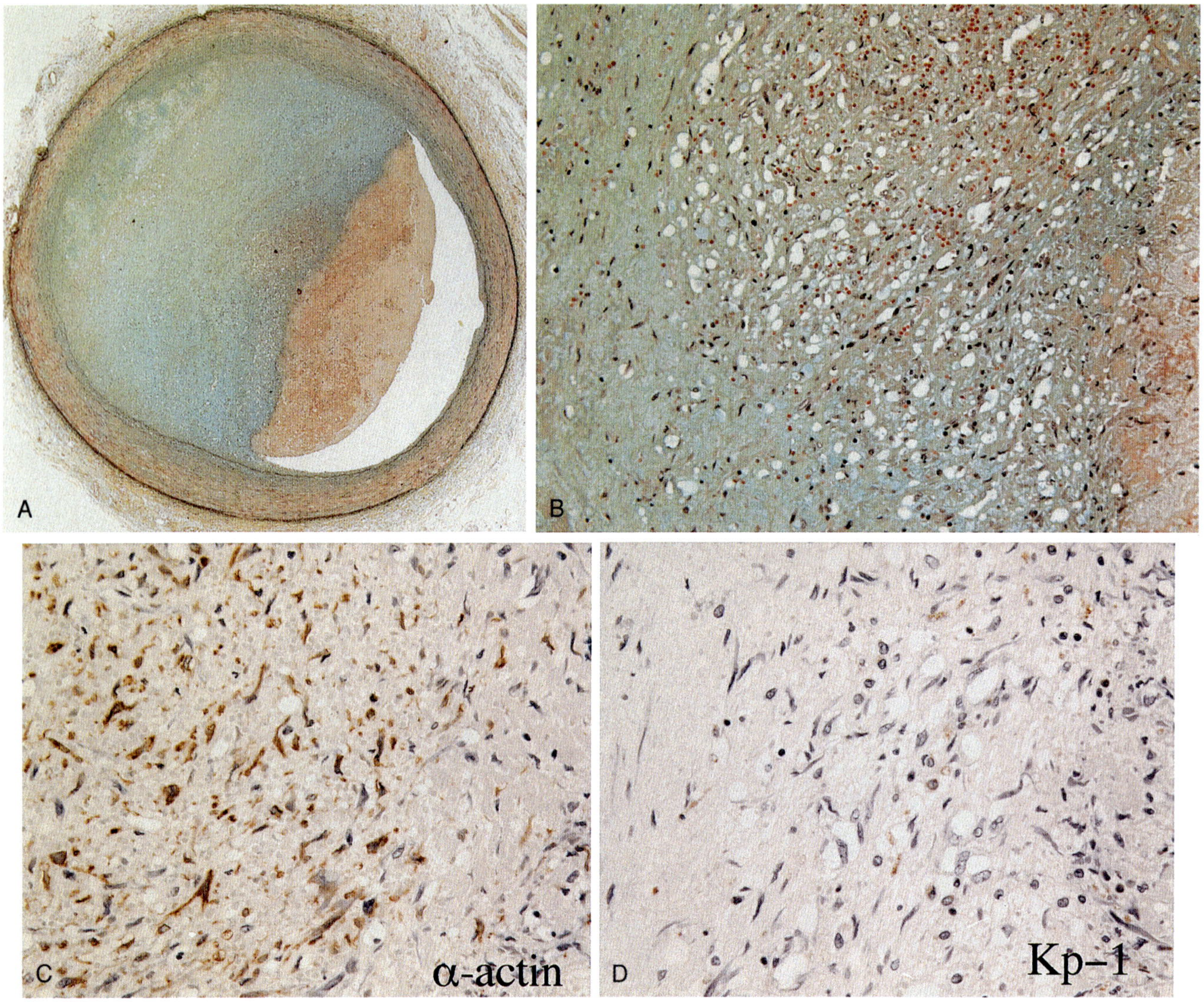

COLOR PLATE 4–3. Acute plaque erosion. Movat pentachrome stains (*A* and *B*) demonstrate luminal thrombus (gray-red) overlaying in a plaque rich in proteoglycans on the surface (blue). A higher magnification of the thrombus region (*B*) shows the smooth muscle cells in the fibrous cap and the proteoglycan-rich (green-blue) matrix. An immunohistochemical stain for alpha (smooth muscle cell) actin demonstrates positivity (brown staining, *C*) with relatively little staining for macrophages (Kp-1, *D*). The lack of hemorrhage into plaque, thin fibrous cap, and macrophages, and the abundance of smooth muscle cells are features that distinguish plaque erosion from plaque rupture. Plaque erosion is the major substrate for atherothrombosis in premenopausal women.

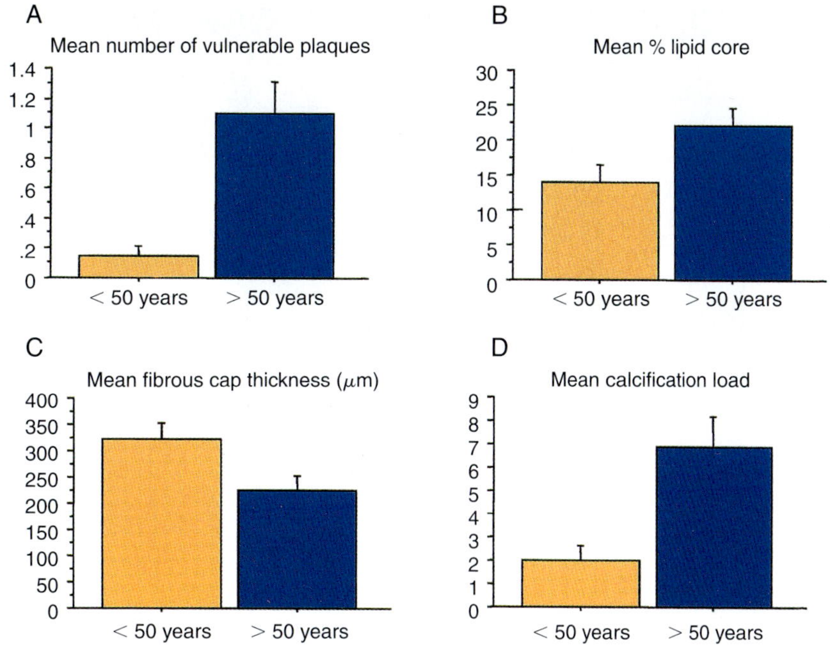

COLOR PLATE 4–4. Characterization of coronary atheromatous plaques seen in women younger and older than 50 years. *A*, Mean numbers of vulnerable plaques in 51 women who died suddenly of severe coronary disease: left bar, mean in women younger than 50 years; right bar, mean in women older than 50 years ($p < .00021$, student's t-test). *B*, Mean lipid core (%) in 51 women who died suddenly of severe coronary disease: left bar, mean % lipid core in women younger than 50 years; right bar, mean in women older than 50 years ($p = .02$, student's t-test). *C*, Mean fibrous cap thickness (μm) in 51 women who died suddenly of severe coronary disease: left bar, the mean thickness in women younger than 50 years; right bar, mean thickness in women older than 50 years ($p = .02$, student's t-test). *D*, Mean calcification score in 51 women who died suddenly of severe coronary disease: left bar, mean calcification score in women younger than 50 years; right bar, mean score in women older than 50 years ($p = .0007$, student's t-test). These results demonstrate that plaques in premenopausal women differ significantly from those in women who are presumably perimenopausal and postmenopausal: The plaques are less lipid rich, with little atrophy of the fibrous caps, which are features predisposing to rupture. The effects of estrogen on plaque morphology are largely unknown.

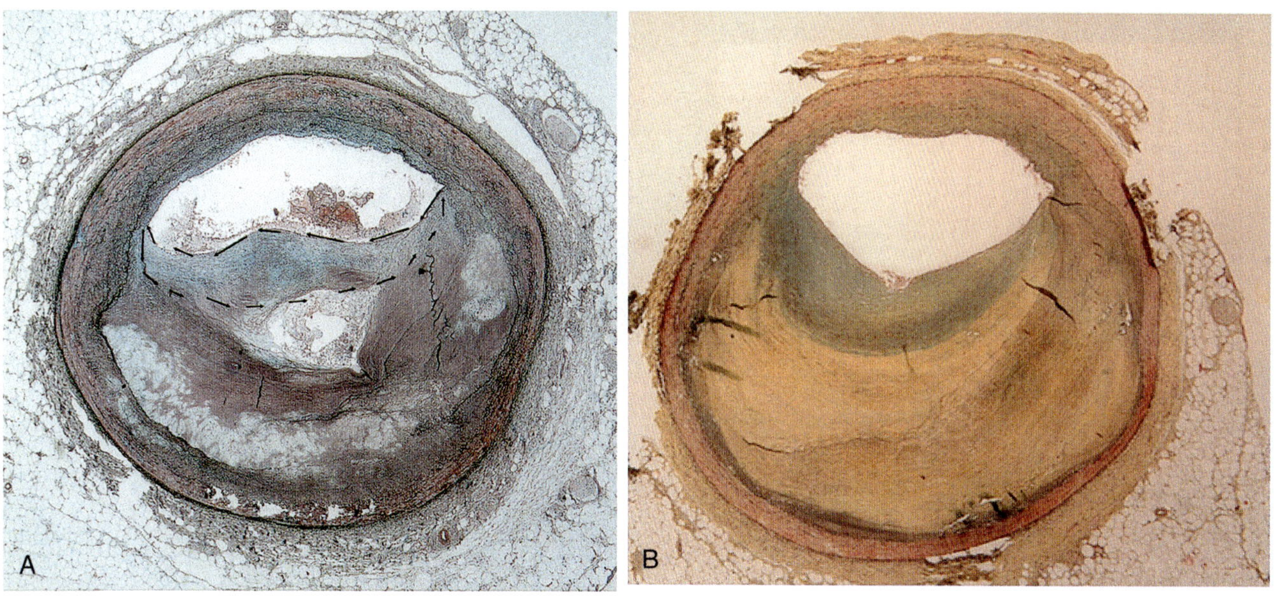

COLOR PLATE 4–5. Healed plaque rupture. *A*, Movat pentachrome stain of a healed rupture showing two separate layers composed of lipid cores and fibrous bands. The most recent fibrous cap (outlined in dotted lines) demonstrates the healing portion of the ruptured plaque. Such layering is not frequently seen in the coronary plaques of women, especially those who are premenopausal. In contrast *(B)*, there is a homogeneous plaque (yellow), lacking in abundant lipid cores and evidence of prior rupture; it has an overlying plaque that is rich in recent proteoglycans and smooth muscle cells (green), representative of a healed plaque erosion. The patient, a 45-year-old woman with three-vessel coronary artery disease, had evidence of a plaque erosion in a different artery.

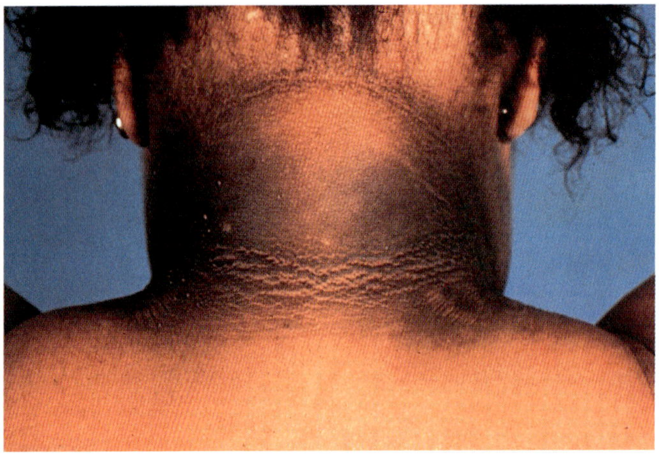

COLOR PLATE 5–1. Acanthosis nigricans

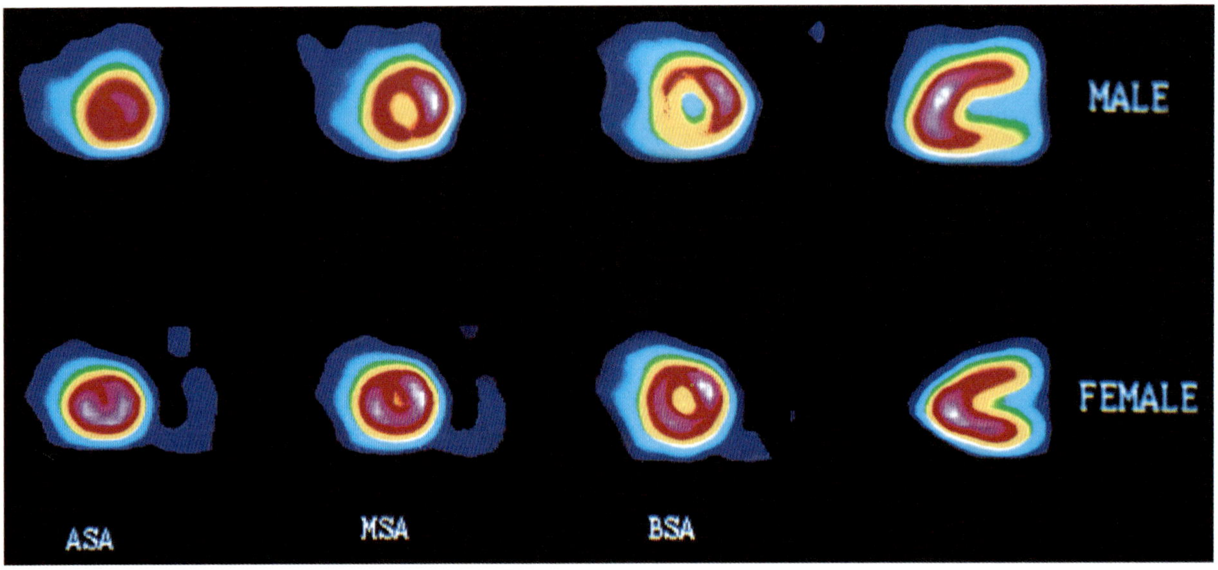

COLOR PLATE 8–1. Representative normal thallium-201 SPECT short-axis sections and a vertical long-axis section in men and women. ASA, apical short-axis; MSA, mid-ventricular short-axis section; BSA, basal short-axis section. (Adapted from McGhie AI, Gould KL, Schelbert HR, Willerson JT: Coronary artery disease—nuclear cardiology. In Willerson JT, Cohn JN [eds]: Cardiovascular Medicine. Churchill Livingstone, New York, 1995, p 475.)

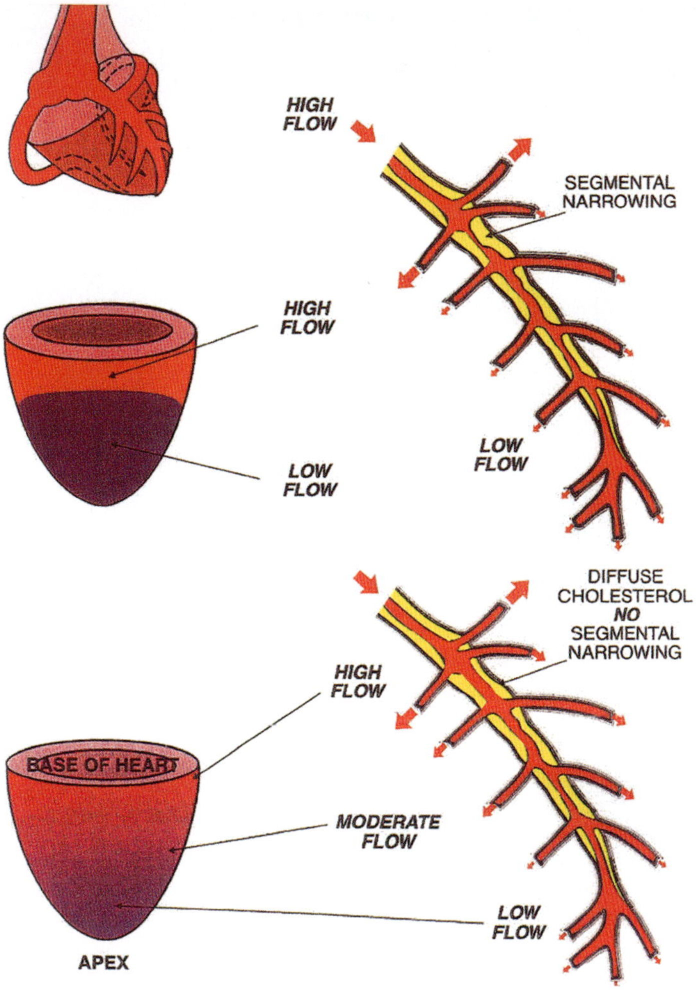

COLOR PLATE 8–2. The segmental perfusion defects caused by localized stenoses, compared with the graded, longitudinal, base-to-apex perfusion abnormality caused by diffuse coronary artery narrowing. (Adapted from Gould KL, Nakagawa Y, Nakagawa N, et al: Frequency and clinical implications of fluid dynamically significant diffuse coronary artery disease manifest as graded, longitudinal base-to-apex myocardial perfusion abnormalities by noninvasive positron emission tomography. Circulation 101:1931, 2000.)

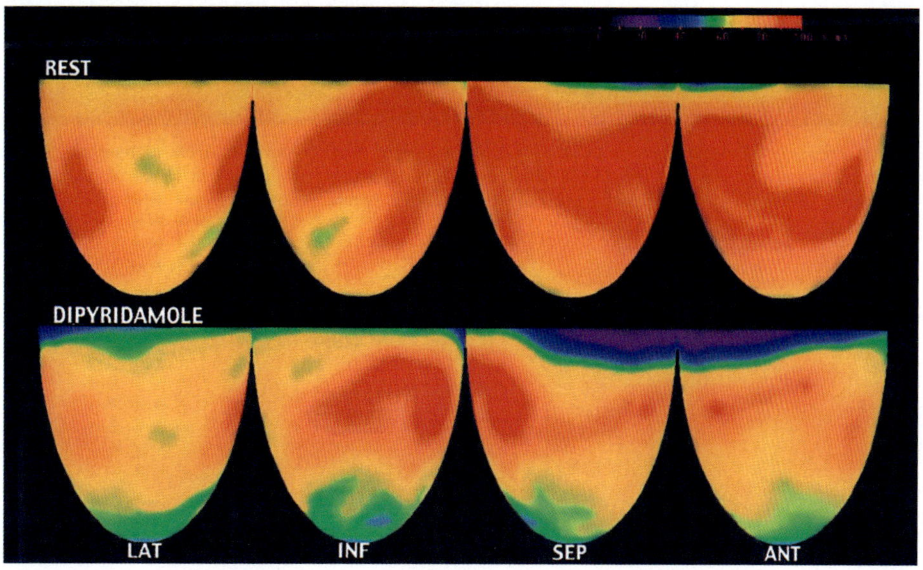

COLOR PLATE 8–3. Positron emission tomography myocardial perfusion images obtained at rest *(upper row)* and after dipyridamole administration *(lower row)*. As shown by the color scale bar, the degree of activity, in descending order, ranges from red (maximal activity) through yellow, green, and blue to black (minimal activity). There is a longitudinal, base-to-apex perfusion gradient characteristic of diffuse coronary athersclerosis without flow-limiting segmental stenosis. ANT, anterior; INF, inferior; LAT, lateral; SEP, septal.

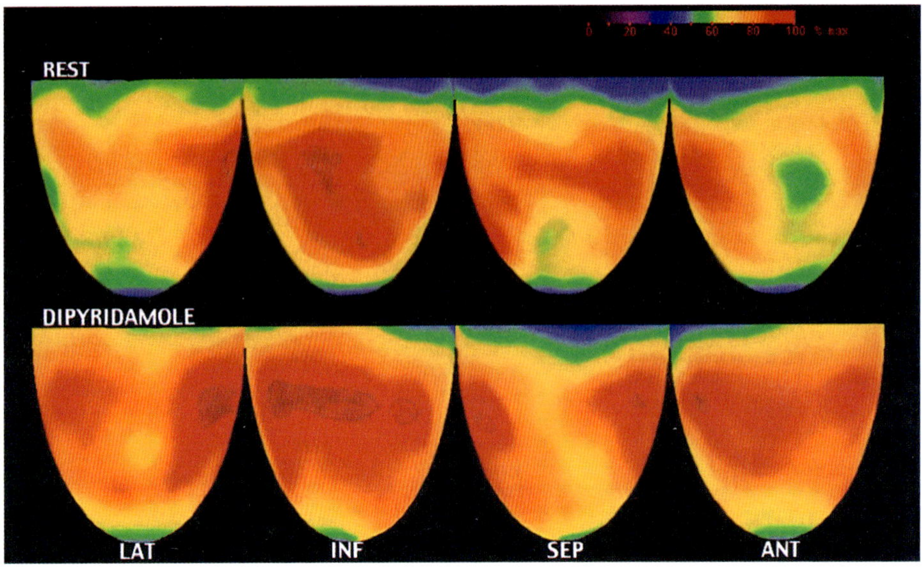

COLOR PLATE 8–4. Positron emission tomography myocardial perfusion images showing abnormal heterogeneous resting perfusion *(upper panel)* that improves after dipyridamole administration *(lower panel)*, reflecting one manifestation of abnormal endothelial function in early coronary atherosclerosis without flow-limiting stenosis. ANT, anterior; INF, inferior; LAT, lateral; SEP, septal.

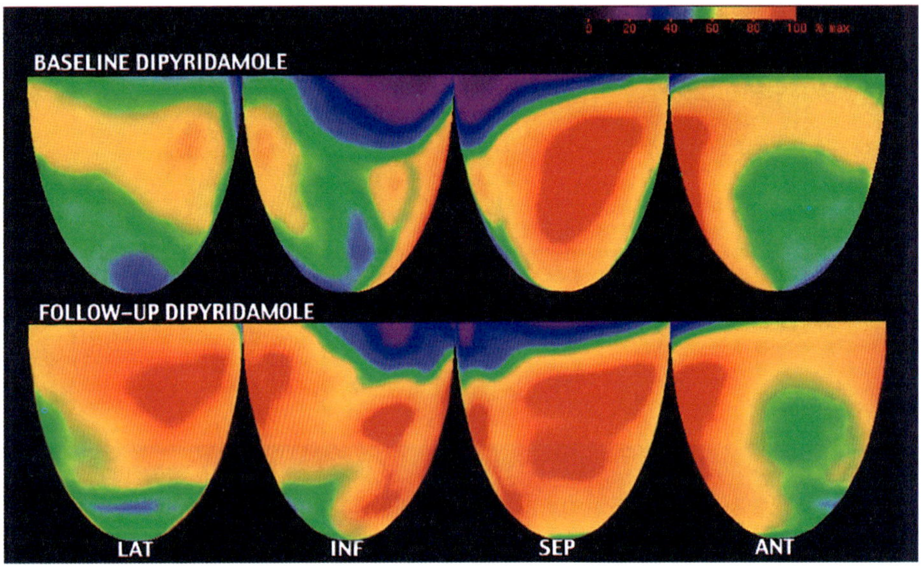

COLOR PLATE 8–5. Positron emission tomography myocardial perfusion images after dipyridamole stress at baseline *(upper row)* and at follow-up examination *(lower row)* after 12 months of vigorous risk-factor treatment, showing an improved myocardial perfusion reserve reflecting regression of coronary artery disease. Blue and green indicate a reduced coronary flow reserve, while yellow, red, and white indicate a progressively better flow reserve. ANT, anterior; INF, inferior; LAT, lateral; SEP, septal.

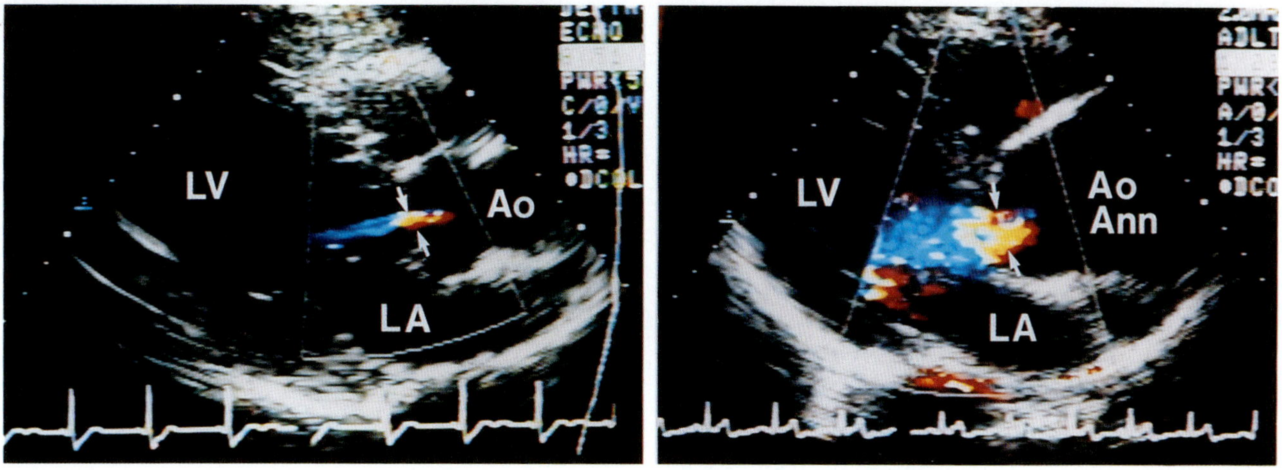

COLOR PLATE 12–1. Color Doppler echocardiographic frames during diastole from the parasternal long-axis view in a patient with mild aortic regurgitation *(left)* and in a patient with severe regurgitation *(right)* who has a large ascending aortic aneurysm. The width of the aortic regurgitation jet in the left ventricular outflow *(between arrows)* provides a good estimate of the severity of regurgitation by color Doppler. (Ao, aorta; Ao Ann, aortic aneurysm; LA, left atrium; LV, left ventricle.) (From Zoghbi WA, Afridi I: Aortic regurgitation. In Crawford MH [ed]: Current Diagnosis and Treatment in Cardiology. Appleton & Lange, Norwalk, Conn, 1995, p 99.)

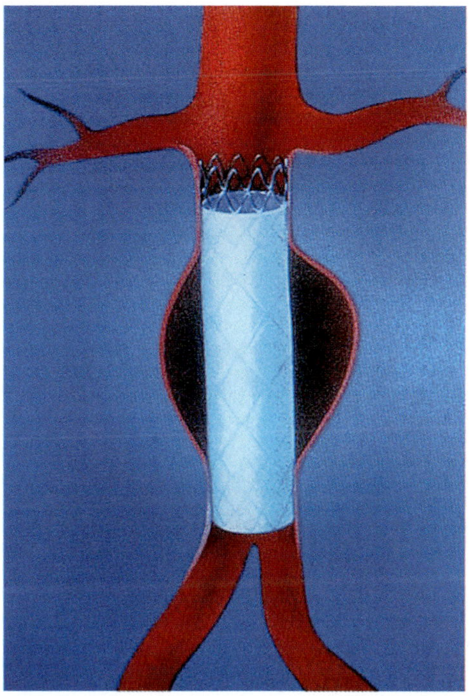

COLOR PLATE 21–1. First-generation abdominal aortic aneurysm stent graft devices. These are made of stiff single tubular components.

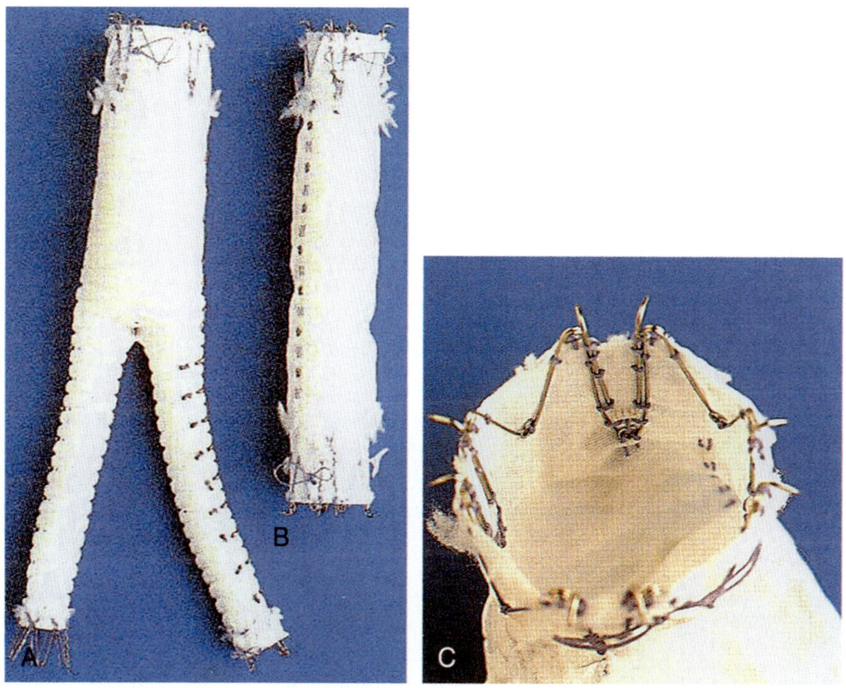

COLOR PLATE 21–2. Bifurcated one-piece *(A)* and tubular *(B)* abdominal aortic aneurysm exclusion grafts. *(C)* Barbs or hooks are used to secure the grafts in position.

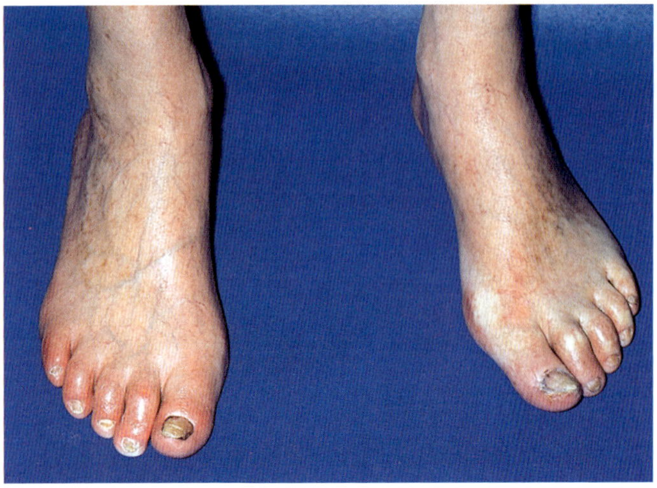

COLOR PLATE 21–3. Dependent rubor is characterized by color changes in the legs when placed in a dependent position. The feet may change color, fluctuating from blue to white and then to red.

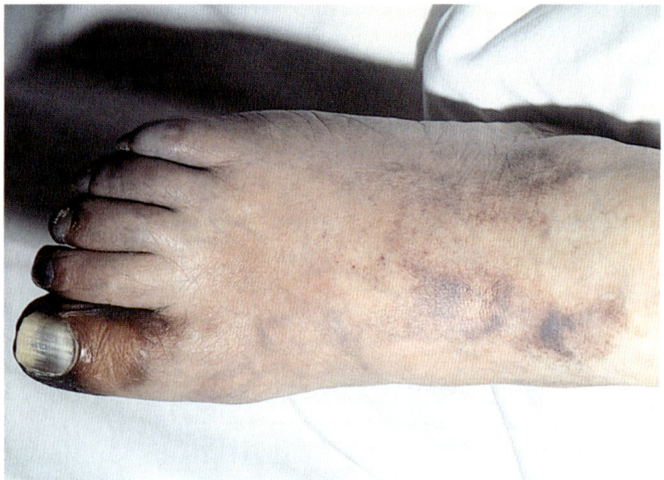

COLOR PLATE 21–4. Cyanosis is evident with a cold ischemic foot. This blue discoloration usually results from acute arterial obstruction, which may cause sudden cessation of blood to the distal circulation.

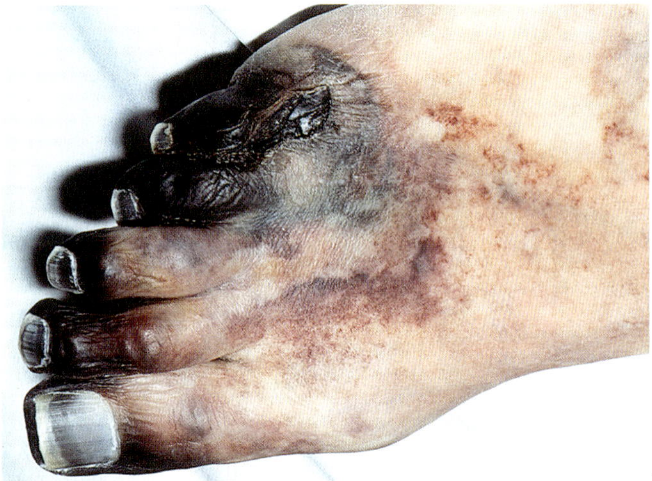

COLOR PLATE 21–5. Critical arterial ischemia results in gangrene and tissue necrosis. Arterial blood flow is often not available, resulting in no or poor tissue perfusion.

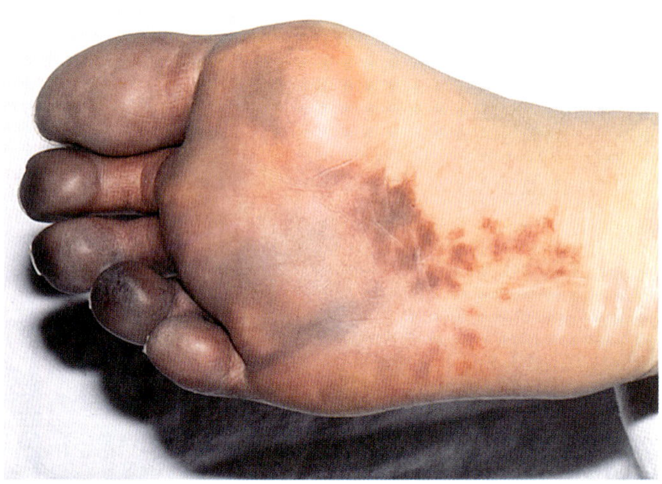

COLOR PLATE 21–6. Distal embolism of thrombosis from abdominal aneurysms is demonstrated with mottled extremities and discoloration of the toes.

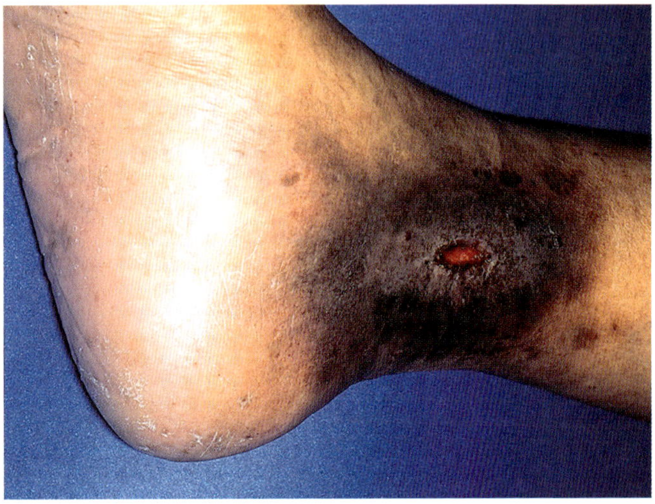

COLOR PLATE 21–7. Venous ulcerations occur on the medial aspect of the leg with tissue demarcation evident as a result of a chronic venous insufficiency.

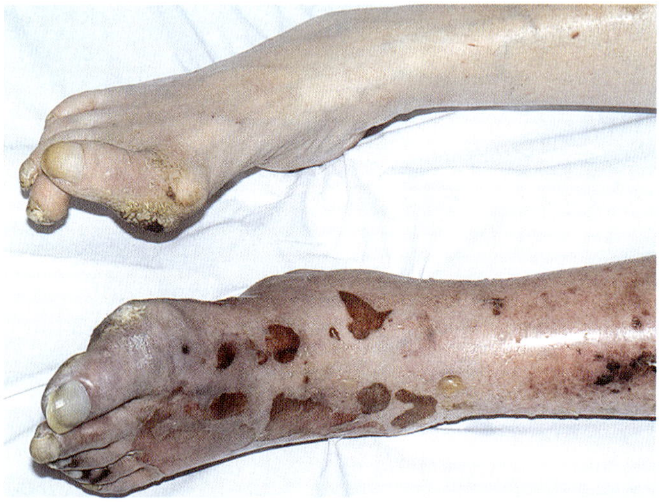

COLOR PLATE 21–8. Venous gangrene is a result of sudden venous occlusion. Swelling, blisters, and bluish discoloration of the extremity result with prolonged occlusion.

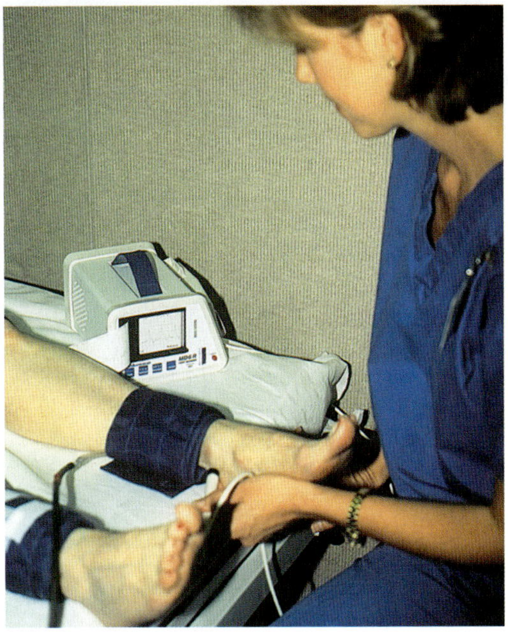

COLOR PLATE 21–9. Segmental blood pressure measurements are performed to determine the blood pressure at specific locations in the extremity. Measuring the ankle/brachial index is a method of determining the severity of obstruction within the leg.

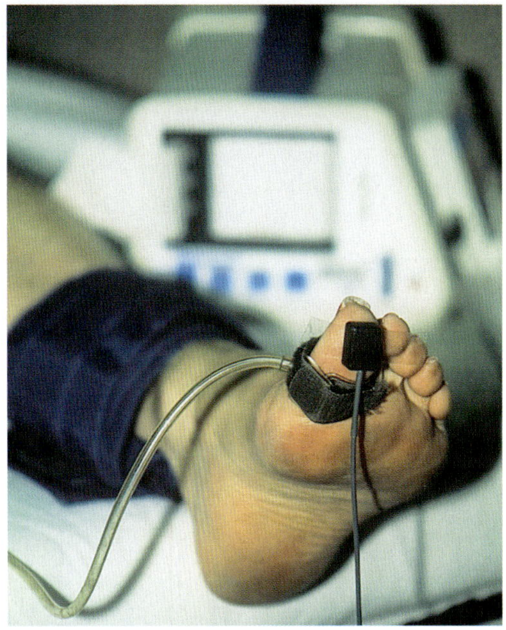

COLOR PLATE 21–10. Toe blood pressures are performed using photoplethysmography. A light-emitting diode reflects signals from moving blood cells. The toe blood pressure is obtained by inflating a digit cuff and observing reappearance of toe blood flow.

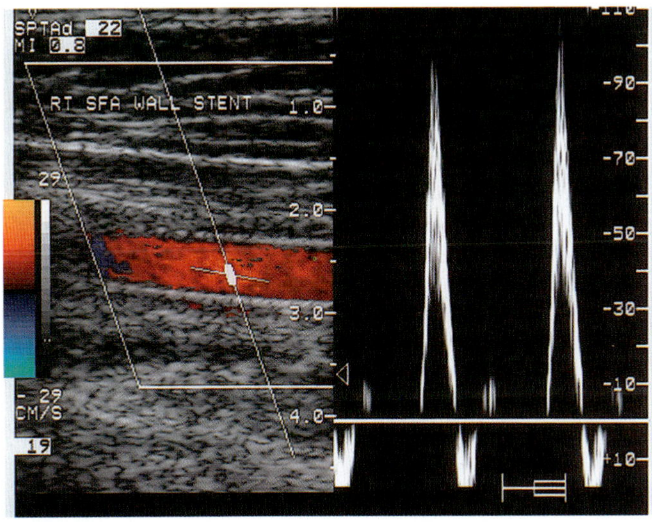

COLOR PLATE 21–11. Duplex ultrasound imaging provides direct visualization of the arterial vessels as well as Doppler blood flow information on the velocity of blood flow in the artery. Obstructive plaque, occlusions, aneurysms, and vessel patency following bypass surgery, PTA, or peripheral stenting can be assessed with this noninvasive technology.

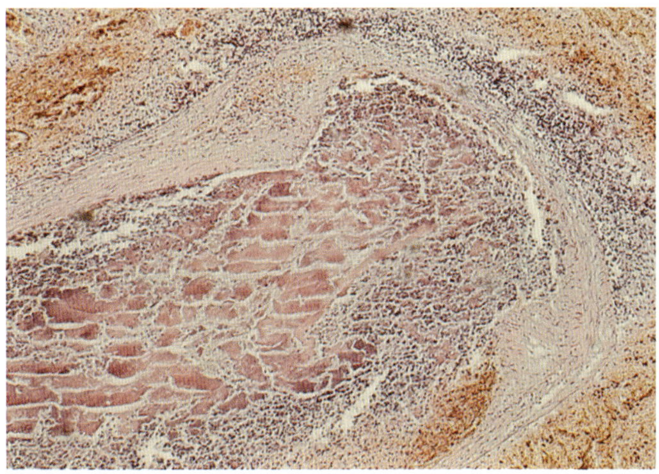

COLOR PLATE 33–1. Septic embolus in a medium-sized pulmonary artery of a 42-year-old intravenous drug user. Note the dense accumulation of inflammatory cells at the periphery of the clot. These cells also invade the vessel wall, including the adventitia. (Hematoxylin and eosin, × 200.)

SECTION I

CARDIOVASCULAR SYSTEM IN WOMEN

CHAPTER 1

Anatomy

L. Maximilian Buja and Margaret O. Uthman

The purpose of this chapter is to present basic information regarding the embryologic development and anatomy of the cardiovascular system with an emphasis on clinically relevant features and points of clinicopathologic correlation.

EMBRYOLOGIC DEVELOPMENT

Basic Embryology

In the 3-week-old fetus, components of splanchnic mesoderm differentiate into a primitive cardiac tube and pericardial cavity, and vascular channels form and link together to form blood vessels.[1–7]

The primitive cardiac tube is formed by the moving together and fusion of two lateral endothelial heart tubes. Subsequently, the epimyocardial mantle and cardiac jelly form. These components differentiate into the endocardium, forming the internal endothelial lining of the heart; the myocardium, forming the muscular wall; and the epicardium or visceral pericardium, covering the outside of the heart. Initially, the cardiac tube is single chambered and is composed of the following portions, extending from caudal to cephalad: the sinus venosus, which is connected to the major veins; the atrium; the ventricle; the bulbus cordis or conus; and the truncus arteriosus, which connects via six pairs of aortic arches to two dorsal aortae (Fig. 1–1).[1–7]

Initially, the single-chambered heart is a straight tube inside the pericardial cavity. Because the bulboventricular portion grows much more rapidly than the pericardial cavity, further elongation in a longitudinal direction cannot occur and the heart tube is forced to bend. The cephalic portion of the loop bends in a ventral and caudal direction and to the right, while the caudal atrial portion moves in a dorsocranial direction and to the left. This process, known as dextro (D)-bulboventricular looping, results in the atrial region coming to be positioned superiorly to the ventricular region and with the cardiac apex pointed to the left (see Fig. 1–1).

During the fourth to seventh week of fetal development, a complex septation process takes place, resulting in a four-chambered heart (Fig. 1–2). Atrial septation begins by the formation of the septum primum, which develops two defects: the ostium primum and the ostium secundum. The septum secundum then grows to the right of the septum primum. The foramen ovale is formed in the midportion as a result of the growth and positioning of the septum primum relative to the septum secundum. The sinus venosus is incorporated into the superior portion of the developing atria. Ventricular septation involves the upward growth of muscular tissue to form the muscular interventricular septum. Endocardial cushion tissue proliferates to form the atrioventricular valves and contributes to the closure of the ostium primum in the atrial septum and the formation of the membranous interventricular septum.

The proximal third of the bulbus cordis forms the trabeculated part of the right ventricle; the midportion, known as the conus cordis, forms the outflow tracts of both ventricles; and the distal part, the truncus arteriosus, forms the roots and proximal parts of the aorta and pulmonary artery. The junction between the primitive ventricle and the bulbus cordis is called the primary interventricular foramen. The primitive ventricle develops into the major component of the definitive left ventricle, and the proximal one third of the bulbus cordis contributes the major component of the definitive right ventricle, as the ventricular septation process occurs.

The separation of the truncus arteriosus by a spiral aorticopulmonary septum establishes aortic and pulmonary channels. Extensive remodeling of the double aortic arch system results in formation of a single aorta with a left-sided aortic arch, a pulmonary trunk with right and left main pulmonary arteries, and the ductus arteriosus, which connects the aortic arch and the left pulmonary artery.

In the fetus, pulmonary vascular resistance is high and systemic vascular resistance is low. The fetal circulation is characterized by right-to-left shunting of blood across the open foramen ovale and the patent ductus arteriosus (Fig. 1–3). After birth, the lungs expand, pulmonary vascular resistance drops, and systemic vascular resistance increases. Functional, followed by fibrous, closure of the foramen ovale and ductus arteriosus ensue, thereby establishing complete separation of the right-sided and left-sided circulations.

Relationship to Congenital Heart Disease

Knowledge of embryologic development of the heart and blood vessels is essential to understanding the pathogenesis of congenital heart disease.[8, 9] The position of the atria follows general body habitus. The anatomic right atrium is defined as the atrium receiving the systemic venous drainage. The anatomic left atrium is defined as the atrium receiving the pulmonary venous drainage. In situs solitus, the right atrium is on the right and the left atrium on the left. In situs inversus, the anatomic right atrium is on the left side and the anatomic left atrium is on the right side of the body. The right and left ventricles are normally connected to the corresponding atria, but the ventricles may be inverted. Inversion of the ventricles is a characteristic of a condition referred to as congenitally corrected transposition of the great vessels. It is associated with levo(L)-bulboventricular looping; hence, the alternative designation of L-transposition. Other positional anomalies include dextrocardia and right-sided aortic arch.

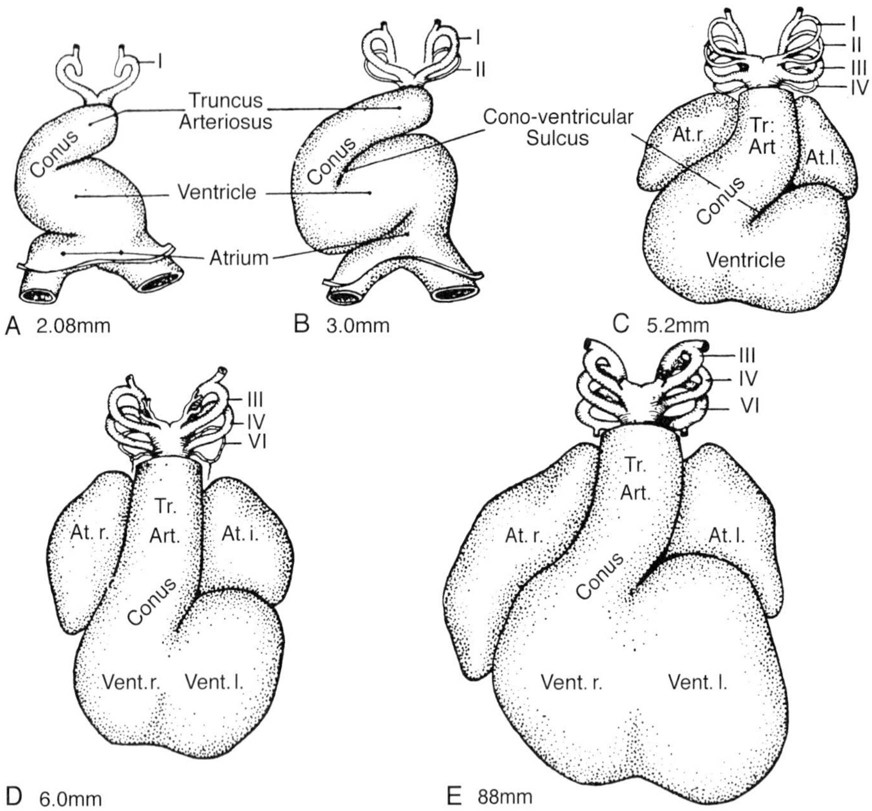

FIGURE 1–1. Ventral views of human embryonic hearts that show bending of cardiac tube and establishment of regional divisions. (At, atrium; l, left; r, right; Tr Art, truncus arteriosus.) (From Kramer TC: The partitioning of the truncus and conus and the formation of the membranous portion of the interventricular septum in the human heart. Am J Anat 71:343, 1942.)

Problems in atrial septation give rise to three types of atrial septal defects: ostium secundum defect, ostium primum defect, and sinus venous defect. Problems in ventricular septation give rise to ventricular septal defects, usually in the region of the membranous septum. Problems in septation of great vessels give rise to congenital complete transposition of the great vessels, or D-transposition, because they occur following normal dextro-bulboventricular looping. Other anomalies include vascular rings, persistent patent ductus arteriosus, and coarctation of the aorta.

Cardiovascular malformations occur in about 0.8% of live births.[10] However, this figure underestimates the incidence of congenital heart disease because cardiac malformations occur 10 times more often in stillborn babies than in liveborn babies. Children with congenital heart disease are predominantly male. However, specific defects have a definite sex preponderance; patent ductus arteriosus and atrial septal defect are more common in girls, but valvular aortic stenosis, congenital aneurysm of the sinus of Valsalva, coarctation of the aorta, tetralogy of Fallot, and congenital complete transposition of the great arteries are more common in boys.[10]

EXTERNAL ANATOMY OF THE HEART AND GREAT VESSELS

Several excellent accounts of the anatomy of the heart and great vessels have been published.[11–17] Normally, the heart is positioned in the mediastinum to the left of the midline, with the cardiac apex pointed to the left. The heart is rotated and tilted in the chest such that most of the anterior surface is composed of the right ventricle, but with the left third occupied by the left ventricle. The right inferior border (obtuse border) is given by the right ventricle, whereas the left lateral border is largely given by the left ventricle. Superior to the right and left ventricles are the right and left auricles of the right and left atria, respectively. The anterior superior surface of the cardiac silhouette is composed of the outflow portion (conus) of the right ventricle and the pulmonary trunk, which extends from right to left as it exits the pericardium. The pulmonary trunk then gives origin to the left and right main pulmonary arteries. The aorta is located posterior to the pulmonary trunk. The aorta extends from the left ventricle and is oriented from left to right as it exits the pericardium. The aorta then curves to the left and inferiorly, creating a left-sided aortic arch from which the right innominate, left common carotid, and left subclavian arteries are sequentially derived. The aorta then courses inferiorly as the descending thoracic aorta.

PERICARDIUM

The pericardial cavity is a narrow, fluid-filled space that surrounds the heart and proximal great vessels. The pericardial lining is a thin layer of connective tissue lined by a single layer of mesothelial cells. There are two divisions. The visceral pericardium covers the epicardium of the heart. The parietal pericardium is the outer layer. The superior reflection or transition of visceral to parietal pericardium occurs approximately 2 to 3 cm superior to the heart, thereby enclosing the proximal aorta and pulmonary trunk in the pericardial cavity. The pericardial cavity normally contains

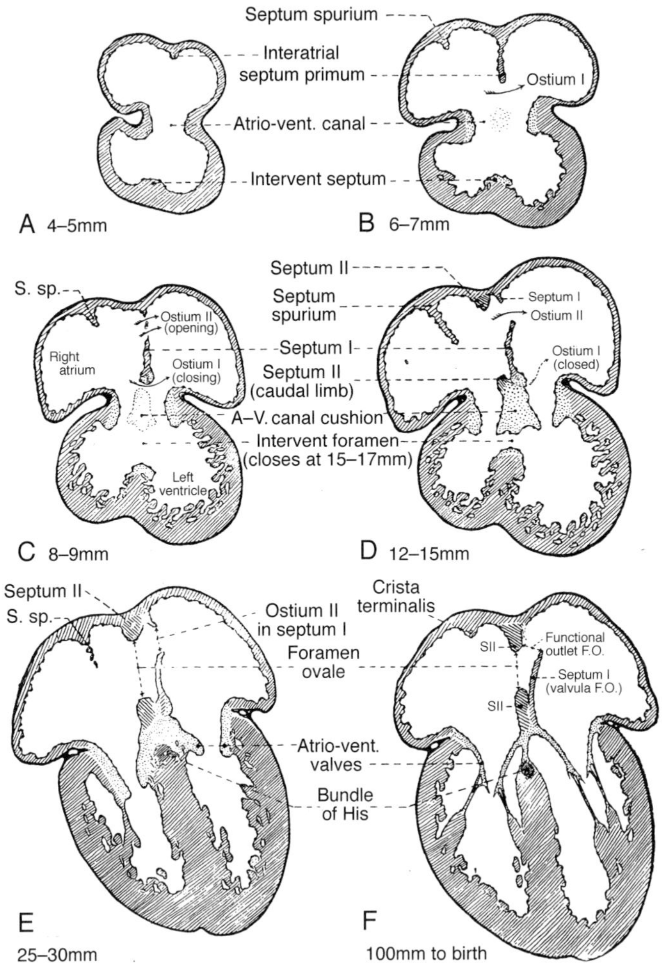

FIGURE 1–2. Sectional plans of an embryonic heart in frontal plane that show the extent of growth of various cardiac septa at several stages of development. These diagrams give a picture of the rate at which partitioning in the human embryo progresses. Stippled areas in the diagrams indicate distribution of endocardial cushion tissue; muscle is shown in diagonal hatching; and epicardium in solid black. The lightly stippled areas in the atrioventricular canal of *B* and *C* indicate the location of dorsal and ventral endocardial cushions of the atrioventricular canal before they have grown sufficiently to fuse with each other in the plane of the diagram. (From Patten BM: Developmental defects at the foramen ovale. Am J Pathol 14: 135, 1938.)

about 20 ml of serous fluid, which serves to lubricate the heart and facilitate its motion.

A variety of inflammatory and neoplastic conditions can affect the pericardium. Hemorrhage into the pericardium may occur as a result of cardiac rupture, usually secondary to acute myocardial infarction, or rupture of the proximal aorta following aortic dissection. Severity of cardiac dysfunction secondary to pericardial disease is influenced by the amount and rapidity of fluid accumulation in the pericardial cavity.

HEART

Basic Structure

Several excellent descriptions of the anatomy of the heart are available.[11–17] The heart consists of three layers: the epicardium, the myocardium, and the endocardium. The epicardium consists of fatty connective tissue and is lined by the visceral pericardium. The myocardium comprises most of the mass of the heart and is composed of cardiac myocytes, vessels, and connective tissue. The cardiac myocytes constitute approximately 80% of the mass but only 20% of the number of cells in the myocardium. The endocardium is composed of the nonvalvular (visceral) and valvular endocardium. The endocardium consists of thin fibrocellular connective tissue, which is lined by a single layer of endothelial cells.

The Coronary Vasculature

The anatomy and physiology of the coronary circulation have been well characterized.[18–25] Normally, the heart is supplied with oxygenated blood by the left and right coronary arteries. These arteries originate via their ostia from the left and right aortic sinuses of Valsalva, which are located just distal to the left and right cusps, respectively, of the aortic valve (Fig. 1–4). The short left coronary artery divides into left anterior descending and left circumflex branches and, occasionally, a left marginal branch. The anterior portion of the left ventricle and interventricular septum are supplied by the left anterior descending coronary artery and its left diagonal and septal branches. The lateral left ventricle is supplied by the left circumflex coronary artery and its circumflex marginal branches. The right coronary artery supplies the right ventricle and, in about 90% of hearts, it extends posteriorly to give rise to the posterior descending coronary artery.

Considerable variation occurs in the anatomic distribution of the coronary arterial branches. However, in most hearts, branches of the left circumflex and right coronary arteries contribute to the blood supply of the posterior left ventricle, creating a so-called balanced circulation. In about 10% of hearts, the right coronary artery is diminutive and the left circumflex coronary artery gives rise to the posterior descending coronary artery and provides the sole blood supply for the posterior left ventricle, creating a so-called left dominant circulation. Rarely, the converse right dominant circulation occurs when the left circumflex is diminutive and the posterior left ventricle is supplied primarily by left ventricular branches of the right coronary artery.

The major artery to the sinoatrial node arises from the proximal right coronary artery in about 60% of hearts and from the left circumflex coronary artery in about 40% of hearts. The major atrioventricular nodal artery originates from the coronary artery that gives rise to the posterior descending branch, which is the right coronary artery in about 90% and the left circumflex coronary artery in about 10% of hearts.

The epicardial coronary arteries deliver oxygenated blood to the myocardial arteries, arterioles, and capillaries. After oxygen and substrate extraction in the myocardium, a small amount of unoxygenated blood flows directly into the ventricular cavities via the thebesian veins, and most blood returns via myocardial venules and veins into the epicardial veins, which drain into the coronary sinus located in the inferoposterior region of the right atrium.

During normal embryologic development, collateral vessels form and connect different components of the coronary

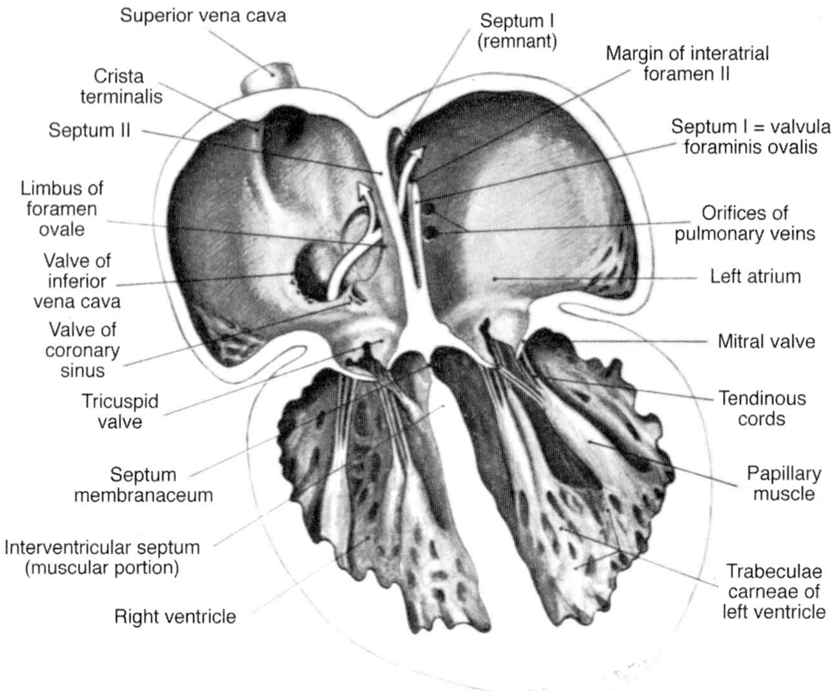

FIGURE 1–3. Schematic drawing that shows the relationship of the septum primum (Septum I) and the septum secundum (Septum II) during the latter part of fetal life. Note that the lower part of the septum primum is situated so that it acts as a one-way valve at the oval foramen in the septum secundum. The split arrow indicates the direction of passage of a considerable part of the blood from the inferior vena cava through the foramen ovale to the left atrium while the remainder eddies back into the right atrium to mingle with the blood being returned by way of the superior vena cava. (From Patten BM: Foundations on Embryology. McGraw-Hill, New York, 1953.)

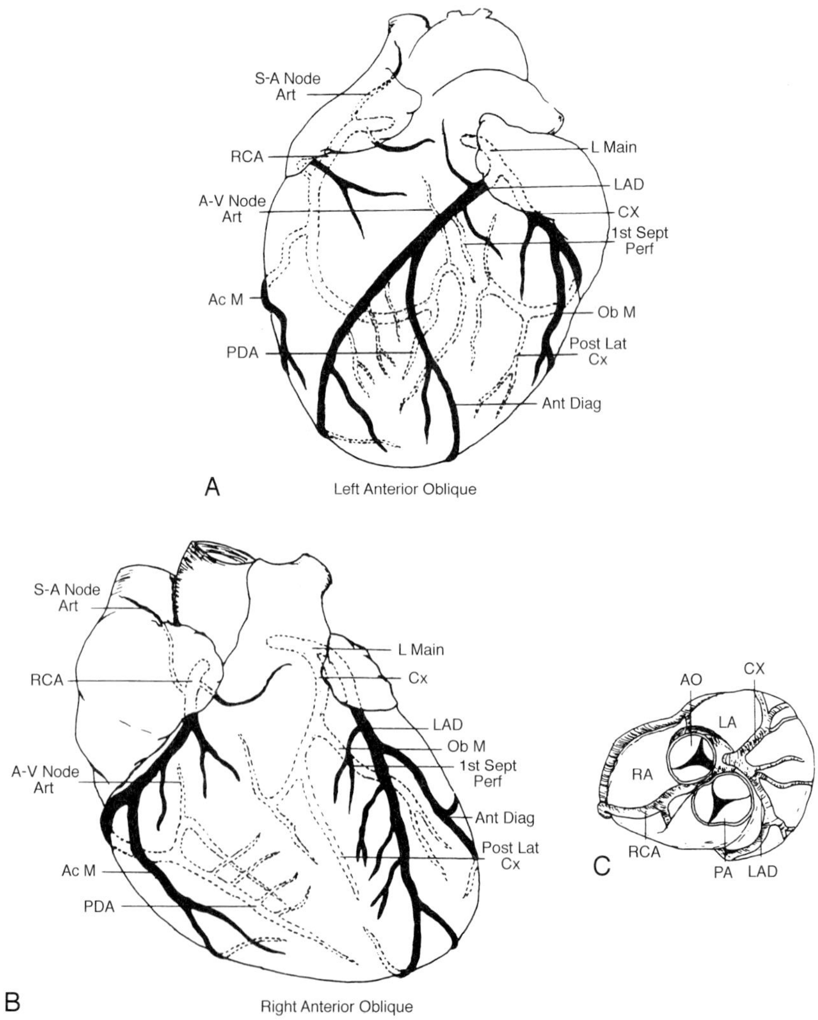

FIGURE 1–4. Left *(A)* and right *(B)* anterior oblique views of the coronary arteries and their distribution, and a cephalad *(C)* view of coronary artery distribution in relation to the great vessels. (S-A, sinoatrial; Art, artery; RCA, right coronary artery; A-V, atrioventricular; AcM, acute marginal; PDA, posterior descending artery; Ant, anterior; Post, posterior; Lat, lateral; Cx, circumflex; ObM, obtuse marginal; Sept, septal; Perf, perforator; LAD, left anterior descending; L, left; Ao, aorta; LA, left atrium; RA, right atrium; PA, pulmonary artery.) (From Boudoulas H, Gravanis MB: Ischemic heart disease. In Gravanis MB [ed]: Cardiovascular Disorders: Pathogenesis and Pathophysiology. Mosby, St. Louis, 1993, p 15.)

arterial circulation.[18–25] The coronary collateral system is composed of four types of vessels: intramural branches of the same coronary artery (homocoronary collaterals); intramural branches of two or more coronary arteries (intercoronary collaterals); atrial branches, which connect with the vasa vasorum of the aorta and other vessels (extracardiac collaterals); and intramural branches, which communicate with the cardiac cavities (arterioluminal vessels). In the normal adult heart, the collateral vessels are thin walled, small channels, usually less than 50 μm in diameter, which contribute little to total coronary blood flow. In response to coronary arterial narrowing and myocardial ischemia, myocardial collateral vessels can increase in diameter into the range of 200 to 600 μm or more, develop muscular media, and transport significant amounts of blood flow. In addition to the collateral vessels described earlier, collateral channels also develop between segments of a coronary artery proximal and distal to a stenosis.

Right and Left Atria and Ventricles

The anatomic features of the right and left atria and ventricles are shown in multiple projections (Figs. 1–5 to 1–8). General characteristics of the anatomic right ventricle are a distinct muscular infundibulum, which separates the right semilunar (pulmonary) valve and the right atrioventricular (tricuspid) valve; a single large anterior papillary muscle; and coarse trabecular muscles (trabeculae carneae cordis) at the apical and inflow portion of the chamber.[11–17] General characteristics of the anatomic left ventricle are a fibrous continuity of the annulus of the left semilunar (aortic) valve and anterior leaflet of left atrioventricular (mitral) valve, two well-developed papillary muscles (anterolateral and posteromedial), and fine trabecular muscles at the apical and inflow portions of the chamber.[11–17]

Cardiac Valves

The heart has four valves: the right semilunar (pulmonic) valve, the right atrioventricular (tricuspid) valve, the left semilunar (aortic) valve, and the left atrioventricular (mitral) valve (Figs. 1–9 and 1–10). The pulmonic and aortic semilunar valves each normally consist of a fibrous connective tissue annulus and three cusps separated by three commissures. The aortic valve cusps are designated as the left, right, and non-coronary cusps. Each semilunar valvular cusp has a ridge about 1 to 2 mm below the free margin, which represents the site of contact of the cusps during valve closure during diastole. The central points of maximal contact are especially prominent and are known as the noduli of Arantius.

The right atrioventricular (tricuspid) valve has a fibrous annulus and three cusps or leaflets separated by three commissures. The leaflets are the lateral, medial, and anterior. The leaflets are anchored to the ventricular muscle by multiple chordae tendineae that extend from the ventricular surfaces of the cusps to the mural ventricular wall, as well as by a well-developed anterior papillary muscle and a diminutive structure, the papillary muscle of the conus.

The left atrioventricular (mitral) valvular apparatus is highly developed and consists of a fibrous annulus, anterior and posterior leaflets, anterior and posterior commissures, multiple chordae tendineae, and anterolateral and posteromedial papillary muscles. The anterior leaflet is a single structure, whereas the posterior leaflet may be divided into two or three scallops. Chordae tendineae from both leaflets extend and attach to both papillary muscles. Chordae have at least three divisions of branching constituting primary, secondary, and tertiary chordae. Abnormal function of the mitral valve can result in abnormalities of the annulus, leaflets, chordae tendineae, papillary muscles, and mural ventricular myocardium.

Ordinarily, the anterior mitral leaflet has a significantly larger area and longer length from the annulus to the free margin than the posterior mitral leaflet, such that the anterior leaflet contributes about two thirds of the area of leaflet tissue involved in closure of the mitral orifice during systole. Expansion of the posterior leaflet to equal the length of the anterior leaflet from the annulus to the free margin is an important anatomic feature of myxomatous degeneration of the mitral valve. Other features include general redundancy

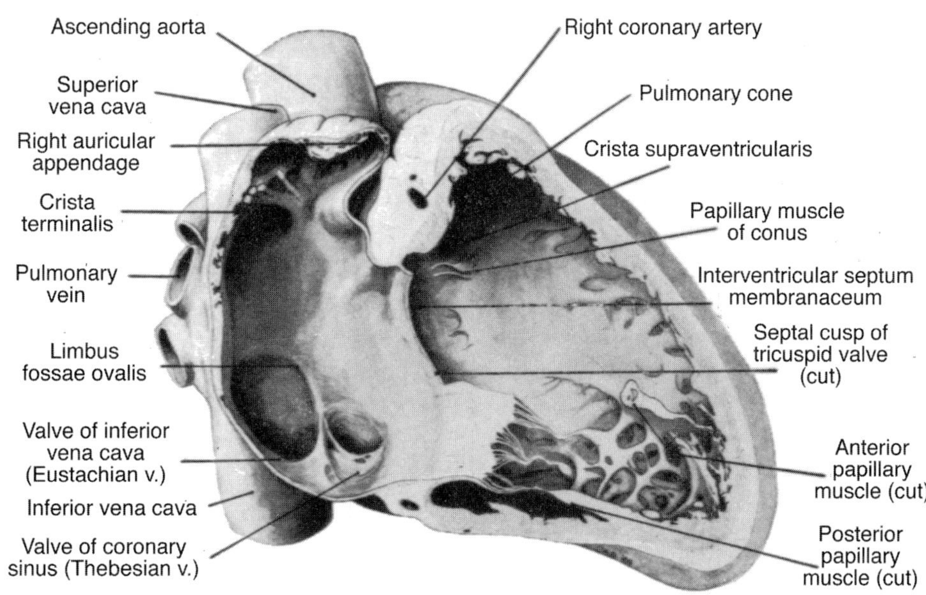

FIGURE 1–5. Right side of the heart opened in a plane approximately parallel to the septa to show the interior of the right atrium and the right ventricle. A segment of the septal leaflet of the tricuspid valve has been cut away to expose more fully the region of the membranous portion of the interventricular septum. (From Barry A, Patten BM: The structure of the adult heart. In Gould SE [ed]: Pathology of the Heart and Blood Vessels, 3rd ed. CC Thomas, Springfield, IL, 1968, p 99. Courtesy of Charles C Thomas, Publisher, Ltd., Springfield, Illinois.)

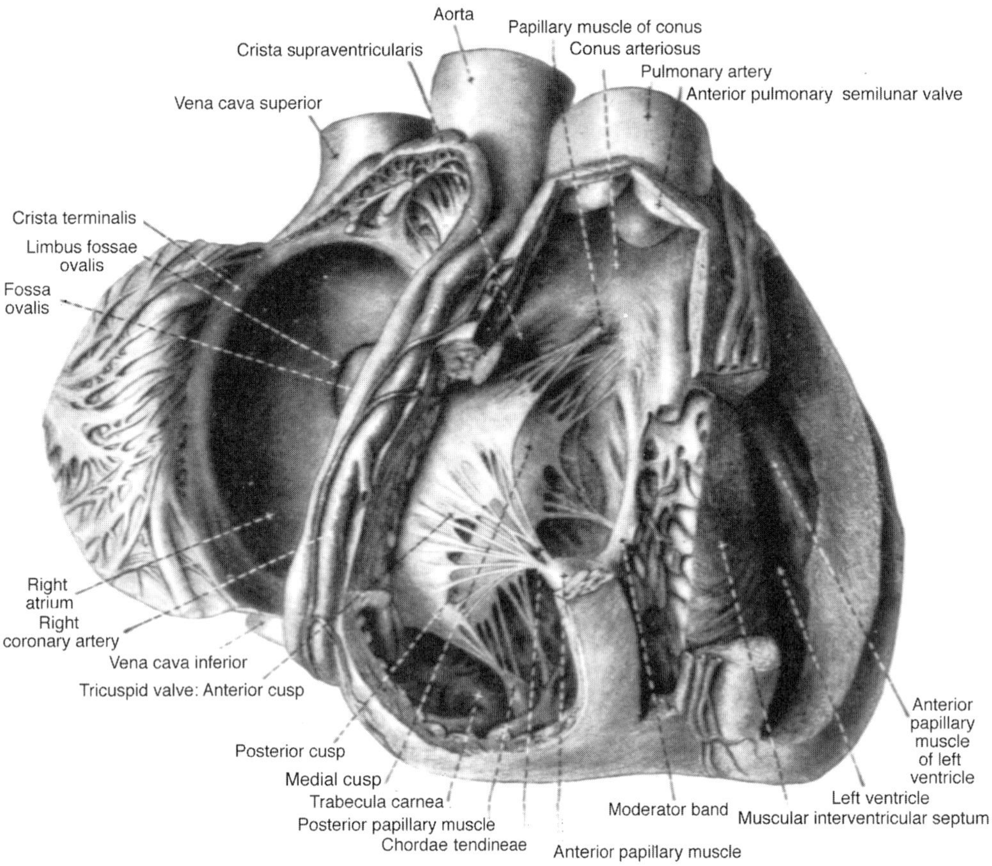

FIGURE 1–6. Ventral view of the heart with the walls of the right atrium and ventricle, which are opened to show their internal configuration. The dissection shows the relations of an unusually well-developed moderator band. In this heart, the position of the foramen ovale is somewhat more cephalic than usual. (From Barry A, Patten BM: The structure of the adult heart. In Gould SE [ed]: Pathology of the Heart and Blood Vessels, 3rd ed. CC Thomas, Springfield, IL, 1968, p 100. Courtesy of Charles C Thomas, Publisher, Ltd., Springfield, Illinois.)

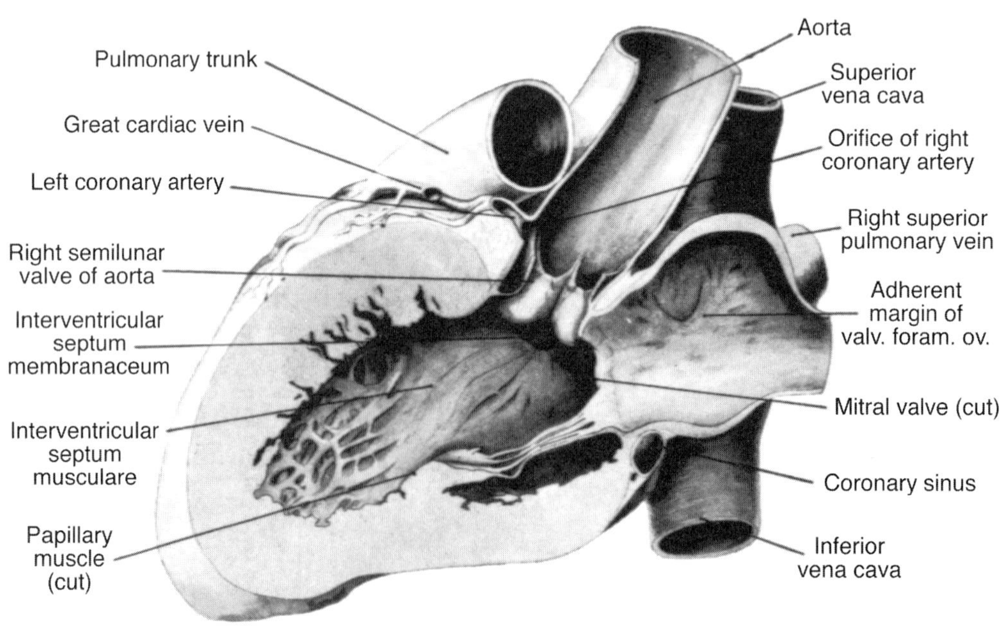

FIGURE 1–7. Left side of the heart opened in a plane approximately parallel to the septa to show the interior of the left atrium and left ventricle. A segment of the anterior leaflet of the mitral valve has been cut away to expose more fully the membranous portion of the interventricular septum and the aortic orifice. (From Barry A, Patten BM: The structure of the adult heart. In Gould SE [ed]: Pathology of the Heart and Blood Vessels, 3rd ed. CC Thomas, Springfield, IL, 1968, p 101. Courtesy of Charles C Thomas, Publisher, Ltd., Springfield, Illinois.)

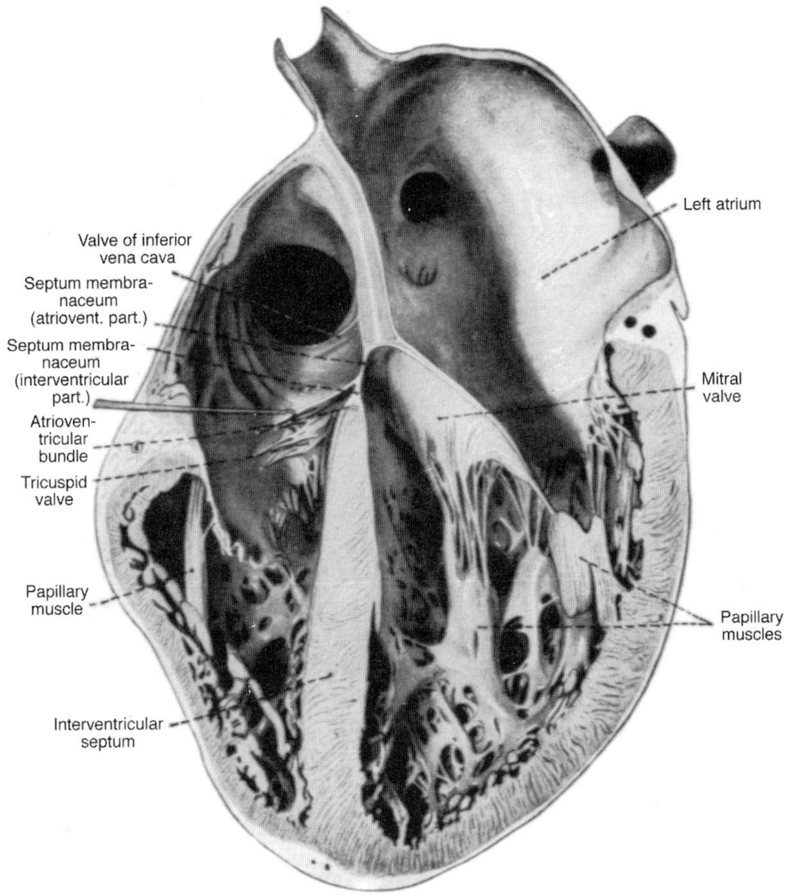

FIGURE 1–8. Frontal section through a heart fixed in diastole, showing a ventral view of the dorsal portion. The plane of dissection passes through the septum membranaceum and both atrioventricular ostia. (From Patten BM: Foundations on Embryology. McGraw-Hill, New York, 1953. Reproduced with permission of The McGraw-Hill Companies.)

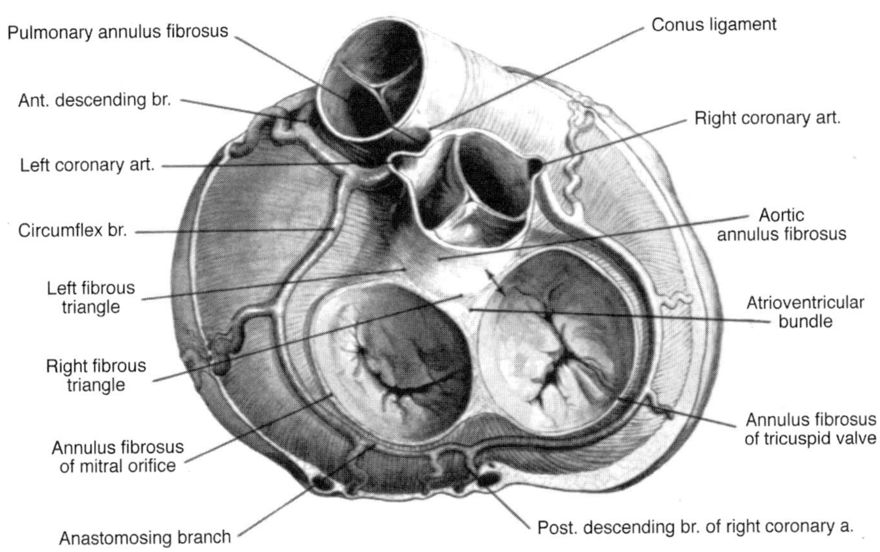

FIGURE 1–9. Ventricular portion of the heart viewed from above with the atria removed to show the four cardiac valves and the fibrous triangles, the annuli fibrosi and the attachment of the ventricular musculature to them. The fatty epicardium has been removed from the atrioventricular sulcus to show the coronary arteries. (From Barry A, Patten BM: The structure of the adult heart. In Gould SE [ed]: Pathology of the Heart and Blood Vessels, 3rd ed. CC Thomas, Springfield, IL, 1968, p 113. Courtesy of Charles C Thomas, Publisher, Ltd., Springfield, Illinois.)

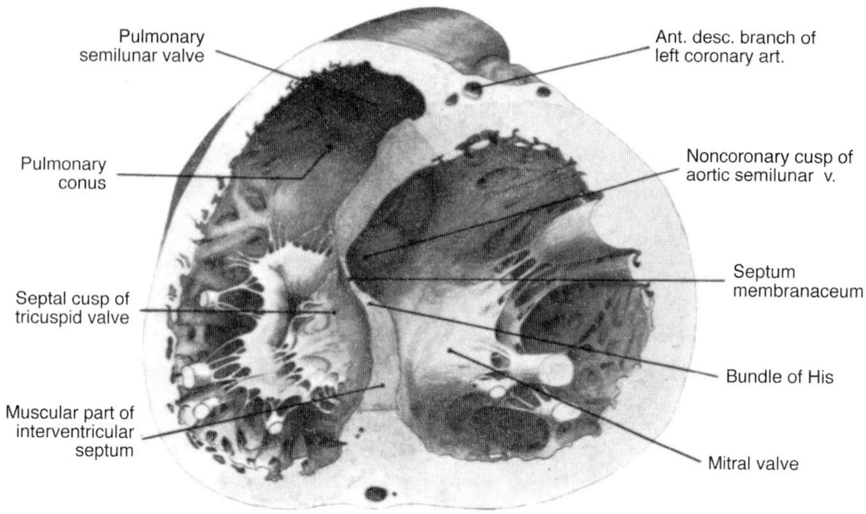

FIGURE 1–10. Interior of the ventricular base of the heart, exposed by removing the apical half of the ventricles. The interventricular septum has been partially cut away to show the interventricular septum membranaceum, and the mitral, the tricuspid, and the aortic valves. (From Barry A, Patten BM: The structure of the adult heart. In Gould SE [ed]: Pathology of the Heart and Blood Vessels, 3rd ed. CC Thomas, Springfield, IL, 1968, p 114. Courtesy of Charles C Thomas, Publisher, Ltd., Springfield, Illinois.)

and thickening of leaflet tissue and chordae tendineae, and a glistening white appearance of leaflets and chordae. These changes are typical of advanced mitral valve prolapse. This condition has an increased frequency in women and may be manifested by arrhythmias and other cardiovascular symptoms.

The most common congenital valvular lesion is a unicuspid or bicuspid aortic valve, which occurs in both men and women.

Conduction System and Cardiac Innervation

Detailed studies have led to clear definition of the anatomy of the cardiac conduction system (Fig. 1–11).[26, 27] The sinoatrial node is embedded in the superficial subepicardium of the superior right atrium at the junction of the superior vena cava and the right auricular appendage. The sinoatrial node contains specialized myocytes that generate electrical impulses and constitute the cardiac pacemaker. The electrical impulses propagate selectively along certain paths in the atria; however, the existence of anatomically distinct conduction pathways in the atria is uncertain. Atrioventricular conduction is accomplished by specialized structures: the atrioventricular node (node of Tawara) and atrioventricular bundle (bundle of His). The atrioventricular node is located in the inferior atrial septum, just anterior and medial to the ostium of the coronary sinus. The specialized conduction tissue then traverses the fibrous tissue separating the atria and ventricles (fibrous skeleton) to connect to the bundle of

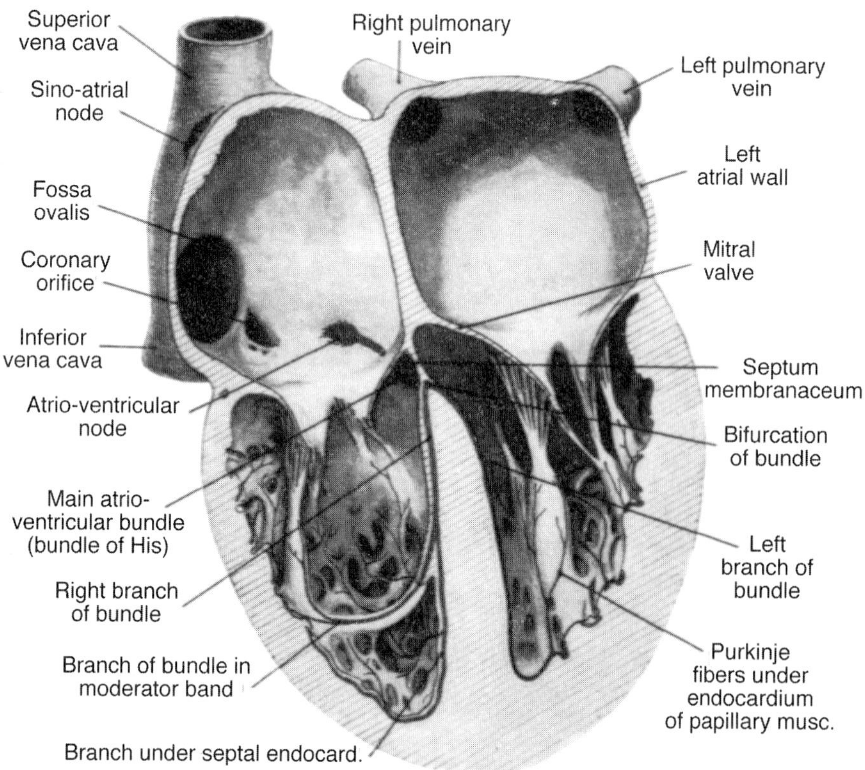

FIGURE 1–11. Schematic diagram of a heart opened frontally that demonstrates the relative locations of the parts of the sinoventricular conduction system. (From Barry A, Patten BM: The structure of the adult heart. In Gould SE [ed]: Pathology of the Heart and Blood Vessels, 3rd ed. CC Thomas, Springfield, IL, 1968, p 121. Courtesy of Charles C Thomas, Publisher, Ltd., Springfield, Illinois.)

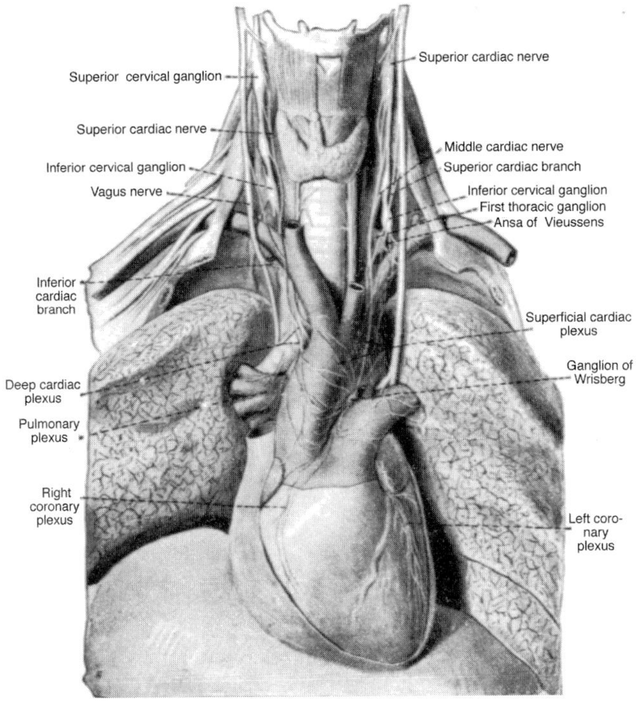

FIGURE 1–12. Ventral view of the heart showing the nerve supply to the heart. (From Barry A, Patten BM: The structure of the adult heart. In Gould SE [ed]: Pathology of the Heart and Blood Vessels, 3rd ed. CC Thomas, Springfield, IL, 1968, p 128. Courtesy of Charles C Thomas, Publisher, Ltd., Springfield, Illinois.)

His, which is located at the apex of the muscular interventricular septum. The bundle of His gives rise to the right and left bundle branches, which extend through the subendocardium of the interventricular septum into the right and left ventricular free walls.

The heart has a dual innervation from the sympathetic (thoracolumbar) and parasympathetic (craniosacral) divisions of the autonomic nervous system (Fig. 1–12).

Cardiac Dimensions and the Effect of Increased Workload, Including Exercise

Several authors have collected data regarding dimensions and measurements of the heart.[11–17] The weight of the heart is proportional to body dimensions, including length and weight. Hudson has developed a useful guide regarding fresh heart weight in men and women.[11] The adult male heart weight is characterized as follows: 0.45% of body weight, average 300 g, range 250 to 350 g. The adult female heart weight is characterized as follows: 0.40% of body weight, average 250 g, range 200 to 300 g. Techniques have been developed for selective determination of right ventricular and left ventricular weights, and ranges have been established for determination of selective enlargement of right and left ventricles, as well as biventricular enlargement. The thickness of the walls of the cardiac chambers are as follows: right and left atria, 0.1 to 0.2 cm; right ventricle, 0.4 to 0.5 cm; left ventricle, 1.2 to 1.5 cm (free wall, excluding papillary muscles and large trabeculae). The average circumferences of the cardiac valves are aortic, 7.5 cm; pulmonic, 8.5 cm; mitral, 10.0 cm; and tricuspid, 12.0 cm.

Cardiac enlargement can occur in response to a pressure load or to a volume load and result in concentric hypertrophy (increased chamber weight and increased chamber wall thickness with normal or reduced chamber volume) or eccentric hypertrophy (increased chamber weight and increased chamber volume with relatively normal chamber wall thickness), respectively (Fig. 1–13).[28–31] Cardiac enlargement is accomplished primarily by an increase in the mass and size of cardiac muscle cells (hypertrophy), accompanied by an increase in the number of connective tissue cells (hyperplasia) and the amount of connective tissue matrix, which maintains the one-to-one ratio of myocytes to capillaries.[28] The process is generically referred to as cardiac hypertrophy. Cardiac hypertrophy may occur in response to repetitive strenuous exercise (physiologic hypertrophy) or to an abnormal load due to a cardiovascular structural or functional abnormality (pathologic hypertrophy). In physiologic cardiac hypertrophy, the critical heart weight of 550 g is not exceeded.[28] Once the heart mass exceeds 550 g, the potential exists for progressive changes leading to irreversible structural alteration of the myocardium and cardiac failure.[28]

The adaptations to increased ventricular load induced by long-term athletic training consist of an increase in left ventricular diastolic cavity dimension, wall thickness, and mass, and collectively, these changes are referred to as athlete's heart.[32] Based on studies in men, athlete's heart is thought to occur routinely in response to strenuous exercise. However, a recently reported study of Italian Olympic athletes has indicated significant gender differences.[33] This study concluded that, although highly trained women athletes frequently demonstrated cardiac dimensional changes as an adaptation to physical training, absolute left ventricular cavity size exceeding normal limits was evident in only a minority (8%) of women athletes and was rarely (1% of athletes) within the range of dilated cardiomyopathy. Athletic training was not a stimulus for substantial increases in absolute left ventricular wall thickness, which was within normal limits for all women athletes. These findings suggest that the clinical differentiation of athlete's heart and hypertrophic cardiomyopathy appears to be a diagnostic dilemma that is limited to male athletes.

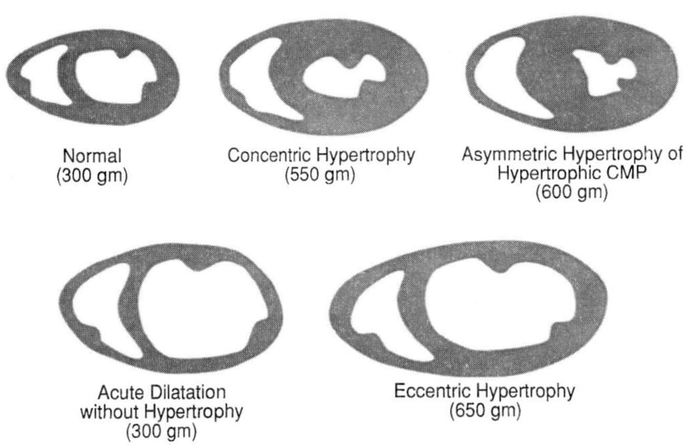

FIGURE 1–13. Patterns of cardiomegaly shown in transverse sections through the cardiac ventricles. Values in parentheses represent corresponding heart weights. (Modified from Buja LM, Petty CS: Heart disease, trauma, and death. In Curran WJ, McGarry AL, Petty CS [eds]: Modern Legal Medicine, Psychiatry, and Forensic Science. F.A. Davis, Philadelphia, 1980, p 191.)

Low fitness has been documented to be an important precursor of mortality from cardiovascular problems.[34] In general, features of low fitness are similar in men and women. In addition to low fitness, smoking was the only other significant independent predictor of cardiovascular mortality in women.[34]

Sudden death in young competitive athletes is fortunately a rare event, usually is precipitated by physical activity, and may be due to a heterogeneous spectrum of cardiovascular disease, most commonly hypertrophic cardiomyopathy in the American population.[35] Sudden death in young competitive athletes is a phenomenon that occurs predominately in men.[35]

VESSELS

Embryologic Development

Governed by a complex genetic program, blood vessel formation begins before the heart starts beating. Beginning around 2 weeks of gestation, blood islands appear in the wall of the yolk sac and extraembryonic vascular channels form in association with them. In addition, a portion of the vasculature of the embryonic body is derived from intraembryonic sources. During the early period of somite formation, networks of small vessels rapidly appear in many regions of the embryo. Some vascular channels coalesce to form larger vessels, and others remain similar to capillaries or disappear. Early vasculogenesis is dynamic, changing in association with growth of the structures that the vascular channels supply.[36, 37]

Embryonic blood vessels form from angioblasts (mesoderm-derived endothelial cell precursors) by (1) coalescence of angioblasts in situ, (2) migration of angioblasts into organs, and (3) sprouting from existing vessels. Several proteins are mitogenic for these cells, including platelet derived growth factor, basic fibroblast growth factor (bFGF), and vascular endothelial growth factor (VEGF), among others.[38–40] These factors appear to be involved in both vasculogenesis (the earliest formation of de novo blood vessels in the embryo) and angiogenesis (the formation of new capillary vessels from pre-existing vessels). Angiogenic factors stimulate the ingrowth of vessels into developing organs. Many of the factors involved in vasculogenesis also play a role in angiogenesis, including angiogenesis in ischemic heart disease and in tumor angiogenesis. The density of microvessels in several solid tumors, including breast cancer, has been shown to have prognostic significance.[41–46]

Genetic defect in these growth factors may lead to malformations in developing embryos. Mutations in one or both VEGF alleles leading to deficiency of VEGF or mutations of either of the two receptors for VEGF result in death of the affected embryo.[40, 47] Recently described angiopoietin-1 is thought to play a role in regulating nonendothelial vessel wall components.[48–51] A genetic mutation of its receptor, tie2, has been demonstrated in congenital venous malformations in which vessel walls are deficient in smooth muscle support.[52]

General Structure of Blood Vessels

Blood vessels of all sizes have some structural features in common, although in the vessels of smallest size, the three tunics (layers) of the vessel wall are greatly simplified (Fig. 1–14). Blood vessels are usually composed of (1) a tunica intima consisting of endothelial cells resting on a basal lamina and lining the interior surface of the vessel; (2) a tunica media composed of concentric layers of smooth muscle with variable amounts of elastic fibers, reticular fibers, and proteoglycans; and (3) a tunica adventitia consisting of collagen and elastic fibers which gradually becomes continuous with the surrounding connective tissue.[53] Nerves, lymphatics, and the vasa vasorum are found in the adventitia. The vasa vasorum (vessels of the vessel) forms a capillary network supplying nutrients to the deep layers of the media of larger arteries and veins. The vasa vasorum takes origin from the vessel it nourishes or from neighboring vessels.

Arteries

Arteries are usually classified according to their size into large elastic arteries and small to medium-sized muscular arteries. The elastic arteries, which include the aorta and its major branches, are sometimes referred to as conducting arteries. They do not contract, but their large elastic tissue component allows them to absorb the pulse wave produced in systole. Elastic recoil of the vascular wall propels blood through the peripheral circulation. They have relatively thin walls compared with their large diameter.

Histologically, the large elastic arteries have a characteristic media formed by numerous concentric elastic lamellae whose number increases with age (about 40 in the newborn, 70 in the adult). However, with aging, the aorta loses some of its elasticity and expands less readily, often becoming progressively tortuous and dilated. The elastic arteries ramify into the muscular arteries.

The muscular arteries, which may vary from 1.0 cm to 0.05 cm in diameter, are capable of contraction. These include most of the named and grossly visible arteries, such as the coronary, renal, and femoral arteries, and are referred to as distributing arteries. A media with circularly or spirally arranged smooth muscle cells and a prominent internal elastic lamina are important histologic features of muscular arteries. Local changes in blood flow are regulated by contraction (vasoconstriction) or relaxation (vasodilatation) of the smooth muscle in the wall of the vessel.

Various hormones and other metabolic substances may have adverse or protective effects on the vasculature. For example, estrogen has an atheroprotective effect in premenopausal women and in postmenopausal women given estrogen replacement.[54] The exact mechanism by which this occurs is unknown, perhaps by indirect modulation of cardiovascular risk factors or by a direct effect on the vessel. Vascular smooth muscle cells have been shown to express estrogen receptors and to respond to estrogen-dependent gene activation. Genes regulating the production of two important vasodilators synthesized by the vessel wall (prostacyclin and nitric oxide) can be up-regulated by estrogen.[55]

In addition to the long-recognized association of hyperlipidemia with atherosclerosis, another condition, hyperhomocysteinemia, has been linked to premature vascular disease and thrombosis.[56–58] Individuals homozygous for the autosomal recessive disorder homocystinuria experience arterial or venous thromboembolic events at an early age and acceler-

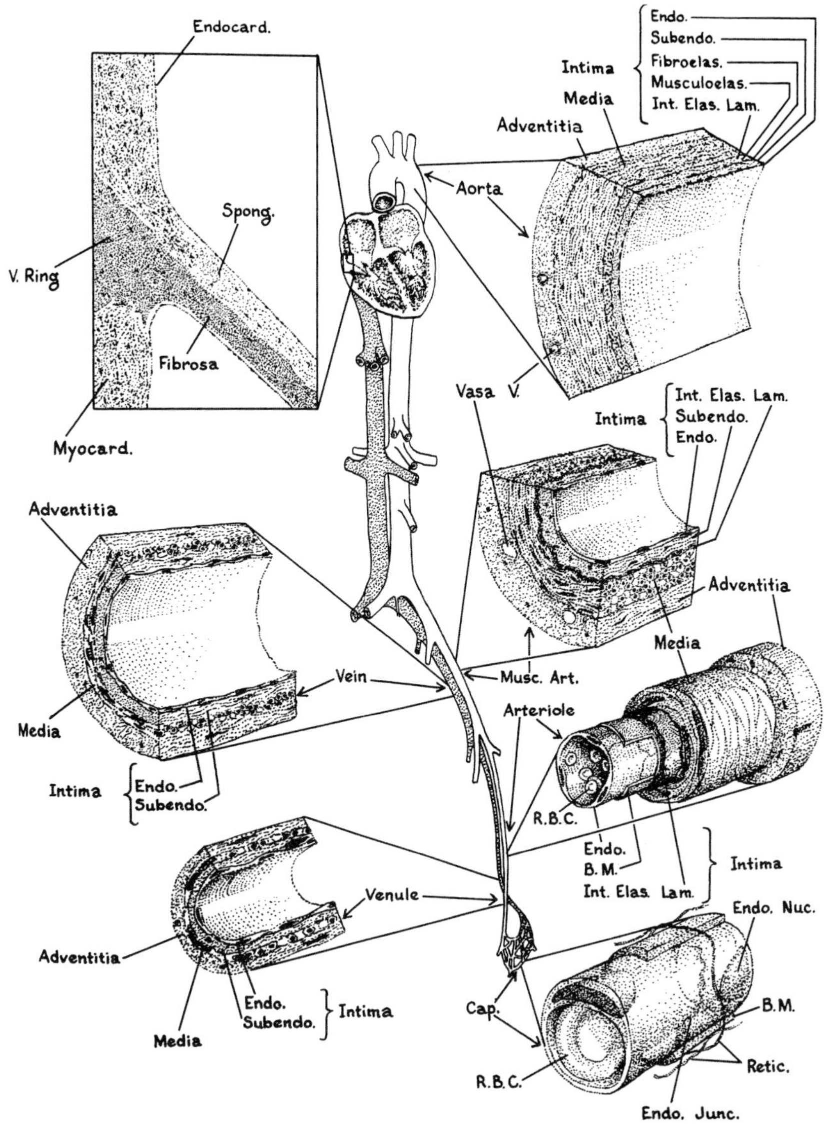

FIGURE 1–14. Histology of the vascular system. (BM, basement membrane; Cap, capillary; Endo, endothelium; Endo Junc, junction between adjacent endothelial cells; Endo Nuc, nucleus of endothelial cell; Endocard, endocardium of right atrium; Fibroelas, fibroelastic layer of aortic intima; Fibrosa, fibrosa of tricuspid valve; Int Elas Lam, internal elastic lamella; Musc Art, muscular artery; Musculoelas, musculoelastic layer of aortic intima; Myocard, myocardium of right ventricle; RBC, red blood cell; Retic, reticulin fibers; Spong, spongiosa of tricuspid valve; Subendo, subendothelial fibrous tissue; V Ring, valve ring of tricuspid valve; Vasa V, vasa vasorum.) (From Fallis BD, Ashworth RD: Textbook of Human Histology. Little, Brown and Co., Boston, 1970, p 65.)

ated atherosclerosis, as well as other abnormalities, including mental retardation and osteoporosis. Even patients with moderate hyperhomocysteinemia have an increased risk of developing premature atherosclerosis. As many as 14% to 30% of patients with premature arterial disease have heterozygous homocystinuria as an independent risk factor for thrombosis.

Microcirculation

The microvasculature is important because of participation in the interchange between the circulation and surrounding tissues. The arterioles are the smallest branches of the arteries, generally smaller than 0.5 mm in diameter with a media composed of one or two circularly arranged layers of smooth muscle cells. Under autonomic and local control, the medial smooth muscle of the arterioles adjust the lumen diameter, thus regulating arterial blood pressure and blood flow into the various capillary beds. The arterioles and small arteries bear the brunt of elevations in blood pressure. Whereas atherosclerosis is a disease largely of elastic and muscular arteries, hypertension is associated with functional and structural changes in the arterioles and small muscular arteries.

Capillaries are composed of a single layer of endothelial cells supported by a thin basement membrane. The lumen of a capillary is the width of a red blood cell, which is 7 to 9 μm. Slow blood flow, large surface area, and a wall a single cell layer thick facilitate the exchange of diffusible substances between the blood and extravascular tissues. Capillaries in different sites vary in the degree of continuity of endothelium and basement membrane; for example, renal glomeruli and bone marrow sinusoids allow more rapid exchange of fluid or passage of cells because of the fenestrated or discontinuous endothelium.

Venules have very thin walls with luminal diameters up to 100 μm. They differ from arterioles in that they have only one or two layers of smooth muscle cells in the media and are lacking an internal elastic lamina. Blood returning to the heart from capillary beds flows initially into the postcapillary venules and then sequentially through collecting venules, then through the small, medium, and large veins.

Veins

Veins are thin-walled vessels with relatively large lumina. When considered as a functional unit, all of the veins can be classified as capacitance vessels because more than 70% of the total blood volume is in this portion of the cardiovascular system at any one time. As with the arteries, it is customary to classify veins into small, medium, and large veins. Veins, particularly those of the legs, may have valves formed by an outfolding of the intima to ensure unidirectional blood flow. The distinction between intima, media, and adventitia is less distinct than in the arteries. The adventitia is the best developed tunic in the veins. Cardiac muscle is present in the adventitia of the vena cava and pulmonary veins for a short distance before they empty into the heart.

The relatively poor support of the media in veins predisposes them to abnormal dilation, compression, and infiltration by tumors. The most common diseases of veins are the development of varicosities and of phlebothrombosis and thrombophlebitis. Varices may occur in any part of the body but share a common pathogenesis—increased pressure of the blood within the vein. In general, varicose veins have narrowing or abnormal dilation, with subsequent incompetence of the venous valves causing venous stasis. Thrombosis may occur, but embolism is rare. In contrast, pulmonary embolism and infarction are potentially fatal complications of thrombophlebitis.

Lymphatics

Fluid from the extravascular tissue spaces is returned to the blood through the lymphatics. With rare exceptions, such as the nervous system and bone marrow, a lymphatic system is found in almost all organs. Lymphatics can be recognized in tissue sections as collapsed, thin-walled, endothelium-lined channels devoid of red blood cells. The lymphatic capillaries originate in the various tissues as thin, blind-ended vessels consisting of a single layer of endothelium. They are held open by numerous microfibrils of the elastic fiber system that also bind them to the surrounding connective tissue. The larger lymphatic vessels have a structure similar to that of veins except that they have thinner walls and a clear-cut separation between the three layers. Like veins, they have numerous internal valves. The thin lymphatic vessels gradually converge and end up as two large trunks—the thoracic duct and the right lymphatic duct—which empty into the junction of the left internal jugular vein and the left subclavian vein. The structure of the large lymphatic ducts is similar to that of a vein, with a reinforcement of smooth muscle in the middle layer.

Although the lymphatics serve as a protective drainage system returning interstitial fluid to the blood, they also provide an important pathway for disease dissemination through transport of bacteria and tumor cells to distant sites.

Obstructive lymphedema may occur following occlusion of a lymphatic vessel with the abnormal accumulation of lymphatic fluid in the affected area. The most common causes of such lymphatic blockage are spread of malignant tumors with the obstruction of either the lymphatic channels or lymph nodes, radical surgical procedures with removal of regional groups of lymph nodes (e.g., the axillary dissection of radical mastectomy), postirradiation fibrosis, filariasis, and postinflammatory thrombosis and scarring of lymphatic channels.

References

1. Patten BM: The development of the heart. In Gould SE (ed): Pathology of the Heart and Blood Vessels, 3rd ed. Charles C Thomas, Springfield, IL, 1968, pp 20–90.
2. Patten BM: Section on heart. In Patten BM (ed): Human Embryology, 2nd ed. McGraw-Hill (Blakiston Division), New York, 1953, pp 656–705.
3. Patten BM: The development of the circulatory system. In Patten BM (ed): Foundations of Embryology. McGraw-Hill, New York, 1958, pp 484–539.
4. Sadler TW: Cardiovascular system. In Langman J (ed): Langman's Medical Embryology, 5th ed. Williams & Wilkins, Baltimore, 1985, pp 168–214.
5. Olson EN, Srivastava D: Molecular pathways controlling heart development. Science 272:671–676, 1996.
6. Patten BM: Developmental defects at the foramen ovale. Am J Pathol 14:135–161, 1938.
7. Kramer TC: The partitioning of the truncus and conus and the formation of the membranous portion of the interventricular septum in the human heart. Am J Anat 71:343–370, 1942.
8. Edwards JE: Congenital malformations of the heart and great vessels. In Gould SE (ed): Pathology of the Heart and Blood Vessels, 3rd ed. CC Thomas, Springfield, IL, 1968, p 262–478.
9. Berry CL: Congenital heart disease. In Pomerance A, Davies MJ (eds): The Pathology of the Heart. Blackwell Scientific Publications, Oxford, 1975, pp 533–578.
10. Friedman WF: Congenital heart disease in infancy and childhood. In Braunwald E (ed): Heart Disease. A Textbook of Cardiovascular Medicine, 4th ed. WB Saunders, Philadelphia, 1992, pp 887–965.
11. Hudson REB: Structure and function of the heart. In Hudson REB (ed): Cardiovascular Pathology, Vol 1. Williams & Wilkins, Baltimore, 1965, pp 1–52.
12. Barry A, Patten BM: The structure of the adult heart. In Gould SE (ed): Pathology of the Heart and Blood Vessels, 3rd ed. CC Thomas, Springfield, IL, 1968, pp 91–130.
13. Patten BM: The cardiovascular system. In Schaeffer JP (ed): Morris' Human Anatomy, 10th ed. Blakiston, Philadelphia, 1942, pp 582–785.
14. Reiner L: Gross examination of the heart. In Gould SE (ed): Pathology of the Heart and Blood Vessels, 3rd ed. CC Thomas, Springfield, IL, 1968, pp 1111–1149.
15. Davies MJ, Pomerance A, Lamb D: Techniques in examination and anatomy of the heart. In Pomerance A, Davies MJ (eds): The Pathology of the Heart. Blackwell Scientific Publications, Oxford, 1975, pp 1–48.
16. Ludwig J, Lie JT: Heart and vascular system. In Ludwig J (ed): Current Methods of Autopsy Practice, 2nd ed. WB Saunders, Philadelphia, 1979, pp 21–50 and 668–673.
17. Silver MM, Freedom RM: Gross examination and structure of the heart. In Silver MD (ed): Cardiovascular Pathology, 2nd ed. Churchill Livingstone, New York, 1991, pp 1–42.
18. James TN: The coronary circulation and conduction system in acute myocardial infarction. Prog Cardiovasc Dis 10:410–446, 1968.
19. Shaper W: The Collateral Circulation of the Heart. American Elsevier Publishing Co, New York, 1971.
20. Crawford T: The anatomy of the coronary arteries. In Crawford T (ed): Pathology of Ischaemic Heart Disease. Butterworths, London, 1977, pp 4–17.
21. Gregg DE, Patterson RE: Functional importance of coronary collaterals. N Engl J Med 303:1404–1406, 1980
22. Willerson JT, Hillis LD, Buja LM: Pathogenesis and pathology of ischemic heart disease. In Willerson JT, Hillis LD, Buja LM (eds): Ischemic Heart Disease: Clinical and Pathophysiological Aspects. Raven Press, New York, 1982, pp 7–83.
23. Marcus ML: The Coronary Circulation in Health and Disease. McGraw-Hill, New York, 1983.
24. Baroldi G: Diseases of extramural coronary arteries. In Silver MD (ed): Cardiovascular Pathology, 2nd ed. Churchill Livingstone, New York, 1991, pp 487–563.
25. Boudoulas H, Gravanis MB: Ischemic heart disease. In Gravanis MB

(ed): Cardiovascular Disorders: Pathogenesis and Pathophysiology. Mosby, St. Louis, 1993, pp 14–16.
26. Lev M: The conduction system. In Gould SE (ed): Pathology of the Heart and Blood Vessels, 3rd ed. Charles C Thomas, Springfield, IL, 1968, pp 180–220.
27. Hudson REB: The conducting system: Anatomy, histology and pathology in acquired disease. In Silver MD (ed): Cardiovascular Pathology, 2nd ed. Churchill Livingstone, New York, 1991, pp 1367–1428.
28. Linzbach AJ: Heart failure from the point of view of quantitative anatomy. Am J Cardiol 5:370–382, 1960.
29. Buja LM, Petty CS: Heart disease, trauma, and death. In Curran WJ, McGarry AL, Petty CS (eds): Modern Legal Medicine, Psychiatry, and Forensic Science. FA Davis, Philadelphia, 1980, pp 187–206.
30. Nguyen ND, Buja LM: The role of ventricular wall stress in cardiac hypertrophy. Cardiovasc Pathol 3:19–31, 1994.
31. Buja LM: Basic pathological processes of the heart: Relationship to cardiomyopathies. In Sperelakis N (ed): Physiology and Pathophysiology of the Heart, 3rd ed. Kluwer Academic Publishers, Boston, 1995, pp 37–53.
32. Huston TP, Puffer JC, Rodney WM: The athletic heart syndrome. N Engl J Med 313:24–32, 1985.
33. Pelliccia A, Maron BJ, Culasso F, et al: Athlete's heart in women. Echocardiographic characterization of highly trained elite female athletes. JAMA 276:211–215, 1996.
34. Blair SN, Kampert JB, Kohl HW III, et al: Influences of cardiorespiratory fitness and other precursors on cardiovascular disease and all-cause mortality in men and women. JAMA 276:205–210, 1996.
35. Maron BJ, Shirani J, Poliac LC, et al: Sudden death in young competitive athletes: Clinical, demographic, and pathological profiles. JAMA 276:199–204, 1996.
36. Carlson BM: Circulatory system. In: Carlson BM (ed): Human Embryology and Developmental Biology. Mosby–Year Book, St. Louis, 1994.
37. O'Rahilly R, Muller F: Human Embryology and Teratology, 2nd ed. Wiley-Liss, New York, 1996.
38. Klagsbrun M, D'Amore PA: Vascular endothelial growth factor and its receptors. Cytokine Growth Factor Rev 7:259–270, 1996.
39. Gendron RL, Tsai FY, Paradis H, Arceci RJ: Induction of embryonic vasculogenesis by bFGF and LIF in vitro and in vivo. Dev Biol 177: 332–346, 1996.
40. Risau W, Flamme I: Vasculogenesis. Ann Rev Cell Dev Biol 11:73–91, 1995.
41. Ware JA, Simons M: Angiogenesis in ischemic heart disease. Nat Med 3:158–164, 1997.
42. Gualandris A, Rusnati M, Belleri M, et al: Basic fibroblast growth factor overexpression in endothelial cells: An autocrine mechanism for angiogenesis and angioproliferative diseases. Cell Growth Differ 7: 147–160, 1996.
43. Gasparini G: Clinical significance of the determination of angiogenesis in human breast cancer: Update of the biological background and overview of the Vincenza studies. Eur J Cancer 32A:2485–2493, 1996.
44. Vermeulen PB, Gasparini G, Fox SB, et al: Quantification of angiogenesis in solid tumours: An international consensus on the methodology and criteria of evaluation. Eur J Cancer 32A:2474–2484, 1996.
45. Ellis LM, Fidler IJ: Angiogenesis and metastasis. Eur J Cancer 32A: 2451–2460, 1996.
46. Axelsson K, Ljung BM, Moore DH II, et al: Tumor angiogenesis as a prognostic assay for invasive breast carcinoma. J Natl Cancer Inst 87: 997–1008, 1995.
47. Carmeliet P, Ferreira V, Breier G, et al: Abnormal blood vessel development and lethality in embryos lacking a single VEGF allele. Nature 380:435–439, 1996.
48. Sato TN, Qin Y, Kozak CA, et al: Tie-1 and tie-2 define another class of putative receptor kinase genes expressed in early embryonic vascular system. Proc Natl Acad Sci U S A 90:9355–9358, 1993.
49. Sato TN, Tozawa Y, Deutsch U, et al: Distinct roles of the receptor tyrosine kinases Tie-1 and Tie-2 in blood vessel formation. Nature 376: 70–74, 1995.
50. Davis S, Aldrich TH, Jones PF, et al: Isolation of angiopoietin-1, a ligand for the TIE2 receptor, by secretion-trap expression cloning. Cell 87:1161–1169, 1996.
51. Suri C, Jone PF, Patan S, et al: Requisite role of angiopoietin-1, a ligand for the TIE2 receptor, during embryonic angiogenesis. Cell 87: 1171–1180, 1996.
52. Vikkula M, Boon LM, Carraway KL III, et al: Vascular dysmorphogenesis caused by an activating mutation in the receptor tyrosine kinase tie2. Cell 87:1181–1190, 1996.
53. Fallis BD, Ashworth RD: Textbook of Human Histology. Little, Brown and Company, Boston, 1970.
54. Mendelsohn ME, Karas RH: Estrogen and the blood vessel wall. Curr Opin Cardiol 9:619–626, 1994.
55. Karas RH, Patterson BL, Mendelsohn ME: Human vascular smooth muscle cells contain functional estrogen receptor. Circulation 89:1943–1950, 1994.
56. Molgaard J, Malinow MR, Lassvik C, et al: Hyperhomocyst(e)inaemia: An independent risk factor for intermittent claudication. J Intern Med 231:273–279, 1992.
57. Wang J, Dudman NP, Wilcken DE, et al: Homocysteine catabolism: Levels of 3 enzymes in cultured human vascular endothelium and their relevance to vascular disease. Atherosclerosis 97:97–106, 1992.
58. Fryer RH, Wilson BD, Gubler D, et al: Homocysteine, a risk factor for premature vascular disease and thrombosis, induces tissue factor activity in endothelial cells. Arterioscler Thromb 13:1327–1333, 1993

CHAPTER 2

Physiology

2.1 Conduction System

Anne Hamilton Dougherty

The heart is a unique muscle capable of generating its own stimulation. The automaticity of specialized cardiac muscle fibers results in rhythmic impulses that are then transmitted to the remainder of the cardiac muscle. The finely orchestrated timing of the conducted impulse produces sequential systole in atrium and ventricle, thus allowing efficient cardiac output.

The primary pacemaker of the heart is the sinus (or sinoatrial [SA]) node, a group of specialized cells located in the sulcus terminalis of the high right atrium, between the superior vena cava and the base of the right atrial appendage (Fig. 2–1). The impulse emitted from the sinus node excites adjacent atrial tissue in a progressive wavefront that produces atrial contraction. The electrical bridge between the atria and ventricles is the atrioventricular (AV) junction, a complex group of structures beginning with the AV node, which transmits the impulse slowly and provides time for active ventricular filling during atrial systole. The impulse then travels throughout the ventricles in a rapid, uniform wavefront by way of the penetrating bundle of His, the bundle branches, and the Purkinje fiber system, the net result of which is synchronized ventricular systole.

CARDIAC ELECTROPHYSIOLOGY

Excitation of cardiac tissue is determined by the flux of ions across cell membranes between intracellular and extracellular spaces. Ion currents are governed by specialized glycoprotein channels in the phospholipid bilayer of the cell membrane, which selectively transport specific ions at critical times in the cardiac cycle. Gating, the response of an ion channel to a stimulus, can be mediated by changes in membrane voltage, chemical signals, receptor activation, or mechanical deformation. The resting (unexcited) membrane potential is maintained primarily by an active, adenosine triphosphate (ATP) dependent sodium-potassium (Na^+/K^+) pump, which maintains a low intracellular sodium concentration. The offsetting potassium ion exchange results in a potential difference between intracellular and extracellular fluid of −90 millivolts (mV) in the Purkinje fibers.[1] Digitalis blocks the sodium-potassium pump.

A stimulus of sufficient amplitude to decrease membrane potential to threshold results in rapid depolarization of the cell and then repolarization back to the resting membrane potential. This cellular cycle is described by the action potential. Figure 2–2 compares the action potentials in atrial and ventricular cells with those in sinus node cells.[2] The corresponding cycles of ion currents from which they result are also described. Purkinje fibers have sodium channel–dependent action potentials similar to those of atrial and ventricular myofibrils. This type of action potential is characterized by a rapid influx of sodium (I_{Na}) with an appropriate stimulus that raises the membrane potential from −90 mV to +30 mV (phase 0). As the membrane potential becomes

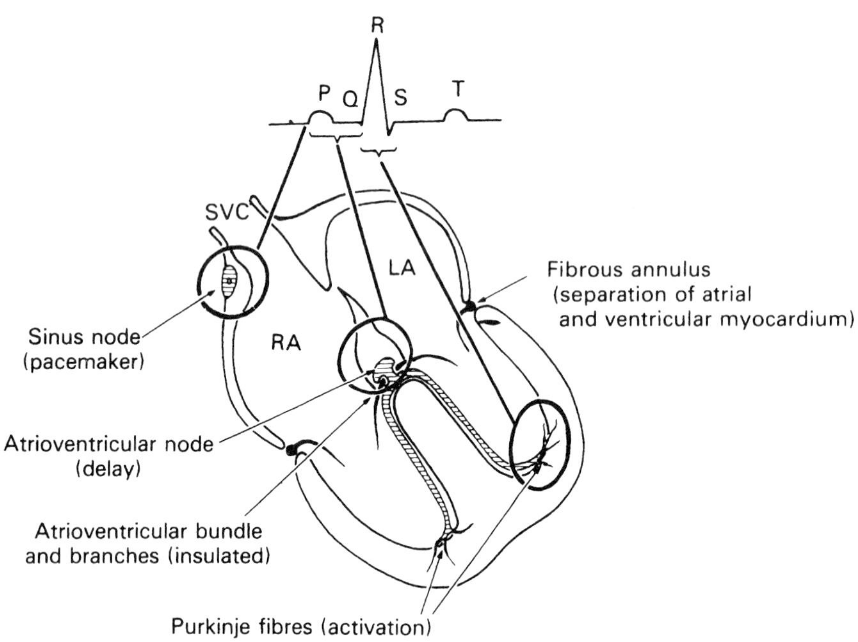

FIGURE 2–1. The conduction system of the heart. The components of the surface electrocardiogram corresponding to their sources are shown. LA, left atrium; RA, right atrium; SVC, superior vena cava. (From Davies MJ, Anderson RH, Becker AE: Anatomy of the conduction tissues. The Conduction System of the Heart. Butterworths, London, 1983, p 9.)

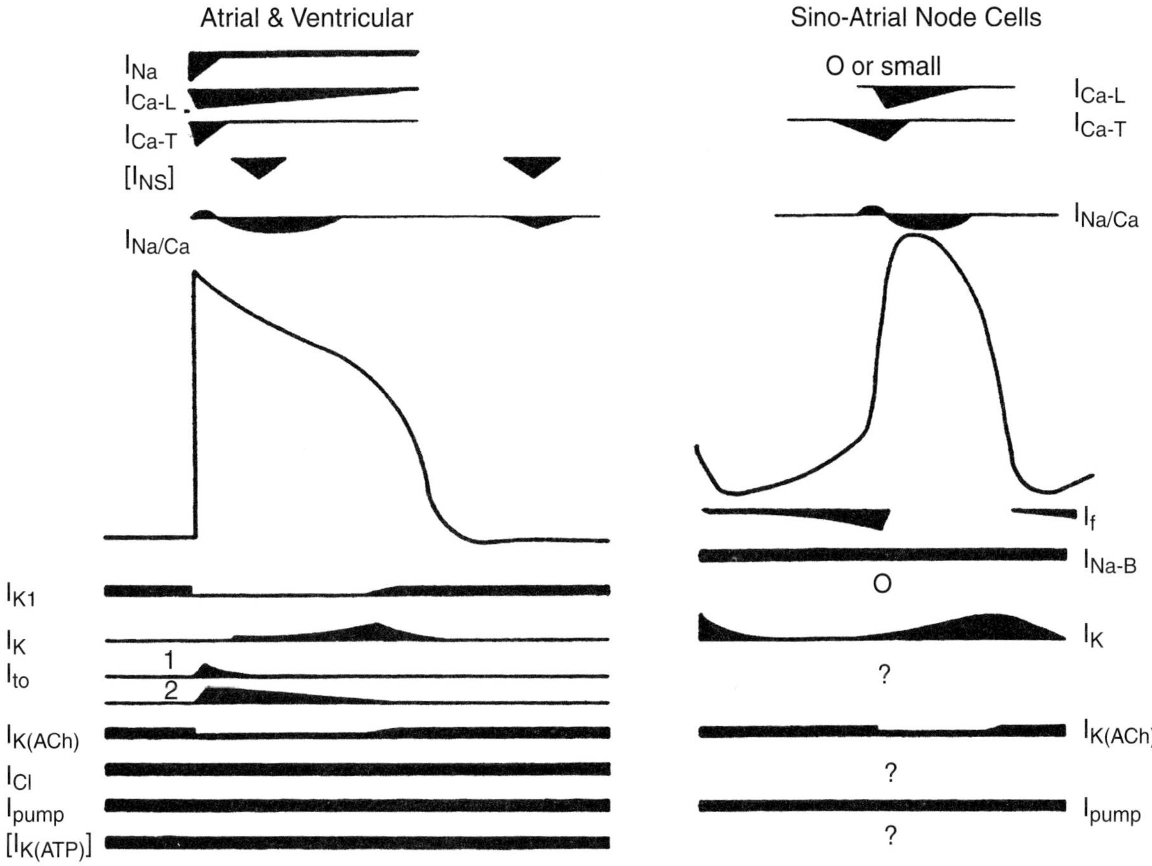

FIGURE 2–2. Currents and channels involved in generating the resting and action potential. The time course of a stylized action potential of atrial and ventricular cells is shown on the left and of sinoatrial node cells on the right. Above and below are the various channels and pumps that contribute the currents underlying the electrical events. Where possible, the approximate time courses of the currents associated with the channels or pumps are shown symbolically without effort to represent their magnitudes relative to each other. The heavy bars for I_{Cl}, I_{pump}, and $I_{K(ATP)}$ only indicate the presence of these channels or pump, without implying magnitude of currents, since that would vary with physiological and pathophysiological conditions. The channels identified by brackets [I_{NS} and $I_{K(ATP)}$] imply that they are active only under pathological conditions. For the sinoatrial node cells, I_{Na} and I_{K1} are small or absent. Question marks indicate that experimental evidence is not yet available to determine the presence of these channels in sinoatrial cell membranes. Although it is likely that other ionic current mechanisms exist, they are not shown here because their roles in electrogenesis are not sufficiently well defined. (From Task Force of the Working Group on Arrhythmias of the European Society of Cardiology: The Sicilian gambit: A new approach to the classification of antiarrhythmic drugs based on their actions on arrhythmogenic mechanisms. Circulation 84:1831, 1991.)

more positive, the sodium current is inactivated, resulting in a brief period of rapid repolarization (phase 1). A slow inward current of calcium (I_{Si}, or I_{Ca-L}) then produces a plateau phase (phase 2), in which the membrane potential hovers near zero. Outward potassium currents (I_K) complete repolarization of the cell during phase 3 and restore the resting membrane potential in phase 4.

Cells capable of automatic behavior are typical of the sinus and AV nodes; however, isolated automatic cells may also be found in other cardiac tissue.[3] These cells have characteristic slow-response action potentials (see Fig. 2–2). Their resting membrane potentials are less negative and stay in the range of −50 to −70 mV. Because sodium channels are sparse in nodal tissue, the slow inward calcium current (rather than sodium influx) produces the upstroke in the action potential, thereby minimizing phases 0 and 1. Spontaneous diastolic depolarization during phase 4 is mediated primarily by activation of inward sodium (I_f) and calcium (I_{Ca-T}) currents and inactivation of the outward potassium (I_K) current. Once threshold potential is attained, cell firing ensues (automaticity). Neurotransmitters modulate I_f and I_K, allowing for autonomic control of heart rate.[2]

The sinus node normally serves as the dominant intrinsic pacemaker of the heart because of its faster rate of spontaneous diastolic depolarization. Cells with slower rates of depolarization during phase 4 (e.g., the AV node) are entrained by impulses conducted from the sinus node. Despite entrainment, these cells retain a latent pacemaker capability that may become manifest during sinus pauses. Ischemia, adrenergic stimuli, and drugs (especially digitalis) may enhance the automaticity of latent pacemakers.

STRUCTURE AND FUNCTION OF THE NORMAL CONDUCTION SYSTEM

The Sinus Node

The sinus node is a collection of specialized myocytes in the superior sulcus terminalis of the high right atrium. Usually spindle-shaped, it measures approximately 1.5 cm by 0.5 cm and surrounds the sinus node artery that flows through its axis. The right coronary artery provides the sinoatrial nodal artery branches in 55% of individuals, and the left coronary artery in 45%.[4] Tightly packed fasciculi of nodal cells are interwoven in a collagen and elastic tissue matrix.[5, 6] The myocytes are small, round, and poorly striated, and they lack intercalated discs. The ratio of nodal cells to fibrous tissue decreases with age, resulting in a relative predominance of fibrous matrix in older people.[7] Transitional cells, which interface with atrial myocytes at intervals, are intermediate in structure between nodal cells and atrial myofibrils; they have a more elongated, parallel arrangement and a higher density of myofibrils and mitochondria. Fibrous septa separate the node from the atrial myocardium in some places, whereas tongues of transitional cells extend into the myocardium in other places.[8]

Sinus nodal electrograms may be recorded with special catheter electrodes in vivo.[9] This technique has proved useful to differentiate between sinus arrest and sinus node exit block. It has also helped document the variability in sinus impulse location. The dominant pacemaker site shifts up to 2 cm along the axis of the sinus node in response to autonomic tone. Superior sites dominate during sympathetic stimulation, whereas inferior sites dominate during vagal stimulation.[10]

The innervation of the sinus node is the richest in the heart. Sympathetic stimulation accelerates heart rate, and vagal stimulation slows it, although parasympathetic influences predominate under most circumstances.[11, 12] Numerous ganglia overlie the node on its epicardial surface, particularly its superior aspect. Parasympathetic nerves, identified by acetylcholinesterase-positive staining, are the most numerous in the sinus node. Sympathetic fibers can be identified from their immunoreactivity with neuropeptide Y and tyrosine hydroxylase. Both sympathetic and parasympathetic nerves are most abundant in the central area of the node.[13] The superficial position of the nodal plexus exposes the node to the effects of pericardial irritation.

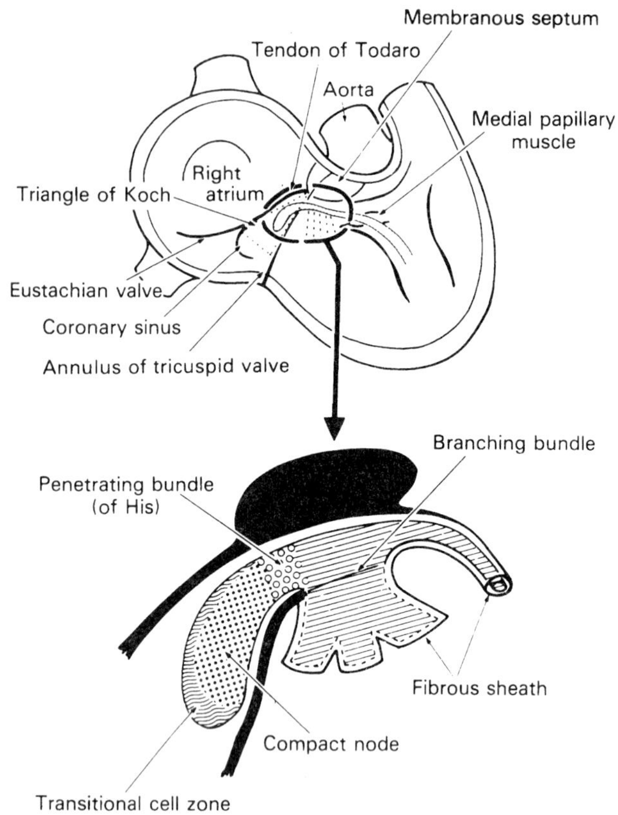

FIGURE 2–3. Location of the AV node at the apex of Koch's triangle. (From Davies MJ, Anderson RH, Becker AE: Anatomy of the conduction tissues. The Conduction System of the Heart. Butterworths, London, 1983, p 9.)

The Atrioventricular Node

The AV node lies in the interatrial septum at the apex of Koch's triangle, an anatomic area with boundaries defined by the tendon of Todaro, the annulus of the tricuspid valve, and the eustachian valve (Fig. 2–3).[8] The atrial impulse is funneled into the AV node by way of its two primary approaches to the compact node. The anterosuperior approach enters the compact node in the anterior interatrial septum near the apex of Koch's triangle. The posteroinferior approach leads from the os of the coronary sinus to the compact node. The compact node, the most visually distinctive portion of the AV node, is an ovoid structure approximately 5 to 6 mm by 3 mm that leads directly to the penetrating bundle of His.[14]

Functionally, the AV node has been divided into three zones: AN, N, and NH. The zones are based upon differences in electrophysiologic properties; however, transitions from zone to zone are gradual.[15–17] The AN zone is primarily composed of long, slender, Purkinje-like cells connected side-to-side by intercalated discs.[18] These cells are highly variable in their resting membrane potentials; action potentials range from fast (sodium channel–dependent) to slow (calcium channel–dependent). The N region, located in the central portion of the compact node, consists of transitional cells—both slender and broad—with irregular, interweaving cell-to-cell connections. These cells have the lowest resting potentials, about −40 to −50 mV, and their action potentials resemble those of the sinus node. Notably, this zone accounts for the greatest conduction delay, which can be as slow as 0.01 to 0.05 m/sec.[19] The NH zone is composed of round or oval transitional cells connected by desmosomes, nexuses or membrane appositions, and P cells (round or oval cells irregularly connected by simple cellular connections). These cells adjoin the large Purkinje-type cells of the bundle of His.

The physiologic conduction delay characteristic of the AV node optimizes ventricular function by allowing atrial systole to augment ventricular filling. Furthermore, AV nodal function is characterized by decremental antegrade conduction, the progressive conduction delay with increasing heart rates or premature impulses. With incremental atrial pacing, second-degree AV block of the Mobitz I or Wenckebach type can be demonstrated (Fig. 2–4). The exact mechanism of conduction slowing is a source of speculation. Some have proposed the following mechanisms: (1) the narrowing of cell diameter from atrial to nodal cells, (2) the complex, interweaving intercellular connections, and (3) specific "braking" action by P cells throughout the node.[18] In a teleologic sense, decremental conduction serves to protect

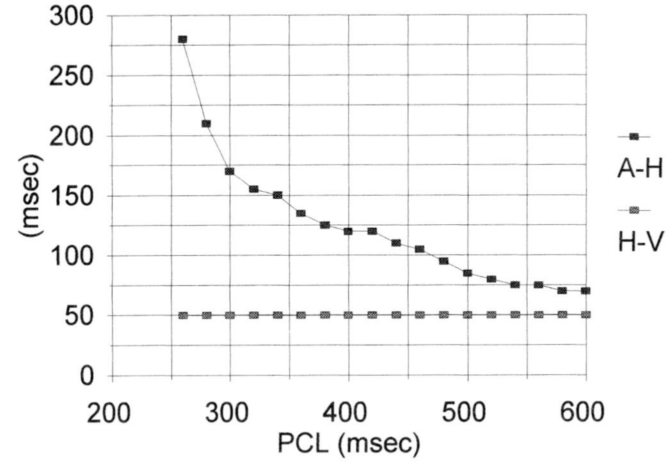

FIGURE 2–4. Decremental conduction in the AV node. The A-H interval measures conduction time from low right atrium through the AV node to the His bundle. The H-V interval represents conduction time from the proximal His bundle to the ventricular myocardial cells. The response of the A-H and H-V intervals to atrial pacing at incremental rates (decreasing pacing cycle lengths, PCL) is shown. Whereas the H-V interval shows little or no change with faster rates (an "all-or-none" phenomenon), the A-H interval decrements are prolonged exponentially until Wenckebach block occurs (in this example, at PCL < 260 msec).

the ventricles from bombardment by excessively rapid or premature atrial impulses during its vulnerable period.

The conduction characteristics of the AV nodes of different individuals form a continuous spectrum that can be described by a bell-shaped curve.[20] James[17] observed that atrial fibers enter the lower portions of the AV node. The Lown-Ganong-Levine syndrome, which consists of a short PR interval and normal QRS complex in patients with tachycardia, was subsequently attributed to a preexcitation syndrome resulting from bypass of the AV node. It is now recognized that patients with Lown-Ganong-Levine syndrome represent a statistical extreme in the continuum of nodal capability: They have physiologically enhanced AV nodal conduction.

Automaticity is also a feature of the AV node.[21] Urthaler and associates[22, 23] demonstrated evidence of two foci of pacemaker activity in the AV junction. The faster of the two foci corresponds to the P cell zone; the slower focus is more distal and serves to produce an escape rhythm during marked sinus bradycardia. Action potentials characteristic of the P cells of the distal node have been recorded during AV junctional rhythm.[24]

Approximately 68% of people with normal antegrade AV node conduction are capable of retrograde atrial activation via the AV node during ventricular pacing or premature ventricular impulses.[25] As the level of antegrade AV nodal dysfunction increases, the fraction of individuals capable of retrograde conduction decreases proportionately. Akhtar and colleagues[26] determined that antegrade AV conduction could be maintained at faster pacing rates than retrograde ventriculoatrial (VA) conduction in 72% of individuals. On the other hand, retrograde conduction intervals are typically shorter than antegrade intervals and less decremental. Furthermore, the site of retrograde block is usually the His-Purkinje system, rather than the AV node as in antegrade Wenckebach block.[27] Compared with antegrade AV conduction, VA conduction intervals are prolonged very little in response to incremental ventricular pacing and extrastimulus testing. Block may occur abruptly in an "all or none" pattern that more closely resembles the behavior of atrial or ventricular nonspecialized myocardium. Other individuals demonstrate decremental retrograde VA conduction, although retrograde decrement is less common than antegrade. The difference between antegrade and retrograde conduction characteristics might reflect either selective retrograde traversal of different approaches or synchronization of the retrograde wavefront in the distal node that results in summation.[28–31]

The AV nodal artery arises from the posterior descending branch of the right coronary artery in 90% of individuals.[4] In the remainder, it arises from the left circumflex artery. Inferior or posterior myocardial infarction may result in transient AV nodal block. However, collateral supply from other penetrating branches of the posterior descending artery and septal perforators usually restores function.[5] Autonomic ganglia are less numerous in the AV node than in the sinus node. They lie in the AV groove inferior to the coronary sinus. Acetylcholinesterase-positive nerve fibers are the most common, particularly in the transitional zone. In the compact AV node, sympathetic and parasympathetic fibers are equally distributed.[13]

Human mapping studies for arrhythmia ablation have underscored the clinical importance of the anterosuperior and posteroinferior approaches to the compact node. They play a critical role in AV nodal reentry tachycardia, the most common form of paroxysmal supraventricular tachycardia.[32, 33] The approaches provide an anatomic site for dual AV nodal function in affected people. The anterosuperior approach is now recognized as the "fast" AV nodal pathway, and the posteroinferior approach as the "slow" pathway (Fig. 2–5). In affected individuals, shifts from the fast pathway to the slow pathway can be demonstrated by incremental atrial

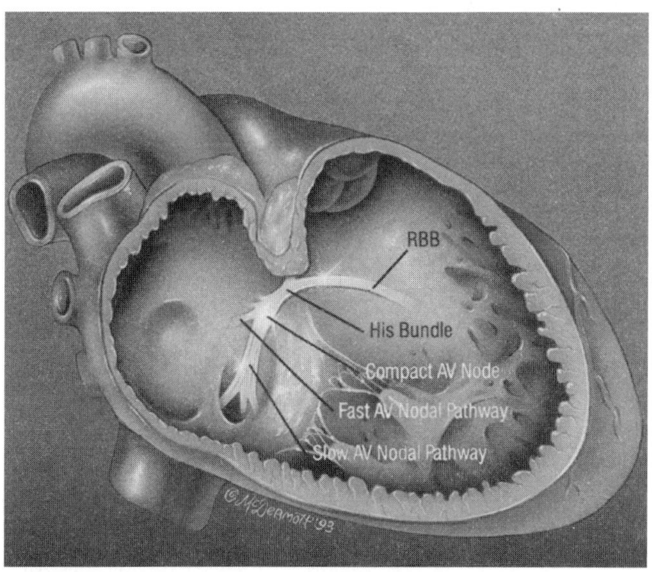

FIGURE 2–5. Approaches to the AV node. Right atrium and ventricle in right anterior oblique view showing the anterosuperior and posteroinferior approaches, which represent the fast and slow AV nodal pathways, respectively. RBB, right bundle branch. (From Moulton K: The AV junction: Evolving concepts in anatomy and physiology. Primary Cardiol 19:22, 1993.)

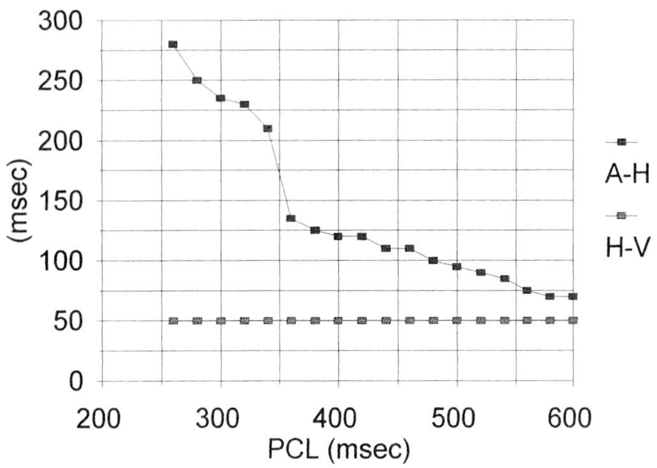

FIGURE 2–6. Dual AV nodal physiology. A discontinuous curve in A-H intervals during incremental atrial pacing indicates a shift from the fast pathway to the slow pathway at 340 msec.

pacing or by refractoriness testing, as shown in Figure 2–6. More importantly, the two pathways form the anatomic substrate for reentry in typical slow-fast or atypical fast-slow AV nodal reentry tachycardia.

Selective radiofrequency catheter ablation of either the fast or the slow pathway can eliminate clinical tachycardia. In a small series, Doig and associates[34] noted that enlargement of the coronary sinus os formed a distinctive "wind sock" configuration in individuals with AV nodal reentry tachycardia. The control subjects had a more narrow tubular morphology. This observation prompted speculation that the anomaly might facilitate the arrhythmia. Potential mechanisms include the stretching of atrial myocardium around the os, which could create areas of slow conduction, and the actual spatial separation of the two approaches, which would lengthen the potential tachycardia cycle.[34] Others have not been able to confirm the correlation between os morphology and clinical arrhythmias.[35]

The His-Purkinje System

As the distal AV node courses atop the interventricular septum and penetrates the annulus fibrosus, it becomes the bundle of His. The common bundle measures approximately 1 cm in length and 1 to 2 mm in diameter.[36] Conduction velocity in the bundle of His is estimated to be 1.5 m/sec.[37] The penetrating bundle then emerges into the left ventricular outflow tract, where it bifurcates into the right and left bundle branches at various locations. The right bundle branch continues as an extension of the penetrating bundle and traverses the myocardium to the base of the medial papillary muscle. It passes subendocardially toward the ventricular apex; then, usually, it crosses over to the right ventricular free wall within the moderator band. Conduction velocities here are estimated to be 2 to 2.5 m/sec.[37]

In contrast to the right bundle, which resembles the common bundle in design, the left bundle branches off in a broad, subendocardial sheet of cells in the left ventricular outflow tract and fans out over the ventricle. The left bundle has been described as having two or three major divisions, or fascicles.[8, 38–42] Perhaps because the physical separation of the fascicles is not discrete, the electrocardiography (ECG) patterns of left anterior and left posterior fascicular blocks do not necessarily correlate with actual anatomic lesions.[5]

Within the bundle of His, typical longitudinal cells gradually become more parallel in orientation and intermingle with progressively fewer P cells throughout its length.[43] The Purkinje cells of the bundle branches are large and vacuolated. The distal ramifications of the right and left bundle branches lose their fibrous sheaths and histologically resemble ventricular myocardial cells.[8] Innervation of the penetrating bundle and bundle branches is more sparse than that of the sinus and AV nodes but more dense than that of either atrial or ventricular myocardium. Most of the nerve fibers in this region are sympathetic.[13]

PATHOLOGIC CONDUCTION PATHWAYS

Wolff-Parkinson-White Syndrome

During human fetal development, atrial and ventricular myocardial fibers communicate until the annulus fibrosus divides them completely.[41] In some individuals, however, remnants of these AV connections persist after birth and are responsible for a variety of supraventricular tachyarrhythmias as well as a risk of sudden cardiac death. Histologically and electrophysiologically, the connections are indistinguishable from atrial myocardial fibers. Accessory AV connections may occur at any location around the AV ring, along the right or left free wall, or in the septum (except in the mitral annular area between the right and left fibrous trigones).[44]

In Wolff-Parkinson-White syndrome, accessory AV connections (Kent bundles) can conduct in either a bidirectional or unidirectional (usually retrograde) manner. In the overt state, antegrade conduction over the accessory pathway during sinus rhythm results in preexcitation of the ventricles and produces a characteristic ECG pattern of a short PR interval with a delta wave on the upstroke of the QRS complex. The preexcited complex is the result of fusion of ventricular activation over the normal and pathologic pathways. Patients with either overt or concealed (retrograde only) Wolff-Parkinson-White syndrome are susceptible to paroxysmal supraventricular tachycardia as a result of reentry between AV node and accessory AV connections by way of intervening atrial and ventricular myocardium. In addition, atrial fibrillation is common and typically produces a very rapid preexcited ventricular response. Heart rates exceeding 250 beats per minute (bpm) can be seen, because the accessory AV connection consists of sodium channel–dependent tissue with little decremental behavior.

Atriofascicular Connections

A less common congenital preexcitation syndrome is characterized by paroxysmal supraventricular tachycardia with left bundle branch block morphology. For five decades, the syndrome was blamed on the anomalous nodoventricular or fasciculoventricular connections described by Mahaim and Benatt[45] in 1938. Elegant electrophysiologic observations by Tchou and colleagues[46] and Haissaguerre and associates,[47]

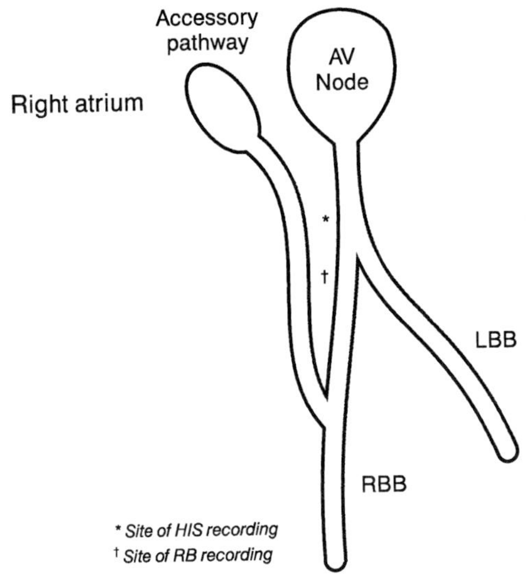

FIGURE 2–7. Diagram of an atriofascicular connection and its relationship to the AV node and His-Purkinje system. LBB, left bundle branch; RBB, right bundle branch. (From Tchou P, Lehmann MH, Jazayeri M, Akhtar M: Atriofascicular connection or a nodoventricular Mahaim fiber? Electrophysiologic elucidation of the pathway and associated reentrant circuit. Circulation 77:837, 1988.)

however, have shown that (at least in most recent cases) the culprit is actually an atriofascicular or AV connection with decremental antegrade conduction (Fig. 2–7). The proximal insertion site is usually mapped to the right lateral atrium and the distal insertion site in the right bundle, or to the anterior right ventricle. No systematic histologic information is available on these structures; however, there have been reports of isolated cases with AV node–like cells at the proximal insertion of the anomalous pathway.[48]

References

1. Gadsby DC: The Na/K pump of cardiac cells. Annu Rev Biophys Bioeng 13:373, 1984.
2. Task Force of the Working Group on Arrhythmias of the European Society of Cardiology: The Sicilian gambit: A new approach to the classification of antiarrhythmic drugs based on their actions on arrhythmogenic mechanisms. Circulation 84:1831, 1991.
3. Vassale M: Cardiac automaticity and its control. In Levy MN, Vassale M (eds): Excitation and Neural Control of the Heart. American Physiological Society, Bethesda, MD, 1982.
4. James TN: Anatomy of the Coronary Arteries. Harper and Row, Hagerstown, MD, 1961.
5. Rossi L: Histopathology of Cardiac Arrhythmias. Lea & Febiger, Philadelphia, 1979.
6. James TN: The sinus node. Am J Cardiol 40:965, 1977.
7. Lev M: Ageing changes in the human sinoatrial node. J Gerontol 9: 1, 1954.
8. Davies MJ, Anderson RH, Becker AE: Anatomy of the conduction tissues. In The Conduction System of the Heart. Butterworths, London, 1983.
9. Yee R, Strauss HC: Electrophysiologic mechanisms: Sinus node dysfunction. Circulation 75(Suppl 3):12, 1987.
10. Kalman JM, Olgin JE, Saxon LA, et al: Electrophysiology of the crista terminalis in normal human atria. Pacing Clin Electrophysiol 19:578, 1996.
11. Levy MN, Zieske H: Autonomic control of cardiac pacemaker activity and atrioventricular transmission. J Appl Physiol 27:465, 1969.
12. Levy MN: Neural control of the heart: The importance of being ignorant. J Cardiovasc Electrophysiol 6:283, 1995.
13. Crick SJ, Wharton J, Sheppard MN, et al: Innervation of the human cardiac conduction system: A quantitative immunohistochemical and histochemical study. Circulation 89:1697, 1994.
14. Anderson RH, Becker AE, Tranum-Jensen J, et al: Anatomico-electrophysiological correlations in the conduction system—a review. Br Heart J 45:67, 1981.
15. Meijler FL, Janse MJ: Morphology and electrophysiology of the mammalian atrioventricular node. Physiol Rev 68:608, 1988.
16. Childres R: The AV node: Normal and abnormal physiology. Prog Cardiovasc Dis 19:361, 1977.
17. James TN: Morphology of the human atrioventricular node, with remarks pertinent to its electrophysiology. Am Heart J 62:756, 1961.
18. Sherf L, James TN, Woods WT: Function of the atrioventricular node considered on the basis of observed histology and fine structure. J Am Coll Cardiol 5:770, 1985.
19. Woods WT, Sherf L, James TN: Structure and function of specific regions in the canine atrioventricular node. Am J Physiol 243:H41, 1982.
20. Jackman WM, Prystowsky EN, Naccarelli GV, et al: Reevaluation of enhanced atrioventricular nodal conduction: Evidence to suggest a continuum of normal atrioventricular nodal physiology. Circulation 67: 441, 1983.
21. Tse WW: Evidence of presence of automatic fibers in the canine atrioventricular node. Am J Physiol 225:716, 1973.
22. Urthaler F, Katholi CR, Macy J, et al: Mathematical relationship between automaticity of the sinus node and the AV junction. Am Heart J 86:189, 1973.
23. Urthaler F, Katholi CR, Macy J, et al: Electrophysiological and mathematical characteristics of the escape rhythm during complete AV block. Cardiovasc Res 8:173, 1979.
24. Kokucun S, Nishimura M, Norma A, et al: The spontaneous action potential of rabbit atrioventricular node cells. Jpn J Physiol 30:529, 1980.
25. Schuilenburg RM: Patterns of V-A conduction in the human heart in the presence of normal and abnormal A-V conduction. In Wellens HJJ, Lie KI, Janse MJ (eds): The Conduction System of the Heart: Structure, Function and Clinical Implications. Lea & Febiger, Philadelphia, 1976, p 485.
26. Akhtar M, Damato AN, Batsford WP, et al: A comparative analysis of antegrade and retrograde conduction patterns in man. Circulation 52: 766, 1975.
27. Narula OS: Retrograde pre-excitation: Comparison of antegrade and retrograde conduction intervals in man. Circulation 50:1129, 1974.
28. Cranefield PF, Hoffman BF: Conduction of the cardiac impulse. II: Summation and inhibition. Circ Res 28:220, 1971.
29. Janse MJ: Influence of the direction of the atrial wave front on A-V nodal transmission in isolated hearts of rabbits. Circ Res 25:439, 1969.
30. Zipes DP, Mendez C, Moe GK: Evidence for summation and voltage dependency in rabbit atrioventricular nodal fibers. Circ Res 32:170, 1973.
31. Wu D: Dual atrioventricular nodal pathways: A reappraisal. Pacing Clin Electrophysiol 5:72, 1982.
32. Moulton K: The AV junction: Evolving concepts in anatomy and physiology. Primary Cardiol 19:22, 1993.
33. Sung RJ, Lauer MR, Chun H: Atrioventricular node reentry: Current concepts and new perspectives. Pacing Clin Electrophysiol 17:1413, 1994.
34. Doig JC, Saito J, Harris L, Downar E: Coronary sinus morphology in patients with atrioventricular junctional tachycardia and other supraventricular tachyarrhythmias. Circulation 92:436, 1995.
35. Weib C, Cappato R, Willems S, et al: Anatomical characteristics of the coronary sinus: Correlation to the presence of AV nodal reentrant tachycardia? Pacing Clin Electrophysiol 19:732, 1996.
36. James TN, Sherf L, Urthaler F: Fine structure of the bundle-branches. Br Heart J 36:1, 1974.
37. Katz AM: Physiology of the Heart. Raven Press, New York, 1977.
38. Tawara S: Das Reizleitungssystem des Saugetierherzens. Gustav Fischer, Jena, 1906.
39. Rosenbaum MB: The hemiblocks: Diagnostic criteria and clinical significance. Mod Concepts Cardiovasc Dis 39:141, 1970.
40. Rossi L: Histopathology of conducting system in left anterior hemiblock. Br Heart J 38:1304, 1976.
41. Rossi L: The pathologic basis of cardiac arrhythmias. Cardiol Clin 1: 1, 1983.

42. Rossi L: His bundle in electrocardiographic semantics of AV block: Anatomoclinical considerations. Pacing Clin Electrophysiol 3:275, 1980.
43. James TN, Isobe JH, Urthaler F: Correlative electrophysiological and anatomical studies concerning the site of origin of escape rhythm during complete atrioventricular block in the dog. Circ Res 45:108, 1979.
44. Cox JL, Gallagher JJ, Cain ME: Experience with 118 consecutive patients undergoing operation for the Wolff-Parkinson-White syndrome. J Thorac Cardiovasc Surg 90:490, 1985.
45. Mahaim I, Benatt A: Nouvelles recherches sur les connexions supérieures de la branche gauche du faisceau de His-Tarawa avec cloison interventriculaire. Cardiologia 1:61, 1938.
46. Tchou P, Lehmann MH, Jazayeri M, Akhtar M: Atriofascicular connection or a nodoventricular Mahaim fiber? Electrophysiologic elucidation of the pathway and associated reentrant circuit. Circulation 77:837, 1988.
47. Haissaguerre M, Cauchemez B, Marcus F, et al: Characteristics of the ventricular insertion of accessory pathways with anterograde decremental conduction properties. Circulation 91:1077, 1995.
48. Guiraudon CM, Guiraudon GM, Kelin GJ: "Nodoventricular" Mahaim pathway: Histologic evidence for an accessory atrioventricular pathway with an AV node–like morphology. Circulation 78(Part 2):II-40, 1988.

2.2 Hematologic and Coagulation Systems

Gerald S. Cyprus

Until the early 1990s, coagulation was perceived to involve a cascade or "waterfall" phenomenon. Evidence has now indicated, however, that the coagulation process is instead "initiated" by interactions among the damaged endothelium, the subsequently exposed tissue factor (TF), and its interaction with factor VII.[1–9] Subsequently, factor VII activates factors X and IX, pathways formerly known as the "common pathway" and the "intrinsic pathway," respectively. Because it is able to activate both arms of the old cascade system, factor VII has been referred to as the "prima ballerina."[10] How factor VII has become the center of the coagulation universe is discussed[1] along with the role of platelets.

Once vascular injury has occurred and the coagulation process has been initiated by endothelial interactions with

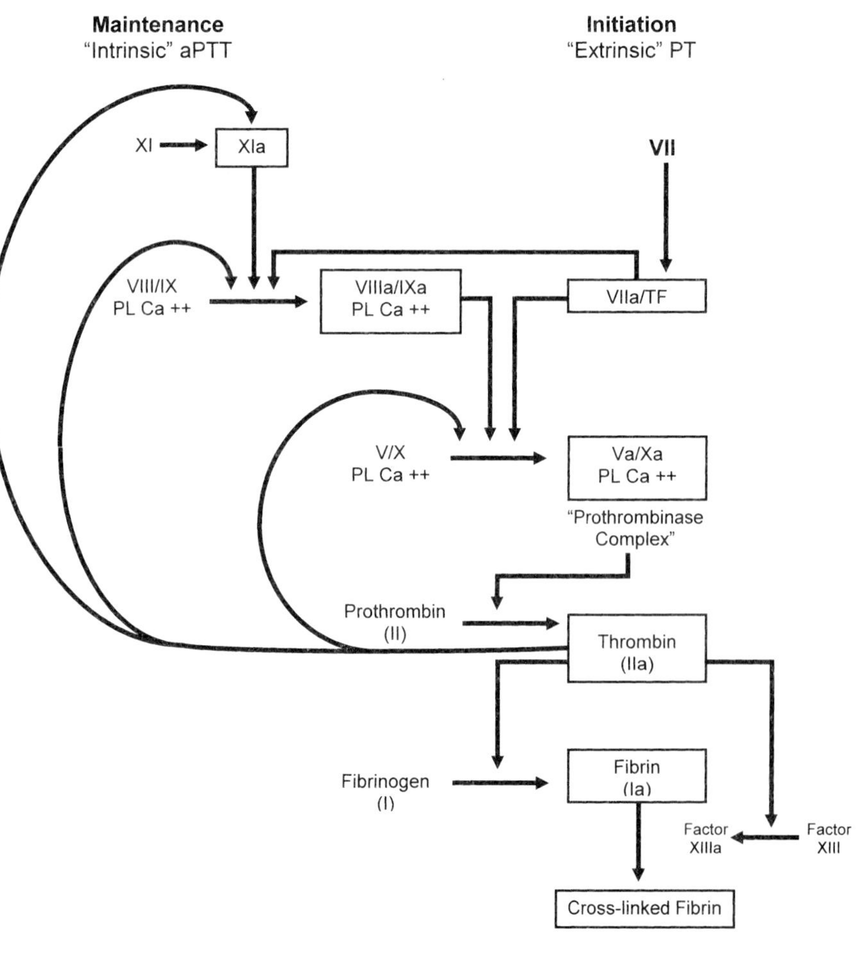

FIGURE 2–8. The coagulation process, which is initiated by endothelial interactions with clotting factors and platelets following vascular injury. Once activated, the coagulation system tends to be self-propagating, with various factors able to stimulate production or activation of others. aPTT, activated partial thromboplastin time; Ca, calcium; PL, platelet; PT, prothrombin time; TF, tissue factor. (From Phillips MD: Advances in the management of hypercoagulable patients [course syllabus], University of Texas at Houston Medical School, Houston, Texas, 1994.)

the other clotting factors and platelets, a delicate balance develops to maintain as well as inhibit the clotting process. The ultimate aim of coagulation is to achieve hemostasis. To prevent overactivity of the clotting process, there exists a set of naturally occurring anticoagulants or inhibitors of clotting, including the protein C and protein S systems, antithrombin III, and the plasminogen or fibrinolytic system.[8]

SYNTHESIS AND FUNCTION

Almost all the clotting factors and regulators are produced in the liver. The exception is TF, which is synthesized in many cells, the most important of which is the endothelial cell. The endothelial cell also synthesizes von Willebrand factor, thrombomodulin, and TF pathway inhibitor. The megakaryocyte synthesizes von Willebrand factor and factor V.

The factors that require vitamin K for synthesis are factors II, VII, IX, and X and proteins C and S. Vitamin K is a necessary cofactor for the carboxylase enzyme. This enzyme converts the precursor molecules that have a single carboxyl group each to molecules with two carboxyls each, allowing the activated molecules to interact with calcium (factor IV).

Each of the aforementioned factors has different specific functions. Some are serine proteases (II, VII, IX, X, XI, XII), cofactors (VIII for IXa, III or TF for VII, V for Xa), or structural proteins (I). Others perform transamidation (XIII), are responsible for platelet adhesion (von Willebrand factor), or serve as regulatory proteins (proteins C and S, thrombomodulin, antithrombin III, and TF pathway inhibitor).

INITIATION OF COAGULATION

As tissue injury occurs, by whatever mechanism (such as rupture of an atherosclerotic plaque, vascular injury from sepsis, or vasculitis), TF is exposed and interacts with factor VII. This TF–factor VII complex is then responsible for initiating the remainder of the clotting sequence (Fig. 2–8).[11] Factor VII activates factor X, which activates factor V; then prothrombin (factor II) is activated to thrombin (IIa), which in turn activates fibrinogen (factor I) to form fibrin (Ia), the final product of the blood clot. Factor XIII cross-links the fibrin via transamidation to finalize the clot.

While the clotting sequence is occurring, TF–factor VII also initiates the other members of the clotting family, namely, factor IX, which in turn interacts with factor X as already described. In addition, the exposure of the vascular surface activates the precursor factors XII (Hageman factor), XI, IX (again), VIII, and, subsequently, the factor X sequence (as noted previously) (Table 2–1). The simplified schematic diagram in Figure 2–9 shows the clotting factors, the laboratory tests of clotting function (prothrombin time, partial thromboplastin time), and the vitamin K–dependent clotting factors.

Once tissue exposure or injury has occurred, followed by activation of TF–factor VII, factor XII, and factor IX, the fourth major promoter of coagulation is the platelet.[12, 13] Platelets first interact with the exposed endothelial surface by adhesion, in which they stick to the surface. This in turn activates the platelets, which release numerous mediators, including platelet-aggregating agents and vasoactive or vasoinhibitory factors. Other mediators are adenosine diphosphate, adenosine triphosphate, and arachidonic acid. Thromboxane A_2 is a potent vasoconstrictor. Prostacyclin (PGI_2) and nitrous oxide, which are produced by the endothelium, contribute to vasodilation. Some of these mediators further propagate the thrombus by causing platelet aggregation and additional release of the granule contents until the platelet plug is created (Fig. 2–10).[14]

The exposed endothelial surface contributes to platelet activation, mainly through the important interaction of von Willebrand factor (part of factor VIII) with the platelet membrane via one of the glycoprotein moieties, known as glycoprotein Ib. Deficiency of this interaction results in a prolonged bleeding time. Thus, bleeding time is prolonged

Table 2–1. SPECIFIC COAGULATION FACTORS AND THEIR SYNONYMS

FACTOR	SYNONYM	AFTER ACTIVATION
I	Fibrinogen	Fibrin
II	Prothrombin	Thrombin
III	Tissue factor	
IV	Calcium	
V	Proaccelerin	
VI		
VII		
VIII-C	Antihemophiliac factor (coagulant)	
VIII-VW	von Willebrand factor	
IX	Christmas factor	
X	Stuart factor	
XI		
XII	Hageman factor	
XIII	Fibrin-stabilizing factor (Laki-Lorand factor)	

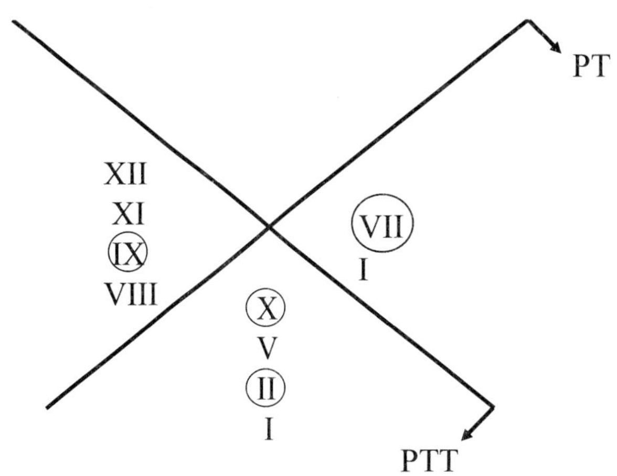

FIGURE 2–9. The "Magic X" illustrates the coagulation factors and the current laboratory measures of coagulation function. The activated partial thromboplastin time (PTT), the time it takes blood to clot after clay is added to ethylenediamine tetraacetic acid–anticoagulated blood, measures the activity of proteins of the intrinsic pathway and everything downstream, including the common pathway. Prothrombin time (PT), the time it takes for thromboplastin to clot blood, measures the activities of the extrinsic pathway, the common pathway complex, and the subsequent propagation phase. Circled numerals represent vitamin K–dependent coagulation factors. Vitamin K–dependent coagulation inhibitors such as proteins C and S are not shown.

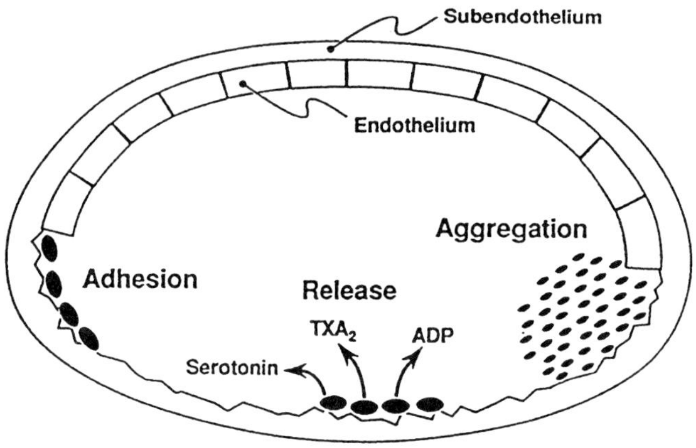

FIGURE 2–10. Platelet thrombus formation. Platelets may be the primary defense against hemorrhage in the arterial circulation, where elevated blood flow limits fibrin deposition (leading to a "white thrombus"). Platelets adhere to exposed subendothelium (adhesion), secrete proaggregatory and vasoactive substances such as serotonin, thromboxane A_2 [TXA_2], and ADP (release), and aggregate to form a plug at the site of vascular endothelial injury ("aggregation"). They also contribute to fibrin ("red thrombus") generation in the venous circulation. The coagulation reactions that result in fibrin production are enhanced by cell surfaces, and platelets are an important site of assembly of the coagulation apparatus. (From Schafer AI, Bridges KR, Kroll MH et al: Hematology Medical Knowledge Self Assessment Program 10:966, 1994.)

in von Willebrand's disease, in which the von Willebrand portion of the factor VIII molecule is defective, but is not prolonged in classic hemophilia, in which the defect is in the coagulant part of factor VIII (rather than the von Willebrand portion of the molecule). Another important interaction with the platelet membrane is the one between fibrinogen and glycoprotein IIb-IIIa.[14]

MAINTENANCE OF COAGULATION

Until the realization of the importance of the interaction of TF with factor VII and its subsequent activation of both factors X and IX, the "intrinsic pathway" was believed to be an important part of the clotting process. The fact that deficiencies of the surface-activating proteins (Hageman factor or factor XII, prekallikrein, and high-molecular-weight kininogen) are not associated with bleeding suggests that the role of the intrinsic system in the initiation of coagulation may not be as critical as initially thought.

Phospholipids, which are critical for the activation of coagulation factors, are found on platelet membranes and membranes from other cells, such as monocytes, activated inflammatory cells, and activated endothelial cells.[15–21] Once the coagulation system has been activated, it tends to be self-propagating; thus, factor Xa can stimulate further activation of factor VII. Likewise, thrombin (factor IIa) stimulates further production or activation of factors V, VIII, XI, and XIII. Calcium is important in the interaction of factor XIa with IX, IXa with X, and Xa with II (see Fig. 2–8).

Table 2–2. COAGULATION REGULATORS OR INHIBITORS

Protein C
Protein S
Thrombomodulin
Antithrombin III
Tissue factor pathway inhibitor
Plasmin
Tissue plasminogen activator and inhibitor
Urokinase

INHIBITION OF COAGULATION

At the same time that the coagulation system is being initiated with the exposed endothelium, TF–factor VII complex, and the platelets and their activation, a complex system of naturally occurring anticoagulants also is being activated (Table 2–2). These anticoagulants ensure that the clotting process is confined to the area of injury and is not disseminated systemically or throughout the vascular tree.[22, 23]

The anticoagulants include proteins C and S, the fibrinolytic system, antithrombin III, and TF pathway inhibitor.[24] Protein C is activated by thrombomodulin in the endothelium. In turn, protein C activates protein S, which then proteolyses factors V and VIII. Protein C then inhibits the tissue plasminogen activator inhibitor; this action essentially produces a double-negative effect: Protein C inhibits an inhibitor, so that tissue plasminogen activator is allowed to act, thereby initiating the plasminogen system (Fig. 2–11). The plasminogen system is initiated by plasminogen activators, such as urokinase (tissue plasminogen activator), that

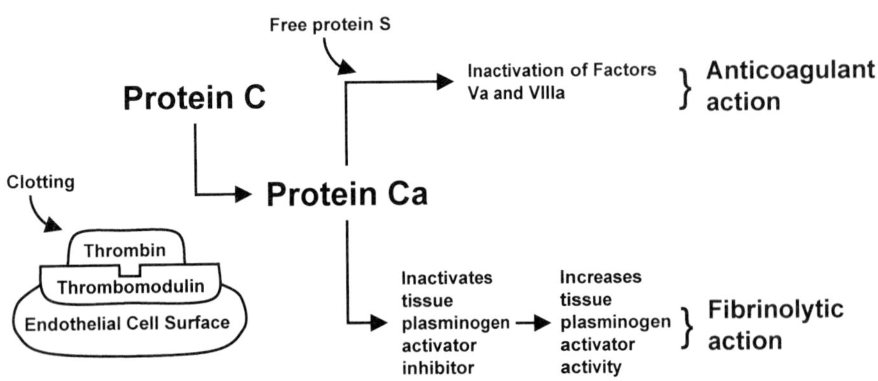

FIGURE 2–11. Thrombin-thrombomodulin model of the anticoagulant and fibrinolytic action of protein C. Thrombin binds to thrombomodulin, a receptor protein on the surface of endothelial cells. The thrombin-thrombomodulin complex rapidly activates protein C. Protein Ca exerts anticoagulant effects by inactivating factors Va and VIIIa, and it facilitates fibrinolysis by neutralizing an inhibitor of plasminogen activator.

convert plasminogen to plasmin.[25] Plasmin in turn lyses fibrin, with the attendant formation of fibrin split products.

The action of antithrombin III is enhanced by interaction with heparin. Heparin-like proteoglycans synthesized by the endothelial cells interact with antithrombin III when the endothelial cell has been injured. Finally, the TF pathway inhibitor downregulates the action of TF–factor VII, thereby decreasing the activation of factors IX and X.[7, 8, 23]

SUMMARY

We now understand the importance of endothelial damage as the initiating event in the clotting process, followed by interaction between TF and factor VII to form the core of coagulation. Thus, the concept of clotting has changed from a cascade process to one of initiation followed by maintenance of the process and the simultaneous activation of regulators or inhibitors of coagulation.

References

1. Mann KG: The coagulation explosion. Ann N Y Acad Sci 714:265, 1994.
2. Rapaport SI: Blood coagulation and its alterations in hemorrhagic and thrombotic disorders. West J Med 158:153, 1993.
3. Sussman II: Normal pathways of coagulation. Semin Hematol 29:157, 1992.
4. Broze GJ: The role of tissue factor pathway inhibitor in a revised coagulation cascade. Semin Hematol 29:159, 1992.
5. McVey JH: Tissue factor pathway [review]. Baillieres Clin Haematol 7: 469, 1994.
6. Carson SD, Brozna JP: The role of tissue factor in the production of thrombin [review]. Blood Coagul Fibrinolysis 4:281, 1993.
7. Broze GJ: Tissue factor pathway inhibitor and the current concept of blood coagulation [review]. Blood Coagul Fibrinolysis 6(Suppl 1): S7, 1995.
8. Abildgaard U: Relative roles of tissue factor pathway inhibitor and antithrombin in the control of thrombogenesis [review]. Blood Coagul Fibrinolysis 6(Suppl 1):S45, 1995.
9. Luchtman-Jones L, Broze GJ: The current status of coagulation [review]. Ann Med 27:47, 1995.
10. Rapaport SI, Rao LV: The tissue factor pathway: How it has become a "prima ballerina." Thromb Haemost 74:7, 1995.
11. Phillips MD: Advances in the management of hypercoagulable patients (Course syllabus), University of Texas at Houston Medical School, Houston, Texas, 1994.
12. Caen JP, Rosa JP: Platelet-vessel wall interaction: From the bedside to molecules. Thromb Haemost 74:18, 1995.
13. Clemetson KJ: Platelet activation: Signal transduction via membrane receptors. Thromb Haemost 74:111, 1995.
14. Schafer AI, Bridges KR, Kroll MH, et al: Hematology[1] Medical Knowledge Self Assessment Program 10:966, 1994. Published by American College of Physicians, Philadelphia.
15. Rickles FR, Hair GA, Zeff RA, et al: Tissue factor expression in human leukocytes and tumor cells. Thromb Haemost 74:391, 1995.
16. Geczy CL: Cellular mechanisms for the activation of blood coagulation. Int Rev Cytol 152:49, 1994.
17. Esmon CT: Cell mediated events that control blood coagulation and vascular injury. Annu Rev Cell Biol 9:1, 1993.
18. Edwards RL, Rickles FR: The role of leukocytes in the activation of blood coagulation. Semin Hematol 29:202, 1992.
19. Altieri DC: Inflammatory cell participation in coagulation. Semin Cell Biol 6:269, 1995.
20. Esmon CT, Fukodome K: Cellular regulation of the protein C pathway. Semin Cell Biol 6:259, 1995.
21. Sims PJ, Wiedmer T: Induction of cellular procoagulant activity by the membrane attack complex of complement. Semin Cell Biol 6:275, 1995.
22. Andree HA, Nemerson Y: Tissue factor: Regulation of activity by flow and phospholipid surfaces [review]. Blood Coagul Fibrinolysis 6:189, 1995.
23. Slack SM, Cui Y, Turitto VT: The effects of flow on blood coagulation and thrombosis. Thromb Haemost 70:129, 1993.
24. Broze GJ: Tissue factor pathway inhibitor. Thromb Haemost 74:90, 1995.
25. Verstraete M: The fibrinolytic system: From Petri dishes to genetic engineering. Thromb Haemost 74:25, 1995.

2.3 Endocrine System

Victor R. Lavis

GENERAL CONSIDERATIONS

The endocrine system serves the function of intercellular communication, which is essential for the adaptation and survival of multicellular organisms. The circulatory system provides a medium for reliable and rapid distribution of endocrine signals. Therefore, it is not surprising that the heart and vasculature are themselves highly regulated by endocrine influences. The heart and vascular endothelia are target organs for many hormones. Additionally, cardiac nerves and muscle are important sources of chemical signals for intercellular communication.

With respect to the cardiovascular system, one may consider the roles of hormones in terms of their effects on (1) development and structure of the heart and vasculature, (2) cardiac rate and rhythm, (3) myocardial function, (4) vascular reactivity, and (5) regulation of the effective volume of intravascular fluids. Additionally, some hormones can influence cardiovascular physiology indirectly, that is, by affecting lipid metabolism in ways that may modify the progression of atherosclerosis.

GROWTH HORMONE AND INSULIN-LIKE GROWTH FACTOR-I

Regulation of Secretion of Growth Hormone

The regulation of the secretion of growth hormone (GH) has been extensively reviewed.[1] Secretion of GH from the somatotrophs of the pituitary is regulated in a dual fashion by hypothalamic peptides. GH-releasing hormone (GHRH) stimulates secretion of GH, and the principal negative regulator is somatostatin (see later).[2] Additionally, certain low-molecular-weight compounds known as GH secretagogues stimulate secretion of GH in a manner that depends on the presence of GHRH but is not mediated by GHRH receptors.[3] A receptor for these secretagogues has been cloned,[4] and a putative endogenous ligand, termed *ghrelin*, has been isolated and characterized as a peptide of gastrointestinal origin.[5] GH and insulin-like growth factor-I (IGF-I) (see later) provide negative feedback regulation at the hypothalamic and pituitary levels.

GH is secreted in a pulsatile fashion, with daily secretory bursts evoked by the onset of slow-wave sleep. Owing to the pulsatility of secretion, there is considerable variability in moment-to-moment levels of GH. Table 2–3 shows some physiologic, pathologic, and pharmacologic influences on GH secretion. In ordinary life, secretion of GH is promoted by stress, exercise, fasting, and ingestion of protein. When integrated over a 24-hour period, GH levels are seen to reach a peak during puberty[6] and then to decline gradually with age.[7, 8] In general, secretion of GH is augmented by gonadal steroids, particularly estrogens.[7] Accordingly, the responses of GH levels to secretory stimuli tend to be higher in premenopausal women than in men.[9] Levels of GH increase during the late follicular phase of the menstrual cycle.[10] In menopausal women, replacement therapy with estrogens increases secretion of GH.[11] Conversely, hypogonadal adults of both sexes have subnormal circulating levels of GH.

In human obesity, secretion of GH is diminished, both spontaneously[12] and in response to a variety of stimuli,[7, 13] but circulating levels of IGF-I (see later) are not diminished. Weight loss restores the normal secretion of GH in obese persons.[13]

Table 2–3. SOME PHYSIOLOGIC, PATHOLOGIC, AND PHARMACOLOGIC INFLUENCES ON THE SECRETION OF GROWTH HORMONE

INFLUENCE	STIMULATORY	INHIBITORY
Physiologic	Slow-wave sleep	Rapid eye movement sleep
	Stress	Normal aging
	Exercise	Increased nonesterified fatty acid levels
	Fasting	
	Ingestion of protein or amino acids	
	Gonadal steroids	
	Puberty	
	Vasopressin	
	Growth hormone–releasing hormone	Somatostatin
Pathologic	Uncontrolled hyperglycemia	Obesity
	Starvation	Hypogonadism
	Uremia	Hypothyroidism
	Acute hypoglycemia	Chronic emotional deprivation
Pharmacologic	α-Adrenergic agonists	α-Adrenergic antagonists
	β-Adrenergic antagonists	β-Adrenergic agonists
	Dopamine agonists	Somatostatin analogues
	Growth hormone secretagogues	Glucocorticoids (pharmacologic doses)

Mechanism of Action of Growth Hormone

GH interacts with plasma membrane receptors that are members of a superfamily including the receptors for prolactin, erythropoietin, and many cytokines.[14–16] The receptors are single-chain transmembrane polypeptides, activated by ligand-induced dimerization. The signaling pathway includes activation of Janus kinase 2 (JAK2), a receptor-associated tyrosine kinase,[17] and selective changes in gene expression mediated by the signal transducers and activators of transcription (STAT) pathway.[14, 16]

Physiologically, many of the actions of GH, including stimulation of linear growth, are mediated by the peptide hormone IGF-I (also known as somatomedin C), circulating levels of which closely parallel integrated secretion of GH. GH stimulates transcription of the gene for IGF-I. Until the age of about 35 years, women have higher circulating levels of IGF-I than men.[9] IGF-I levels are decreased in malnutrition, hepatic disease, hypothyroidism, chronic heart failure, and uncontrolled diabetes.[9, 18] Although circulating IGF-I arises mostly from the liver, IGF-I is produced by a variety of tissues and can act in endocrine, paracrine, and autocrine fashion to evoke a wide spectrum of anabolic, differentiative, mitogenic, and anti-apoptotic activities.[19–22] The IGF-I receptor, found in many cell types, is a plasma membrane–spanning tetramer that bears much structural homology to the insulin receptor. Like the insulin receptor, it signals via its tyrosine kinase activity.[21, 22] Many of the effects of IGF-I on fuel metabolism mimic those of insulin.

Circulating IGF-I is largely bound to high-affinity binding proteins (IGFBPs), of which six have been described to date.[21, 23, 24] The most abundant IGFBP is IGFBP-3, production of which is stimulated by GH. In plasma, most IGF-I exists as a complex with IGFBP-3 and another protein, the acid-labile subunit.[25] The physiology of IGFBPs is complex. Association with IGFBPs can protect IGF-I from degradation and can modulate its interaction with receptors.[21, 23, 24] Evidence suggests that IGFBP-3 may modulate cellular proliferation and apoptosis, independently of its interaction with IGF-I.[21, 24] Conversely, IGFBPs may also prevent IGF-I from gaining access to its receptors. For example, some of the growth retardation observed in patients with poorly controlled type 1 diabetes mellitus may be attributable to elevated IGFBP-1 levels, which are inversely related to insulin action.

Actions of Growth Hormone and Insulin-like Growth Factor-I on the Cardiovascular System

Several discoveries now suggest that the GH/IGF-I system exerts important physiologic influences in adults, including the following[9, 26]:

- Increases in bone density and ratio of lean body mass to fat mass
- Raised basal metabolic rate
- Larger volume of extracellular fluids
- Greater muscular strength and capacity for exercise
- Maintenance of a sense of psychological well-being

The effects of GH and IGF-I on the cardiovascular system have been extensively reviewed.[27, 28]

Hypopituitarism may be regarded as an experiment of nature that illuminates the integrated physiologic effects of the GH/IGF-I axis. Adults with a deficiency of GH exhibit several metabolic and cardiovascular abnormalities.[9, 26, 27] Despite treatment with appropriate replacement doses of cortisol, thyroxine, and sex steroids, patients with hypopituitarism suffer from increased mortality.[29] They have decreases in lean body mass and in strength and exercise capacity,[30] as well as visceral adiposity, inappropriate bradycardia, diastolic dysfunction,[31] and smaller extracellular fluid volume. They also exhibit a number of features of accelerated atherosclerosis, as follows:

1. Elevated levels of circulating triglycerides[32] and low-density lipoprotein (LDL) cholesterol, increased levels of apoprotein B, small dense LDL particles, and decreased high-density lipoprotein (HDL) cholesterol.[9, 33]
2. Reduced arterial compliance.
3. Increased carotid arterial wall thickness.
4. Higher circulating levels of fibrinogen and of plasminogen activator inhibitor-1 (PAI-1).[27]
5. Greater prevalence of hypertension.[32]

Some patients with longstanding hypopituitarism have had dilated cardiomyopathy, which is thought to be related to a deficiency of GH.[34] Treatment of adult patients with hypopituitarism with GH is reported to have many beneficial effects, including increases in lean body mass[35] and exercise capacity,[36] raised HDL levels and reduced LDL levels,[37] increases in renal sodium retention,[38, 39] heart rate, and left ventricular mass, improvements in left ventricular systolic and diastolic function,[30, 40] and reduction of inflammatory mediators linked to atherosclerosis.[41]

Receptors for GH secretagogues have been identified in human myocardium and blood vessels, but their significance has not yet been fully elucidated.[42]

PROLACTIN

Regulation of Secretion of Prolactin

Human prolactin is a 23-kD single-chain peptide with about 40% sequence homology to GH.[43] Secretion of prolactin by the lactotrophs of the anterior pituitary is under tonic inhibitory control by hypothalamic dopamine. Consequently, interruption of the pituitary portal circulation leads to hyperprolactinemia. Hypothalamic thyrotropin-releasing hormone (TRH) acutely stimulates the secretion of prolactin, by acting on a G-protein–coupled plasma membrane receptor,[2, 44] to increase cytosolic free calcium ion (Ca^{2+}) levels. In keeping with a stimulatory effect of TRH, about 40% of women with primary hypothyroidism have increased circulating prolactin levels, although the elevation is usually modest.[45] Pregnancy and treatment with estrogens lead to lactotrophic hyperplasia and sustained hyperprolactinemia. Also, prolactin is secreted in response to mechanical stimulation of the nipples or chest wall as well as to physiologic stress, including epileptic seizures and hypoglycemia. Several drugs increase the prolactin levels (Table 2–4), most commonly by virtue of dopaminergic inhibition.

Table 2–4. DRUGS THAT INCREASE SERUM PROLACTIN LEVELS

CLASS	DRUG
Antihypertensive	Methyldopa
	Verapamil
	Reserpine
Psychotropic	Phenothiazines
	Haloperidol
	Tricyclic antidepressants
	Amoxapine
	Butyrophenones
	Thioxanthenes
	Risperidone
	Monoamine oxidase inhibitors
	Sulpiride
Antiemetic	Metoclopramide
	Phenothiazines
Hormonal	Oral contraceptives
	Replacement estrogens
Nontherapeutic	Cocaine

Adapted from Molitch ME: Pathologic hyperprolactinemia. Endocrinol Metab Clin North Am 21:877, 1992; and Biller BM: Diagnostic evaluation of hyperprolactinemia. J Reprod Med 12 (Suppl): 1095, 1999.

Mechanism of Action of Prolactin

Prolactin interacts with plasma membrane receptors that are members of the class 1 cytokine receptor superfamily. This superfamily also includes receptors for GH and erythropoietin.[14, 16] Signaling occurs via association of the cytoplasmic portion of the receptor with cellular Janus kinases, especially JAK2, and activation of the STAT pathway.[14, 16, 43, 48]

Prolactins are found in all vertebrates. Prolactin receptors are expressed in nearly every tissue in the body, and a very large variety of actions has been described.[48] Physiologically, the most important of these actions, in humans of both sexes, are related to reproduction. This inference is reinforced by studies with knockout mice lacking the prolactin receptor, which appear to be phenotypically normal except for multiple reproductive and mammary abnormalities.[48] Stimulatory effects of prolactin on the immune system have been described, but prolactin is probably not a major physiologic regulator of immunity.[49]

Actions of Prolactin on the Cardiovascular System

Prolactin has been reported to promote renal and intestinal reabsorption of salt and water in animals, but it seems not to have any physiologically important role in regulating extracellular volume in humans.

Prolactin stimulates angiogenesis, promoting the growth of capillaries in the mammary gland as well as the proliferation of vascular smooth muscle cells. Contrarily, one of the products of cleavage of prolactin is a 16-kD N-terminal fragment that has anti-angiogenic properties.[50] The physiologic significance of the effects of prolactin and its cleavage products on angiogenesis remains to be elucidated.

HYPOTHALAMIC-PITUITARY-ADRENAL AXIS: GLUCOCORTICOIDS

Physiology of Hypothalamic-Pituitary-Adrenal Axis

Glucocorticoids are steroids that evoke a panoply of responses. Physiologic glucocorticoid effects are as follows[51]:

- Depletion of circulating lymphocytes and inhibition of inflammatory and immune responses
- Induction of hepatic enzymes that catalyze gluconeogenesis and glycogen synthesis
- Facilitation of excretion of a water load
- Inhibition of secretion of corticotrophin (adrenocorticotropic hormone [ACTH])
- Induction of the rate-limiting enzyme for synthesis of epinephrine in the adrenal medulla
- Maintenance of vascular tone
- Differentiation and maturation of several fetal tissues

Glucocorticoids are essential for the normal response to physiologic stresses, such as fever and hemorrhage. Pharmacologic amounts of glucocorticoids can produce a wide variety of additional effects, including depletion of protein stores, osteoporosis, inhibition of wound healing, hyperglycemia, development of opportunistic infections, redistribution of body fat, hypertension, and psychiatric disorders; some of these effects are extensions of the physiologic effects.

In humans, the principal glucocorticoid is cortisol, which is secreted from the zona fasciculata of the adrenal cortex. The adrenal cortex has essentially no autonomous activity; rather, secretion of cortisol is closely linked to circulating levels of ACTH. Because ACTH is required for maintenance of the zona fasciculata and for secretion of cortisol, a chronic deficiency of ACTH is characterized by adrenal cortical atrophy. ACTH activates adenylyl cyclase, with cyclic adenosine monophosphate (AMP) as the intracellular messenger. In turn, ACTH is secreted in a pulsatile manner from the corticotrophs of the anterior pituitary.

Secretion of ACTH is stimulated by corticotrophin-releasing hormone (CRH), a hypothalamic peptide delivered via the pituitary portal circulation,[2, 51] and by circulating vasopressin. Secretion of ACTH follows a diurnal rhythm, being greatest in the early morning just before awakening. Physiologic "stress" is a powerful stimulus to the secretion of CRH and ACTH. Cortisol and other glucocorticoids inhibit the secretion of ACTH at the hypothalamic and pituitary levels. Chronically high circulating levels of natural or synthetic glucocorticoids lead to long-term suppression of the secretion of CRH and ACTH.

In humans, most circulating cortisol is reversibly bound to a plasma protein, corticosteroid-binding globulin (CBG).[52] Pregnancy and treatment with estrogens increase the level of circulating CBG, but there is no difference in CBG levels between men and nonpregnant women.[52] Because the hypothalamic-pituitary axis is sensitive to the unbound fraction of plasma cortisol, pregnancy and treatment with estrogens are characterized by higher concentrations of total plasma cortisol without a change in the physiologic availability of cortisol to tissues.

Mechanism of Action of Glucocorticoids

Glucocorticoid receptors are members of a superfamily of intracellular proteins that includes receptors for other steroid hormones, vitamin D, retinoids, and 3,5,3′-triiodothyronine (T_3). Receptors in this superfamily are organized into functional domains for ligand binding, dimerization, binding to DNA, and activation of transcription. In the absence of a ligand, glucocorticoid receptors are found in the cytoplasm of target cells, in association with other proteins.[53] Binding of the hormone evokes dissociation, translocation to the nucleus, binding to specific sequences of DNA (glucocorticoid-responsive elements), and alteration of transcription of specific genes.[53–55]

Actions of Glucocorticoids on the Cardiovascular System

With respect to the cardiovascular system, the main physiologic actions of glucocorticoids involve maintenance of vascular tone and regulation of fluid metabolism. A deficiency of glucocorticoids is characterized by hypotension that responds poorly to vasopressors. Overt circulatory collapse, mediated by both volume depletion and myocardial insufficiency, may occur in this situation.[56] Glucocorticoids may contribute to vascular tone by inhibiting the production of prostaglandin I_2 and by stimulating the production of angiotensinogen.[57] Individuals who lack glucocorticoids have inappropriately elevated levels of vasopressin with impaired excretion of free water and hyponatremia.[58, 59] Studies in rats suggest that some of the effects of glucocorticoids on water metabolism may be mediated by increased secretion of atrial natriuretic peptide.[60]

Glucocorticoid receptors in cardiac muscle cells may regulate muscle growth[61] and may induce synthesis of atrial natriuretic peptide.[62] Additionally, it has been proposed that glucocorticoids signal via type I mineralocorticoid receptors (see later) in the heart.[63]

MINERALOCORTICOIDS

Regulation of Secretion of Mineralocorticoids

Mineralocorticoids are steroid hormones that promote the retention of extracellular fluid sodium and the excretion of potassium. In humans, the principal endogenous mineralocorticoid is aldosterone, which is produced by the zona glomerulosa of the adrenal cortex. The secretion of aldosterone is stimulated by loss of extracellular sodium or reduction of effective circulating volume, through mediation of the renin-angiotensin system. Angiotensin II and angiotensin III, peptides derived by sequential cleavage of angiotensin I, interact with receptors on cells of the zona glomerulosa[64]; these receptors are coupled to G proteins and phospholipase C. Also, potassium ions stimulate the secretion of aldosterone directly.[65] Another mineralocorticoid with appreciable physiologic activity is 11-desoxycorticosterone, which is produced by the adrenal zona fasciculata under the influence of ACTH.

Mechanism of Action of Mineralocorticoids

Mineralocorticoid receptors are highly homologous to those for glucocorticoids. Glucocorticoids and mineralocorticoids bind with equal affinity to high-affinity (type I) mineralocorticoid receptors. The hormonal specificity of the mineralocorticoid effector pathway is provided by high local concentrations of type II 11-beta-hydroxysteroid dehydrogenase (11β-HSD), an enzyme that inactivates cortisol by converting it to cortisone.[66, 67] In situations of hereditary or acquired inactivity of type II 11β-HSD, the clinical features are those of excessive mineralocorticoids,[66, 68] owing to the activation of mineralocorticoid receptors by physiologic levels of cortisol. The characteristic cellular action of mineralocorticoids is enhancement of the transepithelial transport of sodium ions, by mechanisms that involve greater synthesis of Na^+/K^+ pump units, enzymes of ATP production, and other proteins whose functions remain to be elucidated.[69, 70]

Actions of Mineralocorticoids on the Cardiovascular System

With respect to the body as a whole, mineralocorticoids promote retention of sodium with maintenance of extracellular fluid volume as well as excretion of potassium. This effect occurs principally at the distal renal tubules, although there are also mineralocorticoid receptors in the colon, sweat glands, and salivary glands,[70] which are all sites for the exchange of fluid and electrolytes. Mineralocorticoids do not directly activate potassium transporters. Excretion of potassium is thought to be consequent to electrochemical gradients established by active transport of sodium. Because potassium ions directly promote the secretion of aldosterone, mineralocorticoids play an important role in preventing hyperkalemia under conditions of potassium loading. Indeed, the major clinical manifestations of an isolated deficiency of mineralocorticoids are hyperkalemia and metabolic acidosis that may be a consequence of the hyperkalemia.

Human myocardium contains type I mineralocorticoid receptors.[71] Because the cardiac activity of 11β-HSD is low, presumably both circulating cortisol and aldosterone can bind to these receptors. Studies in rats suggest that mineralocorticoids can produce myocardial hypertrophy and fibrosis in the context of sodium loading.[72, 73] The demonstration that treatment with spironolactone, a mineralocorticoid receptor antagonist, ameliorates congestive heart failure[74] suggests that cardiac mineralocorticoid receptors are physiologically significant in humans.

VASOPRESSIN

Regulation of Secretion of Vasopressin

Arginine vasopressin (AVP), the human antidiuretic hormone, is a nonapeptide that is synthesized in magnocellular neurons of the supraoptic and paraventricular nuclei of the hypothalamus. Proteolytic cleavage of a ≈23-kD precursor yields AVP and neurophysin II, which are packaged together in secretory granules. The secretory granules are carried to nerve endings in the neurohypophysis by axonal transport.

Vasopressin is secreted into the general circulation in response to increases in plasma osmolality, which are sensed by hypothalamic osmoreceptor cells. The osmotic threshold for secretion is normally about 280 mosm/kg, plasma levels of vasopressin being proportional to osmolality over the range of about 280 to 310 mosm/kg. Over this range, as little as a 1% to 2% change in osmolality evokes a change in the secretion of vasopressin.[75]

Decreases in the blood pressure or effective circulating volume, as sensed by pressure receptors in the carotid sinuses and aortic arch and by volume receptors in the heart and venous system, also stimulate the secretion of vasopressin. At least a 5% to 10% decrease in the effective blood volume or blood pressure is required for activation of vasopressin secretion. In response to volume depletion, plasma vasopressin reaches much higher levels than are attained with purely osmotic stimuli. Additionally, hypovolemia sensitizes vasopressin secretion to osmotic stimuli. Other nonosmotic stimuli of vasopressin secretion are hypoglycemia, hypoxia, nausea, and several drugs, including opiates, nicotine, beta-adrenergic agonists, angiotensin II, carbamazepine, metoclopramide, barbiturates, and some anesthetics. Conversely, alcohol, phenytoin, and alpha-adrenergic agonists inhibit the release of vasopressin.

Mechanism of Action of Vasopressin

Vasopressin interacts with three types of plasma-membrane receptors. V1 receptors signal via changes in intracellular calcium. V1a receptors are located in the liver and vasculature. V1b receptors, also known as V3 receptors, are found in the anterior pituitary, where they promote the secretion of ACTH.

V2 receptors, which are found in renal collecting ducts, signal via G proteins and the adenylyl cyclase–cyclic AMP system. In the kidney, activation of V2 receptors permits reabsorption of water from the collecting ducts by promoting the synthesis and translocation of endosomes containing the water channel protein, aquaporin-2 (AQP-2), into apical plasma membranes. The AQP-2 molecules form channels that facilitate the transepithelial transport of water into the hypertonic medullary interstitium, along an osmotic gradient. In some situations, such as hypokalemia, hypercalcemia, treatment with lithium salts, postobstructive diuresis, and chronic ingestion of hypotonic fluids, renal responsiveness to AVP is blunted, owing in part to reduced intrarenal levels of AQP-2.[76]

Actions of Vasopressin on the Heart and Circulation

AVP, acting via V2 receptors, maintains homeostasis of body fluid osmolality by regulating the renal reabsorption of water. V1 receptors mediate arterial vasoconstriction. However, the physiologic role of AVP in circulatory regulation is complex. Higher levels of AVP are required for vasomotor responses than for maximal urinary concentration. Also, there are regional differences in vascular responses to moderate increases in AVP: Blood flow to skin and muscle is reduced, whereas flow to the kidney and liver is maintained; flow to myocardium is diminished proportionally to the reduction in the cardiac output.[77] Within the kidney, flow is redistributed away from the medulla. Additionally, AVP-mediated vasoconstriction tends to be counterbalanced by an enlarged intravascular fluid volume and by inhibition of the secretion of renin.[78] As a result, a long-term excess of AVP does not result in hypertension.

THYROID HORMONES

Regulation of the Hypothalamic-Pituitary-Thyroid Axis

Synthesis and secretion of thyroid hormones are stimulated by thyrotropin (TSH), a glycoprotein hormone of pituitary origin. The TSH receptor signals through the adenylyl cyclase–cyclic AMP pathway. In turn, synthesis and secretion of TSH are stimulated by thyrotropin-releasing hormone (TRH), a hypothalamic peptide that reaches the pituitary via the pituitary portal circulation. The TRH receptor signals through the adenylyl cyclase–cyclic AMP pathway, leading to hydrolysis of phosphatidylinositol and elevation of intracellular calcium.[2] Secretion of TSH is pulsatile and exhibits a diurnal rhythm, with greater secretion at night, but the physiologic significance of this rhythmicity is questionable because of the extensive binding of circulating thyroid hormones to plasma proteins (see later). The activity of the hypothalamic-pituitary-thyroid axis is regulated principally by feedback inhibition of secretion of TSH by unbound thyroxine (3,5,3′,5′-tetraiodothyronine [T_4]) and (3,5,3′-triiodothyronine [T_3]), exerted at the levels of both the hypothalamus and pituitary.

In humans, about 90% of the hormonal secretion of the thyroid gland is in the form of T_4 (Table 2–5). Circulating T_4 is almost entirely bound reversibly but with very high affinity to plasma proteins, principally thyroxine-binding globulin (TBG), thyroxine-binding prealbumin (transthyretin), and albumin. The system behaves according to the free thyroxine hypothesis, which states that only the tiny unbound fraction (about 0.03%) of circulating thyroxine is available for conversion to T_3 (see later), for exertion of physiologic effects, including inhibition of secretion of TSH, and for degradation. Because of the large buffer of plasma T_4-binding proteins, circulating concentrations of unbound thyroxine exhibit very little temporal variability. Estrogens promote the synthesis and inhibit the degradation of TBG. Consequently, pregnant women[79] and women taking exogenous estrogens, such as oral contraceptives, have elevated concentrations of circulating TBG. Because negative feedback regarding TSH secretion is mediated by the unbound fraction of the circulating thyroid hormones, the thyroid hormonal economy of the individual remains normal in these situations despite the high concentrations of bound thyroxine.

Table 2–5. MOLAR QUANTITIES OF THYROID HORMONES: SECRETION AND TOTAL AND FREE CONCENTRATIONS IN THE CIRCULATION FOR THE TWO MAJOR THYROID HORMONES

VARIABLE	T4	T3
Production rate (nmol/d)	115	48
Thyroidal secretion (nmol/d)	115	10
Concentration in plasma (nmol/L):		
Total	110	2.1
Free	0.03	0.008

Adapted from Robbins J: Thyroid hormone transport proteins and the physiology of hormone binding. In Braverman LE, Utiger RD (eds): Werner and Ingbar's The Thyroid, 7th ed. Lippincott-Raven Publishers, Philadelphia, 1996, pp 96–110; and Chopra IJ: Nature, source, and relative significance of circulating thyroid hormones. In Braverman LE, Utiger RD (eds): Werner and Ingbar's The Thyroid, 7th ed. Lippincott-Raven Publishers, Philadelphia, 1996, pp 111.

Circulating T_4 serves principally as a precursor for conversion to T_3, which is physiologically more active. Conversion of T_4 to T_3 occurs in the liver and target tissues, mediated by 5′-deiodinases. About 80% of the body's T_3 is derived by conversion from T_4, the remaining 20% being secreted directly from the thyroid gland (see Table 2–5). About two thirds of the extrathyroidal T_3 in the body is intracellular.

Mechanism of Action of Thyroid Hormones

T_3 acts by binding to nuclear receptors, proteins that are products of the c-*erb*-A cellular oncogenes. T_3 receptors are members of a superfamily that also includes receptors for glucocorticoids, mineralocorticoids, androgens, estrogens, vitamin D, and retinoids. In humans, there are two genes for T_3 receptors, alpha and beta, each of which codes for two products on the basis of alternative splicing of messenger RNA (mRNA). Only three of the resulting four possible isoforms, $alpha_1$, $beta_1$, and $beta_2$, can bind T_3. The $beta_1$ T_3 receptor is the physiologically predominant isoform in the human myocardium as well as the liver and kidney. The general mechanism of action of T_3 involves the differential regulation of protein synthesis caused by binding of occupied T_3 receptors, probably in the form of receptor dimers, to DNA. T_3 receptors have binding sites for the hormone and for specific sequences (T_3-responsive elements) in the promoter regions of T_3-sensitive genes. Additionally, there may be some actions of thyroid hormones that are not mediated by these T_3 receptors.[82]

Thyroid hormones have multiple and diverse physiologic effects that are exhibited at every stage of life, directly or indirectly involving nearly every organ. Beginning in utero, thyroid hormones are essential for the normal growth and development of many organs, including the central nervous system and skeleton. At all ages, thyroid hormones regulate the whole-body metabolic rate, at least in part by increasing the number or activity of Na^+/K^+-ATPase units in plasma membranes.[83]

Actions of Thyroid Hormones on the Cardiovascular System

Thyroid hormones affect cardiac function directly and indirectly. By virtue of the generalized increase in the turnover of ATP, thyroid hormones augment organismal oxygen consumption and production of heat, leading to compensatory peripheral vasodilatation, renal retention of salt and water, and increased cardiac output.

Additionally, thyroid hormones have a number of direct effects on the heart, the integrated physiologic consequences of which include cardioacceleration and augmentation of both myocardial contractility and relaxation. Many of these effects are mediated by changes in the handling of calcium within the sarcoplasmic reticulum, as well as by cardiac myosin Ca^{2+}-ATPase. Thyroid hormones also increase the expression of other myocardial proteins, including components of Na^+/K^+-ATPase and mitochondrial proteins. Stimulation of cardiac contractility probably contributes significantly to the previously mentioned effects of thyroid hormones on the whole-body metabolism. Treatment of hypothyroidism leads to a proportionally greater augmentation of cardiac work than of cardiac oxygen consumption—that is, to improved myocardial efficiency.[84]

The effects of thyroid hormones on lipoprotein metabolism also can influence the cardiovascular system. In particular, thyroid hormones induce expression of the LDL receptor.[85] Individuals with hypothyroidism, even subclinical hypothyroidism, tend to have elevated levels of LDL cholesterol and a greater risk of atherosclerotic disease.[86]

REGULATION OF EXTRACELLULAR CALCIUM

Hormonal Regulation of Calcium Metabolism

The concentration of calcium in plasma and extracellular fluids ($[Ca^{2+}]_o$) plays a critical role in regulating neuromuscular excitability and conduction. In normal persons, about half of the circulating calcium is complexed tightly with polyvalent anions, including phosphate and anionic proteins. The remainder, termed *ionized calcium*, is available for reversible binding to plasma membranes and for entry into cells via calcium channels. Normally, $[Ca^{2+}]_o$ is tightly regulated by an intricate hormonal system that principally involves parathyroid hormone (PTH) and 1,25-dihydroxyvitamin D ($1,25(OH)_2D$), the active form of vitamin D. Parathyroid hormone–related protein (PTHrP) (see later) and calcitonin are clinically important but do not strongly influence $[Ca^{2+}]_o$.

Parathyroid Hormone and Parathyroid Hormone–Related Protein

PTH is an 84–amino acid polypeptide ($PTH^{1\text{-}84}$), the synthesis and secretion of which are inversely related to $[Ca^{2+}]_o$ over the physiologic range of $[Ca^{2+}]_o$.[87] This relationship is mediated by the interaction of calcium ions with a protein, the calcium receptor (CaR), that is expressed on the surface of parathyroid cells.[88] The structure of the calcium receptor suggests that it signals via a G protein. PTH is degraded within parathyroid cells at a rate that is directly related to $[Ca^{2+}]_o$, thus representing a mechanism by which $[Ca^{2+}]_o$ can regulate the production of physiologically active PTH.[87] Also, the secretion of PTH is stimulated by lithium ions (Li^+) and is inhibited by physiologic concentrations of extracellular magnesium ions (Mg^{2+}). However, severe magnesium depletion inhibits the secretion of PTH. Additionally, $1,25(OH)_2D$ inhibits the proliferation of parathyroid cells as well as the secretion and expression of the gene for PTH, via vitamin D receptors in parathyroid cells.[87] Because PTH acts both to increase the circulating levels of $[Ca^{2+}]$ and to promote the renal formation of $1,25(OH)_2D$, the secretion of PTH is under dual negative-feedback regulation.

$PTH^{1\text{-}84}$ has a circulating half-life of less than 4 minutes, being rapidly metabolized by complex hepatic and renal mechanisms to a variety of smaller peptides.[89] C-terminal fragments account for the great majority of circulating PTH-derived molecules because of their relatively slow degradation and elimination. They do not interact with the classic PTH receptor, and their physiologic role, if any, has not yet been defined. The first 34 amino acids at the N-terminus of PTH ($PTH^{1\text{-}34}$) account for the full activity of the intact hormone at the PTH receptor.[87] However, because the N-terminal products of the cleavage of PTH disappear very rapidly from the circulation, the physiologic effects of circulating PTH on calcium metabolism are attributable mostly to the intact $PTH^{1\text{-}84}$ molecule.

PTHrP was discovered within the last decade to be the agent responsible for the humoral hypercalcemia of malignancy. This protein exhibits limited sequence homology with PTH, at the N-terminus.[90] The gene for PTH is smaller than that for PTHrP and has no intron, so the gene for PTH may have arisen from retroviral activity.

Mechanism of Action of Parathyroid Hormone and Parathyroid Hormone–Related Protein

PTH and PTHrP interact with equivalent affinity with a G protein–coupled receptor, expressed in chondrocytes, osteoblasts, and renal tubular cells.[87] Signal transduction by the PTH/PTHrP receptor is thought to be mediated principally by cyclic AMP, although phosphoinositides, intracellular calcium, and protein kinase C may be additional second messengers.[87] A receptor specific for PTH has been described, but its tissue distribution suggests that it is not related to the regulation of calcium metabolism.[91]

Parathyroid hormone acts in the following three major ways to increase the concentration of ionized calcium in extracellular fluids:

1. Stimulation of mobilization of calcium from bone.
2. Stimulation of renal tubular excretion of phosphorus and fractional reabsorption of calcium, which thereby increases the proportion of circulating calcium in physiologically active ionized form.
3. Activation of renal mitochondrial 25-hydroxyvitamin D 1-hydroxylase, leading to greater formation of $1,25(OH)_2D$ (see later).

Stimulation of osteoclastic bone resorption by PTH appears to be mediated by paracrine signals produced by osteoblasts.[87] This action entails increases in the number as well as activity of osteoclasts.

PTHrP appears to have little or no role in the physiologic regulation of the extracellular calcium concentration in adults. It is widely distributed in fetal tissues[92] and probably has important roles during fetal life, especially stimulation of the transplacental transfer of calcium from mother to fetus.[90] In adults, PTHrP is normally expressed in keratinocytes and is greatly concentrated in milk.[90] It may be important for the mobilization of calcium from the maternal skeleton during lactation.[93]

Mechanism of Action of Vitamin D

The vitamins D are a family of sterol-derived molecules. Although some members of the family (vitamins D_2, the ergocalciferols) are derived from plant sources, the term *vitamin* is a misnomer, because humans can synthesize vitamin D_3 (cholecalciferol) from 7-dehydrocholesterol. Synthesis of vitamin D_3 involves photochemical cleavage of the B ring of the steroid nucleus, which occurs in the skin and requires ultraviolet B light.[94] Aging, residence at higher latitudes, diminished exposure to sunlight, and increased dermal melanin all can place individuals at risk of vitamin D insufficiency.[94] Ergocalciferol and cholecalciferol are equally potent as precursors of physiologically active $1,25(OH)_2D$, which is produced by subsequent hepatic 25-hydroxylation and renal 1α-hydroxylation. Renal 1α-hydroxylation of 25-hydroxyvitamin D is stimulated by PTH (see earlier) and is inhibited by circulating phosphate.[94] The placenta and other tissues can hydroxylate vitamin D at the 1-position, but under normal circumstances, extrarenal production of $1,25(OH)_2D$ probably does not have a role in regulating calcium metabolism.[94]

The physiologic effects of $1,25(OH)_2D$, the active form of vitamin D, on mineral metabolism are (1) induction of gastrointestinal absorption of calcium and phosphorus, (2) promotion of differentiation of bone marrow stem cells into osteoclasts, (3) induction of osteoblastic proteins involved in mineralization, and (4) inhibition of the synthesis of PTH (see earlier).[94]

Vitamin D acts by a mechanism similar to that of steroid hormones. After binding of $1,25(OH)_2D$, activation of the vitamin D receptor (VDR) involves protein phosphorylation, formation of a ternary complex with the retinoic acid receptor, and binding to vitamin D–response elements of the genome.[94] In this manner, $1,25(OH)_2D$ promotes the synthesis of osteocalcin, osteopontin, and alkaline phosphatase by osteoblasts and of calcium-binding protein (CaBP) and other proteins by intestinal epithelial cells.[94] Calcium-binding protein is thought to have a major role in the enhancement of intestinal absorption of calcium by vitamin D. Although the vitamin D receptor is expressed in many tissues, individuals with inactivating mutations of the vitamin D receptor appear normal except for inadequate intestinal absorption of calcium as well as rickets and severe alopecia.[95] Therefore, the essential physiologic actions of vitamin D are apparently confined to the regulation of calcium metabolism and the development of hair.

Physiologic Relevance of Calcitonin

Calcitonin is a 32–amino acid peptide produced in humans by the C cells (parafollicular cells) of the thyroid.[96] In nonmammals, the C cells form a separate organ, the ultimobranchial gland. In neural tissue, alternative splicing of the primary transcript of the calcitonin gene, located on chromosome 11, yields mRNA for calcitonin gene–related peptide (CGRP), a 37–amino acid peptide that appears to function primarily as a neurotransmitter.[97]

Calcitonin binds to G protein–coupled receptors, which are expressed in osteoclasts.[89] These receptors signal via the cyclic AMP pathway and increased intracellular calcium ion ($[Ca^{2+}]$) levels. The hormone rapidly and powerfully inhibits osteoclastic bone resorption. Because serum $[Ca^{2+}]$ is not abnormal in the absence of circulating calcitonin or in states of marked excess (e.g., medullary carcinoma of the thyroid), the hormone is apparently not essential for the regulation of extracellular calcium in adults. Pharmacologic doses of calcitonin are effective for treating pathologic hypercalcemia[98] and for preventing osteoporotic fractures in postmenopausal women.[99]

Actions of Calcitropic Hormones on the Cardiovascular System

The calcitropic hormones influence cardiovascular physiology mainly by means of their effects on the serum calcium concentration. In humans, hypocalcemia has been associated with cardiac conduction defects, and cases of dilated cardiomyopathy have been reported. Epidemiologic studies have suggested that calcemia influences blood pressure and mortality.[100] In observational studies, hypercalcemia and hyperparathyroidism have been linked to increased arterial stiffness,[101] hypertension, and deposition of calcium salts in the heart, but experimental studies have shown that acute infusion of PTH has only minor effects on cardiovascular function.[102]

In animal models and in humans, infusions of PTH or PTHrP have vasodilatory and positive chronotropic effects.[103, 104] Because these effects are observed at pharmacologic concentrations of the peptides, their physiologic significance is open to question. PTHrP, however, may have a role as a paracrine mediator in the cardiovascular system. The PTHrP/PTH receptor is expressed in vascular smooth muscle. PTHrP is expressed in rat vascular smooth muscle cells, in which it can be induced by the vasoconstrictors thrombin, norepinephrine, and endothelin,[105] as well as in secretory granules of rat atrial myocytes.[106] These observations warrant further study.

The vitamin D receptor is expressed in many tissues, including cardiac muscle.[107] In other tissues, $1,25(OH)_2D$ inhibits cellular proliferation and promotes differentiation, but whether vitamin D influences the development or function of the cardiovascular system remains to be determined. As noted previously, individuals who lack functional vitamin D receptors do not have obvious cardiovascular disease.

CGRP and its receptors are found in the brain and extensively throughout the nervous system, including the innervation of the heart and coronary arteries. CGRP is detectable in the circulation, but its physiologic actions are probably mostly paracrine. There are at least two subtypes of CGRP receptors, which are coupled to cyclic AMP. The principal circulatory effects of CGRP are vasodilatation, hypotension, increased atrial contractility, cardioacceleration, and increased coronary blood flow. CGRP is a highly potent vasodilator, with a median effective dose (ED_{50}) of about 50 nM.[97] To date, no human cardiovascular disease has been attributed to an abnormality of CGRP.

SOMATOSTATIN

Physiologic Role of Somatostatin

Somatostatin is a small peptide of either 14 or 28 amino acids, depending on post-translational processing.[2] Somatostatin-14, produced in the hypothalamus and transported to the adenohypophysis by the pituitary portal system, powerfully inhibits the secretion of GH and TSH.[2] Brain somatostatin also has a major role as a neurotransmitter. Somatostatin-28 is produced in the gastrointestinal mucosa and the D cells of the endocrine pancreas. Although somatostatin is found in the peripheral circulation, its major extrapituitary physiologic activities are probably exerted in a paracrine fashion. These actions include (1) inhibition of the secretion of glucagon, insulin, and several intestinal peptides, including somatostatin itself, (2) inhibition of pancreatic exocrine secretion, and (3) inhibition of gastrointestinal motility.

Mechanism of Action of Somatostatin

To date, five different kinds of somatostatin receptors have been identified. These receptors are expressed in a tissue-specific manner and are coupled to G proteins of the G_i class, leading to the inhibition of adenylyl cyclase.[108] Human vascular endothelial cells express somatostatin receptors.[109] Whether somatostatin physiologically regulates the circulation remains to be determined. However, analogues of somatostatin have several potentially important therapeutic uses, including prevention of bleeding from esophageal varices,[110] prevention of restenosis after arterial injury,[111] inhibition of tumor angiogenesis,[112] and inhibition of arterial vasoconstriction.[113]

References

1. Müller EE, Locatelli V, Cocchi D: Neuroendocrine control of growth hormone secretion. Physiol Rev 79:511, 1999.
2. Reichlin S: Neuroendocrinology. In Wilson JD, Foster DW, Kronenberg HM, et al (eds): Williams Textbook of Endocrinology, 9th ed. WB Saunders, Philadelphia, 1998, p 165.
3. Saenger P: Oral growth hormone secretagogues—better than Alice in Wonderland's growth elixir? (editorial). J Clin Endocrinol Metab 81: 2773, 1996.
4. Howard AD, Feighner SD, Cully DF, et al: A receptor in pituitary and hypothalamus that functions in growth hormone release. Science 273:974, 1996.
5. Kojima M, Hosoda H, Date Y, et al: Ghrelin is a growth-hormone-releasing acylated peptide from stomach. Nature 402:656, 1999.
6. Martha PM Jr, Rogol AD, Veldhuis JD, et al: Alterations in the pulsatile properties of circulating growth hormone concentrations during puberty in boys. J Clin Endocrinol Metab 69:563, 1989.
7. Iranmanesh A, Veldhuis JD: Clinical pathophysiology of the somatotropic (GH) axis in adults. Endocrinol Metab Clin North Am 21: 783, 1992.
8. Corpas E, Harman SM, Blackman MR: Human growth hormone and human aging. Endocr Rev 14:20, 1993.
9. DeBoer H, Blok G-J, VanDerVeen EA: Clinical aspects of growth hormone deficiency in adults. Endocr Rev 16:63, 1995.
10. Faria ALS, Bekenstein LW, Booth RA Jr, et al: Pulsatile growth hormone release in normal women during the menstrual cycle. Clin Endocrinol 36:591, 1992.
11. Dawson-Hughes B, Stern D, Goldman J, et al: Regulation of growth hormone and somatomedin-C secretion in postmenopausal women: Effect of physiological estrogen replacement. J Clin Endocrinol Metab 63:424, 1986.
12. Veldhuis JD, Iranmanesh A, Ho KKY, et al: Dual defects in pulsatile growth hormone secretion and clearance subserve the hyposomatotropism of obesity in man. J Clin Endocrinol Metab 72:51, 1991.
13. Williams T, Berelowitz M, Joffe SN, et al: Impaired growth hormone responses to growth hormone-releasing factor in obesity. N Engl J Med 311:1403, 1984.
14. Goffin V, Kelly PA: Prolactin and growth hormone receptors. Clin Endocrinol (Oxf) 45:247, 1996.
15. Cosman D: The hematopoietin receptor superfamily. Cytokine 5:95, 1993.
16. Horseman ND, Yu-Lee LY: Transcriptional regulation by the helix bundle peptide hormones: Growth hormone, prolactin, and hematopoietic cytokines. Endocr Rev 15:627, 1994.
17. Argetsinger LS, Campbell GS, Yang X, et al: Identification of JAK2 as a growth hormone receptor-associated tyrosine kinase. Cell 74: 237, 1993.
18. Reiter EO, Rosenfeld RG: Normal and aberrant growth. In Wilson JD, Foster DW, Kronenberg HM, et al (eds): Williams Textbook of Endocrinology, 9th ed. WB Saunders, Philadelphia, 1998, p 1427.
19. Petley T, Graff T, Jiang W, et al: Variation among cell types in the signaling pathways by which IGF-I stimulates specific cellular responses. Horm Metab Res 31:70, 1999.
20. Prisco M, Romano G, Peruzzi F, et al: Insulin and IGF-I receptors signaling in protection from apoptosis. Horm Metab Res 31:80, 1999.
21. Jones JI, Clemmons DR: Insulin-like growth factors and their binding proteins: Biological actions. Endocr Rev 16:3, 1995.
22. LeRoith D, Werner H, Beitner-Johnson D, et al: Molecular and cellular aspects of the insulin-like growth factor I receptor. Endocr Rev 16:143, 1995.
23. Hwa V, Oh Y, Rosenfeld RG: Insulin-like growth factor binding proteins: A proposed superfamily. Acta Paediatr Suppl 428:37, 1999.
24. Ferry RJ Jr, Katz LEL, Grimberg A, et al: Cellular actions of insulin-like growth factor binding proteins. Horm Metab Res 31:192, 1999.
25. Bach LA, Rechler MM: Insulin-like growth factor binding proteins. Diabetes Rev 3:38, 1995.
26. Cuneo RC, Salomon F, McGauley GA, et al: The growth hormone deficiency syndrome in adults. Clin Endocrinol (Oxf) 37:387, 1992.
27. Sacca L, Cittadini A, Fazio S: Growth hormone and the heart. Endocr Rev 15:555, 1994.
28. Isgaard J, Tivesten Å, Friberg P, et al: The role of the GH/IGF-I axis for cardiac function and structure. Horm Metab Res 31:50, 1999.
29. Bates AS, Van't Hoff W, Jones PJ, et al: The effect of hypopituitarism on life expectancy. J Clin Endocrinol Metab 81:1169, 1996.
30. Cittadini A, Cuocolo A, Merola B, et al: Improved cardiac performance in GH-deficient adults and its improvement after GH replacement. Am J Physiol 267:E219, 1994.
31. Shahi M, Beshyah SA, Sackett D, et al: Myocardial dysfunction in treated adult hypopituitarism: A possible explanation for increased cardiovascular mortality. Br Heart J 67:92, 1992.
32. Rosen T, Eden S, Larson G, et al: Cardiovascular risk factors in adult patients with growth hormone deficiency. Acta Endocrinol 129: 195, 1993.
33. O'Neal D, Hew FL, Sikaris K, et al: Low density lipoprotein particle size in hypopituitary adults receiving conventional hormone replacement therapy. J Clin Endocrinol Metab 81:2448, 1996.
34. Frustaci A, Perrone GA, Gentiloni N, et al: Reversible dilated cardiomyopathy due to growth hormone deficiency. Am J Clin Pathol 97: 503, 1992.
35. Chrisoulidou A, Beshyah SA, Rutherford O, et al: Effects of 7 years of growth hormone replacement therapy in hypopituitary adults. J Clin Endocrinol Metab 85:3762, 2000.
36. Nass R, Huber RM, Klauss V, et al: Effect of growth hormone (hGH) replacement therapy on physical work capacity and cardiac and pulmonary function in patients with hGH deficiency acquired in adulthood. J Clin Endocrinol Metab 80:552, 1995.
37. Beshyah SA, Henderson A, Niththyananthan R, et al: The effects

of short and long term growth hormone replacement therapy in hypopituitary adults on lipid metabolism and carbohydrate tolerance. J Clin Endocrinol Metab 80:356, 1995.
38. Caidahl K, Eden S, Bengtsson B-A: Cardiovascular and renal effects of growth hormone. Clin Endocrinol (Oxf) 40:393, 1994.
39. Cuneo RC, Salomon F, Wilmshurst P, et al: Cardiovascular effects of growth hormone treatment in growth-hormone-deficient adults: Stimulation of the renin-aldosterone system. Clin Sci 81:587, 1991.
40. Valcavi R, Gaddi O, Zini M, et al: Cardiac performance and mass in adults with hypopituitarism: Effects of one year of growth hormone treatment. J Clin Endocrinol Metab 80:659, 1995.
41. Sesmilo G, Biller BMK, Llevadot J, et al: Effects of growth hormone administration on inflammatory and other cardiovascular risk markers in men with growth hormone deficiency. Ann Intern Med 133:111, 2000.
42. Papotti M, Ghe C, Cassoni P, et al: Growth hormone secretagogues binding sites in peripheral human tissues. J Clin Endocrinol Metab 85:3803, 2000.
43. Ben-Jonathan N, Mershon JL, Allen DL, et al: Extrapituitary prolactin: Distribution, regulation, functions, and clinical aspects. Endocr Rev 17:639, 1996.
44. Gershengorn MC: Mechanism of signal transduction by TRH. Ann N Y Acad Sci 553:191, 1989.
45. Honbo KS, Van Herle AJ, Kellett KA: Serum prolactin levels in untreated primary hypothyroidism. Am J Med 64:782, 1978.
46. Molitch ME: Pathologic hyperprolactinemia. Endocrinol Metab Clin North Am 21:877, 1992.
47. Biller BM: Diagnostic evaluation of hyperprolactinemia. J Reprod Med 12(Suppl):1095, 1999.
48. Bole-Feysot C, Goffin V, Edery M, et al: Prolactin (PRL) and its receptor: Actions, signal transduction pathways and phenotypes observed in PRL receptor knockout mice. Endocr Rev 19:225, 1998.
49. Dorshkind K, Horseman ND: The roles of prolactin, growth hormone, insulin-like growth factor-I, and thyroid hormones in lymphocyte development and function: Insights from genetic models of hormone and hormone receptor deficiency. Endocr Rev 21:292, 2000.
50. Struman I, Bentzien F, Lee H, et al: Opposing actions of intact and N-terminal fragments of the human prolactin/growth hormone family members on angiogenesis: An efficient mechanism for the regulation of angiogenesis. Proc Natl Acad Sci 96:1246, 1999.
51. Vale W, Rivier C, Brown MR, et al: Chemical and biological characterization of corticotrophin releasing factor. Recent Prog Hormone Res 39:245, 1983.
52. Brien TG: Human corticosteroid binding globulin. Clin Endocrinol (Oxf) 14:193, 1981.
53. Pratt WB, Toft DO: Steroid receptor interactions with heat shock protein and immunophilin chaperones. Endocr Rev 18:306, 1997.
54. Beato M, Sanchez-Pacheco A: Interactions of steroid hormone receptors with the transcription initiation complex. Endocr Rev 17:587, 1996.
55. Clark JH, Schrader WT, O'Malley BW: Mechanisms of action of hormones that act as transcription-regulatory factors. In Wilson JD, Foster DW, Kronenberg HM, et al (eds): Williams Textbook of Endocrinology, 9th ed. WB Saunders, Philadelphia, 1998, p 55.
56. Bouachour G, Tirot P, Varache N, et al: Hemodynamic changes in acute adrenal insufficiency. Intensive Care Med 20:138, 1994.
57. Stockigt JR, Hewett MJ, Topliss DJ, et al: Renin and renin substrate in primary adrenal insufficiency: Contrasting effects of glucocorticoid and mineralocorticoid deficiency. Am J Med 66:915, 1979.
58. Agus ZS, Goldberg M: Role of antidiuretic hormone in the abnormal water diuresis of anterior hypopituitarism in man. J Clin Invest 50: 1478, 1971.
59. Raff H: Glucocorticoid inhibition of neurohypophysial vasopressin secretion. Am J Physiol 252:R635, 1987.
60. Gardner DG, Hane S, Trachewsky D, et al: Atrial natriuretic peptide mRNA is regulated by glucocorticoids in vivo. Biochem Biophys Res Commun 139:1047, 1986.
61. Sato A, Sheppard KE, Fullerton MJ, et al: CAMP modulates glucocorticoid-induced protein accumulation and glucocorticoid receptor in cardiomyocytes. Am J Physiol 271:E827, 1996.
62. Argentin S, Sun YL, Lihrmann I, et al: Distal cis-acting promoter sequences mediate glucocorticoid stimulation of cardiac atrial natriuretic factor gene transcription. J Biol Chem 266:23315, 1991.
63. Funder JW: Steroids, hypertension and cardiac fibrosis. Blood Press Suppl 2:39, 1995.
64. Blair-West JR, Coghlan JP, Denton DA, et al: A dose-response comparison of the actions of angiotensin II and angiotensin III in sheep. J Endocrinol 87:409, 1980.
65. Davis JO, Urquhart J, Higgins JT Jr: The effects of alterations of plasma sodium and potassium concentration on aldosterone secretion. J Clin Invest 42:597, 1963.
66. White PC, Mune T, Agarwal AK: 11-β hydroxysteroid dehydrogenase and the syndrome of apparent mineralocorticoid excess. Endocr Rev 18:135, 1997.
67. Krozowski ZS, Provencher PH, Smith RE, et al: Isozymes of 11β-hydroxysteroid dehydrogenase: Which enzyme endows mineralocorticoid specificity? Steroids 59:116, 1994.
68. Mune T, Rogerson FM, Nikkilä H, et al: Human hypertension caused by mutations in the kidney isozyme of 11β-hydroxysteroid dehydrogenase. Nat Genet 10:394, 1995.
69. Homsberger J-D, Rossier BC: Aldosterone regulation of gene transcription leading to control of ion transport. Hypertension 19:221, 1992.
70. Garty H: Mechanisms of aldosterone action in tight epithelia. J Membrane Biol 90:193, 1986.
71. Lombes M, Alfaidy N, Eugene E, et al: Prerequisite for cardiac aldosterone activity. Mineralocorticoid receptor and 11β-hydroxysteroid dehydrogenase in the human heart. Circulation 92:175, 1995.
72. Brilla CG, Matsubara LS, Weber KT: Anti-aldosterone treatment and the prevention of myocardial fibrosis in primary and secondary hyperaldosteronism. J Mol Cell Cardiol 25:563, 1993.
73. Young M, Fullertons M, Dilley R, et al: Mineralocorticoids, hypertension, and cardiac fibrosis. J Clin Invest 93:2578, 1994.
74. Pitt B, Zannad F, Remme WJ, et al: The effect of spironolactone on morbidity and mortality in patients with severe heart failure. N Engl J Med 341:709, 1999.
75. Robertson GL: Osmoregulation of thirst and vasopressin secretion: Functional properties and their relationship to water balance. In Schrier RW (ed): Vasopressin. Raven Press, New York, 1985, p 203.
76. Frokiaer J, Marples D, Knepper MA, et al: Pathophysiology of aquaporin-2 in water balance disorders. Am J Med Sci 316:291, 1998.
77. Liard J-F: Effects of arginine vasopressin on regional circulations. In Schrier RW (ed): Vasopressin. Raven Press, New York, 1985, p 59.
78. Reid IA, Golin R, Gregory LC, et al: Vasopressin, the renal nerves, and renin secretion. In Cowley AW Jr, Liard J-F, Ausiello DA (eds): Vasopressin: Cellular and Integrative Functions. Raven Press, New York, 1988, p 447.
79. Glinoer D: The regulation of thyroid function in pregnancy: Pathogenesis of endocrine adaptation from physiology to pathology. Endocr Rev 18:404, 1997.
80. Robbins J: Thyroid hormone transport proteins and the physiology of hormone binding. In Braverman LE, Utiger RD (eds): Werner and Ingbar's The Thyroid, 7th ed. Lippincott-Raven, Philadelphia, 1996, p 96.
81. Chopra IJ: Nature, source, and relative significance of circulating thyroid hormones. In Braverman LE, Utiger RD (eds): Werner and Ingbar's The Thyroid, 7th ed. Lippincott-Raven, Philadelphia, 1996, p 111.
82. Anderson GW, Mariash CN, Oppenheimer JH: Molecular actions of thyroid hormones. In Braverman LE, Utiger RD (eds): Werner and Ingbar's The Thyroid: A Fundamental and Clinical Text, 8th ed. Lippincott Williams & Wilkins, Philadelphia, 2000, p 174.
83. Davis PJ: Cellular actions of thyroid hormones. In Braverman LE, Utiger RD (eds): Werner and Ingbar's The Thyroid: A Fundamental and Clinical Text, 6th ed. JB Lippincott, Philadelphia, 1991, p 190.
84. Bengel FM, Nekolla SG, Ibrahim T, et al: Effect of thyroid hormones on cardiac function, geometry, and oxidative metabolism assessed noninvasively by positron emission tomography and magnetic resonance imaging. J Clin Endocrinol Metab 85:1822, 2000.
85. Diekman MJ, Anghelescu N, Endert E, et al: Changes in plasma low-density lipoprotein (LDL) and high-density lipoprotein cholesterol in hypo- and hyperthyroid patients are related to changes in free thyroxine, not to polymorphisms in LDL receptor or cholesterol ester transfer protein genes. J Clin Endocrinol Metab 85:1857, 2000.
86. Hak AE, Pols HA, Visser TJ, et al: Subclinical hypothyroidism is an independent risk factor for atherosclerosis and myocardial infarction in elderly women: the Rotterdam study. Ann Intern Med 132:270, 2000.
87. Jüppner H, Brown EM, Kronenberg HM: Parathyroid hormone. In Favus MJ (ed): Primer on the Metabolic Bone Diseases and Disorders of Mineral Metabolism, 4th ed. Lippincott Williams & Wilkins, Philadelphia, 1999, p 80.

88. Chattopadhyay N, Mithal A, Brown EM: The calcium-sensing receptor: A window into the physiology and pathophysiology of mineral ion metabolism. Endocr Rev 17:289, 1996.
89. Martin KJ, Hruska KA, Freitag JJ, et al: The peripheral metabolism of parathyroid hormone. N Engl J Med 301:1092, 1979.
90. Strewler GJ, Nissenson RA: Parathyroid-hormone-related protein. In Favus MJ (ed): Primer on the Metabolic Bone Diseases and Disorders of Mineral Metabolism, 4th ed. Lippincott Williams & Wilkins, Philadelphia, 1999, p 88.
91. Osdin TB, Gruber C, Bonner TI: Identification and functional expression of a receptor selectively recognizing parathyroid hormone, the PTH 2 receptor. J Biol Chem 270:15455, 1995.
92. Moseley JM, Hayman JA, Danks JA, et al: Immunohistochemical detection of parathyroid hormone-related protein in human fetal epithelia. J Clin Endocrinol Metab 73:478, 1991.
93. Sowers MF, Hollis BW, Shapiro B, et al: Elevated parathyroid hormone-related peptide associated with lactation and bone density loss. JAMA 276:549, 1996.
94. Holick MF: Vitamin D: Photobiology, metabolism, mechanism of action, and clinical applications. In Favus MJ (ed): Primer on the Metabolic Bone Diseases and Disorders of Mineral Metabolism, 4th ed. Lippincott Williams & Wilkins, Philadelphia, 1999, p 92.
95. Malloy PJ, Pike JW, Feldman D: The vitamin D receptor and the syndrome of hereditary 1,25-dihydroxyvitamin D-resistant rickets. Endocr Rev 20:156, 1999.
96. Deftos LJ, Roos BA, Oates EL: Calcitonin. In Favus MJ (ed): Primer on the Metabolic Bone Diseases and Disorders of Mineral Metabolism, 4th ed. Lippincott Williams and Wilkins, Philadelphia, 1999, p 99.
97. Wimalawansa SJ: Calcitonin gene-related peptide and its receptors: Molecular genetics, physiology, pathophysiology, and therapeutic potentials. Endocr Rev 17:533, 1996.
98. Shane E: Hypercalcemia: Pathogenesis, clinical manifestations, differential diagnosis, and management. In Favus MJ (ed): Primer on the Metabolic Bone Diseases and Disorders of Mineral Metabolism, 4th ed. Lippincott Williams and Wilkins, Philadelphia, 1999, p 183.
99. Chesnut CH, Silverman S, Andriano K, et al: A randomized trial of nasal spray calcitonin in postmenopausal women with established osteoporosis: The Prevent Recurrence Of Osteoporotic Fractures study. Am J Med 109:267, 2000.
100. Leifsson BG, Ahrén B: Serum calcium and survival in a large health screening program. J Clin Endocrinol Metab 81:2149, 1996.
101. Smith JC, Page MD, John R, et al: Augmentation of central arterial pressure in mild primary hyperparathyroidism. J Clin Endocrinol Metab 85:3515, 2000.
102. Barletta G, De Feo ML, Del Bene R, et al: Cardiovascular effects of parathyroid hormone: A study in healthy subjects and normotensive patients with mild primary hyperparathyroidism. J Clin Endocrinol Metab 85:1815, 2000.
103. Shan J, Pang PKT, Lin H-C, et al: Cardiovascular effects of human parathyroid hormone and parathyroid hormone-related peptide. J Cardiovasc Pharmacol 23(Suppl 2):S38, 1994.
104. Wolzt M, Schmetterer L, Dorner G, et al: Hemodynamic effects of parathyroid hormone-related peptide (1–34) in humans. J Clin Endocrinol Metab 82:2548, 1997.
105. Hongo T, Kupfer J, Enomoto H, et al: Abundant expression of parathyroid hormone-related protein in primary rat aortic smooth muscle cells accompanies serum-induced proliferation. J Clin Invest 88:1841, 1991.
106. Deftos LJ, Burton DW, Brandt DW: Parathyroid hormone-like protein is a secretory product of atrial myocytes. J Clin Invest 92:727, 1993.
107. Holick MF: Noncalcemic actions of 1,25-dihydroxyvitamin D_3 and clinical applications. Bone 17:1075, 1995.
108. Benali N, Ferjoux G, Puente E, et al: Somatostatin receptors. Digestion 62(suppl. 1):27, 2000.
109. Curtis SB, Hewitt J, Yakubovitz S, et al: Somatostatin receptor subtype expression and function in human vascular tissue. Am J Physiol Heart Circ Physiol 278:H1815, 2000.
110. Sadowski DC: Use of octreotide in the acute management of bleeding esophageal varices. Can J Gastroenterol 11:339, 1997.
111. Lefkovits J, Topol EJ: Pharmacological approaches for the prevention of restenosis after percutaneous coronary intervention. Prog Cardiovasc Dis 40:141, 1997.
112. Albini A, Florio T, Giunciuglio D, et al: Somatostatin controls Kaposi's sarcoma tumor growth through inhibition of angiogenesis. FASEB J 13:647, 1999.
113. Ruiz E, Del Rio M, Tejerina T: Effect of somatostatin on resistance and on capacitance rabbit isolated arteries. Eur J Pharmacol 388: 255, 2000.

| 2.4 | Autonomic Nervous System

Anne Hamilton Dougherty

The activities of daily living require a broad range of function from the human body and its component organ systems. On the one hand, there must be efficient and seamless anabolism and catabolism at rest to provide for normal growth, development, nutrition, and health without voluntary effort on the part of the individual. On the other hand, the body must be ready, at a moment's notice, to abandon all such vegetative efforts and mobilize the musculoskeletal system to escape internal or external emergencies; this mobilization constitutes the so-called fight-or-flight reaction. In the wide spectrum between these two extremes lie the demands of daily living—work, play, exercise, environmental change, and emotion. The autonomic nervous system (ANS) serves as the central coordinator of bodily processes, orchestrating the dynamic interplay between vegetative and active functions. Thus, the ANS governs blood pressure, distribution of blood flow, expenditure of metabolic energy and visceral smooth muscle activity to accomplish its task.[1] It functions below the level of conscious control, providing homeostasis in most conditions.

ANATOMY AND FUNCTION

The ANS comprises two major divisions, (1) the sympathetic, or thoracolumbar, nervous system and (2) the parasympathetic, or craniosacral, nervous system. The two peripheral divisions are illustrated in Color Plate 2–1.[2] Outflow from the two divisions generally occurs in an antagonistic pattern. For example, sympathetic stimulation increases heart rate, whereas parasympathetic stimulation slows heart rate. Under most circumstances, both the sympathetic and parasympathetic nervous systems are active; the degree of balance between the two determines the overall response.

Visceral afferent fibers carry sensory information, such as pain, pressure, and chemical status, from receptors in the heart, blood vessels, and other organ systems to the ANS. Baroreceptors and chemoreceptors in the aortic arch and carotid sinus are important feedback mechanisms in the regulation of blood pressure, heart rate, and respiration. Impulses from these receptors are carried in the vagus and glossopharyngeal nerves to the brainstem.

Central integration of ANS functions is a subcortical process, occurring at several centers in the brainstem. The hypothalamus, area postrema, and solitary tract regulate blood pressure, heart rate, respiration, temperature, and fluid balance, as well as emotion, sleep, sexual response, and fat and carbohydrate metabolism.[3] The area postrema is rich in receptors for angiotensin II, atrial natriuretic peptide, and endothelin.[4] The medulla oblongata governs respiration. Parasympathetic outflow tracts originate in the midbrain and medulla oblongata. The cortex, limbic system, and neostriatum each modulate these autonomic centers. Cortical input to regulatory centers allows for some voluntary control over autonomic function.

The Sympathetic Nervous System

The efferent unit of both sympathetic and parasympathetic nervous systems consists of a preganglionic fiber, a ganglion, and a postganglionic fiber terminating in the target organ. Preganglionic fibers of the sympathetic nervous system originate in the intermediolateral columns of the spinal cord. All preganglionic neurons are cholinergic, that is, characterized by their neurotransmitter, acetylcholine (ACh). There are three types of sympathetic ganglia: paravertebral, prevertebral, and terminal.[5] Twenty-two pairs of interconnected paravertebral sympathetic ganglia lie along the lateral aspects of the spinal cord, forming the lateral chain. These ganglia serve peripheral blood vessels, sweat glands, and pilomotor muscles. Prevertebral ganglia are found in the abdomen and pelvis, serving the viscera. These include the celiac, superior mesenteric, aorticorenal, and inferior mesenteric ganglia. Terminal ganglia, including the cervical ganglia, which serve the heart, are found in close proximity to the organs they innervate. Postganglionic neurons (effector cells) innervate the viscera, trunk, and limbs. The response of target organs to sympathetic stimulation is described in Table 2–6. Most postganglionic fibers are adrenergic, containing norepinephrine as their neurotransmitter.

Most cardiac ganglia and sympathetic fibers are found in the cardiac conduction system. Details of autonomic innervation of the cardiac conduction system have been mapped and are described earlier in this chapter.[6] Areas most richly innervated with sympathetic fibers are, in order of decreasing magnitude, the sinus (sinoatrial) node, atrioventricular node, and His-Purkinje system, followed by adjacent myocardium.

The adrenal medulla, a neuroendocrine gland, is considered part of the sympathetic nervous system. Derived from the embryonic neural crest, it anatomically resembles sympathetic ganglia. In contrast to other sympathetic ganglia, however, its primary neurotransmitter is epinephrine. The adrenal gland serves as a reservoir of epinephrine and other catecholamines that are secreted systemically to interact with adrenergic receptors throughout the body, as needed. A large epinephrine output can be mobilized within seconds, thus amplifying sympathetic response to crisis.

The Parasympathetic Nervous System

Central parasympathetic preganglionic fibers originate in the midbrain, medulla oblongata, and sacral spinal cord. The midbrain parasympathetic outflow serves the ciliary ganglion of the eye by way of the third cranial nerve. Medullary outflow is important to cardiovascular function, providing the parasympathetic component of the tenth as well as the seventh and ninth cranial nerves. The tenth (vagus) cranial nerve provides long preganglionic fibers to the viscera of the thorax and abdomen, synapsing at the myriad small ganglia immediately adjacent to or within innervated viscera. Afferent fibers from the viscera also return to the medulla by way of the vagus nerve. Sacral parasympathetic outflow innervates the genitourinary tract. Both preganglionic and postganglionic parasympathetic fibers are cholinergic. The response of target organs to parasympathetic stimulation is listed in Table 2–6.

Preganglionic fibers of the parasympathetic nervous system tend to ramify less extensively than fibers of the sympathetic nervous system.[3] Many organs have a 1:1 ratio between preganglionic and postganglionic vagal fibers. (Auerbach's plexus is the exception to this rule, having a ratio of 1:8000.) Postganglionic fibers are short and ramify with sympathetic postganglionic and visceral afferent fibers in complex plexuses, called terminal reticula, at the end organ.

Autonomic Neurotransmission

Excitation of neurons is determined by ion flux across neuronal cell membranes. In the unexcited state, an ATP-dependent sodium-potassium active transport pump in the membrane maintains a sodium concentration gradient between intracellular and extracellular fluid. Diffusion of potassium ions across the membrane results in an intracellular concentration 40 times higher in the axoplasm than in adjacent extracellular fluid, creating a potential difference of −70 mV.[7, 8] A stimulus may depolarize a section of the axonal membrane by triggering a voltage-sensitive sodium channel and producing a rapid sodium influx, which reverses the polarity of the local cell membrane. In sequence, the sodium channel is then rapidly inactivated and a potassium channel is opened to restore the resting negative cell membrane potential.[9] The resulting cycle of depolarization-repolarization constitutes the action potential. Local depolarization of the axon excites adjacent segments of the axon, leading to propagation of the excitatory impulse along the axon. In myelinated fibers, the impulse jumps rapidly between nodes of Ranvier for speedier conduction.

Excitatory and inhibitory impulses are transmitted from neuron to neuron across synapses or from neuron to target cell across neuroeffector junctions by way of chemical neurotransmitters stored in vesicles in the presynaptic axonal terminal (Color Plate 2–2).[2] Depolarization triggers a release of a large quantity of transmitters from vesicles into the intercellular cleft by exocytosis. Neurotransmitter diffuses across the junction and docks with appropriate receptors on the postsynaptic cell membrane, usually resulting in either excitation or inhibition. Local increases in sodium conductance result in depolarization of the cell membrane and propagation of an excitatory impulse along the neuron or target cell. In contrast, inhibitory neurotransmitters may increase permeability to either chloride and other anions or to potassium ions, thereby hyperpolarizing the postsynaptic

Table 2–6. RESPONSE OF THE CARDIOVASCULAR SYSTEM TO AUTONOMIC STIMULATION

EFFECTOR ORGAN	ADRENERGIC RECEPTOR(S)	ADRENERGIC STIMULATION	CHOLINERGIC STIMULATION
Heart			
Sinoatrial node	β_1, β_2	↑ heart rate	↓ heart rate; vagal arrest
Atria	β_1, β_2	↑ contractility and conduction velocity	↓ contractility and duration of action potentials
Atrioventricular node	β_1, β_2	↑ automaticity and conduction velocity	↓ conduction velocity; atrioventricular block
His-Purkinje	β_1, β_2	↑ automaticity and conduction velocity	Little effect
Ventricles	β_1, β_2	↑ contractility, conduction velocity, automaticity, and idioventricular rate	Slight ↓ contractility
Arterioles			
Coronary	α_1, α_2	Constriction	Constriction
	β_2	Dilatation	
Skin and mucosa	α_1, α_2	Constriction	Dilatation
Skeletal muscle	α	Constriction	Dilatation
	β_2	Dilatation	
Cerebral	α_1	Slight constriction	Dilatation
Pulmonary	α_1	Constriction	Dilatation
	β_2	Dilatation	
Abdominal viscera	α_1	Constriction	—
	β_2	Dilatation	
Salivary glands	α_1, α_2	Constriction	Dilatation
Renal	α_1, α_2	Constriction	—
	β_1, β_2	Dilatation	
Veins	α_1, α_2	Constriction	—
	β_2	Dilatation	
Lung			
Tracheal and bronchial muscle	β_2	Relaxation	Contraction
Bronchial glands	α_1	↓ secretion	Stimulation
	β_2	↑ secretion	

Adapted from Lefkowitz RJ, Hoffman BB, Taylor P: Neurotransmission: The autonomic and somatic motor nervous systems. In Hardman JG, Limbird LL (eds): Goodman and Gilman's The Pharmacological Basis of Therapeutics, 9th ed. McGraw-Hill, New York, 1996, p 105.

cell membrane and raising its refractoriness to subsequent excitatory impulses.

ACh, the neurotransmitter of cholinergic transmission, activates two primary types of cholinergic receptors, muscarinic and nicotinic. Nicotinic receptors are sodium-calcium ion channels, the activation of which results in rapid cell depolarization and excitation. Muscarinic receptors interact with G proteins; excitatory or inhibitory responses result from interaction with second messengers (adenylyl cyclase–cyclic AMP), phospholipases, or calcium or potassium channels. Both nicotinic and muscarinic receptors are found in autonomic ganglia. Cardiac cholinergic receptors are muscarinic, inhibiting adenylyl cyclase, activating potassium channels, and resulting in negative chronotropy and inotropy.

The adrenergic family of neurotransmitters includes (1) norepinephrine, the primary transmitter of sympathetic postganglionic fibers, (2) epinephrine, the primary hormone of the adrenal medulla, and (3) dopamine, a catecholamine primarily located in the central nervous system. Like muscarinic receptors, adrenergic receptors couple with G proteins to either stimulate or inhibit second messengers, phospholipases, or ion channels. They are divided into α and β families (see Table 2–6). Vascular and extrathoracic visceral adrenergic receptors are predominantly α type. Epinephrine is the most potent α agonist, followed closely by norepinephrine and distantly by isoproterenol. Beta$_1$ and beta$_2$ receptors differ in their relative responsiveness to epinephrine and norepinephrine. Beta$_1$ receptors are equally responsive to the neurotransmitters and predominate in cardiac tissue; beta$_2$ receptors are much more responsive to epinephrine and predominate in vascular and pulmonary smooth muscle. Antagonists that discriminate between specific receptors are clinically useful in achieving specific actions while minimizing adverse reactions. For example, cardioselective beta-adrenergic blockers selectively affect cardiac beta$_1$ receptors, provoking less bronchospasm than noncardioselective beta-blockers. Isoproterenol is the most potent beta agonist, followed by epinephrine, then norepinephrine.

Coupling of a neurotransmitter with its receptor is a brief event. Once it has served its purpose, the neurotransmitter is then either destroyed or inactivated to make way for more current impulses. ACh is rapidly hydrolyzed by acetylcholinesterase (AChE) in cholinergic junctions. Drugs that oppose AChE potentiate the effects of ACh by prolonging its action. In adrenergic junctions, epinephrine and norepinephrine are inactivated by one of three mechanisms: (1) reuptake into presynaptic axonal terminals, (2) diffusion out of the cleft, and (3) metabolism by monoamine oxidase and catechol *O*-methyltransferase.

CLINICAL ASSESSMENT OF AUTONOMIC NERVOUS SYSTEM FUNCTION

Because of the dynamic and fluid nature of the ANS and its components, the sympathetic and parasympathetic nervous systems, clinical assessment of autonomic function is difficult. Most parameters assess, at most, the level of function at a precise moment. Furthermore, the stress or unnatural setting of the testing situation may introduce unpredictable bias into the results of any in vivo assessment of the ANS.

Pharmacologic and Physiologic Manipulation

The effect of any component of the ANS on a particular cardiovascular parameter can be estimated by administration of a pharmacologic blocker specific to that component. For example, measurement of sinus node recovery time before and after the administration of a beta-adrenergic blocker sheds light on both the preintervention level of beta-adrenergic tone and the sensitivity of the sinus node to adrenergic stimulation. Conversely, administration of a beta-adrenergic agonist also demonstrates the sensitivity of the sinus node to adrenergic stimulation and its capacity to increase the heart rate; however, it provides little information about ambient adrenergic tone. Sympathetic amines have both direct and indirect effects on target tissues; they may activate adrenergic receptors directly or they may stimulate release of norepinephrine from sympathetic nerve endings. Specific receptor agonists and antagonists useful for pharmacologic manipulation of the ANS are listed in Table 2–7.

AChE inhibitors play a unique role in pharmacologic manipulation of the parasympathetic nervous system. They potentiate parasympathetic activity, inhibiting the hydrolysis of ACh at cholinergic synapses. Reversible AChE inhibitors useful in diagnostic and therapeutic contexts include physostigmine, neostigmine, pyridostigmine, and edrophonium.

Simple bedside maneuvers are invaluable in the evaluation of conditions modulated by autonomic tone. Carotid sinus massage stimulates baroreceptors in the carotid body, resulting in a reflex vagal outflow and bradycardia. Carotid sinus hypersensitivity may be demonstrated by the production of a sinus pause of 3 or more seconds in duration or a fall in systolic blood pressure of 50 mm Hg in response to carotid stimulation. Carotid massage is also a particularly useful tool in the differential diagnosis and treatment of supraventricular tachyarrhythmias. For example, gradual slowing of the heart rate in response to massage and gradual acceleration of the heart rate to baseline at completion of massage are consistent with sinus tachycardia; the ventricular response to atrial fibrillation, flutter or tachycardia, also temporarily slows, usually enough to enable the underlying atrial electrocardiogram to be clarified. AV nodal and AV reentry tachycardia may be abruptly terminated with carotid sinus massage when sufficient AV nodal block is produced.

The Valsalva maneuver, when maintained for at least 10 seconds, produces a four-stage response to the effects of increased intrathoracic pressure. Initially, arterial pressure rises with strain and then falls, producing compensatory heart rate acceleration. The third stage begins as the strain is released with a further drop in arterial pressure, followed by an overshoot correction in both pressure and heart rate.

Table 2–7. PHARMACOLOGIC MANIPULATION OF THE AUTONOMIC NERVOUS SYSTEM

RECEPTOR	AGONISTS	ANTAGONISTS
α_1-Adrenergic	Epinephrine Norepinephrine Isoproterenol Phenylephrine	Prazosin
α_2-Adrenergic	Epinephrine Norepinephrine Isoproterenol Clonidine	Yohimbine
β_1-Adrenergic	Isoproterenol Epinephrine Norepinephrine Dobutamine	Propranolol Nadolol Timolol Pindolol Metoprolol Atenolol Esmolol Acebutolol
β_2-Adrenergic	Isoproterenol Epinephrine Norepinephrine Terbutaline	Propranolol Nadolol Timolol Pindolol Labetalol
Dopaminergic	—	Metoclopramide
Nicotinic (neuronal N_N)	Dimethylphenylpiperazinium	Trimethaphan
Muscarinic (M_1)	Oxotremorine	Atropine Scopolamine Pirenzepine
Muscarinic (M_2)	Bethanechol	

Heart Rate Variability

Heart rate variability (HRV) is a noninvasive measure of autonomic influences on the heart that has been shown to be useful in cardiac risk stratification.[10–14] Beat-to-beat variation in R-R intervals, the intervals between individual sinus impulses, can be analyzed from ambulatory ECG recordings in either time domain or frequency domain. In time domain analysis, the standard deviation of all sinus intervals is calculated for a specific period, usually either 5 minutes or 24 hours. Fast Fourier transformation of R-R intervals produces the frequency domain analysis of the periodic oscillations in heart rate. Four different frequency bands may be studied, each representing activity of different components of the ANS. High-frequency (0.15 to 0.4 Hz) bands are mediated by tonic vagal activity.[15, 16] Low-frequency (0.04 to 0.15 Hz) bands are thought to reflect sympathetic activity as well as parasympathetic and baroreceptor activity.[15, 17] Very-low-frequency (0.0033 to 0.04 Hz) and ultra-low-frequency (less than 0.0033 Hz) bands appear to be multifactorial.

Determinants of HRV were examined in the Framingham, Massachusetts, population cohort and their offspring.[18] Older age and higher heart rates were the strongest determinants of poor (reduced) HRV according to both time and frequency domain measures (low- and high-frequency bands). In addition, previous myocardial infarction, diastolic hypertension, congestive heart failure, diabetes mellitus, caffeine consumption, tobacco smoking, and use of beta-adrenergic–blocking and diuretic drugs were associated with lower HRV by two or more measures. Higher HRV values were observed in female subjects and in subjects with systolic hypertension. Of note, HRV measures were also higher with longer ECG recordings and with recordings performed in the morning hours.

Huikuri and associates,[19] studying HRV in middle-aged subjects without heart disease, noted a gender-related dichotomy in frequency domain measures. Like the Framingham group, these researchers found that the high-frequency (vagal) component of HRV was higher in women than in men; in contrast, however, they found that the low-frequency component (mixed) was lower. Women who were taking estrogen replacement therapy had significantly higher values of HRV than those who were not; the higher values were comparable to those in the male subjects studied.

Reduced HRV is associated with higher cardiac mortality and ventricular tachyarrhythmias. Pathophysiologic mechanisms for the marker are not completely elucidated. It appears, however, that the association reflects, in part, the significant role of the ANS in arrhythmogenesis associated with myocardial ischemia.[20–26] Pozzati and colleagues[27] observed a distinct fall in HRV within the 5-minute interval immediately preceding ischemic sudden death in patients experiencing these events during ambulatory ECG monitoring. Low levels of vagal tone reduce the low-frequency component of HRV and are believed to contribute to the higher risk of mortality.[28–30] In an in vitro preparation, physical stretching of the sinus node has also been shown to reduce high-frequency HRV, even after vagal section and beta-blockade.[31] This observation may in part explain the low HRV values observed in clinical conditions with right atrial dilatation, such as congestive heart failure and cardiac transplantation.[32]

In 1978, Wolf and associates[33] observed that patients with acute myocardial infarction demonstrating significant sinus arrhythmia have lower hospital mortality rates. Kleiger and colleagues[10] subsequently studied heart rate variability in the Multicenter Postinfarction Research Group using time domain analysis of 24-hour Holter monitors. These researchers found that the relative risk of mortality was more than five-fold higher in patients with HRV values lower than 50 msec, compared with those whose HRV values exceeded 100 msec.[10] Numerous studies have since demonstrated similar findings using other measures of HRV.[11–13] Particularly when combined with left ventricular ejection fraction and the finding of late potentials on signal-averaged ECG, low HRV is a sensitive, if not specific, marker of the risk of arrhythmic death after myocardial infarction.[11, 14]

After acute myocardial infarction, mortality is nearly twice as high in women as in men.[34–36] It is tempting to postulate that the gender-related differences in baseline HRV reflect underlying differences in autonomic modulation that predispose women to ventricular arrhythmias after myocardial infarction. Nonetheless, in Schwartz's dog model, preinfarction HRV does not predict postinfarction ventricular fibrillation.[37]

Baroreflex Sensitivity

Baroreflex sensitivity (BRS) is an additional clinical tool for assessing ANS function. Like HRV, it measures parasympathetic tone; however, BRS measures primarily the capacity for reflex, rather than tonic, vagal activity. Several maneuvers designed to evoke parasympathetic activity have been studied, the most common of which are administration of phenylephrine and the Valsalva maneuver.[38] Phenylephrine, a powerful vasoconstrictor, increases blood pressure, resulting in stimulation of arterial baroreceptors and reflex parasympathetic outflow. When the Valsalva maneuver is the intervention, heart rate changes are measured in the overshoot phase, wherein a rapid rise in arterial blood pressure stimulates a bradycardic response.[39] In normal middle-aged subjects, BRS is lower in women than in men; however, women taking estrogen replacement therapy after menopause have BRS values comparable to those in men.[19]

Abnormal BRS is associated with enhanced risk of cardiac mortality in both coronary and noncoronary disease conditions. In keeping with observations on HRV, abnormal responsiveness of cardiopulmonary baroreflexes (but not arterial baroreflexes) has been demonstrated in patients with congestive heart failure.[40, 41] Treatment with angiotensin-converting enzyme inhibitors can augment both cardiopulmonary and arterial BRS and can also reduce sympathetic outflow. These effects offer an explanation for the beneficial effect of these agents but do tend to be attenuated over time with long-term therapy.[41, 42] In contrast to HRV, abnormal preinfarction BRS does predict postinfarction ischemia-induced ventricular fibrillation in Schwartz's model.[38] Thus, a finding of low BRS prior to myocardial infarction may identify women with a higher risk of peri-infarction mortality.

β-Adrenergic Receptors

Congestive heart failure results in increased sympathetic outflow and circulating catecholamine levels and, consequently, downregulation of beta-adrenergic receptors.[43] This desensitization of myocardium to catecholamines may contribute further to impairment of contractility. Although the assays are not routinely available, $beta_1$-adrenergic receptor density and receptor mRNA levels may be assessed in specimens of ventricular myocardium on an investigational basis.[44, 45] Engelhardt and associates[45] found that the reduction of $beta_1$-adrenergic receptor mRNA correlates well with the degree of heart failure. Even in mild heart failure (New York Heart Association functional class II), mRNA levels were decreased by 7%, whereas mRNA levels were reduced by 26% in moderate (class III) heart failure and by more than 50% in severe (class IV) heart failure.

Tilt Table Testing

Head-up tilt table testing provides a noninvasive method for evaluating disorders of autonomic tone, particularly neurocardiogenic reflex–mediated (vasovagal) syncope and autonomic neuropathy. Commercially available tables tilt up to 90 degrees and are equipped with safety belts and a foot board, which provide mild weight support during passive standing. ECG and blood pressure are monitored continuously. A standard protocol begins with placement of the patient in the supine position on a tilt table for 20 minutes (or until heart rate and blood pressure are stable). The head of the table is then elevated to an angle of 70 degrees for 20 to 40 minutes or until an endpoint of syncope, bradycardia, or hypotension is reached. The test may be repeated with isoproterenol infusion to increase its sensitivity in reproducing neurocardiogenic reflex–mediated syncope.[46, 47] Furthermore, serial tilt procedures may be used during trials of interventions to predict long-term efficacy.[48]

The normal response to head-up tilt is a slight fall in systolic and diastolic blood pressure (5 to 10 mm Hg) and a commensurate increase in sinus rate of 5 to 10 bpm. A

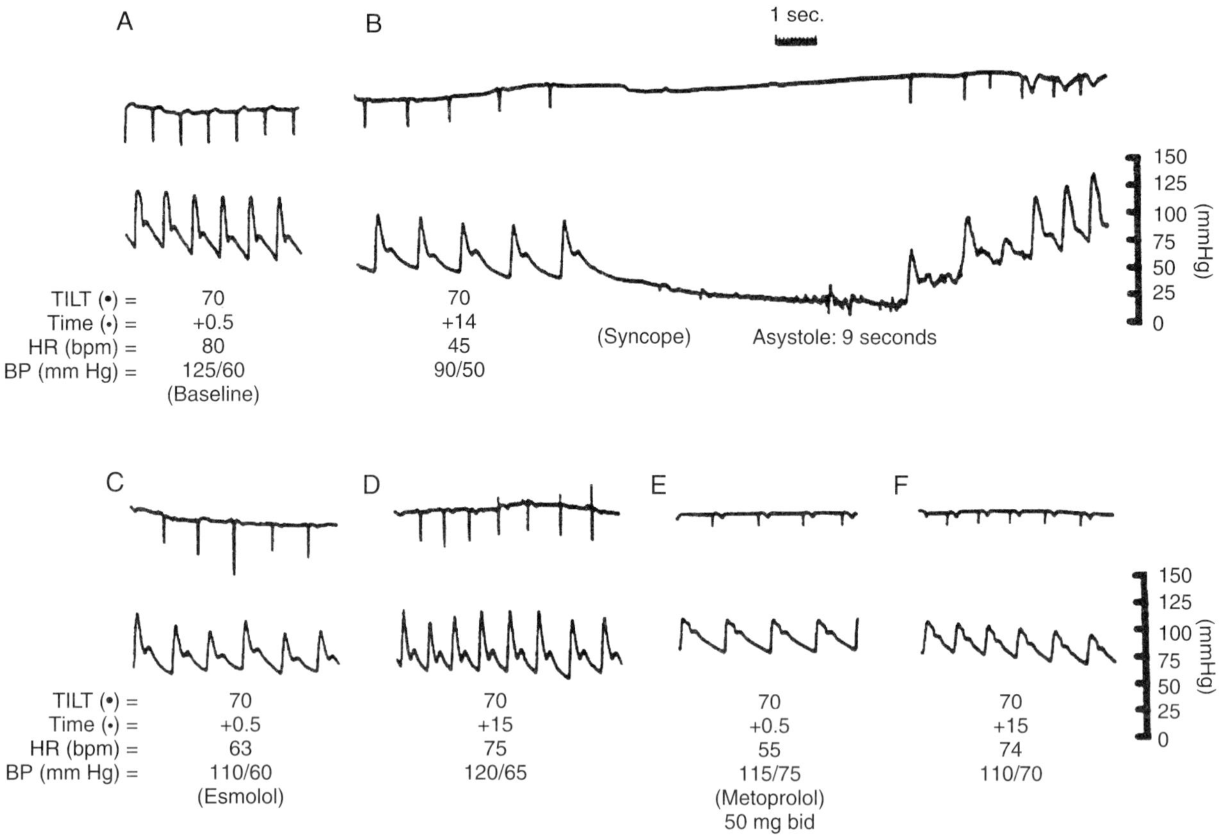

FIGURE 2–12. Serial head-up tilt testing in a patient with neurocardiogenic syncope. Surface ECG lead V_1, arterial pressure, tilt angle and time, heart rate (HR), and blood pressure (BP) are shown from top to bottom in each panel. Panel A demonstrates the initial response to head-up tilt table testing in the baseline state. At 14 minutes (panel B), progressive bradycardia ensues, culminating in a 9-second period of asystole. After resumption of the supine position and stabilization of heart rate and blood pressure, a repeat tilt during esmolol infusion shows a normal response (panels C and D). Repeat testing after 3 days of oral metoprolol also produces a normal response (panels E and F). (From Sra JS, Murthy VS, Jazayeri MR, et al: Use of intravenous esmolol to predict efficacy of oral beta-adrenergic blocker therapy in patients with neurocardiogenic syncope. J Am Coll Cardiol 19:402, 1992. Reprinted with permission from the American College of Cardiology.)

progressive, marked fall in arterial pressure with compensatory tachycardia is seen in secondary orthostatic hypotension. Failure to produce an appropriate compensatory tachycardia in the presence of early orthostatic hypotension suggests chronotropic (sinoatrial) incompetence or autonomic neuropathy. This condition is most often associated with advanced diabetes.

Frank hypotension, bradycardia, or both, especially when reproducing clinical symptoms, constitute a positive test result for neurocardiogenic syncope (Fig. 2–12). Either the cardioinhibitory (bradycardic) or vasodepressor (hypotensive) component may occur alone in some people. The induced cardiovascular collapse is commonly heralded by a relative tachycardia, suggesting a sympathetic surge as the trigger for the paradoxic vagal outpouring. Analysis of frequency domain HRV during tilt testing supports this hypothesis.[49] Overall sensitivity and specificity range from 80% to 90%, depending on the population tested and the protocol used. Baseline tilt testing reproduces syncope in 30% to 50% of individuals with unexplained syncope, but a positive result may be observed in up to 80% of subjects when tilt testing is combined with isoproterenol provocation.[47] The false-positive rate (positive results in subjects with no history of syncope) is approximately 10%. The incidence of syncope in the general population is, however, quite high, this symptom having occurred at least once in 30% to 50% of individuals.[50] Thus, false-positive responses may reflect a predilection for syncope not yet realized.

CONCLUSION

Current methodology for clinical appraisal of the status of the autonomic nervous system is limited. The measurable parameters discussed here are, at best, indirect indicators of instantaneous sympathetic and parasympathetic outflow, a highly dynamic process. We have as yet only a limited view inside the "black box" of the ANS.

References

1. Burnstock G: Evolution of the autonomic innervation of visceral and cardiovascular systems in vertebrates. Pharmacol Rev 21:247, 1969.
2. Lefkowitz RJ, Hoffman BB, Taylor P: Neurotransmission: The autonomic and somatic motor nervous systems. In Hardman JG, Limbird LL (eds): Goodman and Gilman's The Pharmacological Basis of Therapeutics, 9th ed. McGraw-Hill, New York, 1996, p 105.
3. Andresen MC, Kunze DL: Nucleus tractus solitarius—gateway to neural circulatory control. Annu Rev Physiol 56:93, 1994.
4. Ferguson AV: The area postrema: A cardiovascular control centre at the blood-brain interface? Can J Physiol Pharmacol 69:1026, 1991.
5. Elfvin LG, Lindh B, Hokfelt T: The chemical neuroanatomy of sympathetic ganglia. Annu Rev Neurosci 16:471, 1993.

6. Crick SJ, Wharton J, Shepard MN, et al: Innervation of the human cardiac conduction system: A quantitative immunohistochemical and histochemical study. Circulation 89:1697, 1994.
7. Hodgkin AL, Huxley AF: A quantitative description of membrane current and its application to conduction and excitation in nerve. J Physiol 117:500, 1952.
8. Armstrong CM: Voltage-dependent ion channels and their gating. Physiol Rev 72:S5, 1992.
9. Catterall WA: Cellular and molecular biology of voltage-gated sodium channels. Physiol Rev 72:S15, 1992.
10. Kleiger RE, Miller JP, Bigger JT, et al: Decreased heart rate variability and its association with increased mortality after acute myocardial infarction. Am J Cardiol 59:256, 1987.
11. Farrell TG, Bashir Y, Cripps T, et al: Risk stratification for arrhythmic events in postinfarction patients based on heart rate variability, ambulatory electrocardiographic variables and the signal-averaged electrocardiogram. J Am Coll Cardiol 18:687, 1991.
12. Bigger JT, Fleiss JL, Steinman RC, et al: Frequency domain measures of heart period variability and mortality after myocardial infarction. Circulation 85:164, 1992.
13. Barron HV, Lesh MD: Autonomic nervous system and sudden cardiac death. J Am Coll Cardiol 27:1053, 1996.
14. Odemuyima O, Poloniecki J, Malik M, et al: Temporal influences on the prediction of postinfarction mortality by heart rate variability: A comparison with the left ventricular ejection fraction. Br Heart J 71: 521, 1994.
15. Kay SM, Marple SL: Spectrum analysis: A modern perspective. Proc IEEE 69:1380, 1981.
16. Berger RD, Akselrod S, Gordon D, Cohen RJ: An efficient algorithm for spectral analysis of heart rate variability. IEEE Trans Biomed Eng 33:900, 1986.
17. Kamath MV, Ghista DN, Fallen EL, et al: Heart rate variability power spectrogram as a potential noninvasive signature of cardiac regulatory system response, mechanisms, and disorders. Heart Vessels 3:33, 1987.
18. Tsuji H, Venditti FJ, Manders ES, et al: Determinants of heart rate variability. J Am Coll Cardiol 28:1539, 1996.
19. Huikuri HV, Pikkujamsa SM, Airaksinen J, et al: Sex-related differences in autonomic modulation of heart rate in middle-aged subjects. Circulation 94:122, 1996.
20. James RGG, Arnold JMO, Allen JD, et al: The effects of heart rate, myocardial ischemia and vagal stimulation on the threshold for ventricular fibrillation. Circulation 55:311, 1977.
21. El-Sherif N: Reentrant ventricular arrhythmias in the late myocardial infarction period. 6: Effect of the autonomic system. Circulation 58: 103, 1978.
22. Sheridan DJ, Penskoske PA, Sobel BE, Corr PB: Alpha adrenergic contributions to dysrhythmia during myocardial ischemia and reperfusion in cats. J Clin Invest 65:161, 1980.
23. Schwartz PJ, Billman GE, Stone HL: Autonomic mechanisms in ventricular fibrillation induced by myocardial ischemia during exercise in dogs with a healed infarction: An experimental preparation for sudden cardiac death. Circulation 69:780, 1984.
24. Inoue H, Zipes DP: Results of sympathetic denervation in the canine heart: Supersensitivity that may be arrhythmogenic. Circulation 75: 877, 1987.
25. Schwartz PJ, Zuanetti G: Role of the autonomic nervous system in reperfusion arrhythmias. J Mol Cell Cardiol 20(Suppl II):113, 1988.
26. DeLuna AB, Coumel P, Leclercq JF: Ambulatory sudden cardiac death: Mechanisms of production of fatal arrhythmia on the basis of data from 157 cases. Am Heart J 117:151, 1989.
27. Pozzati A, Pancaldi LG, di Pasquale G, et al: Transient sympathovagal imbalance triggers "ischemic" sudden death in patients undergoing electrocardiographic Holter monitoring. J Am Coll Cardiol 27:847, 1996.
28. Vybiral T, Bryg RJ, Maddens ME, et al: Effects of transdermal scopolamine on heart rate variability in normal subjects. Am J Cardiol 65: 604, 1990.
29. Schwartz PJ, La Rovere MT, Vanoli E: Autonomic nervous system and sudden cardiac death: Experimental basis and clinical observations for post-myocardial infarction risk stratification. Circulation 85:I-77, 1992.
30. Fei L, Statters DJ, Hnatkova K, et al: Change of autonomic influence on the heart immediately before the onset of spontaneous idiopathic ventricular tachycardia. J Am Coll Cardiol 24:1515, 1994.
31. Horner SM, Murphy CF, Coen B, et al: Contribution to heart rate variability by mechanoelectric feedback: Stretch of the sinoatrial node reduces heart rate variability. Circulation 94:1762, 1996.
32. Bernardi L, Salvucci F, Suardi R, et al: Evidence for an intrinsic mechanism regulating heart rate variability in the transplanted and the intact heart during submaximal dynamic exercise? Cardiovasc Res 24: 969, 1990.
33. Wolf MM, Varigos GA, Hunt D, Sloman JG: Sinus arrhythmia in acute myocardial infarction. Med J Aust 2:52, 1978.
34. Kannel WB, Sorlie P, McNamara PM: Prognosis after myocardial infarction: The Framingham study. Am J Cardiol 44:53, 1979.
35. Tofler GH, Stone PH, Muller JE, et al: Effects of gender and race on prognosis after myocardial infarction: Adverse prognosis for women, particularly black women. J Am Coll Cardiol 9:473, 1987.
36. Greenland P, Reicher-Reiss H, Goldbourt U, et al: In-hospital and 1-year mortality in 1524 women after myocardial infarction: Comparison with 4315 men. Circulation 83:484, 1991.
37. Hull SSJ, Evans AR, Vanoli E, et al: Heart rate variability before and after myocardial infarction in conscious dogs at high and low risk of sudden cardiac death. J Am Coll Cardiol 16:978, 1990.
38. Schwartz PJ, Vanoli E, Stramba-Badiale M, et al: Autonomic mechanisms and sudden death: New insight from analysis of baroreceptor reflexes in conscious dogs with and without myocardial infarction. Circulation 78:969, 1988.
39. Airaksinen KEJ, Hartikainen JEK, Niemela MJ, et al: Valsalva manoeuver in the assessment of baroreflex sensitivity in patients with coronary artery disease. Eur Heart J 14:1519, 1993.
40. Ferguson DW, Abboud FM, Mark AL: Selective impairment of baroreflex-mediated vasoconstrictor responses in patients with ventricular dysfunction. Circulation 69:451, 1984.
41. Dibner-Dunlap ME, Smith ML, Kinugawa T, Thames MD: Enalaprilat augments arterial and cardiopulmonary baroreflex control of sympathetic nerve activity in patients with heart failure. J Am Coll Cardiol 27:358, 1996.
42. Cody RJ, Franklin FW, Kluger J, Laragh JH: Mechanisms governing the postural response and baroreceptor abnormalities in chronic congestive heart failure: Effects of acute and long-term converting-enzyme inhibition. Circulation 66:135, 1982.
43. Hadcock JR, Malbon CC: Down-regulation of β-adrenergic receptors: Agonist-induced reduction in receptor mRNA levels. Proc Natl Acad Sci U S A 85:5021, 1988.
44. Bristow MR, Minobe WA, Raynolds MV, et al: Reduced beta 1 receptor messenger-RNA abundance in the failing human heart. J Clin Invest 92:2737, 1993.
45. Engelhardt S, Bohm M, Erdmann E, Lohse MJ: Analysis of beta-adrenergic receptor mRNA levels in human ventricular biopsy specimens by quantitative polymerase chain reactions: Progressive reduction of $beta_1$-adrenergic receptor mRNA in heart failure. J Am Coll Cardiol 27:146, 1996.
46. Abi-Samra F, Maloney JD, Fouad-Tarazi FM, et al: The usefulness of head-up tilt testing and hemodynamic investigations in the workup of syncope of unknown origin. Pacing Clin Electrophysiol 11:1202, 1988.
47. Almquist A, Goldenberg IF, Milstein S, et al: Provocation of bradycardia and hypotension by isoproterenol and upright posture in patients with unexplained syncope. N Engl J Med 320:346, 1989.
48. Sra JS, Murthy VS, Jazayeri MR, et al: Use of intravenous esmolol to predict efficacy of oral beta-adrenergic blocker therapy in patients with neurocardiogenic syncope. J Am Coll Cardiol 19:402, 1992.
49. Pruvot E, Vesiin JM, Schlaepfer J, et al: Autonomic imbalance assessed by heart rate variability analysis in vasovagal syncope. Pacing Clin Electrophysiol 17:2201, 1994.
50. Kapoor WN, Karpf M, Wieand S, et al: A prospective evaluation and followup of patients with syncope. N Engl J Med 309:198, 1983.

2.5 Reproductive Life Stages

Shahla Nader

EMBRYOLOGY OF THE FEMALE REPRODUCTIVE ORGANS

Primordial germ cells migrate from protuberances that overlie the mesonephric ducts into gonadal ridges in approximately the fifth week of gestation. At this time, the gonads are bipotential with both cortical and medullary areas; they are composed of germ cells, special epithelia, and mesenchyme.[1] If the bipotential gonad lacks a Y chromosome, it develops into an ovary.[2] Although the developed cortical zone contains the germ cells, the regressing medullary portion forms a compressed nest of tubules and Leydig cells located in the hilus of the ovary.

Beginning in approximately the sixth week of gestation, germ cells undergo rapid mitotic multiplication. By 20 weeks, the number of oogonia peaks at 6 to 7 million[3, 4]; thereafter, the number of germ cells in the ovary decreases irreversibly. The supply of oocytes is essentially depleted by a median age of 52 years (Fig. 2–13).[5]

As oogonia undergo the first meiotic division, they become oocytes. Vascular channels from the deeper medullary areas of the ovary extend into the cortex. Perivascular cells of mesenchymal or epithelial origin migrate into the area and surround the oocyte, thus forming the primordial follicle. During the latter part of gestation, thecal cells surround the follicle. Residual mesenchyme forms the primitive ovarian stroma. These primordial follicles mature variably, with proliferation of granulosa cells, before undergoing atresia.[6] Germ cells are lost during mitosis, meiosis, and atresia after early maturational changes. By birth, only 1 to 2 million germ cells, encased in follicles, remain. During childhood, follicles continue to grow, and occasional antral follicles are found. These follicles also undergo atresia, and by puberty, approximately 300,000 to 400,000 germ cells remain.[7] During the next 4 decades, approximately 500 germ cells develop into mature follicles and are released during ovulation. Thus, more than 99.9% of germ cells are lost to atresia and death.

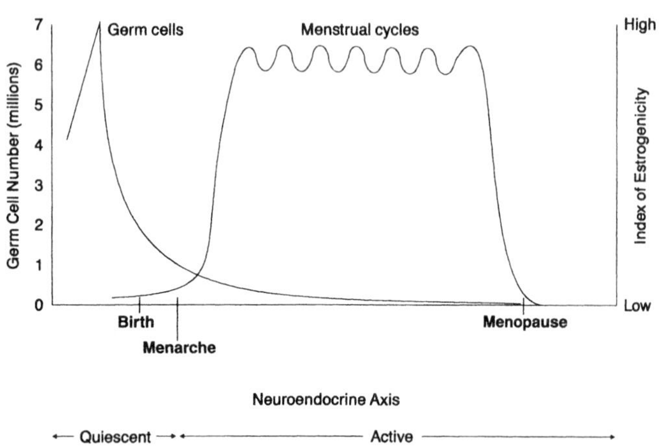

FIGURE 2–13. Germ cell loss and the reproductive life cycle.

The second X chromosome controls the rate of germ cell loss. In chromosomal incompetent gonadal dysgenesis (45,X), such loss is excessively rapid, and the gonads are usually depleted of follicles by birth.

The mesonephric and paramesonephric duct systems lie alongside the bipotential gonad. By the eighth week, one of these duct systems is selected to develop normally; the absence of a functional testis and, thus, the lack of müllerian inhibitory substance allows retention of the müllerian structures.[8] In addition, in the absence of testosterone, the wolffian system regresses. Moreover, in the absence of an androgen effect, the folds of the genital sinus and labioscrotal swellings remain open and form the labia minora and majora. The genital tubercle forms the clitoris, and the urogenital sinus forms the lower vagina. The developing müllerian structures form the fallopian tubes, uterus, and upper vagina. The upper and lower halves of the vagina meet, continuity is established, and development of the internal and external genitalia is completed.

PUBERTY

Childhood maturational changes in ovarian follicles are not associated with significant ovarian hormone production because of the lack of gonadotropin, which stimulates the ovaries to produce hormones. Puberty, which is marked by an increase in hormonal activity, has several components.

Adrenarche

The factors that control adrenarche, which generally precedes menarche by a few years, are not understood. Greater adrenal cortical function, associated with an increase in size of the zona reticularis, causes a rise in the concentration of the androgen dehydroepiandrosterone, its sulfated form, and androstenedione.[9] The result is growth of pubic and axillary hair.

Activation of the Hypothalamic-Pituitary-Gonadotropin Axis

In the first decade of life, secretion of the gonadotropins luteinizing hormone (LH) and follicle-stimulating hormone (FSH) is suppressed to low levels[10] by a highly sensitive negative feedback system and by a central inhibitory influence on the secretion of gonadotropin-releasing hormone (GNRH). A reversal of these mechanisms increases production of gonadotropins and synthesis of ovarian hormones. As a result, the onset of puberty accelerates, and secondary sexual characteristics such as breast development are seen.

Hypothalamic-Pituitary-Ovarian Interactions at Puberty

A fundamental feature of the hypothalamic component of the gonadal axis is the pulsatile release of GNRH from the arcuate nucleus of the hypothalamus.[11] GNRH acts as a self-primer on the gonadotrope cells of the pituitary by upregulating its own receptor. Pulsatile GNRH is necessary to maintain LH pools within the gonadotrope. Increasing levels of gonadotropins stimulate the ovaries to secrete estrogen, which in turn influences the central gonadotropin axis.[12] In addition, greater production of estrogen by the ovaries stimulates further development of the outflow tract and proliferation of the endometrium. Menarche, which is the first episode of endometrial breakdown, occurs at a median age of 12.8 years.

THE MENSTRUAL CYCLE

A woman's ability to reproduce lasts for about 40 years, from approximately age 12 to age 52. During this time, mature oocytes develop and are released from the ovaries in anticipation of fertilization in the fallopian tubes. Ovarian hormones prepare the uterus and its endometrial lining for implantation of a zygote and maintenance of a pregnancy. In the absence of pregnancy, the hormonal activity ceases, and the endometrium is shed through the outflow tract. This decrease in ovarian hormonal activity reactivates the hypothalamic-pituitary axis by means of negative feedback and causes a new wave of folliculogenesis. The entire cycle, called the menstrual cycle, takes approximately 28 days.

The major events of the menstrual cycle involve intricate and carefully orchestrated interactions on the part of several organ systems, as briefly outlined here.

Compartment Systems Involved in the Menstrual Cycle

Hypothalamus

The arcuate nucleus area of the mediobasal hypothalamus houses the GNRH pulse generator, whose rhythmic release of GNRH triggers production and secretion of the gonadotropins LH and FSH from the anterior pituitary (Fig. 2–14). Intermittent stimulation is an obligatory component of the process: The constant infusion of GNRH in women with hypothalamic amenorrhea fails to stimulate continuing gonadotropin secretion, whereas intermittent delivery, at intervals of approximately 60 to 90 minutes, sustains normal gonadotropin levels, leading to oocyte maturation.[13] Indeed, the unreactivity of gonadotrope cells to continuous GNRH stimulation forms the basis of GNRH agonistic analogue therapy in achieving reversible medical hypophysectomy, thus shutting down the reproductive axis. The electrophysiologic manifestation of GNRH pulse generator activity has been demonstrated in rhesus monkeys (Fig. 2–15); abrupt increases in multiunit electrical activity that are synchronous with LH pulses have been recorded from electrodes placed in the mediobasal hypothalamus.[14] GNRH is synthesized and

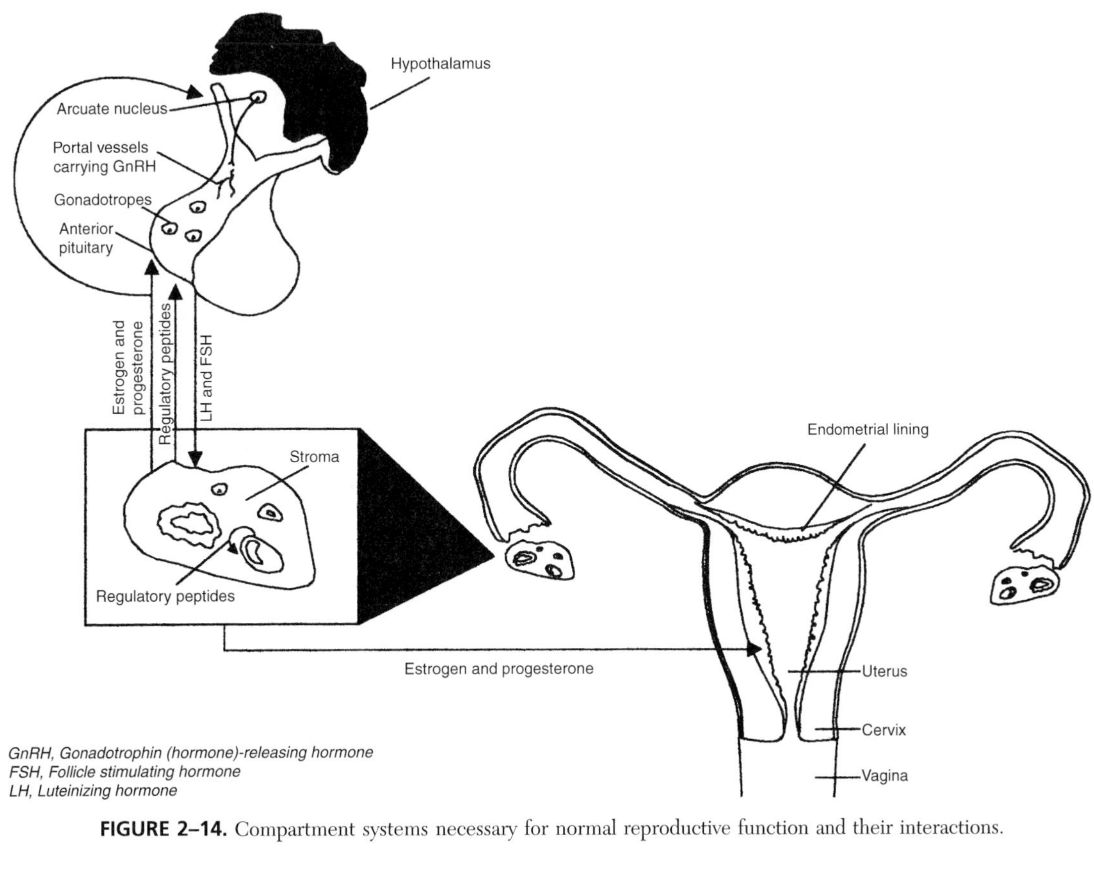

FIGURE 2–14. Compartment systems necessary for normal reproductive function and their interactions.

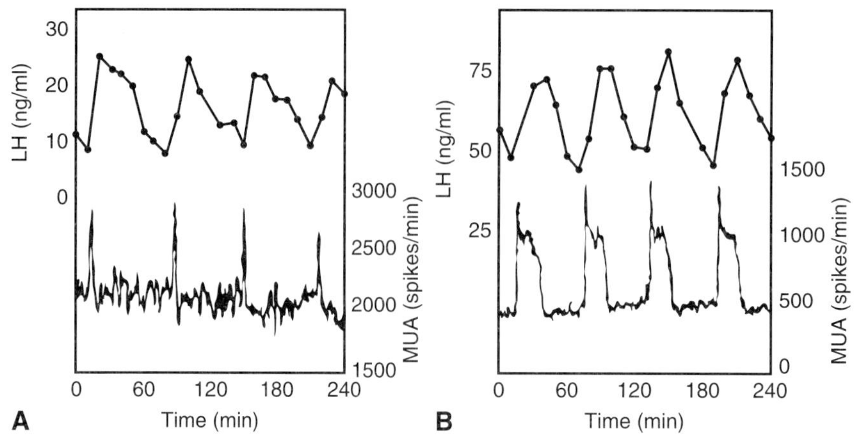

FIGURE 2–15. Volleys of multiunit electrical activity recorded from the mediobasal hypothalamus in a normal monkey on day 5 of the follicular phase (*A*) and in an ovariectomized animal (*B*). (From O'Byrne KT, Chen MD, Nishihara M, et al: Ovarian control of gonadotropin hormone–releasing hormone pulse generator activity in the rhesus monkey: Duration of the associated hypothalamic signal. Neuroendocrinology 57:588, 1993. © Karger, Basel.)

stored in the mediobasal hypothalamus and is released in pulses into the hypophysial-portal circulation.

Various physiologic, pathologic, and pharmacologic factors may modify the periodicity and amplitude of the pulsatile GNRH discharge. Increased levels of circulating estradiol during the follicular phase of the menstrual cycle reduce the amplitude of LH pulses by acting principally at the level of the pituitary. The frequency of the pulses, however, may increase as the follicular phase progresses. Progesterone produced in the luteal phase of the cycle dramatically reduces the frequency of the GNRH pulse generator but proportionally increases the amplitude of the less frequent pulses.[15] The production of endogenous opiates mediates these decelerations, at least in part.[16] Gonadal steroids, opiates, barbiturates, adrenergic blocking agents, stress, intense physical activity, and caloric deprivation also lead to a deceleration of the GNRH pulse generator.[17]

Pituitary

In response to GNRH, the gonadotropes of the anterior pituitary produce the gonadotropins LH and FSH, which are glycoproteins composed of alpha and beta subunits. The alpha subunit is shared, and the beta subunits confer specificity of action. Gonadal hormones can regulate GNRH receptors located on the gonadotrope; binding of the GNRH receptor, which mobilizes extracellular and intracellular Ca^{2+}, is required for its action. Gonadotropin biosynthesis follows exposure to GNRH. Pulsatile exposure to GNRH is important in the maintenance of cellular LH pools. Protein kinase action may be involved in this process.

Whereas the two gonadotropins are produced by the same cells in response to the same stimulus, their metabolic clearance rates are different; the plasma half-life is 60 to 90 minutes for LH and 180 to 200 minutes for FSH. In addition, sex steroids and peptide hormones produced by the ovary and pituitary may modulate the gonadotropin response to GNRH. Inhibin and follistatin reduce FSH secretion, whereas activin increases FSH secretion.[18, 19] Estradiol has both inhibitory and stimulatory effects, as in induction of the midcycle LH surge. Progesterone acts synergistically with estradiol to augment the gonadotropin response to GNRH; this combined effect is important in the orchestration of the midcycle LH surge.

Ovary

Folliculogenesis. The luteal-follicular transition, the point between two menstrual cycles, is characterized by reduced levels of sex steroids and inhibin and, therefore, by raised levels of gonadotropins. FSH stimulation of follicles increases oocyte size and expands the granulosa cell mass. Once initiated, follicular growth progresses to the preantral and then the antral stage, in which the oocyte occupies an eccentric position in the fluid-filled antrum. One follicle becomes dominant by day 5 or 6 of the menstrual cycle and continues to grow as other follicles undergo atresia. Thus, a preovulatory graafian follicle is formed with an estrogen-rich follicular fluid and the highest rates of granulosa cell proliferation (Fig. 2–16).[20]

Hormonogenesis. LH stimulates the production of androgens, predominantly androstenedione, by the thecal cells, which surround follicles that are developing in response to FSH stimulation. The androgens diffuse into the granulosa cell layer, where, under the influence of FSH, they are converted to estradiol. Thus, as the follicular phase of the cycle progresses, circulating concentrations of estradiol increase (Fig. 2–17).[21–23]

Selection of the Dominant Follicle. Under normal circumstances, only one follicle continues its growth until ovulation. The selection of this follicle is in part related to the synergistic action of estradiol on FSH-induced follicular development. The follicle with the highest concentration of estradiol becomes more responsive to FSH. In addition, estradiol and inhibin concentrations suppress FSH, which in turn suppresses growth of the remaining follicles.[24]

Regulatory Peptides. The development of a mature preovulatory graafian follicle normally occurs over the course of approximately 14 days. Various factors affect the development of the preovulatory follicle. The action of gonadotropins is modulated not only by sex steroids but also by local regulatory peptides produced in the ovary in response to

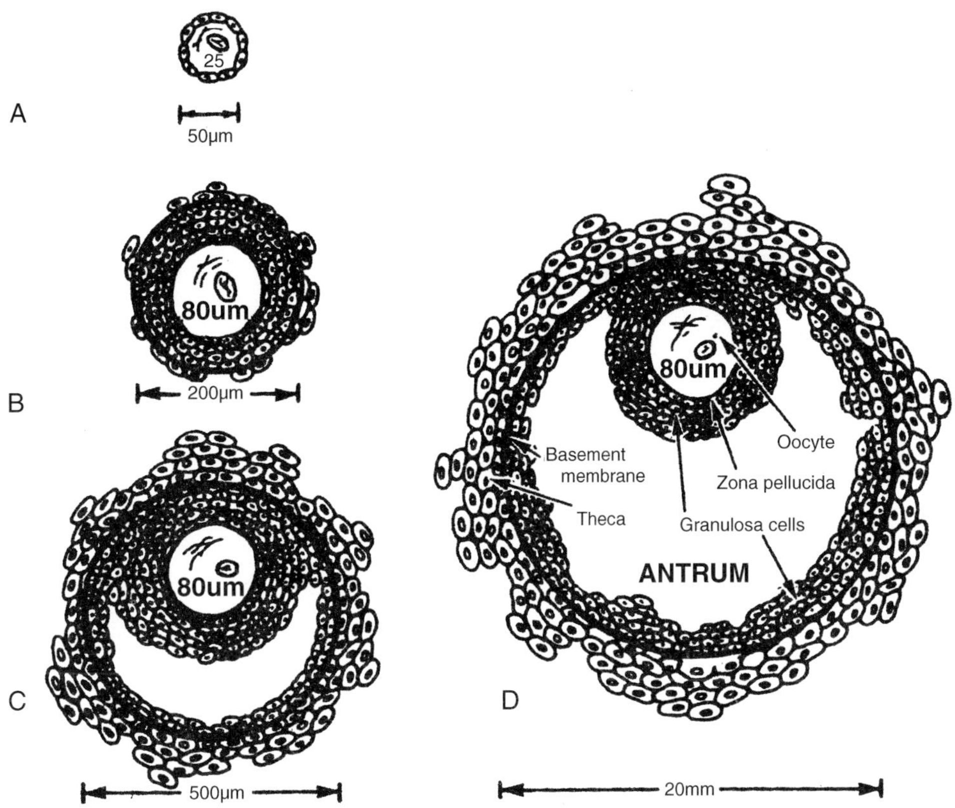

FIGURE 2–16. Follicular development: *A*, Primordial follicle. *B*, Preantral follicle. *C*, Antral follicle. *D*, Preovulatory follicle. (From Fritz MA, Speroff L: The endocrinology of the menstrual cycle: The interaction of folliculogenesis and neuroendocrine mechanisms. Fertil Steril 38:509, 1982.)

gonadotropin stimulation. In addition, production of the following regulatory peptides, by both the ovary and other tissues, may influence the availability of the gonadotropins upon which follicular maturation depends:

1. Inhibin consists of two dissimilar peptides linked by disulfide bonds. FSH stimulates granulosa cells to produce inhibin, which in turn suppresses FSH secretion.[25]
2. Activin stimulates FSH release in the pituitary and augments FSH action in the ovary.[19]
3. Follistatin suppresses FSH activity, probably by binding activin.[19]
4. Insulin-like growth factors, which are similar in structure and function to insulin, mediate growth hormone action. These factors induce the expression of genes responsible for cellular proliferation and differentiation. They may amplify the effect of gonadotropins on follicular development. The availability of these growth factors relates to the concentration of their binding proteins.[26]
5. Other influential peptide hormones: epidermal growth factor, transforming growth factor, fibroblast growth factor, platelet-derived growth factor, and angiogenic growth factor.

Ovulation. The preovulatory follicle produces increasing amounts of estradiol, which peak approximately 24 to 36 hours before ovulation. The ovarian follicle signals ovulation. When the serum concentration of estradiol reaches approximately 200 pg/ml and this concentration is maintained for 36 to 50 hours, the midcycle surge in LH (and, to a lesser degree, FSH) occurs.[27, 28] LH initiates the following important events:

1. Luteinization of granulosa cells, leading to the formation of the corpus luteum and the production of progesterone, which, along with estradiol, maintains the LH surge.
2. Maturation of the oocyte with completion of meiosis I (meiosis is completed after fertilization of the oocyte).
3. Changes in the follicular wall and stimulation of proteolytic enzymes, leading to extrusion of the ovum surrounded by granulosa cells, called the cumulus oophorus.

Prostaglandins participate in this ovulatory process and may promote hyperemia and angiogenesis.[29]

The Corpus Luteum and the Luteal Phase. Luteinization involves an increase in the size of the granulosa cells, vacuolation, and accumulation of a yellow pigment, lutein. The vascularization of the granulosa layer allows sufficient LDL cholesterol to reach the luteal cells; progesterone production depends on the availability of LH and LDL cholesterol. Progesterone levels rise sharply after ovulation, peaking approximately 8 days after the LH surge. Progesterone acts both locally and centrally to suppress growth of new follicles. The life-span of the corpus luteum is approximately 14 days. Its function declines rapidly 9 to 11 days after ovulation. The precise mechanism of luteolysis is unknown but may involve local estrogen, prostaglandins, and oxytocin. In early pregnancy, human chorionic gonadotropin (hCG) produced by the trophoblast maintains the corpus luteum for a few extra weeks, until placental steroidogenesis is well established in the seventh to ninth week of gestation.

Luteal-Follicular Transition. When the hormonal activity of the corpus luteum decreases, the reduced serum concentrations of estradiol, progesterone, and inhibin raise concentrations of gonadotropins, particularly FSH. This rise in FSH allows a new wave of folliculogenesis in the next cycle.[30, 31]

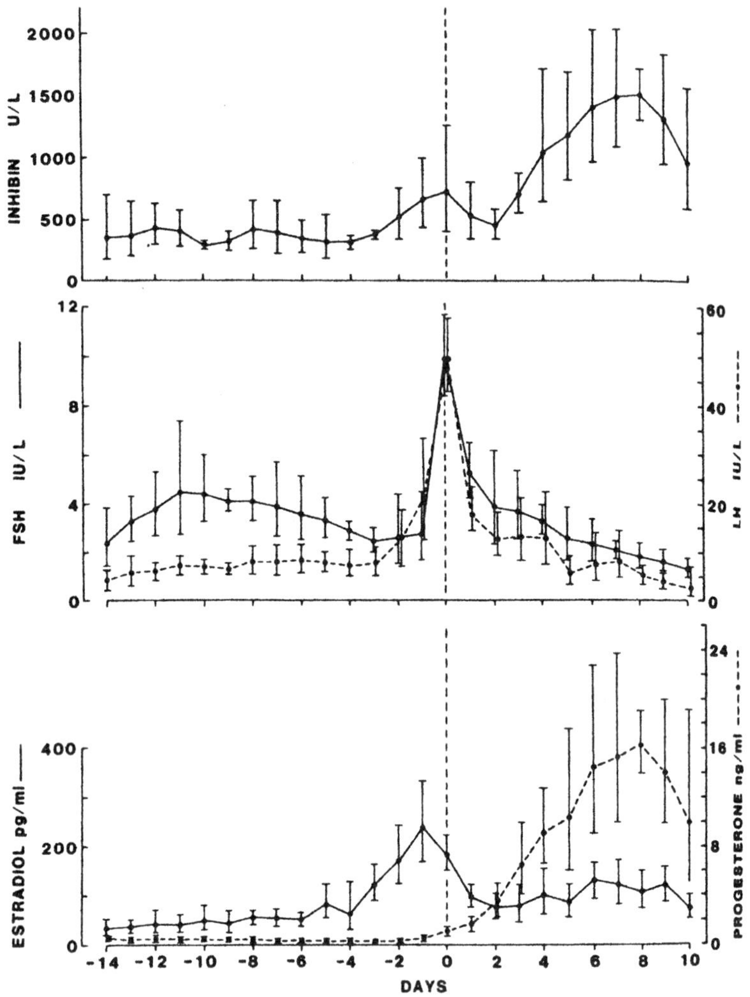

FIGURE 2–17. Plasma concentrations of pituitary gonadotropins, ovarian steroids, and inhibin during the menstrual cycle. Data from ovulatory cycles in 6 normal women are normalized around the LH surge (day 0). (From McLachlan RI, Robertson DM, Healy DL, et al: Circulating immunoreactive inhibin levels during the normal human menstrual cycle. J Clin Endocrinol Metab 65:954, 1987. © The Endocrine Society.)

Timing in the Menstrual Cycle. The GNRH pulse generator sets the hourly pace for intraovarian events, but the ovary determines the length of the menstrual cycle. The duration of the follicular phase is the major determinant of cycle length. The average length of the cycle ranges from 24 to 35 days.

Outflow Tract

The endometrial lining of the uterus can be morphologically divided into the upper functionalis layer and the lower basalis layer. The upper layer undergoes changes in preparation for implantation, and the lower layer provides regenerative endometrium after loss of the upper layer. The endometrium consists of ciliated columnar epithelium, which invaginates to form glands that extend to the base of the endometrial-myometrial border. The blind ends of the glands form the basalis layer. The lamina propria, or endometrial stroma, is a highly cellular connective tissue with an amorphous extracellular matrix. The stroma also responds to hormonal changes.[32] During the follicular phase of the menstrual cycle, the functionalis endometrium responds to rising estradiol concentrations with mitosis in the glands and pseudostratification of nuclei. The stromal cells also undergo mitosis, proliferation, and expansion.[33] The increase in height of the endometrium is readily apparent with transvaginal ultrasound.

After ovulation, the endometrium enters the secretory phase. Glycogen vacuoles appear within the glandular cells, the stroma becomes edematous, and the spiral vessels become prominent and densely coiled. Death of the corpus luteum and decreased levels of estrogen and progesterone initiate three events in the endometrium. First, the spiral arterioles that supply the upper functionalis layer undergo rhythmic vasoconstriction and relaxation, which lead to endometrial ischemia and stasis. Thrombin-platelet plugs appear in the superficial vessels, and the prostaglandin content (prostaglandins $F_{2\alpha}$ and E_2) peaks.[34] The second and third events are tissue loss and extravasation of blood caused by increasing ischemia. A natural cleavage develops between the basalis and functionalis layers. Platelet-thrombin plugs form to limit blood loss, and menstrual flow stops as a result of vasoconstriction, tissue collapse, and vascular stasis.[35] In addition, rising serum levels of estradiol, as the next cycle progresses, induce healing.

Menstrual fluid comprises autolyzed functionalis cells, red cells, inflammatory exudate, and proteolytic enzymes that lyse clots as they form. If the rate of flow is great, clotting occurs. Menstruation usually lasts about 4 to 6 days, resulting in blood loss of about 30 ml. Excessive prostaglandin release may cause dysmenorrhea. The endometrium can be dated according to the histologic changes that occur throughout a hypothetical 28-day cycle.[36] For dating, a biopsy is usually performed a few days before expected menses.

THE LATE REPRODUCTIVE YEARS AND THE PERIMENOPAUSAL TRANSITION

The length of the menstrual cycle tends to shorten once a woman reaches her late 30s. Fewer follicles are recruited in each cycle. Inhibin concentrations are lower, causing serum FSH concentrations to rise, leading to accelerated follicular development and, hence, a shortened follicular phase.[37–39] The decrease in inhibin concentration probably relates to diminished follicular competence, because the better follicles respond earlier in life. This fact may explain the reduced fecundity observed with age. Ovulation continues, however, although luteal progesterone concentrations may be lower.[40]

As menopause approaches, anovulatory cycles may occur, and the cycles may become shorter or longer.[41] At this point, the endometrium is sufficiently estrogen-primed to respond to a progestin challenge, and withdrawal menses are seen. In addition, lack of progesterone in anovulatory cycles may lead to menstruations that differ from the usual ovulatory cycles. During the late reproductive years, ovulatory cycles may be followed by somewhat diminished menstrual flow, and anovulatory cycles may be prolonged, heavy, or light.

As the supply of follicles becomes depleted, gonadotropin stimulation does not initiate follicular estradiol synthesis, and hypoestrogenism ensues. Menopause occurs when menses permanently cease because of the loss of ovarian follicular activity. The climacteric phase of life extends from the late reproductive years, through menopause, into the postmenopausal years. The median age of menopause is 51 to 52 years, with a range of 48 to 55 years.[42] Smoking accelerates menopause by about 1.5 years, and its effect correlates with the number of cigarettes smoked and the duration of smoking.[43] Menses cease abruptly in only a small percentage of women; in most women, irregular cycles precede menopause.

THE CLIMACTERIC

Declining ovarian follicular activity and the loss of endogenous estradiol are associated with several symptoms and outcomes. Many women do not recognize the more insidious symptoms and may be unaware of their association with estrogen deficiency:

Irregularity of Menses

This irregularity was described in the preceding section.

Vasomotor Instability (Hot Flashes and Night Sweats)

Hot flashes are the sudden onset of intense body heat (often perceived as affecting the upper body) with redness of the face, chest, and neck. These episodes may occur frequently and usually last for a few minutes. They originate in the hypothalamus and represent autonomic vasomotor instability related to estrogen withdrawal.[44] Although the timing of the hot flash corresponds to LH pulses, the pituitary does not need to be intact; hot flashes have been observed in women with hypopituitarism. The onset of the hot flash is presumably linked to GNRH secretion, accounting for its association with LH pulses in normal women. Hot flashes dissipate heat through vasodilatation and perspiration in response to hypothalamic thermoregulatory stimuli. Women with gonadal dysgenesis who have not been exposed to estrogen rarely have hot flashes. Norepinephrine and endogenous opiate withdrawal may be involved in the pathogenesis of the hot flash.

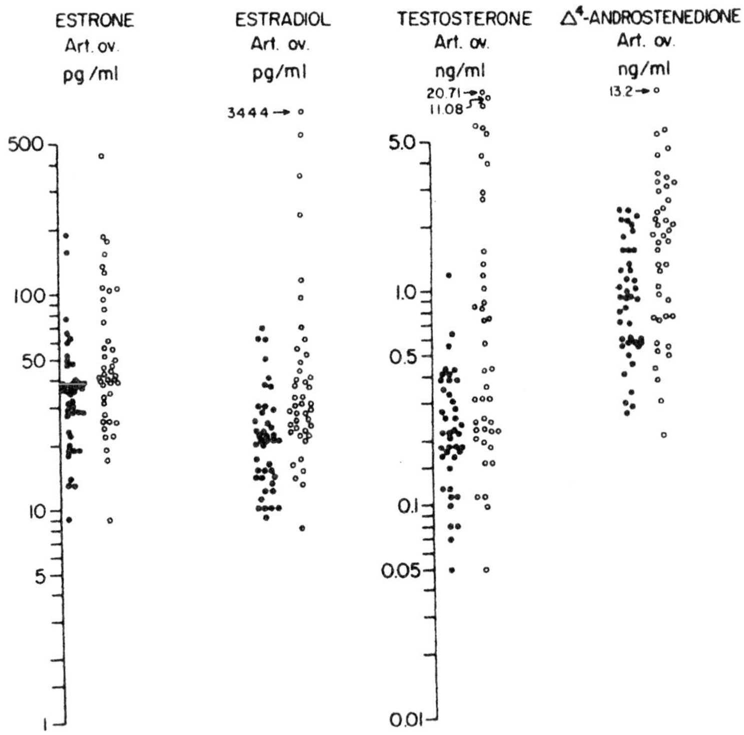

FIGURE 2–18. Concentrations of estrone, estradiol, testosterone, and Δ^4 androstenedione in arterial (Art. ●) and ovarian (ov. ○) vein blood of 42 postmenopausal women undergoing hysterectomy for uterine disease. A gradient was demonstrated for testosterone in 21 subjects and for Δ^4 androstenedione in 16 subjects. (From Longcope C, Hunter R, Franz C: Steroid secretion by the postmenopausal ovary. Am J Obstet Gynecol 138:564, 1980.)

Psychological Symptoms

Headaches, tiredness, lethargy, irritability, anxiety, nervousness, depression, and inability to concentrate are common symptoms experienced by menopausal women. Although not specific to menopause, these symptoms are often alleviated by estrogen replacement. Insomnia and poor sleep are also common symptoms and may be related to frequent night sweats.

Atrophic Changes

Estrogen deficiency reduces skin thickness because of a lower turnover rate of epidermal cells.[45] Vaginal rugae are lost, and the vagina becomes small, atrophic, and susceptible to inflammation caused by trauma or infection. Symptoms include dyspareunia, pruritus, urethritis, and cystitis.

Bone Loss and Cardiovascular Disease

The major long-term consequences of estrogen deprivation are bone loss and cardiovascular disease. The effects of estrogen loss on the cardiovascular system are detailed in Chapter 5.4. Loss of trabecular bone predisposes women to fractures at three common sites: the vertebrae, the distal radius, and the femoral neck. Decreased bone density is related to a higher rate of bone loss; estrogen deficiency accelerates osteoclastic bone resorption.[46] The longer life expectancy of women has increased the relevance of these events.

THE POSTMENOPAUSAL OVARY

The postmenopausal ovary is a viable endocrine organ that responds to gonadotropin stimulation. The ovary contributes little to circulating estrogens, which are almost exclusively derived from the extraglandular conversion of androgens (some of which are of ovarian origin).[47] Under gonadotropin influence, the climacteric ovary contributes 40% of the total production of testosterone and 20% of androstenedione.[48] Thus, the postmenopausal ovary is an endocrine gland capable of producing androgens (Fig. 2–18), but the capacity for androgen production varies.[49]

References

1. Rabinovici J, Jaffe RB: Development and regulation of growth and differentiated function in humans with subhuman primate fetal gonads. Endocr Rev 11:532, 1990.
2. Tho SPT, Layman LC, Lanclos DK, et al: Absence of the testicular determining factor gene SRY in XX true hermaphrodites and presence of this locus in most subjects with gonadal dysgenesis caused by Y aneuploidy. Am J Obstet Gynecol 167:1794, 1992.
3. Gondos B, Bhiraleus P, Hobel CJ: Ultrastructural observations on germ cells in human fetal ovaries. Am J Obstet Gynecol 110:644, 1971.
4. Gondos B, Westergaard L, Byskov A: Initiation of oogenesis in the human fetal ovary: Ultrastructural and squash preparation study. Am J Obstet Gynecol 155:189, 1980.
5. Richardson SJ, Senikas V, Nelson JF: Follicular depletion during the menopausal transition: Evidence for accelerated loss and ultimate exhaustion. J Clin Endocrinol Metab 65:1231, 1987.
6. Himelstein-Braw R, Byskov AG, Peters H, Faber M: Follicular atresia in the infant human ovary. J Reprod Fertil 46:55, 1976.
7. Block E: Quantitative morphological investigations of the follicular system in women: Variations at different ages. Acta Anat 14:108, 1952.
8. Jost A, Vigier B, Prepin J, Perchellet JP: Studies on sex differentiation in mammals. Recent Prog Horm Res 29:1, 1973.
9. Parker LN: Adrenarche. Endocrinol Metab Clin North Am 20:71, 1991.

10. Kenigsberg D, Rosenwaks Z, Hodgen GD: Ovarian follicular maturation, ovulation, and ovulation induction. In de Groot U (ed): Endocrinology. WB Saunders, Philadelphia, 1995, p 2031.
11. Knobil E: The neuroendocrine control of the menstrual cycle. Recent Prog Horm Res 36:53, 1980.
12. Oerter KE, Uriarte MM, Rose SR, et al: Gonadotropin secretory dynamics during puberty in normal girls and boys. J Clin Endocrinol Metab 71:1251, 1990.
13. Reame N, Sauder E, Kelch RP, Marshall JC: Pulsatile gonadotropin secretion during the human menstrual cycle: Evidence for altered frequency of gonadotropin-releasing hormone secretion. J Clin Endocrinol Metab 59:328, 1984.
14. Hotchkiss J, Knobil E: The menstrual cycle and its neuroendocrine control. In Knobil E, Neill JD (eds): The Physiology of Reproduction, 2nd ed. Raven Press, New York, 1994, p 711.
15. Filicori M, Santoro N, Merriam GR, Crowley WF Jr: Characterization of the physiological pattern of episodic gonadotropin secretion throughout the human menstrual cycle. J Clin Endocrinol Metab 62:1136, 1986.
16. Casper RF, Alapin-Rubilovitz S: Progestins increase endogenous opioid peptide activity in postmenopausal women. J Clin Endocrinol Metab 60:34, 1985.
17. Laatikainen T, Raisanen I, Tulenheimo A, Salminen K: Plasma β-endorphin and the menstrual cycle. Fertil Steril 44:206, 1985.
18. Urban RJ, Veldhuis JD, Dufau ML: Estrogen regulates the gonadotropin-releasing hormone-stimulated secretion of biologically active luteinizing hormone. J Clin Endocrinol Metab 72:660, 1991.
19. Halvorson LM, DeCherney AH: Inhibin, activin, and follistatin in reproductive medicine. Fertil Steril 65:459, 1996.
20. Gougeon A: Regulation of ovarian follicular development in primates: Facts and hypotheses. Endocr Rev 17:121, 1996.
21. McNatty KP, Makris A, DeGrazia C, et al: The production of progesterone, androgens and estrogens by granulosa cells, thecal tissue and stromal tissue from human ovaries in vitro. J Clin Endocrinol Metab 49:687, 1979.
22. Hillier SG: Paracrine control of follicular estrogen synthesis. Semin Reprod Endocrinol 9:332, 1991.
23. Shoham Z, Schachter M, Loumaye E, et al: The luteinizing hormone surge—the final stage in ovulation induction: Modern aspects of ovulation triggering. Fertil Steril 64:237, 1995.
24. Hodgen GD: The dominant ovarian follicle. Fertil Steril 38:281, 1982.
25. McLachlan RI, Robertson DM, Healy DL, et al: Circulating immunoreactive inhibin levels during the normal human menstrual cycle. J Clin Endocrinol Metab 65:954, 1987.
26. Giudice LC: Insulin-like growth factors and ovarian follicular development. Endocr Rev 13:641, 1992.
27. Hoff JD, Quigley MB, Yen SSC: Hormonal dynamics at mid cycle: A re-evaluation. J Clin Endocrinol Metab 57:792, 1983.
28. Shoham Z, Schachter M: Estrogen biosynthesis—regulation, action, remote effects, and value of monitoring in ovarian stimulation cycles. Fertil Steril 65:687, 1996.
29. Miyazaki T, Katz B, Dharmarajan AM, et al: Do prostaglandins lead to ovulation in the rabbit by stimulating proteolytic enzyme activity? Fertil Steril 55:1183, 1991.
30. Vermesh M, Kletzky OA: Longitudinal evaluation of the luteal phase and its transition into the follicular phase. J Endocrinol Metab 65: 653, 1987.
31. Hall JE, Schoenfeld DA, Martin KA, Crowley WF Jr: Hypothalamic gonadotropin-releasing hormone secretion and follicle-stimulating hormone dynamics during the luteal follicular transition. J Clin Endocrinol Metab 74:600, 1992.
32. Brenner RM, Slayden OD: Cyclic changes in the primate oviduct and endometrium. In Knobil E, Neill JD (eds): The Physiology of Reproduction, 2nd ed. Raven Press, New York, 1994, p 541.
33. Ferency A, Bergeron C: Histology of the human endometrium: From birth to senescence. In Bulletti C, Gurpide B (eds): The Primate Endometrium. The New York Academy of Sciences, New York, 1991, p 6.
34. Eldering JA, Nag MG, Hoberg LM, et al: Hormonal regulation of prostaglandin production by rhesus monkey endometrium. J Clin Endocrinol Metab 71:596, 1990.
35. Christiaens GCML, Sixma JJ, Haspels AA: Hemostasis in menstrual endometrium: A review. Obstet Gynecol Surv 37:281, 1982.
36. Noyes RW, Hertig AW, Rock J: Dating the endometrial biopsy. Fertil Steril 1:3, 1950.
37. Treloar AE, Boynton RE, Behn BG, Brown BW: Variation of the human menstrual cycle through reproductive life. Int J Fertil 12: 77, 1970.
38. Metcalf MG, Livesay JH: Gonadotrophin excretion in fertile women: Effect of age and the onset of the menopausal transition. J Endocrinol 105:357, 1985.
39. Hughes EG, Robertson DM, Handelsman DJ, et al: Inhibin and estradiol responses to ovarian hyperstimulation: Effects of age with predictive value for in vitro fertilization outcome. J Clin Endocrinol Metab 70:358, 1990.
40. Scott RT Jr, Hofmann GE: Prognostic assessment of ovarian reserve. Fertil Steril 63:1, 1995.
41. Meldrum DR: Female reproductive aging—ovarian and uterine factors. Fertil Steril 59:1,1993.
42. McKinlay SM, Brambilla DJ, Posner JG: The normal menopause transition. Maturitas 14:103, 1992.
43. Midgette AS, Baron JA: Cigarette smoking and the risk of natural menopause. Epidemiology 1:474, 1990.
44. Casper RF, Yen SSC, Wilkes MM: Menopausal flushes: A neuroendocrine link with pulsatile luteinizing hormone secretion. Science 205: 823, 1979.
45. Castelo-Branco C, Duran M, Gonzalez-Merlo J: Skin collagen changes related to age and hormone replacement therapy. Maturitas 15:113, 1992.
46. Lindsay R, Aitken JM, Anderson JB, et al: Long-term prevention of postmenopausal osteoporosis by oestrogen. Lancet 1:1038, 1976.
47. Judd HL, Judd GB, Lucas WE, Yen SS: Endocrine function of the postmenopausal ovary: Concentration of androgens and estrogens in ovarian and peripheral vein blood. J Clin Endocrinol Metab 39:1020, 1974.
48. Adashi E: The climacteric ovary as a functional gonadotrophin-driven androgen-producing gland. Fertil Steril 62:20, 1994.
49. Longcope C, Hunter R, Franz C: Steroid secretion by the postmenopausal ovary. Am J Obstet Gynecol 138:564, 1980.

SECTION

II

CORONARY ARTERY DISEASE

CHAPTER 3

Overview

Kara Thompson and H. Vernon Anderson

The purpose of this chapter is to review specifically the magnitude of the problem of coronary artery disease and call attention to the important but often overlooked differences of gender. Coronary disease is frequently viewed as a disease only of men. Other diseases such as breast and cervical cancers have received much more attention as important illnesses of women. However, coronary disease is the primary cause of death in both men and women in the United States.

Coronary disease typically becomes evident in men in the prime of life, usually in their mid-50s, whereas in women, it generally develops 10 to 20 years later than this. Thus, many studies of this problem have included mostly men, and our knowledge about coronary disease in women has largely been extrapolated from studies primarily focused on men. Although the risk factors for atherosclerosis are similar in men and women, there are enough differences that it is important to address coronary disease in women as a specific issue. The most obvious difference between men and women is the presentation of coronary disease in women in the older, postmenopausal years. Other important gender differences include the less specific clinical manifestations of coronary disease in women, the greater difficulty of diagnosis, and the more severe consequences of myocardial infarction when it occurs in women. These clinical dilemmas emphasize the importance of studying gender-specific aspects of coronary disease.

EPIDEMIOLOGY

Cardiovascular disease is the leading cause of death in women. One of every two women will die of a heart attack, stroke, or other cardiovascular illness.[1] In 1992, 444,000 men and 479,000 women died of cardiovascular disease. Moreover, strokes caused 56,645 deaths in men and 87,124 deaths in women. In comparison, 246,000 women died of cancer of all forms; specifically, 43,100 women died of breast cancer, and 55,900 women died of lung cancer.[2] Thus, more than twice as many women died of cardiovascular disease than cancer. That ratio increases to 10:1 when deaths caused by cardiovascular disease are compared with deaths from accidents, chronic obstructive pulmonary disease, and pneumonia or influenza (Fig. 3–1).

One of the oldest and best sources of data for cardiovascular disease in women is the Framingham Heart Study. In this study, 5127 men and women who were initially free of apparent heart disease were followed prospectively for 26 years. During the study, 752 coronary events occurred in men and 488 in women. Several important observations regarding women and men were noted. In the younger age groups, coronary heart disease was more prevalent in men. The incidence increased rapidly in men until age 45 to 55; then, the incidence increased more gradually. In contrast, the incidence of coronary disease in young women was low and did not increase until later. The difference in the incidence of coronary heart disease in the oldest group of women and the youngest group was 40-fold; the difference between the same groups in men was only sixfold. In the older age groups, the prevalence of coronary disease in women approached that of men (Fig. 3–2).[3]

Once coronary artery disease develops, women do not have a survival advantage over men. In fact, in every age group, women with coronary disease have a higher risk of death from a coronary event than men.[3] Older women are

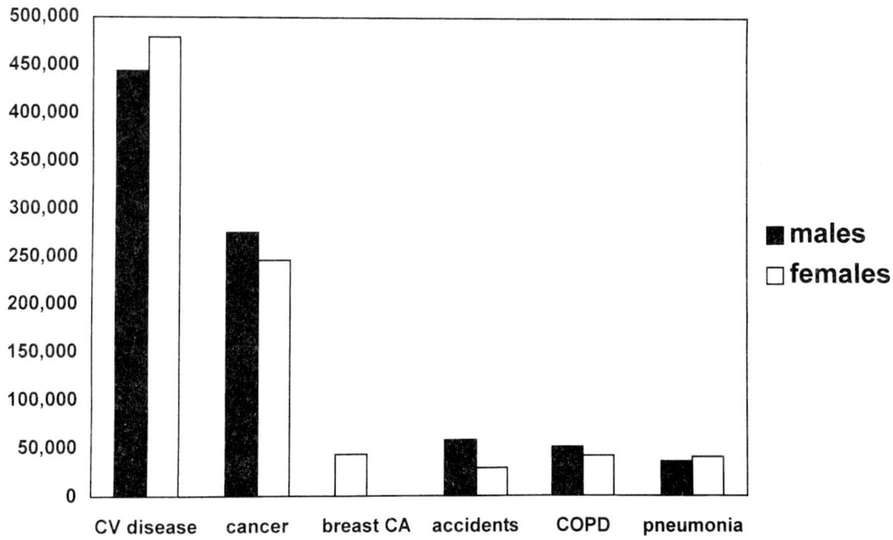

FIGURE 3–1. Causes of death for men and women in 1992. (CA, cancer; COPD, chronic obstructive pulmonary disease; CV, cardiovascular.)

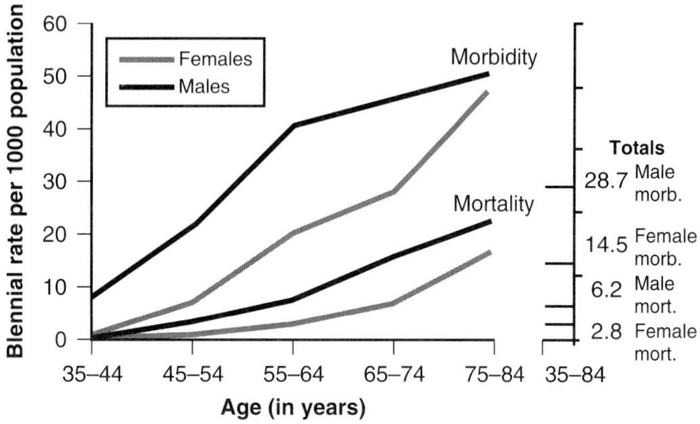

FIGURE 3–2. Incidence of morbidity and mortality from coronary heart disease, a 26-year follow-up from the Framingham Study.

twice as likely as older men to die within weeks after a heart attack. In the first year after a heart attack, 27% of men and 44% of women will die.[2] Free wall and ventricular septal rupture complicate an acute myocardial infarction more often in women than in men.[4] Recurrent myocardial infarction and cardiac failure are also more common in women after a heart attack. In contrast, sudden death is more common in men,[5] and ventricular ectopy after myocardial infarction is associated with increased mortality in men but not in women. However, the risk of death is equal in men and women with ejection fractions less than 35%.[6]

The impact of cardiovascular disease in women is measured not only by death but also by disability and cost. Stroke occurs in 18% of women and 9% of men within 6 years after a heart attack.[2] In 1980, 36% of women between the ages of 55 and 64 who had ischemic heart disease and 55% of those older than 75 were disabled. Of those women who survived strokes in 1980, more than 60% of those older than 55 years were disabled.[7] Although fewer women than men undergo expensive cardiovascular procedures such as coronary angioplasty and coronary artery bypass surgery, women incur more than half of the yearly health-care costs for cardiovascular illnesses.[7]

Although mortality rates for coronary heart disease have decreased for both men and women over the past two decades, coronary disease as a clinical entity is a growing problem in women (Table 3–1; Fig. 3–3). By the year 2015, almost one half of women in the United States will be older than 45 years of age. As the number of older women in the population increases, the absolute number of women with coronary disease will also increase.[7] In 1991, more women than men over the age of 65 died of heart disease.[8, 9] Therefore, a specific program for the prevention and treatment of heart disease in women must be developed.

Table 3–1. DEATHS FROM HEART DISEASE

YEAR	WOMEN	MEN
1986	374,600	390,900
1988	379,800	385,400
1989	365,700	368,200
1990	359,300	360,800
1991	361,000	360,000

RISK FACTORS

Most of the risk factors for coronary artery disease are similar for men and women. These risk factors include diabetes, hyperlipidemia, hypertension, smoking, family history, obesity, and aging. However, the role of estrogen is unique to women.

Data from the Framingham Study suggest that diabetes is a more significant coronary risk factor for women than for men.[10] Asymptomatic hyperglycemia also increases risk in women.[1] In fact, diabetes may negate the protective effect of estrogen in younger women.[11] Intensive treatment of hyperglycemia has been shown to delay the onset and to slow the progression of retinopathy, nephropathy, and neuropathy. However, the effect of intensive treatment of hyperglycemia on the risk of cardiovascular disease requires further study.[12]

Cholesterol profiles of women and men differ with age. Levels of low-density lipoproteins (LDL) are lower in women than in men until the age of 50, when LDL levels increase in women. In women of all ages, high-density lipoproteins (HDL) are about 10 mg/dl higher than in men. In perimenopausal women, levels of lipoprotein(a) increase with age. This change in lipid levels may help explain the increased incidence of coronary artery disease in older women. Epidemiologic studies have confirmed that high cholesterol is a risk factor for coronary disease in women,

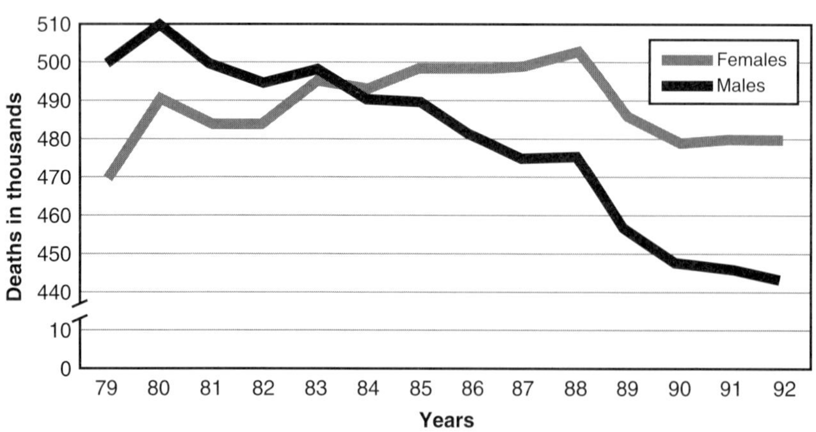

FIGURE 3–3. Cardiovascular disease mortality trends for men and women.

but women have been excluded or included only in small numbers in primary and secondary prevention trials, which have usually included middle-aged men.[1] Women have been enrolled in large numbers in only two secondary prevention studies. In the Scandinavian Simvastatin Survival Study Group, lowering cholesterol levels had a beneficial effect on nonfatal cardiovascular events but did not prevent death in women. The Upjohn Primary Prevention Study, in which 52% of the 2278 participants were women, showed that the use of colestipol was beneficial only in men; however, the statistical power of the study may have been insufficient to detect the effects in women. Thus, the effect of treating hypercholesterolemia on coronary disease risk in women requires further study.[13]

Hypertension is more common in older women than in older men. Although hypertension has been shown to be a risk factor for women, studies of hypertension have included mostly men. Conflicting results have been reported from the few trials that have involved women.

Smoking is an important modifiable risk factor for men and women. Although smoking increases the risk of a first myocardial infarction, the increased risk is eliminated within 2 to 3 years after quitting smoking.[14] However, more men than women have recently quit smoking. In women, the risks of smoking and use of oral contraception are additive.[1]

Family history and obesity, particularly obesity in a truncal distribution, are significant risk factors for both women and men. Family history of coronary disease and a truncal weight distribution, although not modifiable factors, should alert the physician to the possibility of coronary disease in women who have these risk factors.[1]

In women of childbearing age, oral contraceptive pills have been associated with an increased risk of stroke, myocardial infarction, and thromboembolism. Estrogens in these pills enhance both factor VII and fibrinogen in order to create a procoagulant effect. Progestins in contraceptive pills can decrease HDL levels, increase LDL levels, increase blood pressure, and exacerbate glucose intolerance. Estrogens have a favorable effect on lipid profiles; they increase HDL and decrease LDL levels. However, estrogen also increases triglyceride levels. The cardiovascular risk associated with oral contraceptive pills is dose related and is greatest in women smokers older than 40 years of age. Because these studies were done, the formulation of oral contraceptive pills has changed so that minimally effective doses of estrogen and progestin are used. At present, these pills are considered safe in young, nonsmoking women; caution is recommended in women older than 40 years of age and in women who smoke.[1, 11]

In postmenopausal women, estrogen replacement therapy has been associated with a 50% reduction in the risk of coronary heart disease.[7] One possible mechanism for this decreased risk is the favorable effect of low-dose estrogen on lipid profiles. Conjugated estrogens are generally prescribed as replacement therapy in doses of 0.625 mg or 1.25 mg. The higher dose nearly doubles the triglyceride level without significantly improving the HDL and LDL levels when compared with the lower dose.[7] Transdermal estrogen does not change the lipid profile.[1] The addition of progestins to offset the increased risk of endometrial cancer by unopposed estrogen stimulation may attenuate some of the favorable effects of estrogen on lipid profiles. Nevertheless, the combined regimen may still have a beneficial effect on the cardiovascular system.[11] Other benefits from estrogen therapy include vasodilation and a reduction in glucose and insulin levels.[7] In studies of arterial blood flow, estrogen increased endothelium-dependent vasodilation.[15] Controversy exists as to whether estrogen increases risk of breast cancer.[16] Use of progesterone in conjunction with estrogen does not appear to decrease the risk of breast cancer in postmenopausal women.[17] The effect of starting estrogen therapy many years after menopause has not been studied.[18] Estrogen is most beneficial when started soon after menopause and continued for long periods. In the Cardiovascular Health Study of 2955 women aged 65 and older, the postmenopausal use of estrogen reduced LDL levels, increased HDL levels, lowered insulin and glucose levels, and decreased obesity. Past or present estrogen use was associated with less subclinical disease as assessed by carotid intimal-medial thickness, electrocardiographic left ventricular mass, and Doppler filling ratio. This study suggested that postmenopausal estrogen may be beneficial in reducing cardiovascular risks even in elderly women in their 80s.[19]

MANIFESTATIONS

The clinical presentation of coronary disease is often more subtle in women than in men. For example, angina pectoris is a less specific sign of coronary disease in women than in men. Although angina is the most common presentation of coronary disease in women, only one half of women who reported having angina had significant coronary artery disease on angiography in the Coronary Artery Surgical Study, whereas 83% of men with angina had significant disease.[1] In the Framingham Study, women who reported angina had a more favorable prognosis than did men. Because the Framingham data were collected before widespread use of angiography, the more favorable prognosis may be attributed to the absence of coronary artery disease in many of the women who reported having angina. Unfortunately, this observation of a better prognosis in women contributed to the misconception that angina in women is unimportant.[7] In addition, in the Framingham Study, the incidence of sudden death was similar in men and women. More recently, in 1992, 63% of the women and 48% of the men who died suddenly and were found to have coronary disease had had no previous coronary symptoms.[2] The Framingham Study also reported a higher incidence of silent myocardial infarction in women than in men (35% versus 28%).[7]

Noninvasive diagnosis of coronary artery disease is more difficult to achieve in women than in men. Exercise stress testing is associated with a higher false-positive rate in women. This problem may be related to the lower prevalence of coronary artery disease in younger women or to gender-related differences in the electrocardiographic response to exercise.[1] Exercise testing is still useful in evaluating women with chest pain because a normal test is highly predictive for the absence of disease.[7] Specificity with nuclear testing is comparable in women and men, but breast attenuation can be problematic. Although it is more expensive, nuclear testing improves accuracy.[1, 11]

TREATMENT

Medical interventions for coronary artery disease, angina, and myocardial infarction have been studied more thoroughly in men than in women. At the present time, no data indicate gender differences in the benefits associated with the use of beta blockers, angiotensin-converting enzyme (ACE) inhibitors, and nitrates. Long-term use of aspirin has been shown to reduce the risk of myocardial infarction in women.[20] In the Second International Study of Infarct Survival (ISIS-2) trial, aspirin taken in the setting of an acute myocardial infarction was equally effective in men and women.[21] Only 20% to 25% of participants in thrombolytic trials have been women; however, results suggest the risk of bleeding associated with thrombolytics is higher in women. Results from the Thrombosis and Angioplasty in Myocardial Infarction (TAMI), Gruppo Italiano per lo Studio della Sopravvivenza nell'Infarto Miocardico II (GISSI-2), and Global Utilization of Streptokinase and Tissue Plasminogen Activator for Occluded Coronary Arteries (GUSTO-1) trials showed an increased risk of intracerebral hemorrhage in women.[22–24] In GUSTO-1, the increased risk was believed to relate to older age and lower body weight.[24] Use of weight-adjusted, thrombolytic therapy in women has not been studied.[11]

Women undergo fewer invasive cardiac procedures than do men. In one study, 40% of men and only 4% of women with abnormal nuclear stress studies were referred for cardiac catheterization.[1] In 1993, twice as many men as women underwent coronary angioplasty and coronary bypass surgery.[2] In the Coronary Artery Surgery Study, significantly more women than men died after bypass surgery. The women in this study were older than the men, and more women had hypertension, diabetes, and unstable angina.[7] Possible explanations for increased mortality are that women are referred later in the course of disease and they have smaller bodies with proportionally smaller coronary blood vessels for grafting.[1]

SUMMARY

Cardiovascular disease is the primary cause of death in women. Coronary disease generally becomes apparent in women in the postmenopausal years. As the number of older women increases, the problem of coronary artery disease in women will also increase despite the overall decline in coronary heart disease noted during the past two decades. Studies regarding prevention and treatment of coronary disease have largely involved men. In view of the increasing incidence of coronary disease in older women, the less specific signs of coronary disease in women, and the graver prognosis following a coronary event in women, further investigation will need to be devoted specifically to this entity in women.

References

1. Kuhn FE, Rackley C: Coronary artery disease in women: Risk factors, evaluation, treatment, and prevention. Arch Intern Med 153:2626, 1993.
2. Mosca L, Manson JE, Sutherland SE, et al: Cardiovascular disease in women: a statement for healthcare professionals from the American Heart Association. Circulation 96:2468, 1997.
3. Lerner DJ, Kannel WB: Patterns of coronary heart disease morbidity and mortality in the sexes: A 26-year follow-up of the Framingham population. Am Heart J 111:383, 1986.
4. Herman MV, Evans MD, Kay RH: Coronary heart disease and ventricular dysfunction in women. In Eaker ED, Packard B, Wenger NK, et al (eds): Coronary Heart Disease in Women. Haymarket Doyma Inc, New York, 1987, p 198.
5. Kannel WB, Abbott RD: Incidence and prognosis of myocardial infarction in women: The Framingham study. In Eaker ED, Packard B, Wenger NK, et al (eds): Coronary Heart Disease in Women. Haymarket Doyma Inc, New York, 1987, p. 208.
6. Moss AJ, Carleen MS, the Multicenter Postinfarction Research Group: Gender differences in the mortality risk associated with ventricular arrhythmias after myocardial infarction. In Eaker ED, Packard B, Wenger NK, et al (eds): Coronary Heart Disease in Women. Haymarket Doyma Inc, New York, 1987, p 204.
7. Eaker ED, Chesebro JH, Sacks FM, et al: Cardiovascular disease in women: AHA medical/scientific statement. Circulation 88:1999, 1993.
8. Rosamond WD, Chambless LE, Folsom AR, et al: Trends in the incidence of myocardial infarction and in mortality due to coronary heart disease, 1987 to 1994. N Engl J Med 339:861, 1998.
9. McGovern PG, Pankow JS, Shahar E, et al: Recent trends in acute coronary heart disease. N Engl J Med 334:884, 1996.
10. Stokes J III, Kannel WB, Wolf PA, et al: The relative importance of selected risk factors for various manifestations of cardiovascular disease among men and women from 35 to 64 years old: 30 years of follow-up in the Framingham study. Circulation 75:V65, 1987.
11. Fetters JK, Peterson ED, Shaw LJ, et al: Sex-specific differences in coronary artery disease risk factors, evaluation, and treatment: Have they been adequately evaluated? Am Heart J 131:796, 1996.
12. The Diabetes Control and Complications Trial Research Group: The effect of intensive treatment of diabetes on the development and progression of long-term complications in insulin-dependent diabetes mellitus. N Engl J Med 329:977, 1993.
13. Rembold CM: A number needed to treat analysis of the prevention of myocardial infarction and death by anti-dyslipidemic therapy. J Fam Pract 42:577, 1996.
14. Rosenberg L, Palmer JR, Shapiro S: Decline in the risk of myocardial infarction among women who stop smoking. N Engl J Med 322:213, 1990.
15. Anderson HV: Estrogen therapy, atherosclerosis, and clinical cardiovascular events. Circulation 94:1809, 1996.
16. Brinton LA, Schairer C: Estrogen replacement therapy and breast cancer risk. Epidemiol Rev 15:66, 1993.
17. Colditz GA, Hankinson SE, Hunter DJ, et al: The use of estrogens and progestins and the risk of breast cancer in postmenopausal women. N Engl J Med 332:1589, 1995.
18. Wenger NK, Speroff L, Packard B: Cardiovascular health and disease in women. N Engl J Med 329:247, 1993.
19. Manoho TA, Furberg CD, Shemanski L, et al: Associations of postmenopausal estrogen use with cardiovascular disease and its risk factors in older women. Circulation 88:2163, 1993.
20. Manson JE, Stampfer MJ, Colditz GA, et al: A prospective study of aspirin use and primary prevention of cardiovascular disease in women. JAMA 266:521, 1991.
21. ISIS-2 (Second International Study of Infarct Survival) Collaborative Group: Randomised trial of intravenous streptokinase, oral aspirin, both, or neither, among 17,187 cases of suspected acute myocardial infarction. Lancet 2:349, 1988.
22. Topol EJ, Califf RM, George BS, and the Thrombolysis and Angioplasty in Myocardial Infarction (TAMI) Study Group: A multicenter randomized trial of intravenous recombinant tissue plasminogen activator and immediate angioplasty in acute myocardial infarction. N Engl J Med 317:581, 1987.
23. Maggioni AP, Franzosi MG, Santoro E, et al: The risk of stroke in patients with acute myocardial infarction after thrombolytic and antithrombotic treatment. Gruppo Italiano per lo Studio della Sopravvivenza nell'Infarto Miocardico II (GISSI-2), and The International Study Group. N Engl J Med 327:1, 1992.
24. The GUSTO Investigators: An international randomized trial comparing four thrombolytic strategies for acute myocardial infarction. N Engl J Med 329:673, 1993.

CHAPTER 4

Anatomy and Pathophysiology

4.1 Overview

L. Maximilian Buja and Margaret O. Uthman

Coronary artery disease, also known as coronary heart disease or ischemic heart disease, is characterized by relative or absolute impairment of myocardial perfusion of variable duration and severity. Complex interactions between the coronary circulatory system and the myocardium are involved in the pathology of coronary artery disease.[1–3] In most cases, coronary atherosclerosis is present as the underlying anatomic substrate.[1–4]

CORONARY VASCULAR ANATOMY

A more detailed discussion of coronary vascular anatomy is presented in Chapter 1. The heart receives oxygenated blood from the left and right coronary arteries (Fig. 4–1).[1–3] The left main coronary artery gives rise to the left anterior descending coronary artery and its septal and diagonal branches, which supply the anteroseptal and anterolateral left ventricle, respectively. The left main coronary artery also gives rise to the left circumflex coronary artery, which usually supplies the lateral left ventricle, except in the 10% of hearts with a left dominant circulation in which the left circumflex coronary artery also supplies the posterior left and right ventricles. The right coronary artery supplies the right ventricle, and in 90% of hearts, the right coronary artery gives rise to the posterior descending branch, thereby supplying the posterior and posteroseptal left ventricle with oxygenated blood. The left and right atria are supplied from branches of the left and right coronary arteries, respectively. The major blood supply to the atrioventricular node is from the coronary artery and its posterior descending branch, which is the right coronary artery in 90% of cases. The sinoatrial node is supplied primarily from the right coronary artery in 60% of cases and from the left circumflex coronary artery in 40% of cases. Branches of the major coronary arteries are connected by diminutive collaterals that become enlarged and function in response to various stimuli, including intermittent ischemia.[1–3]

The dimensions of the coronary arteries are directly proportional to the mass of the heart up to a critical heart weight of 550 g.[5] Because heart weight depends on body size, hearts in women weigh 50 to 100 g less than hearts in men. Therefore, the coronary arteries in women are generally 0.5 to 1.0 mm smaller in cross-sectional diameter than those in men. Technical challenges related to intervention on smaller coronary arteries likely contribute to the increased morbidity and mortality associated with coronary artery bypass surgery and coronary angioplasty in women.[6, 7]

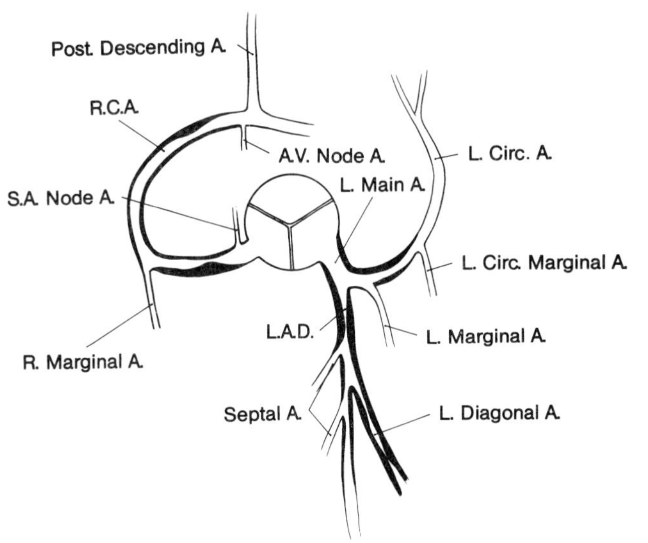

FIGURE 4–1. Diagram of the usual anatomic distribution of the coronary arteries. The dark areas show a typical distribution of atherosclerotic plaques. (A, artery; AV, atrioventricular; Circ, circumflex; L, left; LAD, left anterior descending; Post, posterior; R, right; RCA, right coronary artery; SA, sinoatria.) (From Willerson JT, Hillis LD, Buja LM: Pathogenesis and pathology of ischemic heart disease. In Willerson JT, Hillis LD, Buja LM [eds]: Ischemic Heart Disease: Clinical and Pathophysiological Aspects. Raven Press, New York, 1982, pp 7–83.)

CORONARY ATHEROSCLEROSIS

The lesions of established atherosclerosis are fibrous plaques, which are raised intimal lesions consisting of varying combinations of lipid, cells, and connective tissue matrix (Fig. 4–2).[8–10] Atherogenesis leading to plaque formation involves complex interactions between the vessel wall and soluble and formed elements of the blood.[11–14] The following factors are important in the initiation and growth of plaques: (1) endothelial injury or dysfunction, (2) monocyte and macrophage accumulation, (3) platelet aggregation and attachment, (4) smooth muscle proliferation, (5) influx of T lymphocytes and, possibly, other inflammatory cells, (6) influx of plasma low-density lipoprotein (LDL), (7) oxidation or other local modification of LDL, (8) progressive lipid accumulation in foam cells from uptake of modified LDL and secondary extracellular lipid deposition, and (9) hemodynamic influences related to blood pressure and pattern of blood flow. These factors have been recognized and synthesized into a coherent concept of atherogenesis, known as the response to injury hypothesis.[11–14]

Initially, coronary atherosclerosis develops focally adjacent to branch points in areas of low velocity flow and in areas of

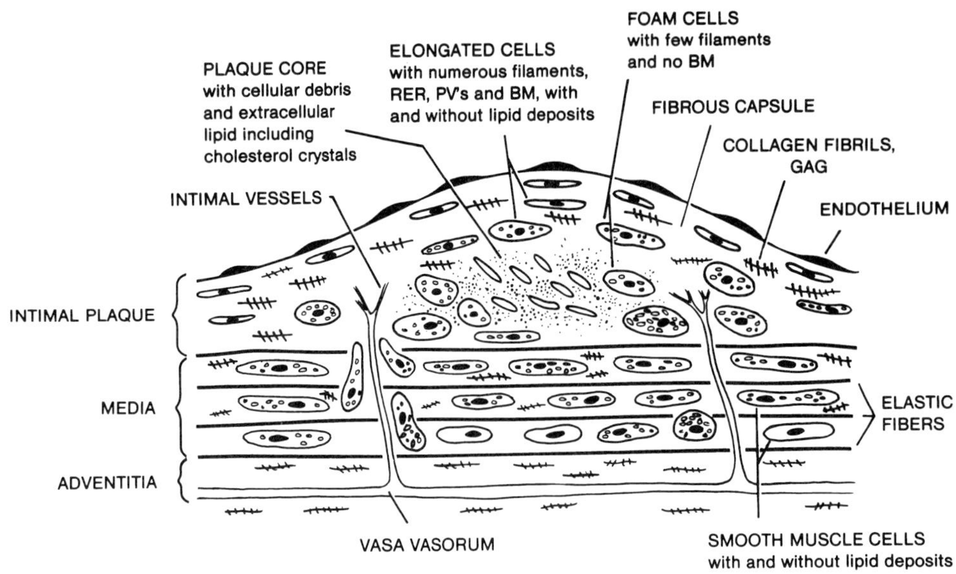

FIGURE 4–2. Schematic diagram of an atherosclerotic plaque. The plaque is lined by endothelial cells and is composed of a fibrous capsule that surrounds a core containing necrotic tissue and extracellular lipid. The plaque is vascularized by vessels derived from the vasa vasorum. Lipid deposits are often present in elongated cells, which are typical of altered smooth muscle cells. These cells contain numerous filaments, rough-surfaced endoplasmic reticulum (RER), pinocytotic vessels (PVs), and a basement membrane (BM). Ovoid foam cells, which have few filaments and no basement membrane, a characteristic consistent with macrophage origin, also possess lipid deposits. Medial smooth muscle cells also may contain lipid deposits. Extracellular components of the plaque include numerous collagen fibrils, deposits of glycosaminoglycans (GAG), and some elastic fibers. (From Buja LM, Kovanen PT, Bilheimer DW: Cellular pathology of homozygous familial hypercholesterolemia. Am J Pathol 97:327–357, 1979.)

low shear stress adjacent to areas of high shear stress.[15] High shear stress may be involved in activating blood elements, which then have increased contact with possibly altered areas of endothelium in the areas of low shear stress and blood flow. These factors initially give rise to typically eccentric plaques in predisposed regions. The zones with the greatest predilection for severe coronary atherosclerosis are the proximal left anterior descending coronary artery, the proximal right coronary artery, and the area of the distal right coronary artery just proximal to the origin of the posterior descending branch (see Fig. 4–1).

As coronary atherosclerosis progresses, extensive remodeling of the vessel wall occurs. In vascular segments with advanced atherosclerosis, all three layers of the arterial wall are involved and exhibit intimal thickening, medial degeneration, adventitial fibrosis, and lymphocyte infiltration.[8–11] At this stage, plaques may be concentric or eccentric. Medial degeneration allows for vascular dilatation, which tends to

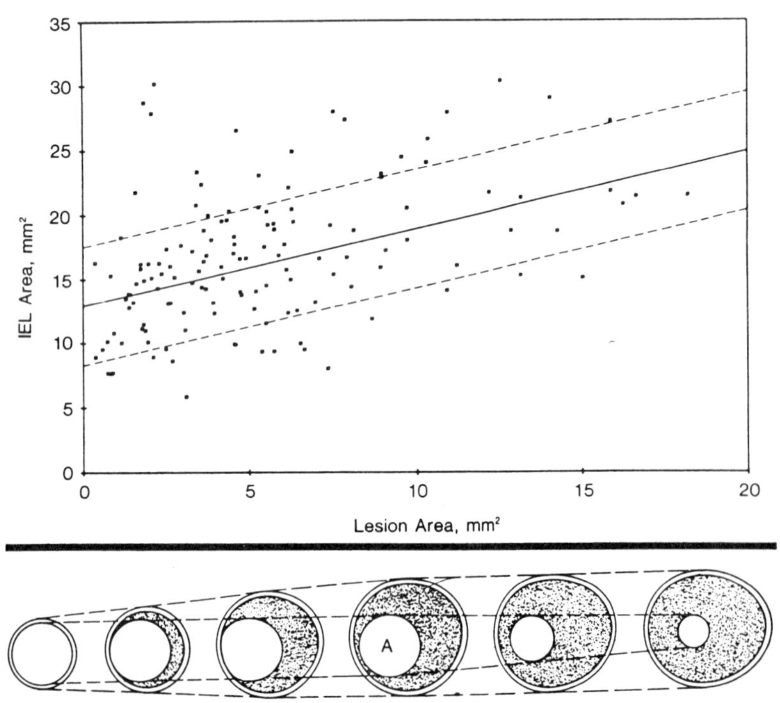

FIGURE 4–3. Compensatory enlargement of human coronary arteries as relates to plaque formation. In the graph, the area encompassed by the internal elastic lamina (IEL area) is plotted against the area of the lesion for sections of the left main coronary artery from 136 adult hearts (obtained postmortem). The IEL area is the potential lumen area if no plaque were present. The IEL area increases linearly as the lesion area increases ($r = .44$; $p < .001$; standard error of 4.8 mm² indicated by the dotted lines above and below the regression line). Below the graph is a diagram of sequential changes in atherosclerotic arteries that may eventually lead to lumen narrowing. Arteries initially enlarge and preserve nearly normal lumen cross section, but the normal lumen area may not be maintained once a lesion occupies more than 40% of IEL area (A). (From Glagov S, Zarins C, Giddens DP, Nu DN: Hemodynamics and atherosclerosis: Insights and perspectives gained from studies of human arteries. N Engl J Med 316:1371–1375, 1987.)

preserve the luminal diameter until growth of atherosclerotic plaque is very advanced (Fig. 4–3).[16] An approximate 50% narrowing of luminal diameter (75% of luminal area) is required to produce a lesion that impairs the increased blood flow required to meet high myocardial oxygen need. An even greater reduction in luminal diameter is needed to impair baseline (resting) myocardial blood flow.[1–3] However, less bulky coronary plaques associated with subcritical coronary stenosis are also subject to acute changes that can lead to sudden coronary thrombotic occlusion.

The extent of anatomic coronary disease in symptomatic patients varies greatly. Notwithstanding, critical coronary stenoses often develop in the presence of multifocal and diffuse disease, which can lead to underestimation of the extent and severity of coronary atherosclerosis on coronary arteriograms (luminograms) (Fig. 4–4).[17]

Complications of Coronary Atherosclerosis

Acute ischemic heart disease is often initiated by secondary changes (complications) that occur in atherosclerotic plaques (Fig. 4–5),[18–20] particularly endothelial injury and disruptions of the plaque surface that lead to fissures, erosion, ulceration, or rupture (Figs. 4–6 to 4–9). These changes predispose the surface to platelet activation, initiation of the coagulation cascade, and formation of mural (nonocclusive) thrombi and occlusive thrombi.[21–28] Coronary lesions at risk for acute changes are atheromatous plaques with thin fibrous capsules and large cores of lipid-rich debris. Hemodynamic trauma, local attachment, and activation of platelets and blood cells, and the cytotoxic effects of plaque contents all contribute to endothelial injury and plaque disruption. The process of injury and disruption can advance to include an influx of blood components, an increase in intraplaque pressure, and an outward rupture of the fibrous capsule. Intraluminal and intramural (intraplaque) thrombus and intraplaque hemorrhage often develop. Intraplaque hemorrhage also can occur without plaque surface changes. Such hemorrhages, which arise from leakage from intraplaque vessels, are rarely clinically significant. Vasospasm induced by vasoactive products released from activated platelets can contribute to coronary occlusion.[18–21] Occasionally, coronary vasospasm occurs as a clinical syndrome in the apparent absence of the plaque changes described above.[18–28]

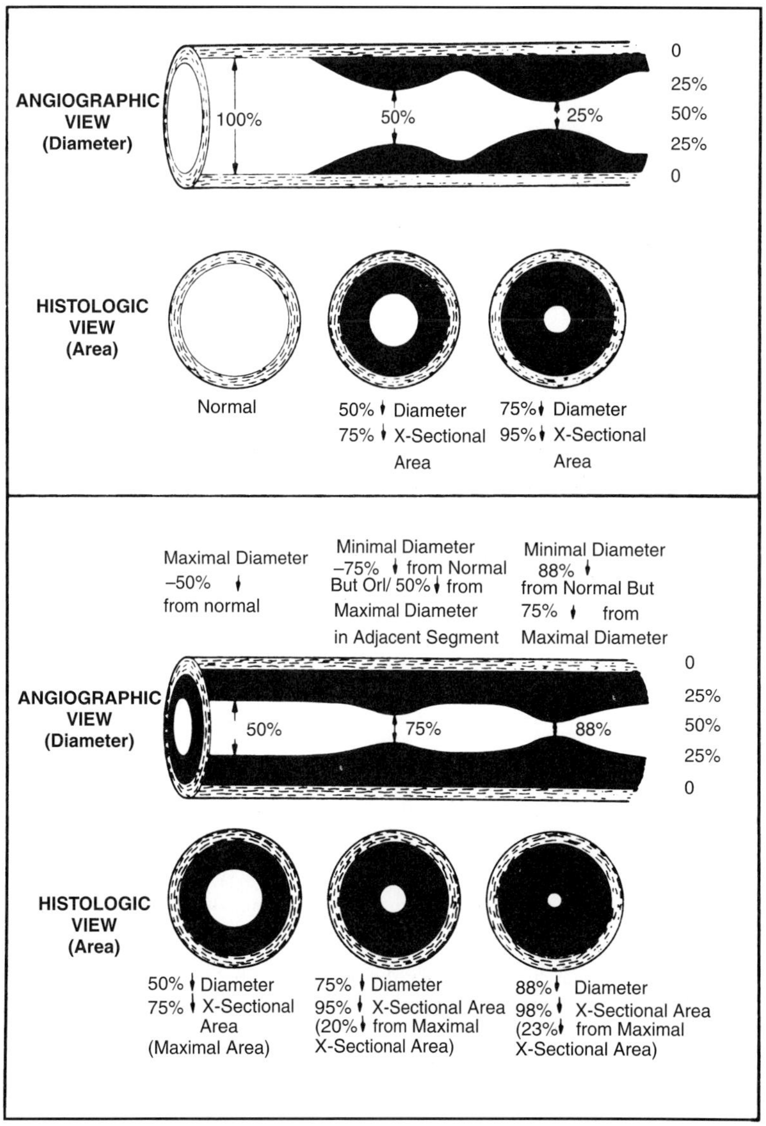

FIGURE 4–4. Relationship between reduction in diameter (as seen by selective coronary arteriography) and cross-sectional area (as seen by histologic examination). *Top*, A coronary artery with a 50% reduction in diameter narrowing has a 75% decrease in cross-sectional area, and a coronary artery with a 75% reduction in diameter narrowing has a 95% reduction in cross-sectional area. *Bottom*, In many patients who undergo coronary arteriography, stenosed segments are not compared with totally normal segments but with segments of the coronary artery that are somewhat diffusely narrowed. Thus, if the least-narrowed segment is actually 50% narrowed, then what appears to be a 50% narrowing in the diameter of an adjacent segment is, in fact, a 75% narrowing and therefore a 95% reduction in cross-sectional area. Similarly, what appears to be a 75% diameter narrowing is actually an 88% diameter narrowing, which corresponds to a 98% reduction in cross-sectional diameter. Because many patients with coronary artery disease have diffuse luminal narrowings in addition to discrete stenoses, the bottom panel more accurately reflects the true clinical situation. (From Arnett EN, Isner JM, Redwood DR, et al: Coronary artery narrowing in coronary heart disease: Comparison of cineangiographic and necropsy findings. Ann Intern Med 91:350–356, 1979.)

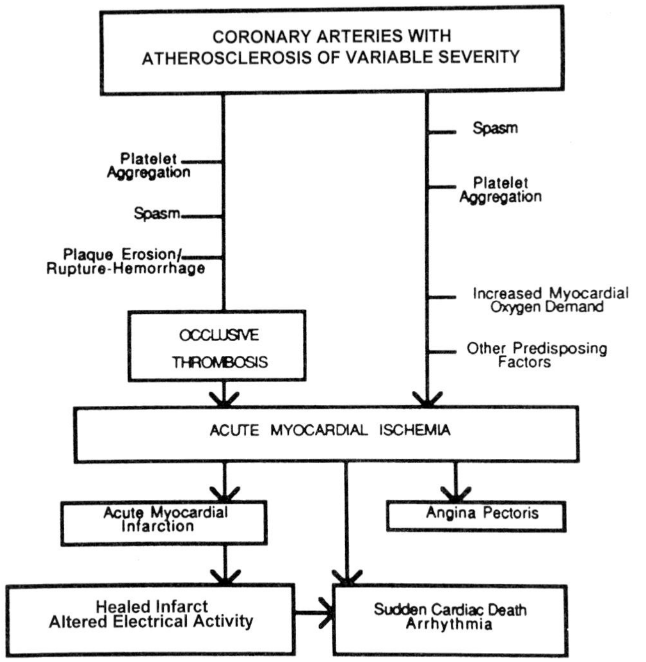

FIGURE 4–5. Pathogenetic mechanisms of acute ischemic heart disease and potential clinical outcomes. (From Buja LM, Hillis LD, Petty CS, Willerson JT: The role of coronary arterial spasm in ischemic heart disease. Arch Pathol Lab Med 105:221–226, 1981.)

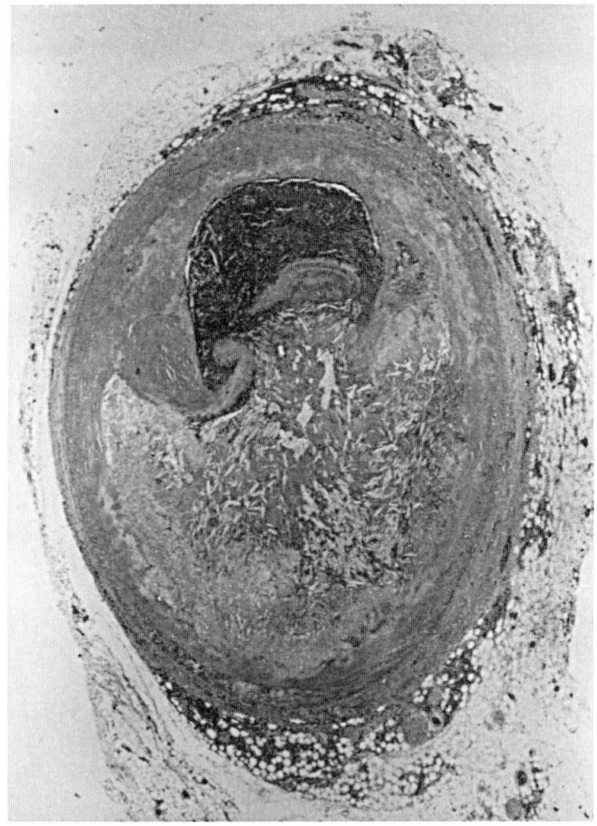

FIGURE 4–7. Histopathologic features of a coronary occlusion with plaque rupture and thrombosis. This atherosclerotic plaque shows rupture of the capsule, outward displacement of plaque contents across the rupture site, and communication with the overlying thrombus. (From Buja LM, Willerson JT: Clinicopathologic correlates of acute ischemic heart disease syndromes. Am J Cardiol 47:343–356, 1981, with permission from Excerpta Medica, Inc.)

NONATHEROSCLEROTIC CORONARY VASCULAR LESIONS

In some cases, the coronary arteries are free of atherosclerosis and the clinical syndrome results from one of a diverse spectrum of coronary lesions, including congenital anomalies, dissection (Fig. 4–10), emboli, and vasculitis (Table 4–1).[29] Isolated coronary artery dissection has an increased incidence in peripartal women.[30]

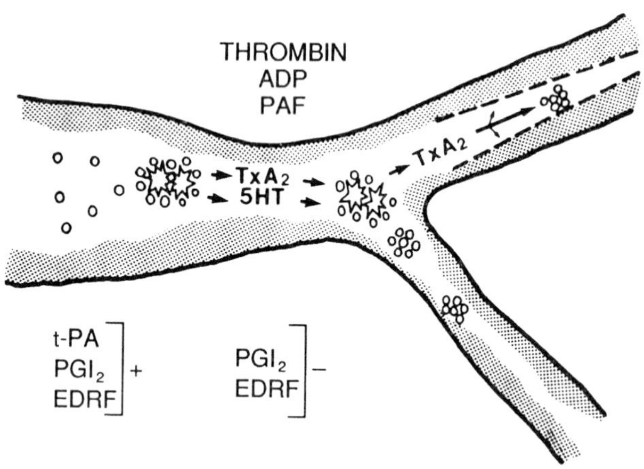

FIGURE 4–6. Schematic diagram indicating the possible mechanisms by which thromboxane A_2 (TxA_2), serotonin (5HT), adenosine diphosphate (ADP), platelet-activating factor (PAF), and thrombin promote platelet aggregation and decrease coronary blood flow in patients with ischemic heart disease. Aggregating platelets (stars) release TxA_2, 5HT, ADP, PAF, and thrombin at sites of coronary artery stenosis and endothelial injury, which causes further platelet aggregation in the coronary artery, dynamic coronary vasoconstriction, and partial or total coronary artery thrombosis. Absence or reductions in endothelially derived relaxing factor (EDRF), prostacylin (PGI_2), and tissue plasminogen activating factor (t-PA) at vascular sites with endothelial injury, and release of endothelins probably contribute to the development of vasoconstriction and thrombosis. (From Willerson JT, Yao S-K, Ferguson JJ, et al: Unstable angina pectoris and the progression to acute myocardial infarction: role of platelets and platelet-derived mediators. Texas Heart Inst J 18:243–247, 1991.)

PATHOLOGIC CORRELATES OF CLINICAL SYNDROMES

The clinical syndromes of acute ischemic heart disease are angina pectoris, sudden cardiac death, and acute myocardial infarction. Ordinary angina pectoris is usually associated with significant atherosclerotic narrowing of one or more of the major coronary arteries.[18–21] Unstable angina pectoris and related syndromes (preinfarction angina, coronary insufficiency) are often associated with coronary atherosclerosis complicated by degeneration of the endothelium and capsule of a plaque (so-called unstable plaque). This coronary atherosclerosis often is superimposed on unstable angina in some patients, platelet aggregates or nonocclusive thrombi are often superimposed on the plaque, and platelet aggregates may be found in the microcirculation of the myocardium.[18–21, 26, 31, 32] Unstable angina pectoris may be a precursor of acute myocardial infarction.[22–28]

Sudden cardiac death is associated with significant atherosclerotic narrowing of at least one coronary artery in 90% of cases.[33–37] Multifocal myocardial scarring or healed infarction

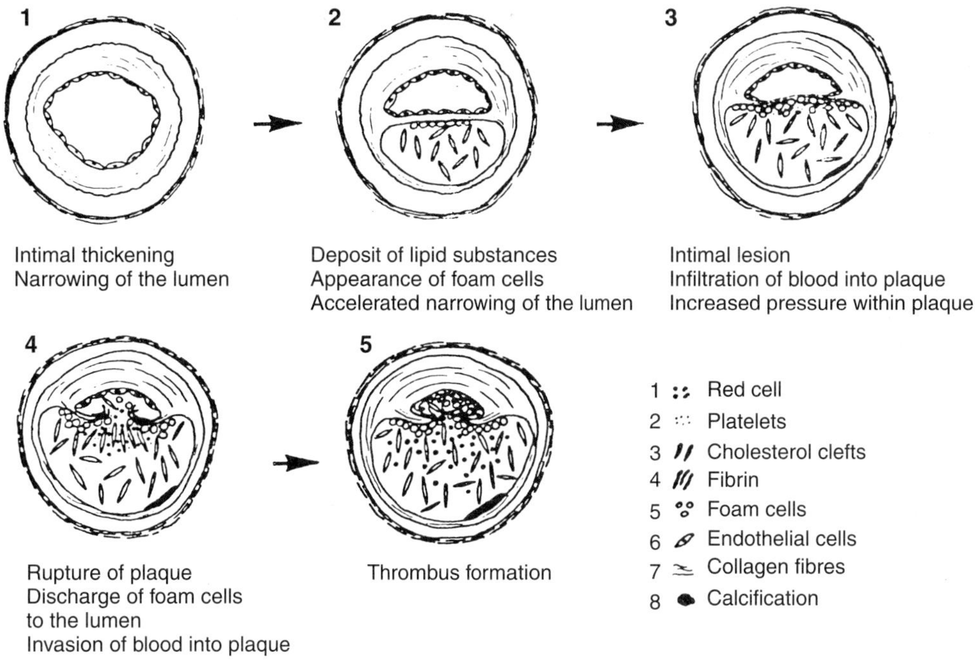

FIGURE 4–8. Postulated sequence of events leading to rupture of a coronary plaque. (From Horie T, Sekiguchi M, Hirosawa K: Coronary thrombosis in pathogenesis of acute myocardial infarction: Histopathological study of coronary arteries in 108 necropsied cases using serial section. Br Heart J 40:152–161, 1978.)

also is common. In most patients, an acute myocardial infarction cannot be seen anatomically. Acute coronary plaque alterations and thrombosis are seen in many cases, although there is significant variation from study to study. Platelet aggregates in the coronary circulation have been documented in a significant subset of patients, particularly in those with a history of unstable angina pectoris.[31, 32] Thus, clinicopathologic studies are consistent with three major mechanisms of sudden cardiac death: ischemia-induced ventricular arrhythmia without acute myocardial infarction, acute myocardial infarction with ventricular arrhythmia, and primary ventricular arrhythmia associated with old myocardial damage and altered electrical conduction (see Fig. 4–5).[33]

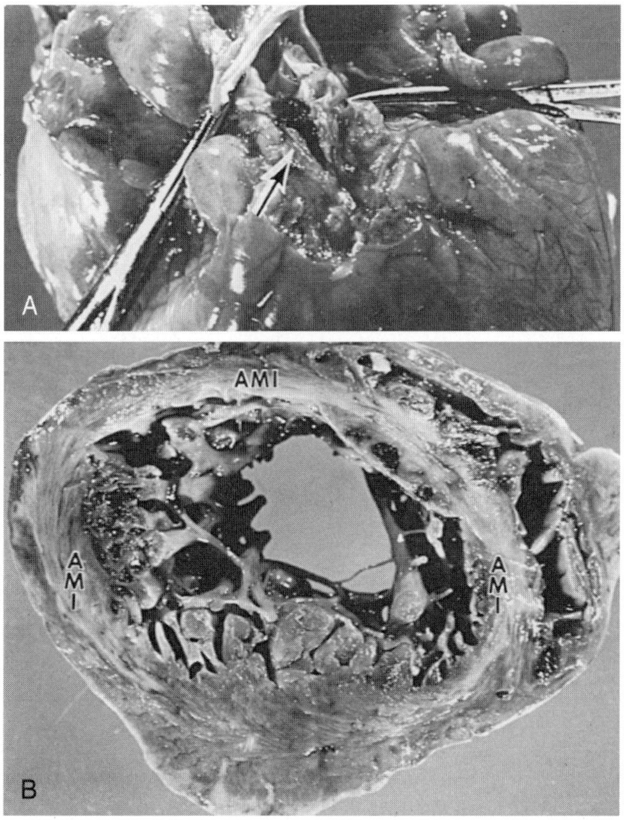

FIGURE 4–9. External view *(A)* and cut section *(B)* of a heart with coronary atherosclerosis, acute thrombosis of the proximal left anterior descending coronary artery *(arrow)*, and a massive acute anterior septal and lateral transmural myocardial infarction (AMI). (From Willerson JT, Hillis LD, Buja, LM: Pathogenesis and pathology of ischemic heart disease. In Willerson JT, Hillis LD, Buja LM [eds]: Ischemic Heart Disease: Clinical and Pathophysiological Aspects. Raven Press, New York, 1982, pp 7–83.)

Table 4–1. CAUSES OF MYOCARDIAL ISCHEMIA AND INFARCTION WITHOUT CORONARY ATHEROSCLEROSIS

CORONARY ARTERY DISEASE OTHER THAN ATHEROSCLEROSIS	
Arteritis	
Luetic	
Granulomatous (Takayasu's disease)	
Polyarteritis nodosa	
Mucocutaneous lymph node (Kawasaki's) syndrome	
Disseminated lupus erythematosus	
Rheumatoid arthritis	
Ankylosing spondylitis	
Trauma to coronary arteries	
Laceration	
Thrombosis	
Iatrogenic	
Coronary mural thickening with metabolic diseases or intimal proliferative disease	
Mucopolysaccharidoses (Hurler's disease)	
Homocystinuria	
Fabry's disease	
Amyloidosis	
Juvenile intimal sclerosis (idiopathic arterial calcification of infancy)	
Intimal hyperplasia associated with contraceptive steroids or with the postpartum period	
Pseudoxanthoma elasticum	
Coronary fibrosis caused by radiation therapy	
Luminal narrowing by other mechanisms	
Spasm of coronary arteries (Prinzmetal's angina with normal coronary arteries)	
Spasm after nitroglycerin withdrawal	
Dissection of the aorta	
Dissection of the coronary artery	
EMBOLI TO CORONARY ARTERIES	
Infective endocarditis	
Prolapse of mitral valve	
EMBOLI TO CORONARY ARTERIES *(Continued)*	
Mural thrombus from left atrium, left ventricle	
Prosthetic valve emboli	
Cardiac myxoma	
Associated with cardiopulmonary bypass surgery and coronary arteriography	
Paradoxical emboli	
Papillary fibroelastoma of the aortic valve ("fixed embolus")	
CONGENITAL CORONARY ARTERY ANOMALIES	
Anomalous origin of left coronary from pulmonary artery	
Left coronary artery from anterior sinus of Valsalva	
Coronary arteriovenous and arteriocameral fistulae	
Coronary artery aneurysms	
MYOCARDIAL OXYGEN DEMAND-SUPPLY DISPROPORTION	
Aortic stenosis, all forms	
Incomplete differentiation of the aortic valve	
Aortic insufficiency	
Carbon monoxide poisoning	
Thyrotoxicosis	
Prolonged hypotension	
HEMATOLOGIC (IN SITU THROMBOSIS)	
Polycythemia vera	
Thrombocytosis	
Disseminated intravascular coagulation	
Hypercoagulability	
Hypercoagulability, thrombosis, thrombocytopenic purpura	
MISCELLANEOUS	
Myocardial contusion	
Myocardial infarction with normal coronary arteries	

Modified from Cheitlin MD, McAllister HA, de Castro CM, et al.: Myocardial infarction without atherosclerosis. JAMA 231:951, 1975. Copyright 1975, American Medical Association.

PATHOGENESIS OF ACUTE MYOCARDIAL ISCHEMIC INJURY AND REPERFUSION EFFECTS

The progression of cell injury in myocardial ischemia following coronary occlusion involves complex metabolic and structural alterations.[38, 39] The extent of membrane damage determines whether ischemic cell injury is reversible. This damage is caused by an excessive accumulation of calcium, degradation or peroxidation of membrane phospholipids, and damage to the cytoskeleton (Fig. 4–11). Recent studies have suggested that apoptosis and necrosis may contribute to muscle cell death induced by coronary occlusion or reperfusion.[40, 41] However, this concept requires confirmation.[42, 43]

After 20 to 30 minutes of coronary occlusion, irreversible myocardial injury begins in the ischemic subendocardium.[44–48] The oxygen demand-supply balance of the subendocardium is normally narrower than that of the subepicardium and, with coronary occlusion, the subepicardium develops a more severe reduction in perfusion (Fig. 4–12). Over the ensuing 3 to 4 hours, irreversible myocardial injury progresses in a wavefront pattern from the subendocardium into the subepicardium of the myocardium-at-risk. In some cases, a slower pattern of myocardial infarction evolves when the previously established coronary collateral perfusion is abundant or when the stimulus for myocardial ischemia is intermittent, as in the case of episodes of intermittent platelet aggregation before occlusive thrombosis. These episodes of intermittent platelet aggregation are often manifested as unstable angina pectoris, which evolves into acute myocardial infarction.

The progression of myocardial ischemia can be pro-

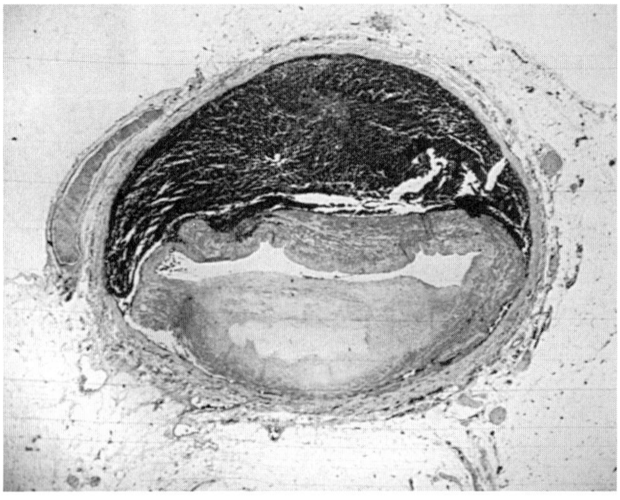

FIGURE 4–10. Spontaneous dissection of the left main coronary artery of a 58-year-old woman with a history of hypertension. (From Dowling GP, Buja LM: Spontaneous coronary artery dissection occurs with and without periadventitial inflammation. Arch Pathol Lab Med 111:470–472, 1987.)

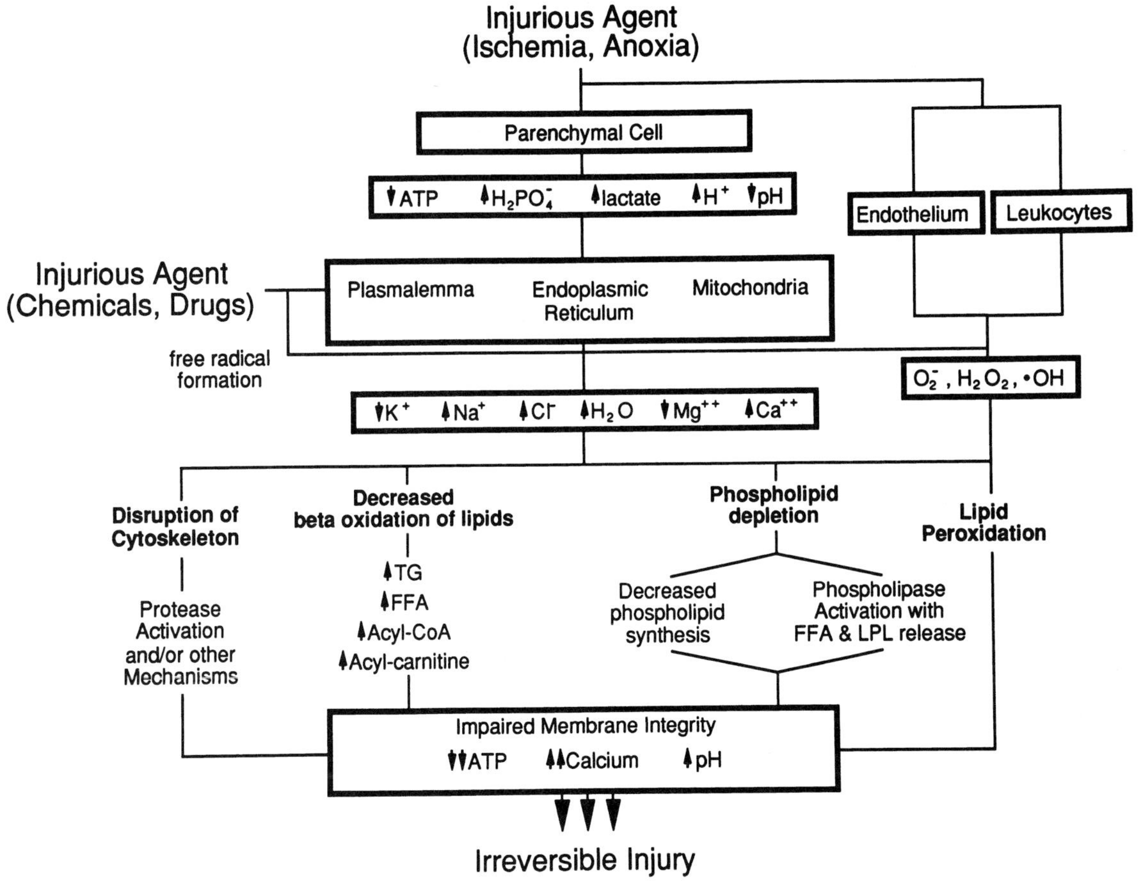

FIGURE 4–11. Postulated sequence of alterations involved in the pathogenesis of irreversible myocardial ischemic injury. Oxygen deficiency induces metabolic changes including decreased ATP, decreased pH, and lactate accumulation in ischemic myocytes. The altered metabolic milieu leads to impaired membrane transport with resulting disturbances in intracellular electrolytes. An increase in cytosolic Ca^{2+} can trigger the activation of proteases and phospholipases, which can result in cytoskeletal damage and an impaired balance in membrane phospholipids. Lipid alterations include increased phospholipid (PL) degradation with release of free fatty acids (FFA) and lysophospholipids (LPL) and decreased phospholipid synthesis. Lipid peroxidation occurs as a result of attacks by free radicals produced in part by the generation of excess electrons (e-) in oxygen-deprived mitochondria. Free radicals may also come from metabolism of arachidonic acid and catecholamines, metabolism of adenine nucleotides by xanthine oxidase in endothelium (species dependent), and activation of neutrophils and macrophages. The irreversible phase of injury appears to be mediated by the severe membrane damage produced by phospholipid loss, lipid peroxidation, and cytoskeletal damage. (From Buja LM: Lipid abnormalities in myocardial cell injury. Trends Cardiovasc Med 1:40–45, 1991, with permission from Elsevier Science.)

foundly influenced by reperfusion, which may occur spontaneously or may be therapeutically induced by thrombolytic therapy or percutaneous transluminal coronary angioplasty.[49–51] The effects of reperfusion are complex and comprise several phenomena including (1) salvage of previously ischemic myocardium, (2) reperfusion injury of previously ischemic myocardium, (3) myocardial stunning, and (4) myocardial preconditioning. Clearly, reperfusion can limit the extent of myocardial necrosis if it is instituted early enough after the onset of coronary occlusion. However, reperfusion changes the pattern of myocardial injury by causing hemorrhage within the severely damaged myocardium and by producing a pattern of myocardial injury characterized by contraction bands and calcification (Fig. 4–13). Reperfusion also accelerates the release of intracellular enzymes and other intracellular constituents from damaged myocardium. This release of factors may lead to a marked elevation of serum levels of myocardial damage markers without necessarily implying further myocardial necrosis.

Although reperfusion can salvage myocardium, it can also cause additional injury. The term reperfusion injury refers to the development of reperfusion-induced damage to myocytes that were injured during an ischemic episode but remained viable. Such injury may involve functional impairment, arrhythmia, or progression to cell death. Clinical documentation of reperfusion-induced necrosis is difficult given the effects of reperfusion on serum markers of necrosis, as discussed earlier. Nevertheless, experimental studies have provided some evidence that reperfusion injury does occur.[49–51] Obviously, the timing of reperfusion is critical to the outcome. The earlier the reperfusion occurs, the greater the potential is for net salvage to exceed damage.

Two other phenomena associated with reperfusion are myocardial stunning and myocardial preconditioning. Myocardial stunning refers to prolonged functional myocardial depression, requiring approximately 24 hours or more for recovery, which develops on reperfusion, even after a relatively brief period of coronary occlusion that is insufficient to cause myocardial necrosis.[49–51] The effects of free radicals and calcium loading have been implicated in the pathogenesis of stunning, as have other components of reperfusion injury.[52–54] Myocardial preconditioning refers to the benefi-

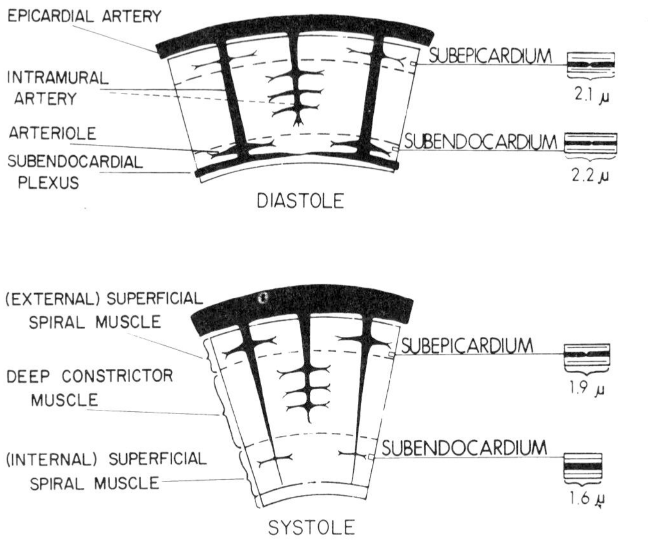

FIGURE 4–12. Cross-section of the left ventricular wall in diastole and systole. Factors that affect the susceptibility of the subendocardium to the development of ischemia include this region's greater dependence on diastolic perfusion and its greater degree of shortening and energy expenditure during systole. (From Bell JR, Fox AC: Pathogenesis of subendocardial ischemia. Am J Med Sci 268:2–13, 1974.)

cial effect, specifically a retardation of the rate of progression of myocardial necrosis with coronary occlusion, induced by prior short intervals of coronary occlusion and reperfusion.[55, 56] Experimental evidence specifically indicates that the extent of myocardial necrosis following 60 to 90 minutes of coronary occlusion is significantly less in animals that have been pretreated with one or more 5-minute intervals of coronary occlusion before the induction of permanent occlusion.[55, 56] However, after 120 minutes of coronary occlusion, infarct size is the same with or without preconditioning. A reduced rate of adenosine triphosphate (ATP) depletion correlates with the beneficial effects of preconditioning.[55, 56] Further studies have suggested that activation of ATP-dependent potassium channels, via adenosine receptors and protein kinase C, may mediate the process of preconditioning, probably by reducing the duration of the action potential and the associated calcium influx.[57]

All of the factors discussed earlier lead to the conclusion that the major determinants of infarct size are the duration and severity of ischemia, the size of the myocardial bed-at-risk, and the amount of collateral blood flow available shortly after coronary occlusion. Infarct size also can be influenced by the major determinants of myocardial metabolic demand: heart rate, wall tension (determined by blood pressure), and myocardial contractility.[58]

PATHOLOGY OF ACUTE MYOCARDIAL INFARCTION

Established myocardial infarcts have distinct central and peripheral regions and a border zone, based on histologic and ultrastructural features (Fig. 4–14).[44–47] In the central zone of severe ischemia, necrotic myocytes exhibit clumped nuclear chromatin, stretched myofibrils with widened I bands, mitochondria containing amorphous matrix (flocculent) densities composed of denatured lipid and protein, linear densities of fused cristae, and defects (holes) in the sarcolemma. In the peripheral region of the infarct, which has some collateral perfusion, many necrotic myocytes exhibit disrupted myofibrils with dense transverse (contraction) bands, mitochondria containing calcium phosphate deposits and amorphous matrix densities, variable amounts of lipid droplets, and clumped nuclear chromatin. A third population of cells at the outermost periphery of the infarct constitutes a border zone; these myocytes contain an excess number of lipid droplets but do not exhibit the features of irreversible injury described above. The pattern of injury seen in the infarcted periphery is also characteristic of myocardial injury produced by temporary coronary occlusion followed by reperfusion. Although some authors have published electron micrographs, which they have interpreted as characteristic

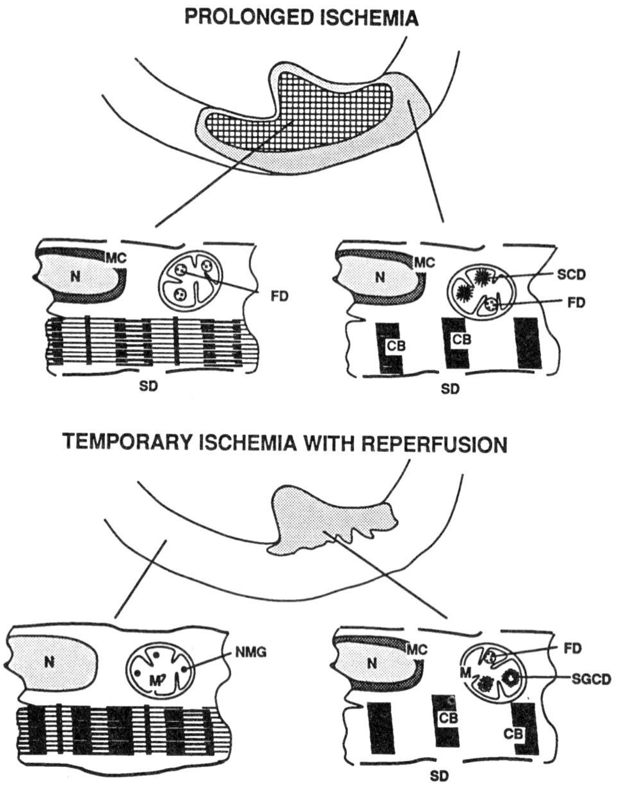

FIGURE 4–13. Schematic diagram comparing pathobiologic features of a transmural infarction produced by permanent coronary occlusion *(upper panel)* and a subendocardial infarction produced by temporary coronary occlusion followed by reperfusion *(lower panel)*. With prolonged coronary occlusion, myocardial necrosis is established in the subendocardium within 40 to 60 minutes, progresses in a wavefront pattern into the subepicardium of the region at risk (risk zone), and is complete in 3 to 6 hours. In prolonged coronary occlusion, the myofibrils of myocytes in the central infarction region are hyperrelaxed compared with those in the normal tissue depicted in the lower panel, and their mitochondria contain flocculent densities of denatured lipid and protein. The myofibrils of myocytes in the peripheral infarction region form contraction bands, and the mitochondria show calcium deposits and flocculent densities. With temporary ischemia and reperfusion, injury is limited to the subendocardium and is characterized by myofibrillar contraction bands and early mitochondrial calcification. (CB, contraction band; FD, flocculent (amorphous) density; MC, marginated chromatin; N, nucleus; NMG, normal matrix granule; SD, sarcolemmal defect; SCD, large spicular calcium deposit; SGCD, small granular calcium deposit.) (From Hagler HK, Buja LM: Subcellular calcium shifts in ischemia and reperfusion. In Piper HM [ed]: Pathophysiology of Severe Ischemic Myocardial Injury. Kluwer Academic Publishers, Dordrecht/Boston/London, 1990, pp 283–296.)

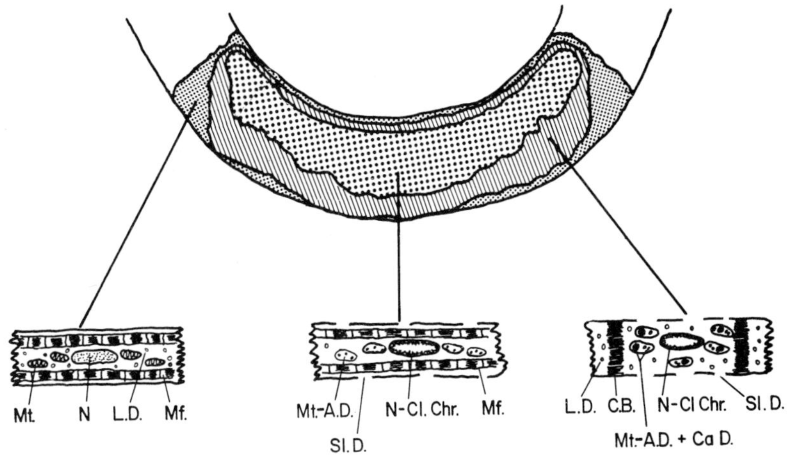

FIGURE 4–14. Patterns of myocardial injury in an acute transmural myocardial infarction. (CB, myofibrillar contraction band; LD, lipid droplet; Mf, myofibril; Mt, mitochondrion; Mt-AD, mitochondrion with amorphous matrix (flocculent) densities; Mt AD + CaD, mitochondrion with amorphous matrix densities and calcium phosphate deposits; N, nucleus; N-Cl Chr, nucleus with clumped chromatin; SlD, sarcolemmal defect.) (From Buja LM: Basic pathological processes of the heart: Relationship to cardiomyopathies. In Sperelakis N [ed]: Physiology and Pathophysiology of the Heart, 3rd ed. Kluwer Academic Publishers, Boston, 1995, p 37.)

of early stages of apoptosis involving ischemic or reperfused myocardium, the full spectrum of morphologic changes characteristic of apoptosis in ischemic or reperfused myocardium has yet to be reported.[39–43]

Myocardial infarcts usually involve the left ventricle (see Fig. 4–9).[1, 59] Right ventricular infarcts occur in association with left ventricular infarcts, particularly posterior transmural left ventricular infarcts. Occasionally, they are isolated entities occurring in association with pulmonary hypertension. Most myocardial infarcts are confined to a single coronary artery and are designated anterior, anteroseptal, lateral, and posteroinferior. Multiregional infarcts also occur. Myocardial infarcts are characterized as subendocardial, when the necrosis is limited to the inner half of the ventricular wall, or transmural, when the necrosis extends from the subendocardium into the outer half of the ventricular wall. On electrocardiogram, the ST-segment elevation–Q wave pattern is seen in transmural infarcts and the ST-segment depression–non-Q wave pattern is seen in subendocardial infarcts.

The overall incidence of occlusive coronary thrombosis and associated plaque fissure or rupture is high (more than 75%) for acute myocardial infarction.[22–28] The thrombus typically involves the major coronary artery in the distribution of the infarcted myocardium. However, the incidence of thrombosis differs significantly with the type of infarct. In autopsy studies, occlusive coronary thrombi are found in more than 90% of cases of transmural myocardial infarction but only in about a third of cases of subendocardial myocardial infarction. Subendocardial infarction without occlusive thrombosis is related to the influence of other factors such as more subtle coronary lesions (platelet aggregation, nonocclusive thrombi) or factors that increase myocardial oxygen demand (aortic stenosis, systemic hypertension, cardiac hypertrophy, excessive stress, or exertion). The relatively frequent occurrence of subendocardial infarction without occlusive thrombosis confirms the increased susceptibility of the subendocardium to ischemic injury.

The major complications of acute myocardial infarction are infarct expansion (shape change leading to stretching and thinning of the ventricular wall), infarct extension (additional necrosis), ventricular aneurysm, cardiogenic shock or recurrent ventricular arrhythmias related to large infarct size (generally greater than 33% to 40% of left ventricular mass), papillary muscle dysfunction, papillary muscle rupture, external cardiac rupture, ventricular pseudoaneurysm (due to sealing off of a relatively slowly evolving rupture), ventricular septal rupture, pericarditis (nonspecific and autoimmune, e.g., Dressler's syndrome), systemic embolization from a left ventricular mural thrombus, and pulmonary thromboembolism.[60]

The risk of infarct rupture is greatest during the first week of myocardial infarction, before significant organization of the necrotic tissue.[60, 61] Healing of a myocardial infarct involves neutrophilic infiltration, followed by formation of granulation tissue, which is grossly visible at approximately 10 days and completely replaces necrotic tissue in 2 to 3 weeks. Thereafter, the granulation tissue is converted to a dense scar; and the healing process is complete in 2 to 3 months.

After multifocal myocardial necrosis or regional infarction, the surviving myocardium undergoes complex changes in response to the myocardial damage. These changes, collectively referred to as myocardial or ventricular remodeling, involve changes in individual myocytes, which include hypertrophy and possibly hyperplasia and apoptosis, and changes in ventricular geometry.[61–64] In patients with milder insults, ventricular remodeling is useful. In patients with more severe insults, ventricular remodeling may be inadequate, and increased wall stress may persist.[65] The result can be chronic ischemic heart disease of variable severity, including the extreme condition of ischemic cardiomyopathy.[65]

References

1. Willerson JT, Hillis LD, Buja LM: Pathogenesis and pathology of ischemic heart disease. In Willerson JT, Hillis LD, Buja LM (eds): Ischemic Heart Disease: Clinical and Pathophysiological Aspects. Raven Press, New York, 1982, pp 7–83.
2. James TN: The coronary circulation and conduction system in acute myocardial infarction. Prog Cardiovasc Dis 10:410–446, 1968.
3. Baroldi G: Diseases of extramural coronary arteries. In Silver MD (ed): Cardiovascular Pathology, 2nd ed. Churchill Livingstone, New York, 1991, pp 487–563.
4. Buja LM: Basic pathological processes of the heart: Relationship to cardiomyopathies. In Sperelakis N (ed): Physiology and Pathophysiology of the Heart, 3rd ed. Kluwer Academic Publishers, Boston, 1995, pp 37–53.
5. Linzbach AJ: Heart failure from the point of view of quantitative anatomy. Am J Cardiol 5:370–382, 1960.

6. Eysmann SB, Douglas PS: Reperfusion and revascularization strategies for coronary artery disease in women. JAMA 268:1903–1907, 1992.
7. Weintraub WS, Wenger NK, Kosinski AS, et al: Percutaneous transluminal coronary angioplasty in women compared to men. J Am Coll Cardiol 24:81–90, 1994.
8. Schwartz CJ, Mitchell JRA: The morphology, terminology and pathogenesis of arterial plaques. Postgrad Med J 38:25–34, 1962.
9. Buja LM, Kovanen PT, Bilheimer DW: Cellular pathology of homozygous familial hypercholesterolemia. Am J Pathol 97:327–357, 1979.
10. Buja LM, Clubb FJ Jr, Bilheimer DW, Willerson JT: Pathobiology of human familial hypercholesterolemia and a related animal model, the Watanabe heritable hyperlipidemic rabbit. European Heart J 11(Suppl E):41–52, 1990.
11. Buja LM, Willerson JT, Murphree SS: Pathobiology of arterial wall injury, atherosclerosis, and coronary angioplasty. In Black AJR, Anderson HV, Ellis SG (eds): Complications of Coronary Angioplasty. Marcel Dekker, New York, 1991, pp 11–33.
12. Munro JM, Cotran RS: The pathogenesis of atherosclerosis: Atherogenesis and inflammation. Lab Invest 58:249–261, 1988.
13. Ross R: The pathogenesis of atherosclerosis: A perspective for the 1990s. Nature 362:801–809, 1993.
14. Libby P, Schoen FJ: Vascular lesion formation. Cardiovasc Pathol 2(Suppl):43S–52S, 1993.
15. Glagov S, Zarins C, Giddens DP, Nu DN: Hemodynamics and atherosclerosis: Insights and perspectives gained from studies of human arteries. Arch Pathol Lab Med 112:1018–1031, 1988.
16. Glagov S, Weisenberg E, Zarins CK, et al: Compensatory enlargement of human atherosclerotic coronary arteries. N Engl J Med 316:1371–1375, 1987.
17. Arnett EN, Isner JM, Redwood DR, et al: Coronary artery narrowing in coronary heart disease: Comparison of cineangiographic and necropsy findings. Ann Intern Med 91:350–356, 1979.
18. Buja LM, Hillis LD, Petty CS, Willerson JT: The role of coronary arterial spasm in ischemic heart disease. Arch Pathol Lab Med 105: 221–226, 1981.
19. Buja LM, Willerson JT: The role of coronary artery lesions in ischemic heart disease: Insights from recent clinicopathologic, coronary arteriographic, and experimental studies. Hum Pathol 18:451–461, 1987.
20. Fuster V, Badimon L, Badimon JJ, Chesebro JH: The pathogenesis of coronary artery disease and the acute coronary syndromes. N Engl J Med 326:242–250, 310–318, 1992.
21. Willerson JT, Yao S-K, Ferguson JJ, et al: Unstable angina pectoris and the progression to acute myocardial infarction: Role of platelets and platelet-derived mediators. Texas Heart Inst J 18:243–247, 1991.
22. Davies MJ, Woolf N, Robertson WB: Pathology of acute myocardial infarction with particular reference to occlusive coronary thrombi. Br Heart J 38:659–664, 1976.
23. Ridolfi RL, Hutchins GM: The relationship between coronary artery lesions and myocardial infarcts: Ulceration of atherosclerotic plaques precipitating coronary thrombosis. Am Heart J 93:468–486, 1977.
24. Horie T, Sekiguchi M, Hirosawa K: Coronary thrombosis in pathogenesis of acute myocardial infarction: Histopathological study of coronary arteries in 108 necropsied cases using serial section. Br Heart J 40: 152–161, 1978.
25. Davies MJ, Fulton WFM, Robertson WB: The relation of coronary thrombosis to ischemic myocardial necrosis. J Pathol 172:99–110, 1979.
26. Buja LM, Willerson JT: Clinicopathologic correlates of acute ischemic heart disease syndromes. Am J Cardiol 47:343–356, 1981.
27. Falk E: Plaque rupture with severe preexisting stenosis precipitating coronary thrombosis: Characteristics of coronary atherosclerotic plaques underlying fatal occlusive thrombi. Br Heart J 50:127–134, 1983.
28. Davies MJ, Thomas AEC: Plaque fissuring—the cause of acute myocardial infarction, sudden ischemic death, and crescendo angina. Br Heart J 53:363–373, 1985.
29. Cheitlin MD, McAllister HA, de Castro CM: Myocardial infarction without atherosclerosis. JAMA 231:951–959, 1975.
30. Dowling GP, Buja LM: Spontaneous coronary artery dissection occurs with and without periadventitial inflammation. Arch Pathol Lab Med 111:470–472, 1987.
31. El-Maraghi N, Genton E: The relevance of platelet and fibrin thromboembolism of the coronary microcirculation with special reference to sudden cardiac death. Circulation 62:936–944, 1980.
32. Davies MJ, Thomas AC, Knapman PA, Hangartner JR: Intramyocardial platelet aggregation in patients with unstable angina pectoris suffering sudden ischemic cardiac death. Circulation 73:418–427, 1986.
33. Buja LM, Willerson JT: Relationship of ischemic heart disease to sudden cardiac death. J Forensic Sci 36:25–33, 1991.
34. Reichenbach DD, Moss NS, Meyer E: Pathology of the heart in sudden cardiac death. Am J Cardiol 39:865–872, 1977.
35. Baroldi G, Falzi G, Mariani F: Sudden coronary death: A postmortem study in 208 selected cases compared to 97 "control" subjects. Am Heart J 98:20–31, 1979.
36. Warnes CA, Roberts WC: Sudden coronary death: Comparison of patients with to those without coronary thrombus at necropsy. Am J Cardiol 54:1206–1211, 1984.
37. Davies MJ, Thomas A: Thrombosis and acute coronary-artery lesions in sudden cardiac ischemic death. N Engl J Med 310:1137–1140, 1984.
38. Buja LM: Lipid abnormalities in myocardial cell injury. Trends Cardiovasc Med 1:40–45, 1991.
39. Buja LM, Eigenbrodt ML, Eigenbrodt EH: Apoptosis and necrosis: Basic types and mechanisms of cell death. Arch Pathol Lab Med 117: 1208–1214, 1993.
40. Gottlieb RA, Burleson KO, Kloner RA, et al: Reperfusion injury induces apoptosis in rabbit cardiomyocytes. J Clin Invest 94:1621–1628, 1994.
41. Kajstura J, Cheng W, Reiss K, et al: Apoptotic and necrotic myocyte cell deaths are independent contributing variables of infarct size in rats. Lab Invest 74:86–107, 1996.
42. Majno G, Joris I: Apoptosis, oncosis, and necrosis: An overview of cell death. Am J Pathol 146:3–15, 1995.
43. Buja LM, Entman ML: Modes of myocardial cell injury and cell death in ischemic heart disease. Circulation 98:1355–1357, 1998.
44. Reimer KA, Jennings RB: The "wavefront phenomenon" of myocardial ischemic cell death: II. Transmural progression of necrosis within the framework of ischemic bed size (myocardium at risk) and collateral flow. Lab Invest 40:633–644, 1979.
45. Reimer KA, Ideker RE: Myocardial ischemia and infarction: Anatomic and biochemical substrates for ischemic cell death and ventricular arrhythmias. Hum Pathol 18:462–475, 1987.
46. Buja LM, Hagler HK, Willerson JT: Altered calcium homeostasis in the pathogenesis of myocardial ischemic hypoxic injury. Cell Calcium 9:205–217, 1988.
47. Hagler HK, Buja LM: Subcellular calcium shifts in ischemia and reperfusion. In Piper HM (ed): Pathophysiology of Severe Ischemic Myocardial Injury. Kluwer Academic Publishers, Dordrecht/Boston/London, 1990, pp 283–296.
48. Bell JR, Fox AC: Pathogenesis of subendocardial ischemia. Am J Med Sci 268:2–13, 1974.
49. Weisfeldt ML: Reperfusion and reperfusion injury. Clin Res 35:13–20, 1987.
50. Hearse DJ, Bolli R: Reperfusion-induced injury: Manifestations, mechanisms and clinical relevance. Trends Cardiovasc Med 1:233–240, 1991.
51. Virmani R, Kolodgie FD, Forman MB, et al: Reperfusion injury in the ischemic myocardium. Cardiovasc Pathol 1:117–130, 1992.
52. Bolli R, Patel BS, Jeroudi MO, et al: Demonstration of free radical generation in "stunned" myocardium of intact dogs with the use of the spin trap alpha-phenyl N-tert-butyl nitrone. J Clin Invest 82:476–485, 1988.
53. Kusuoka H, Porterfield JK, Weisman HF, et al: Pathophysiology and pathogenesis of stunned myocardium: Depressed Ca^{2+} activation of contraction as a consequence of reperfusion-induced cellular calcium overload in ferret hearts. J Clin Invest 79:950–961, 1987.
54. Gao WD, Liu Y, Mellgren R, Marban E: Intrinsic myofilament alterations underlying the decreased contractility of stunned myocardium: A consequence of Ca^{2+}-dependent proteolysis? Circ Res 78:455–465, 1996.
55. Murry CE, Jennings RB, Reimer KA: Preconditioning with ischemia: a delay of lethal cell injury in ischemic myocardium. Circulation 74: 1124–1136, 1986.
56. Murry CE, Richard VJ, Reimer KA, Jennings RB: Ischemic preconditioning slows energy metabolism and delays ultrastructural damage during a sustained ischemic episode. Circ Res 66:913–931, 1990.
57. Liu Y, Gao WD, O'Rourke B, Marban E: Synergistic modulation of ATP-sensitive $K+$ currents by protein kinase C and adenosine: Implications for ischemic preconditioning. Circ Res 78:443–454, 1996.
58. Buja LM: Modulation of the myocardial response to ischemia. Lab Invest 76:1345–1373, 1998.
59. Olsen EGJ: Ischemic disease of the myocardium and its complications. In Silver MD (ed): Cardiovascular Pathology, 2nd ed. Churchill Livingstone, New York, 1991, pp 671–717.
60. Lavie CJ, Gersh BJ: Mechanical and electrical complications of acute myocardial infarction. Mayo Clin Proc 65:709–730, 1990
61. Kajstura J, Zhang X, Reiss X, et al: Myocyte cellular hyperplasia and

myocyte cellular hypertrophy contribute to chronic ventricular remodeling in coronary artery narrowing—induced cardiomyopathy in rats. Circ Res 74:383–400, 1994.
62. Sharov VG, Sabbah HN, Shimoyama H, et al: Evidence of cardiomyocyte apoptosis in myocardium of dogs with chronic heart failure. Am J Pathol 148:141–149, 1996.
63. Narula J, Haider N, Virmani R, et al: Apoptosis in myocytes in end-stage heart failure. N Engl J Med 335:1182–1189, 1996.
64. Nguyen ND, Buja LM: The role of ventricular wall stress in cardiac hypertrophy. Cardiovasc Pathol 3:19–31, 1994.
65. Anversa P, Sonnenblick EH: Ischemic cardiomyopathy: Pathophysiologic mechanisms. Prog Cardiovasc Dis 33:49–70, 1990.

| 4.2 | Pathophysiology, Clinical Recognition, and Diagnosis of Coronary Artery Disease

Renu Virmani, Andrew Farb, Allen P. Burke, and James T. Willerson

Angina pectoris is the clinical term used to describe chest pain resulting from a relative oxygen deficiency in heart muscle. The coronary heart disease syndromes are stable angina pectoris, unstable angina pectoris, variant angina (Prinzmetal's angina), acute myocardial infarction, non–Q-wave infarction (usually nontransmural), and Q-wave infarction (usually transmural). Heberden[1] named this entity when he identified a "disorder of the breast marked with strong and peculiar symptoms and considerable for the kind of danger belonging to it" associated with a "strangling and anxiety," which he suggested should be called "angina pectoris." This description was expanded by Herrick in 1912.[2] Angina is usually described by the patient as a left precordial tightness or ache, provoked by exercise or emotion and relieved by rest. Angina occurs when oxygen demand exceeds supply.[3–7]

PATHOPHYSIOLOGY OF STABLE ANGINA

Most individuals with angina have underlying atherosclerotic coronary artery disease (CAD). However, angina may also develop in some patients with ventricular hypertrophy, left ventricular (LV) outflow obstruction, severe aortic valvular regurgitation or stenosis, cardiomyopathy, or a dilated ventricle or ventricles in whom coronary artery stenosis is not present. This angina occurs because even normal coronary arteries may not adequately supply oxygen to hypertrophied, dilated, or failing heart muscle. On occasion, a limited coronary vasodilator reserve may explain angina, especially in some patients with ventricular hypertrophy associated with LV outflow obstruction, including valvular aortic stenosis and hypertrophic obstructive cardiomyopathy, and in patients with poorly controlled systemic arterial hypertension.[8, 9] Coronary artery vasoconstriction occurring with exercise or stress may also be a contributing factor.[10, 11] Most humans without coronary heart disease or ventricular hypertrophy do not develop angina, probably because the heart is protected from an important imbalance between oxygen supply and demand by other factors that limit physical activity, such as dyspnea and fatigue.

The predisposing pathologic alterations in coronary arteries responsible for angina are atherothrombosis and neointimal fibrous proliferation, that is, atherothrombosclerosis (Color Plate 4–1). The atherothrombosclerosis is more descriptive of the developmental process that has long been called *atherosclerosis* but, in fact, very often includes evidence of thrombosis in the progressive atherosclerotic plaque. Embolic atherosclerotic debris and platelet aggregates almost certainly play a role in more distal coronary artery occlusion and limitation of coronary flow reserve (Fig. 4–15). Severe narrowing of the coronary artery lumen results in a decreased ability of the artery to deliver oxygen, especially when oxygen demand in the heart is increased, as with increases in heart rate, contractile state, myocardial wall tension, or a combination of these.[3–7] Therefore, angina may develop during exercise, cold exposure, or emotional stress or after eating a large meal. Cold exposure decreases oxygen delivery by causing coronary artery vasoconstriction and increased systemic blood pressure, ventricular wall tension, and oxygen demand. Angina may also occur because of extracardiac influences. In particular, severe anemia or carbon monoxide exposure limits the capacity of the blood to carry or release oxygen and may result in angina under conditions that would otherwise be well tolerated. Increases in systemic arterial pressure and consequent dilatation of the heart may result in angina. Increases in heart rate or contractile state, as with hyperthyroidism, pheochromocytoma, and exogenous administration or release of catecholamines, may also lead to angina.

Women may have atypical chest discomfort when they have angina. Although they may describe the pain in classic fashion, they may also describe it as a "peculiar feeling," a knot or a sensation in their chest or neck or left arm that "worries them." An association of symptoms with effort or emotion is typical of stable angina.

PHYSICAL EXAMINATION AND BEDSIDE FINDINGS: STABLE ANGINA

The findings on physical examination in the patient with stable angina pectoris are highly variable. Sometimes, there

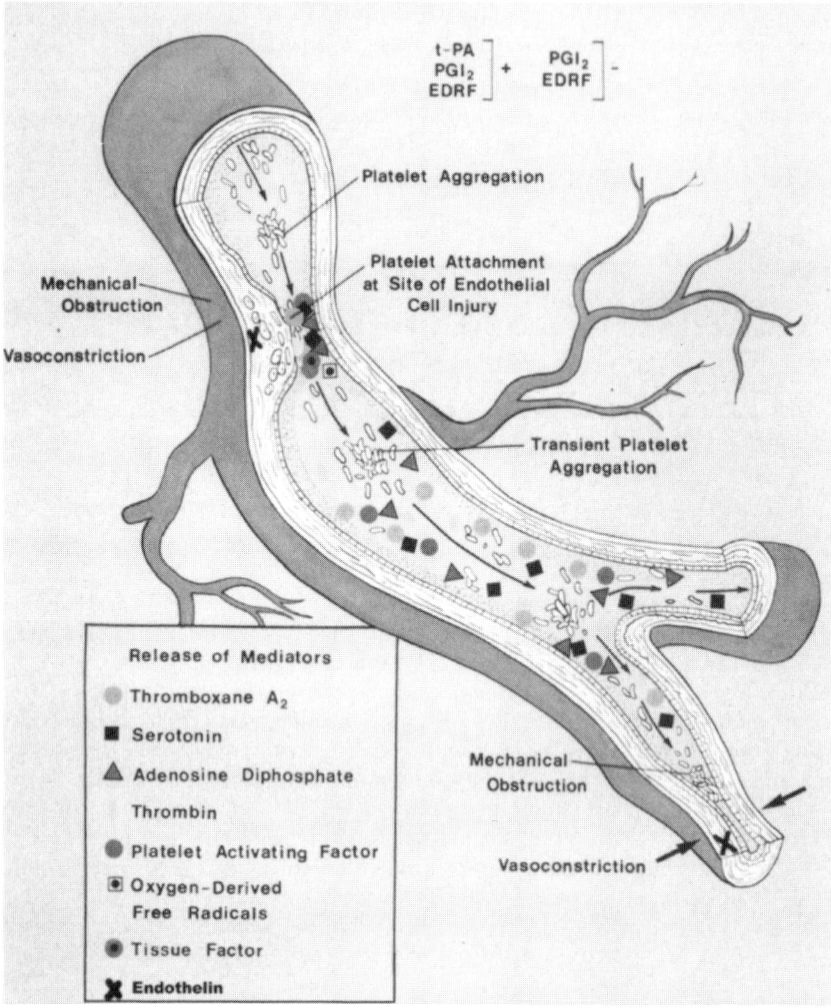

FIGURE 4–15. Probable mechanisms responsible for the conversion from chronic coronary heart disease to acute coronary artery disease syndromes. In this scheme, endothelial injury, generally at sites of atherosclerotic plaques and usually plaque ulceration or fissuring, is associated with platelet adhesion and aggregation, and the release and activation of selected mediators, including thromboxane A_2, serotonin, adenosine, diphosphate, platelet-activating factor, thrombin, oxygen-derived free radicals, and endothelin. Local accumulation of thromboxane A_2, serotonin, platelet-activating factor, thrombin, adenosine diphosphate, and tissue factor promotes platelet aggregation. Thromboxane A_2, serotonin, thrombin, and platelet-activating factor are vasoconstrictors at sites of endothelial injury. The conversion from chronic stable to acute unstable coronary heart disease syndromes is usually associated with endothelial injury, platelet aggregation, accumulation of platelet and other cell-derived mediators, further platelet aggregation, and vasoconstriction, with consequent dynamic narrowing of the coronary artery lumen. In addition to atherosclerotic plaque fissuring or ulceration, other reasons for endothelial injury include flow shear stress, hypertension, immune complex deposition and complement activation, infection, and mechanical injury to the endothelium as it occurs with coronary artery angioplasty and after heart transplantation. Endothelial injury also decreases endothelium-derived relaxing factor (EDRF), which is nitric oxide; prostaglandin I_2 (PGI_2); and tissue-type plasminogen activator (t-PA). (From Willerson JT: Medical treatment of coronary heart disease. In Willerson JT [ed]: Treatment of Heart Diseases. Gower Medical, New York, 1992, p 1.6; modified from Willerson JT, Golino P, Eidt JF, et al: Specific platelet mediators and unstable coronary artery lesions. Experimental evidence and potential clinical implications. Circulation 80:198, 1989, with permission.)

are no localizing or suggestive physical findings. Alternatively, associated risk factors such as systemic arterial hypertension, hyperlipidemia, valvular heart disease, heart failure, or peripheral atherosclerosis result in a specific physical finding, such as elevated blood pressure, a prominent fourth heart sound (S_4), accentuated aortic closure sound, a paradoxically split second heart sound (S_2) (resulting from systemic arterial hypertension during an episode of angina or reflecting left bundle branch block [LBBB]), reduced peripheral pulse (i.e., carotid, femoral, or lower extremity pulse with or without bruit over the artery [atherosclerosis]), murmur of aortic stenosis or mitral insufficiency (the most common valvular heart disease associated with CAD), or a third heart sound (S_3) with heart failure or rapid filling of the ventricle, such as occurs with moderately severe and severe mitral insufficiency. Thus, the patient with coronary heart disease and stable angina may or may not have an enlarged heart, frequent or complex ventricular premature beats, S_4, murmur of mitral insufficiency, S_3 and moist rales, and/or evidence of peripheral vascular disease.

The electrocardiogram (ECG) may be normal, or it may show ST- to T-wave changes, usually ST depression and T-wave flattening or inversion. Changes on ECG often vary on subsequent ECGs, with intermittent normalization and return to the abnormal pattern. The ST- to T-wave depression or inverted T waves may persist for weeks, presumably reflecting chronic ischemia. The ECG may also demonstrate ventricular ectopic beats or evidence of a prior Q-wave myocardial infarction (MI). An echocardiogram may be normal at rest or may show regional or global wall-motion abnormalities, including reduced LV ejection fraction or increased LV dimensions, consistent with myocardial ischemia or infarction, or mitral insufficiency. A chest x-ray study may show a normal-sized or enlarged heart, with or without heart failure. Coronary artery calcification may occasionally be seen on the chest x-ray.

Rapid-speed computed tomography (CT) (or electron beam [EB] CT) or fluoroscopy can be used to identify coronary artery calcification. Several studies[12–16] have shown that coronary calcium assessment using fluoroscopy or EBCT imaging has a sensitivity for significant angiographic stenosis comparable with that of exercise tests when used for symptomatic patients, but the specificity is lower. Symptomatic patients with coronary calcium have at least a fourfold increased risk of death or infarction when compared with patients with less or no coronary calcification. Either the fluoroscopic finding of at least one calcified coronary artery or the EBCT identification of a coronary calcium score exceeding 100 has been shown to be predictive of the presence of advanced coronary plaque and stenosis. These findings may be useful in making subsequent decisions about the need for invasive studies.

In general, greater degrees of calcification in coronary arteries are consistent with greater amounts of atherosclerotic plaque and more advanced coronary luminal diameter narrowing. Assessing coronary artery calcium can be done regardless of the patient's ability to exercise to a maximal level and regardless of the presence or absence of resting electrocardiographic abnormalities. The most valuable finding in the symptomatic patient is a negative EBCT study for coronary calcium. The negative predictive value of such a calcium scan for significant stenosis of a major coronary artery is greater than 90%. Thus, EBCT scanning might be an appropriate first test in individuals with atypical cardiac symptoms in whom the likelihood for ischemic disease is considered to be small by the responsible physician. Patients with a zero or very low calcium score (i.e., <10) may be reassured and further testing may be directed at noncardiac causes of chest pain. On the other hand, if the calcium score is consistent with moderate or severe atherosclerotic plaque development, additional cardiac evaluation, including stress testing with or without perfusion or functional evaluation, may be indicated.

Hemodynamic monitoring typically shows increases in mean pulmonary capillary wedge pressure during episodes of angina pectoris. With the onset of myocardial ischemia, the initial hemodynamic change in the left ventricle is a decrease in myocardial compliance and an increase in stiffness. This results in a sharp increase in mean pulmonary capillary wedge pressure during angina, with a return to baseline as the angina resolves. The change in compliance is followed by ST- to T-wave changes on the ECG, a decline in regional systolic wall thickening, and finally the development of chest pain, with this entire sequence occurring within a few seconds.

Asymptomatic patients differ from symptomatic patients in that the risk of subsequent morbid events is relatively small. Data available at this time are not conclusive regarding whether coronary calcification in asymptomatic individuals can predict short-term risks.[12] Prevalence-risk relationships, however, decrease with age (Fig. 4–16). Although serious overprediction may occur in the young, overprediction is only moderate in the elderly.

PATHOPHYSIOLOGY OF UNSTABLE ANGINA

Angina occuring in a crescendo pattern, with limited physical activity or at rest, is known as *unstable angina.* The chest discomfort is typically milder than that which occurs with acute MI. The pain is usually not severe in character and is described as recurrent chest or epigastric tightness or pressure. Typically, the episodes of angina last less than 30 minutes; they may or may not be associated with nausea. On occasion, however, unstable angina is associated with more severe and prolonged chest pain and nausea, making its differentiation from acute MI at the bedside difficult. In these situations, serial ECGs and measurement of serum creatine kinase (CK) and its relatively specific cardiac isoenzyme, CK-MB, and of troponin I and/or T are needed to distinguish unstable angina from acute MI.

Unstable angina is usually caused by a primary decrease in coronary blood flow and myocardial oxygen delivery that occurs as a consequence of fissuring of atherosclerotic plaque, ulceration, or other injury.[17–20] Fissuring or ulceration is followed by platelet adhesion and aggregation at the site of plaque disruption and by transient thrombosis and dynamic vasoconstriction. Platelet adhesion occurs by platelet attachment to exposed collagen and to von Willebrand binding sites, largely through platelet glycoprotein Ib receptors. Thrombosis and vasoconstriction are promoted by the local accumulation of powerful promoters of platelet aggregation and vasoconstriction at these same sites, including thromboxane A_2, serotonin, adenosine diphosphate, selected leukotrienes, platelet-activating factor, thrombin, oxygen-derived free radicals, and endothelin (see Fig. 4–15).[17–37] Unstable angina may also occur in the individual with a severe coronary artery stenosis or a partially occluded coronary artery when myocardial oxygen demand is increased by emotion,

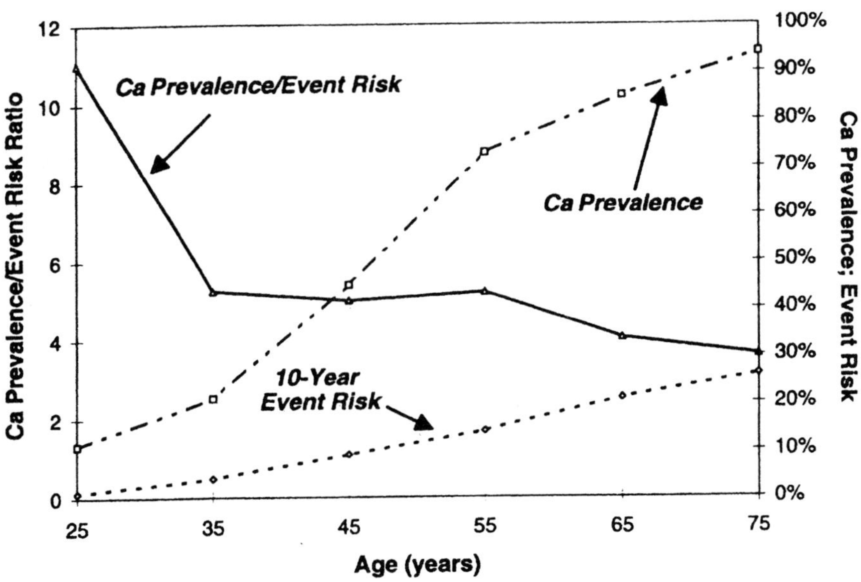

FIGURE 4–16. Coronary artery calcium prevalence, 10-year event risk, and prevalence-risk ratio in asymptomatic men. Event risk and calcium prevalence are plotted against the right axis, and the prevalence-risk ratio is plotted against the left axis. The prevalence-risk curve decreases with age, demonstrating serious overprediction in the young and moderate overprediction in the elderly. (From Wexler L, Brundage B, Crouse J, et al: Coronary artery calcification: pathophysiology, epidemiology, imaging methods, and clinical implications. Circulation 94:1175, 1996, with permission.)

tachycardia, or systemic hypertension. In addition, unstable angina may result from reduced myocardial blood flow associated with severe or progressive coronary artery atherosclerosis, or it may result from dynamic coronary artery constriction associated with coronary artery spasm.[38, 39]

PHYSICAL EXAMINATION AND BEDSIDE FINDINGS: UNSTABLE ANGINA AND NON–Q-WAVE MYOCARDIAL INFARCTION

On physical examination, patients with unstable angina have symptoms similar to those of patients with stable angina, although patients with unstable angina and angina at rest usually are much more concerned about their symptoms. There may not be any localizing finding, or the patient may have an audible S_4, cardiac enlargement, congestive heart failure (CHF), mitral insufficiency, or evidence of peripheral vascular disease.

Between episodes of unstable angina, the resting electrocardiogram (ECG) may be normal or may show ST- to T-wave changes or a prior MI, which is characteristic of patients with stable angina. Typically, however, the ECG demonstrates ST- to T-wave changes during rest angina, usually ST depression, T-wave flattening, or inversion in the electrocardiographic leads, reflecting changes in myocardial perfusion in the culprit artery. Similar electrocardiographic changes are generally found in patients with non–Q-wave MI, thereby making it impossible to distinguish unstable angina and non–Q-wave MI electrocardiographically. On occasion, episodes of unstable angina are not associated with recognizable ST- to T-wave changes on the ECG, but this is unusual.

Other diagnostic findings are also similar to those of patients with stable angina. Echocardiographic findings are as highly variable as those in patients with stable angina, but they may include reversible or fixed reductions in regional wall motion or global left ventricular functional abnormalities. In some patients, reductions in regional wall motion occur with episodes of rest angina and resolve as the angina resolves. Chest x-ray findings in patients with unstable angina also vary greatly from normal-sized hearts to cardiomegaly with congestive heart failure, as is true for patients with stable angina. Hemodynamic findings are also similar to those during episodes of angina in patients with stable angina.

Coronary artery spasm causes abrupt and dynamic decreases in myocardial oxygen delivery, which leads to unstable angina (Fig. 4–17).[38, 39] With a primary decrease in coronary blood flow, there is no association between the development of angina and exertion; in fact, the majority of anginal episodes occur at limited activity or rest. In addition, coronary artery spasm causes little or no change in heart rate or blood pressure before the onset of pain. After the onset of pain, however, blood pressure or heart rate may increase.

In patients with unstable angina, continuous electrocardiographic monitoring often shows transient ST-segment change immediately before the onset of chest pain—either ST-segment elevation indicating transmural ischemia as a consequence of spasm in a major epicardial coronary artery, or platelet-intitiated transient coronary artery thrombosis (see Figs. 4–15 and 4–17), or ST-segment depression.[40, 41] Most commonly, however, the patient with unstable angina has ST-segment depression when subendocardial ischemia develops as a result of transient thrombosis and vasoconstriction-induced narrowing of a coronary artery with flow distribution to the subendocardial region of the heart. In some individuals, ST-segment alterations occur in the absence of chest pain; this is referred to as *silent ischemia.* Silent ischemia has the same prognosis as painful episodes of ischemia.[40–42]

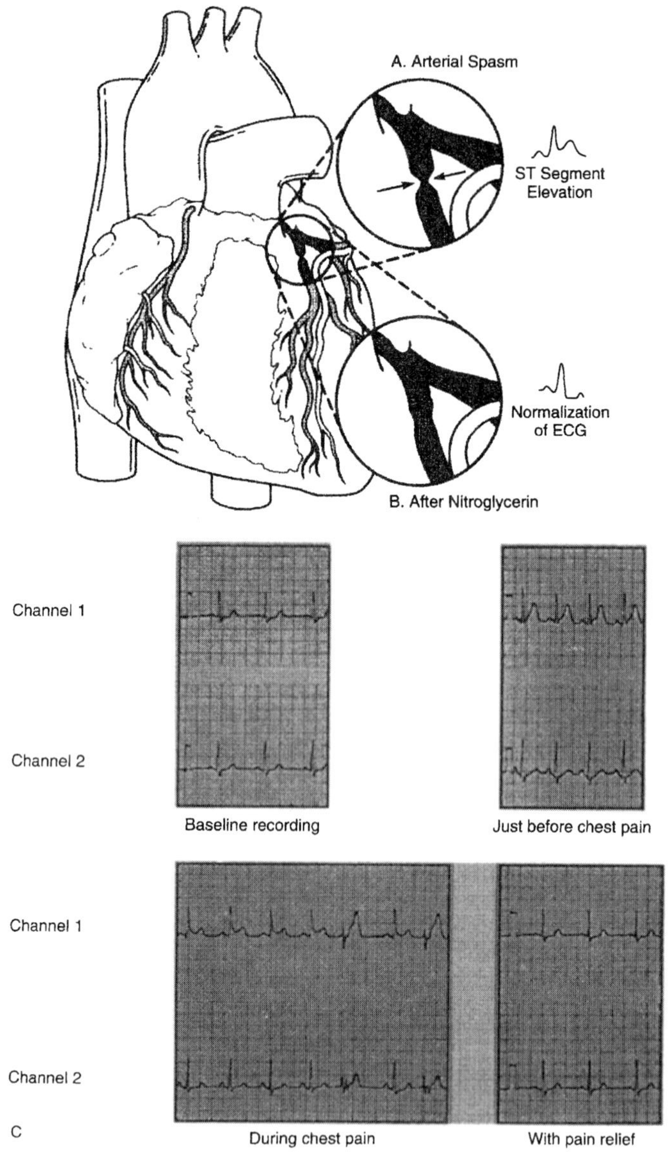

FIGURE 4–17. *A,* Focal obliteration of the coronary artery lumen caused by coronary artery spasm at a spot marked by the arrows. *Inset,* The associated ST-segment elevation that occurs with coronary artery spasm. *B,* Resolution of the coronary artery spasm after administration of nitroglycerin. *Inset,* Normalization of the electrocardiogram (ECG). *C,* Continuous 24-hour Holter recording in a patient with coronary artery spasm before chest pain *(top two panels),* as chest pain begins *(top right panel),* during chest pain *(bottom left panel),* and with pain relief *(bottom right panel)* demonstrating T-wave prominence and ST-segment elevation that occur with coronary artery spasm. (From Willerson JT: Medical treatment of coronary heart disease. In Willerson JT: Treatment of Heart Diseases. Gower Medical, New York, 1992, pp 1.7–1.8, with permission.)

PATHOPHYSIOLOGY OF VARIANT OR PRINZMETAL'S ANGINA

Patients with variant angina pectoris (Prinzmetal's angina) have angina at rest, often in the early morning hours. Variant angina is associated with ST-segment elevation on the ECG and coronary artery spasm, that is, focal obliteration of a coronary artery lumen (see Fig. 4–17).[39, 40]

In their early descriptions, Latham[43] and Osler[44] suggested that typical angina was caused by periodic spasms of a large coronary artery. Subsequently, however, clinical studies with anatomic correlations suggested that fixed atherosclerotic CAD was responsible for typical angina and MI. In 1959, Prinzmetal and coworkers[45] revived interest in coronary arterial spasm when they described a group of individuals with "variant angina." The clinical features of this syndrome are distinctly different from those of typical angina.[38, 45–56] The patients described by Prinzmetal and coworkers[45] usually had chest pain at rest rather than with physical exertion or emotional stimulation. The episodes of pain tended to recur at roughly the same time every day, often during the early morning hours, awakening the patient from sleep. In addition, patients with variant angina usually had ST-segment elevation on the ECG recorded during chest pain (see Fig. 4–17). The episodes of chest pain were sometimes accompanied by atrioventricular block or ventricular ectopic activity, and occasionally, the patients had transient ventricular tachycardia. Finally, the chest discomfort of variant angina was quickly relieved by nitroglycerin, after which the ST-segment elevation resolved. Prinzmetal's patients did not undergo selective coronary arteriography, but Prinzmetal and coworkers[45] hypothesized that patients with variant angina have severe proximal stenosis of one or more large coronary arteries in which spasm occurred periodically.

Since the original description of variant angina by Prinzmetal and coworkers, many observers[45–56] have confirmed the existence of this syndrome and have shown the presence of coronary artery spasm at sites of fixed coronary artery stenosis and in regions of the coronary vasculature where no obvious stenosis exists. In patients with clinically active coronary artery spasm, variant angina can often be induced by ergonovine maleate.[57–67] Other manuvers that have been used to produce coronary artery spasm in susceptible patients include hyperventilation with the administration of an alkaline buffer; cold pressor testing; and the administration of methacholine, a parasympathomimetic agent; acetylcholine; or serotonin.[62, 65–72] We have speculated that endothelial or adventitial injury, often in association with coronary artery stenosis, leads to the accumulation of platelets and white blood cells, mononuclear cells (including mast cells and T cells), and the release of humoral mediators (including serotonin, thromboxane A_2, prostaglandin D_2, thrombin, leukotrienes, platelet-activating factor, endothelin, and/or histamine), which singly or in combination may cause coronary artery spasm (see Figs. 4–15 and 4–17).[30–34] Exposure of tissue factor,[73] accumulation of local inhibitors of thrombolysis, such as the endogenous inhibitor of tissue plasminogen activator (PAI-1),[74] and activation of procoagulant factors, such as factors X and Xa (Fig. 4–18),[75] may also contribute to the development of thrombosis. This is especially likely to be true when endothelial injury decreases vascular concentrations of nitric oxide, tissue plasminogen activator, and prostacyclin (see Fig. 4–15).[31–34] It also seems likely that the endothelium-derived vasoconstrictor, endothelin, may be responsible for coronary artery constriction or spasm in some patients (see Fig. 4–15).[31–40]

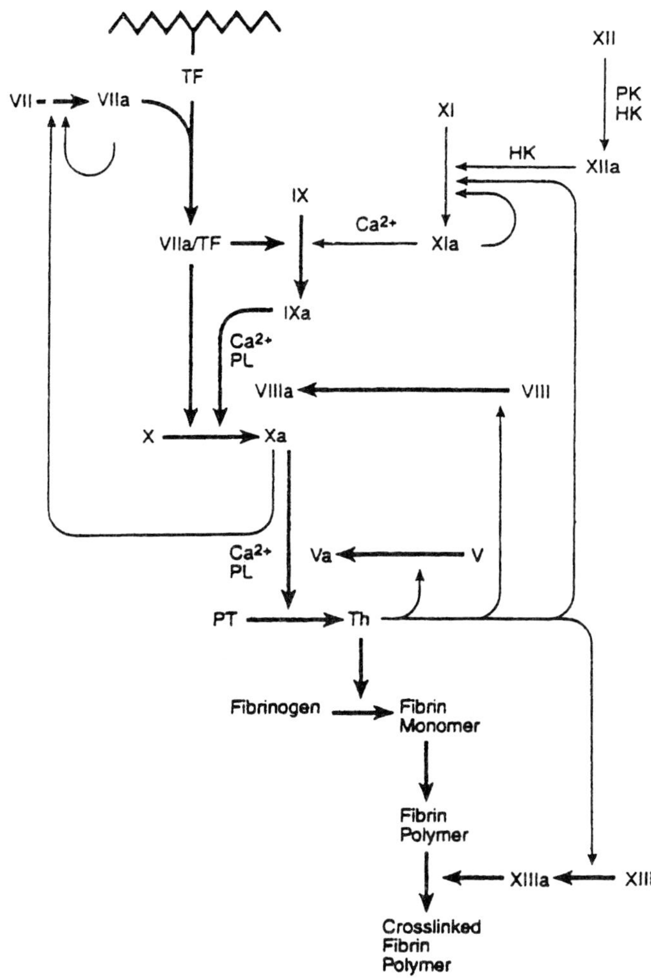

FIGURE 4–18. Role of tissue factors (TF) IX, X, XI, XII, and VIII in the formation of thrombin (Th) and the subsequent role of thrombin in the formation of fibrin. HK, high-molecular-weight; PK, prekallikrein; PL, phospholipid; PT, prothrombin. (From Schafer AI: Coagulation cascade: an overview. In Loscalzo J, Schafer A [eds]: Thrombosis and Hemorrhage. Blackwell Scientific, Boston, 1994, p 7, with permission.)

PATHOPHYSIOLOGY OF ACUTE MYOCARDIAL INFARCTION

Acute MI occurs when severe reductions in coronary blood flow and myocardial oxygen delivery last for more than 20 minutes. The infarct begins on the inner wall or subendocardium of the heart and is confined there for the first 20 minutes to 1 hour (Figs. 4–19 and 4–20). If the coronary artery thrombosis is transient or does not cause complete coronary artery occlusion, the infarct usually remains confined to the subendocardium, and a non–Q-wave MI develops. If the coronary artery occlusion is sustained, the myocardial necrosis progresses vertically outward toward the epicardium in the next 2 to 3 hours becoming a Q-wave, ST-

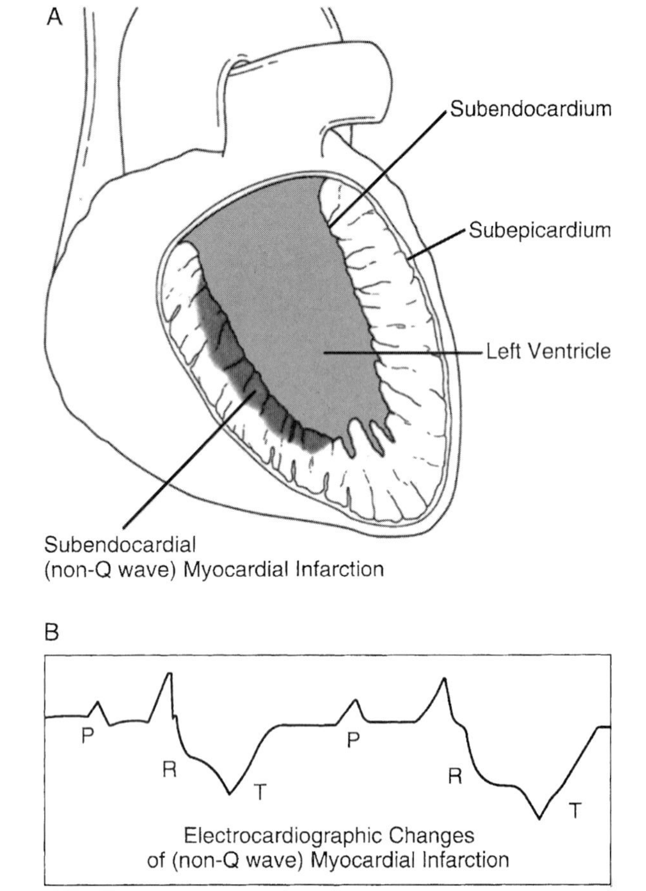

FIGURE 4–19. *A,* Location of myocardial necrosis with subendocardial or non–Q-wave myocardial infarcts and a representation of the typical electrocardiographic changes. *B,* Typical electrocardiogram (ECG) in a patient with acute non–Q-wave MI. With these types of infarcts, the ECG does not provide specific evidence of the presence of the infarct; however, ST-segment depression of varying magnitude and T-wave abnormalities, usually T-wave flattening or inversion, often develop. The only evolution of the electrocardiographic abnormalities is a return to a normal pattern. (From Willerson JT: Medical treatment of coronary heart disease. In Willerson JT: Treatment of Heart Diseases. Gower Medical, New York, 1992, pp 1.10–1.11, with permission.)

elevation, or transmural MI. After Herrick's[2] 1912 description of acute MI caused by coronary artery thrombosis, the role of coronary artery thrombosis in causing MI was debated[76] until arteriography studies by DeWood and colleagues[77] demonstrated that coronary artery thrombosis is virtually always the cause of acute Q-wave myocardial infarcts. Buja and Willerson[78] confirmed the association between thrombosis of the infarct-related coronary artery and the development of acute Q-wave (transmural) MI by detailed clinicopathologic correlations. Ninety percent or more of acute Q-wave infarcts have persistent and occlusive coronary artery thrombosis in the infarct-related coronary artery.[77, 78]

Acute Q-wave MI is usually caused by persistent thrombotic occlusion of a coronary artery, resulting in sustained reductions in coronary blood flow and myocardial oxygen availability. Occasionally, increases in myocardial oxygen demand above the ability of a stenotic coronary artery to deliver oxygen cause MI, often non–Q-wave MI. Such increases in oxygen demand may occur in patients with CAD who have severe systemic arterial hypertension, sustained tachycardia, or both. Sustained reductions in myocardial oxygen delivery, associated with severe systemic arterial hypotension, may also lead to MI, including non–Q-wave MI. Approximately 30% of patients with non–Q-wave MIs have an occlusive thrombus in the infarct-related artery, usually a small coronary artery branch vessel, or in the distal portion of a larger coronary artery.[78–80] Most patients with non–Q-wave MI have transient coronary artery occlusion initiated by platelet aggregation and with associated vasoconstriction, lasting between 30 minutes and 2 hours (see Figs. 4–15 and 4–19).

When critical reductions in myocardial blood flow persist for more than 2 hours, the resultant infarct is usually a transmural, Q-wave MI (see Fig. 4–20). The local accumulation of thromboxane A_2, serotonin, platelet-activating factor, adenosine diphosphate, oxygen-derived free radicals, and endothelin and thrombin activation at sites of endothelial injury contributes to vasoconstriction, platelet aggregation,

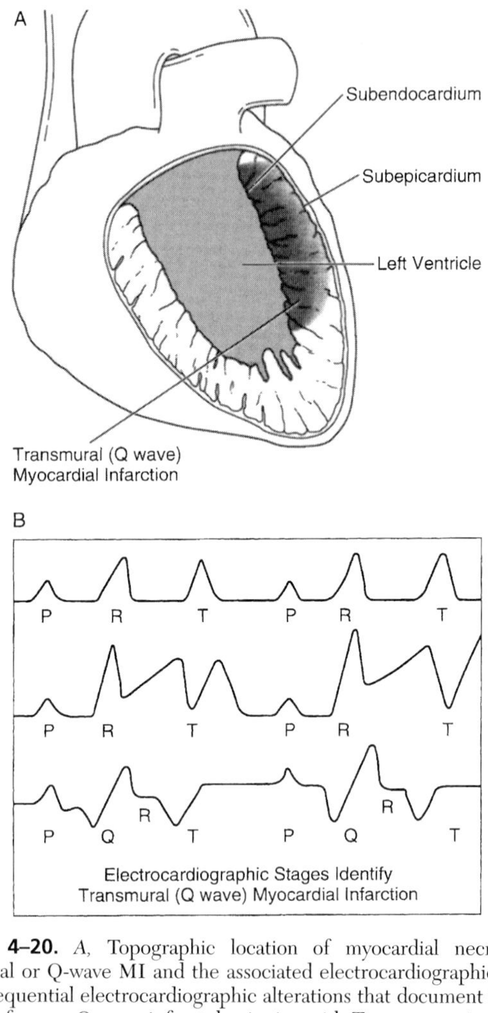

FIGURE 4–20. *A,* Topographic location of myocardial necrosis with transmural or Q-wave MI and the associated electrocardiographic changes. *B,* The sequential electrocardiographic alterations that document the development of a new Q-wave infarct, beginning with T-wave prominence *(top),* followed by hyperactive ST-segment elevation *(middle),* T-wave inversion, and the development of a significant Q-wave (0.04 s in duration) *(bottom).* (From Willerson JT: Medical treatment of coronary heart disease. In Willerson JT: Treatment of Heart Diseases. Gower Medical, New York, 1992, pp 1.12–1.13, with permission.)

and thrombosis (see Fig. 4–15).[32–35] Increases in systemic and local catecholamine concentrations associated with the development of unstable angina and MI also increase platelet aggregation and may contribute to coronary vasoconstriction. Serotonin, adenosine diphosphate, thrombin, and endothelin are mitogens, and they are very likely to contribute to subsequent local fibroproliferation with increases in the neointima, further narrowing the lumen of the endothelium-injured coronary artery.[81] In 30% (or more) of patients with unstable angina and non–Q-wave MIs, there is a rapid anatomic progression in the severity of the coronary luminal diameter narrowing, most likely associated with the inclusion of organized thrombus within the plaque and the fibroproliferation that follows plaque fissuring and ulceration.[81] Reduced fibrinolytic capability at sites of vascular endothelial injury and associated decreases in vascular tissue concentrations of prostacyclin, tissue plasminogen–activating factor, and nitric oxide undoubtedly contribute to coronary artery thrombosis vasoconstriction, and fibroproliferation at these same sites (see Fig. 4–15).[32–34]

We and others[32–34] have suggested that unstable angina, non–Q-wave MI, and Q-wave MI represent a continuum pathophysiologically. The process begins with coronary endothelial injury, usually ulceration or fissuring of atherosclerotic plaque. The degree of coronary artery stenosis at the site of ulceration or fissuring may be mild or severe. Approximately half of these sites have less than 50% narrowing of the luminal diameter.[82] We[32–34] have suggested that the syndrome of unstable angina develops when platelet-fibrin thrombus and associated severe vasoconstriction persist for less than 20 minutes and recur. A non–Q-wave MI occurs when the reduction in coronary blood flow and oxygen delivery to the heart is more prolonged—from 30 minutes to 1–2 hours.[32–34] When inadequate myocardial oxygen delivery persists for more than 2 hours, a Q-wave MI results (see Fig. 4–15).[32–34] When unstable angina and acute MI are viewed in this manner, it is easy to appreciate that patients with unstable angina and non–Q-wave MI have aborted Q-wave MIs, and therefore, they remain at risk for new infarction and its consequences in the ensuing 6 weeks.[78, 79, 83–86] The authors believe that the risk for renewed unstable angina and MI persists until the endothelial injury heals. Other causes of endothelial injury may also lead to this same sequence of events, including endothelial injury associated with systemic arterial hypertension, flow shear stress, smoking, diabetes, infection, aging, immune complex deposition, substance abuse (e.g., cocaine), and the placement of a coronary artery catheter into a coronary artery, especially with the interventional procedures of percutaneous transluminal coronary angioplasty (PTCA) and stent placement.[32–34]

Fissuring and ulceration of plaque most commonly occur in the asymmetric portion or "shoulder region" of a lesion with a thin, lipid-laden fibrous cap. Inflammation at sites of thin fibrous plaques with adjacent lipid cores best predicts atherosclerotic plaque that is unstable and likely to fissure or ulcerate.[17–28] Inflammation in the unstable plaque is characterized by the accumulation of monocyte-derived macrophages, activated T cells, and mast cells. Most likely, proteases released from the infiltrating mononuclear cells contribute to thinning of the fibrous cap through their degradation of collagen and subsequent fissuring and ulceration of atherosclerotic plaque (Fig. 4–21).[26, 32–34, 81–100]

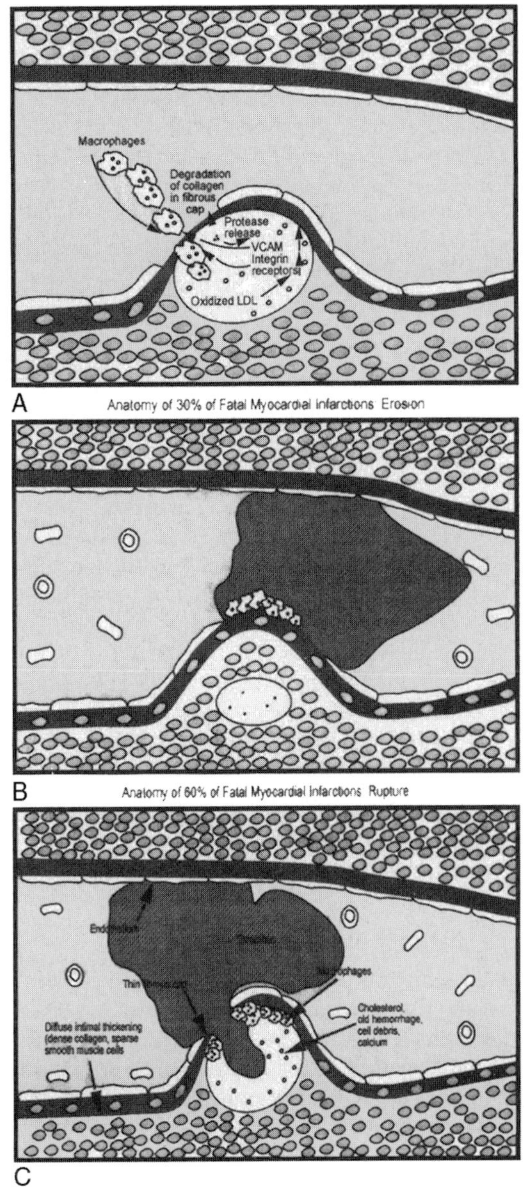

FIGURE 4–21. *A,* Potential mechanisms responsible for atherosclerotic plaque fissuring and ulceration. Oxidized low-density lipoprotein (LDL) within the atherosclerotic plaque promotes the upregulation of vascular cell adhesion molecule (VCAM) and other integrins, resulting in the recruitment of inflammatory cells (primarily monocyte-derived macrophages but including activated T cells and mast cells); subsequent protease release from the mononuclear cells; and degradation of collagen in the fibrous cap, leading to fissuring and ulceration. *B,* Atherosclerotic plaque fissuring, leading to platelet adhesion and aggregation, and thrombosis. *C,* Atherosclerotic plaque ulceration and thrombosis. (From Willerson JT, Maseri A: Pathophysiology and clinical recognition of coronary artery disease syndromes. In Willerson JT, Cohn JN [eds]: Cardiovascular Medicine, 2nd ed. WB Saunders Co, Philadelphia, 2000, p 537, with permission. *B* and *C* drawn with the assistance of Dr. Ward Casscells.)

CLINICAL RECOGNITION OF MYOCARDIAL INFARCTION

History

The patient's history is of the utmost importance in the recognition of acute MI. Typically, patients have very severe chest or epigastric pain that lasts until analgesic medication is administered, usually 30 minutes or longer. The pain is often described as being retrosternal or left precordial—as a heaviness, tightness, or weight on the chest—and is often described as the most severe the individual has ever experienced. The pain is generally associated with nausea and diaphoresis. It may radiate to the back, neck, jaw, or left arm, particularly down its ulnar aspect. Occasionally, the pain occurs only in the back, jaw, left arm, or neck. It usually lasts longer than 30 minutes. In women, however, the pain may be somewhat atypical and less severe (as described for unstable angina). Women may simply "feel poorly" or have discomfort in their neck, jaw, or left arm. The discomfort gradually builds in severity, reaches a peak, and then recedes. Many patients who have acute MIs have unstable angina for hours to days before their infarct. In 10% to 20% of patients with diabetes mellitus, MIs are silent (i.e., painless). Silent MIs also occur in patients who develop CAD after cardiac transplantation (transplant vasculopathy) and occasionally in other individuals with neuromyopathic abnormalities and in some seemingly normal subjects. When a patient, especially one with diabetes, presents with new CHF, ventricular arrhythmias, hypotension, heart murmur of mitral insufficiency, or systemic embolic events, or is resuscitated from sudden death, acute MI should be considered as a possible cause; and serial serum measurements of CK, CK-MB, and troponin I and/or T, and serial ECGs should be ordered immediately.

Physical Examination

Patients with small MIs, particularly non–Q-wave infarcts, may not have any detectable abnormality on physical examination. At the other extreme, patients with extensive damage to the left ventricle (≥40% of the LV mass) often develop "power-failure" complications of their infarct, including cardiogenic shock, severe left ventricular failure, or medically refractory arrhythmias (Fig. 4–22).[101–105]

Inspection and Palpation. Therefore, the findings on physical examination in patients with acute MI depend primarily on the extent of myocardial damage. Most patients are diaphoretic and in obvious discomfort. In those with extensive myocardial damage, mild-to-severe decreases in systemic arterial blood pressure occur. Such decreases may lead to cardiogenic shock, that is, hypotension that results from extensive myocardial damage with evidence that the reduced blood pressure is inadequate for normal systemic perfusion. Patients with cardiogenic shock usually have cool skin, mental confusion, and oliguria. Patients with extensive LV myocardial necrosis may also have an alternating pulse force (pulsus alternans) and frequent premature ventricular beats. If second- or third-degree (complete) atrioventricular block with sinus rhythm is present, the patient will have intermittent cannon *a* waves in the jugular venous pulse. Patients with atrial fibrillation do not have an *a* wave in the jugular venous pulse but instead have an irregularly irregular pulse. Those with major tricuspid insufficiency have prominent *v* waves in their jugular venous pulse. Patients with right ventricular (RV) failure have an increased jugular venous pressure, and they may have hepatomegaly, right upper quadrant tenderness when acute hepatic congestion develops, ascites if the RV failure is severe, and peripheral or sacral edema.

With acute Q-wave MI, a precordial ectopic impulse may sometimes be palpated over the left precordium, typically along the lower left sternal border or between the left sternal border and the apex. This impulse is caused by an increase in regional left ventricular compliance within the area of injury, with a resultant systolic distension or bulging (dyskinesia) of the injured tissue. Over hours to a few days after MI, the compliance of this region decreases (stiffness increases) and the systolic bulging is replaced by reduced (hypokinetic) or absent (akinetic) regional wall motion. If the systolic bulging persists, a ventricular aneurysm may be present.

Auscultation. In most patients with acute and chronic CAD, an S_4 sound can be heard over the middle and lower

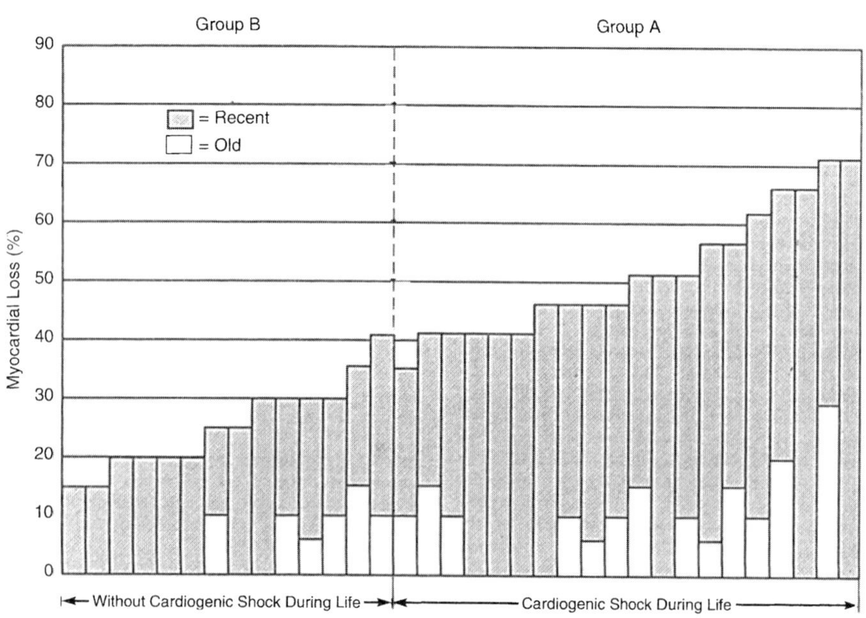

FIGURE 4–22. "Power failure" complications of MI, including cardiogenic shock, occurring in patients with the most extensive myocardial necrosis from their infarcts. (From Page DL, Caulfield JB, Kastor JA, et al: Myocardial changes associated with cardiogenic shock. N Engl J Med 285:133, 1971, with permission. Copyright © 1971 Massachusetts Medical Society. All rights reserved.)

left precordium or at the cardiac apex. S_4 sounds are often soft and are best heard with light application of the bell of the stethoscope. The sounds are caused by a forceful atrial contraction against a ventricle, which has reduced compliance (increased ventricular stiffness) as a consequence of the physiologic effects of CAD.

When the mitral valve apparatus is damaged, a murmur of mitral insufficiency may be audible. These murmurs have variable auscultatory characteristics; they may be ejection in quality, peaking in intensity in mid to late systole, or they may be holosystolic. Intermittent myocardial ischemia with transient dysfunction of the posterior papillary muscle of the mitral valve leads to a murmur of papillary muscle dysfunction typically associated with mild to moderate mitral insufficiency. The murmur of papillary muscle dysfunction usually begins after the first heart sound (S_1), peaks in mid to late systole, and extends up to S_2. It is heard at the cardiac apex and may radiate toward the left sternal border or into the axilla. If it is caused by intermittent myocardial ischemia, the murmur is transient. If caused by infarction of the papillary muscle, the murmur is usually permanent. Rupture of a papillary muscle with acute MI causes severe mitral insufficiency and often a soft apical holosystolic murmur. However, sometimes no audible murmur occurs with a ruptured papillary muscle, even though severe mitral insufficiency develops. Acute mitral insufficiency occurs most commonly in patients with inferior or lateral Q-wave MIs or in those with non–Q-wave MIs.[106–112] Similarly, those with inferior infarcts and structural damage to the tricuspid valve may develop tricuspid insufficiency.

Rupture of the interventricular septum occurs most commonly in patients with acute anterior infarction, although it may also occur in the patient with an inferior MI.[113–122] The murmur caused by a ventricular septal defect (VSD) is located along the lower left sternal border, is holosystolic, and is often associated with a left sternal border systolic thrill. As pulmonary artery pressure and vascular resistance increase, the systolic murmur of a VSD becomes shorter, ultimately disappearing altogether with the development of severe pulmonary hypertension. Functionally large acute VSDs (pulmonary to systemic blood flow ratios of 1.5 to 1 or greater) should be closed by surgical intervention when CHF develops in the patient with MI; otherwise, rapidly progressive CHF and death may ensue. We recommend prompt coronary arteriography and surgical or interventional repair of a VSD with the development of CHF.

S_2 normally splits into two components with inspiration, the earlier aortic and the later pulmonary valve closure sound, because inspiration increases venous return to the right heart and delays pulmonary valve closure. However, this second sound may be paradoxically split (i.e., wider splitting of the second sound during expiration) in patients with angina pectoris, as well as in patients with severe LV failure, systemic arterial hypertension, LBBB or pacing from the right ventricle, and various forms of LV outflow obstruction, including valvular, supravalvular, and subvalvular aortic stenosis (Fig. 4–23). In patients with pulmonary hypertension resulting from LV failure, the pulmonary closure sound is increased in intensity.

A murmur of relative mitral insufficiency occurs when patients have LV failure; a murmur of relative tricuspid insufficiency occurs when patients have right ventricular failure. Mitral and tricuspid murmurs result from spatial abnormalities in the orientation of the papillary muscles of the mitral and tricuspid valves, which are caused by marked dilatation of the left or right ventricles. The mitral and tricuspid insufficiency is usually mild or moderate and diminishes in severity with diuresis.

An S_3 sound occurs in patients with acute MIs who have ventricular filling pressures (LV end-diastolic pressures) of 15 mm Hg or greater and in those with moderate to severe mitral, aortic, or tricuspid valvular insufficiency. An S_3 sound can also be heard in patients with CHF and in those with rapid filling of the ventricles as a consequence of moderate or severe mitral, tricuspid, or aortic valve incompetence. In some young individuals (i.e., those under 30 years of age), S_3 may be heard normally and is a result of rapid ventricular filling.

Pericardial friction rubs are detected in fewer than 10% of patients with acute Q-wave MIs. Patients with audible pericardial friction rubs usually have large transmural MIs and a relatively poor prognosis. If a large pericardial effusion develops, the heart sounds may be distant and the jugular venous pressure elevated. Cardiac tamponade results in the development of hypotension, pulsus paradoxus (reduction of more than 10 mm Hg in systolic blood pressure during inspiration), distant heart sounds, and an elevated jugular venous pressure.

Pulmonary edema occurs in patients with extensive MI, in patients with myocardial ischemia superimposed on extensive previous MI, and in patients who develop mechanical complications of acute MI (acute VSDs, acute mitral insufficiency, or large ventricular aneurysms). Bibasilar or more extensive moist rales usually will be heard in patients who develop LV failure.

Myocardial Stunning and Hibernation

Transient myocardial ischemia followed by reperfusion may lead to protracted recovery of segmental ventricular function, known as myocardial stunning. This is probably caused by cellular calcium overload and generation of free radicals.[123–130] Stunned myocardial segments may contribute to the development of CHF when the area of ischemia or infarction is large. Persistent ischemia can lead to chronic depression of segmental ventricular function, known as myocardial hibernation,[126–130] which may also contribute to CHF. In selected patients who undergo coronary artery revascularization, myocardial hibernation can be reversed, thereby correcting the CHF.

Electrocardiographic Diagnosis

The ECG provides an excellent means for recognizing acute Q-wave MI (Figs. 4–24 to 4–26). The characteristic sequence of electrocardiographic alterations with Q-wave MI includes (1) the initial development of prominent, peaked T waves in the electrocardiographic leads, representing sites of epicardial injury; (2) the development of hyperacute ST-segment elevation; and (3) the development of Q-waves, 0.04 second in duration, or 40% or greater loss of R-wave amplitude. The rapidity with which these electrocardio-

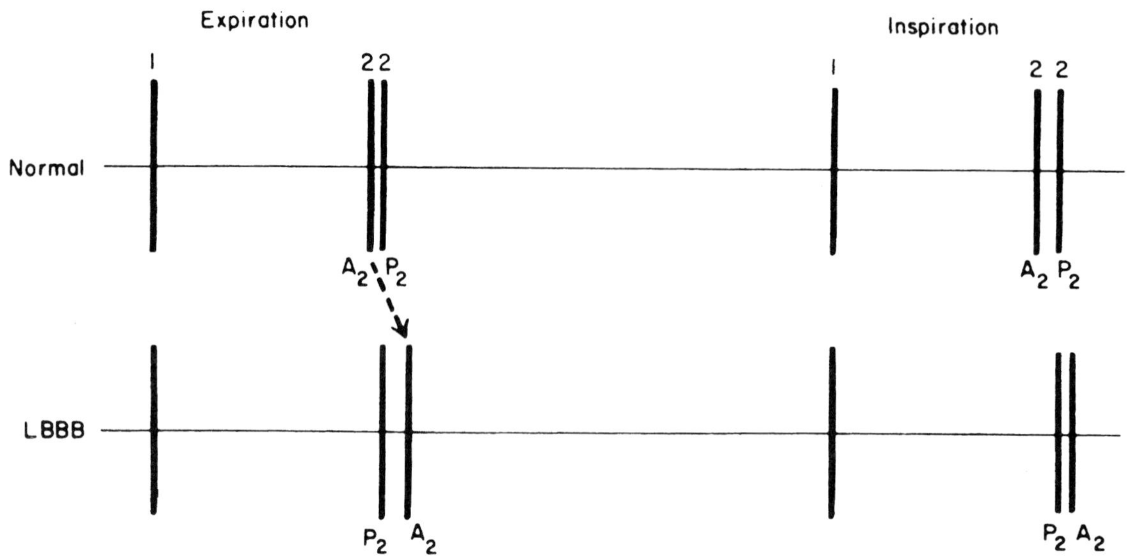

FIGURE 4–23. Normal and paradoxical splitting of the second heart sound: *top* and *bottom,* respectively. Left bundle branch block (LBBB) produces paradoxical splitting of the second heart sound *(bottom)*. (From Willerson JT, Hillis LD, Buja LM: Ischemic Heart Disease: Clinical and Pathophysiological Aspects. Raven, New York, 1982, p 274, with permission.)

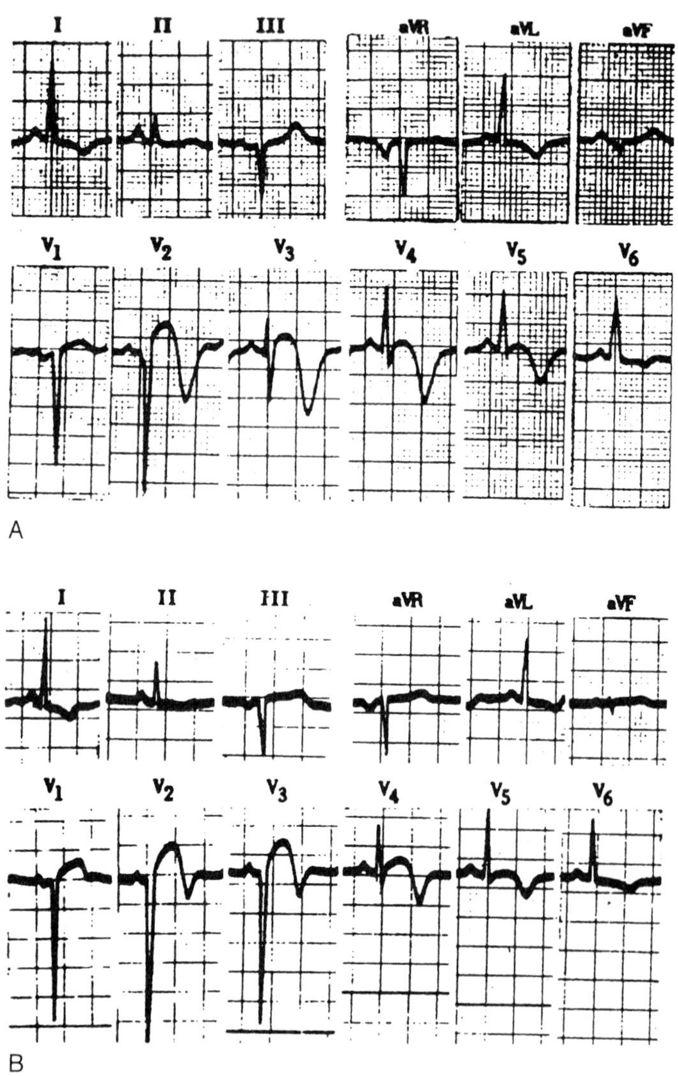

FIGURE 4–24. An evolving Q-wave anterolateral MI *(A)* and the completed evolution of this infarct *(B)*. (From Willerson JT, Hillis LD, Buja LM: Ischemic Heart Disease: Clinical and Pathophysiological Aspects. Raven, New York, 1982, p 275, with permission.)

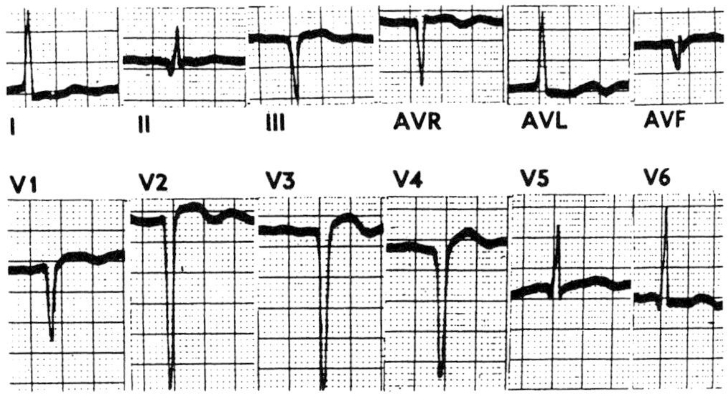

FIGURE 4–25. A completed anteroseptal Q-wave MI is shown by the poor R-wave progression in leads V_1 through V_4. This patient also had a previous inferior Q-wave MI, as shown by the Q-waves in leads II, III, and aVF. (From Willerson JT, Hillis LD, Buja LM: Ischemic Heart Disease: Clinical and Pathophysiological Aspects. Raven, New York, 1982, p 276, with permission.)

graphic changes develop is variable. They can occur within minutes or may be delayed for several hours after onset of symptoms. Some patients with acute MIs have relatively normal ECGs during the first few hours.

In addition to the sometimes variable, time-related evolution of the ECG when an acute Q-wave MI occurs, there are other potential problems in using the ECG to identify acute MI. First, with LBBB, acute anterior MI is not recognizable from the ECG, since the LBBB pattern simulates that of an anterior MI in the left precordial leads. However, if the LBBB pattern is otherwise altered by the presence of diminutive R-wave voltage, S waves, or initial Q waves in leads I, aVL, or V_5 and V_6, the patient may have had a prior anterior and lateral MI. Inferior Q-wave MIs can be recognized in patients with LBBB because the evolution of the inferior Q-wave MI is not altered by LBBB. Abnormal T-wave vectors reversed from the normal pattern—that is, inverted T waves in V_1 to V_3 and/or upright T waves in leads V_4 to V_6—may indicate anterior or lateral ischemia or infarction. Second, in patients who have had previous Q-wave MIs, it is more difficult to recognize new injury in that same general region of the left ventricle. Finally, with rapid electrocardiographic evolution of the MI, it may not be possible to differentiate old from new MI from the ECG alone. ST-segment elevation may also occur under other circumstances: (1) with normal early repolarization; (2) with transient myocardial ischemia, as in Prinzmetal's angina, or with ischemia in an area of previous MI; (3) in some individuals with chronic ventricular aneurysms; (4) transiently, after electrical cardioversion; (5) in the anterior precordial electrocardiographic leads in patients with LBBB; (6) in the anterior precordial leads in some patients with LV hypertrophy; and (7) in an occasional patient with hyperkalemia.

Although the ECG can be used rather reliably to diagnose acute Q-wave MI, it is not as reliable in diagnosing acute non–Q-wave MI. In patients with non–Q-wave MI, the ECG usually shows ST depression and T-wave inversion, and the only evolution is a return to baseline. Unfortunately, subendocardial ischemia, ventricular hypertrophy, tachycardia, severe emotion, electrolyte alterations (especially hypokalemia, and hypomagnesemia, and hypocalcemia), and the use of certain medications (including cardiac glycosides) may produce similar electrocardiographic changes. Indeed, bizarre and deeply inverted T-wave alterations occur in some patients with acute intracerebral hemorrhage. The only useful rule in the electrocardiographic recognition of non–Q-wave MI is that the deeper the ST-segment depression and the longer it lasts, the more likely it is an acute non–Q-wave MI.

Serum Enzyme and Cardiac Intracellular Substance Changes

Changes in cardiac enzyme concentrations and other intracellular myocardial substances are related to the development of acute MI (Fig. 4–27). A previously preferred enzymatic technique was the measurement of CK and, in

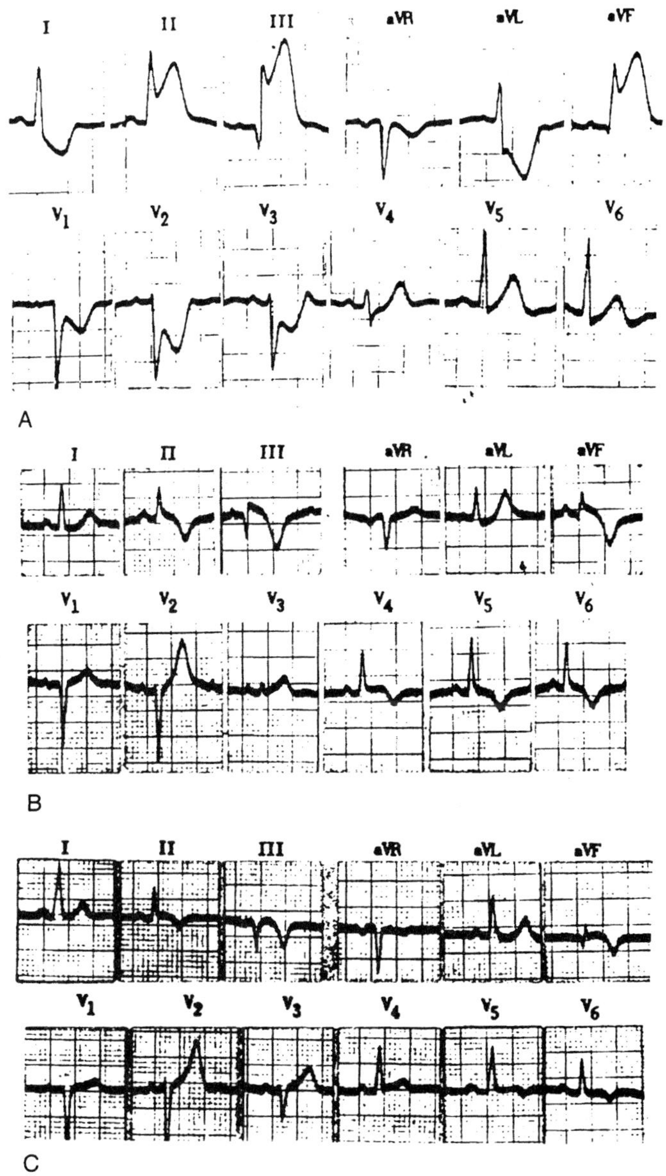

FIGURE 4–26. Evolution of a Q-wave inferior MI. *A*, Note the hyperacute ST-segment elevation in leads II, III, and aVF and the reciprocal changes in leads V_1 through V_4. *B*, Further evolution of the infarct patterns. *C*, Completed evolution of the infarct. (From Willerson JT, Hillis LD, Buja LM: Ischemic Heart Disease: Clinical and Pathophysiological Aspects. Raven, New York, 1982, p 277, with permission.)

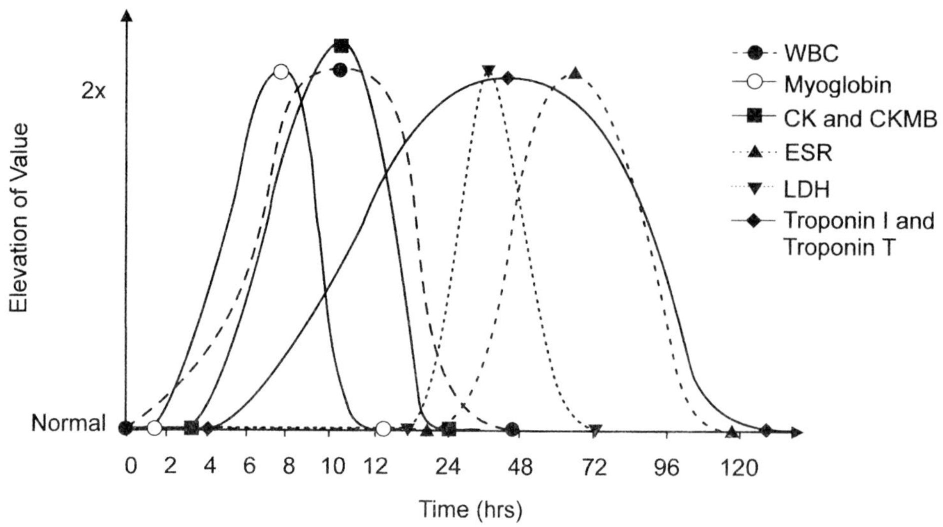

FIGURE 4–27. Typical changes in serial enzymes measured in a patient with an evolving, acute MI. Increases in serum myoglobin concentration are the earliest changes indicative of MI. Note that the white blood cell count (WBC) rises early after infarction and that the serum creatine kinase (CK) and MB isoenzyme of CK (CK-MB) rise before serum troponin I and T. The erythrocyte sedimentation rate (ESR) and lactic dehydrogenase (LDH) rise relatively late after acute MI. (Modified from Willerson JT, Hillis LD, Buja LM: Ischemic Heart Disease: Clinical and Pathophysiological Aspects. Raven, New York, 1982, p 280, with permission.)

particular, the myocardium-specific CK-MB isoenzyme, measured either by spectrophotometry, fluorometry, or radioimmunoassay.[131–146] CK-MB increases in the sera of patients approximately 2 to 3 hours after the onset of acute MI, reaches a peak at 10 to 12 hours, and returns to normal within 24 hours after the event in patients with small infarcts and in those who have reperfusion after thrombolytic therapy or with endogenous thrombolysis. In patients with large infarcts, those not receiving thrombolytic therapy, and those who fail to experience reperfusion after thrombolytic therapy, CK and CK-MB often peak later (e.g., 18 to 24 hours after infarction) and return to normal 30 to 40 hours after the event. Stuttering infarcts, defined as repeated episodes of infarction with recurrent chest pain over hours to days, result in repeated elevations of serum CK and CK-MB.

Radioimmunoassay measurement of alterations in serum myoglobin concentration allows a slightly earlier recognition of acute MI, but there is no means to distinguish myoglobin release from the heart and skeletal muscle when skeletal muscle injury occurs. Therefore, in the patient with skeletal muscle damage from trauma, intramuscular injection, recent surgery, cardioversion, heat exposure, excess consumption of alcohol, or primary skeletal muscle disorders, determining the presence of MI is not possible by measurement of serum myoglobin. However, in the patient without skeletal muscle injury, measurement of serum myoglobin by radioimmunoassay provides a sensitive and relatively rapid means to detect MI within 1 to 2 hours of the event. Myoglobin is released from injured myocardial cells within 1 to 2 hours, peaks within 4 to 6 hours, and returns to normal values within 10 to 12 hours.

Radioimmunoassay measurement of alterations in the serum concentration of the light chain of myosin may also allow a relatively early and precise recognition of acute MI.[137, 138] In the past, serum transaminase values were measured, but these values are nonspecific and, at present, are not used to detect MI. Serial serum measurements of lactic dehydrogenase (LDH) and LDH isoenzymes have also been used to diagnose acute MI. There are five LDH isoenzymes. Increases in LDH isoenzymes 1 and 2 are consistent with MI: when LDH-1 and/or LDH-2 elevations represent more than 50% of the total, acute MI may have occurred. Increases in LDH levels occur 18 to 30 hours after MI and usually return to normal within 48 to 72 hours. Therefore, LDH measurements may detect MI in some patients who do not come to the hospital immediately and in others in whom it is not possible to rely on changes in CK and CK-MB to detect an infarction. More recent studies have indicated that damaged heart muscle releases the proteins troponin I and T, which increase in the circulation within 6 to 8 hours after the onset of chest pain and remain elevated for 2 or 3 days (see later).

Measurements of CK isoforms, as well as myoglobin, have proved useful in detecting reperfusion after thrombolytic therapy or after release of an experimental coronary artery occlusion.[140–144] The conversion of CK isoform from CKMM-1 to CKMM-2 in the peripheral circulation appears to correlate with successful reperfusion therapy. Staccato increases in serum myoglobin in the first 4 to 6 hours after MI are indicative of reperfusion, as are rapid peaking of increases in serum and CK-MB (within 10 to 12 hours from symptom onset).

Three troponin subunits regulate muscle contraction by modulating the calcium-dependent interaction of actin and myosin: the tropomyosin-binding subunit T, the calcium-binding subunit C, and the actomyosin-adenosine triphosphatase (ATPase)-inhibiting subunit I. Troponin I exists in three isoforms: slow-twitch, fast-twitch, and cardiac. Cardiac troponin I (cTn-I) is the 26.5-kDa isoform of the muscle subunit and is genetically and structurally distinct from that produced in extracardiac muscle.

Previous studies have shown that cTn-I and cardiac troponin T (cTn-T) correlate with acute myocardial necrosis in the general population.[139, 145, 146] Both substances are increased in the systemic circulation within 6 to 8 hours after acute MI or other forms of myocardial necrosis, and they often remain elevated for at least 2 to 3 days. However, in patients with renal failure, spurious cTn-T elevations and increases in CK-MB can occur.[147] Recent studies have shown that cTn-I accurately predicts myocardial injury in patients wih renal failure. A study conducted by Martin and coworkers[147] evaluated 56 patients (mean age, 62) with acute or chronic renal failure or end-stage renal disease, assessing the sensitivity and specificity of cTn-I for detecting myocardial injury in these patients. Patients admitted with suspected MI were evaluated over a 6-month period. There were an equal number of men and women. Further cardiac testing, including echocardiography, stress testing, or arteriography, was performed at the discretion of the primary physician. The sensitivity and specificity for CK-MB were 44% and 56%, whereas they were 94% and 100% for cTn-I. In this study, elevated cTn-I levels were associated with increased short-term mortality and an ability to risk-stratify patients with severe renal failure and true myocardial injury. Troponin T values were slightly elevated in patients with renal disease, although not necessarily outside the normal range. In these patients, troponin I values appeared to be more reliable in infarct detection.[147]

Myocardial Scintigraphy

Radionuclide myocardial scintigraphy techniques can also be useful in identifying acute MI.[148–160] These techniques allow visualization of the region or regions of acute MI (infarct-avid imaging technique) or identification of areas of severely decreased myocardial perfusion (myocardial perfusion imaging technique). The prototype infarct-avid imaging agent, technetium 99m (^{99m}Tc) stannous pyrophosphate, accumulates in irreversibly damaged myocardium 1 to 5 days after MI and can detect acute MIs 3 g or larger more than 90% of the time. With successful reperfusion, MI may be detected within 2 to 3 hours of the event. An antimyosin antibody labeled with technetium or iodine, which binds to myosin with myocyte membrane injury and MI, can also be used for imaging. It has the same sensitivity in MI detection as pyrophosphate, but it does not accumulate in bone. Thallium 201 (^{201}Tl) and Tc-sestamibi are myocardial perfusion imaging agents that accumulate in the myocardium in direct proportion to blood flow. When used within 24 hours after acute MI, their sensitivities for infarct detection are approximately 90%. ^{99m}Tc-sesamibi provides information similar to that of ^{201}Tl, but it also allows for an evaluation of regional systolic function, including systolic wall thickening. The size of the initial ^{201}Tl or ^{99m}Tc-sestamibi defect after acute MI appears to have prognostic significance, as do persistently abnormal pyrophosphate scintigrams, that is, those that remain abnormal for 3 months or longer after MI. Large MIs, as detected by extensive perfusion defect or by pyrophosphate or antimyosin uptake, and persistently abnormal pyrophosphate scintigram, are associated with an increased risk for future coronary events and heart failure.

In addition to these imaging techniques, the cardiovascular blood pool can be identified with technetium-labeled erythrocytes to characterize the impact of acute MI on regional and global ventricular function by dynamic myocardial scintigraphy. This latter technique allows measurement of ventricular ejection fraction, ventricular volumes, regional wall motion, left-to-right shunts (i.e., VSDs), and valvular insufficiency (including mitral or tricuspid regurgitation) and the identification of ventricular aneurysms.

Echocardiography

Two-dimensional (or three-dimensional) echocardiographic measurements can be used to detect intramyocardial masses and to evaluate global and segmental ventricular functional alterations in patients with acute MI.[161–165] Transthoracic and transesophageal two-dimensional echocardiography can also be used to detect left ventricular thrombi in patients with acute MIs.[163–165] Patients with acute anterior Q-wave MIs more frequently develop left ventricular mural thrombi acutely (10% to 40%). These patients have an increased risk for systemic embolic events, requiring that they receive anticoagulants unless there is some exceptional contraindication. Transthoracic and transesophageal Doppler echocardiography can also be used to detect and estimate the severity of mitral insufficiency and VSDs, to identify ventricular aneurysms and pseudoaneurysms, and to assess the extent of wall motion abnormality in patients who have had an infarction.[166–183] Detection of these abnormalities is often important, especially in patients with a low-output state, hypotension, or heart failure, because proper medical management or surgical repair may save the patient's life.

Cardiac Rupture

Pseudoaneurysms (false aneurysms) developing after MI represent partial tears in the left ventricle and a risk for complete rupture. They are distinguished from true aneurysms by demonstration—on two-dimensional echocardiography, angiography, radionuclide ventriculography, or magnetic resonance imaging—of communication with the true left ventricle by a narrow channel or neck. True LV aneurysms communicate with the left ventricular cavity by an imperceptible pathway. False LV aneurysms may rupture spontaneously and should be surgically corrected as soon as they are identified. Patients at greatest risk for heart rupture after MI are those with a first MI who have systemic arterial hypertension and elderly patients. To minimize this risk, blood pressure elevations should be prevented in patients after MI. When myocardial rupture occurs after MI, most patients die suddenly of exsanguination or cardiac tamponade. A few develop tamponade with a sealing of the tear by a blood clot in the pericardial space. Although blood does not usually clot in the pericardial space, it may clot in the patient with extensive MI as a consequence of the loss of segmental wall motion in the infarcted segment. Thus, continued bleeding is prevented, providing the observant physician an opportunity to recognize the development of an enlarging pericardial effusion with early tamponade and to intervene surgically to correct the tamponade and repair the myocardial rupture. The pericardial fluid/thrombosis is best evacuated with the circulation supported by cardiopulmonary bypass rather than by pericardiocentesis before instituting bypass. The classic finding in the patient with sudden myocardial rupture is the development of electromechanical dissociation (EMD), i.e., blood pressure is lost, and the patient becomes unresponsive but has continuing electrical activity on the ECG for the subsequent few seconds to minutes. EMD not only occurs with myocardial rupture but may also occur with a large anteroseptal infarct, pericardial tamponade of any etiology, and severe systemic hypoxemia or acidosis.

Further Detail of Pathology of Coronary Heart Disease

Morphologic changes of atherosclerosis are heterogeneous and vary somewhat by clinical syndrome. In stable angina, the coronary arteries almost always show more than 75% cross-sectional area luminal narrowing, equivalent to 50% diameter reduction.[184] The plaque consists of either a calcified lipid-rich fibrous plaque (40%) or a predominantly pure fibrous lesion (60%).[184] The lumen may be either eccentric (24%) or concentric (76%).[184] Luminal acute thrombi from either a plaque rupture or plaque erosion are infrequent, occurring in less than 10% of cases.[184–187] However, recanalized thrombi have been described in 79% of patients with isolated stable angina,[184, 186] and iron deposition (a marker of plaque hemorrhage) within plaques is seen in 77% of cases. To our knowledge, sex differences in plaque morphology in patients with stable angina have not been reported.

In unstable angina, angiography of coronary arteries demonstrates 50% diameter reduction in most patients, and angioscopy shows luminal thrombi in over 70%.[188] Morphologic studies have shown the presence of organized thrombi in more than 90% of patients with unstable angina.[189] In two studies reported by Roberts and colleagues, plaque hemorrhage was seen in 64%; plaque rupture occurred in 36%, and thrombi were seen in 29%.[189, 190] The atherosclerotic plaque often shows the presence of a necrotic core, and the majority of the severely narrowed arteries are calcified.[190] Again, differences in plaque morphology in men and women have not been reported.

There is greater agreement between clinical and morphologic studies in acute myocardial infarction than in stable and unstable angina. In patients with electrocardiographic evidence of acute myocardial infarction, angiograms demonstrate thrombi in 90% of patients.[191, 192] Angiographic studies have characterized the plaque lesions, which are highly predictive of the presence of thrombus.[192] At the sites of thrombi, the degree of underlying luminal diameter reduction is often less than 50%.[192, 193] Although sites of severe stenosis (>75% cross-sectional luminal narrowing) are more prone to thrombosis than less involved arteries, there are many more sites that are not severely narrowed. Therefore, the total number of lesions with thrombosis will be greater at sites away from severe stenosis. In necropsy studies, the frequency of thrombi has varied from 50% to 90%. This variability can partly be explained by the duration of symptoms to death.[194] Davies reports the presence of plaque rupture of a thin fibrous cap and an overlying thrombus in 75% of patients who die suddenly.[195] Analysis of morphologic characteristics of atherosclerotic plaques from patients with acute myocardial infarction has suggested that plaques are rich in lipids and are often calcified.[196] Plaque hemorrhage is seen in 90% of cases.[190]

Plaque Rupture and Plaque Erosion

Until recently, it was reported that symptomatic thrombotic coronary artery disease was caused solely from plaque rupture of a thin fibrous plaque.[193, 197] We have recently demonstrated that thrombi in sudden coronary death may occur from two distinctly different plaque morphologies: plaque rupture and plaque erosion.[197] In plaque rupture, a thin fibrous cap—which overlies a large, necrotic core that is heavily infiltrated by foamy macrophages—is disrupted, allowing a direct communication of luminal blood with the highly thrombogenic lipid core (Color Plate 4–2). In plaque erosion, a thrombus overlies a base rich in smooth muscle cells within a proteoglycan-rich matrix (Color Plate 4–3). The necrotic core is often absent; when present, it is an insignificant part of the plaque that does not communicate with the thrombus. Plaque rupture accounts for 60% of thrombi in patients with sudden death, whereas plaque erosion accounts for 40%.

Plaque erosion is generally seen in younger individuals, more frequently women. Lesions are less often calcified and are more often nonocclusive and eccentric, as compared to lesions of plaque rupture.[197] Arbustini and coworkers[198] reported that 291 of 298 patients (98%) with myocardial infarction documented by ECG changes and cardiac enzymes had coronary thrombi at autopsy. Of these, 25% (74 patients) demonstrated plaque erosion. Plaque erosion was found in 37% of women with thrombi but only 18% of men with thrombi.[198]

Pathology of Atherosclerotic Plaques in Sudden Coronary Death in Men

We have correlated the association of risk factors to plaque morphology in sudden coronary death.[199] In 113 men, we determined the risk factors at autopsy by biochemical analysis of serum for total cholesterol (TC), high-density lipoprotein (HDL) cholesterol, TC/HDL ratio, and serum thiocyanate, a surrogate marker for smoking. Red cell glycosylated hemoglobin was used to determine presence of glucose intolerance (>8%). We observed that risk factors were present in 96.5% of cases of sudden coronary death. Smoking was a predictor of acute thrombosis and thrombi from plaque rupture and correlated with high total cholesterol, low HDL cholesterol, and a high TC/HDL–cholesterol ratio. We also observed that as cholesterol rose, so did the number of vulnerable plaques. A vulnerable plaque was defined as a plaque with a large necrotic core and a thin fibrous cap (<65 μm) that was heavily infiltrated by macrophages.[199]

Pathology of Atherosclerotic Plaques in Sudden Coronary Death in Women

In women, risk factors also have a distinct effect on plaque morphology and vary with menopausal status. We have observed that plaque erosion is highly correlated with cigarette smoking in women and is the most frequent type of coronary thrombus seen in women younger than 50 years.[200] In contrast, plaque rupture is the more frequent mode of coronary thrombosis in women older than 50 years and is correlated with elevated serum total cholesterol.

We assessed the underlying percent stenosis with plaque rupture or erosion in men and women and found no significant differences. For plaque rupture, the underlying percent stenosis in men was 71 ± 13% compared with 77 ± 8% in women; in erosion, the underlying percent stenosis was 68 ± 17% in men compared with 68 ± 16% in women. Therefore, coronary angiography would not be sensitive in detecting the presence of a potential lethal erosive lesion. In fact, as many as 70% of plaque erosion lesions in men and women are seen in arteries with ≤70% cross-sectional area narrowing (equivalent to <50% diameter reduction); in plaque rupture, less than 50% of cases have borderline luminal narrowing, which would be missed on routine angiography. Therefore, new tools for the detection of patients at risk for plaque erosion and rupture are urgently needed.

We have shown in autopsy samples that vulnerable plaques occur more frequently in women older than 50 years than in those younger than 50 years (Color Plate 4–4). The morphologic characteristics of calcification and the lipid core were also studied. The extent of calcification in coronary arteries with 50% or greater narrowing was determined on a six-point scale: 0, no calcification; 1+, microcalcifications less than 20 μm in diameter; 2+, foci of calcification greater than 20 μm involving one quadrant of the plaque; 3+, calcification involving 2 quadrants; 4+, calcification involving 3 quadrants; and 5+, calcification involving the entire circumference of the coronary artery. A mean calcification score was calculated for each heart, and the mean was compared between women younger and older than 50. Similarly, the lipid core was measured in each plaque, as well as the thickness of the fibrous cap. The percent area occupied by the lipid core was calculated and the mean determined for women younger and older than 50 years. Comparison of coronary plaques that were more than 50% narrowed in cross-sectional area in women younger and older than 50 years showed several differences (see Color Plate 4–4). These can be summarized as follows: (1) the mean percent lipid core is smaller in women younger than 50 years; (2) the fibrous cap is thicker in women younger than 50 years; and (3) the mean calcification index is less in women younger than 50 years.

Therefore, it appears that women younger than 50 years are largely protected from the development of lesions of plaque rupture, but they are not protected from developing plaque erosion. Because the underlying mechanisms of plaque rupture and plaque erosion are poorly understood, it is unknown what possible hormonal effects are important in plaque instability. We postulate that vasospasm may be important in the genesis of plaque erosion, because the internal elastic lamina (IEL) area of erosion lesions is smaller than that of plaque rupture lesions. The effect of the components of cigarette smoke on vasospasm and thrombosis in the setting of plaque erosion is an area open for study.

Healed Plaque Rupture

We studied in detail the coronary trees of men and women who died suddenly of coronary atherosclerotic disease and divided the culprit lesions into those with luminal thrombi (plaque rupture and erosion) and stable plaques with or without healed myocardial infarction.[201] The stable lesions were further divided into those that showed healed plaque rupture and those that were fibrocalcific. We decided to evaluate each coronary segment that was more than 50% narrowed to determine if plaque progression could occur from repeated silent plaque ruptures. Healed plaque ruptures in men and women who died suddenly were morphologically characterized by Sirius red staining, followed by visualization under polarized light. The areas of healed plaque rupture showed a deep necrotic core with discontinuity of the overlying fibrous cap (staining yellow pink under polarized light, collagen type I), with an overlying proteoglycan-rich matrix with interspersed smooth muscle cells (type III collagen that stained green under polarized light). On routine sections, healed areas of rupture were identified as layers of collagen; these areas can be distinguished from stable plaque without healed rupture (Color Plate 4–5). We examined all epicardial arteries with more than 50% luminal narrowing in 142 men who died suddenly. Healed plaque ruptures were present in 75% of 44 hearts with acute plaque rupture (mean, 1.5 ± 1.2 ruptures per heart), 55% of hearts without acute thrombi (mean, 1.3 ± 1.4), and 20% of 23 hearts with acute erosion.[201] By univariate analysis, healed ruptures were associated with healed myocardial infarcts (1.7 ± 1.4 in hearts with healed infarcts versus 1.0 ± 1.2, p = .0007), increased cholesterol/HDL ratio (p < .0001), increased body mass index (BMI) (p = .0003), and increased glycohemoglobin (p = .04). By multivariate analysis, healed ruptures were associated with TC/HDL ratio (p < .00001), glycohemoglobin (p = .01), and BMI (p = .05) and were independent of smoking, age, number of sections examined, and hypertension. Mean luminal narrowing was 77 ± 9% for healed ruptures, compared with 69 ± 12% for acute ruptures. In women, healed plaque ruptures were infrequently observed; when present, they occurred more frequently in women older than 50 years (38% of women >50 years vs. 4% of women <50 years, p = .015) and in women with healed myocardial infarction. Thus, we can conclude that healed plaque ruptures are more frequent in patients with acute plaque rupture and those with healed myocardial infarction. The underlying risk factors most predictive of healed lesions are hypercholesterolemia, glucose intolerance, and higher BMI.

Mann and Davies[202] reported that healed plaque ruptures were a frequent finding in 31 men who died suddenly of coronary artery disease. The incidence of healed plaque rupture increased with increasing stenosis: from 16% in arteries with 0% to 20% narrowing, to 18% in arteries with 21% to 50% narrowing, to 73% in arteries with greater than 50% narrowing. The difference in incidence of healed ruptures between arteries with less than and greater than 50% narrowing was highly significant (p < .0001).[202] We also observed that the greater the number of healed plaque rupture sites in a localized area, the greater the likelihood of greater percent stenosis.[201] Our data agree with those of Mann and Davies[202] and suggest that plaque growth is episodic, occurs suddenly (often silently), and is a major cause of plaque progression. Our data also suggest that, as a mechanism of plaque progression in women, healed ruptures are likely significant after menopause.

References

1. Heberden W: Some account of a disorder of the breast. Med Trans R Coll Phys II London, 1772, pp 59–67.

2. Herrick JB: Certain features of sudden obstruction of the coronary arteries. Trans Assoc Am Phys 59:2015, 1912.
3. Sarnoff SJ, Braunwald E, Welch GHJ: Hemodynamic determinants of oxygen consumption of the heart with special reference to the tension-time index. Am J Physiol 192:148, 1958.
4. Rude RE, Izquierdo C, Buja LM, Willerson JT: Effects of inotropic and chronotropic stimuli on acute myocardial ischemic injury. I. Studies with dobutamine in the anesthetized dog. Circulation 65:1321, 1982.
5. Rude RE, Izquierdo C, Bush LR, et al: Effects of inotropic and chronotropic stimuli on acute myocardial ischemic injury. II. Studies with dopamine and ouabain in the barbiturate-anesthetized dog. J Cardiovasc Pharmacol 5:717, 1983.
6. Rude RE, Bush LR, Izquierdo C, et al: Effects of inotropic and chronotropic stimuli on acute myocardial ischemic injury. III. Influences of basal heart rate. Am J Cardiol 53:1688, 1984.
7. Sonnenblick EH, Ross J Jr, Braunwald E: Oxygen consumption of the heart. Newer concepts of its multifactorial determination. Am J Cardiol 22:328, 1968.
8. Marcus ML, Doty DB, Hiratzka LF, et al: Decreased coronary reserve: A mechanism for angina pectoris in patients with aortic stenosis and normal coronary arteries. N Engl J Med 307:1362, 1982.
9. Marcus ML, Mueller TM, Eastham CL: Effects of short- and long-term left ventricular hypertrophy on coronary circulation. Am J Physiol 241:H358, 1981.
10. Berkenboom GM, Abramowicz M, Vandermoten P, Degre SG: Role of alpha-adrenergic coronary tone in exercise-induced angina pectoris. Am J Cardiol 57:195, 1986.
11. Gage JE, Hess OM, Murakami T, et al: Vasoconstriction of stenotic coronary arteries during dynamic exercise in patients with classic angina pectoris: Reversibility by nitroglycerin. Circulation 73:865, 1986.
12. Wexler L, Brundage B, Crouse J, et al: Coronary artery calcification: Pathophysiology, epidemiology, imaging methods, and clinical implications. Circulation 94:1175, 1996.
13. Agatston AS, Janowitz WR, Hildner FJ, et al: Quantification of coronary artery calcium using ultrafast computed tomography. J Am Coll Cardiol 15:827, 1990.
14. Detrano R, Hsiai T, Wang S, et al: Prognostic value of coronary calcification and angiographic stenoses in patients undergoing coronary angiography. J Am Coll Cardiol 27:285, 1996.
15. Secci A, Wong N, Tang W, et al: Electron beam computed tomographic coronary calcium as a predictor of coronary events: Comparison of two protocols. Circulation 96:1122, 1997.
16. Arad Y, Spadaro LA, Goodman K, et al: Predictive value of electron beam computed tomography of the coronary arteries. 19-month follow-up of 1173 asymptomatic subjects. Circulation 93:1951, 1996.
17. Constantinides P: Plaque fissuring in human coronary thrombosis. J Atheroscler Res 6:1, 1966.
18. Davies MJ, Thomas AC: Plaque fissuring—the cause of acute myocardial infarction, sudden ischaemic death, and crescendo angina. Br Heart J 53:363, 1985.
19. Falk E: Plaque rupture with severe preexisting stenosis precipitating coronary thrombosis. Characteristics of coronary atherosclerotic plaques underlying fatal occlusive thrombi. Br Heart J 50:127, 1983.
20. Buja LM, Willerson JT: Clinicopathologic correlates of acute ischemic heart disease syndromes. Am J Cardiol 47:343, 1981.
21. Davies MJ, Fulton WF, Robertson WB: The relation of coronary thrombosis to ischaemic myocardial necrosis. J Pathol 127:99, 1979.
22. Buja LM, Willerson JT: The role of coronary artery lesions in ischemic heart disease: Insights from recent clinicopathologic, coronary arteriographic, and experimental studies. Hum Pathol 18:451, 1987.
23. Buja LM, Tofe AJ, Kulkarni PV, et al: Sites and mechanisms of localization of technetium-99m phosphorus radiopharmaceuticals in acute myocardial infarcts and other tissues. J Clin Invest 60:724, 1977.
24. Davies MJ, Thomas AC, Knapman PA, Hangartner JR: Intramyocardial platelet aggregation in patients with unstable angina pectoris suffering sudden ischemic cardiac death. Circulation 73:418, 1986.
25. Willerson JT, Hillis LD, Buja LM: Ischemic heart disease: Clinical and pathophysiological aspects. Raven, New York, 1982.
26. Fuster V, Badimon L, Badimon JJ, Chesebro JH: The pathogenesis of coronary artery disease and the acute coronary syndromes. N Engl J Med 326:310, 1992.
27. Fuster V, Lewis A: Mechanisms leading to myocardial infarction: Insights from studies of vascular biology. Circulation 91:256, 1995.
28. Libby P: Molecular bases of the acute coronary syndromes. Circulation 91:2844, 1995.
29. Ashton JH, Ogletree ML, Michel IM, et al: Cooperative mediation by serotonin S2 and thromboxane A2/prostaglandin H2 receptor activation of cyclic flow variations in dogs with severe coronary stenoses. Circulation 76:952, 1987.
30. Golino P, Ashton JH, Buja JM, et al: Local platelet activation causes vasoconstriction of large epicardial canine coronary arteries in vivo. Thromboxane A2 and serotonin are possible mediators. Circulation 79:154, 1989.
31. Bush LR, Campbell WB, Kern K, et al: The effects of alpha 2-adrenergic and serotonergic receptor antagonists on cyclic blood flow alterations in stenosed canine coronary arteries. Circ Res 55:642, 1984.
32. Willerson JT, Hillis LD, Winniford M, Buja LM: Speculation regarding mechanisms responsible for acute ischemic heart disease syndromes. J Am Coll Cardiol 8:245, 1986.
33. Willerson JT, Campbell WB, Winniford MD, et al: Conversion from chronic to acute coronary artery disease: Speculation regarding mechanisms. Am J Cardiol 54:1349, 1984.
34. Willerson JT, Golino P, Eidt J, Campbell WB, Buja LM: Specific platelet mediators and unstable coronary artery lesions. Experimental evidence and potential clinical implications. Circulation 80:198, 1989.
35. Hirsh PD, Hillis LD, Campbell WB, et al: Release of prostaglandins and thromboxane into the coronary circulation in patients with ischemic heart disease. N Engl J Med 304:685, 1981.
36. Eidt JF, Allison P, Noble S, et al: Thrombin is an important mediator of platelet aggregation in stenosed canine coronary arteries with endothelial injury. J Clin Invest 84:18, 1989.
37. van den Berg EK, Schmitz JM, Benedict CR, et al: Transcardiac serotonin concentration is increased in selected patients with limiting angina and complex coronary lesion morphology. Circulation 49:116, 1989.
38. Maseri A, Severi S, Nes MD, et al: "Variant" angina: One aspect of a continuous spectrum of vasospastic myocardial ischemia. Pathogenic mechanisms, estimated incidence and clinical and coronary arteriographic findings in 138 patients. Am J Cardiol 42:1019, 1978.
39. Dalen JE, Ockene IS, Alpert JS: Coronary spasm, coronary thrombosis and myocardial infarction: A hypothesis concerning the pathophysiology of acute myocardial infarction. Am Heart J 104:1119, 1982.
40. Gottlieb SO, Weisfeldt ML, Ouyang P, et al: Silent ischemia as a marker for early unfavorable outcomes in patients with unstable angina. N Engl J Med 314:1214, 1986.
41. Fleg JL, Gerstenblith G, Zonderman AB, et al: Prevalence and prognostic significance of exercise-induced silent myocardial ischemia detected by thallium scintigraphy and electrocardiography in asymptomatic volunteers. Circulation 81:428, 1990.
42. Weiner DA, Ryan TJ, McCabe CH, et al: Significance of silent myocardial ischemia during exercise testing in patients with coronary artery disease. Am J Cardiol 59:725, 1987.
43. Latham M: The Collected Works of Dr. P.M. Lathan. Vol 1. New Sydenham Society, London, 1876.
44. Osler W: The Lumleian lectures on angina pectoris. Lancet 1:697, 1910.
45. Prinzmetal M, Kennamer R, Merliss R: Angina pectoris. I. A variant form of angina pectoris. Am J Med 27:375, 1959.
46. Hillis LD, Braunwald E: Coronary-artery spasm. N Engl J Med 299: 695, 1978.
47. Silverman ME, Flamm MD: Variant angina pectoris. Anatomic findings and prognostic implications. Ann Intern Med 75:339, 1971.
48. Cheng TO, Bashour T, Kelser GA, et al: Variant angina of Prinzmetal with normal coronary arteriograms. A variant of the variant. Circulation 47:476, 1973.
49. Wiener L, Kasparian H, Duca PR, et al: Spectrum of coronary arterial spasm. Clinical, angiographic, and myocardial metabolic experience in 29 cases. Am J Cardiol 38:945, 1976.
50. Dhurandhar RW, Watt DL, Silver MD, et al: Prinzmetal's variant form of angina with arteriographic evidence of coronary arterial spasm. Am J Cardiol 30:902, 1972.
51. Oliva PB, Potts DE, Pluss RG: Coronary arterial spasm in Prinzmetal angina. Documentation by coronary arteriography. N Engl J Med 288: 745, 1973.
52. Maseri A, Mimmo R, Chierchia S: Coronary artery spasm as a cause of acute myocardial ischemia in man. Chest 68:625, 1975.
53. Higgins CB, Wexler L, Silverman JF, Schroeder JS: Clinical and arteriographic features of Prinzmetal's variant angina: Documentation of etiologic factors. Am J Cardiol 37:831, 1976.
54. Maseri A, Parodi O, Severi S, Pesola A: Transient transmural reduction of myocardial blood flow demonstrated by thallium-201 scintigraphy, as a cause of variant angina. Circulation 54:280, 1976.

55. McLaughlin PR, Doherty PW, Martin RP, et al: Myocardial imaging in a patient with reproducible variant angina. Am J Cardiol 39:126, 1977.
56. Berman ND, McLaughlin PR, Huckell VF, et al: Prinzmetal's angina with coronary artery spasm. Angiographic, pharmacologic, metabolic, and radionuclide perfusion studies. Am J Med 60:727, 1976.
57. Ricci DR, Orlick AE, Doherty PW, et al: Reduction of coronary blood flow during coronary artery spasm occurring spontaneously and after provocation by ergonovine maleate. Circulation 57:392, 1978.
58. Nelson C, Nowak B, Childs H, et al: Provocative testing for coronary arterial spasm: Rationale, risk, and clinical illustrations. Am J Cardiol 40:624, 1977.
59. Schroeder JS, Bolen JL, Quint RA, et al: Provocation of coronary spasm with ergonovine maleate. New test with results in 57 patients undergoing coronary arteriography. Am J Cardiol 40:487, 1977.
60. Curry RC Jr, Pepine CJ, Sabom MB, et al: Effects of ergonovine in patients with and without coronary artery disease. Circulation 56: 803, 1977.
61. Heupler FA, Proudfit WL, Razavi M, et al: Ergonovine maleate provocative test for coronary arterial spasm. Am J Cardiol 41:631, 1978.
62. Helfant RH: Coronary arterial spasm and provocative testing in ischemic heart disease. Am J Cardiol 41:787, 1978.
63. Buxton A, Goldberg S, Hirshfeld JW, et al: Refractory ergonovine-induced coronary vasospasm: Importance of intracoronary nitroglycerin. Am J Cardiol 46:329, 1980.
64. Scherf D, Perlman A, Schlachman M: Effect of dihydroergonovine on the heart. Proc Soc Exp Biol Med 71:420, 1949.
65. Heupler FA Jr: Provocative testing for coronary arterial spasm: Risk method, and rationale. Am J Cardiol 46:335, 1980.
66. Fester A: Provocative testing for coronary arterial spasm with ergonovine maleate. Am J Cardiol 46:338, 1980.
67. Cipriano PR, Guthaner DF, Orlick AE, et al: The effects of ergonovine maleate on coronary arterial size. Circulation 59:82, 1979.
68. Endo M, Hirosawa K, Kaneko N, et al: Prinzmetal's variant angina. Coronary arteriogram and left ventriculogram during angina attack induced by methacholine. N Engl J Med 294:252, 1976.
69. Yasue H, Horio Y, Nakamura N, et al: Induction of coronary artery spasm by acetylcholine in patients with variant angina: Possible role of the parasympathetic nervous system in the pathogenesis of coronary artery spasm. Circulation 74:955, 1986.
70. Raizner AE, Chahine RA, Ishimori T, et al: Provocation of coronary artery spasm by the cold pressor test. Hemodynamic, arteriographic and quantitative angiographic observations. Circulation 62:925, 1980.
71. Mudge GH Jr, Grossman W, Mills RM Jr, et al: Reflex increase in coronary vascular resistance in patients with ischemic heart disease. N Engl J Med 295:1333, 1976.
72. Yasue H, Nagao M, Omote S, et al: Coronary arterial spasm and Prinzmetal's variant form of angina induced by hyperventilation and Tris-buffer infusion. Circulation 58:56, 1978.
73. Nemerson Y: The phospholipid requirement of tissue factor in blood coagulation. J Clin Invest 47:72, 1968.
74. Hamsten A, Wiman B, de Faire U, Blomback M: Increased plasma levels of a rapid inhibitor of tissue plasminogen activator in young survivors of myocardial infarction. N Engl J Med 313:1557, 1985.
75. Schafer AI: Coagulation cascade: An overview. In Loscalzo J, Schafer AJ (eds): Thrombosis and Hemorrhage. Blackwell Scientific, Boston, 1993, p 3.
76. Chandler AB, Chapman I, Erhardt LR, et al: Coronary thrombosis in myocardial infarction. Report of a workshop on the role of coronary thrombosis in the pathogenesis of acute myocardial infarction. Am J Cardiol 34:823, 1974.
77. DeWood MA, Spores J, Notske R, et al: Prevalence of total coronary occlusion during the early hours of transmural myocardial infarction. N Engl J Med 303:897, 1980.
78. Buja LM, Willerson JT: Clinicopathologic correlates of acute ischemic heart disease syndromes. Am J Cardiol 47:343, 1981.
79. Gibson RS, Beller GA, Gheorghiade M, et al: The prevalence and clinical significance of residual myocardial ischemia 2 weeks after uncomplicated non–Q-wave infarction: A prospective natural history study. Circulation 73:1186, 1986.
80. Falk E: Unstable angina with fatal outcome: Dynamic coronary thrombosis leading to infarction and/or sudden death. Autopsy evidence of recurrent mural thrombosis with peripheral embolization culminating in total vascular occlusion. Circulation 71:699, 1985.
81. Haft JI, Haik BJ, Goldstein JE, Brodyn NE: Development of significant coronary artery lesions in areas of minimal disease. A common mechanism for coronary disease progression. Chest 94:731, 1988.
82. Little WC, Constantinescu M, Applegate RJ, et al: Can coronary angiography predict the site of a subsequent myocardial infarction in patients with mild-to-moderate coronary artery disease? Circulation 78:1157, 1988.
83. The RISC Group: Risk of myocardial infarction and death during treatment with low dose aspirin and intravenous heparin in men with unstable coronary artery disease. Lancet 336:827, 1990.
84. Lewis HD, Davis JW, Archibald DG, et al: Protective effects of aspirin against acute myocardial infarction and death in men with unstable angina. Results of a Veterans Administration Cooperative study. N Engl J Med 309:396, 1983.
85. Freeman MR, Williams AE, Chisholm RJ, Armstrong PW: Intracoronary thrombus and complex morphology in unstable angina. Relation to timing of angiography and in-hospital cardiac events. Circulation 80:17, 1989.
86. Sherman CT, Litvack F, Grundfest W, et al: Coronary angioscopy in patients with unstable angina pectoris. N Engl J Med 315:913, 1986.
87. Libby P, Hansson GK: Involvement of the immune system in human atherogenesis: Current knowledge and unanswered questions. Lab Invest 64:5, 1991.
88. Hansson GK, Jonasson L, Seifert PS, Stemme S: Immune mechanisms in atherosclerosis. Arteriosclerosis 9:567, 1989.
89. Gerrity RG: The role of the monocyte in atherogenesis: I. Transition of blood-borne monocytes into foam cells in fatty lesions. Am J Pathol 103:181, 1981.
90. Jonasson L, Holm J, Skalli O, et al: Regional accumulations of T cells, macrophages and smooth muscle cells in the human atherosclerotic plaque. Arteriosclerosis 6:131, 1986.
91. Parthasarathy S, Printz DJ, Boyd D, et al: Macrophage oxidation of low density lipoprotein generates a modified form recognized by the scavenger receptor. Arteriosclerosis 6:505, 1986.
92. Forman MB, Oates JA, Robertson D, et al: Increased adventitial mast cells in a patient with coronary spasm. N Engl J Med 313:1138, 1985.
93. Carry M, Korley V, Willerson JT, et al: Increased urinary leukotriene excretion in patients with cardiac ischemia. In vivo evidence for 5-lipoxygenase activation. Circulation 85:230, 1992.
94. Henney AM, Wakeley PR, Davies MJ, et al: Localization of stromelysin gene expression in atherosclerotic plaques by in situ hybridization. Proc Natl Acad Sci USA 88:8154, 1991.
95. Nikkari ST, O'Brien KD, Ferguson M, et al: Interstitial collagenase (MMP-1) expression in human carotid atherosclerosis. Circulation 92: 1393, 1995.
96. Sukhova G, Schönbeck U, Rabkin E, et al: Evidence for increased collagenolysis by interstitial collagenases-1 and -3 in vulnerable human atheromatous plaques. Circulation 99:2503, 1999.
97. Galis ZS, Muszynski M, Sukhova GK, et al: Increased expression of vascular matrix metalloproteinases induced in vitro by cytokines and in regions of human atherosclerotic lesions. Ann N Y Acad Sci 748: 501, 1995.
98. Moreno PR, Falk E, Palacios IF, et al: Macrophage infiltration in acute coronary syndromes. Implications for plaque rupture. Circulation 90: 775, 1994.
99. Henney AM, Wakeley PR, Davies MJ, et al: Localization of stromelysin gene expression in atherosclerotic plaques by in situ hybridization. Proc Natl Acad Sci USA 88:8154, 1991.
100. Rajavashisth TB, Xu XP, Jovinge S, et al: Membrane type 1 matrix metalloproteinase expression in human atherosclerotic plaques: Evidence for activation by proinflammatory mediators. Circulation 99: 3103, 1999.
101. Page DL, Caulfield JB, Kastor JA, et al: Myocardial changes associated with cardiogenic shock. N Engl J Med 285:133, 1971.
102. Alonso DR, Scheidt S, Post M, Killip T: Pathophysiology of cardiogenic shock: Quantification of myocardial necrosis, clinical, pathologic, and electrocardiographic correlation. Circulation 48:588, 1973.
103. Willerson JT, Curry GC, Watson JT, et al: Intraaortic balloon counterpulsation in patients in cardiogenic shock, medically refractory left ventricular failure, and/or recurrent ventricular tachycardia. Am J Med 58:183, 1975.
104. Platt MR, Willerson JT, Watson JT, et al: The use of AVCO intraaortic balloon circulatory assistance for patients with cardiogenic shock, severe left ventricular failure and refractory, recurrent ventricular tachycardia. In Norman JC (ed): Coronary Artery Medicine and Surgery: Concepts & Controversies. Appleton-Century-Crofts, New York, 1975, pp 401–409.
105. Sehapayak G, Watson JT, Curry GC, et al: Late development of intractable ventricular tachycardia after acute myocardial infarction. J Thorac Cardiovasc Surg 67:818, 1974.

106. Austen WG, Sanders CA, Averill JH, Friedlich AL: Ruptured papillary muscle. Report of a case with successful mitral valve replacement. Circulation 32:597, 1965.
107. Nishimura RA, Schaff HV, Shub C, et al: Papillary muscle rupture complicating acute myocardial infarction: Analysis of 17 patients. Am J Cardiol 51:373, 1983.
108. Ballester M, Tasca R, Marin L, et al: Different mechanisms of mitral regurgitation in acute and chronic forms of coronary heart disease. Eur Heart J 4:557, 1983.
109. Barbour DJ, Roberts WC: Rupture of a left ventricular papillary muscle during acute myocardial infarction: Analysis of 22 necropsy patients. J Am Coll Cardiol 8:558, 1986.
110. Meister SG, Helfant RH: Rapid bedside differentiation of ruptured interventricular septum from acute mitral insufficiency. N Engl J Med 287:1024, 1972.
111. Coma-Canella I, Gamallo C, Onsurbe PM, Jadraque LM: Anatomic findings in acute papillary muscle necrosis. Am Heart J 118:1188, 1989.
112. Come PC, Riley MF, Weintraub R, et al: Echocardiographic detection of complete and partial papillary muscle rupture during acute myocardial infarction. Am J Cardiol 56:787, 1985.
113. Radford MJ, Johnson RA, Daggett WM, et al: Ventricular septal rupture: A review of clinical and physiologic features and an analysis of survival. Circulation 64:545, 1981.
114. Moore CA, Nygaard TW, Kaiser DL, et al: Postinfarction ventricular septal rupture: The importance of location of infarction and right ventricular function in determining survival. Circulation 74:45, 1986.
115. Bansal RC, Eng AK, Shakudo M: Role of two-dimensional echocardiography, pulsed, continuous wave color flow Doppler techniques in the assessment of ventricular septal rupture after myocardial infarction. Am J Cardiol 65:852, 1990.
116. Cummings RG, Reimer KA, Califf R, et al: Quantitative analysis of right and left ventricular infarction in the presence of postinfarction ventricular septal defect. Circulation 77:33, 1988.
117. Mann JM, Roberts WC: Acquired ventricular septal defect during acute myocardial infarction: Analysis of 38 unoperated necropsy patients and comparison with 50 unoperated necropsy patients without rupture. Am J Cardiol 62:8, 1988.
118. Edwards BS, Edwards WD, Edwards JE: Ventricular septal rupture complicating acute myocardial infarction: Identification of simple and complex types in 53 autopsied hearts. Am J Cardiol 54:1201, 1984.
119. Jones MT, Schofield PM, Dark JF, et al: Surgical repair of acquired ventricular septal defect. Determinants of early and late outcome. J Thorac Cardiovasc Surg 93:680, 1987.
120. Norell MS, Gershlick AH, Pillai R, et al: Ventricular septal rupture complicating myocardial infarction: Is earlier surgery justified? Eur Heart J 8:1281, 1987.
121. Miller DC, Stinson EB: Surgical management of acute mechanical defects secondary to myocardial infarction. Am J Surg 141:677, 1981.
122. Lader E, Colvin S, Tunick P: Myocardial infarction complicated by rupture of both ventricular septum and right ventricular papillary muscle. Am J Cardiol 52:423, 1983.
123. Heyndrickx GR, Millard RW, McRitchie RJ, et al: Regional myocardial functional and electrophysiological alterations after brief coronary occlusion in conscious dogs. J Clin Invest 56:978, 1975.
124. Bush LR, Buja LM, Tilton G, et al: Effects of propranolol and diltiazem alone and in combination on the recovery of left ventricular segmental function after temporary coronary occlusion and long-term reperfusion in conscious dogs. Circulation 72:413, 1985.
125. Ellis SG, Henschke CI, Sandor T, et al: Time course of functional and biochemical recovery of myocardium salvaged by reperfusion. J Am Coll Cardiol 1:1047, 1983.
126. Braunwald E, Kloner RA: The stunned myocardium: Prolonged, postischemic ventricular dysfunction. Circulation 66:1146, 1982.
127. Rahimtoola SH: The hibernating myocardium. Am Heart J 117:211, 1989.
128. Fedele FA, Gewitz H, Capone RJ: Metabolic response to prolonged reduction of myocardial blood flow distal to a severe coronary artery stenosis. Circulation 78:729, 1988.
129. Marban E: Myocardial stunning and hibernation. The physiology behind the colloquialisms. Circulation 83:681, 1991.
130. Schaefer S, Schwartz GG, Gober JR, et al: Relationship between myocardial metabolites and contractile abnormalities during graded regional ischemia. Phosphorus-31 nuclear magnetic resonance studies of porcine myocardium in vivo. J Clin Invest 85:706, 1990.
131. Roberts R, Sobel BE, Parker CW: Radioimmunoassay for creatine kinase isoenzymes. Science 194:855, 1976.
132. Roberts R, Sobel BE: Editorial: Isoenzymes of creatine phosphokinase and diagnosis of myocardial infarction. Ann Intern Med 79:741, 1973.
133. Willerson JT, Stone MJ, Ting R, et al: Radioimmunoassay of creatine kinase-B isoenzyme in human sera: Results in patients with acute myocardial infarction. Proc Natl Acad Sci USA 74:1711, 1977.
134. Stone MJ, Willerson JT, Gomez-Sanchez CE, Waterman MR: Radioimmunoassay of myoglobin in human serum. Results in patients with acute myocardial infarction. J Clin Invest 56:1334, 1975.
135. Stone MJ, Waterman MR, Murray G, et al: Serum myoglobin level as diagnostic test in patients with acute myocardial infarction. Br Heart J 39:375, 1977.
136. Gilkeson G, Stone MJ, Waterman M, et al: Detection of myoglobin by radioimmunoassay in human sera: Its usefulness and limitations as an emergency room screening test for acute myocardial infarction. Am Heart J 95:70, 1978.
137. Trahern CA, Gere JB, Krauth GH, Bigham DA: Clinical assessment of serum myosin light chains in the diagnosis of acute myocardial infarction. Am J Cardiol 41:641, 1978.
138. Khaw BA, Gold HK, Fallon JT, Haber E: Detection of serum cardiac myosin light chains in acute experimental myocardial infarction: Radioimmunoassay of cardiac myosin light chains. Circulation 58:1130, 1978.
139. Katus HA, Remppis A, Neumann FJ, et al: Diagnostic efficiency of troponin T measurements in acute myocardial infarction. Circulation 83:902, 1991.
140. Stone MJ, Waterman MR, Poliner LR, et al: Myoglobinemia is an early and quantitative index of acute myocardial infarction. Angiology 29:386, 1978.
141. Ellis AK, Little T, Mausud AR, et al: Early noninvasive detection of successful reperfusion in patients with acute myocardial infarction. Circulation 78:1352, 1988.
142. Puleo PR, Perryman MB, Bresser MA, et al: Creatine kinase isoform analysis in the detection and assessment of thrombolysis in man. Circulation 75:1162, 1987.
143. Abendschein D, Seacord LM, Nohara R, et al: Prompt detection of myocardial injury by assay of creatine kinase isoforms in initial plasma samples. Clin Cardiol 11:661, 1988.
143. Abendschein D, Seacord LM, Nohara R, et al: Prompt detection of myocardial injury by assay of creatine kinase isoforms in initial plasma samples. Clin Cardiol 11:661, 1988.
144. Mair J, Morandell D, Genser N, et al: Equivalent early sensitivities of myoglobin, creatine kinase MB mass, creatine kinase isoform ratios, and cardiac troponins I and T for acute myocardial infarction. Clin Chem 41:1266, 1995.
145. Adams JE III, Bodor GS, Davila-Roman VG, et al: Cardiac troponin I. A marker with high specificity for cardiac injury. Circulation 88: 101, 1993.
146. Cummins B, Auckland MI, Cummins P: Cardiac-specific troponin-I radioimmunoassay in the diagnosis of acute myocardial infarction. Am Heart J 113:1333, 1987.
147. Martin GS, Becker BN, Schulman G: Cardiac troponin-I accurately predicts myocardial injury in renal failure. Nephrol Dial Transplant 13:1709, 1998.
148. Bonte FJ, Parkey RW, Graham KD, et al: A new method for radionuclide imaging of myocardial infarcts. Radiology 110:473, 1974.
149. Willerson JT, Parkey RW, Stokely EM, et al: Infarct sizing with technetium-99m stannous pyrophosphate scintigraphy in dogs and man: Relationship between scintigraphic and praecordial mapping estimates of infarct size in patients. Cardiovasc Res 11:291, 1977.
150. Parkey RW, Bonte FJ, Meyer SL, et al: A new method for radionuclide imaging of acute myocardial infarction in humans. Circulation 50: 540, 1974.
151. Willerson JT, Parkey RW, Bonte FJ, et al: Technetium stannous pyrophosphate myocardial scintigrams in patients with chest pain of varying etiology. Circulation 51:1046, 1975.
152. Wackers FJ III, Schoot JB, Sokole EB, et al: Noninvasive visualization of acute myocardial infarction in man with thallium-201. Br Heart J 37:741, 1975.
153. Wackers FJ, Sokole EB, Samson G, et al: Value and limitations of thallium-201 scintigraphy in the acute phase of myocardial infarction. N Engl J Med 295:1, 1976.
154. Silverman KJ, Becker LC, Bulkley BH, et al: Value of early thallium-201 scintigraphy for predicting mortality in patients with acute myocardial infarction. Circulation 61:996, 1980.
155. Wheelan K, Wolfe C, Corbett J, et al: Early positive technetium-99m stannous pyrophosphate images as a marker of reperfusion after

thrombolytic therapy for acute myocardial infarction. Am J Cardiol 56:252, 1985.
156. Parkey RW, Kulkarni PV, Lewis SE, et al: Effect of coronary blood flow and site of injection on Tc-99m PPi detection of early canine myocardial infarcts. J Nucl Med 22:133, 1981.
157. Dec GW, Palacios I, Yasuda T, et al: Antimyosin antibody cardiac imaging: Its role in the diagnosis of myocarditis. J Am Coll Cardiol 16:97, 1990.
158. Johnson LL, Seldin DW, Becker LC, et al: Antimyosin imaging in acute transmural myocardial infarctions: results of a multicenter clinical trial. J Am Coll Cardiol 13:27, 1989.
159. Carrio I, Berna L, Ballester M, et al: Indium-111 antimyosin scintigraphy to assess myocardial damage in patients with suspected myocarditis and cardiac rejection. J Nucl Med 29:1893, 1988.
160. Buja LM, Poliner LR, Parkey RW, et al: Clinicopathologic study of persistently positive technetium-99 stannous pyrophosphate myocardial infarction. Circulation 56:1016, 1977.
161. Nixon JV, Narahara KA, Smitherman TC: Estimation of myocardial involvement in patients with acute myocardial infarction by two-dimensional echocardiography. Circulation 62:1248, 1980.
162. Sheiban I, Casarotto D, Trevi G, et al: Two-dimensional echocardiography in the diagnosis of intracardiac masses: A prospective study with anatomic validation. Cardiovasc Intervent Radiol 10:157, 1987.
163. Stratton JR, Resnick AD: Increased embolic risk in patients with left ventricular thrombi. Circulation 75:1004, 1987.
164. Spirito P, Bellotti P, Chiarella F, et al: Prognostic significance and natural history of left ventricular thrombi in patients with acute anterior myocardial infarction: A two-dimensional echocardiographic study. Circulation 72:774, 1985.
165. Schnittger I: Cardiac and extracardiac masses: Echocardiographic evaluation. In Marcus ML, Schelbert HR, Skorton DJ, et al (eds): Cardiac Imaging: A Companion to Braunwald's Heart Disease. WB Saunders, Philadelphia, 1991, pp 511–537.
166. Pearlman AS, Otto CM: The use of Doppler techniques for quantification evaluation of valvular regurgitation. Eur Heart J 8(Suppl C): 35–43, 1987.
167. Pearson AC, Labovitz AJ, Mrosek D, et al: Assessment of diastolic function in normal and hypertrophied hearts: Comparison of Doppler echocardiography and M-mode echocardiography. Am Heart J 113: 1417, 1987.
168. Stein PD, Sabbah HN, Albert DE, Snyder JE: Continuous-wave Doppler for the noninvasive evaluation of aortic blood velocity and rate of change of velocity: Evaluation in dogs. Med Instrum 21: 177, 1987.
169. Rokey R, Kuo LC, Zoghbi WA, et al: Determination of parameters of left ventricular diastolic filling with pulsed Doppler echocardiography: Comparison with cineangiography. Circulation 71:543, 1985.
170. Loeppky JA, Greene ER, Hoekenga ED, et al: Beat-by-beat stroke volume assessment by pulsed Doppler in upright and supine exercise. J Appl Physiol 50:1173, 1981.
171. Aschenberg W, Schluter M, Kremer P, et al: Transesophageal two-dimensional echocardiography for the detection of left atrial appendage thrombus. J Am Coll Cardiol 7:163, 1986.
172. Nellessen U, Daniel WG, Matheis G, et al: Impending paradoxical embolism from atrial thrombus: Correct diagnosis by transesophageal echocardiography and prevention by surgery. J Am Coll Cardiol 5: 1002, 1985.
173. Lee W, Schiller NB: Transesophageal echocardiography in clinical cardiology. In Marcus ML, Schelbert HR, Skorton DJ, et al (eds): Cardiac Imaging: A Companion to Braunwald's Heart Disease. WB Saunders, Philadelphia, 1991, pp 605–616.
174. Nordrehaug JE, Johannessen KA, von der Lippe G: Usefulness of high-dose anticoagulants in preventing left ventricular thrombus in acute myocardial infarction. Am J Cardiol 55:1491, 1985.
175. Halperin JL, Fuster V: Left ventricular thrombus and stroke after myocardial infarction: Toward prevention or perplexity? J Am Coll Cardiol 14:912, 1989.
176. Weintraub WS, Ba'albaki HA: Decision analysis concerning the application of echocardiography to the diagnosis and treatment of mural thrombi after anterior wall acute myocardial infarction. Am J Cardiol 64:708, 1989.
177. Ascah KJ, Stewart WJ, Jiang L, et al: Doppler-two-dimensional echocardiographic method for quantitation of mitral regurgitation. Circulation 72:377, 1985.
178. Mintz GS, Kotler MN, Segal BL, Parry WR: Two-dimensional echocardiographic recognition of ruptured chordae tendineae. Circulation 57:244, 1978.
179. Spain MG, Smith MD, Grayburn PA, et al: Quantitative assessment of mitral regurgitation by Doppler color flow imaging: Angiographic and hemodynamic correlations. J Am Coll Cardiol 13:585, 1989.
180. Gillam LD, Hogan RD, Foale RA, et al: A comparison of quantitative echocardiographic methods for delineating infarct-induced abnormal wall motion. Circulation 70:113, 1984.
181. Guyer DE, Foale RA, Gillam LD, et al: An echocardiographic technique for quantifying and displaying the extent of regional left ventricular dyssynergy. J Am Coll Cardiol 8:830, 1986.
182. Gatewood RP, Nanda NC: Differentiation of left ventricular pseudoaneurysm from true aneurysm with two dimensional echocardiography. Am J Cardiol 46:869, 1980.
183. Kerber RE: Echocardiography in coronary artery disease: Myocardial ischemia and infarction. In Marcus ML, Schelbert HR, Skorton DJ, et al (eds): Cardiac Imaging: A Companion to Braunwald's Heart Disease. WB Saunders, Philadelphia, 1991, pp 594–603.
184. Hangartner JR, Charleston AJ, Davies MJ, Thomas AC: Morphological characteristics of clinically significant coronary artery stenosis in stable angina. Br Heart J 56:501, 1986.
185. Virmani R, Roberts WC: Extravasated erythrocytes, iron and fibrin in atherosclerotic plaques of coronary arteries in fatal coronary heart disease and their relation to luminal thrombus: Frequency and significance in 57 necropsy patients and in 2958 five mm segments of 224 major epicardial coronary arteries. Am Heart J 105:788, 1983.
186. Davies MJ: A macro and micro view of coronary vascular insult in ischemic heart disease. Circulation 82:II38, 1990.
187. Arbustini E, Grasso M, Diegoli M, et al: Coronary atherosclerotic plaques with and without thrombus in ischemic heart syndromes: A morphologic, immunohistochemical, and biochemical study. Am J Cardiol; 68:36B, 1991.
188. Silva JA, Escobar A, Collins TJ, et al: Unstable angina. A comparison of angioscopic findings between diabetic and non-diabetic patients. Circulation 92:1731, 1995.
189. Roberts WC, Kragel AH, Gertz SD, et al: The heart in fatal unstable angina pectoris. Am J Cardiol 68:22B, 1999.
190. Kragel AH, Gertz SD, Roberts WC: Morphologic comparison of frequency and types of acute lesions in the major epicardial coronary arteries in unstable angina pectoris, sudden coronary death and acute myocardial infarction. J Am Coll Cardiol 18:801, 1991.
191. DeWood MA, Leimgruber PP, Shields JP, et al: Thrombosis in acute myocardial infarction and sudden death: Angiographic aspects. Cardiovasc Clin 18:195, 1987.
192. Ambrose JA, Tannenbaum MA, Alexopoulos D, et al: Angiographic progression of coronary artery disease and the development of myocardial infarction. J Am Coll Cardiol 12:56, 1988.
193. Falk E, Shah PK, Fuster V: Coronary plaque disruption. Circulation 92:657, 1995.
194. Farb A, Tang AL, Burke AP, et al: Sudden coronary death: Frequency of active coronary lesions, inactive coronary lesions, and myocardial infarction. Circulation 92:1702, 1995.
195. Davies MJ: Anatomic features in victims of sudden coronary death. Coronary artery pathology. Circulation 85:I19, 1992.
196. Burke AP, Taylor A, Farb A, et al: Coronary calcification: Insights from sudden coronary death victims. Z Kardiol 89 Suppl 2:49, 2000.
197. Farb A, Burke AP, Tang AL, et al: Coronary plaque erosion without rupture into a lipid core. A frequent cause of coronary thrombosis in sudden coronary death. Circulation 93:1354, 1996.
198. Arbustini E, Dal Bello B, Morbini P, et al: Plaque erosion is a major substrate for coronary thrombosis in acute myocardial infarction. Heart 82:269, 1999.
199. Burke AP, Farb A, Malcom GT, et al: Coronary risk factors and plaque morphology in men with coronary disease who died suddenly [see comments]. N Engl J Med 336:1276, 1997.
200. Burke AP, Farb A, Malcom GT, et al: Effect of risk factors on the mechanism of acute thrombosis and sudden coronary death in women. Circulation 97:2110, 1998.
201. Burke AP, Kolodgie FD, Farb A, et al: Healed plaque ruptures and sudden coronary death: evidence that subclinical rupture has a role in plaque progression. Circulation 103:934, 2001.
202. Mann J, Davies MJ: Mechanisms of progression in native coronary artery disease: Role of healed plaque disruption. Heart 82:265, 1999.

CHAPTER 5

Risk Factors

5.1 Overview

William K. Vaughn

The onset and severity of coronary heart disease (CHD) differ between women and men. However, risk factors for CHD have been studied more extensively in men. Only since the 1980s have they been studied in large, carefully designed clinical trials in women. Many factors (including oral contraceptive use, menopause, hormone replacement therapy [HRT], and cultural and social roles) contribute to the sex difference and may act synergistically with known CHD risk factors (smoking, elevated cholesterol levels, and obesity) to increase risk.

CIGARETTE SMOKING

Cigarette smoking is associated with a higher risk of cardiovascular disease in both men and women.[1] Studies have shown that after a person quits smoking, the risk returns to near-normal levels.[1] Studies have also shown that among current smokers, there is a dose-response relationship between the relative risks of fatal CHD and of nonfatal myocardial infarction (MI).[1] In women, the risk of CHD has been independently related to smoking after adjustments for weight, menopausal status, estrogen use, family history of MI, and personal history of diabetes, hypertension, or hypercholesterolemia.[1, 2]

Other studies have shown a positive interaction between smoking and the use of oral contraceptives, particularly in younger women.[3, 4] Goldbaum and associates[3] demonstrated a linear increase in the relative risk (RR) for CHD among women smokers who did not use oral contraceptives. The RR ranged from 3.4 for light smokers (1–24 cigarettes per day) to 7 for heavy smokers (25 or more cigarettes per day). In contrast, these researchers demonstrated a nonlinear increase in RR among women smokers who did use oral contraceptives.[3] That risk ranged from 4.5 for light smokers to 39 for heavy smokers. Rosenberg and colleagues[4] obtained similar results: For women smokers who had never used oral contraceptives, the RR was 2.0 for light smokers and 4.8 for heavy smokers. For women smokers who did use oral contraceptives, the RR was 3.1 for light smokers and 23 for heavy smokers.

Wilson and associates[2] studied cardiovascular disease among postmenopausal women who used estrogen. These researchers found an increased rate of CHD (RR, 4.2), MI (RR, 3.2), and angina pectoris (RR, 5.2) in women smokers who use estrogen. Among nonsmokers, the relative risks for these diseases were greater than 1 but not statistically significant.

DIABETES

Several large studies have shown a substantial increase in the incidence and mortality of CHD in diabetics. In some studies, the rise in incidence and mortality was higher in women than in men.

The Evans County cohort study analyzed data on 1165 subjects classified as diabetic, probably diabetic, or nondiabetic.[5] Results were adjusted for potential confounding variables (age, systolic blood pressure, cholesterol and triglyceride levels, body mass, and smoking). Standardized CHD risk ratios were similar for men and women; the standardized risk ratio was approximately 2.4 for diabetic men and women.

The Chicago Heart Association Detection Project in Industry used multivariate Cox regression analysis to evaluate data from 39,572 middle-aged men and women employed by various companies in Chicago.[6] Variables included diabetes, age, serum cholesterol, smoking, systolic blood pressure, echocardiographic abnormalities, and education. Diabetes was associated with a higher risk of death due to CHD, and this association was greater in women than in men (RR in diabetic women, 3.09; RR in diabetic men, 1.58).

The Tecumseh Study examined the relationship between diabetes, gender, and CHD.[7, 8] It demonstrated a relationship between diabetic status and increased risk of death from CHD, even though multivariate analysis showed that the interaction was neither statistically significant nor large.[8]

Barrett-Connor and Wingard[9] studied 1657 adult residents of Rancho Bernardo, California. After adjusting for age, heart disease, risk factors, and exogenous sex hormones, they found that diabetic patients had a higher all-cause mortality rate than nondiabetic patients. The risk ratio was 2.2 in women and 1.5 in men. Unlike other studies, this study showed diabetes to be an independent risk factor for CHD mortality in men and women; however, it did not demonstrate a higher risk in women.

Diabetes is clearly a very powerful risk factor for CHD. However, it can be controlled by appropriate diet or treatment with oral medicine or insulin injections.

MENOPAUSE AND HORMONE REPLACEMENT THERAPY

Premenopausal women have a much lower incidence and mortality of CHD than both men and postmenopausal women who are not receiving estrogen replacement therapy. Earlier in life, these rates are much lower in women than in men. However, the difference between men and women narrows with increasing age. By the sixth to seventh decade of life, the incidence and mortality of CHD in men and women are similar.[10–13] These findings suggest that premenopausal women have a mechanism that protects against CHD.

Dallongeville and associates[11] studied 22,100 women to determine the relationship among CHD risk factors, menopause, and HRT. They found that postmenopausal women had significantly higher levels of cholesterol (6.23 versus 5.93 mmol/L), triglycerides (1.23 versus 1.14 mmol/L), apolipoprotein (apo) B (1.26 versus 1.19 g/L), apo A-I (1.8 versus 1.74 g/L), and diastolic blood pressure (78.7 versus 77.5 mm Hg). When the investigators compared postmenopausal women who were not receiving HRT with postmenopausal women who were receiving combined HRT, these differences were reversed, and the combined therapy group had lower lipid levels and blood pressure.

Matthews and colleagues[14] studied 541 premenopausal women for 5 years to assess biologic changes occurring at menopause. Women who entered menopause but did not receive hormone therapy had significantly higher levels of total cholesterol, triglycerides, apo A-I, and apo A-II. Furthermore, women who received HRT experienced substantial increases in triglycerides, apo A-I, and apo A-II from baseline to follow-up.

Hong and associates[15] studied the effects of estrogen replacement therapy in 90 women undergoing elective diagnostic coronary angiography. Of the 90 women, 18 were receiving estrogen replacement therapy and 72 were not. Risk factors (body mass index, hypertension, diabetes, smoking, family history, exercise, and alcohol use) were similar in the two groups. However, high-density lipoprotein (HDL) cholesterol levels were higher in the group receiving estrogen replacement therapy.

In summary, these studies show that menopause raises the risk of death due to cardiovascular disease. This higher risk is mediated through changes in various risk factors. HRT can modify these changes in risk factors to provide a healthier risk profile for postmenopausal women.

LIPIDS, APOLIPOPROTEINS, AND LIPOPROTEINS

Many epidemiologic studies and clinical trials have studied the relationship between variations in lipid levels and subsequent development of CHD. These studies have shown that increases in total cholesterol and its subfractions (except for HDL cholesterol) increase the risk of CHD.[16, 17]

Unfortunately, most of these studies have involved only men, usually of middle age. Extrapolating their findings to women may be inappropriate because (1) estrogen reduction (as occurs at menopause) modifies lipid profiles so that they increase the risk of CHD and (2) HRT after surgical or natural menopause modifies lipid profiles in women so that they mimic premenopausal profiles.

In later studies, some investigators[18–22] have attempted to define the relationship between lipid subspecies (i.e., the lipoprotein fragment Lp(a), apo A1, apo B, apo (a), and apo E) and CHD. Schwartzkopff and colleagues[18] studied 939 Chinese patients, 716 of whom had no history of CHD and 223 of whom had had an MI. MI sufferers of both sexes had significantly higher triglyceride, total cholesterol, and apo B levels than controls. In addition, women had higher low-density lipoprotein (LDL) cholesterol levels and higher LDL-HDL ratios than men. In a nested case-control study, Coleman and associates[22] studied a small group of 51 cases and 201 controls from the Guernsey Study. They found a strong positive relationship between cholesterol levels and risk of ischemic heart disease as well as a closer association between cholesterol levels and disease than between apo B levels and disease.

Kronmal and colleagues[23] studied the relationships between total cholesterol, HDL cholesterol, and LDL cholesterol and all-cause mortality in both men and women. In men, these researchers found a strong positive relationship between cholesterol level and all-cause mortality at age 40 years and a negative relationship between these two variables at age 80 years. In women younger than 70 years, they found a slight positive relationship between high cholesterol levels and all-cause mortality. However, in women older than 80 years, Kronmal and colleagues[23] found an association between higher levels of cholesterol and lower mortality. Unfortunately, these comparisons were based on unadjusted mortality, and survivor bias cannot be ruled out.

Kark and associates[21] studied Jewish patients (age range, 25–64 years) from Jerusalem who had had a first MI. In particular, they studied the relationship between Lp(a) values and CHD in women and the association of apo A phenotypes with risk. They found that men and women who were regular smokers or who had hypertension, hypercholesterolemia, or diabetes were at higher risk for a first MI. In women, Lp(a) values did not differ significantly between patients and controls, regardless of whether the results were adjusted.

In both men and women, total serum cholesterol, LDL cholesterol, and HDL cholesterol levels are strong predictors of the development of CHD. However, in women, these relationships may be mediated by age, menopausal status, and HRT. In addition, the impact of Lp(a) and apo A isoforms are predictors of risk for CHD independent of ethnicity and cultural background.[19]

HYPERTENSION AND OBESITY

Numerous studies have provided substantial evidence that hypertension (both systolic and diastolic) is a major independent risk factor for CHD in both men and women.[8, 24–26] Fiebach and associates,[27] analyzing data from a cohort of 121,700 female nurses, found that cardiovascular deaths were significantly more common among subjects who had high blood pressure. The age-adjusted RR was significant: 6.3 for coronary death and 4.1 for nonfatal MI. Because the role of obesity was confounded by the prevalence of high blood pressure in this study, the interaction between relative weight and high blood pressure was examined further; however, no significant interaction was found.

In a prospective, 12-year longitudinal study of 1462 Swedish women, subjects who were receiving antihypertensive therapy at the baseline visit had a much higher cumulative incidence of MI than did women with newly diagnosed or no hypertension at baseline.[26] Mortality was significantly higher than expected in the treatment-at-baseline group but not in the newly diagnosed and nonhypertensive groups.

Systolic and diastolic hypertension are important risk factors for cardiovascular morbidity and mortality. Although obesity is related to the prevalence of hypertension in women, concurrent obesity and hypertension do not appear to interact to raise the risk of cardiovascular disease.

FAMILY HISTORY

It has been widely documented that children of parents with early-onset CHD have a greater risk of experiencing the disease. This tendency toward greater risk is also found in subjects whose first-degree relatives have CHD. Several studies in the United Kingdom,[28] Italy,[29] and Spain[30] have confirmed the importance of family history as an independent risk factor for CHD and MI. Using logistic regression to adjust simultaneously for blood pressure, smoking, angina, and lipid levels, Grech and colleagues[28] showed family history to be an important risk factor for CHD. They also demonstrated that the number of diseased arteries was generally greater in patients with a family history of CHD and that the number of relatives with a history of CHD was directly related to the prevalence of CHD.

Roncaglioni and associates[29] studied MI in 916 patients and 1106 hospitalized control subjects from hospitals involved in the Gruppo Italiano per lo Studio della Sopravvivenza nell'Infarto Miocardico-2 (GISSI-2) trial. Using logistic regression, the investigators showed that risk (1) increased twofold to fourfold in patients with a family history of MI and (2) rose with the number of relatives with a history of MI. Just as important, the interaction of family history with the risk factors of smoking and a high cholesterol level also raised the risk. The RR increased from 6.2 to 14.0 in patients with a family history of MI. Similar increases resulted from the interaction of family history and cholesterol levels. The relative risk rose from 4.8 in patients with high cholesterol but no family history of heart disease to 8.3 in those with a family history of heart disease. These results were the same regardless of sex.

In a case-control study of 168 patients and 251 hospitalized control subjects, La Vecchia and associates[31] studied risk factors for MI in young women. The relative risk was 3.2 (after age adjustment only) and was 3.1 (after multivariate adjustment) for subjects who had more than one first-degree relative with a history of early CHD. The investigators concluded that family history, cigarette smoking, diabetes, and hypertension independently increase the risk of MI in young women and that the use of oral contraceptives marginally raises the risk of MI.

BEHAVIORAL CHARACTERISTICS AND PSYCHOSOCIAL FACTORS

First postulated in the 1950s, the relationship between type A behavior and an increased incidence of CHD has been studied extensively. Friedman and Rosenman,[32] in 1959, were the first to develop the concept of type A behavior and to relate it to cardiovascular events. Later, Haynes and associates[33] analyzed data from 1674 coronary disease–free individuals from the Framingham Study who were monitored for more than 8 years to determine the incidence of CHD. These researchers showed that scores on type A behavior, suppressed hostility, tension, and anxiety symptoms scales were higher in women and men with CHD.

Indicators of psychosocial risks and their relationship to MI and mortality have also been studied. O'Connor and associates[34] studied 340 patients who had had a first MI and an equal number of age-, sex-, and community-matched control subjects. They found that the type A personality was associated with a higher risk of nonfatal MI (odds ratio, 1.57; $p = 0.008$). The results were similar for men and women and were not statistically significant after multivariate adjustment. O'Connor and associates[34] also investigated modes of expressing anger and their relationship with cardiovascular risk factors; they found a positive, but not statistically significant, relationship between the two variables (odds ratio, 1.33; $p = 0.065$).

Gorkin and colleagues[35] studied psychosocial predictors of mortality in 1498 patients enrolled in the randomized Cardiac Arrhythmia Suppression Trial-1 (CAST-1). The psychosocial predictors (e.g., social, physical, and emotional functioning) were taken from the General Health Survey of the Rand Corporation. When the analysis included the entire population, there was no relationship between any of these potential psychosocial predictors and mortality. When the analysis was restricted to patients who received placebo only, however, level of social support was a highly significant predictor of mortality.

In a case-control study, Werlin and associates[36] examined the relationship between several variables (type A behavior, health locus of control, sleep problems, and alcohol consumption) and MI. Using multivariate analysis, they found no relationship between type A behavior and MI in either men (288 cases and 283 controls) or women (55 cases and 129 controls). However, these investigators did find that external health locus of control and sleep problems significantly raised the risk of MI in men (both before and after multivariate adjustment), whereas only sleep problems did so in women.

Conflicting results have been obtained regarding the relationship between psychosocial risk factors and both MI and death after cardiac arrhythmia. It is unknown whether the higher risk of such behavior patterns in type A personality modifies lipid profiles and therefore mediates CHD. However, Werlin and associates[36] have shown that health locus of control and sleep problems may be independently related to MI.

CONCLUSION

Large studies have shown that risk factors for the development of CHD are similar in men and women. However, the interactions between those risk factors are clearly more important in women. For example, the interaction between smoking and oral contraceptive use is synergistic. Many studies have shown that, even though premenopausal women seem to be protected against the development of CHD, this protection rapidly dissipates after menopause. Shortly after menopause, women have the same risk of developing CHD as men. HRT may reduce this risk. Fortunately, many of the risk factors for CHD (i.e., cigarette smoking, diabetes, HRT, high lipid levels, and hypertension) are under the direct control of the patient and physician. Women should therefore be encouraged to reduce these risk factors whenever possible.

References

1. Willett WC, Green A, Stampfer MJ, et al: Relative and absolute excess risks of coronary heart disease among women who smoke cigarettes. N Engl J Med 317:1303, 1987.

2. Wilson PWF, Garrison RJ, Castelli WP: Postmenopausal estrogen use, cigarette smoking, and cardiovascular morbidity in women over 50. N Engl J Med 313:1038, 1985.
3. Goldbaum GM, Kendrick JS, Hogelin GC, Gentry EM: The relative impact of smoking and oral contraceptive use on women in the United States. JAMA 258:1339, 1987.
4. Rosenberg L, Kaufman DW, Helmrich SP, et al: Myocardial infarction and cigarette smoking in women younger than 50 years of age. JAMA 253:2965, 1985.
5. Heyden S, Heiss G, Bartel AG, Hames CG: Sex differences in coronary mortality among diabetics in Evans County, Georgia. J Chronic Dis 33: 265, 1980.
6. Pan WH, Cedres LB, Liu K, et al: Relationship of clinical diabetes and asymptomatic hyperglycemia to risk of coronary heart disease mortality in men and women. Am J Epidemiol 123:504, 1986.
7. Butler WJ, Ostrander LD Jr, Carman WJ, Lamphiear DE: Diabetes mellitus in Tecumseh, Michigan: Prevalence, incidence, and associated conditions. Am J Epidemiol 116:971, 1982.
8. Butler WJ, Ostrander LD Jr, Carman WJ, Lamphiear DE: Mortality from coronary heart disease in the Tecumseh Study: Long-term effect of diabetes mellitus, glucose tolerance and other risk factors. Am J Epidemiol 121:541, 1985.
9. Barrett-Connor E, Wingard DL: Sex differential in ischemic heart disease mortality in diabetics: A prospective population-based study. Am J Epidemiol 118:489, 1983.
10. Barrett-Connor EL, Cohn BA, Wingard DL, Edelstein SL: Why is diabetes mellitus a stronger risk factor for fatal ischemic heart disease in women than in men? JAMA 265:627, 1991.
11. Dallongeville J, Marecaux N, Isorez D, et al: Multiple coronary heart disease risk factors are associated with menopause and influenced by substitutive hormonal therapy in a cohort of French women. Atherosclerosis 118:123, 1995.
12. Grodstein F, Stampfer M: The epidemiology of coronary heart disease and estrogen replacement in postmenopausal women. Prog Cardiovasc Dis 8:199, 1994.
13. Gorodeski GI: Impact of the menopause on the epidemiology and risk factors of coronary artery disease in women. Exp Gerontol 29:357, 1994.
14. Matthews KA, Meilahn E, Kuller LH, et al: Menopause and risk factors for coronary heart disease. N Engl J Med 321:641, 1989.
15. Hong MK, Romm PA, Reagan K, et al: Effects of estrogen replacement therapy on serum lipid values and angiographically defined coronary artery disease in postmenopausal women. Am J Cardiol 69:176, 1992.
16. Hearn JA, DeMaio SJ Jr, Roubin GS, et al: Predictive value of lipoprotein(a) and other serum lipoproteins in the angiographic diagnosis of coronary artery disease. Am J Cardiol 66:1176, 1990.
17. Stensvold I, Urdal P, Thürmer H, et al: High-density lipoprotein cholesterol and coronary cardiovascular and all-cause mortality among middle-aged Norwegian men and women. Eur Heart J 13:1155, 1992.
18. Schwartzkopff W, Schleicher J, Pottins I, et al: Lipids, lipoproteins, apolipoproteins, and other risk factors in Chinese men and women with and without myocardial infarction. Atherosclerosis 82:253, 1990.
19. Sandholzer C, Saha N, Kark JD, et al: Apo(a) isoforms predict risk for coronary heart disease: A study in six populations. Arterioscler Thromb 12:1214, 1992.
20. Murai A, Miyahara T, Fujimoto N, et al: Lp(a) lipoprotein as a risk factor for coronary heart disease and cerebral infarction. Atherosclerosis 59:199, 1986.
21. Kark JD, Sandholzer C, Friedlander Y, Utermann G: Plasma Lp(a), apolipoprotein(a) isoforms and acute myocardial infarction in men and women: A case-control study in the Jerusalem population. Atherosclerosis 98:139, 1993.
22. Coleman MP, Key TJA, Wang DY, et al: A prospective study of obesity, lipids, apolipoproteins and ischemic heart disease in women. Atherosclerosis 92:177, 1992.
23. Kronmal RA, Cain KC, Ye Z, Omenn GS: Total serum cholesterol levels and mortality risk as a function of age: A report based on the Framingham data. Arch Intern Med 153:1065, 1993.
24. Gilbert BW: ACE inhibitors and regression of left ventricular hypertrophy. Clin Cardiol 15:711, 1992.
25. Vester EG, Kuhls S, Ochiulet-Vester J, et al: Electrophysiological and therapeutic implications of cardiac arrhythmias in hypertension. Eur Heart J 13(Suppl D):70, 1992.
26. Sigurdsson JA, Bengtsson C, Lapidus L, et al: Morbidity and mortality in relation to blood pressure and antihypertensive treatment. Acta Med Scand 215:313, 1984.
27. Fiebach NH, Hebert PR, Stampfer MJ, et al: A prospective study of high blood pressure and cardiovascular disease in women. Am J Epidemiol 130:646, 1989.
28. Grech ED, Ramdale DR, Bray CL, Faragher EB: Family history as an independent risk factor of coronary artery disease. Eur Heart J 13: 1311, 1992.
29. Roncaglioni MC, Santoro L, D'Avanzo B, et al: Role of family history in patients with myocardial infarction: An Italian case-control study. Circulation 85:2065, 1992.
30. Castro-Beiras A, Muñiz J, Fernández-Fuertes I, et al: Family history as an independent risk factor for ischemic heart disease in a low incidence area (Galicia, Spain). Eur Heart J 14:1445, 1993.
31. La Vecchia C, Franceschi S, Decarli A, et al: Risk factors for myocardial infarction in young women. Am J Epidemiol 125:832, 1987.
32. Friedman M, Rosenman RH: Association of specific overt behavior pattern with blood and cardiovascular findings. JAMA 16:1286, 1959.
33. Haynes SG, Feinleib M, Kannel WB: The relationship of psychosocial factors to coronary heart disease in the Framingham Study. III: Eight-year incidence of coronary heart disease. Am J Epidemiol 111:37, 1980.
34. O'Connor NJ, Manson JE, O'Connor GT, Buring JE: Psychosocial risk factors and non-fatal myocardial infarction. Circulation 92:1458, 1995.
35. Gorkin L, Schron EB, Brooks MM, et al: Psychosocial predictors of mortality in the Cardiac Arrhythmia Suppression Trial-1 (CAST-1). Am J Cardiol 71:263, 1993.
36. Werlin CLM, Rosengren A, Wilhelmsen LW: Behavioral characteristics in patients with myocardial infarction: A case-control study. J Cardiovasc Risk 2:247, 1995.

5.2 Lipids and Atherosclerosis

John A. Farmer and Antonio M. Gotto, Jr.

The age-adjusted death rates for coronary atherosclerosis have decreased significantly in the United States since 1970. However, the incidence and prevalence of coronary disease has not decreased, which has led to an increase in the morbidity and mortality associated with coronary atherosclerosis in the older population group. The decline in age-adjusted death rates for coronary atherosclerosis has been less striking in women than in men.[1] Instituting preventive measures in women has been hampered by the general perception that women are protected from the complications of coronary heart disease (CHD). However, coronary atherosclerosis is the most common cause of mortality among women in the United States, accounting for approximately 250,000 deaths in 1995. The process of atherosclerosis appears to be similar in men and women, but comparison of the two sexes reveals significant differences in the risk factor profile and prevalence of lipoprotein distribution.

RISK FACTORS IN WOMEN

The concept of the identification and modification of risk factors as a means to decrease subsequent morbidity and mortality rates from coronary heart disease has gained acceptance, using the principles of evidence-based medicine. Evidence-based medicine requires clinical decisions to be made using data from clinical trials that have demonstrated a reduction in morbidity and mortality following risk factor modification. Coronary atherosclerosis in women is predominantly a disease of the elderly, with symptomatic manifestations occurring approximately 10 years later in women than in men. Additionally, analysis of the Framingham Study database reveals that myocardial infarction (MI) occurs approximately 20 years later in women than in men.[2] The incidence of CHD increases significantly in middle-aged women and has been correlated with intimal thickness determinations by carotid ultrasonography in the Atherosclerosis Risk in Communities (ARIC) study.[3] The Cholesterol Lowering Atherosclerosis Study (CLAS) also supports the premise that carotid disease can act as a surrogate for predicting coronary events and provides a noninvasive screening test for both women and men.[4]

Several risk factors contribute to an increased risk for CHD in women. Diabetes, for example, raises the risk for a symptomatic cardiac event in women by sevenfold, essentially eliminating any gender-mediated protection. The use of tobacco products represents a significant modifiable risk factor that appears to exert a dramatic effect: Approximately half of all cardiac events in women are related to smoking.[5] Hypertension appears to be a strong predictor of CHD in women and may raise the risk for coronary mortality by as much as tenfold.

The role of obesity as an independent risk factor is controversial, because higher body mass index is also commonly associated with sedentary lifestyle, poor nutritional habits, glucose intolerance, and hypertension. Moreover, women who manifest truncal obesity appear to be at significant risk for CHD; thus, in women, the waist-hip ratio can predict mortality better than body mass index.[6] Women are frequently less physically active than men, but physically active women may reduce their risk of CHD by 50% to 60% compared with individuals who have a sedentary lifestyle.

Low-dose oral contraceptives may be safely administered to women without eliciting a significant risk factor profile. However, high-dose formulations have been associated with a significantly higher risk for acute MI in women who smoke.[7] Furthermore, high-dose oral contraceptives have been associated with increased circulating levels of low-density lipoprotein (LDL) cholesterol, which is accompanied by decreased levels of high-density lipoprotein (HDL) cholesterol, glucose intolerance, and a propensity for blood clotting. The third-generation low-dose oral contraceptives have essentially eliminated the adverse effects on metabolic parameters.

Finally, dyslipidemia is a major modifiable risk factor for CHD in both men and women. Data demonstrating the clinical efficacy of lowering LDL cholesterol levels for women in both angiographic and clinical trials are emphasized in this discussion.

PLASMA LIPOPROTEINS

Lipid metabolism encompasses the synthesis, transport, and functional activities of plasma lipoproteins (Table 5–1). Lipoproteins, a family of circulating particles that have a similar chemical structure, consist of a nonpolar core composed of cholesteryl ester and triglyceride and a polar surface coat composed of unesterified cholesterol, phospholipid, and apolipoproteins. Apolipoproteins stabilize the lipoprotein particle, activate enzymes involved in the degradation of circulating lipids, and interact with receptors that allow the recognition, binding, and removal of lipoproteins from the circulation.

Chylomicrons

Chylomicrons, triglyceride-rich particles formed in the lacteals of the lymphatic system of the intestinal wall, are the initial particles of exogenous lipid transport. These large particles are synthesized from dietary fat and transport free fatty acids as a potential energy source for muscle and other peripheral tissues. Chylomicrons are metabolized through the action of lipoprotein lipase, which is activated by apo C-II on the chylomicron surface. The resulting chylomicron remnant has a relatively short half-life in the circulation.

Very-Low-Density Lipoproteins

Very-low-density lipoprotein (VLDL) is a triglyceride-rich particle produced predominantly in the liver. VLDL particles are smaller than chylomicrons and are the initial particles of endogenous lipid transport. VLDL and the subsequent lipoproteins in its lipid cascade transport endogenous triglyceride to the periphery, where it may be used for energy or stored for future use. VLDL is metabolized through the action of lipoprotein lipase, which is activated by apo C-II on the VLDL surface. The resulting particle is intermediate-density lipoprotein (IDL).

Intermediate-Density Lipoproteins

IDLs are rich in both triglyceride and cholesterol. IDL particles are either removed from the circulation by the B/E receptor, through the recognition and binding of apo E on the IDL surface, or they may be further metabolized through the action of hepatic lipase, which removes fatty acids, C apolipoproteins, and apo E from the IDL particle to form LDL. Approximately 30% to 40% of IDL particles are transformed into LDL.

Low-Density Lipoproteins

LDL is a relatively small particle that carries approximately 70% of circulating cholesterol. The LDL core is composed almost entirely of cholesteryl ester, with only a minimal amount of triglyceride. Apo B-100 is the sole apolipoprotein of LDL; each LDL particle has one apo B-100 molecule on its surface.

LDL may be further classified into seven subgroups according to size and density. For clinical purposes, however, two subclass patterns have been identified. LDL subclass pattern A is characterized by a preponderance of large,

Table 5–1. CLASSIFICATION AND PROPERTIES OF PLASMA LIPOPROTEINS

LIPOPROTEIN CLASS	MAJOR LIPIDS	APOLIPOPROTEINS	DENSITY (g/ml)	DIAMETER (Å)	ELECTROPHORETIC MOBILITY
Chylomicrons	Dietary triglyceride, cholesteryl ester	A-I, A-II, A-IV, B-48, C-I, C-II, C-III, E	<0.95	800–5000	Origin
Chylomicron remnants	Dietary cholesteryl ester	B-48, E	<1.006	>300	Origin
VLDL	Endogenous triglyceride	B-100, C-I, C-II, C-III, E	<1.006	300–800	Pre-beta
IDL	Cholesteryl ester, triglyceride	B-100, E	1.006–1.019	250–350	Broad-beta
LDL	Cholesteryl ester	B-100	1.019–1.063	180–280	Beta
HDL_2	Cholesteryl ester	A-I, A-II, C-I, C-II, C-III, E	1.063–1.125	90–120	Alpha
HDL_3	Cholesteryl ester	A-I, A-II, C-I, C-II, C-III, E	1.125–1.210	50–90	Alpha

HDL, high-density lipoprotein; IDL, intermediate-density lipoprotein; LDL, low-density lipoprotein; VLDL, very-low-density lipoprotein.
From: Farmer JA, Gotto AM Jr: Dyslipidemia and other risk factors for coronary artery disease. In Braunwald E (ed): Heart Disease: A Textbook of Cardiovascular Medicine, 5th ed. WB Saunders, Philadelphia, 1997, 1126.

buoyant LDL particles; LDL subclass pattern B is characterized by a preponderance of small, dense LDL particles and is associated with a threefold-increased risk for MI.[8] LDL subclass pattern B has been reported in approximately 25% of females and 37% of males, but in only 13% of premenopausal females and 17% of males aged 6 to 19 years.[9] Although the mechanism by which LDL subclass pattern B increases atherosclerotic risk has not been established, small, dense LDL has been reported to be more susceptible to in vitro oxidation than large, buoyant LDL.[10] Small, dense LDL particles frequently occur in the presence of hypertriglyceridemia, as triglyceride from the triglyceride-rich lipoproteins is exchanged for cholesteryl ester in LDL through the action of cholesteryl ester transfer protein (CETP).

Approximately 75% of LDL particles are removed from the circulation through recognition and binding of apo B-100 by the B/E receptor. (B/E receptors are generated within the hepatocyte and transported to the coated pit on the cell surface, where they protrude into the circulation, allowing recognition of circulating lipoproteins whose surfaces contain apo B-100 or apo E.) The number of B/E receptors is not fixed and can be upregulated or downregulated in response to the amount of intracellular cholesterol. A rise in intracellular cholesterol decreases the activity of these receptors and restores normal cholesterol homeostasis. Estrogen activates a promoter region on the B/E receptor gene, which activates transcription and increases LDL removal. In postmenopausal women, B/E receptor activity diminishes if estrogen is not replaced. As a result, LDL cholesterol concentration rises and may exceed that of age-matched men.

LDL modified chemically, such as by oxidation or acetylation, is susceptible to removal by scavenger receptors on macrophages. Unlike the B/E receptor, the scavenger receptor is not downregulated as intracellular cholesterol increases, and as the scavenger receptor continues to take up LDL, the macrophage is converted into a lipid-laden foam cell.

Lipoprotein (a)

Lipoprotein (a) (Lp[a]) is identical to LDL with the addition of an apo(a) molecule attached to the apo B-100 molecule by a disulfide bond. Circulating concentration of Lp(a) is primarily determined by genetic factors and varies among racial groups. In white people, the distribution of Lp(a) concentration is highly skewed and in most individuals is less than 20 mg/dl, whereas in black people, the distribution is gaussian. In addition to genetic influences, conditions such as renal insufficiency and hormonal status may alter Lp(a) concentration. Lp(a) concentration increases after menopause, and estrogen administration may reduce circulating concentrations of Lp(a).[11] Lp(a) concentration greater than 30 mg/dl is generally considered elevated.

Lp(a) binds to the B/E receptor but is not effectively cleared because of decreased binding affinity. This impairment of receptor-mediated clearance has important therapeutic implications, because lipid-regulating drugs whose primary mechanism is the upregulation of the B/E receptor, such as bile acid resins and 3-hydroxy-3-methylglutaryl coenzyme A (HMG CoA) reductase inhibitors, have little or no effect on Lp(a) concentration.

Diet and exercise do not appear to affect Lp(a) concentration. In addition to estrogen, nicotinic acid[12] and bezafibrate[13] have been reported to decrease Lp(a) concentration. The effect of lowering elevated Lp(a) concentration has not been studied in clinical trials of lipid-regulating therapy.

High-Density Lipoprotein

HDL is synthesized by the liver and intestine as a discoidal precursor particle composed of phospholipid, unesterified cholesterol, and apolipoproteins. Through the action of lecithin-cholesterol acyltransferase (LCAT) on the phospholipid and cholesterol, the particle gradually assumes a spherical shape with a core of cholesteryl ester. This mature particle, HDL_3, receives additional phospholipid and cholesterol from the redundant surface layer of hydrolyzed triglyceride-rich lipoproteins and from cell membranes. Through the continued action of LCAT, HDL_3 is converted to HDL_2, which is a larger, more cholesterol-rich particle. HDL_3 cholesterol concentrations are roughly the same in women and men. The well-documented higher HDL cholesterol concentration in women results largely from an increase in HDL_2 cholesterol.

ROLE OF LIPIDS IN ATHEROGENESIS

The positive curvilinear relation between cholesterol, particularly LDL cholesterol, and CHD has been established in epidemiologic, genetic, experimental, and interventional studies.[14] The relationship between coronary mortality rates and cholesterol is valid for both men and women. Although blood cholesterol concentrations are useful in population studies, total cholesterol alone does not adequately discriminate potential risk in an individual patient, and the measurement of lipid subfractions—LDL cholesterol, HDL cholesterol, and total triglyceride—is recommended by the U.S. National Cholesterol Education Program (NCEP) for more precise risk assessment.[14] Chylomicrons and VLDL do not appear to be atherogenic, but their hydrolyzed remnants may increase CHD risk. Cholesterol from chylomicron remnants downregulates B/E receptor activity and so decreases LDL clearance from the circulation. IDL has been shown to predict progression of atherosclerotic lesions.[15, 16]

Abnormal lipoproteins, such as oxidized LDL and small, dense VLDL, are removed from the circulation by the scavenger receptor on activated macrophages. Because this receptor is not downregulated as intracellular cholesterol accumulates, macrophages may become lipid-laden foam cells, the primary component of the fatty streak thought to be the initial atherosclerotic lesion. Atherosclerotic lesions appear to develop in response to endothelial injury.[17] Oxidized LDL is cytotoxic and may cause endothelial injury, or endothelial injury may be caused by factors such as shear stress and hypercholesterolemia.[18] Endothelial dysfunction may be reversed by lipid lowering.[19–21]

The mechanism by which Lp(a) influences atherosclerotic risk is multifactorial and poorly understood. Because of the structural similarity between apo(a) and plasminogen, Lp(a) may interfere with the generation of plasmin[22] and may provide a link between atherosclerosis and thrombosis. Lp(a) has been found deposited in the arterial wall, especially in areas with atherosclerotic lesions.[23] Lp(a) appears to be more susceptible to oxidation than LDL[24] and may be more susceptible to uptake by the scavenger receptor.

HDL is inversely related to risk for CHD.[25] Each 1-mg/dl increase in HDL cholesterol decreases CHD risk approximately 3% in women and 2% in men.[26] Although the underlying mechanisms have not been completely elucidated, a commonly accepted hypothesis is reverse cholesterol transport, the posited process by which HDL is thought to remove cholesterol from peripheral cells and return it to the liver. Other possible mechanisms are enhanced endothelial repair,[27] greater prostacyclin stabilization,[28] and protection against LDL oxidation.[29]

EVIDENCE FOR INTERVENTION

A large number of clinical trials have established the efficacy of lipid lowering by several interventions.[30] However, women have typically been underrepresented in these trials, even though CHD is the leading cause of death in both women and men in the United States.[31] Many of the early trials were conducted exclusively in men, and no published primary-prevention studies (studies conducted in subjects without known CHD) have included women. Although most later secondary-prevention studies (studies conducted in subjects with known CHD) have enrolled both women and men, this discussion is limited to studies in which results in women have been analyzed separately.

Trials Whose Primary Endpoint Was Clinical Events

Program on the Surgical Control of the Hyperlipidemias

In the Program on the Surgical Control of the Hyperlipidemias (POSCH), 838 patients (including 78 women) with prior MI were randomly assigned to receive either partial ileal bypass surgery or usual care.[32] All subjects received dietary instruction. Eligible patients were 30 to 64 years old and had, after a dietary trial, either a total cholesterol level of 220 mg/dl or higher or, in patients with a total cholesterol level of 200 to 219 mg/dl, an LDL cholesterol level of 140 mg/dl or higher. The primary endpoint was death from any cause, but angiographic studies were performed at 3, 5, and 7 or 10 years.

At 5-year follow-up, in comparison with control patients, patients who had undergone bypass surgery had lower levels of total cholesterol (by 23%) and LDL cholesterol (by 38%), and higher levels of HDL cholesterol (by 4%) and triglyceride (by 20%). At 10-year follow-up, total mortality was 22% lower and CHD mortality was 28% lower in the surgery group than in the control group, but these differences were not statistically significant. However, the combined endpoint of CHD death or nonfatal MI was significantly lower (by 35%) in the surgery group. Angiographic results, expressed as a global change score, showed significant reductions in progression in patients undergoing surgery at each follow-up visit: 28% of patients undergoing surgery had progression compared with 41% of control patients at 3 years; 37% compared with 65%, respectively, at 5 years; 48% compared with 77%, respectively, at 7 years; and 55% compared with 85%, respectively, at 10 years. Angiographic change between baseline and 3-year follow-up studies was significantly associated with subsequent total mortality and CHD mortality.[33]

Among the women at 5-year follow-up, patients undergoing surgery had lower levels of total cholesterol (by 24%) and LDL cholesterol (by 36%) and higher levels of HDL cholesterol (by 8.5%) and triglyceride (by 2.5%) compared with control patients.[34] The incidence of clinical events among women was not significantly different in the two treatment groups because of the relatively small number of women; however, in the surgery group, the combined endpoint of CHD death and nonfatal MI was 31% lower, the proportion of patients undergoing coronary artery bypass grafting (CABG) during the trial was 30% lower, and the proportion of patients undergoing percutaneous transluminal coronary angioplasty (PTCA) during the trial was 58% lower than in the control group. Five women in the surgery group and two women in the control group died. Angiographic change, as indicated by global change score, showed disease progression in fewer women in the surgery group at each follow-up visit: 19% of women in the surgery group had progression compared with 32% of women in the control group at 3 years; 29% compared with 57%, respectively, at 5 years; 35% compared with 75%, respectively, at 7 years; and 55% compared with 100%, respectively, at 10 years. The difference was significant only at 5 years.

Scandinavian Simvastatin Survival Study

The Scandinavian Simvastatin Survival Study (4S) randomly assigned 4444 patients with a history of angina pectoris or MI (including 827 women evenly divided between treatment groups) to receive placebo or simvastatin at a dosage titrated to reduce total cholesterol to 116 to 201 mg/dl.[35] The initial 20 mg/day simvastatin dosage was increased to 40 mg/day in 37% of patients and decreased to 10 mg/day in two patients. Eligible subjects were 35 to 70 years of age; premenopausal women with childbearing potential were excluded. The lipid criteria for entry in the study were total cholesterol 212 to 309 mg/dl and triglyceride 221 mg/dl or lower after dietary instruction. The primary endpoint was total mortality. The secondary endpoint was major coronary events (coronary death, nonfatal MI, resuscitated cardiac arrest, and definite silent MI) analyzed by time to first event. Median follow-up was 5.4 years.

In simvastatin subjects, the total cholesterol level was reduced by 25%, LDL cholesterol by 35%, and triglyceride by 10%, and the HDL cholesterol level was increased by 8%. The placebo group showed 1% increases in total cholesterol and both LDL and HDL cholesterol levels, and a 7% increase in triglyceride level. Simvastatin therapy reduced total mortality by 30% when compared with placebo. Additionally, simvastatin therapy significantly reduced the incidence of coronary mortality by 42% when compared with placebo. In women, simvastatin therapy reduced the incidence of major coronary events by 35% when compared with placebo, but the total mortality and coronary mortality were similar in the two treatment groups, owing to the relatively small number of female patients.

Cholesterol and Recurrent Events Trial

In the Cholesterol and Recurrent Events (CARE) trial, 4159 patients with previous MI (including 576 women) were randomly assigned to receive pravastatin, 40 mg/day, or placebo.[36] Women accounted for 14% of each treatment group. Eligible subjects were 21 to 75 years of age; women were required to be postmenopausal. The lipid criteria for entry in the study were plasma total cholesterol less than 240 mg/dl, and LDL cholesterol 115 to 174 mg/dl while the patient was following an NCEP Step I diet.[14] In patients with LDL cholesterol greater than or equal to 175 mg/dl during the trial, the Step II diet was initiated. If LDL cholesterol remained greater than or equal to 175 mg/dl, cholestyramine, 8 to 16 g/day as needed, was assigned in addition to the randomized study drug. The primary endpoint was fatal CHD (including fatal MI, sudden death, death during coronary intervention, and death from other coronary causes) or nonfatal MI. Major coronary events (fatal CHD, nonfatal MI, CABG, and PTCA) were monitored separately in women and men. Median follow-up was 5.0 years.

Compared with the placebo group, the pravastatin group had lower levels of total cholesterol (by 20%) and LDL cholesterol (by 28%), higher HDL cholesterol levels (by 5%), and lower triglyceride levels (by 14%). Among all patients, the primary endpoint was significantly lower (by 24%) in the pravastatin group. With pravastatin, the rate of major coronary events was significantly lower (by 46%) among women but was only 20% lower among men.

Trials Whose Primary Endpoint Was Angiographic

University of California, San Francisco, Arteriosclerosis Specialized Center of Research Intervention Trial

The University of California, San Francisco, Arteriosclerosis Specialized Center of Research (UCSF-SCOR) intervention trial was conducted in 72 patients aged 19 to 72 years with heterozygous familial hypercholesterolemia (FH), including 41 women evenly divided between the treatment groups.[37] Lipid criteria for entry in the trial were LDL cholesterol greater than 200 mg/dl and triglyceride less than 275 mg/dl with diet in patients with tendinous xanthomas. For patients without tendinous xanthomas, criteria were LDL cholesterol greater than 250 mg/dl or both LDL cholesterol greater than 200 mg/dl and a first-degree relative with tendinous xanthomas. Patients were randomly assigned to receive placebo or various binary and ternary combinations of colestipol, 15 to 30 g/day; nicotinic acid, less than or equal to 7.5 g/day; and lovastatin, 40 to 60 mg/day. During the course of the study, the control group was offered colestipol, 15 g/day. All patients received dietary instruction. The primary endpoint was a mean within-patient change in percent area stenosis. Quantitative coronary angiography was performed at baseline and at a mean of 26 months later.

In the combination-drug group, LDL cholesterol decreased by 38%, HDL cholesterol increased by 28%, and triglyceride decreased by 19%. The primary endpoint indicated regression. Angiographic studies showed that stenosis decreased by 1.53 percentage points in the combination-drug group and increased by 0.80 percentage points in the placebo group; the difference between groups was statistically significant. Only one clinical coronary event occurred in a patient receiving placebo.

Changes in LDL cholesterol and HDL cholesterol concentrations were similar in men and women. LDL cholesterol decreased by 38% in both women and men, and HDL cholesterol increased by 27% in women and by 29% in men. Triglyceride levels were reduced 25% in women and 11% in men, but the difference was not statistically significant. Among women, the mean percent area stenosis decreased by 2.06 percentage points in patients receiving combination-drug therapy and increased by 1.07 percentage points in control patients; the difference was statistically significant ($p = 0.05$). Although men also had angiographic improvement with combination-drug therapy, the difference between treatment groups was not statistically significant.

Canadian Coronary Atherosclerosis Intervention Trial

In the Canadian Coronary Atherosclerosis Intervention Trial (CCAIT), 331 patients with angiographically demonstrated diffuse CHD, including 62 women, were randomly assigned to receive placebo or lovastatin at a dosage titrated to decrease LDL cholesterol to 90 to 130 mg/dl.[38] The initial 20 mg/day lovastatin dosage was increased to 40 mg/day in 41 patients and to 80 mg/day in 33 patients (mean lovastatin dosage, 36 mg/day). Eligible subjects were 21 to 70 years of age; women were required to be without childbearing potential. Lipid criteria for entry into the trial were total cholesterol 220 to 300 mg/dl and triglyceride 500 mg/dl or lower. All subjects were counseled in the Step I diet. The primary endpoint was a coronary change score, defined as the per-patient mean change in minimum luminal diameter for all lesions measured. The proportions of patients with progression, regression, and new lesions, and the numbers of clinical coronary events (cardiac death, MI, and unstable angina) were monitored. Quantitative coronary angiography was performed at baseline and at 2 years.

The lovastatin group showed reductions in total cholesterol (of 21%) and LDL cholesterol (of 29%), a rise in HDL cholesterol (of 7%), and a reduction in triglyceride (of 8%). The placebo group had reductions in total cholesterol (of 1%) and LDL cholesterol (of 2%), a rise in HDL cholesterol (of 3%), and a rise in triglyceride (of 4%). Significantly less angiographic progression was seen in the lovastatin group (decrease of 0.05 mm in mean minimum luminal diameter) than in the placebo group (decrease of 0.09 mm). Progression without regression was seen in significantly fewer patients taking lovastatin (33% compared with 50% of those receiving placebo). The rates of regression without progression were similar in the two groups. New lesions developed in significantly fewer patients taking lovastatin (16% compared with 32% in the placebo group). Clinical coronary events occurred less often in the lovastatin group (15 events in 14 subjects) than in the placebo group (20 events in 18 subjects), but the difference was not statistically significant.

In women, the mean lovastatin dosage was 34.3 mg/day. Total cholesterol was reduced by 24% and LDL cholesterol by 32%, which represented slightly, but not significantly, greater reductions than were seen in men.[39] The mean change in coronary score among the women was the same as that in the overall population, but the difference between treatment groups was not statistically significant. Significantly fewer women in the lovastatin group (28%) had progression than in the placebo group (59%). Furthermore, new lesions developed in significantly fewer women in the lovastatin group (4%) than in the placebo group (45%). Clinical coronary events occurred in equal numbers of women in each treatment group.

Pravastatin Limitation of Atherosclerosis in the Coronary Arteries Trial

The Pravastatin Limitation of Atherosclerosis in the Coronary Arteries (PLAC I) trial was conducted in 408 patients (including 62 women) with CHD as evidenced by recent MI, recent PTCA, or at least one coronary lesion causing 50% or greater stenosis.[40] Lipid criteria for entry in the study were LDL cholesterol 130 to 190 mg/dl and triglyceride 350 mg/dl or lower while the patient was following an American Heart Association Type 1 diet. Patients were randomly assigned to receive pravastatin, 40 mg/day, or placebo. The primary endpoint was a change in mean luminal diameter as determined by quantitative coronary angiography performed at baseline and at 3-year follow-up. Clinical events monitored were nonfatal and fatal MI, cardiac death, MI, PTCA, CABG, nonfatal completed stroke, and noncardiovascular death.

Mean changes from baseline were reductions of 19% in total cholesterol and 28% in LDL cholesterol, a rise of 7% in HDL cholesterol, and a reduction of 8% in triglycerides in the pravastatin group; and rises of 2% in total cholesterol, 1% in LDL cholesterol, 2% in HDL cholesterol, and 9% in triglycerides in the placebo group. The change in mean luminal diameter was not significantly different in treatment groups (decrease of 0.02 mm/year in the pravastatin group compared with a decrease of 0.04 mm/year in the placebo group). However, the decrease in minimum luminal diameter was significantly smaller in the pravastatin group (0.03 mm/year) than in the placebo group (0.05 mm/year). Moreover, significantly fewer fatal or nonfatal MIs occurred in patients taking pravastatin (8) compared with those receiving placebo (17).

In a subgroup analysis of the women, there were no MIs in the pravastatin group, compared with four MIs in the placebo group; the difference was statistically significant. Among women, there were five events in five pravastatin patients compared with 12 events in five placebo patients.

DYSLIPIDEMIAS

Abnormalities of circulating lipid or lipoprotein concentrations may occur as a result of primary genetic disorders or secondary to conditions such as obesity, diet, drugs, and metabolic disturbances. In addition, diseases such as diabetes mellitus, myxedema, nephrotic syndrome, and obstructive jaundice are commonly associated with lipid abnormalities.

Fredrickson Classification of Hyperlipidemias

The Fredrickson classification of hyperlipidemias characterizes dyslipidemias according to which lipoprotein concentrations are elevated (Table 5–2). The system is not diagnostic, does not differentiate between primary and secondary dyslipidemias, and does not include HDL and Lp(a). Nevertheless, it remains useful in characterizing phenotypic patterns of dyslipidemia in patients.

Type I Hyperlipidemia

Type I hyperlipidemia is characterized by marked elevations of chylomicrons, even in fasting blood specimens. The presence of chylomicrons is determined by a creamy supernatant layer of lipid on refrigerated serum; the supernatant occupies approximately 50% of the sample. Type I hyperlipidemia may be genetic, or it may be secondary to diseases such as systemic lupus erythematosus and multiple myeloma.

Table 5–2. FREDRICKSON CLASSIFICATION OF THE HYPERLIPIDEMIAS*

PHENOTYPE	LIPOPROTEIN(S) ELEVATED	PLASMA CHOLESTEROL LEVEL	PLASMA TRIGLYCERIDE LEVEL	ATHEROGENICITY	RELATIVE FREQUENCY†
I	Chylomicrons	Normal to ↑	↑↑↑↑	None seen	<1%
IIa	LDL	↑↑	Normal	+++	10%
IIb	LDL and VLDL	↑↑	↑↑	+++	40%
III	IDL	↑↑	↑↑↑	+++	<1%
IV	VLDL	Normal to ↑	↑↑	+	45%
V	VLDL and chylomicrons	↑ to ↑↑	↑↑↑↑	+	5%

IDL, intermediate-density lipoprotein; LDL, low-density lipoprotein; VLDL, very-low-density lipoprotein.
*The Fredrickson classification does not consider levels of HDL cholesterol. It is not an etiologic classification and does not differentiate primary and secondary hyperlipidemias.
†Approximate percentages of U.S. patients with hyperlipidemias.
From International Lipid Information Bureau: The ILIB Lipid Handbook for Clinical Practice. International Lipid Information Bureau, Houston, 1995, with permission.

Type II Hyperlipidemia

Type IIa hyperlipidemia is characterized by elevated LDL; type IIb is characterized by elevations in both LDL and VLDL. Type II hyperlipidemia may be caused by genetic conditions, such as familial hyperlipidemia or familial combined hyperlipidemia (FCH), or by a variety of secondary causes.

Type III Hyperlipidemia

Type III hyperlipidemia is characterized by elevated IDL concentration. Cholesterol and triglyceride concentrations are elevated to roughly the same extent, and an abnormally high cholesterol-triglyceride concentration is found in VLDL. The disorder occurs most often in individuals homozygous for apo E_2, an isoform of apo E characterized by decreased affinity for the B/E receptor, but usually requires additional metabolic or environmental factors for clinical expression.

Type IV Hyperlipidemia

Type IV hyperlipidemia is characterized by elevated VLDL concentration. The serum appears diffusely turbid in these patients. Type IV hyperlipidemia may be a primary disorder or may be secondary to causes such as diabetes, obesity, hypertension, and consumption of a high-fat diet.

Type V Hyperlipidemia

Type V hyperlipidemia is characterized by elevations in both chylomicrons and VLDL. Examination of the serum reveals a creamy white supernatant of chylomicrons over a turbid layer of VLDL. Type V hyperlipidemia may be a primary disorder or may be secondary to diabetes, obesity, or excessive alcohol intake.

Genetic Hyperlipidemias

The realization that a number of genetic abnormalities express themselves in lipid abnormalities, combined with greater availability of genetic tools, has greatly expanded knowledge of primary dyslipidemias. A variety of genetic diseases involving lipid structure and metabolism have been elucidated, the more common of which are discussed here.

Familial Hypercholesterolemia

Familial hypercholesterolemia (FH) is inherited as an autosomal dominant defect that results in decreased function or production of the B/E receptor.[41] As a result, apo B– and apo E–mediated clearance of lipoproteins is impaired, and circulating LDL cholesterol concentration is increased.

Patients with heterozygous FH, which occurs in approximately 1 in 500 people in the United States, have half the normal number of functioning B/E receptors, and total cholesterol concentration may be 350 to 500 mg/dl. Clinical features include tendinous xanthomas and corneal arcus, and CHD symptoms are typically present by age 60 in women and age 50 in men. As in women without FH, CHD risk markedly accelerates after menopause.

In patients with homozygous FH, which occurs in approximately 1 in 1 million individuals in the United States, virtually no competent B/E receptors are present, and total cholesterol concentration is 700 to 1200 mg/dl. Severe premature atherosclerosis is the rule. Other clinical features are cutaneous and tendinous xanthomas and corneal arcus. CHD symptoms are typically present before age 20 in women and men, and MI has been reported by age 2 years.

Polygenic Hypercholesterolemia

Polygenic hypercholesterolemia is the most common genetic cause of type IIa hyperlipidemia.[42] The underlying genetic abnormality has not been elucidated. The disorder may represent a combination of several mild to moderate metabolic conditions that together result in dyslipidemia. The exact prevalence is not known but is thought to be 1% to 5% of the U.S. population. Diagnosis is difficult, because cholesterol concentrations in this disorder are commonly not as high as in FH, and tendinous xanthomas are not seen.

Familial Defective Apolipoprotein B-100

Familial defective apo B-100 results from a genetic abnormality in the apo B-100 molecule that impairs its binding to normal B/E receptors. LDL cholesterol concentrations may approximate those found in heterozygous FH, but tendinous xanthomas are not seen. Specific diagnosis requires molecular analysis of apo B-100. The prevalence is approximately 1 in 700 among whites in the United States.

Familial Combined Hyperlipidemia

Familial combined hyperlipidemia may present as type IIa, type IIb, or type IV hyperlipidemia, and expression may vary within a person over time. Prevalence is approximately 1% in the United States. The disorder is associated with a higher risk for CHD. The underlying defect is thought to be hepatic overproduction of apo B-100. Transmission may be monogenic, and environmental influences such as diet, obesity, and medication could account for the various phenotypic expressions. Transmission may also be polygenic, and the particular abnormality inherited could account for the phenotype expressed.

Familial Hypertriglyceridemia

Familial hypertriglyceridemia may present as type IV or type V hyperlipidemia. Clinical manifestations are usually not seen until the affected individual reaches adulthood. In the type IV phenotype, which has a prevalence of approximately 1 in 300 individuals in the United States, blood triglyceride concentration is typically 200 to 500 mg/dl, and CHD risk may be increased. In the rare type V phenotype, triglyceride concentration is typically greater than 1000 mg/dl, total cholesterol may also be elevated, and CHD risk is higher.

Dysbetalipoproteinemia

In dysbetalipoproteinemia, or type III hyperlipidemia, both cholesterol and triglyceride concentrations are elevated, and the risk for premature coronary and peripheral atherosclerosis is increased. The prevalence of the disorder is approximately 1 in 5000 people in the United States. Clinical signs may include tuberoeruptive xanthomas and palmar xanthomas. Although the disorder most often occurs in people homozygous for apo E_2, other metabolic or environmental factors are usually needed for full clinical expression. Apo E_2 has diminished affinity for the B/E receptor, resulting in impaired clearance of remnants of chylomicron and VLDL lipolysis. The remnant particles can then be taken up by the macrophages, which become lipid-laden foam cells as uptake continues.

Familial Chylomicronemia

Familial chylomicronemia is a rare condition characterized by triglyceride concentration greater than 1000 mg/dl. The underlying cause may be a deficiency of lipoprotein lipase or its activator apo C-II[43] or the presence of an inhibitor to lipoprotein lipase.[44] The disorder is typically diagnosed in childhood. Severe pancreatitis is common, but CHD risk does not appear to be increased.

TREATMENT OF DYSLIPIDEMIA

The National Cholesterol Education Program (NCEP) stratifies treatment of dyslipidemia according to the risk status of each patient. Because patients with established CHD are at highest risk for a CHD event, the NCEP recommends the most aggressive program for lowering LDL cholesterol in these patients. Treatment for patients without established CHD is further stratified according to risk status. Positive risk factors in the NCEP's algorithm for primary prevention are as follows:

1. Age: in women, age 55 years or more or premature menopause without estrogen replacement therapy; in men, age 45 years or more.
2. Family history of premature CHD: definite MI or sudden death before age 65 in mother or other first-degree female relative or before age 55 in father or other first-degree male relative.
3. Current cigarette smoking.
4. Hypertension: 140/90 mm Hg or higher confirmed on several occasions, or the use of antihypertensive medication.
5. Low HDL cholesterol (<35 mg/dl confirmed on several occasions).
6. Diabetes mellitus.

High HDL cholesterol (60 mg/dl or higher confirmed on several occasions) is a negative risk factor in the NCEP algorithm and is subtracted from the number of positive risk factors.

Dietary Therapy

Excess intake of saturated fat and cholesterol increases intracellular cholesterol concentration and decreases B/E receptor activity. Restriction of saturated fat and cholesterol consumption reduces circulating LDL cholesterol concentration by increasing B/E receptor activity. The institution and success of dietary therapy requires considerable time, effort, and expertise, which may be difficult for the physician to provide. Nutritionists and dietitians can promote patient adherence to therapy by performing close monitoring, providing follow-up, and collecting and analyzing food records. In addition to dietary modification, therapy should include regular physical exercise and weight control.

In patients without CHD, the NCEP recommends instituting a Step I diet (Table 5–3) if LDL cholesterol is ≥160 mg/dl and two or more other risk factors are present; the goal in these patients is LDL cholesterol less than 160 mg/dl (Table 5–4). In patients without CHD and a net of fewer than two risk factors, the NCEP recommends instituting a Step I diet if LDL cholesterol is 130 mg/dl or higher; the goal in these patients is LDL cholesterol less than 130 mg/dl. If LDL cholesterol remains above the treatment goal for patients without known CHD in either of these risk categories, the Step II diet should be initiated. The Step II diet is the initial therapy in patients with CHD and LDL cholesterol greater than 100 mg/dl; the treatment goal in these patients is LDL cholesterol 100 mg/dl or lower.

In general, the Step I diet decreases total cholesterol by

Table 5–3. DIETARY THERAPY FOR HIGH BLOOD CHOLESTEROL

NUTRIENT	STEP I DIET*	STEP II DIET
Total fat	≥30% of total calories	
Saturated fat	8–10% of total calories	<7% of total calories
Polyunsaturated fat	≤10%	
Monounsaturated fat	≤15%	
Carbohydrates	≥55% of total calories	
Protein	≈15% of total calories	
Cholesterol	<300 mg/d	<200 mg/d
Total calories	Sufficient to achieve and maintain desirable weight	

*Recommended eating pattern for all healthy Americans aged 2 years or older.

From National Cholesterol Education Program: Second report of the expert panel on detection, evaluation, and treatment of high blood cholesterol in adults (Adult Treatment Panel II). Circulation 89:1333, 1994.

5% to 7% in patients previously consuming a typical Western diet, and the Step II diet reduces total cholesterol by 10% to 20% from pretreatment values.[45]

Pharmacologic Therapy

With patients for whom adherence to maximal dietary therapy does not adequately lower LDL cholesterol, adding a lipid-regulating drug to the diet should be considered (Table 5–5). An adequate trial of diet is usually 6 months, but a shorter trial may be warranted in patients who have severe hypercholesterolemia that is not expected to respond adequately to diet alone or who are known to have CHD. Women appear to have a response to pharmacologic agents similar to that of men. Because atherosclerosis is a chronic disease, some people may benefit from a more intense attempt to lower cholesterol by hygienic measures before drugs are initiated.

Pharmacologic agents should be initiated only after careful consideration of the patient's clinical status and risk factor profile as well as of the risk-benefit ratio of a therapy that will likely be lifelong. Because younger patients without CHD are at lower risk for CHD events, the NCEP recommends delaying drug therapy in premenopausal women and in men younger than 35 years unless LDL cholesterol is 220 mg/dl or higher, except in patients with additional risk. Clinical judgment should be used to determine whether to initiate drug therapy in patients with CHD whose LDL cholesterol level is 100 to 129 mg/dl with diet.

Table 5–4. CHOLESTEROL LEVELS FOR DIETARY THERAPY IN ADULTS

	LDL CHOLESTEROL LEVEL (mg/dl)	
RISK	Initiation Level	Goal
Without CHD, <2 other risk factors	≥160	<160
Without CHD, ≥2 other risk factors	≥130	<130
With CHD or other atherosclerotic disease	>100	≤100

CHD, coronary heart disease; LDL, low-density lipoprotein.

From National Cholesterol Education Program: Second report of the expert panel on detection, evaluation, and treatment of high blood cholesterol in adults (Adult Treatment Panel II). Circulation 89:1333, 1994.

Table 5–5. CHOLESTEROL LEVELS FOR DRUG THERAPY IN ADULTS

	LDL CHOLESTEROL LEVEL (mg/dl)	
RISK	Consideration Level	Goal
Without CHD, <2 other risk factors	≥190*	<160
Without CHD, ≥2 other risk factors	≥160	<130
With CHD or other atherosclerotic disease	≥130†	≤100

CHD, coronary heart disease; LDL, low-density lipoprotein.

*In younger patients (men aged <35 years and premenopausal women) with LDL cholesterol 190–220 mg/dl, drug therapy may be delayed if other risk is absent.

†In patients with CHD and LDL cholesterol 100–130 mg/dL, the physician should exercise clinical judgment in deciding whether to initiate drug therapy.

From: Farmer JA, Gotto AM Jr: Dyslipidemia and other risk factors for coronary artery disease. In Braunwald E (ed): Heart Disease: A Textbook of Cardiovascular Medicine, 5th ed. WB Saunders, Philadelphia, 1997, p 1126.

If LDL cholesterol is not adequately lowered after 3 months of pharmacologic monotherapy, the addition of a second lipid-regulating agent may be considered. Combination-drug therapy may reduce both adverse effects and cost, thereby improving patient compliance. Clinical judgment should be used to determine whether to initiate combination-drug therapy in patients with CHD whose LDL cholesterol level is 100 to 129 mg/dl with single-drug therapy.

Effective pharmacologic intervention requires the precise determination of the lipid abnormality and the exclusion of secondary causes. Although no currently available pharmacologic agent affects a single lipid subfraction, individual agents should be selected on the basis of whether the predominant action is to lower cholesterol or triglyceride.

Agents Whose Predominant Effect Is on Cholesterol

3-Hydroxy-3-Methylglutaryl Coenzyme A Reductase Inhibitors

The introduction of the 3-hydroxy-3-methylglutaryl coenzyme A (HMG CoA) reductase inhibitors represented a dramatic breakthrough in the management of dyslipidemic patients. These agents have been proved safe and effective and are considered first-line pharmacologic therapy by many experts. Fluvastatin, lovastatin, pravastatin, simvastatin, and atorvastatin are currently available in the United States.

Mechanisms of Action. Despite different chemical characteristics, the HMG CoA reductase inhibitors share a common mechanism of action: the partial inhibition of HMG CoA reductase, which is the rate-limiting enzyme in cholesterol biosynthesis. The reduction in circulating total cholesterol and LDL cholesterol is caused not only by the decrease in synthesis but also by greater B/E receptor activity, because the receptor is upregulated in response to lowered intracellular cholesterol levels. Greater receptor activity enhances clearance of VLDL, IDL, and LDL particles. HDL cholesterol may be mildly increased through an undetermined mechanism.

Efficacy. Fluvastatin, 20 to 40 mg/day; lovastatin, 10 to 80 mg/day; pravastatin, 10 to 40 mg/day; or simvastatin, 10 to 40 mg/day decreases LDL cholesterol approximately 20%

to 40%. Triglyceride may be decreased 10% to 20%, and HDL cholesterol may be increased 5% to 15%. No effect on Lp(a) concentration has been demonstrated. The greatest effect per milligram occurs at lower dosages; the dose-response curve is blunted as the dosage increases. Because cholesterol synthesis varies diurnally, with peak net quantitative synthesis occurring at approximately midnight, the HMG CoA reductase inhibitors are typically administered once a day in the evening.

Adverse Effects and Drug Interactions. Despite the early concern that reduced cholesterol production might adversely affect cell membrane stability or steroidogenesis and the demonstrated increase in lens opacities in experimental animals treated with earlier inhibitors of cholesterol synthesis,[46] the HMG CoA reductase inhibitors have been established as safe and effective lipid-regulating agents during more than 10 years of clinical use. The major clinically significant adverse effects are hepatic abnormalities and myopathy.

Liver function abnormalities, defined as transaminase concentrations more than three times the upper limit of normal on two successive determinations, have been reported in less than 1% of patients receiving HMG CoA reductase inhibitor therapy.[47] Most transaminase elevations occur in the first 4 to 12 months of treatment. Clinical hepatitis has not been demonstrated with these agents.

Rhabdomyolysis induced by HMG CoA reductase inhibitors has been reported in approximately 0.1% of patients receiving these agents as monotherapy.[48] Incidence is increased when an HMG CoA reductase inhibitor is administered in combination with cyclosporine,[49] a fibric acid derivative,[50] erythromycin,[51] or nicotinic acid.[52] Risk for myopathy also appears to be greater in patients with underlying renal insufficiency. The cause of muscle pain and higher creatine kinase levels is unknown but may be secondary to a reduction in ubiquinone or hypocholesterolemia-induced cell membrane instability. This membrane instability, though rarely severe, can result in frank rhabdomyolysis with myoglobinuria and renal failure. However, myositis is generally self-limited and resolves with discontinuation of the medication.

Rare instances of thrombocytopenia and arthralgias have been reported with the use of HMG CoA reductase inhibitors, but a cause-and-effect relationship has not been definitely established.[53] Lovastatin administered with warfarin has been reported to prolong prothrombin time.[54]

Bile Acid Resins

Bile acid resins were among the first pharmacologic agents used for lipid-regulating therapy. Much evidence has been generated concerning the efficacy and safety of these compounds in clinical practice. Cholestyramine and colestipol are the currently available agents, and modifications in their formulations have been made in an attempt to increase palatability and compliance. The use of these agents as monotherapy has decreased with the advent of the HMG CoA reductase inhibitors, and the bile acid resins are now more commonly used in combination regimens.

Mechanisms of Action. Cholestyramine and colestipol are highly charged polycationic compounds that bind the cholesterol-rich bile acids within the gastrointestinal tract and prevent their reabsorption by the distal ileum, resulting in greater fecal loss of bile acids secondary to interruption of the enterohepatic circulation.[55] The bile acid pool normally recirculates approximately 10 times per day. The administration of a bile acid resin decreases the normal recirculation. The reduction in intrahepatic cholesterol concentration stimulates the activity of 7-alpha-hydroxylase, the rate-limiting enzyme in bile acid synthesis, and increases the conversion of cholesterol into bile acids. In addition, LDL cholesterol concentration in the plasma compartment is reduced through the upregulation of the B/E receptor in response to the reduction in intrahepatic cholesterol. However, the initial cholesterol-lowering effect of the resins is blunted by the compensatory increase in HMG CoA reductase activity and the resulting rise in cholesterol synthesis, thereby returning LDL cholesterol toward pretreatment concentrations.[56]

Efficacy. The practical efficacy of cholestyramine and colestipol is predominantly a function of patient compliance. Cholestyramine, 4 to 24 g/day, or colestipol, 5 to 30 g/day, reduces LDL cholesterol by approximately 15% to 30% and increases HDL cholesterol by approximately 3% to 5%. Triglyceride concentration is usually not affected but may rise in patients with underlying metabolic defects that predispose to hypertriglyceridemia. No effect on Lp(a) has been demonstrated.

Adverse Effects and Drug Interactions. Patient compliance may be limited by adverse effects frequently associated with bile acid resins. The major side effects are gastrointestinal, including constipation, which may be ameliorated by increasing fluid and fiber intake or by concomitant administration of stool softeners. Because bile acid resins are not absorbed into the circulation, they are not usually associated with systemic side effects. Because of nonspecific binding by these agents, however, decreased absorption of concomitantly administered medications, such as digitalis,[57] thiazide diuretics,[58] thyroid hormone,[59] warfarin,[60] and beta blockers,[61] may necessitate dose separation to maintain adequate therapeutic levels.

Agents Whose Predominant Effect Is on Triglyceride

Nicotinic Acid

Nicotinic acid is a B vitamin that has lipid-regulating effects when used in doses far exceeding the amount required to prevent pellagra.

Mechanisms of Action. Nicotinic acid decreases hepatic VLDL production by reducing both synthesis and release. Consequently, production of lipoproteins resulting from VLDL metabolism, IDL and LDL, is also decreased. In addition, nicotinic acid has peripheral effects on the mobilization of free fatty acids.[62] Free fatty acids are produced in peripheral adipocytes and transported to the liver, where they form the synthetic substrate for VLDL production. The peripheral effect of nicotinic acid leads to reduction of the metabolic precursors of triglyceride synthesis and the subsequent incorporation of triglyceride into VLDL. However, the quantitative long-term effect of nicotinic acid on free fatty acids remains controversial.

Efficacy. Nicotinic acid has beneficial effects on all the major lipid subfractions except chylomicrons. Effective clinical use of this agent requires a concerted effort by both patient and physician to achieve a maximally effective dosage with a minimum of significant side effects. Nicotinic acid is generally increased gradually to a total dosage of at least 1.5 g/day. Optimization of the dose-effect relation occurs at a dosage of 2 to 6 g/day. At this dosage, the LDL cholesterol level diminishes by approximately 10% to 25%, the HDL cholesterol level rises by approximately 15% to 35%, and the triglyceride level decreases by approximately 20% to 50%. Unlike most lipid-regulating drugs, nicotinic acid also decreases Lp(a) concentration.[12] Nicotinic acid may be effective in treating familial defective apo B-100,[63] which is not effectively treated by agents whose predominant effect is to increase B/E receptor activity.

Adverse Effects and Drug Interactions. Administration of nicotinic acid is associated with adverse effects of varying clinical severity. Before receiving nicotinic acid, the patient should be told of potential adverse effects and their relative frequency, with emphasis on the self-limited nature of some of the potential problems.

Dermatologic complications, such as flushing, are virtually universal with nicotinic acid therapy. Flushing, which results from peripheral vasodilation, may occasionally be severe enough to cause systemic hypotension. Flushing and pruritus may be minimized by starting therapy with low doses of nicotinic acid taken with meals and taken along with aspirin to partially inhibit the prostaglandin-mediated mechanism underlying this complication. Although rare, acanthosis nigricans may occur after prolonged use of nicotinic acid.

The use of nicotinic acid may result in several metabolic abnormalities that are of clinical importance in patients at risk for CHD. Commonly, glucose tolerance is adversely altered by nicotinic acid use, and care should be used in administration of this agent to patients with known or potential diabetes. This complication may be minimized through alteration of hypoglycemic agent dosages or intensification of dietary therapy. Nicotinic acid is not contraindicated in diabetic patients, although failure to control the induced metabolic abnormalities may reduce the benefits of nicotinic acid therapy. Nicotinic acid also has adverse effects on uric acid concentration and may precipitate gout.

Gastrointestinal side effects of nicotinic acid range from mild gastric irritation to exacerbation of peptic ulcer disease. Drug-induced hepatotoxicity and fulminant hepatic necrosis[64] have been reported with the use of this agent, but these hepatic effects appear to be more common with sustained-release preparations.[65] Liver function tests should be performed intermittently, and any sudden, unexplained fall in cholesterol concentration may be a clinical indication of nicotinic acid–induced hepatotoxicity.

Myositis may rarely occur with nicotinic acid monotherapy[66] and is somewhat more common with coadministration of an HMG CoA reductase inhibitor.[67]

Fibric Acid Derivatives

The fibric acid derivatives have a long history of clinical use in the treatment of dyslipidemia. Clofibrate, whose use has decreased dramatically in the United States, and gemfibrozil are currently available in the United States; fenofibrate has been approved in the United States, and marketing of this drug has just begun. Bezafibrate, ciprofibrate, and fenofibrate are available in other countries.

Mechanism of Action. Although the fibric acid derivatives differ in chemical structure, they appear to have similar mechanisms of action. Their predominant effect is increased catabolism of VLDL as a result of greater lipoprotein lipase activity. HDL cholesterol is also higher because of increased transfer of components of hydrolyzed triglyceride-rich lipoproteins.[68] The fibric acid derivatives may also have minor peripheral effects that reduce hepatic synthesis of VLDL.

Efficacy. Gemfibrozil, 1200 mg/day, or clofibrate, 2000 mg/day, decreases triglyceride levels by approximately 20% to 50% and increases HDL cholesterol levels by approximately 10% to 15%. LDL cholesterol generally decreases by approximately 10% to 15%, but the effect of fibric acid derivatives on LDL cholesterol concentration is variable and depends on pretreatment triglyceride concentration and the number and functioning of B/E receptors. Greater VLDL catabolism in a patient with receptor abnormalities may result in higher LDL cholesterol concentration with administration of a fibric acid derivative. However, gemfibrozil[69] and bezafibrate[70] have been shown to reduce the concentration of small, dense LDL particles, so the rise in LDL cholesterol with fibric acid derivative therapy may reflect shifting of the LDL subclass pattern to a less atherogenic phenotype.

The fibric acid derivatives have also been shown to have nonlipid benefits. Gemfibrozil decreases platelet aggregability and reactivity in response to epinephrine.[71] Gemfibrozil also reduces activity of plasminogen activator inhibitor-1 (PAI-1),[72] thereby providing the potential for enhanced intravascular fibrinolysis. Fibrinogen concentration, which has been correlated in epidemiologic studies with risk for CHD,[73] has been shown to be reduced by bezafibrate administration.[74]

Adverse Effects and Drug Interactions. As a class, the fibric acid derivatives are generally well tolerated and are not associated with serious adverse effects. Approximately 5% of patients have clinically insignificant effects, usually gastrointestinal. Mild liver function abnormalities may occur but are usually limited to elevations of alanine transaminase and aspartate transaminase. Rhabdomyolysis is exceedingly rare with monotherapy using a fibric acid derivative, but risk for myopathy is increased when one of these agents is coadministered with an HMG CoA reductase inhibitor, as previously described. Fibric acid derivatives increase the anticoagulant activity of warfarin; when these agents are coadministered, prothrombin time and international normalized ratio should be monitored intermittently to ensure adequate coagulation.

Estrogen

At menopause, LDL cholesterol increases and HDL cholesterol may decrease. Estrogen replacement therapy provides an alternative to lipid-regulating drug therapy in some postmenopausal women. Although estrogen does not have a U.S. Food and Drug Administration indication for lipid regulation or reduction of CHD risk, estrogen replacement therapy has beneficial effects on the lipid profile. However, in controlled clinical trials, HRT has not been shown to definitely reduce cardiovascular events in postmenopausal women.

The Postmenopausal Estrogen/Progestin Interventions (PEPI) trial, a multicenter, double-blind trial, was conducted in 875 healthy postmenopausal women aged 45 to 64 years. Patients were randomly assigned to receive (1) estrogen, 0.625 mg/day, (2) estrogen, 0.625 mg/day, plus cyclic medroxyprogesterone acetate (MPA), 10 mg/day for 12 days/month, (3) estrogen, 0.625 mg/day, plus consecutive MPA, 2.5 mg/day, (4) estrogen, 0.625 mg/day, plus cyclic micronized progesterone, 200 mg/day for 12 days/month, or (5) placebo.[75] Compared with the placebo, active treatment decreased LDL cholesterol significantly and increased HDL cholesterol significantly. Although the improvement in HDL cholesterol was significantly greater with estrogen alone than with estrogen plus MPA, estrogen alone also raised the risk for endometrial hyperplasia. Patients randomly assigned to receive estrogen plus micronized progesterone had the most benefit without a greater risk for endometrial hyperplasia.

Mechanism of Action. The mechanism of action by which estrogen replacement therapy alters lipid concentrations is complicated and may vary. Estrogen stimulates a promoter region on the B/E receptor gene, resulting in upregulation of the B/E receptor and greater clearance of particles removed by the B/E receptor. The mechanism by which estrogen raises HDL cholesterol concentration has not been elucidated and may be multifactorial. Estrogen has been demonstrated to increase the production of apo A-I ,[76] the major apolipoprotein on HDL. Hepatic production of VLDL is promoted by estrogen therapy,[77] and the cumulative effect on circulating triglyceride concentration is determined by the equilibrium established between greater removal of apo B–containing lipoproteins by the upregulated B/E receptor and increased VLDL production.

Efficacy. Orally administered conjugated estrogen, 0.625 mg/day, or micronized estradiol, 2 mg/day, decreases LDL cholesterol by approximately 15% and increases HDL cholesterol by up to 15%. Triglyceride concentration may rise, particularly in patients with elevated triglycerides. Lp(a) concentration may be reduced[11]; estrogen combined with progesterone has been reported to decrease Lp(a) by 50%.[78]

Despite the demonstrable improvement in effect of hormone replacement therapy in the form of estrogen on circulating lipid levels, clinical trials have been disappointing. The Heart and Estrogen/Progestin Replacement Study (HERS) evaluated 2763 women with known coronary disease who were postmenopausal and had an intact uterus. Conjugated equine estrogen (0.625 mg) in combination with 2.5 mg of methoxyprogesterone was compared with placebo. The women, whose mean age was 66.7 years, were followed for 4.1 years for the incidence of the primary outcome of nonfatal myocardial infarction or coronary heart disease death. Hormone replacement therapy resulted in an 11% reduction in low-density lipoprotein combined with a 10% increase in high-density lipoprotein when compared with the placebo group. However, the overall rate of coronary heart disease events was not decreased by hormone replacement therapy. Subsequent statistical analysis revealed that, despite the overall null effect, there was a statistically significant time trend, with more coronary heart disease events occurring in the group randomized to receive estrogen/progesterone at 1 year and fewer events in years 4 to 5. Additionally, thromboembolic events were also increased by hormone replacement therapy.[79]

Further evaluation of the HERS database for cerebrovascular events (stroke incidence and stroke death over 4.1 years) demonstrated no significant effect on the risk of stroke in postmenopausal women with known coronary disease.[80] The clinical data obtained in the HERS study is substantiated by angiographic data. The Estrogen Replacement and Atherosclerosis (ERA) trial demonstrated that estrogen replacement with or without progestin did not significantly alter the angiographic progression of atherosclerotic disease in postmenopausal women who had known coronary artery disease when compared with placebo.[81] The implications of the HERS and ERA trials would be that estrogen replacement therapy should not be used in women with documented atherosclerosis in an attempt to decrease the early risk of coronary event rates.

Adverse Effects and Drug Interactions. Postmenopausal use of unopposed estrogen raises the risk for endometrial cancer and should be used with caution in women who have not undergone hysterectomy. Coadministration of a progestational agent markedly reduces the risk for endometrial malignancy. Estrogen may increase risk of breast cancer, but the data are controversial.

References

1. Mosca L, Manson JE, Sutherland SE: Cardiovascular disease in women: A statement for health care professionals from the American Heart Association. Circulation 96:2468, 1997.
2. Murabito JM: Women and cardiovascular disease: Contributions from the Framingham Heart Study. J Am Med Wom Assoc 50:35, 1995.
3. Chambless LE, Heiss G, Folsom AR: Association of coronary artery disease incidents with carotid arterial wall thickness and major risk factors. Am J Epidemiol 146:483, 1997.
4. Hodis HN, Mack WJ, La Bree L: The role of carotid artery intima-media thickness in predicting clinical coronary events. Ann Intern Med 128:262, 1998.
5. Douglas PS: Coronary artery disease in women. In Braunwald E (ed): Heart Disease: A Textbook of Cardiovascular Medicine, 5th ed. WB Saunders, Philadelphia, 1997, p 1704.
6. Rexrode KM, Carey EJ, Henneken CH: Abdominal adiposity and coronary heart disease in women. JAMA 280:1843, 1998.
7. Henekens CH: Risk factors for coronary heart disease in women. Cardiol Clin 16:1, 1998.
8. Austin MA, Breslow JL, Hennekens CH, et al: Low-density lipoprotein subclass patterns and risk of myocardial infarction. JAMA 260:1917, 1988.
9. Austin MA, King MC, Vranizan KM, et al: Inheritance of low-density lipoprotein subclass patterns: Results of complex segregation analysis. Am J Hum Genet 43:838, 1988.
10. Dejager S, Bruckert E, Chapman MJ: Dense low density lipoprotein subspecies with diminished oxidative resistance predominate in combined hyperlipidemia. J Lipid Res 34:295, 1993.
11. Gotto AM Jr: Postmenopausal hormone-replacement therapy, plasma lipoprotein[a], and risk for coronary heart disease [editorial]. J Lab Clin Med 123:800, 1994.
12. Carlson LA, Hamsten A, Asplund A: Pronounced lowering of serum levels of lipoprotein Lp(a) in hyperlipidaemic subjects treated with nicotinic acid. J Intern Med 226:271, 1989.
13. Bimmermann A, Boerschmann C, Schwartzkopff W, et al: Effective therapeutic measures for reducing lipoprotein(a) in patients with dyslipidemia: Lipoprotein(a) reduction with sustained-release bezafibrate. Current Therapeutic Research: Clinical and Experimental 49:635, 1991.
14. National Cholesterol Education Program: Second report of the expert panel on detection, evaluation, and treatment of high blood cholesterol in adults (Adult Treatment Panel II). Circulation 89:1333, 1994.

15. Krauss RM, Lindgren FT, Williams PT, et al: Intermediate-density lipoproteins and progression of coronary artery disease in hypercholesterolaemic men. Lancet 2:62, 1987.
16. Phillips NR, Waters D, Havel RJ: Plasma lipoproteins and progression of coronary artery disease evaluated by angiography and clinical events. Circulation 88:2762, 1993.
17. Ross R: Factors influencing atherogenesis. In Schlant RC, Alexander RW (eds): The Heart: Arteries and Veins, 8th ed. McGraw-Hill, New York, 1994, p 989.
18. Steinberg D, Witztum JL: Lipoproteins and atherogenesis: Current concepts. JAMA 264:3047, 1990.
19. Egashira K, Hirooka Y, Kai H, et al: Reduction in serum cholesterol with pravastatin improves endothelium-dependent coronary vasomotion in patients with hypercholesterolemia. Circulation 89:2519, 1994.
20. Treasure CB, Klein JL, Weintraub WS, et al: Beneficial effects of cholesterol-lowering therapy on the coronary endothelium in patients with coronary artery disease. N Engl J Med 332:481, 1995.
21. Anderson TJ, Meredith IT, Yeung AC, et al: The effect of cholesterol-lowering and antioxidant therapy on endothelium-dependent coronary vasomotion. N Engl J Med 332:488, 1995.
22. Loscalzo J, Weinfeld M, Fless GM, et al: Lipoprotein(a), fibrin binding, and plasminogen activation. Arteriosclerosis 10:240, 1990.
23. Beisiegel U, Niendorf A, Wolf K, et al: Lipoprotein(a) in the arterial wall. Eur Heart J 11(Suppl E):174, 1990.
24. Naruszewicz M, Selinger E, Davignon J: Oxidative modification of lipoprotein(a) and the effect of beta-carotene. Metabolism 41:1215, 1992.
25. Gordon T, Castelli WP, Hjortland MC, et al: High density lipoprotein as a protective factor against coronary heart disease: The Framingham Study. Am J Med 62:707, 1977.
26. Gordon DJ, Probstfield JL, Garrison RJ, et al: High-density lipoprotein cholesterol and cardiovascular disease: Four prospective American studies. Circulation 79:8, 1989.
27. Kuhn FE, Mohler ER, Satler LF, et al: Effects of high-density lipoprotein on acetylcholine-induced coronary vasoreactivity. Am J Cardiol 68: 1425, 1991.
28. Aoyama T, Yui Y, Morishita H, et al: Prostacyclin stabilization by high density lipoprotein is decreased in acute myocardial infarction and unstable angina pectoris. Circulation 81:1784, 1990.
29. Mackness MI, Abbott C, Arrol S, et al: The role of high-density lipoprotein and lipid-soluble antioxidant vitamins in inhibiting low-density lipoprotein oxidation. Biochem J 294:829, 1993.
30. Gotto AM Jr: Lipid lowering, regression, and coronary events: A review of the Interdisciplinary Council on Lipids and Cardiovascular Risk Intervention, Seventh Council Meeting. Circulation 92:646, 1995.
31. American Heart Association: 1997 Heart and Stroke Statistical Update. American Heart Association, Dallas, 1996.
32. Buchwald H, Varco RL, Matts JP, et al: Effect of partial ileal bypass surgery on mortality and morbidity from coronary heart disease in patients with hypercholesterolemia: Report of the Program on the Surgical Control of the Hyperlipidemias (POSCH). N Engl J Med 323: 946, 1990.
33. Buchwald H, Matts JP, Fitch LL, et al, for the Program on the Surgical Control of the Hyperlipidemias (POSCH) Group: Changes in sequential coronary arteriograms and subsequent coronary events. JAMA 268:1429, 1992.
34. Buchwald H, Campos CT, Matts JP, et al: Women in the POSCH trial: Effects of aggressive cholesterol modification in women with coronary heart disease. The POSCH Group. Program on the Surgical Control of the Hyperlipidemias. Ann Surg 216:389, 1992.
35. Scandinavian Simvastatin Survival Study Group: Randomised trial of cholesterol lowering in 4444 patients with coronary heart disease: The Scandinavian Simvastatin Survival Study (4S). Lancet 344:1383, 1994.
36. Sacks FM, Pfeffer MA, Moye LA, et al, for the Cholesterol and Recurrent Events Trial Investigators: The effect of pravastatin on coronary events after myocardial infarction in patients with average cholesterol levels. N Engl J Med 335:1001, 1996.
37. Kane JP, Malloy MJ, Ports TA, et al: Regression of coronary atherosclerosis during treatment of familial hypercholesterolemia with combined drug regimens. JAMA 264:3007, 1990.
38. Waters D, Higginson L, Gladstone P, et al: Effects of monotherapy with an HMG-CoA reductase inhibitor on the progression of coronary atherosclerosis as assessed by serial quantitative arteriography: The Canadian Coronary Atherosclerosis Intervention Trial. Circulation 89: 959, 1994.
39. Waters D, Higginson L, Gladstone P, et al, for the CCAIT Study Group: Effects of cholesterol lowering on the progression of coronary atherosclerosis in women: A Canadian Coronary Atherosclerosis Intervention Trial (CCAIT) Substudy. Circulation 92:2404, 1995.
40. Pitt B, Mancini GBJ, Ellis SG, et al, for the PLAC I Investigators: Pravastatin limitation of atherosclerosis in the coronary arteries (PLAC I): Reduction in atherosclerosis progression and clinical events. J Am Coll Cardiol 26:1133, 1995.
41. Goldstein JL, Hobbs HH, Brown MS: Familial hypercholesterolemia. In Scriver CR, Beaudet AL, Sly WS, Valle D (eds): The Metabolic and Molecular Bases of Inherited Disease, 7th ed. McGraw-Hill, New York, 1995, p 1981.
42. Grundy SM: Multifactorial etiology of hypercholesterolemia: Implications for prevention of coronary heart disease. Arterioscler Thromb 11: 1619, 1991.
43. Santamarina-Fojo S, Brewer HB Jr: The familial hyperchylomicronemia syndrome: New insights into underlying genetic defects. JAMA 265: 904, 1991.
44. Brunzell JD, Miller NE, Alaupovic P, et al: Familial chylomicronemia due to a circulating inhibitor of lipoprotein lipase activity. J Lipid Res 24:12, 1983.
45. Kris-Etherton PM, Krummel D, Russell ME, et al: The effect of diet on plasma lipids, lipoproteins, and coronary heart disease. J Am Diet Assoc 88:1373, 1988.
46. Kirby TJ: Cataracts produced by triparanol (MER-29). Trans Am Ophthalmol Soc 65:494, 1967.
47. Bradford RH, Shear CL, Chremos AN, et al: Expanded Clinical Evaluation of Lovastatin (EXCEL) Study results. I: Efficacy in modifying plasma lipoproteins and adverse event profile in 8245 patients with moderate hypercholesterolemia. Arch Intern Med 151:43, 1991.
48. Tobert JA, Shear CL, Chremos AN, et al: Clinical experience with lovastatin. Am J Cardiol 65:23F, 1990.
49. Corpier CL, Jones PH, Suki WN, et al: Rhabdomyolysis and renal injury with lovastatin use. Report of two cases in cardiac transplant recipients. JAMA 260:239, 1988.
50. Pierce LR, Wysowski DK, Gross TP: Myopathy and rhabdomyolysis associated with lovastatin-gemfibrozil combination therapy. JAMA 264: 71, 1990.
51. Spach DH, Bauwens JE, Clark CD, et al: Rhabdomyolysis associated with lovastatin and erythromycin use. West J Med 154:213, 1991.
52. Tobert JA: Efficacy and long-term adverse effect pattern of lovastatin. Am J Cardiol 62:28J, 1988.
53. Mantell G, Burke T, Staggers J: Extended clinical safety profile of lovastatin. Am J Cardiol 66:11B, 1990.
54. Ahmad S: Lovastatin: Warfarin interaction. Arch Intern Med 150: 2407, 1990.
55. Moore RB, Crane CA, Frantz ID Jr: Effect of cholestyramine on the fecal excretion of intravenously administered cholesterol-4-^{14}C and its degradation products in a hypercholesterolemic patient. J Clin Invest 47:1664, 1968.
56. Grundy SM, Ahrens EH Jr, Salen G: Interruption of the enterohepatic circulation of bile acids in man: Comparative effects of cholestyramine and ileal exclusion on cholesterol metabolism. J Lab Clin Med 78: 94, 1971.
57. Bazzano G, Bazzano GS: Digitalis intoxication: Treatment with a new steroid-binding resin. JAMA 220:828, 1972.
58. Hunninghake DB, King S, LaCroix K: The effect of cholestyramine and colestipol on the absorption of hydrochlorothiazide. Int J Clin Pharmacol Ther Toxicol 20:151, 1982.
59. Northcutt RC, Stiel JN, Hollifield JW, et al: The influence of cholestyramine on thyroxine absorption. JAMA 208:1857, 1969.
60. Gallo DG, Bailey KR, Sheffner AL: The interaction between cholestyramine and drugs. Proc Soc Exp Biol Med 120:60, 1965.
61. Hibbard DM, Peters JR, Hunninghake DB: Effects of cholestyramine and colestipol on the plasma concentrations of propranolol. Br J Clin Pharmacol 18:337, 1984.
62. Grundy SM, Mok HY, Zech L, et al: Influence of nicotinic acid on metabolism of cholesterol and triglycerides in man. J Lipid Res 22: 24, 1981.
63. Schmidt EB, Illingworth DR, Bacon S, et al: Hypolipidemic effects of nicotinic acid in patients with familial defective apolipoprotein B-100. Metabolism 42:137, 1993.
64. Mullin GE, Greenson JK, Mitchell MC: Fulminant hepatic failure after ingestion of sustained-release nicotinic acid. Ann Intern Med 111: 253, 1989.

65. Rader JI, Calvert RJ, Hathcock JN: Hepatic toxicity of unmodified and time-release preparations of niacin. Am J Med 92:77, 1992.
66. Litin SC, Anderson CF: Nicotinic acid–associated myopathy: A report of three cases. Am J Med 86:481, 1989.
67. Reaven P, Witztum JL: Lovastatin, nicotinic acid, and rhabdomyolysis [letter]. Ann Intern Med 109:597, 1988.
68. Simpson HS, Williamson CM, Olivecrona T, et al: Postprandial lipemia, fenofibrate and coronary artery disease. Atherosclerosis 85:193, 1990.
69. Tilly-Kiesi M, Tikkanen MJ: Low density lipoprotein density and composition in hypercholesterolaemic men treated with HMG CoA reductase inhibitors and gemfibrozil. J Intern Med 229:427, 1991.
70. Eisenberg S, Gavish D, Oschry Y, et al: Abnormalities in very low, low, and high density lipoproteins in hypertriglyceridemia: Reversal toward normal with bezafibrate treatment. J Clin Invest 74:470, 1984.
71. Todd PA, Ward A: Gemfibrozil: A review of its pharmacodynamic and pharmacokinetic properties, and therapeutic use in dyslipidemia. Drugs 36:314, 1988.
72. Andersen P, Smith P, Seljeflot I, et al: Effects of gemfibrozil on lipids and haemostasis after myocardial infarction. Thromb Haemost 63:174, 1990.
73. Ernst E: Plasma fibrinogen—an independent cardiovascular risk factor. J Intern Med 227:365, 1990.
74. Bo M, Bonino F, Neirotti M, et al: Hemorrheologic and coagulative pattern in hypercholesterolemic subjects treated with lipid-lowering drugs. Angiology 42:106, 1991.
75. Writing Group for the PEPI Trial: Effects of estrogen or estrogen/progestin regimens on heart disease risk factors in postmenopausal women: The Postmenopausal Estrogen/Progestin Interventions (PEPI) trial. JAMA 273:199, 1995.
76. Brinton EA: Oral estrogen replacement therapy in postmenopausal women selectively raises levels and production rates of lipoprotein A-I and lowers hepatic lipase activity without lowering the fractional catabolic rate. Arterioscler Thromb Vasc Biol 16:431, 1996.
77. Sacks FM, Walsh BW: Sex hormones and lipoprotein metabolism. Curr Opin Lipidol 5:236, 1994.
78. Soma MR, Osnago-Gadda I, Paoletti R, et al: The lowering of lipoprotein[a] induced by estrogen plus progesterone replacement therapy in postmenopausal women. Arch Intern Med 153:1462, 1993.
79. Hulley S, Grady D, Bush T, et al: Randomized trial of estrogen plus progestin for secondary prevention of coronary heart disease in postmenopausal women. Heart and Estrogen/progestin Replacement Study (HERS) Research Group. JAMA 280:650, 1998.
80. Simon JA, Hsia J, Cauley JA, et al: Postmenopausal hormone replacement therapy and the risk of stroke: The Heart and Estrogen-Progestin Replacement Study (HERS). Circulation 103:638, 2001.
81. Herrington DM, Reboussin DM, Brosnihan B, et al: Effects of estrogen replacement on the progression of coronary artery atherosclerosis. N Engl J Med 343:522, 2000.

5.3 Diabetes Mellitus

Philip R. Orlander

Diabetes mellitus is a complex metabolic syndrome characterized by abnormalities in insulin secretion and action and resulting in hyperglycemia. Diabetes is associated with abnormalities in numerous metabolic pathways, including lipid metabolism, fibrinolysis, coagulation, and platelet function, all of which may contribute to a rise in cardiovascular disease risk. Epidemiologic studies have demonstrated that diabetes mellitus frequently aggregates with other known cardiovascular risk factors but is also a major independent risk factor for cardiovascular disease.[1–3] In fact, the previously noted metabolic abnormalities are now known to be associated with insulin resistance, a known risk factor for the development of diabetes as well as heart disease.[4–6]

Long-term follow-up of women with diabetes, who were screened as part of the Nurses' Health Study cohort,[2] and men with diabetes, who were screened as part of the Multiple Risk Factor Intervention Trial (MRFIT),[3] demonstrates that diabetic persons have an excess cardiovascular mortality rate at every stratum of blood pressure, cholesterol, and smoking in comparison with women and men who do not have diabetes (Fig. 5–1). Although absolute risk is magnified at the highest strata, the relative risk of individuals with diabetes compared with those without diabetes is actually higher in the absence of other known cardiovascular risk factors. Almost 80% of hospitalizations for the chronic complications of diabetes are related to cardiovascular disease, the most common cause of death in people with diabetes (Fig. 5–2).[7] The impact of diabetes can be expected to rise substantially as the population ages and the prevalence of diabetes rises.

Diabetes appears to amplify the background cardiovascular risk in every population studied, but women with diabetes are affected disproportionately (Fig. 5–3).[8–11] It is the only condition that increases the rates of heart disease in women compared with those in men. In several population-based studies, age-adjusted cardiovascular mortality rates in diabetic men are twice those of nondiabetic men, and premenopausal diabetic women have death rates as high as, or higher than, those of nondiabetic men.[2, 9, 11–13]

Diabetes is commonly underrecorded on death certificates. After correction of ischemic heart disease death rates through the use of the National Mortality Follow-Back Survey data among persons aged 45 to 64, black women with diabetes were almost seven times more likely to die from ischemic heart disease than similar women without diabetes, and white women with diabetes were nine times more likely to die from ischemic heart disease than similar women without diabetes.[12] Although the corrected rates of death due to ischemic heart disease were higher for men with diabetes than for women with diabetes, the percentage of deaths attributable to diabetes was higher in women than in men. Almost 29% of the deaths in women aged 45 to 64 years who died of ischemic heart disease were attributable to diabetes.

Women with diabetes in all age categories generally have lower high-density lipoprotein (HDL) cholesterol levels, higher blood pressure and triglyceride levels, and a greater likelihood of left ventricular hypertrophy than women without diabetes.[9, 11, 14] Even modest impairments in glucose tolerance, associated with hyperinsulinemia and insulin resistance, are associated with a greater prevalence of cardiovascular risk factors years prior to the development of clinical

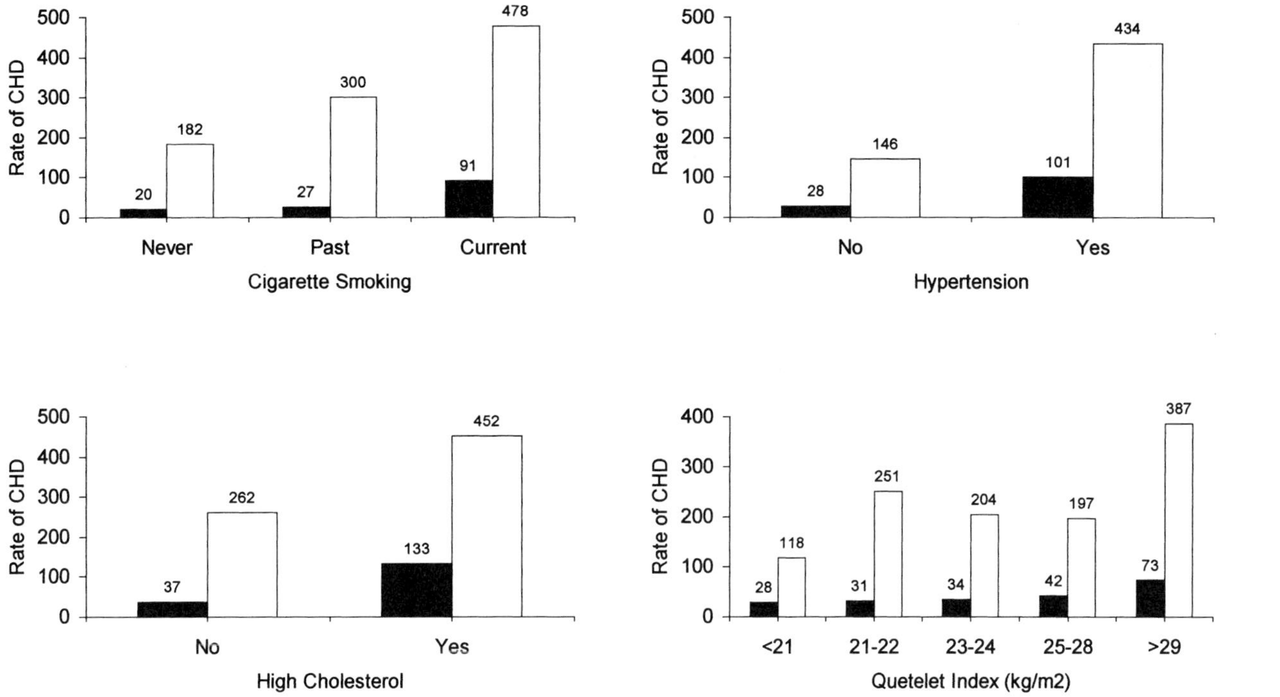

FIGURE 5–1. Age-adjusted rates of nonfatal myocardial infarction and fatal coronary heart disease (combined) per 100,000 person-years in relation to diabetes status, as modified by the presence or absence of other coronary risk factors in the Nurses' Health Study. Solid black bars indicate subjects without diabetes; open bars indicate subjects with diabetes (From Manson JE, Colditz GA, Stampfer MJ, et al: A prospective study of maturity-onset diabetes mellitus and risk of coronary heart disease and stroke in women. Arch Intern Med 151:1141, 1991.)

diabetes (Fig. 5–4).[6, 15, 16] The role of hormone replacement therapy (HRT) in modifying insulin sensitivity, lipid measurements, and cardiovascular risk among postmenopausal women with diabetes needs to be determined, especially in light of recent studies demonstrating an adverse impact of estrogen therapy on women with coronary disease.[17]

DEFINITION AND PREVALENCE AMONG WOMEN

Definition

In 1997, the Expert Committee on the Diagnosis and Classification of Diabetes Mellitus issued revised criteria that

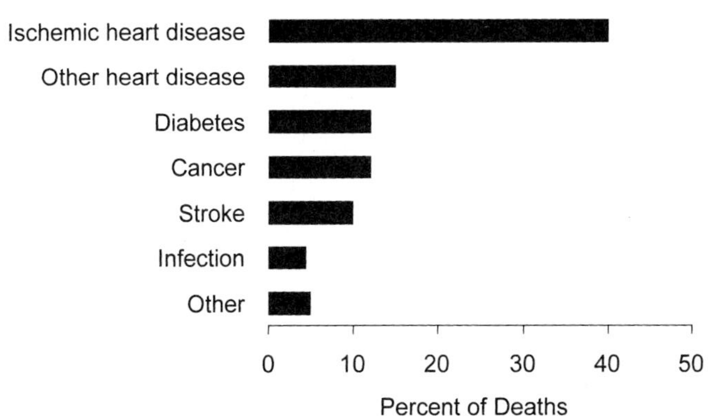

FIGURE 5–2. Mortality in people with diabetes: Causes of death (From Geiss LS, Herman WH, Smith PJ: Mortality in non-insulin dependent diabetes. In Harris MI, Cowie CC, Stern MP, et al [eds]: Diabetes in America, 2nd ed. [NIH publication 95-1468]. National Institutes of Health, Washington, DC, 1995, pp 233.)

lowered the fasting glucose threshold for diagnosis and discouraged the routine use of the oral glucose tolerance test.[18] The rationale for these changes was based on epidemiologic data regarding the relationship of metabolic control to the risk of microvascular complications of diabetes, and the desire to increase the ease and frequency of testing while reducing the cost. The fasting glucose level of $\geq$126 mg/dl correlates well with a 2-hour post-glucose load of $\geq$200 mg/dl during a 75-g oral glucose tolerance test (OGTT). However, it is recognized that this approach does lead to slightly lower prevalence rates of diabetes when compared with the OGTT.

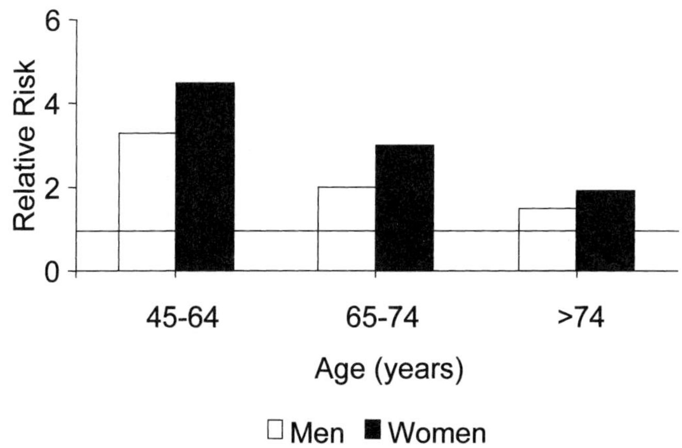

FIGURE 5–3. Mortality in people with diabetes: U.S. population. (From Ford ES, DeStefano F: Risk factors for mortality from all causes and from coronary heart disease among persons with diabetes. Findings from the National Health and Nutrition Examination Survey I Epidemiologic Follow-up Study. Am J Epidemiol 133:1220, 1991.)

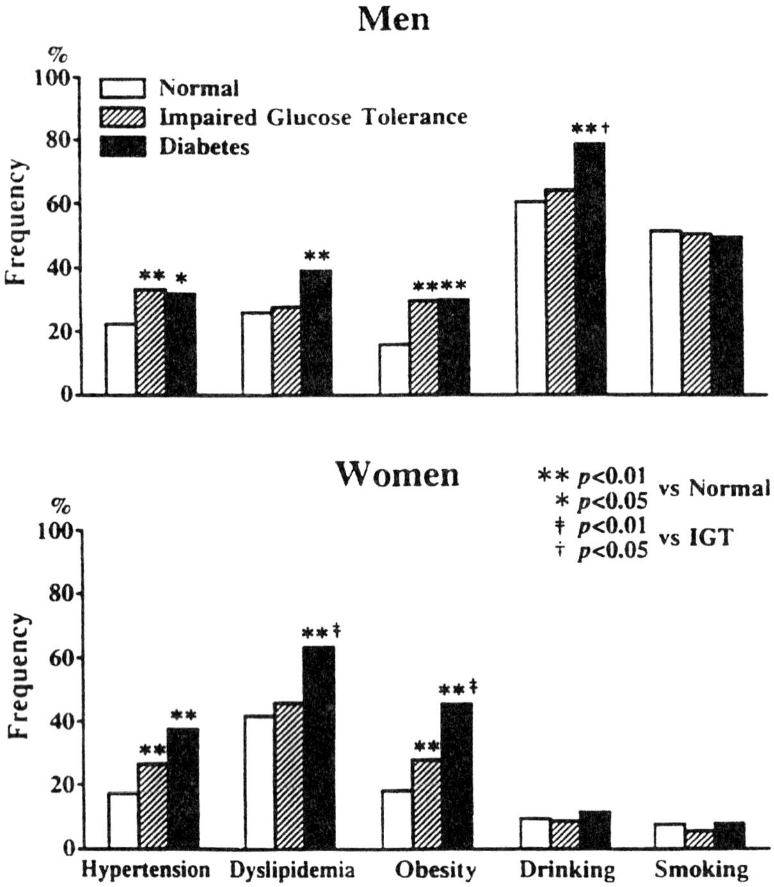

FIGURE 5–4. Age-adjusted frequencies of cardiovascular risk factors by glucose tolerance in Japanese women: The Hisayama Study. Hypertension = 160/95 or more, dyslipidemia-cholesterol 220 mg/dl or higher, obesity = BMI 2504 kg/m^2 or more. (From Fujishima M, Kiyohara Y Kato I, et al: Diabetes and cardiovascular disease in a prospective population survey in Japan: The Hisayama Study. Diabetes 45[Suppl 3]:S14, 1996.)

The revised criteria for the diagnosis of diabetes includes the following categories: Normal fasting glucose (<110 mg/dl), impaired fasting glucose (IFG) (≥110 mg/dl and <126 mg/dl), and diabetes (fasting plasma glucose of ≥126 mg/dl after at least an 8-hour fast and *confirmed on a subsequent day,* **or** symptoms of diabetes plus a casual plasma glucose level ≥ 200 mg/dl, **or** a 2-hour plasma glucose ≥ 200 mg/dl during an OGTT.

Fasting plasma glucose levels are more strongly associated with the microvascular complications of diabetes than with the macrovascular consequences of the disease.[19] The older criteria issued by the WHO includes the category of impaired glucose tolerance, defined by a 2-hour post-glucose load plasma glucose level of >140 mg/dl and <200 mg/dl.[18] In a meta-analysis of over 22,000 individuals with a median follow-up of 8.8 years, 2-hour post-glucose load plasma glucose values were more predictive of all-cause and cardiovascular mortality when compared with fasting plasma glucose values.[19] The results were similar in men and women, with and without diabetes. Individuals with impaired glucose tolerance are generally obese, insulin resistant, and at an increased risk of developing diabetes.[21, 22] Thus, subtle degrees of glucose intolerance confer an increased cardiovascular risk. Further refinements of the diagnostic criteria for glucose intolerance may better predict this increased cardiovascular risk.

All types of diabetes mellitus confer an increased risk of cardiovascular disease. Type 1, or insulin-dependent diabetes mellitus (IDDM), results from destruction of the β cells of the pancreas. Type 1 diabetes is relatively rare, accounting for only 5% to 10% of all cases of diabetes. It occurs most commonly in children and adolescents, but people of all ages are susceptible. Type 1 diabetes is associated with organ-specific antibodies (islet cell antibodies, anti–glutamic acid decarboxylase [anti-GAD] antibodies, anti-insulin antibodies) in more than 80% of patients.[23]

Possible causes of type 1 diabetes include autoimmune phenomena and environmental triggers such as viruses and exposure to foreign proteins (cow's milk during the perinatal period).[24] The concordance of identical twins with type 1 diabetes is approximately 30% to 50%, demonstrating the strong but not exclusive importance of genetics in the presentation of this disease. Several HLA- and non–HLA-associated genes have been described that increase the risk for the development of type 1 diabetes.

Although the destruction of β cells may progress over months to years, the presentation of frank hyperglycemia is generally sudden and clinically obvious. Ketosis is common at presentation, and urgent insulin administration is generally indicated. Therefore, at least in children and adolescents, the clinical onset of the disease is acute and characteristic, the incidence in different populations is known and varies dramatically by geography, and the time from presentation to chronic complications, such as microvascular or macrovascular disease, is well defined. In adults, however, β cell destruction is slower, the clinical presentation is less explosive, and the incidence is less well known.

It is sometimes difficult to differentiate type 1 and type 2 diabetes (non–insulin-dependent diabetes mellitus or NIDDM) in adults. One way of distinguishing type 1 from type 2 diabetes in adults is by body habitus. A thin individual who is continuing to lose weight with poor glucose control is probably insulin deficient. Ketosis or ketoacidosis would also imply insulin deficiency. The presence of islet cell antibodies and low C peptide measurements would confirm the diagnosis of type 1 diabetes. There is no consistent sex difference between boys and girls or men and women for type 1 diabetes.

Type 2 diabetes is a heterogeneous group of disorders characterized by significant insulin resistance associated with variable degrees of impairment in insulin secretion. Type 2 occurs most commonly in people older than 40 years but can appear at any age. Approximately 90% of all patients with diabetes are classified as having type 2, and at least 80% to 90% of people with type 2 diabetes are obese.[25, 26] There is frequently a long preclinical period between the onset of hyperglycemia and the clinical diagnosis.[27] Thus, chronic complications of diabetes, such as retinopathy, may already be present at the time of diagnosis.

Strong environmental and genetic effects on the development of type 2 diabetes have been described. Monozygotic twins have a concordance for type 2 diabetes that approaches 90%. Several genes have been described that are associated with a particular form of diabetes in children, maturity-onset diabetes of youth (MODY), but these genes are not associated with type 2 diabetes.[28] A concerted search of the genome is beginning to describe genes that may explain some of the higher prevalence of type 2 diabetes in certain populations.[29]

The primary defect in type 2 diabetes is not known. Longitudinal population studies have demonstrated insulin resistance, hyperinsulinemia, and subtle defects in insulin secretion to be present for years prior to the development of diabetes.[15, 16] These metabolic abnormalities have been used to accurately predict the risk of future development of diabetes. The components of the insulin resistance syndrome, also referred to as syndrome X, include many of the metabolic abnormalities seen in patients with diabetes, such as dyslipidemia, abnormal fibrinolysis, hypertension, and accelerated atherogenesis (Table 5–6).[30, 31] The presence of any one of these disorders, even in the absence of any glucose intolerance, may indicate an insulin-resistant state, and the patient should be evaluated for the presence of other cardiovascular risk factors. A clinical clue to the diagnosis of the insulin resistance syndrome is the presence of acanthosis nigricans, a hyperpigmented skin lesion typically found on the dorsal surface of the neck and back, and intertriginous and extensor areas such as the axillae, elbows, and knees (Color Plate 5–1).

Table 5–6. COMPONENTS OF THE INSULIN RESISTANCE SYNDROME

Hypertension
Dyslipidemia
Phenotype B (small dense LDL particles, decreased HDL, elevated triglycerides)
Dysfibrinolysis
Elevated PAI-1, decreased tPA
Glucose intolerance

HDL, high-density lipoprotein; LDL, low-density lipoprotein; PAI-1, plasma activator inhibitor-1; tPA, tissue plasminogen activator.

Table 5–7. MANIFESTATIONS OF THE INSULIN RESISTANCE SYNDROME IN WOMEN

Central obesity
Increased waist-hip ratio
Acanthosis nigricans
Ovarian hyperandrogenism
Hirsutism
Acne
Polycystic ovarian syndrome

In women, hyperinsulinemia and insulin resistance are associated with ovarian hyperandrogenism and result in central distribution of visceral fat, hirsutism, acne, menstrual irregularities, and ovarian cysts (Table 5–7).[32–34] Ovarian androgen production, principally testosterone, is stimulated by increased insulin secretion. Biochemical abnormalities of this syndrome include elevated dehydroepiandrosterone sulfate, reduced sex hormone binding globulin (SHBG) with resultant increases in free testosterone, and decreased HDL cholesterol. The greater waist girth and waist-hip ratio commonly found in this syndrome substantially raise the risk of diabetes and cardiovascular disease.[35] Additional risks of this syndrome in women are infertility and endometrial cancer, due to ovulatory dysfunction and unopposed estrogen action, respectively. Medications that reduce insulin resistance, such as metformin and thiazolidenediones, have been shown to reduce insulin and free testosterone levels as well as improve the lipid profile.[33, 34, 36] The development and use of medications that improve insulin sensitivity may prove useful in preventing or delaying the consequences of insulin resistance, including the development of diabetes, cardiovascular disease, and reproductive disorders.[37]

The metabolic and cardiovascular stresses of pregnancy are well known.[38] The higher insulin resistance related to the changing hormonal milieu may precipitate glucose intolerance. Gestational diabetes is defined as a transient metabolic disorder that occurs only during pregnancy and resolves after delivery. Affected patients probably have limited β cell reserve and cannot tolerate any increase in insulin resistance. Approximately 3% to 5% of pregnant women have gestational diabetes. Criteria for diagnosis of gestational diabetes differ from those for diabetes in nonpregnant adults. All pregnant women should be screened for diabetes between the 24th and 28th week of gestation, and women at a high risk of diabetes should be screened earlier.

Women with a history of gestational diabetes are at an increased risk for development of diabetes in later life. A small percentage (5% to 10%) will develop type 1 diabetes, but the majority will develop type 2 diabetes (30% to 50% over 5 years, or approximately 7% per year). The best discriminator for the future development of diabetes is an abnormal result of an oral glucose tolerance test performed 6 weeks postpartum. In one study, 80% of Mexican-American women who had impaired glucose tolerance postpartum were diagnosed with type 2 diabetes within 5 years (Fig. 5–5).[39] This population is being investigated in clinical trials designed to test preventive strategies, including diet, exercise, and pharmacologic intervention.

It is sometimes difficult to determine whether a pregnant woman has preexisting diabetes or gestational diabetes.[40] Approximately 2% to 4% of pregnant women have undiag-

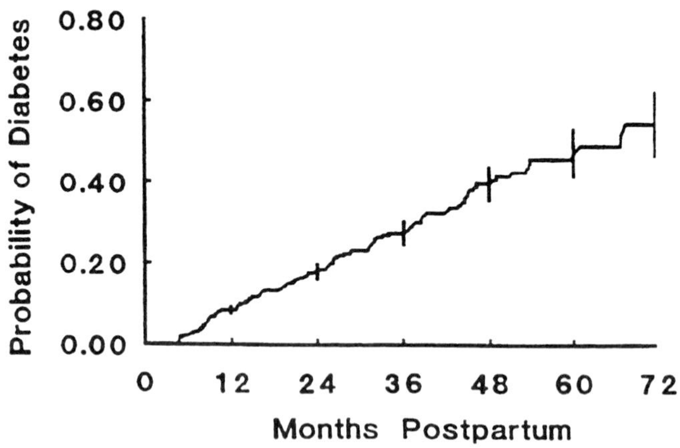

FIGURE 5–5. Cumulative incidence rates of type 2 diabetes as determined by life table analysis in 671 Hispanic women with recent gestational diabetes. The women were initially tested 4 to 16 weeks postpartum and did not have diabetes at that time. They returned for at least one additional oral glucose tolerance test within 7.5 years. (From Kjos SL, Peters RK, Ziang A, et al: Predicting future diabetes in Latino women with gestational diabetes: Utility of early postpartum glucose tolerance testing. Diabetes 44: 586, 1995.)

nosed preexisting diabetes that is discovered during routine pregnancy screening. These women are at risk for the development of chronic complications of diabetes during the pregnancy and require active surveillance for the development of proliferative retinopathy, eclampsia, progressive renal dysfunction, and cardiovascular disease.

The babies of women with preexisting diabetes whose disease is not metabolically controlled during the first 6 weeks of gestation are at increased risk of fetal death and congenital malformations (8% to 12% in patients with preexisting diabetes versus approximately 2% for the general population).[39] Women with preexisting complications of diabetes, such as retinopathy and nephropathy, are at a particularly high risk for rapid progression of eye and kidney disease, some effects of which may be irreversible. Intrauterine growth retardation and placental vasculopathy are also more common in this group. Preconception counseling should be given, and effective contraception should be initiated and continued until good metabolic control is attained.[41] The babies of women with either type 1 or 2 diabetes who attain a glycosylated hemoglobin (HbA_{1c}) level within 1% of the normal range are not at a higher risk of congenital malformations.

Angiotensin-converting enzyme (ACE) inhibitors are contraindicated during pregnancy because of their effects on the fetal kidney. Nevertheless, control of hypertension remains critical. The consequences of hyperglycemia later in the pregnancy include perinatal complications such as macrosomia and fetal hypoglycemia. Children with birth weights less than 2.5 kg (intrauterine growth retardation or small for gestational age) or greater than 4 kg are at increased risk for development of diabetes and premature cardiovascular disease as adults.[40]

Prevalence of Glucose Intolerance and Its Risk Factors Among Women

In 1996, it was estimated that approximately 16 million people in the United States had diabetes, 1 million with type 1 diabetes, 7.5 million with diagnosed type 2 diabetes, and an additional 7.5 million people with undiagnosed type 2 diabetes (Fig. 5–6). The total annual economic cost of diabetes is increasing rapidly and was estimated at 91.8 billion dollars in 1992, compared with $20.4 billion in 1987. One of every seven health care dollars is spent on diabetes care, and 63 cents of that dollar goes to hospital care.[25, 42]

There are strong ethnic differences in the prevalence of diabetes. Type 1 diabetes, although relatively rare, is most commonly seen in white people and is rare in Hispanics and Asians. On the other hand, the prevalence of type 2 diabetes is lowest in white people and substantially increased in Native Americans, Mexican-Americans, blacks, and peoples who have experienced rapid changes in lifestyle or environment (e.g., Asians who have migrated to the United States, Pacific Islanders).[43]

In most populations, the prevalence of type 2 diabetes is slightly higher among women than among men. In the general U.S. population, about 55% of adults diagnosed with diabetes are women.[25] On the basis of data from the Hispanic Health and Nutrition Examination Survey (HHANES)[44] and the National Health and Nutrition Examination Survey (NHANES II), the age-standardized rate of total diabetes (diagnosed and undiagnosed combined) in women relative to the rate in men is 1.3 for non-Hispanic whites, 1.2 for blacks, 1.1 for Mexican-Americans, and 1.0 for Puerto Ricans. This slight predominance persists among very-high-risk populations such as Native American populations, in which 13.2% of women and 11% of men have type 2 diabetes. These differences represent differing distributions of risk factors for diabetes (obesity, physical activity, parity, and genetics).

The prevalence of type 2 diabetes increases with age (Fig. 5–7). In the general U.S. population, the prevalence of diabetes is approximately 3%, but among individuals older than 65 years, the prevalence is 10%.[25] An additional 11% have impaired glucose tolerance. In the high-risk populations, however, diabetes develops at a younger age as well as at a higher rate.[43–46] Among Pima Indians, the cumulative lifetime risk of developing type 2 diabetes continues to increase over time; for Pima Indian women aged 55 to 64

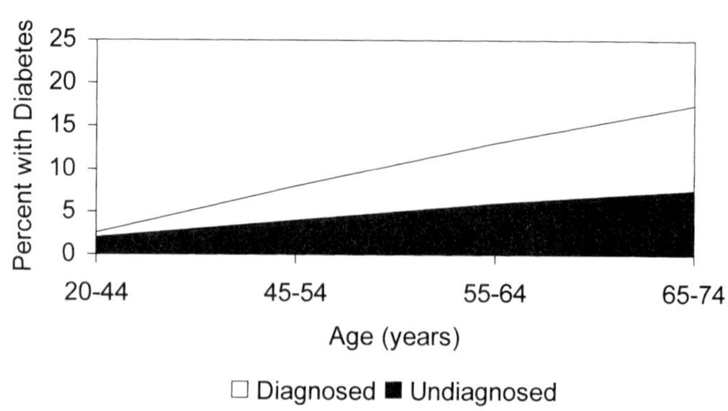

FIGURE 5–6. Percent of diagnosed and undiagnosed NIDDM in adults, U.S. 1976 to 1980. Diagnosed NIDDM was determined by medical history and undiagnosed NIDDM by oral glucose tolerance test using WHO criteria for a representative sample of U.S. adults aged 20 to 74 years in the 1976 to 1980 Second National Health and Nutrition Examination Survey. (From Harris MI, Hadden WC, Knowler WC, Bennett PH: Prevalence of impaired glucose tolerance and plasma glucose levels in the U.S. population age 20 to 74 years. Diabetes 36:523, 1987.)

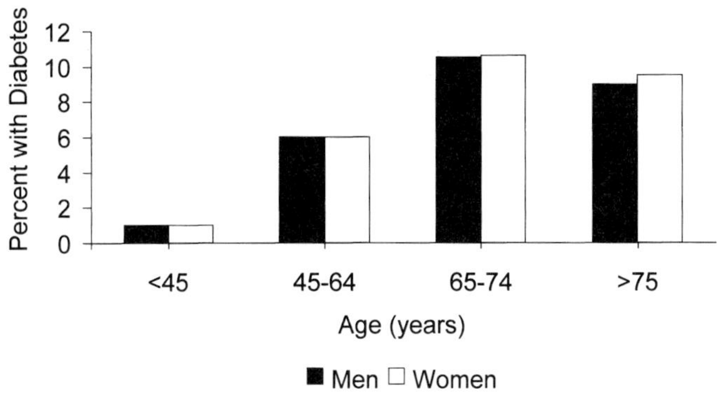

FIGURE 5–7. Percent of the population with diagnosed diabetes by age and sex, U.S., 1991 to 1993. (From Kenny SJ, Aubert RE, Geiss LS: Prevalence and incidence of NIDDM. In Harris MI [ed]: Diabetes in America, 2nd ed. National Institutes of Health; NIH publication 95-1468, Washington, DC, 1995, p 50.)

years, the prevalence is greater than 80%, the highest known rate in the world.[46] The risk of chronic complications of diabetes rises as individuals are exposed to this abnormal metabolic milieu for a longer duration.

Obesity is a major risk factor for the development of type 2 diabetes. The dramatic increase in the prevalence of obesity in the United States has important health consequences for women.[47] In the Nurses' Health Study,[48] relatively minor increases in weight, and in the Iowa Women's Study,[49] wide fluctuations of weight over time were strongly associated with cardiovascular mortality. The NHANES, conducted on 30,000 people from 1991 to 1994, noted that the prevalence of obesity, as defined by a body mass index (BMI) greater than 25 (BMI is calculated by dividing the height in meters by the square of the weight in kilograms), was 59% in men and 49% in women, an increase of 8% in both sexes over the previous 10 years. The prevalence of obesity is particularly high in Mexican-American, black, and Native American women and is strongly related to the growing prevalence of type 2 diabetes in these populations.[50] Mean BMI among persons with type 2 diabetes is higher in women (range, 30.4–33.7) than in men (range, 26.9–32.7) and is highest in Native Americans. Among women with type 2 diabetes, severe obesity, as denoted by a BMI of 30 or more, is seen in 60% to 71% of Native Americans, 65.4% of blacks, and 52.2% of Mexican-Americans, the lowest rates being seen among non-Hispanic whites in Rancho Bernardo, California (19.0%), and Japanese-American women (18.2%).

The amount of abdominal visceral adipose tissue, as measured from waist circumference, waist-hip ratio, subscapular skin folds, or computed tomography (CT), is a critical correlate of the insulin resistance syndrome and is significantly associated with more cardiovascular risk indicators among women than among men (Fig. 5–8).[35, 47, 51–53] Waist circumference is an easy and reliable measurement that correlates with increases in fasting and post-glucose insulin and glucose levels, raised triglyceride levels, and diminished HDL cholesterol levels. Han and associates[51] reported that, in a population of Dutch men and women aged 20 to 59 years, waist circumference exceeding 94 cm in men and 80 cm in women correctly identified subjects with BMIs of 25 or higher as well as men with waist-hip ratios of 0.95 or higher and women with waist-hip ratios of 0.80 or higher, the majority of whom were identified as having at least one cardiovascular risk factor. Larger waist circumferences (especially >100 cm) are most likely to identify individuals with higher total and cardiovascular mortality. Measures of visceral adiposity with the use of CT identified individuals at risk for type 2 diabetes even when BMI was less than 25.[45] Bengtsson and colleagues,[54] who monitored women in Gothenburg, Sweden, for 20 years, found that abdominal obesity and hypertriglyceridemia, both hallmarks of the insulin resistance syndrome, were independently predictive of total mortality and death from myocardial infarction (MI) but that, unlike in men, cholesterol was not. Insulin resistance increases with age, but in a cross-population study, insulin resistance was found to be more closely associated with abdominal adiposity than with age.[53, 55]

The combination of the major risk factors for diabetes—age, obesity, and ethnicity—has resulted in a major public health epidemic in certain geographic areas. In some urban populations, postmenopausal black women have a prevalence of type 2 diabetes that approaches 25%.[56] Because of the serious health consequences of diabetes and the high prevalence, screening has been recommended for populations at increased risk (Table 5–8). Individuals with the following factors would be considered at increased risk:

- First-degree relative with type 2 diabetes
- Age more than 45 years
- History of gestational diabetes

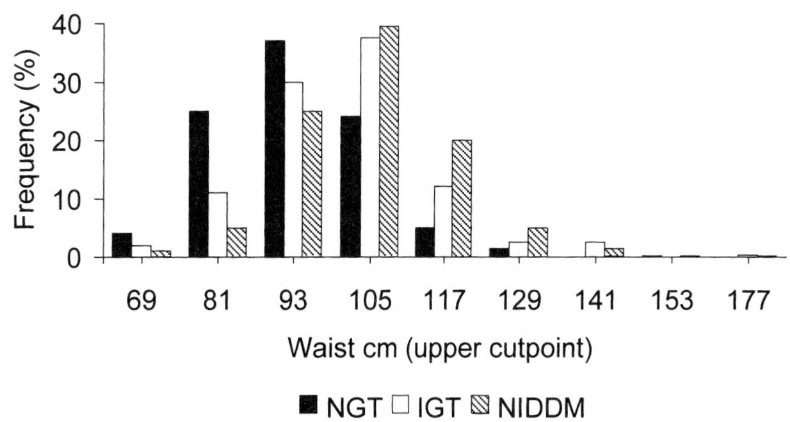

FIGURE 5–8. Frequency distribution of minimum waist girth (cm) by glucose tolerance status. Black bars indicate individuals with normal glucose tolerance, white bars indicate individuals with impaired glucose tolerance, and shaded bars indicate individuals with diabetes in the Insulin Resistance and Atherosclerosis Study. (From Karter AJ, Mayer-Davis EJ, Selby JV, et al: Insulin sensitivity and abdominal obesity in African-American, Hispanic, and non-Hispanic white men and women: the Insulin Resistance and Atherosclerosis Study. Diabetes 45:1547, 1996.)

Table 5–8. RISK FACTORS FOR TYPE 2 DIABETES

Age >45 years
Family history of type 2 diabetes
History of gestational diabetes
Impaired glucose tolerance
Birth weight >4 kg or <2.5 kg
Hispanic-, African-, Asian-, or Native-American heritage

- Previous history of glucose intolerance at times of stress, such as glucocorticoid use, illness, and surgery
- Birth weight of children greater than 4 kg
- Membership in an ethnic group with a high rate of diabetes

Sedentary lifestyle and personal birth weight greater than 4 kg or less than 2.5 kg are also thought to increase risk for diabetes.

The presence of the following findings on physical examination should trigger further evaluation:

- Obesity (especially central adiposity)
- Hypertension
- Acanthosis nigricans
- Hirsutism
- Signs of virilization
- Any findings suggestive of the chronic complications of diabetes (neuropathy, foot ulcers, retinopathy)

The screening test of choice is a fasting plasma glucose test. Fasting is defined as no food consumption for more than 8 hours. A value greater than 110 mg/dl should merit further evaluation. Persons with more than one risk factor should be retested in 3 years even if the fasting plasma level is less than 110 mg/dl. Note that different methods have different ranges (capillary vs. venipuncture) and that a variety of medications and medical illnesses can transiently elevate glucose levels.

A fasting lipid profile and measurement of urinary albumin would also be appropriate. People at risk for glucose intolerance frequently exhibit elevated triglyceride and lowered HDL cholesterol levels. A glycosylated hemoglobin (HbA_{1c}) value greater than 6% is also suggestive of glucose intolerance but may not be reliable for diagnostic purposes.

A screening questionnaire developed by the Centers for Disease Control and Prevention (CDC) includes age >45 years, >120 percent ideal body weight, sedentary lifestyle, first-degree relative with diabetes, and history of delivering a baby weighing more than 4 kg as risk factors. This questionnaire has a sensitivity of 73% and is meant to be followed by a blood screening test.[42]

RISK OF CARDIOVASCULAR DISEASE AMONG WOMEN WITH DIABETES

Diabetes is associated with an increased risk of fatal and nonfatal ischemic heart disease, peripheral vascular disease, hypertension, and stroke. Among individuals hospitalized with acute MI in Corpus Christi, Texas, approximately 65% of the Mexican-American women and 40% of the non-Hispanic white women had a diagnosis of diabetes (Fig. 5–9).[125] Using the Rose questionnaire for angina and MI and the oral glucose tolerance test for the diagnosis of diabetes, the NHANES II, conducted from 1976 to 1980, reported a higher prevalence of both angina and MI in women aged 35 to 74 years who had either previously diagnosed or newly diagnosed diabetes, in comparison with similarly studied diabetic men.[11] Both men and women with diabetes had a higher prevalence of a history of ischemic heart disease than nondiabetic individuals, but the difference began at age 35 years for diabetic women and at age 55 years for diabetic men. Of all the diabetic adults interviewed who were aged 45 to 64 years, 11.2% reported complaints of angina, 21.8% had other cardiac-related complaints, and 22.3% had seen a cardiologist within the past year. On the basis of the 1989–1991 National Hospital Discharge Surveys regarding heart disease discharge diagnoses in adults older than 55 years, the risk ratio of women with and without diabetes was consistently higher for all ischemic heart disease diagnoses than the risk ratio of men with and without diabetes. In the Rancho Bernardo, California, study, a clustering of cardiovascular risk factors was more common in women than in men, possibly explaining the higher risk in women.[14]

The diagnosis of ischemic heart disease in women with diabetes is confounded by a high rate of silent myocardial ischemia and infarction. Autonomic denervation of the heart is a common consequence of diabetes and contributes to the increased frequency of silent ischemia. Silent ST-segment depression and coronary perfusion abnormalities are twice as common among patients with diabetes than among similar patients without diabetes during exercise testing and thallium scintigraphy.[57, 58] In the previously mentioned population-based study of non-Hispanic whites living in Rancho Bernardo, California, 13.7% of the women with type 2 diabetes and 20.9% of the men with type 2 diabetes had evidence of silent ischemia or infarction related to abnormal electrocardiographic (ECG) changes without corresponding symptoms.[59] CHD, diagnosed from either the history or ECG, was found to be present in 43.1% of men and 41.9% of women with type 2 diabetes.

Similar prevalences were found in Hispanic and non-Hispanic men and women in San Luis Valley, Colorado,[60] and in Japanese-American men and women in King County, Washington,[61, 62] with the association of glucose intolerance

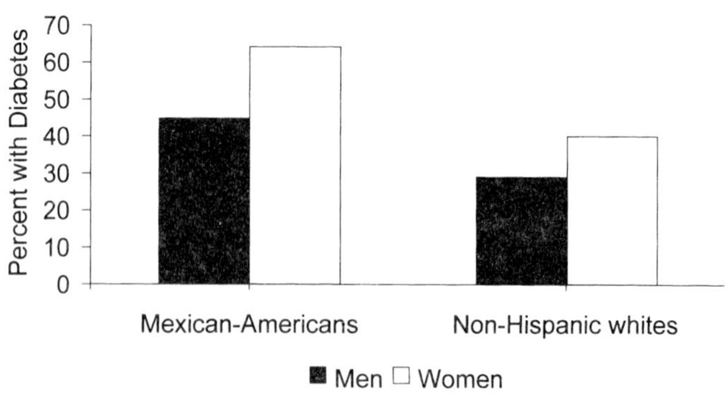

FIGURE 5–9. Percent of men and women with diagnosed diabetes at the time of hospitalization for acute myocardial infarction among Mexican-Americans and non-Hispanic whites: The Corpus Christi Heart Project. (Adapted from Orlander PR, Goff DC, Morrissey M, et al: The relation of diabetes to the severity of acute myocardial infarction and post-myocardial infarction survival in Mexican-Americans and non-Hispanic whites: The Corpus Christi Heart Project. Diabetes 43:897, 1994.)

and CHD in women being as great as or greater than that in men. As in patients with type 2 diabetes, approximately 50% of the diagnosed coronary disease in patients with type 1 diabetes followed at the Joslin Clinic was silent ischemia.[63]

Type of Diabetes and Age as Cardiovascular Risk Factors

It is difficult to distinguish among the effects of aging, the duration of diabetes, and the type of diabetes on the development of ischemic heart disease. According to the 1989 National Health Interview Survey, self-reported heart disease in individuals with diabetes increased with age, but the difference between those with and without diabetes was greatest in younger people, especially those using insulin. There is a 20-fold increase in the risk of CHD among subjects with type 1 diabetes between the ages of 25 and 40 years, but the attained age is more important than the age at diagnosis, the duration, or the metabolic control.[64–66] Symptomatic coronary disease is unusual in patients with type 1 diabetes before age 30 years, even if the onset of the disease was in early childhood. Still, data from the Pittsburgh Epidemiology of Diabetes Complications Study show an association between fatal cardiovascular disease and the duration of type 1 diabetes.

Women with type 1 diabetes appear to have different risk factors for the development of cardiovascular disease from those in similar men. In the prospective Pittsburgh Epidemiology of Diabetes Complications Study, sex-specific Cox proportional hazards models showed that for women with type 1 diabetes, duration of disease, hypertension, waist-hip ratio, physical activity, and depressive symptomatology were all significant independent predictors of CHD, and nephropathy status did not enter the model.[66] In contrast, for men with type 1 diabetes, HDL cholesterol, fibrinogen, hypertension, and smoking were significantly associated with the onset of CHD, but the addition of nephropathy status to the model replaced all the risk factors except for HDL cholesterol. Thus, the effect of renal disease was stronger in men, but the cluster of physical activity, waist-hip ratio, and depressive symptomatology were more important in women.[66]

In subjects with type 2 diabetes, the onset of disease is less clear, and because the patients are generally older, aging and other cardiovascular risk factors probably play a more important role than in type 1 diabetes. The Nurses' Health Study reported a twofold higher risk among women with type 1 diabetes than in women with type 2 diabetes (age-adjusted risk ratios for type 1 and type 2 diabetes were 12.2 and 6.7, respectively, in comparison with nondiabetic women).[2] In this study, longer duration of type 2 diabetes was associated with a higher risk of CHD, even after age adjustment (Fig. 5–10).

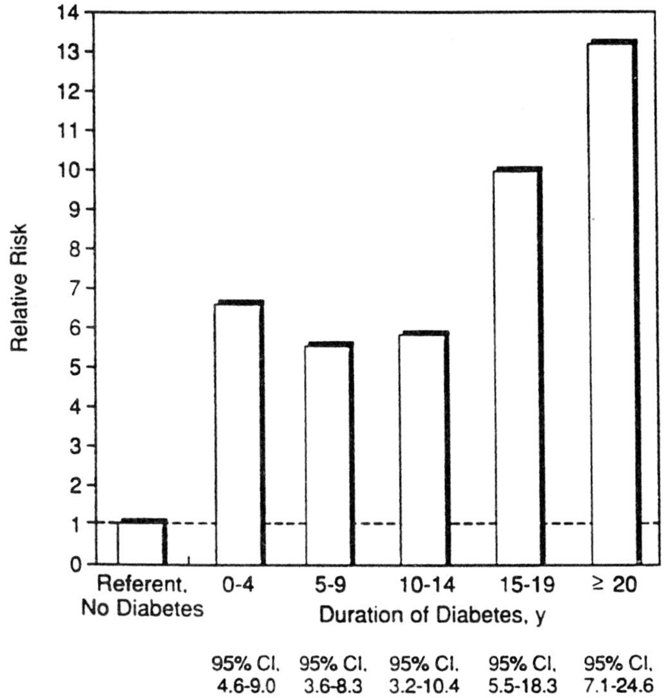

FIGURE 5–10. Age-adjusted relative risks of nonfatal myocardial infarction and fatal coronary heart disease (combined) in relation to duration of type 2 diabetes in the Nurses' Health Study. (From Manson JE, Colditz GA, Stampfer MJ, et al: A prospective study of maturity-onset diabetes mellitus and risk of coronary heart disease and stroke in women. Arch Intern Med 151:1141, 1991.)

Metabolic Control of Diabetes as a Risk Factor

There is a stepwise increase in CHD risk in patients with normal glucose tolerance, impaired glucose tolerance, newly diagnosed diabetes, and previously known diabetes, suggesting a role of long-term glycemic control in the pathogenesis of macrovascular disease.[67] Observations from the Diabetes Control and Complications Trial (DCCT) in type 1 diabetes[20] and from a similar study in Japanese men with type 2 diabetes (the Kumamoto study)[68] demonstrate a decrease in cardiac risk associated with improved glucose control in patients undergoing intensive insulin treatment. However, the total number of events in these generally healthy populations was small, limiting the clinical and statistical significance. Jackson and associates[69] in England and Beks and colleagues[70] in the Netherlands found a significant association between fasting and 2-hour postprandial plasma glucose levels and the presence of vascular disease in adults without previously known diabetes. In the Rancho Bernardo and Framingham studies, glycohemoglobin was significantly related to prevalent cardiovascular disease in women with and without diabetes but not in men.[71, 72] Glycosylated hemoglobin was also related to hypertension and to the ratio of serum total cholesterol to HDL cholesterol. The relative odds of cardiovascular disease increased 1.39-fold for each 1% rise in HbA_{1c}. The relationship was not affected by therapy with medications, such as β blockers and thiazide diuretics, that would affect glucose tolerance, and there was no relationship between heart disease and casual blood glucose measurements. Thus, in these studies, the relationship between glycemia, as measured by HbA_{1c}, and heart disease was robust and independent of other risk factors in older women.

Kuusisto and associates[73] noted an increase in cardiovascular mortality related to metabolic control of diabetes in an elderly Finnish population (Fig. 5–11). However, the direct toxic effect of glucose on endothelial tissue remains contro-

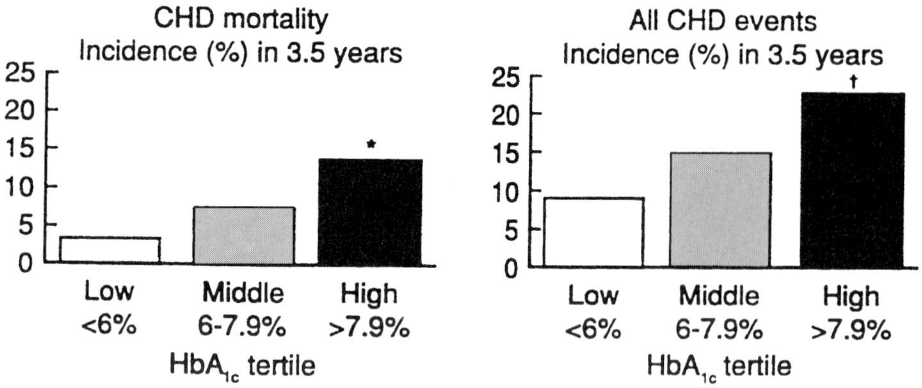

FIGURE 5–11. HbA_{1c} predicts coronary heart disease in type 2 diabetes. The 3.5-year incidence of CHD deaths with respect to median glycohemoglobin. $GHbA_{1c}$, glycohemoglobin. (From Kuusisto J, Mykkänen L, Pyörälä K, Laakso M: NIDDM and its metabolic control predict coronary heart disease in elderly subjects. Diabetes 43: 960, 1994.)

versial, raising the possibility that other associated factors, such as insulin, proinsulin, growth hormone, and insulin-like growth factors (e.g., insulin-like growth factor-1) may play an important role in the promotion of CHD in patients with type 2 diabetes.[74, 75]

The United Kingdom Prospective Diabetes Study (UKPDS) was a randomized clinical trial conducted between 1977 and 1997 that followed 5102 patients with newly diagnosed diabetes type 2 over an average of 10 years to determine if intensive pharmacotherapy to lower blood glucose levels would result in a reduced rate of microvascular and cardiovascular complications.[75a, 75b] In addition to lifestyle and diet modification, therapeutic modalities included monotherapy and combination therapy with metformin, sulfonylureas, and insulin, as well as antihypertensives (captopril vs. atenolol). The subjects assigned to intensive therapy achieved a median hemoglobin A_{1c} (HbA_{1c}) of 7.0% compared with 7.9% in the subjects assigned to conventional therapy. A continuous relationship was noted between glycemia and microvascular complications, with a 1% improvement in HbA_{1c} associated with a 25% reduction in complications.[75a] No threshold effect was noted, such that any improvement in glucose control was associated with a reduction in microvascular complications, such as retinopathy. A 16% reduction in fatal and nonfatal myocardial infarction and sudden death was noted, but this did not attain statistical significance ($p = 0.052$). Albeit weaker, a continuous association was demonstrated between glucose control and cardiovascular complications, with again no threshold effect noted. A prospective observational study was also conducted by the same investigators and yielded similar results, with a 1% reduction in mean HbA_{1c} associated with a 21% reduction in risk for any diabetes-related endpoint ($p < .0001$), a 21% reduction in deaths related to diabetes ($p < .0001$), a 14% reduction in myocardial infarction ($p < .0001$), a 12% reduction in strokes ($p = .035$), a 16% reduction in heart failure ($p = .021$), and a 37% reduction in microvascular complications ($p < .0001$).[75c] However, even at near normal levels of glycohemoglobin, the relative risk of myocardial infarction was 2 to 3 times that of microvascular complications, whereas in the group with the highest levels of glycemia (HbA_{1c} >10%) the risks were similar.

All hypoglycemic agents were similarly effective in controlling glucose levels, and there was no difference in cardiovascular outcome based on therapy with either diet alone, sulfonylureas, or insulin.[75c] A smaller group of obese patients treated with metformin alone had a significant decrease in cardiovascular morbidity.[75b] There was a progressive deterioration in glucose control and an increase in weight over the time course of the study, regardless of the initial therapy, with patients assigned to insulin gaining the most weight and patients assigned to metformin gaining the least.[75a, 75b] However, only 25% of the patients were at the goal of <7% HbA_{1c} after 9 years of study using monotherapy, suggesting the need for combination therapy to achieve glycemic goals.[75d]

Relationship of Diabetes to Other Cardiovascular Risk Factors

Hypertension

The mechanisms for the development of hypertension differ according to the type of diabetes, with the prevalence of hypertension in people with type 1 diabetes primarily related to the development of diabetic nephropathy. Hypertension is much more common among people with type 2 diabetes and has been associated with the insulin-resistant state.[76] According to the WHO criteria for hypertension (blood pressure ≥160/95 mm Hg), 63% of people with type 2 diabetes have hypertension, with 45% having poorly controlled hypertension. According to the criteria from the Joint National Committee on Detection, Evaluation, and Treatment of High Blood Pressure (blood pressure ≥140/90 mm Hg), 74% of people with type 2 diabetes have hypertension, and about 60% have uncontrolled hypertension.[50] The prevalence of hypertension among women with type 2 diabetes who are between 45 and 64 years of age is higher (65.7%) than among similarly diabetic men (55.2%), whereas the prevalence of hypertension is lower among nondiabetic women than among men with normal glucose tolerance. In persons with diabetes, the prevalence of hypertension is highest among blacks (71.3%) and lowest among Mexican-Americans (37.5%).[50] Coexisting hypertension has been shown to have a synergistic effect with diabetes in causing myocardial interstitial fibrosis and diastolic dysfunction.

The UKPDS clinical trial demonstrated a reduction in both microvascular and macrovascular complications with improved blood pressure control.[75e, 75f] There was a significant decrease in the rate of strokes, diabetes-related deaths, and heart failure achieved with a median blood pressure of 144/82 mm HG compared with 154/87 mm HG over approximately 8 years of follow-up.[75e] Similar findings were noted in a contemporaneous observational study performed by the same investigators, with the lowest risk at systolic pressures of <120 mm Hg.[75g] Each decrease of 10 mm Hg in mean systolic blood pressure was associated with reductions in risk of 12% for any complication related to diabetes ($p<.0001$), 15% for deaths related to diabetes ($p<.0001$), 11% for myocardial infarction ($p<.0001$), and 13% for microvascular complications ($p<.0001$). Myocardial infarction occurred twice as frequently as microvascular complications at each level of blood pressure. All of these associations persisted after adjustment for recognized cardiovascular risk factors. Atenolol and captopril were similarly effective.[75f]

Dyslipidemia

Blood lipid levels are commonly abnormal in patients with diabetes. These individuals have higher numbers of both glycosylated lipid particles and particles modified by free radical formation and peroxidation in their blood.[77] Glycation of apolipoprotein B (apo B) is increased in diabetic individuals, causing impaired recognition of low-density lipoprotein (LDL) by its receptor and increasing the half-life of LDL particles. In contrast, glycation of HDL increases its clearance and thereby decreases its half-life. Glycation can cause greater oxidation of LDL within the vessel wall. Oxidized LDL is preferentially taken up by macrophages and by endothelial cells. Chisolm and associates[77] have demonstrated that in streptozocin-treated diabetic rats, the lipid fractions very-low-density lipoprotein (VLDL) and LDL had increased amounts of peroxidized particles that were cytotoxic to vascular endothelial cells and smooth muscle cells. The toxicity of the lipid particles was decreased by pretreating the animals with antioxidants such as vitamin E. Increased levels of circulating oxidized lipids correlate with triglyceride levels and glycohemoglobin levels. Women with type 1 diabetes tend to have greater concentrations of oxidized lipoproteins.[78]

Lipid patterns are different among people with type 1 and type 2 diabetes. Patients with uncontrolled type 1 diabetes have decreased lipoprotein lipase activity, which results in diminished clearance and greater production of VLDL particles, normal or lower LDL cholesterol levels, and decreased HDL cholesterol levels. Intensive insulin therapy, as demonstrated in DCCT, resulted in significant lowering of LDL cholesterol and improvement in HDL cholesterol levels.[20] Careful analysis of the individual lipoprotein particles, however, demonstrates compositional abnormalities that are not corrected even after 6 months of intensive insulin therapy. These abnormalities include an increase in the amount of triglycerides in many of the particles, including the VLDL particles.

In patients with type 2 diabetes, the most common abnormalities are an increase in free fatty acid production by the liver associated with decreased clearance peripherally.[79, 80] This results in a rise in triglyceride levels and a fall in HDL cholesterol. In addition, many of the particles are abnormal. Plasma VLDL particles are larger, with higher triglyceride content. These particles may be less easily converted to LDL and thus are picked up by macrophages to form foam cells. The LDL particles are small and dense. Even among normolipidemic individuals with type 2 diabetes, the LDL B subclass pattern (small, dense LDL particles, higher plasma triglyceride levels, lower HDL cholesterol levels) was twice as common as among age-matched controls with similar lipid levels.[80] The clearance of triglyceride-rich lipoproteins was slowed in subjects with the LDL subclass pattern B. Indices of diabetic control, such as fasting and glycohemoglobin levels, were similar regardless of the LDL subclass pattern, suggesting that insulin, its precursors, or insulin resistance may play a primary role.

Total HDL cholesterol is reduced in patients with type 2 diabetes, and HDL_2 is reduced more than HDL_3. Diabetic patients with CHD have lower HDL_2 levels than diabetic patients without CHD. All of these lipid abnormalities may be present years before the occurrence of clinical hyperglycemia and have been associated with hyperinsulinemia and the insulin-resistant state.[16, 79, 81] The prevalence of subclass pattern B rises progressively from 5.6% of women with no manifestations of the insulin resistance syndrome to 100% in women with more than three components.[81]

More than 50% of subjects with type 2 diabetes mellitus have dyslipidemia. Mean total cholesterol concentration, based on the NHANES II and HHANES data for patients aged 20 to 74 years, is higher in people with type 2 diabetes (232 mg/dl) and impaired glucose tolerance (228 mg/dl) than in people with normal glucose tolerance (208 mg/dl), with the largest differences occurring in people aged 20 to 44 years.[50] Total cholesterol, LDL cholesterol, and triglyceride levels were higher in women with diabetes than in men with diabetes, and were highest among non-Hispanic white women.[82] Among patients with diabetes, women were more likely than men to have total cholesterol levels greater than 240 mg/dl (43.7% vs. 37.4%, respectively), LDL cholesterol levels greater than 160 mg/dl (43.8% vs. 30.9%, respectively), and fasting triglyceride levels greater than 250 mg/dl (22.2% vs. 13.9%, respectively). More than 11% of the women with type 2 diabetes had HDL levels less than 35 mg/dl, a remarkably low value in women because of the salutary effect of estrogen on HDL cholesterol.

Abnormalities of Coagulation and Fibrinolysis

Diabetes predisposes people to abnormalities in various pathways involved in coagulation, hemostasis, and fibrinolysis.[75, 83–87] These abnormalities include elevated levels of kallikrein, factors VIII and XI, and von Willebrand factor. Patients with diabetes have lower antithrombin III activity and an acquired protein C deficiency. Fibrinolysis is impaired because such patients have increased plasminogen activator inhibitor–1 (PAI-1) activity and decreased levels of tissue plasminogen activator (tPA).[85–87] In the MONICA study, insulin resistance was highly correlated with reduced measures of fibrinolytic activity. PAI-1 activity was elevated in men and women with insulin resistance, and tPA was inversely correlated.[85]

Lp(a) is a macromolecular complex with a unique glycoprotein, apo(a), that is linked to apo B. It combines structural elements of the lipoprotein and blood clotting systems and is associated with premature CHD and stroke. Lp(a) has marked homology with plasminogen and competes with binding for the plasminogen receptor, thus inhibiting fibrinolysis. Lp(a) levels are frequently found to be elevated in people with type 2 diabetes. It remains controversial whether improved glycemic control has any effect on Lp(a) levels.[88–89]

Smoking, Alcohol, and Sedentary Lifestyle

Individuals with diabetes smoke less frequently and drink less alcohol than nondiabetic persons, with women generally smoking less often than men.[50] However, the frequency of self-reported physical activity is lower among women with diabetes.[50]

Presence of Microvascular Disease

In all patients with diabetes, regardless of its type, identical microvascular lesions develop in the retina, kidney, and nerves, thus supporting the primacy of glucose control.[90] Average serum glucose levels are generally lower in patients with type 2 diabetes than in those with type 1 diabetes; thus, the individual risk of complications is thought to be lower in patients with type 2 diabetes. However, type 2 diabetes is tenfold more prevalent, resulting in high absolute numbers of complications in patients with both disorders. Diabetes is the most common cause of blindness in adults, end-stage renal disease, and nontraumatic amputations.

The epidemiology of the complications of diabetes is different for different organ systems. Retinopathy rarely develops until the disease has been present for 5 years; at least background retinal changes are found in more than 80% of patients with type 1 diabetes and 40% to 70% of patients with type 2 diabetes after 10 years.[90, 91] However, about 20% of patients with type 2 diabetes have evidence of diabetic retinopathy at initial presentation because of a long delay in diagnosis (Fig. 5–12).[27, 91, 92] The cumulative lifetime risk of retinopathy approaches 100% with longer duration of disease. There is no sex difference in the rate of diabetic retinopathy, but older women have higher rates of legal blindness, nonwhite women having the highest rates.[93] In addition to affecting vision, retinopathy is an important indicator of the state of the arterial and arteriolar system. The presence of retinopathy, in men and women, is strongly predictive of cardiovascular disease and higher rate of death.[94]

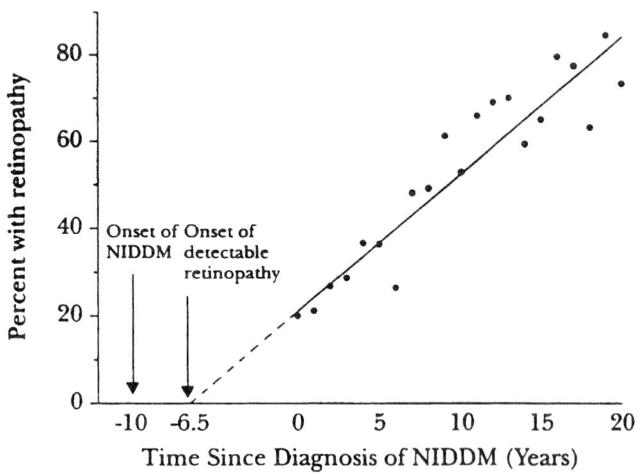

FIGURE 5–12. Estimated time of onset of retinopathy and of NIDDM, Wisconsin, 1980–1982. Data points are prevalence of any retinopathy in a representative sample of subjects with NIDDM according to time since diagnosis of diabetes. Line is linear regression of the data (R^2 = 0.89) to estimate time at which detectable retinopathy first began. Onset of NIDDM is believed to occur some years before evidence of detectable retinopathy. (From Harris MI, Klein RE, Welborn TA, et al: Onset of NIDDM occurs at least 4–7 years before clinical diagnosis. Diabetes Care 15:815, 1992.)

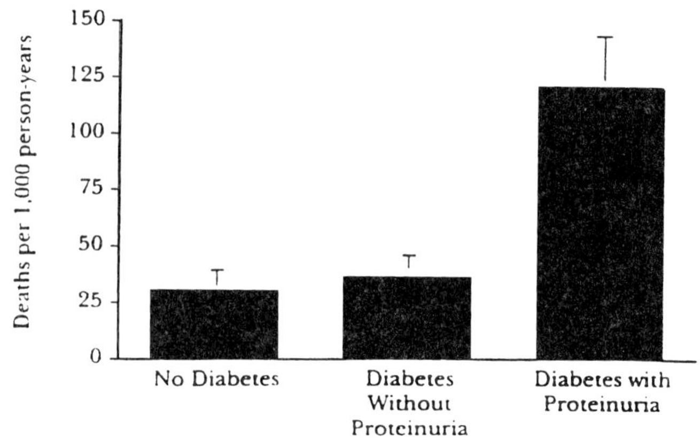

FIGURE 5–13. Mortality in Pima Indians age 45 years or older, by diabetes and proteinuria status. (From Nelson RG, Pettit DJ, Carraher MJ, et al: Effect of proteinuria on mortality in NIDDM. Diabetes 37:1499, 1988.)

Clinical nephropathy is rarely seen until 10 to 15 years after the onset of diabetes, is almost always preceded by retinopathy, and is seen in only a portion of patients over the long term (approximately 40% of those with type 1 diabetes and 20% of those with type 2 diabetes). Incipient diabetic renal disease is characterized by increased glomerular filtration rates and microalbuminuria.[95] Microalbuminuria is defined as urinary excretion of 30 to 300 mg albumin per gram of creatinine. Microalbuminuria is affected by exercise, ambient glucose level, and intercurrent illness. Day-to-day variation in albuminuria in an individual can approach 50%. Therefore, an average of three measurements is recommended for determination of this disorder. Yearly screening can be performed by measurement of spot urine specimens for urinary albumin and creatinine ratios. Microalbuminuria correlates histologically with mesangial changes and is predictive of increased proteinuria and progressive renal dysfunction if untreated. Most people also have hypertension coincident with microalbuminuria.

Diabetic patients with incipient and clinical nephropathy have a higher risk of cardiovascular disease and higher mortality, similar to those with retinopathy (Fig. 5–13).[95, 96] This issue has been studied in several different cohorts with both type 1 and type 2 diabetes, although in the Pittsburgh cohort, nephropathy with type 1 diabetes was more closely associated with coronary disease among men than among women.[66, 97, 98] The mortality was threefold higher among a cohort with type 1 diabetes mellitus and microalbuminuria, and even higher among the diabetic patients with proteinuria greater than 1 gram per day.[98–102] Nearly all of the difference in mortality associated with either type of diabetes, primarily cardiovascular, is found in people with proteinuria.

Patients with microalbuminuria have elevated total cholesterol and triglyceride levels and reduced HDL cholesterol levels. This pattern is seen even when the creatinine clearance is in the normal range. In fact, increased lipid levels may be a risk factor for urinary albumin and progression of renal disease. Microalbuminuria appears to be a risk factor for heart disease in older people without diabetes, especially in the presence of hyperinsulinemia.[103] It is possible that the proteinuria is associated with lipid or blood pressure changes that may promote atherogenesis. Another possibility is that the permeability found in the glomerulus may be a more generalized phenomenon, with higher permeability in all the vasculature leading to greater penetration by lipids into the intima and the formation of foam cells.

Reduced protein intake (0.8 g protein/kg body weight) and rigorous blood pressure control, especially with angiotensin-converting enzyme (ACE) inhibitors, are effective in reducing proteinuria, delaying progression of renal disease, and reducing the frequency of dialysis or transplantation.[104] Similar trends have been demonstrated in patients with type 1 and type 2 diabetes and in patients with incipient and clinical nephropathy. ACE inhibitors are important in the treatment of congestive heart failure and have been shown to decrease cardiovascular morbidity and mortality in patients with diabetes.[105]

Ethnic differences are seen in the frequency of the occurrence of complications.[106] Native Americans, Mexican-Americans and blacks are at increased risk for retinopathy and nephropathy.[43] The reason for this finding is not clear but may be related to delay in diagnosis, limited access to care, poorer metabolic control, and different rates of hypertension in comparison with the general U.S. population.

Presence of Other Macrovascular Disease

There is a strong relationship between diabetes and subclinical vascular disease, in both the carotid arteries and the lower extremities. In the Framingham Study, the 2-year incidence of carotid or femoral bruits or nonpalpable pedal pulses was higher among diabetic than nondiabetic people.[107] The 2-year incidence of stroke was higher in women with both carotid bruits and diabetes than in similarly affected men. The presence of a nonpalpable pedal pulse or femoral bruit and diabetes was also associated with a substantially higher risk of stroke among women than among men.

Most ischemic strokes in diabetic patients are due to occlusion of small paramedial penetrating arteries. The occlusions cause small infarcts within the white matter of the brain.[108] Diabetes is associated with a 2.5-fold higher risk of stroke, affecting up to 13% of all patients with diabetes who are older than 65 years.[109] The risk ratio of stroke for women with diabetes in the Nurses' Health Study was 4.1 (95% CI, 2.8–6.1),[2] compared with 1.9 for men in the Honolulu Heart Program.[110] The risk of fatal and nonfatal stroke was also higher for women in the Rancho Bernardo study (risk ratio, 2.0 for women and 1.5 for men, both with diabetes).[109] The higher prevalence of diabetes and hypertension among blacks contributes to the greater risk of stroke.

In the Atherosclerosis Risk in Communities (ARIC) study, there was a direct relationship of carotid artery thickness with both blood glucose levels and diagnosed diabetes, for both black and white men and women.[111] The 30-year follow-up of the Framingham Study found that blood glucose level was an independent risk factor for stroke in multiple logistic regression analysis among women but not men.[107] A higher blood glucose level at hospital admission predicts a poorer prognosis after stroke or MI, regardless of whether the patient has a prior diagnosis of diabetes.

The risk factors for stroke—hypertension, hypercholesterolemia, and smoking—also contribute to the higher frequency of peripheral vascular disease among people with diabetes. Clinical lower extremity arterial disease is 10-fold more common among patients with diabetes and, when compounded with the presence of peripheral neuropathy and susceptibility to infection, commonly leads to foot ulcers, gangrene, and amputation.[112] Peripheral vascular disease is more diffuse and distal in patients with diabetes than in those without it and has a predilection to be concentrated below the knee. Calcified arteries are common in patients with diabetes, causing noncompressible vessels and unreliable ankle-brachial systolic pressure measurements. Medial artery calcification, detected by radiography, is an independent risk factor for cardiovascular mortality in patients with type 2 diabetes.[113] Angioplasty is, therefore, only modestly successful. Perioperative mortality for revascularization of the limb is high, and because of coexisting CHD, the 3-year survival rate is less than 50%. In patients with diabetes, the rates of lower extremity vascular disease and amputation are slightly higher among men than among women.[112]

Endogenous and Exogenous Insulin

Insulin is a potent growth factor, known to stimulate smooth muscle proliferation in vessel walls. It has both vasodilator and vasocontrictive properties, depending on the experimental model. Population studies conducted by Haffner and associates[16] and McPhillips and colleagues[74] demonstrate that hyperinsulinemia may be present 10 to 15 years prior to the development of diabetes. During the 1970s, three prospective population-based studies of insulin and cardiovascular disease found insulin levels to be an independent predictor of cardiovascular disease in men.[114–116] Since that time, multiple studies have been conducted to explore this association. Although an independent association among insulin levels, insulin resistance, and the prevalence of cardiovascular risk factors has been confirmed in men and women,[5] no study has yet found a significant association between insulin levels and the development of cardiovascular disease and mortality among women. Differences in study design, ethnic differences in insulin secretion and resistance, and methodologic difficulties in measuring insulin resistance may all contribute to the lack of significant findings.

There are no consistent data supporting the contention that exogenous insulin promotes atherogenesis. In the DCCT, young adults with type 1 diabetes randomly assigned to intensive insulin therapy had a significant 34% reduction in LDL cholesterol and a nonsignificant 41% reduction in cardiac events.[20] The number of events in this otherwise healthy population was too small to approach statistical significance. In a similarly designed study, the Stockholm Diabetes Intervention Study, people with type 1 diabetes randomly assigned to an intensive insulin regimen with excellent glucose control (mean HbA_{1c} 7.1%) maintained over 10 years were found to have less macroangiopathic disease than the group assigned to conventional insulin therapy (mean HbA_{1c} 8.2%).[117] Subjects with higher levels of glycemia had significantly stiffer arteries and thicker intima-media in the common carotid arteries. Thus, in patients with type 1 diabetes, intensive insulin therapy with improved glucose control reduces cardiovascular risk.

The role of exogenous insulin in people with type 2 diabetes is controversial. Janka and colleagues[118] noted an association between insulin use and a higher risk of heart disease in patients with type 2 diabetes treated with insulin. However, this association may be a reflection of more advanced vascular disease in patients with poorly controlled diabetes. In the University Group Diabetes Program, no differences in cardiovascular mortality were noted during 9 to 13 years of follow-up among groups receiving dietary, low-dose insulin, and high-dose insulin therapy.[119] Similar results were noted in the UKPDS.[75a] In a randomized prospective study of diabetic patients presenting with an acute MI, Malmberg and associates[120] tested the hypothesis that immediate and intensive insulin therapy, during and after the index hospitalization, would improve cardiovascular morbidity. The overall mortality after 1 year was 19% in the group receiving intensive insulin therapy and 26% in the control group ($p < .05$). However, in the 2-year feasibility trial of the Veterans Affairs Cooperative Study on Glycemic Control and Complications in Type 2 Diabetes, there were 61 new cardiovascular events in 40 patients, the majority occurring in men treated with intensive insulin therapy.[121] On the basis of these preliminary data, adequate control of hyperglycemia should be the primary goal, with insulin therapy used as necessary.

PROGNOSIS OF HEART DISEASE AMONG WOMEN WITH DIABETES

In 1994, diabetes was the seventh leading cause of death in the US, but ranked higher as a leading cause of death among women than among men, and was the fourth leading cause of death among women who were African-American, American Indian, Hawaiian, Filipino, or of Hispanic origin.[121a] African-American women had the highest age-adjusted diabetes-related death rates among the ethnic groups. Between 1980 and 1994, the number of deaths for which diabetes was listed as the underlying cause increased 27%, with the highest rates occurring in minorities and the elderly.

The presence of diabetes dramatically reduces survival after MI.[13, 122–125] In the Corpus Christi Heart Project, the 28-day case fatality rate was twice as great among people with diabetes, and the long-term mortality (44 months) rate was 60% greater among diabetic patients than among nondiabetic patients (Fig. 5–14).[125] In the Framingham Study, women with diabetes were three times more likely to have a second MI within 2 years than women without diabetes ($p < .001$) and were at an increased risk for death within 2 years after infarction (risk ratio, 2.6 for diabetic women vs. 1.8 for diabetic men).[13]

The size of the infarct is not a predictor of the higher morbidity or mortality seen in patients with diabetes. Comparison studies of subjects with and without diabetes have indicated that infarcts of similar size result in a higher

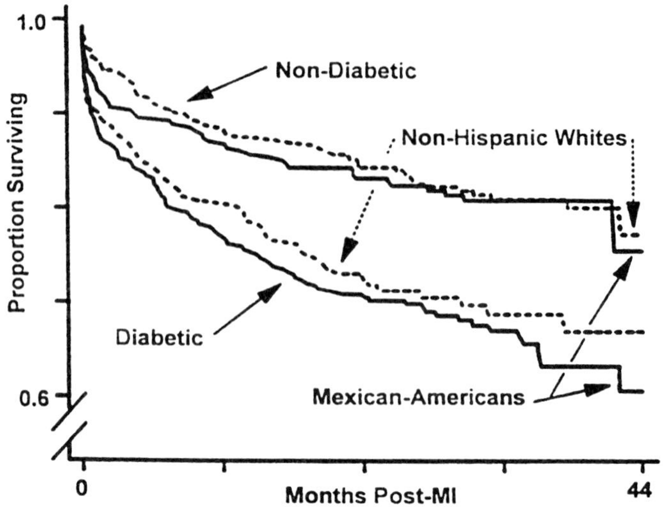

FIGURE 5–14. Proportion of patients hospitalized with acute myocardial infarction surviving 0–44 months by diabetes status and ethnicity in the Corpus Christi Heart Project. (From Orlander PR, Goff DC, Morrissey M, et al: The relation of diabetes to the severity of acute myocardial infarction and post-myocardial infarction survival in Mexican-Americans and non-Hispanic whites: The Corpus Christi Heart Project. Diabetes 43:897, 1994.)

morbidity and mortality in patients with diabetes. For example, Jaffe and colleagues[126] quantified infarct size according to enzyme elevation and found that congestive heart failure was twice as common in patients with diabetes as in those without (31.2% vs. 15.7%) despite smaller enzyme elevations. Takahashi and associates[127] found regional wall motion abnormalities more commonly in the noninfarcted left ventricle among diabetic patients.

In the Corpus Christi Heart Project, examination of the coronary angiograms performed after MI suggested that diabetic patients, in contrast to nondiabetic patients, had more diffuse CHD but probably similar infarct sizes; in addition, they had more frequent congestive heart failure, poorer prognostic scores, and longer hospitalizations.[125] These results are consistent with those of the Multicenter Investigation of the Limitation of Infarct Size (MILIS).[128] Despite having similar or even smaller infarct sizes and similar left ventricular ejection fractions in comparison with the 415 nondiabetic subjects, the 85 diabetic subjects in this study experienced a higher incidence of heart failure and death. Women treated with insulin were at a particularly high risk for postinfarction heart failure.[128] The risk of in-hospital death among diabetic patients in this study was greater in women than in men (risk ratio, 2.6 for women vs. 1.6 for men).

These data suggest that abnormalities other than CHD may be playing a role in the cardiac function of patients with diabetes. Echocardiography, exercise testing, and radionuclide angiography have demonstrated myocardial dysfunction in children, adolescents, and young adults with type 1 diabetes.[129, 130] Comparison studies of young adults with type 1 diabetes and age- and sex-matched healthy controls note an increase in diastolic dysfunction more than twice as frequently as systolic dysfunction and occurring after as few as 8 years after diagnosis. It remains unclear whether these differences are related to a metabolic cardiomyopathy or to differences in physical activity of the two groups. Patients with poorly controlled diabetes have excessive delivery of lipid substances to the myocardium, which could impair carbohydrate utilization in the Krebs cycle and decrease production of adenosine triphosphate.[131] In the Framingham Study, women with diabetes, but not men, had significantly increased left ventricular wall thickness and mass, independent of hypertension.[10] Despite the strong association between microvascular disease and macrovascular disease in people with diabetes, there is no convincing autopsy evidence that microvascular disease of the heart contributes to the cardiac dysfunction.[132]

Subjects with diabetic autonomic neuropathy have an inability to adjust the ejection fraction to changes in posture and volume.[133, 134] Lack of heart rate variability is predictive of both mortality and left ventricular failure. Zola and associates[135] found that 91% of patients with longstanding type 1 diabetes had cardiac autonomic neuropathy, of whom 59% had depressed left ventricular function in the absence of CHD. Such patients experience orthostatic hypotension, painless ischemia, and silent MIs, and may have malignant hypertension after hypoglycemia. Simple bedside tests of the autonomic nervous system can be useful in predicting cardiovascular risks, especially in relationship to anesthesia and surgery. These bedside maneuvers include tilting, hyperventilation, and Valsalva maneuver, all of which should normally result in greater variations in the R-R interval on ECG. Individuals with diabetic autonomic neuropathy do not have these variations.

The high frequency of congestive heart failure after MI in women with diabetes should alert physicians to be especially vigilant for the signs and symptoms of both systolic and diastolic dysfunction and to seriously consider early use of ACE inhibitors in such patients.

Despite strong ethnic differences in the prevalence of diabetes, the impact of the disease on cardiovascular morbidity and mortality appears unrelated to ethnicity. In the Corpus Christi Heart Project, diabetes had similar adverse effects on survival after hospitalization for MI in both Mexican-Americans and non-Hispanic white subjects.[125] However, women received fewer cardiovascular drugs than men, and Mexican-American patients received fewer cardiovascular drugs than non-Hispanic white patients.[136] Beta blockers were prescribed rarely, even though these agents are efficacious in reducing mortality and reinfarction in patients with type 2 diabetes.[137, 138] Diabetic patients included in other clinical trials, such as the Hypertension Detection and Follow-up Program,[139] the Helsinki Heart Study,[140] 4S,[141] and the Early Detection and Treatment of Diabetic Retinopathy Study,[142] received benefits similar to those seen in the nondiabetic patients when both groups were treated with standard antihypertensive, hypolipidemic, and aspirin therapy.

Estrogen replacement therapy was less commonly prescribed for diabetic women who were admitted for acute MIs than for nondiabetic women.[136] The effect of estrogens in preventing heart disease is now controversial based on the adverse effects of estrogen replacement on postmenopausal women with CHD noted in HERS.[17]

Despite aggressive interventionist care, patients with diabetes continue to have a worse prognosis than patients without the disease. In patients with established CHD, those who also have diabetes show a poor response to angioplasty. In the Bypass Angioplasty Revascularization Investigation, patients with type 1 or type 2 diabetes who were treated with oral agents or insulin had a 5-year mortality rate of 35% after initial revascularization with percutaneous transluminal coronary angioplasty, which was significantly greater than the 19% mortality seen in diabetic patients treated with coronary artery bypass grafting.[143, 144] Mortality in both groups was considerably greater than the 9% mortality associated with these procedures in nondiabetic patients or diabetic patients treated with diet only. These findings suggest that people with diabetes have a greater vulnerability of vessels subjected to the injury of angioplasty, possibly related to the abnormal clotting mechanisms and fibrinolysis found in such patients.[75] Restenosis rates in diabetic patients who have received coronary stents is also higher than in nondiabetic patients. At 4-month follow-up, Carrozza and associates[145] reported that patients with diabetes had smaller lumen diameter, higher percentage stenosis, and a greater restenosis rate than patients without diabetes, suggesting higher rates of intimal hyperplasia within the stent due to diabetes.

Women with acute MI receive thrombolytic therapy less often and with longer delays than men.[135, 146, 147] Granger and associates[148] found that, after thrombolytic therapy for acute MI, diabetic patients had twice the risk of having another infarction prior to hospital discharge than similarly treated nondiabetic patients. Among patients treated with thrombolytic agents, the risk of in-hospital death was higher in women with diabetes (risk ratio, 3.8 for diabetic women vs. 3.2 for diabetic men). After coronary artery bypass surgery, early mortality was not significantly greater among individuals with diabetes, but long-term mortality (mean follow-up, 7.4 years) was greater (risk ratio, 1.87).[149]

The especially adverse outcomes related to diabetes emphasize the importance of preventive measures that would reduce the risk of development of diabetes, its cardiovascular consequences, and its other chronic complications. Key features of preventive strategies would include early clinical recognition of the insulin resistance syndrome, treatment of obesity (by means of a multidisciplinary approach using nutritionists, exercise physiologists, psychologists, and possibly pharmacotherapists), strict glucose control (with self-monitoring of blood glucose and measurement of glycohemoglobin), close surveillance and treatment of hypertension and dyslipidemias, smoke cessation programs, and frequent foot and eye examinations with routine referral to podiatrists and ophthalmologists. The addition of aspirin and antioxidant therapy (e.g., vitamin E) may also be prudent in certain people.

SUMMARY

Women, especially nonwhite women, have a higher prevalence of obesity and type 2 diabetes than men. Gestational diabetes is predictive of the development of later diabetes. Women with diabetes have a higher prevalence of other cardiovascular risk factors, such as hypertension and lipid abnormalities, than men. Diabetic women with CHD are at a high risk for recurrent infarction, congestive heart failure, other vascular disease, and death. Acute treatment of MI is less effective in women with diabetes, and angioplasty may be detrimental. Cardioprotective therapy is less commonly administered to women. Early detection and treatment of the insulin-resistant state may prevent or delay the development of diabetes and its associated cardiovascular risk factors, and early aggressive treatment of hyperglycemia and other coexisting cardiovascular risk factors may prevent or delay the higher morbidity and mortality associated with diabetes.[139]

References

1. Raman M, Nesto RW: Heart disease in diabetes mellitus. Endocrinol Metab Clin North Am 25:425, 1996.
2. Manson JE, Colditz GA, Stampfer MJ, et al: A prospective study of maturity-onset diabetes mellitus and risk of coronary heart disease and stroke in women. Arch Intern Med 151:1141, 1991.
3. Stamler J, Vaccaro O, Neaton JD, et al: Diabetes, other risk factors, and 12-yr cardiovascular mortality for men screened in the Multiple Risk Factor Intervention Trial. Diabetes Care 16:434, 1993.
4. Eriksson J, Franssila-Kallunki A, Ekstrand A, et al: Early metabolic defects in persons at increased risk for NIDDM. N Engl J Med 321: 337, 1989.
5. Howard G, O'Leary DH, Zaccaro D, et al: Insulin sensitivity and atherosclerosis. Circulation 93:1809, 1996.
6. Després J-P, Lamarche B, Mauriege P, et al: Hyperinsulinemia as an independent risk factor for ischemic heart disease. N Engl J Med 334: 952, 1996.
7. Geiss LS, Herman WH, Smith PJ: Mortality in non-insulin dependent diabetes. In Harris MI, Cowie CC, Stern MP, et al (eds): Diabetes in America, 2nd ed (NIH Publication No. 95–1468). National Institutes of Health, Washington, DC, 1995, p 233.
8. Orchard TJ: The impact of gender and general risk factors on the occurrence of atherosclerotic vascular disease in NIDDM. Ann Med 28:323, 1996.
9. Goldschmid MG, Barrett-Connor E, Edelstein SL, et al: Dyslipidemia and ischemic heart disease mortality among men and women with diabetes. Circulation 89:991, 1994.
10. Kannel WB, Wolf PA, Garrison RJ (eds): The Framingham Study: An Epidemiological Investigation of Cardiovascular Disease (NIH Publication No. 87-2703). U.S. Department of Health and Human Services, National Heart, Lung, and Blood Institute, Washington, DC, 1987.
11. Wingard DL, Barrett-Connor E: Heart disease and diabetes. In Harris MI, Cowie CC, Stern MP, et al (eds): Diabetes in America, 2nd ed (NIH Publication No. 95-1468). National Institutes of Health, Washington, DC, 1995, p 429.
12. Will JC, Casper M: The contribution of diabetes to early deaths from ischemic heart disease: US gender and racial comparisons. Am J Public Health 86:576, 1996.
13. Abbott RD, Donahue RP, Kannel WB, Wilson PWF: The impact of diabetes on survival following myocardial infarction in men vs women. JAMA 260:3456, 1988.
14. Wingard DL, Barrett-Connor E, Criqui MH, Suarez L: Clustering of heart disease risk factors in diabetic compared to nondiabetic adults. Am J Epidemiol 117:19, 1983.
15. Edwards KL, Austin MA, Newman B, et al: Multivariate analysis of the insulin resistance syndrome in women. Arterioscler Thromb 14: 1940, 1994.
16. Haffner SM, Stern MP, Hazuda HP, et al: Cardiovascular risk factors in confirmed prediabetic individuals. JAMA 263:2893, 1990.
17. Hulley S, Grady D, Bush T, et al: Randomized trial of estrogen plus progestin for secondary prevention of coronary heart disease in postmenopausal women. HERS Research Group. JAMA 280:605, 1998.
18. Report of the Expert Committee on the Diagnosis and Classification of Diabetes Mellitus. Diabetes Care 20:1183, 1997.
19. DECODE Study Group: Glucose tolerance and cardiovascular mortality: Comparison of fasting and 2-hour diagnostic criteria. Arch Intern Med 161:397, 2001.
20. Diabetes Control and Complications Trial Research Group: The effect of intensive treatment of diabetes on the development and progression of long-term complications in insulin dependent diabetes mellitus. N Engl J Med 329:977, 1993.
21. Haffner SM, Stern MP, Mitchell BD, et al: Incidence of type II diabetes in Mexican-Americans predicted by fasting insulin and glucose levels, obesity, and body fat distribution. Diabetes 39:283, 1990.
22. Harris MI, Hadden WC, Knowler WC, Bennett PH: Prevalence of diabetes and impaired glucose tolerance and plasma glucose levels in U.S. population aged 20–74 yr. Diabetes 36:523, 1987.
23. Dorman JS, McCarthy BJ, O'Leary LA, Koehler AN: Risk factors for insulin dependent diabetes. In Harris MI, Cowie CC, Stern MP, et al (eds): Diabetes in America, 2nd ed (NIH Publication No. 95-1468). National Institutes of Health, Washington, DC, 1995, p 165.
24. Gerstein HC: Cow's milk exposure and type I diabetes mellitus: A critical overview of the clinical literature. Diabetes Care 17:13, 1994.
25. Kenny SJ, Aubert RE, Geiss LS: Prevalence and incidence of NIDDM. p 47. In Harris MI, Cowie CC, Stern MP, et al (eds): Diabetes in America, 2nd ed (NIH Publication No. 95-1468). National Institutes of Health, Washington, DC, 1995.
26. Stern MP: Primary prevention of type II diabetes mellitus. Diabetes Care 14:399, 1991.
27. Harris MI, Klein RE, Welborn TA, et al: Onset of NIDDM occurs at least 4–7 years before clinical diagnosis. Diabetes Care 15:815, 1992.
28. Froguel P, Zouali H, Vionnet N, et al: Familial hyperglycemia due to mutations in the glucokinase gene. N Engl J Med 328:697, 1993.
29. Hanis CL, Bjoerwinkle E, Chakraborty R, et al: A genome-wide search for the human non–insulin dependent (type 2) diabetes genes reveals a major susceptibility locus on chromosome 2. Nature Genetics 13: 161, 1996.
30. Bierman EL: Atherogenesis in diabetes. Arteriosclerosis Thrombosis 12:647, 1992.
31. Reaven GM: Banting Lecture 1988: Role of insulin resistance in human disease. Diabetes 37:1595, 1988.
32. Andersson B, Marin P, Lissner L, et al: Testosterone concentrations in women and men with NIDDM. Diabetes Care 17:405, 1994.
33. Berkowitz K, Peters R, Kjos SL, et al: Effect of troglitazone on insulin sensitivity and pancreatic β-cell function in women at high risk for non insulin dependent diabetes mellitus. Diabetes 45:1572, 1996.
34. Dunaif A, Scott D, Finegood D, et al: The insulin sensitizing agent troglitazone improves metabolic and reproductive abnormalities in the polycystic ovary syndrome. J Clin Endocrinol Metab 81:3299, 1996.
35. Karter AJ, Mayer-Davis EJ, Selby JV, et al: Insulin sensitivity and abdominal obesity in African-American, Hispanic, and non-Hispanic white men and women: The insulin resistance and atherosclerosis study. Diabetes 45:1547, 1996.
36. Defronzo RA, Goodman AM, and the Multicenter Metformin Study Group: Efficacy of metformin in patients with NIDDM. N Engl J Med 333:541, 1995.
37. Nolan JJ, Ludvik B, Beerdsen P, et al: Improvement in glucose tolerance and insulin resistance in obese subjects treated with troglitazone. N Engl J Med 331:1188, 1994.
38. Buchanan TA, Coustan DR: Diabetes mellitus. In Burrows GN, Ferris TF (eds): Medical Complications During Pregnancy, 4th ed. WB Saunders, Philadelphia 1994, p 29.
39. Kjos SL, Peters RK, Ziang A, et al: Predicting future diabetes in Latino women with gestational diabetes: Utility of early postpartum glucose tolerance testing. Diabetes 44:586, 1995.
40. Buchanan TA: Pregnancy in pre-existing diabetes. In Harris MI, Cowie CC, Stern MP, et al (eds): Diabetes in America, 2nd ed (NIH Publication No. 95-1468). National Institutes of Health, Washington, DC, 1995, p 719.
41. Kitzmiller JL, Buchanan TA, Kjos S, et al: Pre-conception care of diabetes, congenital malformations, and spontaneous abortions. Diabetes Care 19:514, 1996.
42. Rubin RJ, Altman WM, Mendelson DN: Health care expenditures for people with diabetes mellitus, 1992. J Clin Endocrinol Metab 78: 809A, 1994.
43. Carter JS, Pugh JA, Monterrosa A: Non-insulin dependent diabetes mellitus in minorities in the United States. Ann Intern Med 125: 221, 1996.
44. Flegal KM, Ezzati TM, Harris MI, et al: Prevalence of diabetes in Mexican-Americans, Cubans, and Puerto Ricans for the Hispanic Health and Nutrition Examination Survey, 1982–84. Diabetes Care 14(Suppl 3):628, 1991.
45. Fujimoto WY: Diabetes in Asian and Pacific Island Americans. In Harris MI, Cowie CC, Stern MP, et al (eds): Diabetes in America,

2nd ed (NIH Publication No. 95-1468). National Institutes of Health, Washington, DC, 1995, p 661.
46. Gohdes D: Diabetes in North American Indians and Alaskan natives. In Harris MI, Cowie CC, Stern MP, et al (eds): Diabetes in America, 2nd ed (NIH Publication No. 95-1468). National Institutes of Health, Washington, DC, 1995, p 683.
47. Folsom AR, Kaye SA, Sellers TA, et al: Body fat distribution and 5 year risk of death in older women. JAMA 269:483, 1993.
48. Manson JE, Willett WC, Stampfer MJ, et al: Body weight and mortality among women. N Engl J Med 333:677, 1995.
49. Folsom AR, French SA, Zheng W, et al: Weight variability and mortality: The Iowa women's study. Int J Obesity 20:704, 1996.
50. Cowie CC, Harris MI: Physical and metabolic characteristics of persons with diabetes. In Harris MI, Cowie CC, Stern MP, et al (eds): Diabetes in America, 2nd ed (NIH Publication No. 95-1468). National Institutes of Health, Washington, DC, 1995, p 117.
51. Han TS, van Leer EM, Seidell JC, Lean ME: Waist circumference action levels in the identification of cardiovascular risk factors: Prevalence study in a random sample. BMJ 311:1401, 1995.
52. Pouliot MC, Després J-P, Lemieux S, et al: Waist circumference and abdominal sagittal diameter: Best simple anthropometric indexes of abdominal visceral adipose tissue accumulation and related cardiovascular risk in men and women. Am J Cardiol 73:460, 1994.
53. Weidner MD, Gavigan KE, Tundall GL, et al: Which anthropometric indices of regional adiposity are related to the insulin resistance of aging? Int J Obesity 19:325, 1995.
54. Bengtsson C, Bjorkelund C, Lapidus L, Lissner L: Associations of serum lipid concentrations and obesity with mortality in women: 20 year follow up of participants in prospective population study. BMJ 307:1385, 1993.
55. Kohrt WM, Kirwan JP, Staten MA, et al: Insulin resistance in aging is related to abdominal obesity. Diabetes 42:273, 1993.
56. Tull ES, Roseman JM: Diabetes in African Americans. In Harris MI, Cowie CC, Stern MP, et al (eds): Diabetes in America, 2nd ed (NIH Publication No. 95-1468). National Institutes of Health, Washington, DC, 1995, p 613.
57. Nesto R, Watson F, Kowalchuk G, et al: Silent myocardial ischemia and infarction in diabetics with peripheral vascular disease: Assessment by dipyridamole thallium-201 scintigraphy. Am Heart J 120: 1073, 1990.
58. Langer A, Freeman M, Josse R, et al: Metaiodobenzylguanidine imaging in diabetes mellitus: Assessment of cardiac sympathetic denervation and its relation to autonomic dysfunction and silent myocardial ischemia. J Am Coll Cardiol 25:610, 1995.
59. Scheidt-Nave C, Barret-Connor E, Wingard DL: Resting electrocardiographic abnormalities suggestive of asymptomatic ischemic heart disease associated with NIDDM in a defined population. Circulation 81:899, 1990.
60. Rewers M, Shetterly JM, Baxter J, et al: Prevalence of coronary heart disease in subjects with normal and impaired glucose tolerance and NIDDM in a biethnic Colorado population: The San Luis Valley Diabetes Study. Am J Epidemiol 12:1321, 1992.
61. Fujimoto WY, Leonetti DL, Kinyoun JL, et al: Prevalence of complications among 2nd generation Japanese-American men with diabetes, impaired glucose tolerance and normal glucose tolerance. Diabetes 36:730, 1987.
62. Fujimoto WY, Leonetti DL, Bergstrom RW, et al: Glucose intolerance and diabetic complications among Japanese-American women. Diabetes Res Clin Pract 13:119, 1991.
63. Krolewski AS, Kosinski EJ, Warram JH, et al: Magnitude and determinants of coronary artery disease in juvenile onset IDDM. Am J Cardiol 59:750, 1987.
64. Dorman JS, La Porte RE, Kuller LH, et al: The Pittsburgh IDDM morbidity and mortality study: Mortality results. Diabetes 33:271, 1984.
65. Portuese E, Orchard TJ: Mortality in IDDM. In Harris MI, Cowie CC, Stern MP, et al (eds): Diabetes in America, 2nd ed (NIH Publication No. 95-1468). National Institutes of Health, Washington, DC, 1995, p 221.
66. Lloyd CE, Kuller LH, Ellis D, et al: Coronary artery disease in IDDM: Gender differences in risk factors but not risk. Arterioscler Thromb Vasc Biol 16:720, 1996.
67. Andersson DKG, Svärdsudd K. Long-term glycemic control relates to mortality in type II diabetes. Diabetes Care 18:1534, 1995.
68. Ohkuba Y, Kishikawa H, Araki E, et al: Intensive insulin therapy prevents the progression of diabetic microvascular complications in Japanese patients with NIDDM: A randomized prospective 6 year study. Diabetes Res Clin Pract 28:103, 1995.
69. Jackson CA, Yudkin JS, Forrest RD: A comparison of the relationships of the glucose tolerance test and the glycated haemoglobin assay with diabetic vascular disease in the community: The Islington Diabetes Survey. Diabetes Res Clin Pract 17:111, 1992.
70. Beks PJ, Mackay AJC, de Nelling JND, et al: Peripheral arterial disease in relation to glycaemic level in elderly Caucasian population: The Hoorne Study. Diabetologia 38:86, 1995.
71. Singer DE, Nathan DM, Anderson KM, et al: Association of HbA_{1c} with prevalent cardiovascular disease in the original cohort of the Framingham Heart Study. Diabetes 41:202, 1992.
72. Park S, Barrett-Connor E, Wingard DL, et al: GHb is a better predictor of cardiovascular disease than fasting or postchallenge plasma glucose in women without diabetes: The Rancho Bernardo Study. Diabetes Care 19:450, 1996.
73. Kuusisto J, Mykkanen L, Pyörälä K, Laakso M: NIDDM and its metabolic control predict coronary heart disease in elderly subjects. Diabetes 43:960, 1994.
74. McPhillips JB, Barrett-Connor E, Wingard DL: Cardiovascular disease risk factors prior to the diagnosis of impaired glucose tolerance and non-insulin dependent diabetes. Am J Epidemiol 131:443, 1990.
75. Sobel BE: Potentiation of vasculopathy by insulin: Implications from an NHLBI Clinical Alert. Circulation 93:1613, 1996.
75a. UKPDS: Intensive blood-glucose control with sulfonylureas or insulin compared with conventional treatment and risk of complications in patients with type 2 diabetes (UKPDS 33). Lancet 352:837, 1998.
75b. UKPDS: Effects of intensive blood-glucose control with metformin on complications in overweight patients with type 2 diabetes (UKPDS 34). Lancet 352:854, 1998.
75c. Stratton IM, Adler AI, Neil HAW, et al: Association of glycemia with macrovascular and microvascular complications of type 2 diabetes (UKPDS 35): Prospective observational study. BMJ 321:405, 2000.
75d. UKPDS Group: Glycemic control with diet, sulfonylurea, metformin, or insulin in patients with type 2 diabetes mellitus: Progressive requirement for multiple therapies (UKPDS 49). JAMA 281:2005, 1999.
75e. UKPDS: Tight blood pressure control and risk of macrovascular and microvascular complications in type 2 diabetes (UKPDS 38). BMJ 317:703, 1998.
75f. UKPDS: Efficacy of atenolol and captopril in reducing risk of both macrovascular and microvascular complications in type 2 diabetes (UKPDS 39). BMJ 317:713, 1998.
75g. Adler AI, Stratton IM, Neil HAW, et al: Association of systolic blood pressure with macrovascular and microvascular complications of type 2 diabetes (UKPDS 36): Prospective observational study. BMJ 321: 412, 2000.
76. Reaven GM, Lithell H, Landsberg L: Hypertension and associated metabolic abnormalities—the role of insulin resistance and the sympathoadrenal system. N Engl J Med 334:374, 1996.
77. Chisolm G, Irwin K, Penn M: Lipoprotein oxidation and lipoprotein-induced cell injury in diabetes. Diabetes 41(Suppl 2):61, 1992.
78. Evans RW, Orchard TJ: Oxidized lipids in insulin dependent diabetes mellitus: A sex-diabetes interaction. Metabolism 43:1196, 1994.
79. Modan M, Or J, Karasik A, et al: Hyperinsulinemia, sex, and risk of atherosclerotic cardiovascular disease. Circulation 84:1165, 1991.
80. Feingold KR, Grunfeld C, Pang M, et al: LDL subclass phenotypes and triglyceride metabolism in NIDDM. Arterioscler Thromb 12: 1496, 1992.
81. Selby JV, Austin MA, Newman B, et al: LDL subclass phenotypes and the insulin resistance syndrome in women. Circulation 88:381, 1993.
82. Cowie CC, Howard BV, Harris MI: Serum lipoproteins in African-Americans and whites with NIDDM in the US population. Circulation 90:1185, 1994.
83. Kwaan H: Changes in blood coagulation, platelet function and plasminogen-plasmin system in diabetes. Diabetes 41(Suppl 2):31, 1992.
84. Bruno G, Cavallo-Perin P, Bargero G: Association of fibrinogen with glycemic control and albumin excretion rate in patients with NIDDM. Ann Intern Med 125:653, 1996.
85. Lindahl B, Asplund K, Eliasson M, Evrin PE: Insulin resistance syndrome and fibrinolytic activity: The Northern Sweden Monica study. Int J Epidemiol 25:291, 1996.
86. McGill JB, Schneider DJ, Arfken CL, et al: Factors responsible for impaired fibrinolysis in obese subjects and NIDDM patients. Diabetes 43:104, 1994.
87. Nordt TK, Sawa H, Fujii S, Sobel BE: Induction of plasminogen activator inhibitor type-1 (PAI-1) by proinsulin and insulin in vivo. Circulation 91:764, 1995.

88. Wolffenbuttel BH, Leurs PB, Sels JP, et al: Improved blood glucose control by insulin therapy in type 2 diabetic patients has no effect on lipoprotein(a) levels. Diabet Med 10:427, 1993.
89. Nakata H, Horita K, Eto M: Alteration of lipoprotein(a) concentration with glycemic control in NIDDM without diabetic complications. Metabolism 42:1323, 1993.
90. Clark CM Jr, Lee DA: Prevention and treatment of the complications of diabetes mellitus. N Engl J Med 332:1210, 1995.
91. Davis MD: Diabetic retinopathy. Diabetes Care 15:1844, 1992.
92. Klein R, Klein BEK, Moss SE, et al: The Wisconsin epidemiological study of diabetic retinopathy. III: Prevalence and risk of diabetic retinopathy when age at diagnosis is greater than 30 years. Arch Ophthalmol 102:527, 1984.
93. Klein R, Klein BEK: Vision disorders in diabetes. In Harris MI, Cowie CC, Stern MP, et al (eds): Diabetes in America, 2nd ed (NIH Publication No. 95-1468). National Institutes of Health, Washington, DC, 1995, p 293.
94. Hanis CL, Chu HH, Lawson K, et al: Mortality of Mexican-Americans with NIDDM: Retinopathy and other predictors in Starr County, Texas. Diabetes Care 16:82, 1993.
95. Alzaid AA: Microalbuminuria in patient with NIDDM: An overview. Diabetes Care 19:79, 1996.
96. Borch-Johnsen K, Kreiner S: Proteinuria: Value as predictor of cardiovascular mortality in IDDM. BMJ 294:165, 1987.
97. Klein R, Klein BEK, Moss S: Incidence of gross proteinuria in older-onset diabetes: A population-based perspective. Diabetes 42:381, 1993.
98. Massant JWC, Elliott TG, Hill RD, et al: Prognostic significance of microalbuminuria in IDDM: 23 year follow up. Kidney Int 41: 836, 1992.
99. Mogensen CE: Microalbuminuria predicts clinical proteinuria and early mortality in maturity onset diabetes. N Engl J Med 310:356, 1984.
100. Nelson RG, Pettit DJ, Carraher MJ, et al: Effect of proteinuria on mortality in NIDDM. Diabetes 37:1499, 1988.
101. Nathan DM: Long-term complications of diabetes mellitus. N Engl J Med 328:1676, 1993.
102. Savage S, Estachio RO, Jeffers B, Schrier RW: Urinary albumin excretion as a predictor of diabetic retinopathy, neuropathy, and cardiovascular disease in NIDDM. Diabetes Care 19:1243, 1996.
103. Kuusisto J, Mykkanen L, Pyorala K, et al: Hyperinsulinemic microalbuminuria: A new risk factor for coronary heart disease. Circulation 90:831, 1995.
104. Lewis EJ, Hunsicker LG, Bain RP, et al: The effect of angiotensin-converting enzyme inhibition on diabetic nephropathy. N Engl J Med 329:1456, 1993.
105. Moye L, Pfeffer M, Wun C, et al, for the SAVE Investigators: Uniformity of captopril benefit in the SAVE study: Subgroup analysis. Survival and Ventricular Enlargement Study. Eur Heart J 15(Suppl B): 2, 1994.
106. Stern MP, Haffner SM: Type II diabetes and its complications in Mexican-Americans. Diabetes Metab Rev 6:29, 1990.
107. Abbott RD, Brand FN, Kannel WB: Epidemiology of some peripheral arterial findings in diabetic men and women: Experiences from the Framingham Study. Am J Med 88:376, 1990.
108. McCall AL: The impact of diabetes on the CNS. Diabetes 41:557, 1992.
109. Barret-Conner E, Khaw K-T: Diabetes mellitus: An independent risk factor for stroke? Am J Epidemiol 128:116, 1988.
110. Abbott RD, Donahue RP, MacMahon SW, et al: Diabetes and risk of stroke: The Honolulu Heart Program. JAMA 257:949, 1987.
111. Folsom AR, Eckfeldt JH, Weitzman S, et al: Relation of carotid artery wall thickness to diabetes mellitus, fasting glucose and insulin, body size, and physical activity. Stroke 25:66, 1994.
112. Reiber GE, Boyko EJ, Smith DG: Lower extremity foot ulcers and amputations in diabetes. p. 409. In Harris MI, Cowie CC, Stern MP, et al (eds): Diabetes in America, 2nd ed (NIH Publication No. 95-1468). National Institutes of Health, Washington, DC, 1995.
113. Lehto S, Niskanen L, Suhonen M, et al: Medial artery calcification: A neglected harbinger of cardiovascular complications in NIDDM. Arterioscler Thromb Vasc Biol 16:978, 1996.
114. Welborn TA, Wearne K: Coronary heart disease incidence and cardiovascular mortality in Busselton with reference to insulin and glucose concentration. Diabetes Care 2:154, 1979.
115. Pyörälä K: Relationship of glucose tolerance and plasma insulin to incidence of coronary heart disease. Diabetes Care 2:131, 1979.
116. Ducimetiere P, Eschwege E, Papoz L, et al: Relationship of plasma insulin to the incidence of myocardial infarction and coronary heart disease mortality in a middle aged population. Diabetologia 19:205, 1980.
117. Jensen-Urstad KJ, Reichard PG, Rosfors JS, et al: Early atherosclerosis is retarded by improved long-term blood glucose control in patients with IDDM. Diabetes 45:1253, 1996.
118. Janka HU, Ziegler AG, Standl E, et al: Daily insulin dose as a predictor of macrovascular disease in insulin treated NIDDM. Diabet Metab 13:359, 1987.
119. Genuth S: Exogenous insulin administration and cardiovascular risk in non-insulin dependent and insulin-dependent diabetes mellitus. Ann Intern Med 124(1 Part 2):104, 1996.
120. Malmberg K, Ryden L, Hamsten A, et al: Effects of insulin treatment on cause specific one year mortality and morbidity in diabetic patients with acute myocardial infarction. Eur Heart J 17:1337, 1996.
121. Abraira C, Colwell JA, Nuttall FQ, for the VA CSDM Group: Veterans Affairs Cooperative Study on glycemic control and complications in type II diabetes (VA CSDM). Diabetes Care 18:1113, 1995.
121a. Geiss LS (ed): Diabetes Surveillance, 1997. US Department of Health and Human Services, Atlanta, 1997.
122. Jacoby RM, Nesto RW: Acute myocardial infarction in the diabetic patient: Pathophysiology, clinical course and prognosis. J Am Coll Cardiol 20:736, 1992.
123. Kober L, Torppedersen C, Ottesen M, et al: Influence of gender on short- and long-term mortality after acute myocardial infarction. Am J Cardiol 77:1052, 1996.
124. Mitchell BD, Hazuda HP, Haffner SM, et al: Myocardial infarction in Mexican-Americans and non-Hispanic whites: The San Antonio Heart Study. Circulation 83:45, 1991.
125. Orlander PR, Goff DC, Morrissey M, et al: The relation of diabetes to the severity of acute myocardial infarction and post-myocardial infarction survival in Mexican-Americans and non-Hispanic whites: The Corpus Christi Heart Project. Diabetes 43:897, 1994.
126. Jaffe AS, Spadaro JJ, Schechtman K, et al: Increased congestive heart failure after myocardial infarction of modest extent in patients with diabetes mellitus. Am Heart J 108:31, 1984.
127. Takahashi N, Iwasaka T, Sugiura T, et al: Left ventricular regional function after acute anterior myocardial infarction in diabetic patients. Diabetes Care 12:630, 1989.
128. Stone PH, Muller JE, Hartwell T, et al: The effect of diabetes mellitus on prognosis and serial left ventricular function after acute myocardial infarction: The MILIS study group. J Am Coll Cardiol 14:49, 1989.
129. Baum VC, Levitsky LL, Englander RM: Abnormal cardiac function after exercise in IDDM children and adults. Diabetes Care 10:319, 1987.
130. Raev DC: Which left ventricular function is impaired earlier in the evolution of diabetic cardiomyopathy? An echocardiographic study of young type I diabetic patients. Diabetes Care 17:633, 1994.
131. Taegtmeyer H, Passmore JM: Defective energy metabolism of the heart in diabetes. Lancet 1(8421):139, 1985.
132. Waller B, Palumbo P, Roberts W: Status of the coronary arteries at necropsy in diabetes mellitus with onset after age 30 years. Am J Med 69:498, 1980.
133. Zarich S, Waxman S, Freeman R, et al: Effect of autonomic nervous system dysfunction on the circadian pattern of myocardial ischemia in diabetes mellitus. J Am Coll Cardiol 24:968, 1994.
134. Lehtinen JM, Niskanen L, Hyvonen K, et al: Nerve function and its determinants in patients with newly diagnosed type II diabetes mellitus and in control subjects: A 5-year follow-up. Diabetologia 36: 68, 1993.
135. Zola B, Kahn JK, Juni JE, Vinik AI: Abnormal cardiac function in diabetic patients with autonomic neuropathy in the absence of ischemic heart disease. J Clin Endocrinol Metab 63:208, 1986.
136. Herholz H, Goff DC, Ramsey DJ, et al: Women and Mexican-Americans receive fewer cardiovascular drugs following myocardial infarction than men and non-Hispanic whites: The Corpus Christi Heart Project, 1988–1990. J Clin Epidemiol 49:279, 1996.
137. Gunderson T, Kjekshus J: Timolol treatment after myocardial infarction in diabetic patients. Diabetes Care 6:285, 1983.
138. Malmberg K, Herliz J, Hjalmarson A, et al: Effects of metoprolol on mortality and late infarction in diabetics with suspected acute myocardial infarction: Retrospective data from two large studies. Eur Heart J 10:423, 1989.

139. Barrett-Connor E: Intervention in patients with diabetes mellitus: Will it prevent heart disease. In Higgins MW, Luepker RV (eds): Trends in Coronary Heart Disease Mortality. Oxford University Press, New York, 1988, p 119.
140. Koskinen P, Mänttäri M, Manninen V, et al: Coronary heart disease incidence in NIDDM patients in the Helsinki Heart Study. Diabetes Care 15:820, 1982.
141. Scandinavian Simvastatin Survival Study Group: Randomized trial of cholesterol lowering in 4444 patients with coronary heart disease: The Scandinavian Simvastatin Survival Study (4S). Lancet 344:1383, 1994.
142. ETDRS Investigators: Aspirin effects on mortality and morbidity in diabetes mellitus: Early Treatment Diabetic Retinopathy Study. JAMA 268:1292, 1992.
143. Bypass Angioplasty Revascularization Investigation (BARI) Investigators: Comparison of coronary bypass surgery with angioplasty in patients with multivessel disease. N Engl J Med 335:217, 1996.
144. Stein B, Weintraub W, Gebhart SP: Influence of diabetes mellitus on early and late outcome after percutaneous transluminal coronary angioplasty. Circulation 91:979, 1995.
145. Carrozza J, Kuntz R, Fishman R, et al: Restenosis after arterial injury caused by coronary stenting in patients with diabetes mellitus. Ann Intern Med 118:344, 1993.
146. Weaver WD, White HD, Wilcox RG, et al: Comparisons of characteristics and outcomes among women and men with acute myocardial infarction treated with thrombolytic therapy. JAMA 275:777, 1996.
147. Zuanetti G, Latini R, Maggioni A, et al, on behalf of the GISSI-2 Investigators: Influence of diabetes on mortality in acute myocardial infarction: Data from the GISSI-2 study. J Am Coll Cardiol 22: 1788, 1993.
148. Granger C, Califf R, Young S, et al: Outcome of patients with diabetes mellitus and acute myocardial infarction treated with thrombolytic agents. J Am Coll Cardiol 21:920, 1993.
149. Risum O, Abdelnoor M, Svennevig JL, et al: Diabetes mellitus and morbidity and mortality risks after coronary artery bypass surgery. Scand J Thorac Cardiovasc Surg 30:71, 1996.

| 5.4 | Role of Hormone Replacement in Coronary Artery Disease

H. Vernon Anderson

Atherosclerotic cardiovascular disease is rare in women before menopause, when estrogen levels are higher, but after menopause, when estrogen levels fall, the incidence of atherosclerotic disease is equal to or greater than that in men. This linkage between atherosclerotic disease and estrogen levels is reinforced by the observation that women who undergo surgical or chemical oophorectomy early in life have an accelerated rate of atherosclerosis. The cardiovascular benefits of estrogens may be partially or even completely preserved after menopause by exogenous hormone replacement (HRT), which refers to the use of estrogens with or without the concomitant use of progestins. However, many issues of HRT are controversial and unresolved. Results of completed large clinical trials are under scrutiny, and those of several other ongoing clinical trials are anticipated within the next few years.

MECHANISMS

Estrogens (of which there are several) have a variety of actions on the cardiovascular system. Some of these actions are opposed to some extent by progestins. Probably the best-established mechanism of estrogen's effect on cardiovascular disease involves alterations in lipid profiles. These alterations reflect the biologic actions of estrogens on lipid metabolism in the liver. The plasma levels of total cholesterol, low-density lipoprotein (LDL), and lipoprotein(a) [Lp(a)] are lower before menopause than after; in contrast, the levels of high-density lipoprotein (HDL) are higher before menopause. Thus, after menopause, total cholesterol, LDL, and Lp(a) increase and HDL decreases.[1, 2] Experimental and clinical studies directly link these lipid changes with atherogenesis.

Exogenous estrogens can reestablish the lower-risk lipid pattern seen before menopause.[3, 4] However, progestins, which can attenuate some of the lipid changes caused by estrogens, may interfere with some of the protective benefits of estrogen therapy. Progestins are commonly used either cyclically or consecutively with estrogen to prevent estrogen's unopposed stimulation of uterine and breast tissues, which can induce hyperplasia and potentially lead to tumor development.

THE POSTMENOPAUSAL ESTROGEN/ PROGESTIN INTERVENTIONS TRIAL

In the Postmenopausal Estrogen/Progestin Interventions Trial (PEPI),[5] the largest and latest trial, 875 women aged 45 to 64 years were randomly assigned to one of five treatment groups: placebo, conjugated equine estrogens (CEE), CEE plus cyclic medroxyprogesterone acetate (MPA), CEE plus consecutive MPA, and CEE plus cyclic micronized progesterone (MP). The PEPI investigators monitored blood pressure and levels of total cholesterol, HDL, LDL, triglyceride, serum insulin, and fibrinogen over 3 years. They reported that systolic and diastolic blood pressure and serum levels of insulin did not change significantly over the 3-year period and did not vary with treatment assignment.

Fibrinogen levels rose slightly in women assigned to the placebo group and diminished slightly in women receiving any of the active treatments (0.10 g/L versus 0.06 g/L, respectively; $p < .001$). Fibrinogen levels decreased similarly among the five active treatment groups. Total cholesterol decreased by approximately 2% in women in the placebo group, by 4% in women in the CEE and CEE plus MP groups, and by 6% in women in the CEE plus consecutive and CEE plus cyclic MPA groups (Fig. 5–15). Furthermore, LDL levels decreased and HDL levels increased in most treatment groups.

These sorts of changes in lipid levels have been associated with reductions both in atherosclerosis and in cardiovascular events. For example, in a carefully performed study, Waters and colleagues[6] randomly assigned 62 women with diffuse but not severe coronary disease to treatment with lovastatin (an HMG CoA reductase inhibitor that lowers cholesterol) or placebo. After 2 years, the women receiving active treatment showed less progression of coronary disease and fewer new lesions as seen on quantitative coronary arteriography than the placebo-treated patients. Unfortunately, small studies such as this one are not powerful enough to detect significant changes in clinical event rates. However, the large clinical trials of lipid-lowering agents have demonstrated conclusively that reductions in cholesterol lower the rate of clinical events.[7,8]

OTHER VASCULAR EFFECTS

In addition to its effects on lipid profiles, HRT has other potentially beneficial vascular effects. Estrogens have systemic and coronary arterial vasodilator activities. These activities may be mediated by endothelium-dependent mechanisms, such as via nitric oxide, suggesting that estrogen may directly affect endothelial cell function; however, the exact mechanisms for these effects are unknown. Some experimental evidence suggests that calcium channel blockade may be one mechanism for estrogen-induced vasodilation. Estrogens also have antioxidant properties. Furthermore, they alter the circadian variation in the fibrinolytic factors PAI-1 and tPA.[9]

CLINICAL EVIDENCE

More than 30 clinical trials have shown the benefits of HRT after menopause.[10] In a comprehensive meta-analysis, the

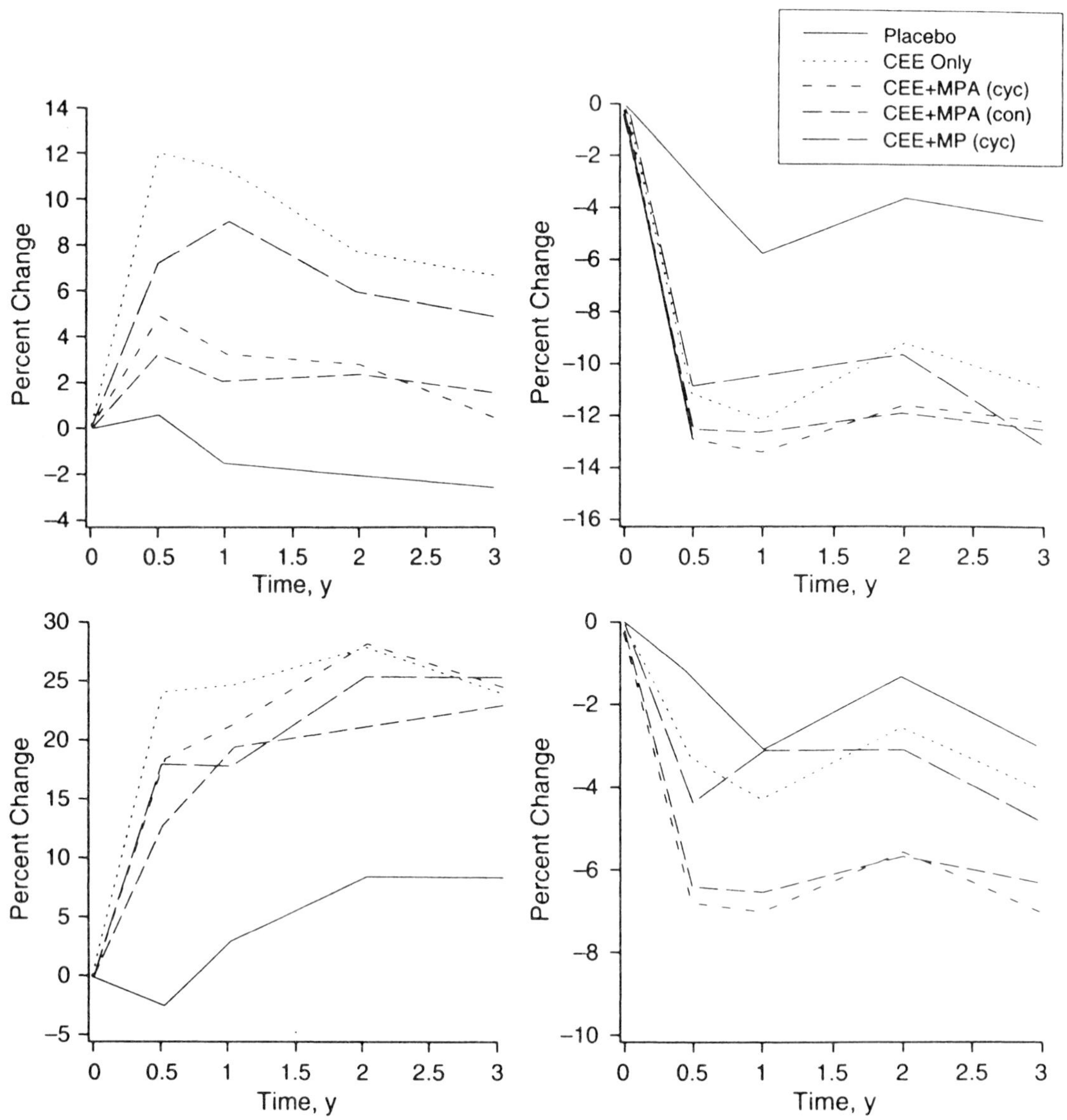

FIGURE 5–15. Lipid changes according to randomized assignment of therapy in the PEPI trial. The four graphs illustrate mean percent change from baseline for HDL *(top left panel)*, LDL *(top right panel)*, triglycerides *(bottom left panel)*, and total cholesterol *(bottom right panel)*. (From The Writing Group for the PEPI Trial: Effects of estrogen or estrogen/progestin regimens on heart disease risk factors in postmenopausal women. JAMA 273:199, 1995.)

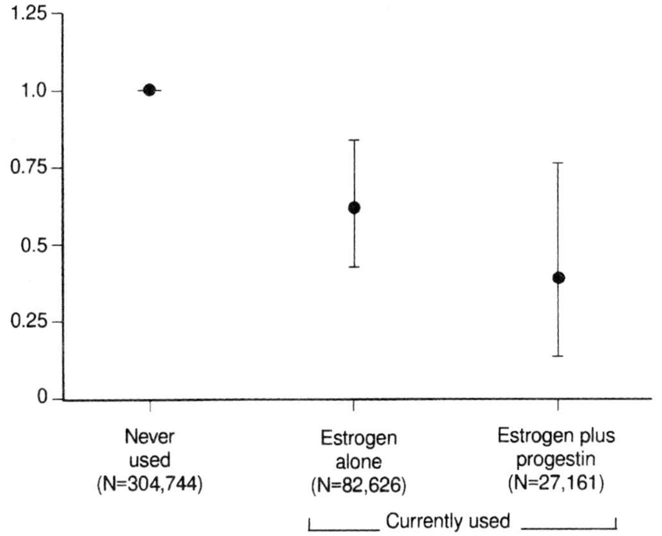

FIGURE 5–16. Relative risks of developing cardiovascular disease according to hormone use for women in the Nurses' Health Study. (From Grodstein F, Stampfer MJ, Manson JE, et al: Postmenopausal estrogen and progestin use and the risk of cardiovascular disease. N Engl J Med 335:453, 1996. Copyright © 1996 Massachusetts Medical Society. All rights reserved.)[11]

relative risk for developing cardiovascular events in women who use HRT after menopause is about 50% of that in women who do not use HRT. For example, in the Nurses' Health Study, more than 59,000 women between the ages of 30 and 55 years, none of whom had evidence of cardiovascular disease at entry, were followed for up to 16 years.[11] After adjustment for age and risk factors, the women who used only estrogens had a relative risk of 0.6 (95% CI, 0.43–0.83) (Fig. 5–16) for development of significant CAD. Women who used estrogen plus progestin had a relative risk of 0.39 (0.19 to 0.78). Former users who had stopped taking HRT had a relative risk of eventual cardiovascular mortality that was intermediate, at 0.85 (0.72 to 1.01) compared with women who had never used HRT. Moreover, this risk clearly increased as the interval since last hormone use lengthened. These results support those of a prior observational population study in which the relative risk of MI in women who used combined estrogen plus progesterone was 0.68.[12]

RISKS

Estrogens can have a number of deleterious effects. One significant effect is stimulation of hyperplasia in breast and uterine tissues, which may lead to cancer in these organs. In addition, estrogen use increases the risk of thrombosis, especially peripheral deep venous thrombosis or pulmonary embolism. This risk is further increased in women who smoke.[10]

The hyperplasia and prothrombotic effects of estrogens are dose-related; during the 1970s and 1980s, recommended doses were reduced because of these associated risks. The current recommended dose of estrogen, 0.625 mg/day of conjugated equine estrogens, reduces LDL levels to the same extent as the former, higher dose of 1.25 mg/day, but without producing the same degree of hyperplasia and risk of thrombosis. The lower dose of estrogen appears to confer as much protection from coronary disease as the higher dose.

Nevertheless, the question remains whether or not the additional risk of breast or uterine cancer is outweighed by the benefit of reducing deaths from CHD. The PEPI trial reported on this question. Adenomatous or atypical uterine hyperplasia developed in 34% of women using estrogen alone and in only 1% of women using estrogen plus progesterone. In women who had not undergone hysterectomy, 36% of those using estrogen alone stopped HRT, whereas 11% to 15% of women using estrogen plus progesterone and only 8% of those using placebo stopped HRT. Of the 875 women in the PEPI trial, breast cancer developed in eight and uterine cancer in two during the 3 years of follow-up. No relationship to treatment assignment was shown for these small numbers of cancer cases. Importantly, hysterectomy was associated with the use of estrogen alone without progesterone ($p = .04$).

CONCLUSIONS

A balance between a decreased risk of coronary disease and an increased risk of breast or uterine cancers is not easy to achieve. For women who do not otherwise have a higher risk of breast or uterine cancer, which includes most postmenopausal women, HRT may be beneficial in increasing life expectancy and diminishing coronary events. In contrast, if a woman *does* have an increased risk of breast or uterine cancer, the potential benefit of HRT is less clear. In most patients, the level of cardiovascular protection provided by HRT outweighs the risks of malignancies.[13] However, each patient should be individually assessed as a candidate for HRT. For those women who are not candidates for HRT, aggressive lowering of cholesterol should be considered as an alternative cardiovascular preventive strategy.[14] More information will become available as additional clinical trials are completed. For the present, HRT should be considered in all postmenopausal women who do not have contraindications for this therapy.

References

1. Akahoshi M, Soda M, Nakashima E, et al: Effects of menopause on trends of serum cholesterol, blood pressure, and body mass index. Circulation 94:61, 1996.
2. Posner BM, Cupples LA, Miller DR, et al: Diet, menopause, and serum cholesterol levels in women: The Framingham study. Am Heart J 125:483, 1993.
3. Nabulsi AA, Folsom AR, White A, et al: Association of hormone replacement therapy with various cardiovascular risk factors in postmenopausal women. N Engl J Med 328:1069, 1993.
4. Haines C, Chung T, Chang A, et al: Effect of oral estradiol on Lp(a) and other lipoproteins in postmenopausal women: A randomized, double-blind, placebo-controlled study. Arch Intern Med 156:866, 1996.
5. The Writing Group for the PEPI trial: Effects of estrogen or estrogen/progestin regimens on heart disease risk factors in postmenopausal women. JAMA 273:199, 1995.
6. Waters D, Higginson L, Gladstone P, et al: Effects of cholesterol lowering on the progression of coronary atherosclerosis in women: A Canadian Coronary Atherosclerosis Intervention Trial (CCAIT) Substudy. Circulation 92:2404, 1995.
7. Gotto AM: Lipid lowering, regression, and coronary events: A review of the Interdisciplinary Council on Lipids and Cardiovascular Risk Intervention, Seventh Council Meeting. Circulation 92:646, 1995.

8. Scandinavian Simvastatin Survival Study Group: Randomised trial of cholesterol lowering in 4444 patients with coronary heart disease: The Scandinavian Simvastatin Survival Study (4S). Lancet 344:1383, 1994.
9. Katz RJ, Hsia J, Walker P, et al: Effects of hormone replacement therapy on the circadian pattern of atherothrombotic risk factors. Am J Cardiol 78:876, 1996.
10. Grodstein F, Stampfer M: The epidemiology of coronary heart disease and estrogen replacement in postmenopausal women. Prog Cardiovascular Dis 38:199, 1995.
11. Grodstein F, Stampfer MJ, Manson JE, et al: Postmenopausal estrogen and progestin use and the risk of cardiovascular disease. N Engl J Med 335:453, 1996.
12. Psaty BM, Heckbert SR, Atkins D, et al: The risk of myocardial infarction associated with the combined use of estrogens and progestins in postmenopausal women. Arch Intern Med 154:1333, 1994.
13. Col NF, Eckman MH, Karas RH, et al: Patient-specific decisions about hormone replacement therapy in postmenopausal women. JAMA 277: 1140, 1997.
14. Guetta V, Cannon RO 3rd: Cardiovascular effects of estrogen and lipid-lowering therapies in postmenopausal women. Circulation 93:1928, 1996.

5.5 The Role of Oral Contraceptives

Janice L. B. Byrne

The availability of oral steroid contraceptives in 1960 revolutionized birth control options for women in both industrialized and developing nations. With control of fertility comes opportunity. In industrialized nations, the planning for and limitation of family size enable women to pursue career options both within and outside the home and liberate many single parents from a never-ending cycle of poverty. In developing nations, regulation of fertility has a significant impact on maternal and infant morbidity and mortality. Currently, about three quarters of the world's population lives in developing nations, accounting for 85% of all births, 95% of all infant and childhood deaths, and 99% of all maternal mortality. A woman who becomes pregnant in a developing country has a chance of dying from obstetrical complications 200-fold that of a pregnant woman in an industrialized country.[1] The additional burden of restrictive abortion laws and a lack of safe abortions further increase risks to women living in areas without access to effective and safe contraception. Indeed, even in industrialized countries, among women aged 15 to 44 years, rates of death from all causes are consistently higher in pregnant women than in women who use oral contraceptives. Even among smokers who use oral contraceptives, death rates are lower than for pregnant women up to age 40 years.[2]

Throughout the world, nearly half of all married women of reproductive age use some form of fertility regulation. Lactational suppression of ovulation may be partially effective as a contraceptive, particularly in calorie-deprived women, but women in most developing countries rely heavily on female sterilization or an intrauterine device (IUD) for contraception. In industrialized nations, women are more likely to use barrier methods (condoms, diaphragm) or oral contraceptives, although sterilization is overall the most common method of birth control for married couples. Worldwide, approximately 15% of the 400 million women of reproductive age use oral contraceptives. Of this 15%, half live in the United States, Brazil, Germany, and France.[3]

As a society becomes more affluent, fertility rates decline. This stems in part from the trend toward delayed marriages and childbirth and in part from voluntary limitation of family size. As women enter the work force in greater numbers and remain in active careers for longer periods prior to starting families, there is a need for more effective, reversible contraception. The aging post–World War II "baby boomer" generation has seen an increase in births of babies to women through their late 40s. In some cases, with the availability of assisted reproductive technologies, even postmenopausal women have achieved successful pregnancies. This trend toward delayed childbirth has resulted in the use of contraception for longer periods and until later in life than seen previously. Especially for the mature woman, the choice of appropriate contraception as well as the decision whether to attempt pregnancy should involve a comprehensive review of a woman's overall medical health and risk factors for disease, including cardiovascular disease.

TRENDS IN THE UNITED STATES

By 1965, approximately 24% of married U.S. women using birth control used oral steroid contraceptives. (When birth control pills were first marketed, single women could not legally purchase them in many states; thus, the reference to "married women" in most early reports of their use.) By 1970, the use of oral contraceptives had increased to 36% of married women using birth control by 1970 and had plateaued at 20% of all childbearing women by 1976.[4, 5] In 1975, reports in the medical literature of a link between oral contraceptive use and fatal myocardial infarction (MI) and stroke led to widespread panic among consumers and physicians alike, and use of prescribed oral contraceptives dropped dramatically.[6, 7] In the same year, reports of a higher incidence of endometrial cancer in postmenopausal women taking high doses of unopposed estrogen caused a concern about the potential carcinogenic risk of estrogen.

In the early 1980s, only about 20% of married women using contraception (12% of all women of childbearing age) were using oral steroid contraceptives.[4] By 1995, 26% of U.S. married women aged 15 to 50 years who were in need of contraception used oral steroid contraceptives; 24% had undergone some form of permanent sterilization. Overall, 80% of women in the United States use oral steroid contraceptives at some time in their reproductive lives. During a woman's years of maximal fertility, oral contraceptives are the most common method of birth control, with use peaking at age 20 to 24 years. By age 35 to 44 years, more than half of all women or their husbands are surgically sterile, for either contraceptive or medical reasons.[8, 9]

The tremendous need for reliable contraception and the sheer magnitude of use of birth control pills have resulted in extensive research into their safety and efficacy. Despite these efforts, questions about rare but serious events often raise doubts and obscure more rational and practical concerns. Thus, women who might otherwise benefit from the use of oral contraceptives instead find themselves at risk for an unintended pregnancy.

DEVELOPMENT OF THE ORAL STEROID CONTRACEPTIVE

Estradiol is the most potent naturally occurring estrogen and the major estrogen secreted by the ovary. The 1938 discovery that the addition of an ethinyl group at position 17 created an orally active form of the sex steroid paved the way for the development of oral steroid contraceptives.[8] Ethinyl estradiol, a very potent oral estrogen, is one of the two forms of estrogen contained in every birth control pill. Mestranol is found only in the older, higher-dose pills (>50 μg). Metabolism of ethinyl estradiol varies from individual to individual and even within an individual over time. It is the estrogen content of the birth control pill that has major clinical importance. Thrombosis, one of the most serious potential side effects of oral steroid contraceptives, is directly related to estrogen dose. Thrombosis is of particular concern in women with personal or family histories of clotting disorders; an important risk factor for thrombosis during pregnancy or during oral contraceptive use is activated protein C resistance caused by factor V Leiden mutations.[10]

Ethisterone, an orally active derivative of testosterone, also became available in the 1930s. It was not until the 1950s, however, that the removal of the 19 carbon from ethisterone changed its major hormonal effect from that of an androgen compound to that of a progestational agent, norethindrone. These compounds, the 19-nortestosterones, retained some androgenic properties, although their major effect was progestational. Minimal estrogenic activity was associated with the earlier (higher) doses of these compounds at the time of initial development. As with the estrogen component of steroid contraceptives, serious side effects have been associated with the higher doses of the progestins used in old formulations rather than with the particular progestin itself. Currently, the estrogen content in all oral contraceptives in routine usage is limited to the lower dose (average 30–35 μg of ethinyl estradiol).

MECHANISM OF ACTION OF ORAL STEROID CONTRACEPTIVES

The first oral contraceptive pills on the U.S. market contained significantly higher doses of hormones than today's pills: 150 μg of estrogen and as much as 10 mg of progestin. Today, the two major categories of oral contraceptives are the combination oral steroid contraceptives and the progestin-only "minipills." Combination oral contraceptives contain both a synthetic estrogen (ethinyl estradiol) and a synthetic progestational agent of the female hormone progesterone (progestogen or progestin). The progestin-only minipill contains small amounts of progestogens without estrogen.

The so-called first-generation combination oral contraceptives contained 50 μg or more of estrogen plus a progestogen, whereas second-generation pills (less than 50 μg) incorporated a new progestational agent, levonorgestrel. Subsequently, third-generation pills containing newer progestogens—desogestrel, gestodene, and norgestimate—have been introduced. Combination oral contraceptives are administered daily for 21 days of a 28-day cycle. The last 7 days are the period of withdrawal bleeding known as menstruation.

The primary mechanism of action of combination oral contraceptives is to inhibit the midcycle gonadotropin surge[8] by directly affecting the pituitary, thus interfering with the release of gonadotropin-releasing hormone. The combination pill also affects the hypothalamus, decreasing the release of luteinizing hormone (LH) and follicle-stimulating hormone (FSH) and thus preventing ovulation. Other effects are a thickening of the cervical mucus (making sperm penetration more difficult), an alteration of the motility of the uterus and fallopian tubes (impairing transport of the egg and the sperm), and a reduction in the glycogen production of the endometrium (thereby decreasing energy availability for blastocyst survival). There may also be some alteration in ovarian responsiveness to gonadotropin stimulation.

Pills containing a progestogen only do not consistently inhibit ovulation and are associated with a high incidence of irregular bleeding or "breakthrough bleeding" episodes. The addition of the estrogen component in combination birth control pills helps to stabilize the endometrium, preventing irregular or breakthrough bleeding during a cycle. The estrogen in combination pills can also potentiate the action of the progestational agent, thus enabling a consistent reduction in the dosage of progestational agents in combination pills. The progestin in a combination pill induces the decidual reaction within the endometrium to inhibit egg implantation, increases the thickness of cervical mucus to resist sperm penetration, and decreases motility within the fallopian tubes.

Typical use of combination oral contraceptives results in approximately a 3% failure rate during the first year of use. However, highly motivated women who use the pill correctly could expect a failure rate as low as 0.1%.[3] The efficacy is significantly decreased in the progestin-only minipill.

NONCONTRACEPTIVE ACTIONS OF ORAL CONTRACEPTIVES

Although protection from pregnancy and regulation of fertility are the most obvious benefits of the appropriate use of oral steroid contraceptives, many noncontraceptive benefits can be major factors in the decision to use oral contraceptives. There is a clear association between a reduced risk of endometrial and ovarian cancers and the use of oral contraceptives. With respect to endometrial cancer, the rate of development is 50% less in women who have ever used combination pills. This protection increases with duration of use and persists for 10 or more years following discontinuation of use.[11]

Epithelial ovarian cancer is perhaps the most lethal of gynecologic cancers because of its characteristic late presentation at the time of diagnosis. It is known that pregnancy and lactation are associated with a lower risk of ovarian cancer, suggesting that suppression of ovulation may be the mechanism behind this protection. The Cancer and Steroid Hormone (CASH) study conducted by the Centers for Disease Control and Prevention (CDC) and the National Institutes of Health (NIH) demonstrated that oral contraceptive users reduce their risk for ovarian cancer by 40% compared with nonusers. As with endometrial cancer, the protective effect appears to last for 10 or more years after discontinuation of oral contraceptive use and increases with duration of use.[12]

The effect on cervical cancer, however, is less clear, and some studies have suggested a possible higher risk for cervical cancer with oral contraceptive use. Possible explanations include greater sexual activity in younger pill users, increased exposure to larger numbers of sexual partners, and sexual experiences at an earlier age, all of which are known risk factors for cervical cancer. Another potential explanation is that women who seek birth control prescriptions from their physicians have Papanicolaou smears more frequently and thus also have higher rates of (and earlier) detection of cervical cancer.[13]

Although oral contraceptives alone do not protect against sexually transmitted disease, they offer some protective influence on the upper genital tract against pelvic inflammatory disease. Perhaps this influence is due to a thick, viscid mucus within the cervix that decreases the transmission of bacteria to the upper tract. Menstrual regulation, including treatment of dysmenorrhea and irregular heavy bleeding with resultant anemia in chronic anovulatory cycles, is also treated with oral contraceptive therapy. Hyperandrogenic disorders are associated with increased insulin resistance and metabolic abnormalities related to cardiovascular disease risks. The hirsutism and chronic anovulatory bleeding in women with these disorders is often managed by oral contraceptive therapy, with either neutral or beneficial effects on their metabolic profiles.[14] Although not a primary treatment for acne, estrogen-dominant pill formulations also improve blemish-prone individuals with hyperandrogen conditions as well. Furthermore, as women approach the perimenopausal years, oral contraceptive therapy may reduce the incidence of anovulatory cycles and the resultant unpredictable cycle length and bleeding patterns that may appear. Finally, nonsmokers older than 35 years may frequently be treated with oral contraceptives until ovarian failure ensues, at which time HRT may be substituted.[15, 16]

THE PERIMENOPAUSAL YEARS

The highest birth rate ever recorded in the United States occurred within the 20-year period following World War II. Women of that generation are now in the midst of their own childbearing years, with the oldest women of this group now approaching menopause. Today, most women can expect to live approximately one third of their lives after menopause, a fact that has tremendous health consequences for the future.[17]

The perimenopause phase is characterized by declining ovarian function directly related to falling hormone levels. Symptoms resulting from the diminished hormone levels include menstrual irregularities, vasomotor symptoms (hot flushing, drenching sweats, sleep disruption), vaginal atrophy, infertility, decreased bone mass, and higher risk for heart disease. Women who experience premature menopause and who do not receive HRT are also at a known higher risk for coronary heart disease (CHD). Furthermore, as women age, many experience higher incidences of chronic medical conditions such as hypertension and glucose intolerance, which are also risk factors for heart disease.

As long as ovulation (however irregular) continues in the perimenopausal period, pregnancy may still occur, and thus, effective contraception is needed. Low-dose oral contraceptives can prevent pregnancy and treat many of the symptoms associated with declining ovarian function in the perimenopausal years. Careful assessment of other risk factors should take place prior to use of any medical therapy, including oral contraceptives; smoking in particular should be strongly discouraged in perimenopausal women.

CARDIOVASCULAR DISEASE

CHD continues to be the leading cause of death in the United States, and it is now the most common cause of death in both women and men. It is generally accepted that CHD is a multifactorial disease and that the relative contribution of each risk factor varies among studies and populations. Epidemiologically, the major coronary risk factors are cholesterol, smoking, diabetes, and hypertension. The physician-patient relationship established during the course of routine medical care offers invaluable opportunities to educate the patient regarding a healthy lifestyle. Information about smoking cessation, exercise, dietary modification, and stress reduction can be incorporated into routine visits and can have significant impact on reducing the risk of CHD in women using oral steroid contraceptives.[18–21] Active intervention may also identify women for whom other choices of contraception may be more appropriate and may affect long-term health risks. CHD, although rare in women of reproductive age, may become a more common concern owing to the present trend toward pregnancy and childbirth in the later reproductive years.

Considerable evidence supports the hypothesis that ovarian hormones suppress the development of atherosclerosis and CHD in women. Indeed, women who have premature ovarian failure from either a surgical or medical cause are at risk for earlier CHD (similar to the incidence in men) if they do not receive HRT. Although atherosclerosis is a major cause of progressive CHD and MI, other less common causes—coronary artery spasm, connective tissue diseases, coronary artery dissection, small vessel coronary disease, emboli, hypertrophic cardiomyopathy, hemoglobin abnormalities, homocystinuria, thrombocytosis, and metabolic abnormalities—are proportionately more prevalent in younger women. Cigarette smoking has also been identified as a major risk factor in the pathogenesis of CHD; the amount and duration of cigarette smoking progressively elevate the risk. Diabetes and hypertension are also independent risk factors.

Although there is no consistent interpretation regarding the mechanism by which estrogen appears to protect from cardiovascular disease, considerable experimental data support this hypothesis. The finding of estrogen receptors in the arterial wall presents perhaps the strongest evidence for a direct estrogen effect on the vascular tree.[22] Estrogen-mediated vasodilatation may be especially important in atherosclerotic vessels. Estrogen inhibits the formation of atherosclerotic plaques, primarily via reduction of plasma cholesterol levels, and it also has antioxidant and lipophilic properties.

Cynomolgus macaque monkeys have been used extensively for research in CHD because of the similarity to humans of their lipoprotein profiles and relative protection from premenopausal CHD accompanied by a postmenopausal acceleration of disease. This same monkey model also illustrates many of the estrogen deficiency disorders commonly seen in humans and thus makes a good model for studying perimenopausal and postmenopausal states. If estrogen is truly cardioprotective because it inhibits the progression of atherogenesis and all of its sequelae, the extent of disease at the onset of estrogen deficiency may be a primary determinant of the risk for the progression of disease and the associated clinical sequelae (e.g., MI). An interesting phenomenon in the macaque monkey model is the exacerbation of coronary artery atherosclerosis due to ovarian dysfunction caused by chronic social stress.[23, 24] Also of interest, monkeys that were clinically estradiol deficient and that were treated with exogenous estrogen via oral contraceptives had less iliac artery atherosclerosis than untreated animals. The implications for humans is that premenopausal normalization of ovarian function or estradiol levels or both could perhaps suppress early onset or progression of atherogenesis, which in the postmenopausal estrogen-deficient state would be more apt to become clinically significant.[24]

The risks and benefits of using any prescribed medication must always be balanced against the risks and benefits of not using it. For example, women with a history of cardiac disease (including CHD) or renal disease are at high risk for fatal complications during pregnancy. Women with these conditions should be strongly counseled about avoiding pregnancy, either by voluntary surgical sterilization or a reliable progestin-only method such as implants or injectable progestins. If these methods are not acceptable, the risks associated with low-dose combination oral contraceptive pills are almost certainly lower than the risks associated with pregnancy.

Oral steroid contraceptives are some of the most widely prescribed and extensively studied medications on the market today, yet few medications are surrounded by such a level of emotional controversy about their prescribed use. The first-generation oral contraceptives, containing an average of 80–100 μg of estrogen combined with a progestogen, were linked to an increased risk for venous thromboembolism (including deep venous thrombosis and pulmonary embolism), stroke, and MI, largely on the basis of studies conducted in the United States and the United Kingdom in the 1960s and 1970s.[6, 7] These risks were associated with current use of the pills and declined to baseline population risks within a month of cessation of their use, implying an acute process such as thrombosis as the cause. A higher risk for stroke and MI was largely confined to smokers and women older than 35 years. In addition to the association of clotting abnormalities, adverse effects on carbohydrate and lipid metabolism seen with the first-generation pills continued to raise concerns about the potential for the pill's contribution to atherosclerosis. This effect was primarily limited to those pill combinations containing progestogens derived from 19-nortestosterone (ethisterone) and was not seen with progestogens derived from progesterone.

Primarily out of concern for the dose-related side effect profile of estrogen, combination contraceptives were developed with progressively decreasing amounts of estrogen. Today, all formulations of birth control pills in routine use contain less than 50 μg of estrogen, with some containing as little as 20 μg of estrogen. Similarly, in an attempt to decrease progestogen-related side effects, amounts of progestins were decreased by 10-fold in the newer preparations. The second-generation contraceptives, containing less than 50 μg of estrogen combined with levonorgestrel, were found to be as efficacious as the first-generation pills in preventing pregnancy, but with a fraction of the pill-related side effects. Likewise, the concern over the risks of venous thrombosis–related events was also reduced. The third-generation oral contraceptives containing the "new" progestogens (desogestrel, gestodene, and norgestimate) were hailed as a breakthrough in the safety and efficacy of combined oral contraceptives. Extensive study showed that these new progestins caused minimal perturbation of the lipid and carbohydrate metabolism compared with previous pills.[25, 26]

Upon their release in the United States in the early 1990s, third-generation oral contraceptives were highly prescribed, especially among women at high risk for carbohydrate intolerance and lipid disorders. However, in late 1995, a report issued by the British Committee on Safety of Medicines warned about then-unpublished epidemiologic data regarding a greatly increased risk for venous thromboembolism among users of the contraceptives that contained desogestrel and gestodene.[27, 28] Factor V Leiden mutation was an especially high risk.[29] A widespread "pill" scare ensued, not unlike the scare following the warnings regarding MI with first-generation pills, and a concomitant increase in unintended pregnancy and abortion resulted, especially in the United Kingdom. Following publication of these studies, Planned Parenthood Federation of America has maintained a formal recommendation that third-generation oral contraceptives be prescribed only to women who do not tolerate other formulations. There are several potential explanations for the increased risk for venous thromboembolism seen in these studies, including the practice of prescribing the "newer, safer" pills to women at higher risk.[30]

The WHO's collaborative study, a multinational case-control study of premenopausal women of reproductive age conducted from 1989 to 1993, evaluated 2998 women with first episodes of idiopathic venous thromboembolism. The relative risk (RR) estimate for oral contraceptive users compared with nonusers was increased fourfold in Europe. Comparison of users of third- and second-generation oral contraceptives with nonusers shows the RR estimate to be significantly elevated in third-generation users (RR, 3.1). For third-generation versus second-generation use, the RR estimate was 2.2.[31]

Concerning MI, the numbers obviously are low in premenopausal, reproductive-age women. The Transnational study examined 153 women after their first MI.[32] After controlling for factors such as duration of oral contraceptive use and smoking, the researchers found that the RR estimate for current users of third-generation oral contraceptives (containing desogestrel or gestodene) compared with nonusers was close to 1. For users of second-generation oral contraceptives compared with nonusers, the RR was significantly elevated to 3.1. This study was the basis for many claims of the greater safety of third-generation oral contraceptives.

The WHO collaborative study also examined ischemic and hemorrhagic stroke.[33] For ischemic stroke, the overall RR for current oral contraceptive users was three times higher in Europe; however, these estimates were lower in younger women and for pill formulations containing lower doses of estrogen. Statistically, there was no significant difference between second- and third-generation progestogens. The risk of stroke was significantly increased (fivefold) for women who smoked and used birth control pills, and increased 10-fold for users with a history of hypertension. The risk of hemorrhagic stroke also rose among oral contraceptive users who smoked or had a history of hypertension. In general, pill formulations with less than 50 μg of estrogen had no influence on the risk of stroke unless other risk factors, such as smoking and hypertension, were present.[34]

SUMMARY

Cardiovascular disease is rare in women of reproductive age, although the trend toward pregnancy and childbirth in the later reproductive years may sometimes be associated with increased risks. A thorough medical evaluation to determine individual risk factors is recommended before prescription of any medication, and this principle also applies to oral steroid contraceptives. The risks of rare medical complications must be weighed against the very real risks of unintended pregnancy. In addition, the noncontraceptive benefits must also be considered in the equation. Although no medication is risk-free, the newer, low-dose combination oral contraceptives clearly have a favorable risk-benefit ratio and side effect profile, especially compared with first-generation birth control pills. The increased risk of cardiovascular disease seen in the older studies of oral contraceptive users does not appear to relate to modern contraceptive use. In women without other risk factors for heart disease (smoking or hypertension), prior or current oral contraceptive use does not appear to increase the risk of MI or stroke.[30, 33–36] Finally, the importance of fertility regulation for the welfare and advancement of women in both industrialized and developing nations cannot be underestimated. The availability of effective and safe contraceptive methods is vital. Apart from surgical sterilization, oral steroid contraceptives remain one of the safest and most effective forms of contraception available today.

References

1. Diczfalusy E: The worldwide use of steroidal contraception. Int J Fertil 8(Suppl)34:56, 1989.
2. Harlap S, Kost K, Forrest JD: Preventing Pregnancy, Protecting Health: A New Look at Birth Control Choices in the United States. Alan Guttmacher Institute, New York, 1991.
3. Trussel J, Hatcher RA, Cates W Jr, et al: Contraceptive failure in the United States: An update. Stud Fam Plann 21:51, 1990.
4. Bachrach CA: Contraceptive practice among American women, 1973–1982. Fam Plann Perspect 16:253, 1984.
5. Mosher WD: Contraceptive utilization. Vital and Health Statistics, Series 23, No. 7 (DHHS Publication No. PHS 81), 1983.
6. Mann JI, Vessey MP, Thorogood M, Doll SR: Myocardial infarction in young women with special reference to oral contraceptive practice. BMJ 2(5965):241, 1975.
7. Mann JI, Inman WH: Oral contraceptives and death from myocardial infarction. Br Med J 2(5965):245, 1975.
8. Speroff L, Glass RH, Kase NJ: Clinical Gynecologic Endocrinology and Infertility, 5th ed. Williams & Wilkins, Baltimore, 1994.
9. Hatcher RA, Trussell J, Stewart F, et al: Contraceptive Technology, 16th ed. Irvington Publishers, New York, 1994.
10. Hirsch DR, Mikkola KM, Marks PW, et al: Pulmonary embolism and deep venous thrombosis during pregnancy or oral contraceptive use: Prevalence of factor V Leiden. Am Heart J 131:1145, 1996.
11. The Cancer and Steroid Hormone Study of the Centers for Disease Control and Prevention and the National Institute of Child Health and Human Development: Combination oral contraceptive use and the risk of endometrial cancer. JAMA 257:796, 1987.
12. Cancer and Steroid Hormone Study of the Centers for Disease Control and Prevention and National Institute of Child Health and Human Development: The reduction in risk of ovarian cancer associated with oral contraceptive use. N Engl J Med 316:650, 1987.
13. Kaunitz AM: Oral contraceptives and gynecologic cancer: An update for the 1990s. Am J Obstet Gynecol 167(4 Pt 2):1171, 1992.
14. Burkman RT Jr: The role of oral contraceptives in the treatment of hyperandrogenic disorders. Am J Med 98:130S, 1995.
15. Sulak PJ, Haney AF: Unwanted pregnancies: Understanding contraceptive use and benefits in adolescents and older women. Am J Obstet Gynecol 168(6 Pt 2):2042, 1993.
16. Thorneycroft IH: Noncontraceptive benefits of modern low-dose oral contraceptives. Adv Contracept 8(Suppl 1):5, 1992.
17. Sulak PJ: The perimenopause: A critical time in a woman's life. Int J Fertil Menopausal Stud 41:85, 1996.
18. Flint PM, Lapane KL, Barbour MM, et al: Cardiovascular risk profiles of oral contraceptive users and non-users: A population-based study. Prev Med 24:586, 1995.
19. Raitakari OT, Porrka KV, Rasanen L, Viikari JS: Relations of life-style with lipids, blood pressure and insulin in adolescents and young adults: The Cardiovascular Risk in Young Finns Study. Atherosclerosis 111: 237, 1994.
20. Haskell WL, Alderman EL, Fair JM, et al: Effects of intensive multiple risk factor reduction on coronary atherosclerosis and clinical cardiac events in men and women with coronary artery disease: The Stanford Coronary Risk Intervention Project. Circulation 89:975, 1994.
21. Godsland IF: Interaction of oral contraceptive use with the effects of age, exercise habits and other cardiovascular risk modifiers on metabolic risk markers. Contraception 53:9, 1996.
22. Karas RH, Patterson BL, Mendelsohn ME: Human vascular smooth muscle cells contain functional estrogen receptor. Circulation 89:1943, 1994.
23. Kaplan JR, Adams MR, Anthony MS, et al: Dominant social status and contraceptive hormone treatment inhibit atherogenesis in premenopausal monkeys. Arterioscler Thromb Vasc Biol 15:2094, 1995.
24. Clarkson TB, Kaplan JR, Shively CA, et al: Benefits of exogenous estrogen in inhibiting stress-related coronary artery atherosclerosis. Br J Obstet Gynaecol 103:73, 1996.
25. Godsland IF, Crook D, Wynn V: Clinical and metabolic considerations of long-term oral contraceptive use. Am J Obstet Gynecol 166(6 Pt 2): 1955, 1992.
26. Godsland IF, Crook D: Update on the metabolic effects of steroidal contraceptives and their relationship to cardiovascular disease risk. Am J Obstet Gynecol 170(5 Pt 2):1528, 1994.
27. World Health Organization Collaborative Study of Cardiovascular Disease and Steroid Hormone Contraception: Effect of different progestagens in low oestrogen oral contraceptives on venous thromboembolic disease. Lancet 346(8990):1582, 1995.
28. Jick H, Jick SS, Gurewich V, et al: Risk of idiopathic cardiovascular death and nonfatal venous thromboembolism in women using oral

contraceptives with differing progestogen components. Lancet 346(8990):1589, 1995.
29. Bloemenkamp KW, Rosendaal FR, Helmerholst FM, et al: Enhancement by factor V Leiden mutation of risk of deep-vein thrombosis associated with oral contraceptives containing a third-generation progestagen. Lancet 346(8990):1593, 1995.
30. Rosenberg L, Palmer JR, Sands MI, et al: Modern oral contraceptives and cardiovascular disease. Am J Obstet Gynecol 177:707, 1997.
31. World Health Organization Collaborative Study of Cardiovascular Disease and Steroid Hormone Contraception: Acute myocardial infarction and combined oral contraceptives: Results of an international multicentre case control study. Lancet 349(9060):1202, 1997.
32. Lewis MA, Spitzer WO, Heinemann LAJ, et al: Third generation oral contraceptives and risk of myocardial infarction: An international case-control study. BMJ 312:88, 1996.
33. World Health Organization Collaborative Study of Cardiovascular Disease and Steroid Hormone Contraception: Venous thromboembolic disease and combined oral contraceptives: Results of international multicentre case control study. Lancet 346(8990):1575, 1995.
34. Petitti DB, Sydney S, Bernstein A: Stroke in users of low-dose oral contraceptives. N Engl J Med 335:8, 1996.
35. Grimes DA: The safety of oral contraceptives: Epidemiologic insights from the first 30 years. Am J Obstet Gynecol 166(6 Pt 2):1950, 1992.
36. Colditz GA : Oral contraceptive use and mortality during 12 years of follow-up: The Nurses' Health Study. Ann Intern Med 120:821, 1994.

CHAPTER

6 Behavioral Barriers to Health

6.1 Smoking

Susan Wilansky

Research over the last 50 years on smoking and coronary heart disease (CHD) has documented a strong association between smoking behavior and increased risks for most types of CHD in men[1, 2]; women were presumed to be relatively protected against CHD until menopause.[1, 3] As the incidence of CHD has risen rapidly in women in recent decades, researchers have increasingly questioned whether data on male smokers and CHD risks can be extrapolated to women. Although it is less complete, the available epidemiologic and case-controlled research on smoking and CHD risks in women shows that smoking is highly predictive for fatal and nonfatal CHD,[4] coronary spasm,[5] peripheral occlusive arterial disease,[2, 6] stroke,[7, 8] and angina.[9]

Several studies have estimated that between 60% and 90% of all fatal and nonfatal CHD events in women can be attributed to smoking, with the increase in risk related to the level of tobacco consumption.[10] In women, as in men, risks for acute manifestations of CHD decline precipitously after smoking cessation,[8, 11–13] although atherosclerotic changes in the cardiovascular system are ameliorated but never completely eliminated in former smokers.[14] Therefore, a substantial decrease in smoking prevalence in women would decrease excess CHD risk commensurably and potentially would reduce CHD deaths among women more effectively than any other preventive effort.[10, 14]

Despite similar associations between smoking and increased risks of CHD in women and men, salient differences in their smoking patterns and relative risks for specific manifestations of CHD should be considered in trying to maximize the cardiovascular health of individual women and in planning strategies to decrease CHD incidence among women in the general population.

SMOKING PROFILE AND PREVALENCE IN WOMEN

Changing Trends

Despite large differences in the current prevalence of smoking among women in different countries,[15–19] the *trends* in smoking behavior among women are quite similar in most countries: Women are smoking in increasing numbers, at younger ages, and more heavily than previous groups of women did,[19] and smoking is significantly more common among women with less education and lower socioeconomic status (Fig. 6–1).[20] About a quarter to one third of adult women in the United States now smoke.[10, 20]

Although the overall prevalence of smoking among women has rarely reached that among men in many countries, the gap is narrowing rapidly. Young women more frequently are becoming smokers, and women's rates of smoking cessation continue to lag far behind men's.[10] Young women in most Western countries are now equally likely or more likely to smoke than are their male counterparts.[14, 20] Among high school seniors in the United States, the percentage of women who smoked consistently exceeded that of men from 1976 until 1990, when the smoking prevalence for male and female high school seniors converged at approximately 18%.[20]

The age at which women begin smoking is steadily decreasing. Initial experimentation with cigarettes peaks during preadolescence, and some girls adopt regular smoking habits by about age 15.[21, 22] As a result, the number of women who smoke from teenage years through adult life is steadily increasing, and the full impact of long-term smoking on

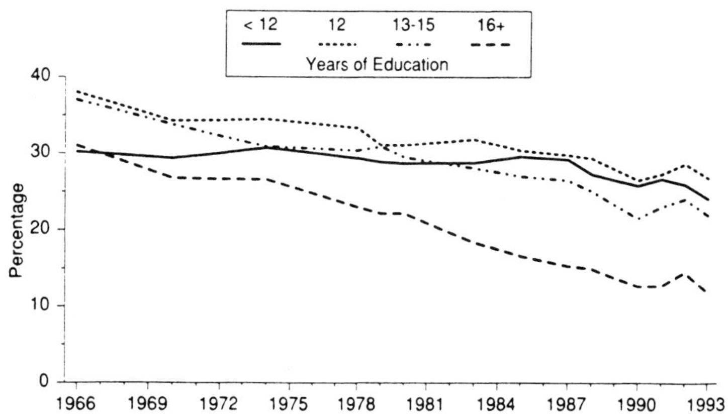

FIGURE 6–1. Percentage of women aged 25 years or older who are current cigarette smokers, by education—United States, 1965–1993. Note that estimates since 1992 incorporate some-day smoking. (Modified from Husten CG, Chrismon JH, Reddy MN: Trends and effects of cigarette smoking among girls and women in the United States, 1965–1993. J Am Med Womens Assoc 51:11–18, 1996.)

the cardiovascular health of women may not yet be fully apparent.

Women's Perceptions of Smoking

Smoking can carry very different connotations for women than it does for men. In preadolescent girls, the strongest predictors of smoking initiation are social factors—having a parent or best friend who smokes and being aware of a cigarette brand name.[21] Although the impact of advertising on smoking behavior is still controversial, several studies show that cigarette advertising in the last 30 years has substantially reinforced the positive views of smoking already held by many women.[23, 24] Beginning with the introduction of Virginia Slims as a women's cigarette in 1968, major tobacco companies have capitalized on existing ideas by associating smoking with women's liberation, social and economic success, healthy outdoor activities, sexual attraction, and independence.[23, 24] Adolescent girls are particularly susceptible to the positive images of smoking projected by advertising.[22, 24]

Women also view smoking as a means of controlling weight[24, 25] and dealing with stress, anger, anxiety, and pressure at work.[21, 26] Women are also more likely than men to report that they cannot find alternative means for dealing with these reactions.[27]

It may be difficult to counterbalance these positive perceptions of smoking because women consistently underestimate the health risks of smoking and because women's magazines, the vehicles most likely to influence women to stop smoking, carry stories on the hazards of smoking in inverse proportion to the amount of revenue they derive from cigarette advertising.[28]

Ease of Cessation

Historically, women have been less successful than men in stopping smoking.[10, 13] The youngest groups of female smokers, aged 12 to 24, report the same level of dependence on cigarettes (75%) as older women with long-established smoking habits. More worrisome is the fact that 54% of women who smoke fewer than six cigarettes a day reported feeling dependent on cigarettes, and female smokers of all ages reported greater dependence on cigarettes (75%) than did male smokers (67%). More than 80% of women reported an inability to quit smoking despite repeated efforts, compared with 75% of men.[20] This apparently greater smoking dependence may be attributed as much to women's social and psychological dependence on smoking as to a physical dependence on nicotine.

Because many women identify smoking with favorable images of themselves, the habit is seen as a successful strategy for coping with pressures at work and at home, and they report greater dependence on cigarettes and greater difficulty quitting than do men; therefore, the prevalence of smoking among women will probably continue to rise. In many countries, the proportion of women who smoke may soon exceed the proportion of men who smoke. The potential impact of these smoking trends on CHD death rates in women can best be appreciated by noting the greater increases in relative risks for CHD in female smokers than in male smokers.

CORRELATIONS BETWEEN SMOKING AND CORONARY HEART DISEASE

Relative Risks

Almost all research on smoking and CHD in women, whether case controlled or prospective, concludes that smoking is an important risk factor for CHD in women (Fig. 6–2).[29] The association between myocardial infarction (MI) incidence and smoking behavior in women has been especially well documented.[4, 7, 9, 10, 16–19, 30–34] The total incidence of MI may be lower for women than for men,[18] but smoking increases the *relative* risk of MI for women at twice the rate it does for men, regardless of other CHD risk factors.[9, 18, 35] The link between cigarette smoking and a substantial increase in risk for nonfatal MI in women is of particular concern because nonfatal MI is such a strong predictor for subsequent death from acute CHD.[31]

Smoking appears to increase CHD risk disproportionately in women, especially young women, for whom smoking is the single most predictive risk factor for MI and sudden cardiac death.[19] After multivariate adjustment for all other risk factors for CHD, the relative risks for deaths from cardiovascular disease (CVD), ischemic heart disease (IHD), and stroke remain substantially higher for female smokers than for male smokers.[18] Because smoking is even more closely associated with increased CHD risk in women than it is in men, smoking is considered a particularly strong predictor of CHD in women.[7]

Smoking as an Independent Risk Factor for Coronary Heart Disease

In studies involving both women and men, smoking corresponds with increased risk for CHD independent of other risk factors, adding to but not multiplying the increased risks for CHD associated with genetic predisposition, personal behavior, and environmental circumstances.[7, 33] However, research on CHD in women only has produced conflicting evidence on the combined effects of smoking and other risk factors on CHD incidence in women. Some studies have documented a multiplicative effect of smoking and other risk factors, especially with the use of oral contraceptives.

Some researchers report no interaction between smoking and use of oral contraceptives,[33] some show that oral contraceptive use increases CHD risk only in women who smoke,[36] and others find that women who used oral contraceptives and smoked heavily had a risk of a first MI 23 to 39 times greater than that in women who used oral contraceptives and did not smoke.[4, 19, 37] Estrogen replacement therapy is associated with an equal decrease in risk for CHD in both smokers and nonsmokers, indicating that smoking should not preclude the use of estrogen replacement therapy for postmenopausal women.[38]

A number of studies show that cigarette smoking is associated with other conditions considered to be independent

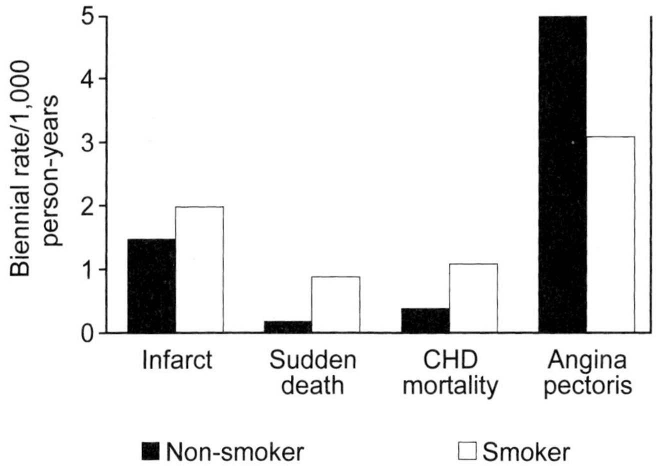

FIGURE 6–2. Smoking and risk for different manifestations of coronary heart disease (CHD) among women in the Framingham study. (Modified from Kannel WB, McGee DL, Castelli WP: Latest perspectives on cigarette smoking and cardiovascular disease: The Framingham Study. J Cardiac Rehabil 4:267–277, 1984.)

risk factors for CHD, including unfavorable shifts in high-density lipoprotein (HDL) to low-density lipoprotein (LDL) ratios (Fig. 6–3),[2, 18] increased prevalence of diabetes,[39] and a shift in distribution of fat toward abdominal accumulation.[40] Thus, smoking may indirectly as well as directly augment risks for CHD in women.

Dose-Response Relationship Between Smoking and Increased Coronary Heart Disease Risk

Most studies on CHD in men and women identify a dose-response relationship between elevated risks for CHD and age at smoking initiation, quantity smoked daily, and depth of inhalation. CHD risks associated with smoking are highest for women who start smoking before the age of 15.[11] For MI, risk patterns in women have a closer dose-dependent relationship with inhalation and quantity of tobacco smoked daily than with lifetime history of smoking.[4, 35] Current smoking is a considerably stronger risk factor for MI in women than it is for men,[18] despite the fact that women tend to smoke less tobacco than men do on a daily basis.[18, 35]

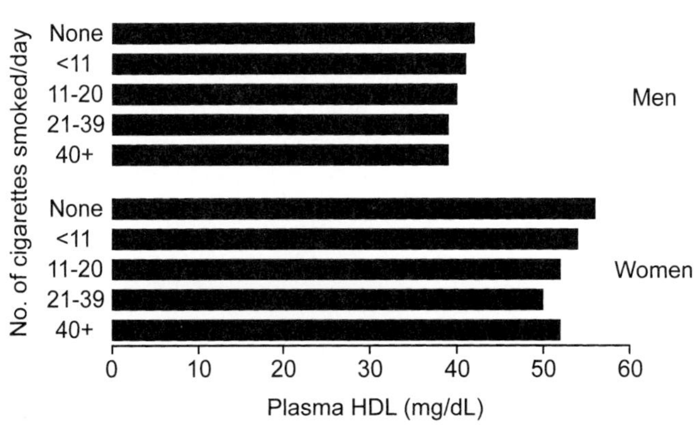

FIGURE 6–3. The effect of cigarette smoking on plasma high-density lipoproteins in men and women. HDL, high-density lipoproteins. (Modified from Kannel WB, McGee DL, Castelli WP: Latest perspectives on cigarette smoking and cardiovascular disease. The Framingham Study. J Cardiac Rehabil 4:267–277, 1984.)

Smoking decreases the age at first MI in both men and women by as many as 10 years if they are heavy smokers.[32] However, preinfarction smoking appears to have little effect on the mortality rate for cardiac causes subsequent to the first MI because most patients stop smoking after an infarction and the greatest risks of CHD reverse shortly after smoking cessation.[32] Women as a group tend to develop heart disease about 10 years later than men do,[10] but the decreased age at first MI associated with heavy smoking among women could easily erase this gap in age at onset of heart disease, counteracting any protection from MI that women are thought to enjoy because of their premenopausal status.

Tobacco Consumption

The risk for first MI in women and men combined increases 2% to 3% for every gram of tobacco smoked per day,[35] but the dose-dependent relationship between MI and current smoking levels is even more marked in women than in men.[18] Smoking increases the risk for CHD in women at every level of tobacco consumption, and even very light smokers have a greatly increased risk of fatal CHD or nonfatal MI compared with women who are nonsmokers. Women who smoke one to four cigarettes a day have a twofold increase in risk, and those who smoke up to 15 cigarettes a day have a threefold increase.[29] For women who smoke more than 25 cigarettes a day, the age-adjusted risk of CHD ranges from an estimated 5 to 21 times the risk found in women who do not smoke.[17–19, 30] Smoking accounts for about 58% of fatal and nonfatal CHD among the lightest smokers and for 91% among heavy smokers. More than 80% of deaths from CHD in women who smoke heavily can be attributed to cigarette smoking.[9]

Inhalation

Inhalation is even more strongly associated with MI incidence than the quantity smoked. The incidence of MI among smokers who inhale is two times greater than that among smokers who do not inhale. Women who inhale while smoking a small quantity of tobacco (1 to 14 g/day) are at greater risk for initial MI than are heavy smokers (≥30 g/day) who do not inhale (Fig. 6–4).[35]

Low-Yield Cigarettes

Women smoke low-yield cigarettes more frequently than men do, perhaps with the belief that low-yield cigarettes are safer than other cigarettes.[13, 41, 42] With such a clear dose-response relationship between current levels of smoking and risk for CHD, one might expect women who smoke low-yield cigarettes to have lower CHD risks, but, paradoxically, women of all ages who smoke low-yield cigarettes appear to have an equal or *higher* risk of developing CHD than do women who smoke regular cigarettes.[35, 41]

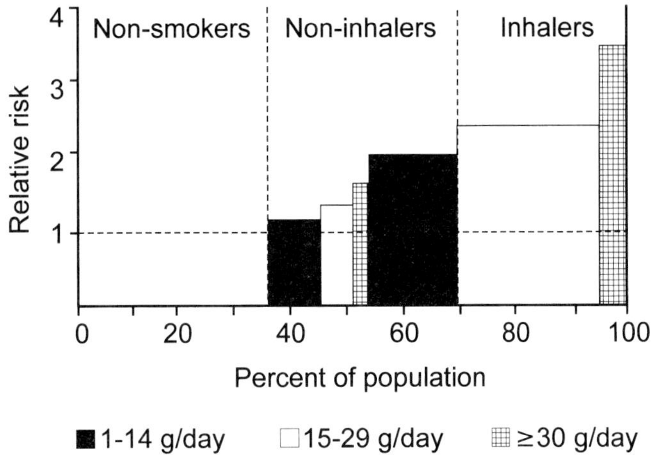

FIGURE 6–4. Estimated effects of tobacco smoking on risk of first acute myocardial infarction. Horizontal scale represents distribution of smoking groups in study population.

The association between depth of inhalation and MI risk may explain this observation. Low-yield cigarettes have the same tobacco and nicotine content as regular cigarettes but are engineered to deliver less smoke in a normal puff. Smokers who switch to low-yield cigarettes tend to compensate for the lower levels of nicotine delivered by each puff by increasing the number of cigarettes they smoke, puffing more frequently, or inhaling more deeply,[42] thereby maintaining blood levels of nicotine and carboxyhemoglobin comparable to those in regular smokers.[2] Any type of cigarette that encourages women to inhale more deeply, such as low-yield and mentholated[43] cigarettes, will substantially increase women's risk of a first MI.

ENVIRONMENTAL TOBACCO SMOKE

Inhalation of environmental tobacco smoke has been compared with light smoking and associated with a measurable increase in incidence of CHD. The strength of this connection is hotly debated[44, 45] because of the difficulty in measuring exposure levels and controlling for confounding risk factors.[46, 47] Nevertheless, of the 14 available epidemiologic studies on environmental tobacco smoke, 13 reported an increased risk of about 20% for death from CHD among those who never smoked and were regularly exposed to cigarette smoke, but there appears to be no relationship between CHD incidence and years of exposure.[48] The patterns of increased risk associated with exposure to environmental smoke strongly parallel the risk patterns observed in active smokers: Increases in CHD risks for both groups are more strongly associated with levels of current exposure than cumulative exposure, and women who otherwise have the lowest risks for CHD show the greatest increases in relative risk.[47, 48]

MECHANISMS OF SMOKING ON PROCESSES OF CONGESTIVE HEART DISEASE

The exact mechanisms of smoking involved in the processes of CHD are still debated, but most researchers concur that smoking invokes acute cardiovascular reactions and contributes to atherosclerotic changes in the cardiovascular system.

Smoking has a notable antiestrogenic effect, altering estrogen metabolism in both premenopausal and postmenopausal women, significantly lowering estrogen levels for women at all ages[49–51] in a dose-response manner,[52] and decreasing the age at menopause in smokers by 1 to 2 years.[53] Because estrogen is instrumental in protecting the endothelium in arterial walls, this antiestrogenic effect of smoking may account for the relatively greater risk of CHD associated with smoking in women than in men.[18]

Smoking also increases the metabolism of cardiovascular drugs (i.e., their clearance from the body is faster). Thus, physicians may need to prescribe higher doses of these drugs for patients who smoke.

Intense nicotine intake immediately raises norepinephrine levels in the blood[29] and increases both heart rate and diastolic and systolic aortic pressures for at least 20 minutes after smoke inhalation.[54, 55] These effects, combined with impairment of coronary vasoreactivity, may trigger coronary spasm and lead to myocardial ischemia and fatal cardiac arrhythmia.[5, 30, 55]

Smoking as few as two cigarettes increases platelet aggregation, hematocrit and hemoglobin concentrations, and fibrinogen levels,[1, 29, 55, 56] all of which increase the risk of thrombosis. The shared tendency of smoking and oral contraceptives to increase thrombosis may explain the increased risk of MI in women who concurrently smoke and use oral contraceptives.[4]

Animal and human studies show that smoking impairs endothelial function[57] and accelerates atherosclerosis and plaque development.[1, 44, 55] Smoking decreases HDL levels and raises LDL levels, increases levels of fibrinogen, and increases plasma viscosity. As a result, smokers develop new plaques at twice the rate of nonsmokers, and the plaques in smokers tend to have a higher lipid content and a thinner fibrous cap than those in nonsmokers, enhancing the chances of plaque rupture in smokers.[1, 55]

SMOKING CESSATION

Benefits

Because smoking appears to increase risk of CHD through both short-term effects (thrombosis, coronary spasm, and arrhythmia) and long-term effects (HDL/LDL ratios and atherosclerotic changes), the benefits of smoking cessation are divided between short-term and long-term improvements in relative risks. Case-control studies tend to report shorter intervals for reversal of CHD risks than do cohort studies.[12]

The excess risk of acute episodes of CHD among smokers drops by 30% to 60% within the first year after cessation regardless of age, presence of other CHD risk factors, duration of smoking, or amount previously smoked.[11–13, 29, 30] The excess risk of acute CHD associated with smoking is commonly viewed as reversible, even if different studies report that the period required for the risks in former smokers to match those in nonsmokers varies from 3 to 15 years.[12, 13] Although excess risks for acute CHD can virtually be eliminated by smoking cessation, atherosclerotic degeneration and aortic calcification are far less affected.

Methods

Nicotine Patch

Nicotine replacement therapy in the form of either chewing gum or transdermal patches maintains a constant blood nicotine level that, although lower than the level produced by smoking, is sufficient to counteract the withdrawal symptoms that afflict two thirds of smokers who are trying to quit.[58] Several studies have shown that the use of 24-hour transdermal patches doubles the rates of sustained abstinence from smoking at 12 months.[59, 60] Smokers with a low to moderate dependence on nicotine and those who have been motivated to stop smoking by a CHD event use nicotine patches most successfully, maintaining smoking abstinence for 1 year at twice the rate attained by heavily dependent smokers.[59] Even in patients who continue to smoke, patches lead to lower blood nicotine levels, most likely because patients who use patches smoke fewer cigarettes.[58]

In one study, patients who used patches and abstained from smoking for 6 weeks had a significant decrease in heart rate, systolic blood pressure, and LDL and a significant increase in HDL and triglycerides, all indicating an improvement in risk levels.[25]

Contrary to popular belief, nicotine patches can be used in high-risk patients who have existing atherosclerotic vascular disease without increasing the frequency of subsequent cardiovascular events, but the effectiveness of patches in patients who are heavily dependent on nicotine is questionable.[58]

Counseling

Because the social and cultural associations with smoking are so strong and because smokers who try to stop are subject to psychological withdrawal as well as nicotine withdrawal, nicotine replacement therapy by itself is relatively ineffective. Even though studies on the effect of counseling combined with patch use have reported only a 25% success rate among smokers attempting to quit,[60] campaigns to reduce smoking among women may be more successful if they directly address and counteract the positive connotations smoking holds for women: independence, adulthood, low weight, sexual attractiveness, social and professional success, and sophistication. Counselors should also recognize that women are more likely than men to use smoking as a way to deal with stress, anger, and anxiety,[21, 26, 27]

Long-term abstinence from smoking is best predicted by smoking behavior in the first 2 weeks of a quit attempt or even during the first day; those who abstain on the first day are 10 times more likely to sustain long-term abstinence.[60] Thus, health-care providers may best assist smokers who are trying to quit by motivating them in their initial decision to stop smoking and by dealing intensely with the social and psychological aspects of smoking during the first few days or weeks of quit attempts, in addition to treating these patients' physical withdrawal symptoms.[26]

CONCLUSION

Smoking is already a major contributor to CHD incidence in women, and it promises to be an increasingly serious risk factor for CHD in women as increasing numbers of women worldwide begin to smoke at ever-younger ages. The most effective way to eliminate the smoking-associated risk of CHD in women is to prevent the initiation of smoking by publicizing the CHD risks associated with smoking and by counteracting the positive images of smoking that surround young people today. For patients who already smoke, cessation offers an almost complete reversal of smoking-related risks for CHD, with substantial benefits accruing immediately and long-term benefits appearing within 5 to 10 years. At both the overall population and individual patient levels, health-care providers who address the social and psychological aspects of smoking for women will be most successful in permanently influencing their smoking behaviors, thereby permanently lowering their risks for CHD.

References

1. McGill HC Jr: The cardiovascular pathology of smoking. Am Heart J 115:250, 1988.
2. Kannel WB, McGee DL, Castelli WP: Latest perspectives on cigarette smoking and cardiovascular disease: The Framingham Study. J Cardiac Rehabil 4:267, 1984.
3. Barrett-Connor E: Sex differences in coronary heart disease. Why are women so superior? The 1995 Ancel Keys Lecture. Circulation 95: 252, 1997.
4. Rosenberg L, Kaufman DW, Helmrich SP, et al: Myocardial infarction and cigarette smoking in women younger than 50 years of age. JAMA 253:2965, 1985.
5. Caralis DG, Deligonul U, Kern MJ, et al: Smoking is a risk factor for coronary spasm in young women. Circulation 85:905, 1992.
6. Fowkes FG, Housley E, Riemersma RA, et al: Smoking, lipids, glucose intolerance, and blood pressure as risk factors for peripheral atherosclerosis compared with ischemic heart disease in the Edinburgh Artery Study. Am J Epidemiol 135:331, 1992.
7. Janghorbani M, Hedley AJ, Jones RB, et al: Gender differential in all-cause and cardiovascular disease mortality. Int J Epidemiol 22: 1056, 1993.
8. Kawachi I, Colditz GA, Stampfer MJ, et al: Smoking cessation and decreased risk of stroke in women. JAMA 269:232, 1993.
9. Willett WC, Green A, Stampfer MJ, et al: Relative and absolute excess risks of coronary heart disease among women who smoke cigarettes. N Engl J Med 317:1303, 1987.
10. Meilahn EN, Becker RC, Corrao JM: Primary prevention of coronary heart disease in women. Cardiology 86:286, 1995.
11. Kawachi I, Colditz GA, Stampfer MJ, et al: Smoking cessation in relation to total mortality rates in women. A prospective cohort study. Ann Intern Med 119:992, 1993.
12. Kawachi I, Colditz GA, Stampfer MJ, et al: Smoking cessation and time course of decreased risks of coronary heart disease in middle-aged women. Arch Intern Med 154:169, 1994.
13. Rosenberg L, Palmer JR, Shapiro S: Decline in the risk of myocardial infarction among women who stop smoking. N Engl J Med 322:213, 1990.
14. Schenck-Gustafsson K: Risk factors for cardiovascular disease in women: Assessment and management. Eur Heart J 17(Suppl D):2, 1996.
15. Gupta R, Gupta KD, Sharma S, et al: Influence of cessation of smoking on long term mortality in patients with coronary heart disease. Indian Heart J 45:125, 1993.
16. Waldron I: Recent trends in sex mortality ratios for adults in developed countries. Soc Sci Med 36:451, 1993.
17. La Vecchia C, Franceschi S, Decarli A, et al: Risk factors for myocardial infarction in young women. Am J Epidemiol 125:832, 1987.
18. Njolstad I, Arnesen E, Lund-Larsen PG: Smoking, serum lipids, blood

pressure, and sex differences in myocardial infarction. A 12-year follow-up of the Finnmark Study. Circulation 93:450, 1996.
19. Brezinka V, Padmos I: Coronary heart disease risk factors in women. Eur Heart J 15:1571, 1994.
20. Husten CG, Chrismon JH, Reddy MN: Trends and effects of cigarette smoking among girls and women in the United States, 1965-1993. J Am Med Womens Assoc 51:11, 1996.
21. Charlton A, Blair V: Predicting the onset of smoking in boys and girls. Soc Sci Med 29:813, 1989.
22. Pierce JP, Lee L, Gilpin EA: Smoking initiation by adolescent girls, 1944-1988. An association with targeted advertising. JAMA 271:608, 1994.
23. O'Keefe AM, Pollay RW: Deadly targeting of women in promoting cigarettes. J Am Med Womens Assoc 51:67, 1996.
24. Davis RM: Current trends in cigarette advertising and marketing. N Engl J Med 316:725, 1987.
25. Allen SS, Hatsukami D, Gorsline J, Group TNS: Cholesterol changes in smoking cessation using the transdermal nicotine system. Transdermal Nicotine Study Group. Prev Med 23:190, 1994.
26. Wilhelmsen L: Antismoking counselling: Methods of helping hypertensive patients to stop smoking. J Hypertens Suppl 8:S25, 1990.
27. LaCroix AZ: Psychosocial factors and risk of coronary heart disease in women: An epidemiologic perspective. Fertil Steril 62(Suppl 2): 133S, 1994.
28. Warner KE, Goldenhar LM, McLaughlin CG: Cigarette advertising and magazine coverage of the hazards of smoking. A statistical analysis. N Engl J Med 326:305, 1992.
29. Wilhelmsen L: Coronary heart disease. Epidemiology of smoking and intervention studies of smoking. Am Heart J 115:242, 1988.
30. Hanson MJ: Modifiable risk factors for coronary heart disease in women. Am J Crit Care 3:177, 1994.
31. Hennekens CH, Buring JE: Smoking and coronary heart disease in women [editorial]. JAMA 253:3003, 1985.
32. Gottlieb S, Falavollita J, McDermott M, et al: Cigarette smoking and the age at onset of a first non-fatal myocardial infarction. Coron Artery Dis 5:687, 1994.
33. Jensen G, Nyboe J, Appleyard M, et al: Risk factors for acute myocardial infarction in Copenhagen, II: Smoking, alcohol intake, physical activity, obesity, oral contraception, diabetes, lipids, and blood pressure. Eur Heart J 12:298, 1991.
34. Seeman T, Mendes de Leon C, Berkman L, et al: Risk factors for coronary heart disease among older men and women: A prospective study of community-dwelling elderly. Am J Epidemiol 138:1037, 1993.
35. Nyboe J, Jensen G, Appleyard M, et al: Smoking and the risk of first acute myocardial infarction. Am Heart J 122:438, 1991.
36. Miller VT: Lipids, lipoproteins, women and cardiovascular disease. Atherosclerosis 108(Suppl):S73, 1994.
37. Hennekens CH, Evans D, Peto R: Oral contraceptive use, cigarette smoking and myocardial infarction. Br J Family Planning 5:66, 1979.
38. Ginsburg GS, Douglas PS: Why cardiologists should be interested in estrogen [editorial]. Am J Cardiol 78:559, 1996.
39. Rimm EB, Manson JE, Stampfer MJ, et al: Cigarette smoking and the risk of diabetes in women. Am J Public Health 83:211, 1993.
40. Shimokata H, Muller DC, Andres R: Studies in the distribution of body fat. III. Effects of cigarette smoking. JAMA 261:1169, 1989.
41. Palmer JR, Rosenberg L, Shapiro S: "Low yield" cigarettes and the risk of nonfatal myocardial infarction in women. N Engl J Med 320: 1569, 1989.
42. Benowitz NL: Health and public policy implications of the "low yield" cigarette [editorial]. N Engl J Med 320:1619, 1989.
43. McCarthy WJ, Caskey NH, Jarvik ME, et al: Menthol vs nonmenthol cigarettes: Effects on smoking behavior. Am J Public Health 85:67, 1995.
44. Glantz SA, Parmley WW: Passive and active smoking. A problem for adults [editorial]. Circulation 94:596, 1996.
45. Weiss ST: Cardiovascular effects of environmental tobacco smoke. Circulation 94:599, 1996.
46. Steenland K: Passive smoking and the risk of heart disease. JAMA 267: 94, 1992.
47. Kawachi I, Colditz GA, Speizer FE, et al: A prospective study of passive smoking and coronary heart disease. Circulation 95:2374, 1997.
48. Steenland K, Thun M, Lally C, et al: Environmental tobacco smoke and coronary heart disease in the American Cancer Society CPS-II Cohort. Circulation 94:622, 1996.
49. Michnovicz JJ, Hershcopf RJ, Naganuma H, et al: Increased 2-hydroxylation of estradiol as a possible mechanism for the anti-estrogenic effect of cigarette smoking. N Engl J Med 315:1305, 1986.
50. Friedman AJ, Ravnikar VA, Barbieri RL: Serum steroid hormone profiles in postmenopausal smokers and nonsmokers. Fertil Steril 47: 398, 1987.
51. Baron JA, Adams P, Ward M: Cigarette smoking and other correlates of cytologic estrogen effect in postmenopausal women. Fertil Steril 50: 766, 1988.
52. Khaw K, Tazuke S, Barrett-Connor E: Cigarette smoking and levels of adrenal androgens in postmenopausal women. N Engl J Med 318: 1705, 1988.
53. McKinlay SM, Bifano NL, McKinlay JB: Smoking and age at menopause in women. Ann Intern Med 103:350, 1985.
54. Stefanadis C, Tsiamis E, Vlachopoulos C, et al: Unfavorable effect of smoking on the elastic properties of the human aorta. Circulation 95: 31, 1997.
55. Waters D, Lespérance J, Gladstone P, et al: Effects of cigarette smoking on the angiographic evolution of coronary atherosclerosis: A Canadian Coronary Atherosclerosis Intervention Trial (CCAIT) Substudy. Circulation 94:614, 1996.
56. Celermajer DS, Adams MR, Clarkson P, et al: Passive smoking and impaired endothelium-dependent arterial dilatation in healthy young adults. N Engl J Med 334:150, 1996.
57. McVeigh GE, Lemay L, Morgan D, et al: Effects of long-term cigarette smoking on endothelium-dependent responses in humans. Am J Cardiol 78:668, 1996.
58. Joseph AM, Norman SM, Ferry LH, et al: The safety of transdermal nicotine as an aid to smoking cessation in patients with cardiac disease. N Engl J Med 335:1792, 1996.
59. Richmond RL, Kehoe L, de Almeida Neto AC: Effectiveness of a 24-hour transdermal nicotine patch in conjunction with a cognitive behavioural programme: One year outcome. Addiction 92:27, 1997.
60. Westman EC, Behm FM, Simel DL, et al: Smoking behavior on the first day of a quit attempt predicts long-term abstinence. Arch Intern Med 157:335, 1997.

6.2 Obesity

James K. Alexander

Current estimates indicate an increasing prevalence of overweight among women in the United States.[1] In the National Health and Nutrition Examination Survey III (NHANES III), conducted between 1988 and 1991, 35% of women aged 20 to 74 years were classified as overweight based on their having a body mass index (BMI = weight/height^2) greater than 27.3 kg/m^2 (approximately 120% of "desirable weight") (Fig. 6–5). Unadjusted prevalence of obesity among non-Hispanic white women was 32.9%; among Hispanics, 46.7%; and among blacks, 48.6%. Thus, nearly half of Hispanic and black women surveyed were overweight. These figures contrast with the data collected in NHANES II (1976–1980), when 27.1% of women were estimated to be overweight.

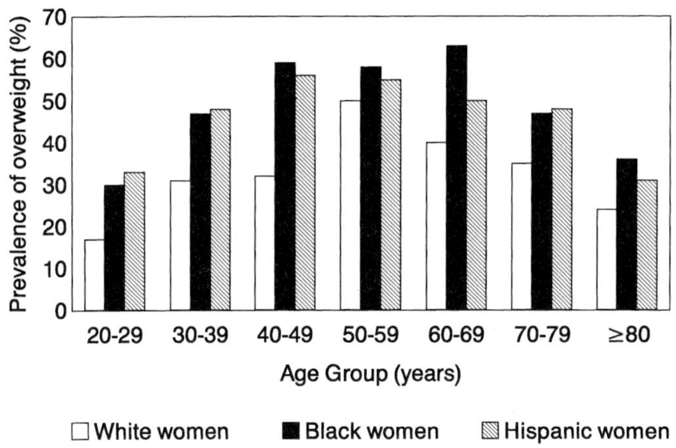

FIGURE 6–5. Unadjusted prevalence of overweight by age and race/ethnicity for women aged 20 years or older—United States, 1988–1991. (Modified from Kuczmarski RJ, Flegal KM, Campbell SM, Johnson CL: Increasing prevalence of overweight among US adults. The National Health and Nutrition Examination Surveys, 1960 to 1991. JAMA 272:205, 1994. Copyright 1994, American Medical Association.)

Yearly weight gain is highest in younger women. Among women aged 25 to 34, 37% gained 5% to 15% of their body weight over a 10-year period.[2] Furthermore, black women are more likely to gain weight than are white women. In a 1991 10-year survey of a cohort of U.S. women aged 30 to 55 (black women, 535; white women, 2976), the incidence of major weight gain (10 kg or more) was 17.3% in blacks and 11.7% in whites.[3] In addition, there appears to be a negative correlation between weight gain and both education and income levels.[4]

Although the development of obesity is more frequent in adulthood, 70% of children who are obese as preadolescents (ages 10 to 13 years) remain obese as adults.[5] Thus, from a preventive standpoint, the power of BMI levels in childhood (ages 1 to 18 years) to predict BMI levels in adults (age 35 years) is important (Fig. 6–6).[6] For women, the correlation between the two increased from ages 1 through 18 years, with exceptions from ages 1 through 3 and 10 through 13.[6] Childhood obesity has become more common in the United States during the last 20 years. Recent estimates indicate that, overall, 27.1% of 6- to 11-year-olds and 21.9% of 12- to 18-year-olds are obese, with a higher obesity incidence in girls (25.5%) than in boys (18.3%).[7] The timing of the menarche may also have preventive implications. In a study of 16,000 white women, the timing of the menarche (early, 11 years or younger; intermediate, 12 to 13 years; late, 14 years or older) was related to subsequent weight gain and obesity in adulthood.[8] An estimated 26% of early maturers were obese by age 30, compared with 15% of intermediate and late maturers.

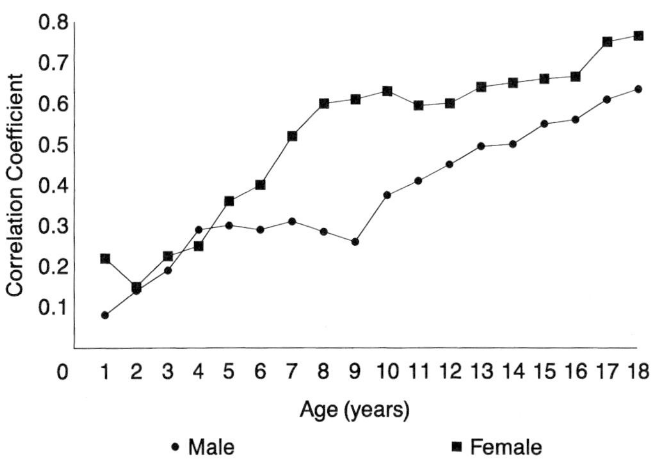

FIGURE 6–6. Correlation coefficients between body mass index at age 35 years and childhood body mass index from 1 to 18 years. (Modified from Guo SS, Roche AF, Chumlea WC, et al: The predictive value of childhood body mass index values for overweight at age 35. Am J Clin Nutr 59: 810, 1994.)

CORONARY MORTALITY AND MORBIDITY

By examining the relationship between obesity and coronary disease in women, it may be determined whether obesity has an impact on the initiation or progression of coronary heart disease (CHD) and, if so, by what mechanism or mechanisms. Approaches to this issue have involved (1) long-term epidemiologic or cross-sectional studies designed to assess manifestations of the disease in relation to some measure of total body fat or visceral adiposity; (2) examination of the association of obesity with other conditions or factors that have been identified as predictors of the incidence of coronary disease in population surveys (coronary risk factors); and (3) an attempt to prove or disprove that visceral adiposity itself gives rise to a unique causal atherogenic mechanism, possibly humoral or metabolic (i.e., that obesity by itself is a risk factor for CHD).

A pattern of conflicting results has characterized studies on the impact of obesity on overall mortality as well as on coronary morbidity and mortality.[9, 10] Data on women are relatively few, particularly data with a specific focus on coronary morbidity and mortality. However, two aspects of past epidemiologic studies deserve attention. First, the validity of conclusions from a number of studies has been questioned because of failure to control for smoking, small cohort size, length of follow-up, and failure to eliminate early death and misclassification biases.[11, 12] Second, some studies had inappropriate control for intermediate risk factors. That is, conclusions were drawn regarding the impact of obesity on mortality rate after controlling for conditions such as hypertension, dyslipidemia, and diabetes. However, these conditions are not confounding; rather, they are intermediate risk factors that are influenced by obesity and through which CHD may be conditioned. A number of studies in women have been limited by one or more of these factors.[11]

In light of these considerations, several epidemiologic studies may be cited as noteworthy in that they involve large numbers of women, control for smoking, have few potential flaws, and focus on CHD mortality and/or morbidity. In the 1979 American Cancer Study, Lew and Garfinkel reported CHD mortality in 419,060 women (ages 30 to 89 years) from 1959 to 1972 and related mortality ratios to weight index. Women at 90% to 109% of average weight were used as the reference category.[13] For women aged 40 to 69 years, the coronary mortality rate was significantly increased among those at 120% to 129% of average weight or more.

A report of the Consultation Bureau Project on Cardiovascular Diseases in the Netherlands recorded relative risk of CHD death as a function of BMI in 25,540 women (ages 30 to 54 years) during an average of 12 years of follow-up. A BMI between 18.5 and 24.9 kg/m^2 was used as the reference category.[14] In this study, the hazard ratio for CHD mortality in women with a BMI in the range of 25 to 30 kg/m^2 was about double that in the reference category. Twenty-eight percent of CHD deaths in women were calculated to be attributable to adiposity.

In the Nurses' Health Study, the association between BMI and CHD mortality rates was examined during 16 years of follow-up in a cohort of 115,195 U.S. women (ages 30 to 55 years) who were free from CHD at entry into the study.[15] Using a BMI of over 19 kg/m^2 as the reference category, the relative risk of death due to CHD increased: 1.7 for a BMI of 25 to 27 kg/m^2, 3.1 for a BMI of 27 to 29 kg/m^2, 4.6 for a BMI of 29 to 32 kg/m^2, and 5.8 for a BMI above 32 kg/m^2. Furthermore, a weight gain of 10 to 19 kg since age 18 was associated with a relative risk of death from CHD of 2.6; a gain of more than 20 kg was associated with a relative risk of 7.4. However, in a separate report based on this study, examination of the incidence of CHD (defined as nonfatal myocardial infarction or fatal CHD), using a BMI above 21 kg/m^2 as the reference category and controlling for age, menopausal status, postmenopausal hormone use, parental history of CHD, and smoking, yielded somewhat reduced levels of relative risk: 1.46 for a BMI of 23 to 25 kg/m^2, 2.06 for a BMI of 25 to 29 kg/m^2, and 3.56 for a BMI above 29 kg/m^2.[16] Comparison of relative risk for women who gained weight after age 18 with those who did not yielded relative risk levels of 1.64 for an 8- to 10.9-kg gain, 1.92 for an 11- to 19-kg gain, and 2.65 for a gain of over 20 kg. Thus, weight gain after 18 years of age was a strong predictor of CHD risk (Fig. 6–7). Among women who did not currently smoke, 46% of the CHD incidence in this group could be attributed to excess body weight; 30% of that could be attributed to their weight gain after age 18. In another prospective study with a 15-year follow-up of 8373 women (ages 30 to 59 years), the mortality rate for CHD was positively associated with BMI.[17] Among lean women with a BMI above 22.5 kg/m^2, the age-adjusted CHD mortality rate was 2/10,000 person-years, increasing to 10 with a BMI of 22.5 kg/m^2 and 13 with a BMI above 22.5 kg/m^2.

The First National Health and Nutrition Examination Survey I (NHANES I) was a prospective study of 1259 white women (ages 65 to 74 years) and had a mean follow-up of 14 years.[18] Data from this survey were adjusted for smoking and age and related BMI to the incidence of CHD. The incidence of CHD included a hospital discharge diagnosis of CHD and coronary death. Compared with those women with a reference BMI of 21 kg/m^2, women with a BMI above 29 kg/m^2 had a relative risk of 1.5, and women with a BMI of 23 to 24 kg/m^2 had a lower relative risk of 0.6. Among those women with a BMI above 29 kg/m^2 and whose weight had been stable before entry into the study, relative risk was increased to 2.8 as compared with those whose BMI was less than 23 kg/m^2. For those who had lost more than 7.7% of their maximum weight at some time before entry into the study, the relative risk curve was J-shaped, with no change for those who had a BMI above 29 kg/m^2 as compared with those with a BMI below 23 kg/m^2, but with double the risk for those who had a BMI of 23 to 24 kg/m^2. Therefore, duration of obesity conferred increased risk.

Information pointing to the regional distribution of adipose tissue, namely intra-abdominal visceral adiposity (mesenteric and omental fat), as a factor in relation to CHD morbidity and mortality is considerable.[19–22] However, data relating to women are few. In epidemiologic studies, the waist-to-hip ratio (WHR) is the most widely used index for the measure of abdominal visceral adiposity. The WHR is a measurement of the circumference of the abdomen at the smallest area between the lower rib cage and the umbilicus, divided by the largest hip circumference measurement at the posterior extension of the buttocks.[23] In a longitudinal study of 1462 women (ages 38 to 60 years) over a 12-year period, univariate analysis showed a significant positive association between WHR and the incidence of myocardial infarction, angina pectoris, and death—more so than with BMI or sum of skinfold thickness.[24] A 5-year cohort study of 41,837 women (98% white) in the Iowa Women's Health Study sought to determine if BMI and WHR are risk factors for overall and CHD deaths in women aged 55 to 69 years.[25]

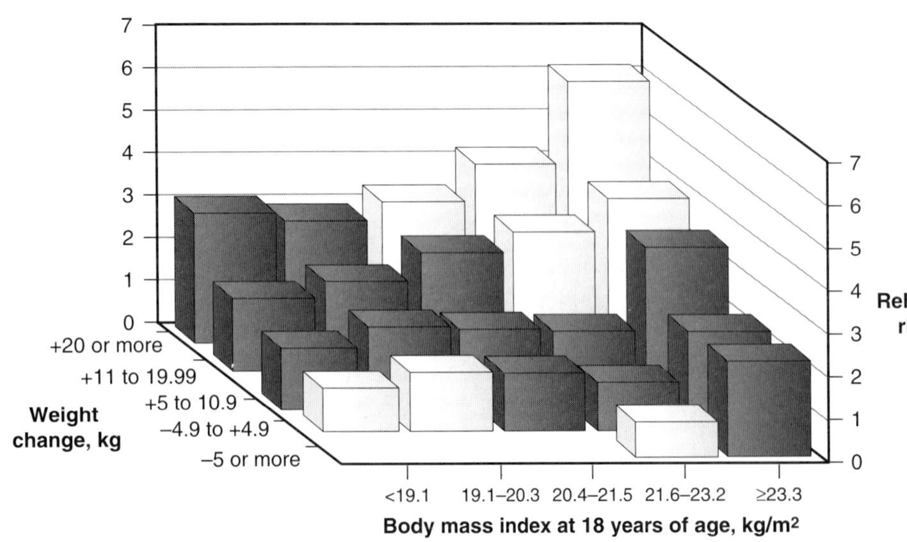

FIGURE 6–7. Data from the Nurses' Health Study. (From Willett WC, Manson JE, Stampfer MJ, et al: Weight, weight change, and coronary heart disease in women. JAMA 273:461, 1995. Copyright 1995, American Medical Association.)

For both smokers and nonsmokers, BMI analysis gave a J-shaped association for coronary death. However, for WHR, risk of coronary death was positively associated, increasing monotonically across each quintile. Women in the fifth quintile had a greater than threefold increased risk than women in the first quintile. It is interesting that the women at highest risk were those with a low BMI and a high WHR. In the Nurses' Health Study,[15] the WHR was a stronger predictor of CHD death than was BMI among women who had never smoked. Relative risk rose progressively for increasing quintiles of WHR as follows: 1.0, 2.8, 2.2, 3.7, 8.7. Thus, truncal obesity has greater prognostic impact on coronary disease than does BMI.

OBESITY AND CORONARY RISK FACTORS

A variety of CHD risk factors have been identified.[26] For purposes of this discussion, consideration will be limited to obesity and its relationship to hypertension, dyslipidemia, and diabetes.

The association between hypertension and overweight is well recognized and documented by large-scale population studies. For example, the nationwide Community Hypertension Evaluation Clinic screening program surveyed 399,416 women (356,091 white; 38,325 black). The study defined overweight as being 125% or more of the desirable weight and defined hypertension as having a diastolic blood pressure of over 95 mm Hg. Overweight white women aged 20 to 39 were found to have a hypertension frequency of 111/1000, compared with 41/1000 for women in the normal weight category; for ages 40 to 64, these frequencies were 353/1000 and 222/1000.[27] For black women, the corresponding frequencies were 201/1000 and 102/1000 for ages 20 to 39 and 539/1000 and 412/1000 for ages 40 to 64.

Correlation of indices of obesity and blood pressure levels tends to be better in women than in men,[28–30] disappearing after middle age.[28] Weight gain in adulthood increases the risk of hypertension.[31] The degree of upper body fat, as assessed by skinfold thickness, also correlates with blood pressure in overweight[32] and nonobese[33] women.[34] In addition, a positive association between WHR and blood pressure has been reported in healthy obese women[35] as well as the prevalence of hypertension in black women.[36] However, total fat mass, which correlates reasonably well with BMI, appears to be more closely associated with blood pressure levels than with relative measures of body fat, as indicated by waist circumference or skinfold thickness.[37] In older women, WHR may also be associated with alterations in plasma lipids, but not with hypertension when effects of BMI are held constant.[38] Thus, the impact of truncal obesity may be more strongly related to metabolism than to hypertension. The mechanism or mechanisms of obesity-induced hypertension have not been clearly elucidated.

Obesity is frequently associated with a pattern of atherogenic dyslipidemia, which is usually more pronounced in those with abdominal adiposity.[39] Abdominal adiposity in women is associated with high levels of plasma triglycerides[40] and low levels of high-density lipoproteins (HDLs),[41] which may predispose women to atherogenesis.[42] Total blood cholesterol concentrations do not correlate well with body fat mass or regional fat distribution.[43] However, with abdominal adiposity there is a preponderance for the more atherogenic, small, dense low-density lipoprotein (LDL) fraction[44] in both men and women. These lipid alterations appear to be due (at least partly) to delivery of large quantities of free fatty acids to the portal vein, with lipolytic stimulation of excessive visceral fat depots. High fatty acid content in the portal vein increases hepatic gluconeogenesis, increases production of atherogenic lipoproteins, decreases clearance of hepatic insulin, and induces hyperinsulinemia.[45] In obese women with low levels of intra-abdominal fat, increased plasma triglyceride and insulin levels may be the only metabolic disorders identified. However, obese women with high levels of intra-abdominal fat have more numerous disorders, including increased LDL cholesterol, LDL apoprotein B, and glucose and insulin levels during glucose tolerance testing and reduced HDL cholesterol, HDL/LDL cholesterol ratios, and HDL apoprotein A-1/LDL apoprotein B ratios.[43, 46] There is no correlation between abdominal fat deposition and plasma HDL cholesterol levels in nonobese women, suggesting that obesity in women must be present before some of these metabolic alterations take place.[46] It appears that sex hormone levels may play a role in the regulation of plasma HDL cholesterol in abdominal obesity,[46] but mechanisms other than sex hormone levels are also involved in the association of fat distribution with lipoprotein levels in women.[47]

The association of obesity with non–insulin-dependent diabetes mellitus is well recognized.[48] However, body fat distribution is more important than BMI in its effect on glucose and insulin metabolism.[25, 49] Hyperinsulinemia and insulin resistance develop with visceral adiposity because of increased pancreatic secretion and diminished hepatic insulin extraction.[43, 50] This leads to glucose intolerance and, with the proper genetic susceptibility, to non–insulin-dependent diabetes mellitus.[46]

A clustering of risk factors often occurs with obesity. For example, the Consultation Bureau Project of Cardiovascular Diseases in the Netherlands[14] found that increasing BMI was associated with increasing prevalence of hypertension and dyslipidemia. In the Swedish Obese Subjects (SOS) Study of severely obese persons, 78% of women had at least one of the following risk factors: elevated insulin, triglyceride, glucose, cholesterol, or blood pressure levels, or a decreased HDL level.[51] In the San Antonio Heart Study, 80% of obese subjects had hypertension and abnormal glucose tolerance.[52] In children with central obesity, alterations in blood pressure and carbohydrate and lipid metabolism continue into young adulthood, before a clustering of risk factors and the manifestations of CHD appear in adulthood.[53]

OBESITY AS AN INDEPENDENT RISK FACTOR FOR CHD

Epidemiologic studies have used multivariate analysis to control for various CHD risk factors in an effort to determine whether the presence of obesity alone has an impact on the incidence of coronary morbidity and mortality. Results of these studies have been inconsistent.[9] Stallones[54] notes that this is due partly to difficulty in interpreting complex interactions among weight and diet, physical activity, or other conditions. The interactions are not easily summarized by available mathematical models, and little attention has been given to the question of whether these predictors are equally valid in obese and nonobese subjects. In addition, studies interpreted as establishing obesity itself as an independent risk factor are subject to misclassification and confounding factors. In the Framingham Study, for example, obesity was related to mortality and morbidity rates after controlling for smoking, diabetes, hypertension, and lipid levels and was judged an independent risk factor.[55] But the residual variance due to obesity has two potential explanations[12]: (1) Measurements were imperfect and control for traditional risk factors was incomplete, and (2) obesity exerts damaging effects via mechanisms other than those controlled for in the study.

Visceral adiposity appears to be the closest approximation to an independent risk factor for CHD. It is possible to link diabetes, hypertriglyceridemia, reduced fibrinolysis, and hypertension to elevated portal-free fatty acid concentrations because of an increased visceral adipose tissue depot.[51] However, excess visceral adiposity is not limited to obese subjects, as determined by BMI. Some normal-weight individuals with excess intra-abdominal mass have the same metabolic profile of risk factors as those associated with the insulin-resistant syndrome.[46, 51] Furthermore, visceral adiposity is a heterogeneous condition, and not every viscerally obese subject will be at increased risk for CHD. Visceral adiposity appears to exacerbate a genetically predetermined sensitivity to diabetes, dyslipidemia, and CHD, which accounts for the heterogeneous outcome.[42] Accordingly, obesity, defined as a BMI of over 30 kg/m^2, and abdominal obesity, defined in men as a waist circumference of over 102 cm and in women as a circumference of over 88 cm, are categorized by the American Heart Association and the American College of Cardiologists as predisposing coronary risk factors.[56]

WEIGHT LOSS, RISK FACTORS, AND PROGNOSIS

Weight loss usually has a favorable effect on CHD risk factors in obese subjects. In 50% or more of hypertensive, obese individuals, sustained weight reduction is associated with decreased blood pressure.[57, 58] In a study largely composed of women, decreased blood pressure tended to occur early in the course of weight reduction.[59] Decreased blood pressure usually accompanies a modest or significant weight loss,[60] and blood pressure tends to plateau over a period of months.[61] The systolic and diastolic decrease per kilogram of weight loss may average 1 to 4 mm Hg and 1 to 2 mm Hg, respectively, although variability among subjects is considerable.[59] Although restricting salt intake may enhance the effect, blood pressure reduction through weight loss may occur independently of a salt-restricted diet,[62, 63] and in women, weight loss has an effect that is distinct from energy restriction.[60, 63, 64]

A meta-analysis of the effects of weight reduction on blood lipids and lipoproteins in obese subjects indicates that a significant lowering of total cholesterol, LDL, very low density lipoprotein (VLDL), and triglyceride levels may accompany weight loss.[65] An increase in HDL levels may occur in subjects who are relatively "stable." Although the effect on HDL levels may be modest, weight loss is usually more effective for raising HDL levels and lowering triglyceride levels than for lowering LDL levels,[66] particularly for patients who have undergone gastric bypass surgery for severe obesity.[67] There may be poor correlation between alterations in the lipid profile and large amounts of weight loss after gastric surgery.[68] Small amounts of weight loss in moderately overweight women who lose weight through diet and exercise may effect no change in HDL levels, whereas only a modest decline may be recorded in association with a dietary regimen alone.[69]

In view of the potential for decrement in HDL levels with dietary regimens that involve caloric restriction and decreased intake of saturated fats and cholesterol,[70] and the fact that HDL levels appear to be a more accurate predictor of CHD risk in women,[71] exercise should be incorporated into the weight reduction protocol.[69] Although diet and exercise studies of premenopausal women have demonstrated favorable modifications of plasma lipids, studies in postmenopausal and older women have not resulted in consistent changes, possibly due to degree of weight loss. In one study of overweight, postmenopausal women (ages 53.8 ± 2.5 years) who had a weight loss of 8 to 10 kg on regimens of either diet alone or diet plus exercise, the ratio of HDL to LDL increased 20% to 30% in both groups[72]; however, the diet-plus-exercise group lost more fat. In another study of moderately obese older women (ages 65.6 ± 3.3 years) who were on a similar protocol and had a lesser weight loss of 4 to 6 kg, lipid levels remained unchanged.[73] Weight reduction of about 5 kg in obese (BMI, 33 kg/m^2) premenopausal women has been found to be associated with decrements in lipoprotein(a), particularly in those with control levels above 25 mg/dl.[74]

Obesity is associated with diminished binding of insulin to its cell membrane receptor, and this inhibited binding is reversed by caloric restriction.[75] In obese subjects with non–insulin-dependent diabetes mellitus, weight loss leads to restoration of normal fasting glucose levels, lower glycosylated hemoglobin values, decreased fasting insulin levels, and decreased insulin resistance.[76–78] Those with the highest fasting glucose levels tend to respond more vigorously, and those who do respond usually do so after a modest weight reduction of 2 to 3 kg.[79, 80] Therefore, some evidence does suggest that weight loss improves prognosis in obese patients with diabetes.[81]

A review of risk factor alterations in obese subjects with weight loss indicates that salutary effects commonly involve a combination of several factors to varying degrees.[60] In subjects with abdominal obesity, weight loss may effect preferential reduction in visceral fat and WHR.[82] This may be a factor of considerable importance in view of the higher incidence of CHD risk factors in these subjects.[49, 50] During weight reduction, adolescent girls with abdominal obesity exhibit more beneficial changes in the CHD risk profile than do girls with gluteal-femoral obesity.[83]

Despite the evidence that weight reduction usually has a favorable impact on CHD risk factors in obese women, its effect on CHD morbidity and mortality rates has not yet been clearly established. However, some evidence suggests a favorable effect. Long-term weight reduction to "acceptable" levels for insurance purposes is associated with decreased CHD mortality rate in obese men and women.[84–86] A long-term interventional study is needed to provide more definitive information.[12]

CONCLUSIONS

Current estimates indicate an increasing prevalence of overweight among women in the United States. For women with relatively stable weight, a BMI above 27 kg/m^2 is associated with a significantly increased risk for CHD, as is a weight gain of more than 10 kg after age 18. Failure to demonstrate a linear correlation between an index of obesity (such as BMI) and CHD suggests that coronary risk may not be a direct function of total body fat or lean body mass, but of some other factor that influences that relationship. That is, if only certain subgroups of obese subjects are at increased risk, the subgroup risk may be diluted below the level of statistical detection when the group as a whole is considered.[12]

Identification of a subgroup of obese persons with a specific pattern of fat distribution has clarified, to some extent, the relation between weight and CHD. A pattern of visceral adiposity, reflected by abdominal (central) adiposity and WHR, has a higher correlation with CHD morbidity and mortality than do measures of total fat mass (BMI) or of subcutaneous fat (skinfold thickness). Visceral adiposity also predisposes obese patients to the development of established CHD risk factors such as dyslipidemia and diabetes mellitus. Although excess total body fat, as assessed by BMI, is also associated with a higher incidence of dyslipidemia and diabetes mellitus, the impact of truncal obesity appears to be greater in relation to these metabolic factors. Reported findings are not uniform, but the incidence of hypertension appears to correlate more closely with absolute fat mass than with regional fat distribution.

Obesity per se, as indicated by indices of overweight or total fat mass, has not been established as a risk factor for CHD, and was not listed as such in the National Cholesterol Education Program Report.[87] The presence of visceral adiposity is perhaps the closest approximation to an independent risk factor for obesity, but this is not limited to subjects with excess total body fat. Based on current information, the effect of obesity in relation to CHD is determined by its association with a variety of intermediate factors, the impact of which has not yet been well characterized, either qualitatively or quantitatively.

Although weight reduction may have a favorable effect on risk factors for CHD, interventional studies are needed to affirm the efficacy and the degree of weight reduction necessary in relation to CHD risk. Current studies greatly emphasize the importance of weight-gain prevention as opposed to weight reduction.

References

1. Kuczmarski RJ, Flegal KM, Campbell SM, Johnson CL: Increasing prevalence of overweight among US adults. The National Health and Nutrition Examination Surveys, 1960 to 1991. JAMA 272:205, 1994.
2. Williamson DF: Descriptive epidemiology of body weight and weight change in US adults. Ann Intern Med 119:646, 1993.
3. Williamson DF, Kahn HS, Byers T: The 10-y incidence of obesity and major weight gain in black and white US women aged 30-55. Am J Clin Nutr 53(suppl):1515S, 1991.
4. Kuczmarski RJ: Prevalence of overweight and weight gain in the United States. Am J Clin Nutr 55(suppl):495S, 1992.
5. Epstein L: New developments in childhood obesity. In Stunkard AJ, Wadden TA (eds): Obesity: Theory and Therapy, 2nd ed. Raven Press, New York, 1993, p 301.
6. Guo SS, Roche AF, Chumlea WC, et al: The predictive valve of childhood body mass index values for overweight at age 35. Am J Clin Nutr 59:810, 1994.
7. Gortmaker SL, Dietz WH Jr, Sobol AM, Wehler CA: Increasing pediatric obesity in the United States. Am J Dis Child 141:535, 1987.
8. Garn SM, LaVelle M, Rosenberg RR, Hawthorne VM: Maturational timing as a factor in female fatness and obesity. Am J Clin Nutr 43:879, 1986.
9. Barrett-Connor EL: Obesity, atherosclerosis, and coronary artery disease. Ann Intern Med 103:1010, 1985.
10. Troiano RP, Frongillo EA Jr, Sobal J, Levitsky DA: The relationship between body weight and mortality: A quantitative analysis of combined information from existing studies. Int J Obes Relat Metab Disord 20:63, 1996.
11. Manson JE, Stampfer MJ, Hennekens CH, Willett WC: Body weight and longevity. A reassessment. JAMA 257:353, 1987.
12. Sjostrom LV: Mortality of severely obese subjects. Am J Clin Nutr 55(Suppl):516S, 1992.
13. Lew EA, Garfinkel L: Variations in mortality by weight among 750,000 men and women. J Chronic Dis 32:563, 1979.
14. Seidell JC, Verschurenn WM, van Leer EM, Kromhout D: Overweight, underweight, and mortality. A prospective study of 48,287 men and women. Arch Intern Med 156:958, 1996.
15. Manson JE, Willett WC, Stampfer MJ, et al: Body weight and mortality among women. N Engl J Med 333:677, 1995.
16. Willett WC, Manson JE, Stampfer MJ, et al: Weight, weight change, and coronary heart disease in women. JAMA 273:461, 1995.
17. Jousilahti P, Tuomilehto J, Vartiainen E, et al: Body weight, cardiovascular risk factors, and coronary mortality. Circulation 93:1372, 1996.
18. Harris TB, Ballard-Barbasch R, Madans J: Overweight, weight loss, and risk of coronary heart disease in older women. The NHANES I Epidemiologic Follow-Up Study. Am J Epidemiol 137:1318, 1993.
19. Larsson B, Svardsudd K, Welin L, et al: Abdominal adipose tissue distribution, obesity and risk of cardiovascular disease and death: A 13 year follow up of participants in the study of men born in 1913. Br Med J (Clin Res Ed) 288:1401, 1984.
20. Bjorntorp P, Sjostrom L: Adipose tissue dysfunction and its consequences. In Cryer A, Van R (eds): New Perspectives in Adipose Tissue. Butterworths, London, 1985.
21. Donahue RP, Abbott RD, Bloom E, et al: Central obesity and coronary heart disease in men. Lancet 1:821, 1987.
22. Bjorntorp P: Abdominal fat distribution and disease: An overview of epidemiological data. Ann Med 24:15, 1992.
23. Caro JF: Clinical review 26: Insulin resistance in obese and nonobese man. J Clin Endocrinol Metab 73:691, 1991.
24. Lapidus L, Bengtsson C, Larsson B, et al: Distribution of adipose tissue and risk of cardiovascular disease and death: A 12 year follow up of participants in the population study of women in Gothenburg, Sweden. Br Med J (Clin Res Ed) 289:1257, 1984.
25. Folsom AR, Kaye SA, Sellers TA, et al: Body fat distribution and 5-year risk of death in older women. JAMA 269:483, 1993.
26. Higgins M, Lenfant C: Multiple risk factors: What is next? In Gotto AM, Lenfant C, Caapano AL, Paoletti R (eds): Multiple Risk Factors in Cardiovascular Disease. Kluwer Academic Publishers, Norwell, MA, 1995, p 7.
27. Stamler R, Stamler J, Riedlinger WF, et al: Weight and blood pressure. Findings in hypertension screening of 1 million Americans. JAMA 240:1607, 1978.
28. Johnson AL, Cornoni JC, Cassel JC, et al: Influence of race, sex, and weight on blood pressure behavior in young adults. Am J Cardiol 35:523, 1975.
29. Kannel WB, Brand N, Skinner JJ Jr, et al: The relation of adiposity to blood pressure and development of hypertension. The Framingham Study. Ann Intern Med 67:48, 1967.
30. Voors AW, Webber LS, Frerichs RR, Berenson GS: Body height and body mass as determinants of basal blood pressure in children—The Bogalusa Heart Study. Am J Epidemiol 106:101, 1977.
31. Hsu PH, Mathewson FA, Rabkin SW: Blood pressure and body mass index patterns—A longitudinal study. J Chronic Dis 30:93, 1977.
32. Weinsier RL, Norris DJ, Birch R, et al: The relative contribution of body fat and fat pattern to blood pressure level. Hypertension 7:578, 1985.
33. Despres JP, Tremblay A, Theriault G, et al: Relationships between body fatness, adipose tissue distribution, and blood pressure in men and women. J Clin Epidemiol 41:889, 1988.
34. Blair D, Habicht JP, Sims EA, et al: Evidence for an increased risk for

hypertension with centrally located body fat and the effect of race and sex on this risk. Am J Epidemiol 119:526, 1984.
35. Kalkoff RK, Hartz AH, Rupley D, et al: Relationship of body fat distribution to blood pressure, carbohydrate tolerance, and plasma lipids in healthy obese women. J Lab Clin Med 102:621, 1983.
36. Svec F, Rivera M, Huth M: Correlation of waist to hips ratio to the prevalence of diabetes and hypertension in black females. J Natl Med Assoc 82:257, 1990.
37. Spiegelman D, Israel RG, Bouchard C, Willett WC: Absolute fat mass, percent body fat, and body-fat distribution: Which is the real determinant of blood pressure and serum glucose? Am J Clin Nutr 55:1033, 1992.
38. Stevens J, Gautman SP, Keil JE: Body mass index and fat patterning as correlates of lipids and hypertension in an elderly, biracial population. J Gerontol 48:M249, 1993.
39. Ostlund RE Jr, Staten M, Kohrt WM, et al: The ratio of waist-to-hip circumference, plasma insulin levels, and glucose intolerance as independent predictors of the HDL_2 cholesterol level in older adults. N Engl J Med 322:229, 1990.
40. Krotkiewski M, Bjorntorp P, Sjostrom L, Smith U: Impact of obesity on metabolism in men and women. Importance of regional adipose tissue distribution. J Clin Invest 72:1150, 1983.
41. Despres JP, Allard C, Tremblay A, et al: Evidence for a regional component of body fatness in the association with serum lipids in men and women. Metabolism 34:967, 1985.
42. Bouchard C, Despres JP, Mauriege P: Genetic and nongenetic determinants of regional fat distribution. Endocrinol Rev 14:72, 1993.
43. Peiris AN, Sothmann MS, Hoffman RG, et al: Adiposity, fat distribution and cardiovascular risk. Ann Intern Med 110:867, 1989.
44. Terry RB, Wood PD, Haskell WL, et al: Regional adiposity patterns in relation to lipids, lipoprotein cholesterol, and lipoprotein subfraction mass in men. J Clin Endocrinol Metab 68:191, 1989.
45. Bjorntorp P: "Portal" adipose tissue as a generator of risk factors for cardiovascular disease and diabetes. Arteriosclerosis 10:493, 1990.
46. Despres JP, Moorjani S, Lupien PJ, et al: Regional distribution of body fat, plasma lipoproteins, and cardiovascular disease. Arteriosclerosis 10: 497, 1990.
47. Soler JT, Folsom AR, Kaye SA, Prineas RJ: Associations of abdominal adiposity, fasting insulin, sex hormone binding globulin, and estrone with lipids and lipoproteins in post-menopausal women. Atherosclerosis 79:21, 1989.
48. Health implications of obesity. National Institutes of Health Consensus Development Conference, 11-13 February 1985. Ann Intern Med 103: 977, 1985.
49. Kissebah AH, Vydelingum M, Murray R, et al: Relation of body fat distribution to metabolic complications of obesity. J Clin Endocrinol Metab 54:254, 1982.
50. Peiris AN, Mueller RA, Smith GA, et al: Splanchnic insulin metabolism in obesity. Influence of body fat distribution. J Clin Invest 78:1648, 1986.
51. Sjostrom LV: Morbidity of severely obese subjects. Am J Clin Nutr 55(Suppl):508S, 1992.
52. Mitchell BD, Stern MP, Hoffner SM, et al: Risk factors for cardiovascular mortality in Mexican Americans and non-Hispanic whites. San Antonio Heart Study. Am J Epidemiol 131:423, 1990.
53. Srinivasan SR, Bao W, Berenson GS: Coexistence of increased levels of adiposity, insulin, and blood pressure in a young adult cohort with elevated very-low-density lipoprotein cholesterol: The Bogalusa Heart Study. Metabolism 42:170, 1993.
54. Stallones RA: Epidemiologic studies of obesity. Ann Intern Med 103: 1003, 1985.
55. Hubert HB, Feinlieb M, McNamara PM, Castelli WP: Obesity as an independent risk factor for cardiovascular disease: A 26-year follow-up of participants in the Framingham Heart Study. Circulation 67: 968, 1983.
56. Grundy SM, Pasternak R, Greenland P, et al: Assessment of cardiovascular risk by use of multiple-risk-factor assessment equations: A statement for health care professionals from the American Heart Association and the American College of Cardiology. Circulation 100:1481, 1999.
57. Rissanen A, Pietinen P, Siljamaki-Oransuu U, et al: Treatment of hypertension in obese subjects: Efficacy and feasibility of weight and salt reduction programs. Acta Med Scand 218:149, 1985.
58. Reisin E: Weight reduction in the management of hypertension: Epidemiologic and mechanistic evidence. Can J Physiol Pharmacol 64:818, 1986.
59. Schotte D, Stunkard AJ: The effects of weight reduction on blood pressure in 301 obese subjects. Arch Intern Med 150:1701, 1990.
60. Goldstein DJ: Beneficial health effects of modest weight loss. Int J Obes Rel Metab Disord 16:397, 1992.
61. Cohen N, Flamenbaum W: Obesity and hypertension. Demonstration of a "floor" effect. Am J Med 80:177, 1986.
62. Reisin E, Abel R, Modan M, et al: Effect of weight loss without salt restriction on the reduction of blood pressure in overweight hypertensive patients. N Engl J Med 298:1, 1978.
63. Staessen J, Fagard R, Lijnen P, Amery A: Body weight, sodium intake and blood pressure. J Hypertens Suppl 7:S19, 1989.
64. Weinsier RL, James LD, Darnell BE, et al: Obesity-related hypertension: Evaluation of the separate effects of energy restriction and weight reduction on hemodynamic and neuroendocrine status. Am J Med 90: 460, 1991.
65. Dattilio AM, Kris-Etherton PM: Effects of weight reduction on blood lipids and lipoproteins: a meta-analysis. Am J Clin Nutr 56:320, 1992.
66. Margolis S, Dobs AS: Nutritional management of plasma lipid disorders. J Am Coll Nutr 8(suppl):33S, 1989.
67. Barakat HA, Carpenter JW, McLendon VD, et al: Influence of obesity, impaired glucose tolerance, and NIDDM on LDL structure and composition. Possible link between hyperinsulinemia and atherosclerosis. Diabetes 39:1527, 1990.
68. Kelly TM, Jones SB: Changes in serum lipids after gastric bypass surgery. Lack of a relationship to weight loss. Int J Obes 10:443, 1986.
69. Wood PD, Stefanick ML, Williams PT, Haskell WL: The effects on plasma lipoproteins of a prudent weight-reducing diet, with or without exercise, in overweight men and women. N Engl J Med 325:461, 1991.
70. Krauss RM: Regulation of high density lipoprotein levels. Med Clin North Am 66:403, 1982.
71. Bush TL, Fried LP, Barrett-Connor E: Cholesterol, lipoproteins, and coronary heart disease in women. Clin Chem 34:B60, 1988.
72. Svendsen OL, Hassager C, Christiansen C: Effect of an energy-restrictive diet, with or without exercise, on lean tissue mass, resting metabolic rate, cardiovascular risk factors, and bone in overweight postmenopausal women. Am J Med 95:131, 1993.
73. Fox AA, Thompson JL, Butterfield GE, et al: Effects of diet and exercise on common cardiovascular disease risk factors in moderately obese older women. Am J Clin Nutr 63:225, 1996.
74. Sonnichsen AC, Richter WO, Schwandt P: Reduction of lipoprotein (a) by weight loss. Int J Obes 14:487, 1990.
75. Archer JA, Gorden P, Roth J: Defect in insulin binding to receptors in obese man. Amelioration with calorie restriction. J Clin Invest 55: 166, 1975.
76. Savage PJ, Bennion LJ, Flock EV, et al: Diet-induced improvement of abnormalities in insulin and glucagon secretion and in insulin receptor binding in diabetes mellitus. J Clin Endocrinol Metab 48:999, 1979.
77. Hughes TA, Gwynne JT, Switzer BR, et al: Effects of caloric restriction and weight loss on glycemic control, insulin release and resistance, and atherosclerotic risk in obese patients with type II diabetes mellitus. Am J Med 77:7, 1984.
78. Franssila-Kallunki A, Rissanen A, Ekstrand A, et al: Effects of weight loss on substrate oxidation, energy expenditure, and insulin sensitivity in obese individuals. Am J Clin Nutr 55:356, 1992.
79. Wing RR, Shoemaker M, Marcus MD, et al: Variables associated with weight loss and improvements in glycemic control in type II diabetic patients in behavioral weight control programs. Int J Obes 14:495, 1990.
80. Watts NB, Spanheimer RG, DiGirolamo M, et al: Prediction of glucose response to weight loss in patients with non-insulin-dependent diabetes mellitus. Arch Intern Med 150:803, 1990.
81. Lean ME, Powrie JK, Anderson AS, Garthwaite PH: Obesity, weight loss and prognosis in type 2 diabetes. Diabet Med 7:228, 1990.
82. Leenen R, van der Kooy K, Deurenberg P, et al: Visceral fat accumulation in obese subjects: Relation to energy expenditure and response to weight loss. Am J Physiol 263:E913, 1992.
83. Wabitsch M, Hauner H, Heinze E, et al: Body-fat distribution and changes in atherogenic risk-factor profile in obese adolescent girls during weight reduction. Am J Clin Nutr 60:54, 1994.
84. Dublin LI: Relation of obesity to longevity. N Engl J Med 248:971, 1953.
85. Shephard WP, Marks HH: Life insurance looks at the arteriosclerosis problem. Minn Med 38:736, 1955.
86. Society of Actuaries, Build and Blood Pressure Study. Vol 1, Chicago 1959.
87. The Expert Panel II. Summary of the second report of the National Cholesterol Education Program (NCEP) Expert Panel on Detection, Evaluation, and Treatment of High Blood Cholesterol in Adults. JAMA 269:3015, 1993.

CHAPTER 7

Clinical Recognition: Risk Assessment Screening

Leslee J. Shaw, Eric D. Peterson, and Daniel B. Mark

Since the 1990s, reports of differences in the management of men and women with suspected coronary disease have raised the issue of "gender bias."[1] Initial attempts to explain these differences focused on the possibility that physicians took an inappropriately less aggressive approach to the diagnosis and treatment of women. Later studies of diagnostic evaluation have suggested that gender-based differences relate to variations in the underlying pretest probability of coronary disease and to atypical symptoms in women. In addition, some evidence indicates that the gender gap in treatment of coronary disease reflects the overtreatment of men rather than the undertreatment of women. Research has focused attention on the important epidemiologic and biologic differences that may translate into differences in management for women and men.

For many reasons, women who present with suspected cardiac symptoms pose a management dilemma for primary care physicians. First, coronary disease is less prevalent in women than in men. In the Framingham Heart Study, only 17% of women with chest pain had a cardiac event during 14 years of follow-up, compared with 44% of men.[2] Further, chest pain symptoms are more often characterized as atypical in women. Despite a lower prevalence of coronary artery disease (CAD) in women, nearly 500,000 women die each year of this disease.[3] Research has now been focused on women, but the majority of our knowledge about the effectiveness of diagnostic and therapeutic methods for the management of CAD is derived from studies performed mostly in men.

This chapter considers three main topics. First, methodologic issues that are important in studying the effects of gender on the diagnosis and treatment of coronary disease are reviewed. Next, the problems of screening asymptomatic women are examined. Finally, diagnostic and prognostic risk stratification in symptomatic women is considered.

METHODOLOGIC CONSIDERATIONS IN RISK ASSESSMENT

Risk assessment involves the use of available patient data to predict the probability of important future adverse outcomes. Because all clinical management is based on risk assessment (either explicit or implicit), the appropriateness of gender-related differences in practice patterns may be examined through the use of formal quantitative tools to assess a woman's diagnostic and prognostic risk.

The methods most often used by clinicians for risk assessment are informal heuristics, or "rules of thumb." These informal rules have limited usefulness, however, because usually only a few of the relevant risk factors are considered, and the relative importance of these factors is often not weighed correctly. Over the last two decades, clinical researchers have developed statistical models to estimate more accurately the risk of cardiovascular disease and its outcomes. A useful risk stratification model must take into account the available information and the options in patient management at each stage of the evaluation process. An initial evaluation model should include only data from the initial history, physical examination, and laboratory studies for the patient at presentation. Results of subsequent decisions, including diagnostic testing and a therapeutic trial, can be used to revise or update the initial risk assessment. At each stage of the evaluation, physicians must understand the effect of gender on the predictive value of each risk marker.

Determining whether gender alters the importance of the major prognostic factors in coronary disease can be difficult. Observed differences in outcome in individual studies may be related to (1) the type of analysis, (2) chance (because of the small number of women), (3) confounding factors, including variations in disease severity, (4) biases inherent in referral populations, or (5) true biologic differences related to the underlying risk in women.

Analytical Approaches to Studying Gender-Based Issues

Gender-based differences in treatment or outcome can be evaluated with two methods, subgrouping and modeling. Each has important advantages and disadvantages.

Subgrouping creates subsets of the study population on the basis of characteristics of interest, such as gender. The major advantage to subgrouping is that it is easily understood and mirrors the way clinicians tend to think. In theory, at least, subgrouping is appropriate when the investigator does not want to make an assumption about the difference between the groups before the study begins. However, subgrouping has important statistical limitations. Statistical power is lost when smaller sample sizes are used, and thus, the likelihood of false-negative results (type II error) is increased. Furthermore, because the statistical analysis is performed in each subgroup, the likelihood of a type I error (a higher false-positive rate) is increased. Identifying risk factors in a group of men and a separate group of women requires performance of the same statistical test in each group.

The modeling technique used for examining gender differences involves pooling data from men and women and applying regression models with specific tests for interactions by gender. An interaction by gender is said to be present when the factor in question (e.g., diabetes) has a different relationship to the outcome being studied depending on the patient's gender. A major advantage of this type of analysis is that it preserves all of the available statistical power from the entire patient data set for estimating the overall importance of the risk factor. The chance of a false-positive result may also be reduced by applying appropriate regression rules and diagnostic tests.[4] A potential disadvantage of this type of analysis is that the test for interaction in a regression model is relatively conservative. In other words, the empirical data would have to contain strong gender-based differences for an interaction term to reach statistical significance. In addition, the results of a regression model are less clinically intuitive and do not mirror the way clinicians tend to think about patient management.

Ideally, the subgroup and pooling or modeling techniques can serve complementary purposes. For example, regression analysis in a pooled data set may uncover a significant gender interaction with a particular characteristic, such as diabetes or exercise time. Then, subgroup analyses by gender may be presented to describe more clearly the differences evident in these characteristics.

Statistical Power

Another critical factor in evaluating gender-related differences is the ability of a study to detect outcome differences when a true difference exists (i.e., the statistical power of the analysis). Almost all reports comparing outcomes by gender have been limited to small, statistically underpowered samples. Women have been inadequately represented in large multicenter trials[5] and in studies of noninvasive testing.[6] For example, published reports on the prognostic value of exercise treadmill testing have included an average of 32 women per study. Slightly more women have been reported in studies of stress myocardial perfusion imaging (average 110) and radionuclide angiography (average 230), but because of the lower risk of cardiac events, these numbers are insufficient to compare test accuracy by gender. Thus, the true accuracy of screening in women by noninvasive testing is poorly defined because of the lack of female representation.

Confounding Clinical Factors

When an apparent relationship between a potential risk factor and an outcome of interest is actually caused by the influence of a second risk factor that is correlated with both the first risk factor and the outcome, epidemiologists refer to the second risk factor as a *confounding* factor. For example, obesity has been identified in some studies as a risk factor for development of coronary heart disease, but this relationship is confounded by the associations between obesity and diabetes, hypertension, and hyperlipidemia (the true risk factors for this outcome). In most cases, gender-related comparisons have not controlled for a uniform set of variables within the regression analyses. Thus, reported differences in outcome may be caused by a true gender-related difference or by confounding factors that were not accounted for in the data set being studied.

Women tend to be older and to have more unstable or atypical symptoms than men when they present for cardiac care.[2] Women also present more often with diabetes and other comorbid conditions. These differences could explain the lower short- and long-term cardiac event-free survival rates in women.[7, 8] Thus, the risk associated with female gender may be explained by a different distribution of risk factors common to both men and women. For example, the National Heart, Lung, and Blood Institute PTCA Registry reported that women were three times more likely to die in hospital after angioplasty.[9] A meta-analysis of published reports showed that the risk of perioperative mortality is more than two times higher in women than in men.[10] In contrast, adjusted late survival after coronary revascularization is similar in women and men.[11, 12] Differences in the severity of presenting symptoms and degree of comorbidity may explain variations in gender-based short-term outcome. Not all studies measure and can adjust for all relevant disease severity and comorbidity factors, which may explain why gender is an independent predictor of short-term outcome in some but not all studies.[7–12]

Referral Bias

Epidemiologic concerns (listed previously) affect the perceptions of physicians and their referral patterns. For example, indications for coronary artery bypass surgery were established on the basis of studies performed mostly in men. In fact, only 86 women were included in a 1994 report by Yusuf and colleagues[13] of pooled randomized controlled trials of bypass surgery versus medical treatment. Later reports suggest that women are referred less often for cardiac procedures, including noninvasive testing, cardiac catheterization, angioplasty, and bypass surgery.[14–16] Because physicians may think that noninvasive techniques for risk stratification are less accurate in women, they often proceed directly to more expensive diagnostic techniques, such as cardiac catheterization and imaging tests. However, in a relatively unselected population of symptomatic women, catheterization is likely to yield no evidence of obstructive coronary disease in 33% to 50% of subjects.[17]

Mark and associates[14] examined whether women undergoing exercise testing for evaluation of angina were less likely than men to be referred for catheterization. As in previous studies, these researchers found that women were referred less often for catheterization than men. They also found that the lower rate of catheterization in women resulted from the referring physician's lower estimate of disease risk before and after noninvasive testing. In a later study, men were referred for catheterization after stress perfusion imaging more often than women, but when the data were stratified by the amount of abnormally perfused myocardium (in the setting of severe ischemia), women were actually referred for catheterization more often than men. Because of the higher "hard" event rate in the female cohort, this latter referral pattern was considered appropriate.[18]

Absolute versus Relative Risk

Evaluation of potential differences between risk stratification strategies in women and men requires an understanding of

Table 7–1. CORONARY ARTERY DISEASE PREDICTION CHART: ASYMPTOMATIC PATIENTS WITHOUT KNOWN CORONARY ARTERY DISEASE

1. FIND POINTS FOR EACH RISK FACTOR

Age (Females), y				Age (Males), y				HDL Cholesterol		Total Cholesterol		Systolic Blood Pressure			
Age	*Pts*	*Age*	*Pts*	*Age*	*Pts*	*Age*	*Pts*	*HDL-C*	*Pts*	*Total-C*	*Pts*	*SBP*	*Pts*	**Other**	**Pts**
30	−12	47–48	5	30	−2	57–59	13	25–26	7	139–151	−3	98–104	−2	Cigarettes	4
31	−11	49–50	6	31	−1	60–61	14	27–29	6	152–166	−2	105–112	−1	Diabetic—male	3
32	−9	51–52	7	32–33	0	62–64	15	30–32	5	167–182	−1	113–120	0	Diabetic—female	6
33	−8	53–55	8	34	1	65–67	16	33–35	4	183–199	0	121–129	1	ECG-LVH	9
34	−6	56–60	9	35–36	2	68–70	17	36–38	3	200–219	1	130–139	2		
35	−5	61–67	10	37–38	3	71–73	18	39–42	2	220–239	2	140–149	3		
36	−4	68–74	11	39	4	74	19	43–46	1	240–262	3	150–160	4	0 pts for each NO	
37	−3			40–41	5			47–50	0	263–288	4	161–172	5		
38	−2			42–43	6			51–55	−1	289–315	5	173–185	6		
39	−1			44–45	7			56–60	−2	316–330	6				
40	0			46–47	8			61–66	−3						
41	1			48–49	9			67–73	−4						
42–43	2			50–51	10			74–80	−5						
44	3			52–54	11			81–87	−6						
45–46	4			55–56	12			88–96	−7						

2. SUM POINTS FOR ALL RISK FACTORS

___ +	___ +	___ +	___ +	___ +	___ +	___ =	___
Age	HDL-C	Total-C	SBP	Smoker	Diabetes	ECG-LVH	Point Total

NOTE: *Minus points subtract from total.*

3. LOOK UP RISK CORRESPONDING TO POINT TOTAL / **4. COMPARE WITH AVERAGE 10-YEAR RISK**

	Probability			Probability			Probability			Probability			Probability	
Pts	*5 Yr*	*10 Yr*	*Pts*	*5 Yr*	*10 Yr*	*Pts*	*5 Yr*	*10 Yr*	*Pts*	*5 Yr*	*10 Yr*	*Age*	*Women*	*Men*
≤1	<1%	<2%	10	2%	6%	19	8%	16%	28	19%	33%	30–34	<1%	3%
2	1%	2%	11	3%	6%	20	8%	18%	29	20%	36%	35–39	<1%	5%
3	1%	2%	12	3%	7%	21	9%	19%	30	22%	38%	40–44	2%	6%
4	1%	2%	13	3%	8%	22	11%	21%	31	24%	40%	45–49	5%	10%
5	1%	3%	14	4%	9%	23	12%	23%	32	25%	42%	50–54	8%	14%
6	1%	3%	15	5%	10%	24	13%	25%				55–59	12%	16%
7	1%	4%	16	5%	12%	25	14%	27%				60–64	13%	21%
8	2%	4%	17	6%	13%	26	16%	29%				65–69	9%	30%
9	2%	4%	18	7%	14%	27	17%	31%				70–74	12%	24%

C, cholesterol; ECG-LVH, electrocardiographic left ventricular hypertrophy; HDL, high-density lipoprotein; Pts, points; SBP, systolic blood pressure.

From Califf RM, Armstrong PW, Carver JR, et al: 27th Bethesda Conference: Matching the intensity of risk factor management with the hazard for coronary disease events. Task Force 5: Stratification of patients into high, medium and low risk subgroups for purposes of risk factor management. J Am Coll Cardiol 27:1007, 1996.

the difference between absolute risk and relative risk. Absolute risk is illustrated by the following statement: 5 per 100 more individuals with factor X will die in the next year than individuals without it. Relative risk can be stated as follows: Factor X increases the 1-year mortality rate threefold. Absolute risk is the sum of all the influences of relative risks operating in an individual.

In most analyses of patients with coronary disease, gender has been significantly correlated with absolute risk. In contrast, gender may not always influence relative risk. The concept of absolute risk and relative risk may be illustrated with the Framingham Coronary Risk Score (Table 7–1).[19] The total number of points determines a patient's absolute risk for development of coronary disease, but the number of points applied for a given systolic blood pressure or cholesterol reading is determined by the relative risk associated with either risk marker. According to Table 7–1, neither systolic blood pressure nor total cholesterol is affected by gender. However, the number of points received for age differs for women and men. For example, a 68-year-old woman would receive the same number of points as a 52-year-old man. The total of the risk factor scores on this table would then determine a given patient's absolute risk; a 68-year-old woman with hypertension and hypercholesterolemia would be at lower risk than a man of similar age with these risk factors.

Understanding the difference between relative risk and absolute risk may also help determine the clinical appropriateness of some procedures. For example, if the relative risks of mortality after coronary artery bypass surgery compared with medical treatment differ for women and men, then clinicians might need to develop separate guidelines for selecting men and women for bypass surgery. However, if the reduction in mortality from coronary bypass surgery is the same for men and women once body size or coronary artery diameter and other baseline factors are accounted for, guidelines for appropriate treatment should be based on absolute risk levels irrespective of gender.

Because of age-related differences in the onset of coronary disease between women and men, assessment of clinical risk becomes the decisive step in subsequent treatment and clinical decision making. A systematic approach to the assessment of clinical risk in women is described in the rest of this chapter. First, multiple variables from the clinical history and physical examination data are integrated into an overall assessment of a woman's risk for coronary disease and cardiac events. The use of a noninvasive stress test in the next step depends on whether that test would add enough information beyond that obtained from the clinical history to warrant the added cost to the patient.

ASSESSING CARDIAC RISK IN WOMEN

As women age, the risk of coronary disease and its complications increases (Fig. 7–1). The diagnostic and prognostic questions posed by clinicians also change with a patient's age and the presence of cardiac symptoms. Established cardiac risk factors become increasingly important in an asymptomatic population without known coronary disease, for whom treatment is aimed at primary prevention and control of the clinical sequelae of longstanding metabolic or hemodynamic abnormalities. Predictive models in asymptomatic populations address the likelihood of development of coronary disease or clinical symptoms (see Table 7–1).[20]

When a woman presents with chest pain, the type and duration of symptoms are important factors in assessing diagnosis and prognosis. As the underlying cardiac risk increases, the identification of high-risk coronary disease becomes more important than the assessment of *significant* disease (i.e., stenosis 75% or more in a major epicardial coronary artery). In populations with known coronary disease, certain symptoms, including those of unstable chest pain or heart failure, substantially increase the predicted risk (Table 7–2).[19] Other factors associated with mortality are a history of noncardiac atherosclerosis (vascular or cerebrovascular disease), myocardial infarction (MI), and revascularization. In higher-risk populations, a principal goal of risk assessment is to identify patients who may benefit from percutaneous or surgical interventions that improve cardiac survival. In lower-risk, symptomatic women, diagnostic and prognostic assessments should focus on opportunities for symptom relief and secondary prevention (Table 7–3).[21, 22]

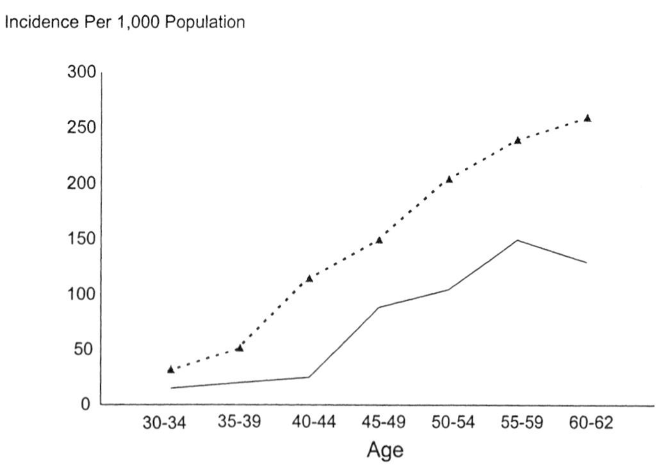

FIGURE 7–1. Incidence of coronary disease by age groups ranging from 30 to 62 years. Women *(solid line)* have a lower incidence of coronary disease than men *(dotted line)* across all age groups. (From Levy D, Wilson DW, Anderson KM, et al: Stratifying the patient at risk from coronary disease: New insights from the Framingham Heart Study. Am Heart J 119:712, 1990.)

Assessment of Diagnosis and Prognosis in Asymptomatic Women

Screening for latent coronary disease is a major public health challenge, given that half of all sudden cardiac deaths and acute MIs occur in asymptomatic patients.[23] Thus, screening is an important first step in prevention. Accurately identifying high-risk, asymptomatic individuals is extremely difficult, however, because of the limitations of available screening tools.[24] For example, before an acute coronary event, many asymptomatic patients who are at risk have only "insignificant" coronary plaques that do not cause ischemia and cannot be detected by stress testing.[25, 26] Furthermore, although the total number of cardiac events in asymptomatic patients on a national level is high, the overall risk of cardiac death in individual asymptomatic women and men is quite low.[19, 20] The prevalence of CAD is about 3% in asymptomatic women (increasing after menopause) and 5% to 12% in men.[27] Another limitation to screening in women is the lower sensitivity and specificity of diagnostic tests.[28, 29] Hlatky and associates[28] reported that the sensitivity of exercise treadmill testing is lower in women than in men, even after adjustments are made for age, treadmill performance, and severity of coronary disease.

The limitations to testing largely relate to the lower prevalence of disease and the severity of disease in women. Part of this problem is explained by Bayes' rule, which states that the probability that a positive test result is a true-positive result (i.e., that underlying disease is present) relates to the prevalence of disease in the screened population.[27] When the clinical risk is low, an abnormal test result does not substantially improve diagnostic or prognostic prediction. For example, in one report of patients undergoing exercise treadmill testing, the post-test risk estimates of disease and survival for patients who had low pretest risk remained low (<5%) for patients with an abnormal test result.[30] In most cases, abnormal test results were false-positive results, whereas most patients with coronary disease actually had false-negative test results.

Epstein and colleagues[31] illustrated the problems involved in screening asymptomatic individuals in a hypothetical example involving the screening of 10,000 asymptomatic subjects who underwent an assessment of cardiovascular risk factors plus an exercise test to classify them into low and high risk strata (see Fig. 7–1). Approximately 5% of screened patients would be identified as high-risk, with an annual

Table 7–2. RISK OF CARDIAC EVENT, STROKE, OR CARDIOVASCULAR DEATH IN WOMEN WITH EXISTING CORONARY DISEASE

1. FIND POINTS FOR EACH RISK FACTOR

Age		Total-C,	Points by HDL cholesterol									Systolic BP	
Age, y	*Points*	mm Hg	*25*	*30*	*35*	*40*	*45*	*50*	*60*	*70*	*80*	*mm Hg*	*Points*
35	0	160	4	3	3	2	2	1	1	0	0	100	0
40	1	170	4	3	3	2	2	2	1	1	0	110	0
45	2	180	4	3	3	2	2	2	1	1	0	120	1
50	3	190	4	4	3	3	2	2	1	1	1	130	1
55	4	200	4	4	3	3	2	2	2	1	1	140	2
60	5	210	4	4	3	3	3	2	2	1	1	150	2
65	6	220	5	4	4	3	3	2	2	1	1	160	2
70	7	230	5	4	4	3	3	3	2	2	1	170	3
75	7	240	5	4	4	3	3	3	2	2	1	180	3
		250	5	4	4	4	3	3	2	2	1	190	3
		260	5	5	4	4	3	3	2	2	1	200	3
Other	**Points**	270	5	5	4	4	3	3	2	2	2	210	4
		280	5	5	4	4	3	3	3	2	2	220	4
Diabetes	3	290	5	5	4	4	4	3	3	2	2	230	4
Smoking	3	300	6	5	4	4	4	3	3	2	2	240	4
												250	4

2. SUM POINTS FOR ALL RISK FACTORS

___ + ___ + ___ + ___ + ___ + ___ = ___
Age HDL-C Total-C SBP Smoker Diabetes Point Total

NOTE: *Minus points subtract from total.*

3. LOOK UP RISK CORRESPONDING TO POINT TOTAL

Total Points	2-Yr Probability	Total Points	2-Yr Probability
0	0	14	10
2	1	16	15
4	1	18	23
6	1	20	35
8	2	22	51
10	4	24	68
12	6	26	85

4. COMPARE WITH AVERAGE 2-YEAR RISK IN PTS WITH CVD

Age	Probability
35–39	<1
40–44	<1
45–49	<1
50–54	4
55–59	6
60–64	8
65–69	12

BP, blood pressure; C, cholesterol; CVD, cardiovascular disease; HDL, high-density lipoprotein; SBP, systolic blood pressure.

From Califf RM, Armstrong PW, Carver JR, et al: 27th Bethesda Conference: Matching the intensity of risk factor management with the hazard for coronary disease events. Task Force 5: Stratification of patients into high, medium and low risk subgroups for purposes of risk factor management. J Am Coll Cardiol 27:1007, 1996.

mortality rate of 0.72%. By contrast, the annual mortality in low-risk patients was 0.06%. However, the high-risk subgroup accounted for only 25% of all cardiac deaths.

This example emphasizes the imperfect nature of diagnostic tests. Although these tests do provide incremental information, the patient's true diagnosis often remains unknown. Consequently, probability tools are often used to express the level of uncertainty before and after use of a screening test.

Multivariable Risk Assessment in Asymptomatic Women

Although routine diagnostic testing to screen for coronary disease risk is not recommended for asymptomatic women, an overall assessment of cardiac risk, an important part of preventive health care services, should be used to determine the necessity for modifying risk factors. Multivariable risk assessments (see Table 7–1) have been developed to predict the probability of coronary disease in asymptomatic patients.[32]

The Framingham Coronary Risk Score demonstrates that the risk of cardiac events is a function of an entire set of risk factors operating in concert (increasing or decreasing cardiac risk).[32] A cholesterol level of 250 mg/dl, which may be associated with a higher risk in an older woman, is a lower risk in a younger, normotensive, nondiabetic woman. In an older woman, the risk of a cardiac event is increased fourfold by such a cholesterol level, and aggressive modification of the risk factor should proportionally reduce the risk. In contrast, modifying the risk factor in the younger woman may result in a lessened benefit. Except for age and diabetes, the major cardiac risk factors have similar prognostic importance in women and men.[32, 33]

Assessment of Probability of Coronary Disease in Symptomatic Women

A woman's description of her symptoms provides important clues about their cause.[22, 34–37] Because most of our knowledge of the clinical presentation of coronary disease has been

Table 7–3. IMPORTANT VARIABLES USED IN DIAGNOSTIC AND PROGNOSTIC RISK ASSESSMENTS

CHARACTERISTIC	ANY DISEASE	SEVERE DISEASE	LEFT MAIN DISEASE	SURVIVAL
History				
Age	X	X	X	X
Gender	X	X	X	X
Chest pain				
Type	X	X	X	X
Frequency		X		X
Course		X		X
Nocturnal		X		
Length of time present		X	X	
Diabetes	X	X		
Smoking	X	X		
Hyperlipidemia	X	X		
Hypertension		X		
Prior infarction	X	X		X
Peripheral or cerebral vascular disease		X		X
Congestive heart failure severity				X
Physical examination				
Carotid bruit		X	X	X
Ventricular gallop				X
Electrocardiogram				
Significant Q waves	X	X		X
ST-T–wave changes	X	X		X
Conduction abnormalities				X
Premature ventricular contractions				X
Chest radiograph				
Cardiomegaly				X

From Pryor DB, Shaw LK, Harrell FE Jr, et al: Estimating the likelihood of severe coronary artery disease. Am J Med 90:552, 1991.

defined predominantly in men, our definitions of "typical" symptoms may not reflect the "typical" symptoms in a woman with ischemia. In general, older patients have more atypical symptoms. Because the onset of coronary disease is later in women, the frequency of atypical symptoms is expected to be greater. A synthesis of several large observational series reveals that women do present with atypical symptoms of chest pain that occur more often at rest or without exertion.[15, 36–38]

The two main goals of clinical assessment in symptomatic women are the establishment of a diagnosis and an estimation of prognosis. To estimate the likelihood that a woman's symptoms are related to myocardial ischemia associated with significant underlying coronary disease, the clinician must know the key clinical risk factors and how they interact. The probability of coronary disease is related to the following five major factors[27, 34, 35]:

1. The physician's overall grading of a patient's symptoms (i.e., typical, atypical, or nonanginal).
2. Evidence of prior MI.
3. The patient's sex.
4. The patient's age.
5. The number of major cardiac risk factors present.

The probability of significant coronary disease in symptomatic women referred for cardiac catheterization is approximately 30% to 40%.[34, 39] In contrast, symptomatic men had twice the rate of significant coronary disease in the Coronary Surgery Study and Duke Databank for Cardiovascular Disease registries.[34, 39]

Several integrated predictive models of clinical history and physical examination variables have been developed from large patient registries to estimate the risk of significant and severe disease.[25, 32, 35, 37, 38] From the Duke Databank for Cardiovascular Disease, Pryor and colleagues[34, 35] developed diagnostic models to predict significant and severe CAD. Although these models were developed in patients who had undergone cardiac catheterization, they have since been validated in outpatient, community-based populations.[40] Most of the factors used to estimate the likelihood of coronary disease in the Duke diagnostic models have the same importance in women and men, but age is an exception. A synthesis of these models shows that gender is an independent predictor of coronary disease, even after adjustment for a variety of clinical risk markers. Consequently, separate nomograms have been developed to estimate the likelihood of significant coronary disease in men and women. For example, a 60-year-old woman with typical angina has a 50% chance of having significant coronary disease, whereas a man of similar age has a 90% chance of having significant coronary disease.

Age is also a key factor in the estimation of severe coronary disease. The prevalence of severe, multivessel coronary disease is about 20% for women and 40% for men referred for coronary angiography.[34, 39] This estimation of severe coronary disease may be the rate-limiting factor in a clinician's decision to refer a patient for cardiac catheterization; therefore, the accuracy of this estimation is critical to establishment of an appropriate referral pattern.[14] A multivariable nomogram for estimating severe coronary disease has been developed from women referred to Duke for diagnostic catheterization.[35]

These clinical risk estimates are beneficial because they can help determine who requires additional noninvasive testing. Because of the age-related lower prevalence of coronary disease in women, more women are likely to require and benefit from additional testing to improve diagnostic certainty than men of similar age. Thus, guidelines for the use of noninvasive testing may be based on these pretest risk estimates.

Assessment of Prognosis in Symptomatic Women

Prognostic assessment requires the clinician to decide how likely it is that a given patient will die from cardiac causes or have an MI, particularly during the next 6 to 12 months. Understanding prognosis and its assessment is essential for appropriate referral for medical or surgical intervention.[41] The following major prognostic variables are provided by the initial clinical history:

1. The presence and extent of left ventricular dysfunction (as evidenced by prior MI, congestive heart failure symptoms, or cardiomegaly on a chest radiograph).
2. The likelihood of underlying significant or severe coronary disease.
3. The course and frequency of the patient's angina.
4. The patient's age.

Multivariable Prognostic Risk Assessment

Several large observational series have developed integrated clinical history and physical examination models from the population-based Framingham Heart Study to predict a patient's risk of cardiac events, stroke, or cardiovascular death.[19, 42] Table 7–3 has been developed to estimate the 2-year probability of cardiac events in women with overt coronary disease. These estimates may differ from those derived from referral or symptomatic populations. From the Duke Databank, the risk of mortality at 1 year in women referred for cardiac catheterization may be estimated from information given in Table 7–4, which consists of the woman's age and symptoms as well as comorbidity that can increase her risk of cardiac death.[19]

CONCLUSION

Nearly 500,000 women die each year of CAD, yet a review of current evidence reveals that most of our diagnostic knowledge is derived from studies of men. The underrepresentation of women in published reports may reflect the atypical symptoms and the lower prevalence of disease in women. Assessing patient risk is a critical step at each stage of patient management. Using clinical risk indices derived from large cohorts of women, a physician may accurately estimate the risk of significant and extensive coronary disease and cardiac events. From this initial clinical estimation, the physician may determine whether a woman needs additional tests or, for the high-risk patient, should be referred for coronary angiography. Furthermore, decisions about which risk factors, if any, need to be modified are best based on a comprehensive estimation of risk. Additional studies are needed to incorporate information on estrogen status and

Table 7–4. RISK OF MORTALITY AT 1 YEAR IN WOMEN: CLINICAL HISTORY VARIABLES

1. FIND POINTS FOR EACH RISK FACTOR

Age (years)		Anginal Characteristics		Comorbid Factors	
Age	*Points*	*Pain Type*	*Points*	*Factor*	*Points**
20	0	Nonanginal pain	3	Cerebrovascular disease	28
30	12	Atypical angina	35	Peripheral vascular disease	22
40	25	Typical angina		Diabetes	38
50	38	Stable	63	Prior myocardial infarction	8
60	50	Progressive	71	Hypertension	3
70	62	Unstable	78	Mitral regurgitation	
80	75			Mild	9
90	87			Severe	59
100	100				

2. SUM POINTS FOR ALL RISK FACTORS

_______ + _______ + _______ = _______
Age Pain Score Comorbidity Point Total

3. LOOK UP RISK CORRESPONDING TO POINT TOTAL

Total Points	Probability of 1-Year Death	Total Points	Probability of 1-Year Death
102	1%	244	30%
129	2%	258	40%
146	3%	271	50%
167	5%	282	60%
195	10%	293	70%
225	20%	304	80%

*0 points for each "No."
Adapted from Califf RM, Armstrong PW, Carver JR, et al: 27th Bethesda Conference: Matching the intensity of risk factor management with the hazard for coronary disease events. Task Force 5: Stratification of patients into high, medium and low risk subgroups for purposes of risk factor management. J Am Coll Cardiol 27:1007, 1996.

comorbidity and thereby improve current diagnostic and prognostic risk estimates.

References

1. Tobin JN, Wassertheil-Smoller S, Wexler JP, et al: Sex bias in considering coronary bypass surgery. Ann Intern Med 107:19, 1987.
2. Lerner DJ, Kannel WB: Patterns of coronary heart disease morbidity and mortality in the sexes: A 26-year follow-up of the Framingham population. Am Heart J 111:383, 1986.
3. National Center for Health Statistics: Vital statistics of the United States. In Statistical Abstracts of the United States. National Center for Health Statistics, Washington, DC, 1992, p 84.
4. Harrell FE Jr, Lee KL, Mark DB: Multivariable prognostic models: Issues in developing models, evaluating assumptions and adequacy, and measuring and reducing errors. Stat Med 15:361, 1996.
5. Maynard C, Selker HP, Beshansky JR, et al: The exclusion of women from clinical trials of thrombolytic therapy: Implications for developing the thrombolytic predictive instrument database. Med Decis Making 15:38, 1995.
6. Shaw LJ, Peterson ED, Johnson LL: Noninvasive stress testing in coronary artery disease in women: What all physicians need to know. In Charney P (ed): American College of Physicians Women's Health Series. Philadelphia, 1999, p 327.
7. Fetters JK, Peterson ED, Shaw LJ. et al: Sex-specific differences in coronary artery disease risk factors, evaluation, and treatment: Have they been adequately evaluated? Am Heart J 131:796, 1996.
8. Vaccarino V, Krumholz HM, Berkman LF, et al: Sex differences in mortality after myocardial infarction: Is there evidence for an increased risk for women? Circulation 91:1861, 1995.
9. Holmes DR Jr, Holubkov R, Vlietstra RE, et al: Comparison of complications during percutaneous transluminal coronary angioplasty from 1977 to 1981 and from 1985 to 1986: The National Heart, Lung, and Blood Institute Percutaneous Transluminal Coronary Angioplasty Registry. J Am Coll Cardiol 12:1149, 1988.
10. Davis K: Coronary artery bypass surgery in women. In Eaker ED, Packer B, Wenger NK, et al (eds): Coronary Heart Disease in Women. Haymarket Doyma, New York, 1987, p 247.
11. Eaker ED, Kronmal R, Kennedy JW, et al: Comparison of the long-term, post-surgical survival of women and men in the Coronary Artery Surgery Study (CASS). Am Heart J 117:71, 1989.
12. Rahimtoola SH, Bennett AJ, Grunkemeier GL, et al: Survival at 15 to 18 years after coronary bypass surgery for angina in women. Circulation 99(5 Pt 2):II71, 1993.
13. Yusuf S, Zucker D, Peduzzi P, et al: Effect of coronary artery bypass graft surgery on survival: Overview of 10-year results from randomized trials by the Coronary Artery Bypass Graft Surgery Trialists Collaboration. Lancet 344:563, 1994.
14. Mark DB, Shaw LK, DeLong ER, et al: Absence of sex bias in the referral of patients for cardiac catheterization. N Engl J Med 330: 1101, 1994.
15. Shaw LJ, Miller DD, Romeis JC, et al: Gender differences in the noninvasive evaluation and management of patients with suspected coronary artery disease. Ann Intern Med 120:559, 1994.
16. Ayanian JZ, Epstein AM: Differences in the use of procedures between women and men hospitalized for coronary heart disease. N Engl J Med 325:221, 1991.
17. Shaw LJ, Kesler K, Peterson ED, et al: Long-term prognostic implications of abnormal stress electrocardiographic or myocardial perfusion scintigraphic measures in patients with angiographically insignificant coronary artery disease. J Am Coll Cardiol 27:78A, 1996.
18. Hachamovitch R, Berman DS, Kiat H, et al: Gender-related differences in clinical management after exercise nuclear testing. J Am Coll Cardiol 26:1457, 1995.
19. Califf RM, Armstrong PW, Carver JR et al: 27th Bethesda Conference: Matching the intensity of risk factor management with the hazard for coronary disease events. Task Force 5: Stratification of patients into high, medium and low risk subgroups for purposes of risk factor management. J Am Coll Cardiol 27:1007, 1996.
20. Furberg CD, Hennekens CH, Hulley SB, et al: 27th Bethesda Conference: Matching the intensity of risk factor management with the hazard for coronary disease events. Task Force 2: Clinical epidemiology: The conceptual basis for interpreting risk factors. J Am Coll Cardiol 27: 976, 1996.
21. Peterson ED, Shaw LJ, Oddone E: An empirical approach to evaluation of chest pain in women. J Clin Outcomes 2:9, 1996.
22. Pryor DB, Shaw LK, McCants CB, et al: Value of the history and physical in identifying patients at increased risk for coronary artery disease. Ann Intern Med 118:81, 1993.
23. Kannel WB, Feinleib M: Natural history of angina pectoris in the Framingham study: Prognosis and survival. Am J Cardiol 29:154, 1972.
24. Coplan NL, Fuster V: Limitations of the exercise test as a screen for acute cardiac events in asymptomatic patients. Am Heart J 119: 987, 1990.
25. Fuster V: Mechanisms leading to myocardial infarction: Insights from studies of vascular biology [erratum published in Circulation 91:256, 1995.]. Circulation 90:2126, 1994.
26. Fuster V, Badimon L, Badimon JJ, et al: The pathogenesis of coronary artery disease and acute coronary syndromes (1). N Engl J Med 326; 242, 1992.
27. Diamond GA, Forrester JS: Analysis of probability as an aid in the clinical diagnosis of coronary artery disease. N Engl J Med 300:1350, 1979.
28. Hlatky MA, Pryor DB, Harrell FE Jr, et al: Factors affecting sensitivity and specificity of exercise electrocardiography: Multivariable analysis. Am J Med 77:64, 1984.
29. Weiner DA, Ryan TJ, McCabe CH, et al: Exercise stress testing correlations among history of angina, ST segment response, and prevalence of coronary artery disease in the Coronary Artery Surgery Study (CASS). N Engl J Med 301:230, 1979.
30. Shaw LJ, Kesler K, Peterson ED, et al: The Duke Treadmill Score is an accurate predictor of the extent of coronary artery disease and 5-year survival. Circulation 92(Suppl 1):I271, 1995.
31. Epstein SE, Quyymi AA, Bonow RO: Sudden cardiac death without warning: Possible mechanisms and implications for screening asymptomatic populations. N Engl J Med 321:320, 1989.
32. Anderson KM, Wilson PWF, Odell PM, et al: An updated coronary risk profile: A statement for health professionals. Circulation 83:356, 1991.
33. Bush TL, Criqui MH, Cowan LD, et al: Cardiovascular disease mortality in women: Results from the lipid research clinics follow-up study. In Eaker ED, Packard B, Wenger NK (ed): Coronary Heart Disease in Women. Haymarket Doyma, New York, 1987, p 106.
34. Pryor DB, Harrell FE Jr, Lee KL, et al: Estimating the likelihood of significant coronary artery disease. Am J Med 75:771, 1983.
35. Pryor DB, Shaw LK, Harrell FE Jr, et al: Estimating the likelihood of severe coronary artery disease. Am J Med 90:552, 1991.
36. Douglas PS, Ginsburg GS: The evaluation of chest pain in women. N Engl J Med 334:1311, 1996.
37. Holdright DR, Fox KM: Characterization and identification of women and angina pectoris. Eur Heart J 17:510, 1996.
38. Shaw LJ, Miller DD, Romeis JC, et al: Prognostic value of noninvasive risk stratification and coronary revascularization in younger and older patients referred for evaluation of suspected coronary artery disease. J Am Geriatr Soc 44:1190, 1996.
39. Chaitman BR, Bourassa MG, Davis K, et al: Angiographic prevalence of high-risk coronary artery disease in patient subsets (CASS). Circulation 64:360, 1981.
40. Gray D, Hampton JR, Shaw LK, et al: Successful international application of a predictive model of coronary diseases. Circulation 86:I41, 1992.
41. Mark DB: Assessment of prognosis in patients with coronary artery disease. In Roubin GS, Califf RM, O'Neill WW, et al (eds): Interventional Cardiovascular Medicine: Principles and Practice. Churchill Livingstone, New York, 1994, p 165.
42. Levy D, Wilson DW, Anderson KM, et al: Stratifying the patient at risk from coronary disease: New insights from the Framingham Heart Study. Am Heart J 119:712, 1990.

CHAPTER

8 Noninvasive Diagnostic Testing

8.1 Exercise Testing in Women

Rollo P. Villareal and James T. Willerson

The predominant perception for many years has been that coronary artery disease (CAD) is less common and has a benign prognosis in women. Both perceptions are incorrect. CAD is the single leading cause of death and morbidity among women in the United States today, accounting for roughly 30% of all deaths.[1] Most U.S. women fear and can quote the one in nine incidence of breast cancer, but few realize that one in two women succumb to cardiovascular disease (CVD). Data from the American Heart Association and the Framingham Heart Study show that although the mortality of CVD in men has steadily declined, the rate for women has remained relatively stable.[1, 2]

There is an age-related increase in the incidence of CVD in women.[1–3] It is true that a lower incidence is observed in the younger and premenopausal woman, but convergence with the incidence of CAD in men is seen in postmenopausal women. By the age of 75 years, the rates of cardiovascular morbidity and mortality in men and women are equivalent. As the population ages and women's life expectancy lengthens, the significance of CVD increases.

Various gender-related differences have been demonstrated in morbidity and mortality associated with coronary syndromes and with revascularization in women and men. On the whole, women more commonly present with atypical chest pain, non–Q-wave myocardial infarctions (MIs), and nonfatal and silent MIs.[4–7] They have a higher mortality after MI as well as higher rates of reinfarction and clinical congestive heart failure.[8–11] Women are less likely to be evaluated noninvasively, to be referred for coronary angiography, and to undergo percutaneous or surgical revascularization.[12–20] Among patients who undergo revascularization, women fare worse than men.[21, 22] In the Coronary Artery Surgery Study (CASS), the operative mortality for women was 4.5%, compared with 1.9% for men.[23] Angioplasty registries likewise demonstrate a higher procedural mortality for women.[24–28]

The critical role of noninvasive testing in women is thus to diagnose CAD accurately in a population with a lower prevalence of disease prior to the development of more severe clinical manifestations, when therapeutic interventions have a higher risk and poorer outcomes. This subchapter focuses on the role of exercise testing in the assessment of CAD in women.

EXERCISE TESTING: THE ISSUE OF ACCURACY

Standard exercise electrocardiography (ECG) is the most commonly used and least costly of the noninvasive methods for the evaluation of patients with known or suspected ischemic heart disease. Its reported limitations in women include lower sensitivity and specificity and a higher false-positive rate than in men, but these differences may be explained, at least in part, by differences in disease prevalence and in the ischemic response to exercise.

Profant and colleagues[29] were the first to observe that exercise-induced ST depression was more common in normal women than in men. Wu and associates[30] reported a high incidence of false-positive results in women younger than 45 years, but this incidence decreased with patient age.[30] In a classic study, Sketch and associates[31] first described a low specificity for exercise ECG, reporting false-positive rates of 67% for women and 8% for men.[31] However, the prevalence of significant CAD as detected by coronary angiography in this group of patients was 8% for women and 53% for men. This finding strongly suggests that the lower incidence of CAD in women accounts for the lower post-test probability of disease and a less accurate test. Koppes and associates[32, 33] combined the results of four early studies and reported false-positive rates of 24% to 35% for women. Amsterdam and colleagues[34] reviewed the exercise ECG data of 96 men and 65 women who underwent treadmill testing and had normal coronary angiograms. These researchers reported a 15% false-positive rate for women and an 11% rate for men.

Weiner and coworkers[35] reported on the treadmill results from the CASS trial, which at the time had the largest female cohort (n = 580).[35] The sensitivity and specificity of exercise ECG were 76% and 64%, respectively, for women compared with 80% and 74%, respectively, for men (n = 1465). A 3% false-positive rate was reported for men, and a 14% rate for women. However, when the same population was matched for differences in baseline demographics and clinical characteristics, the differences in the false-positive rates were no longer detected.

Kwok and associates[36] performed a meta-analysis of 19 studies involving 3721 women who underwent exercise treadmill testing and confirmatory coronary angiography. The weighted mean sensitivity was 61%, and specificity was 70%. In the 10 studies that included men, sensitivity and specificity of such testing were 70% and 77%, respectively. These figures are consistent with an earlier, larger meta-analysis, performed by Gianrossi and colleagues,[37] of 147 studies involving 24,074 patients (mostly men), which yielded a weighted sensitivity of 68% and a specificity of 77% for exercise treadmill testing. Table 8–1 summarizes the findings of selected studies on exercise treadmill testing in women.[31, 35, 38–55]

Overall, these data demonstrate that the exercise ECG is less accurate in women than in men. Conversely, these data also show that the false-negative rate for women is low (12%

Table 8–1. SELECTED EXERCISE ELECTROCARDIOGRAM STUDIES

AUTHORS	YEAR	n	SENSITIVITY (%)	SPECIFICITY (%)
Sketch et al[31]	1975	56	45	78
Detry et al[38]	1977	47	80	63
Barolsky et al[39]	1979	92	60	68
Weiner et al[35]	1979	580	76	64
Guiteras et al[40]	1982	112	79	66
Friedman et al[41]	1982	60	32	75
Hung et al[42]	1984	92	75	59
Hlatky et al[43]	1984	613	57	86
Weiner et al[44]	1985	109	59	81
Masini et al[45]	1988	83	72	52
Sawada et al[46]	1989	57	29	83
Pratt et al[47]	1989	200	69	56
Robert et al[48]	1991	250	61	59
Chae et al[49]	1993	243	27	79
Richardson et al[50]	1995	62	91	51
Severi et al[51]	1994	122	71	46
Chikamori et al[52]	1995	132	82	54
Lee et al[53]	1995	188	65	71
Morise et al[54]	1995	660	51	76
Marwick et al[55]	1995	161	77	56

to 22%) and is comparable to that for men (12% to 40%). These findings suggest that routine treadmill testing, although less specific and with a higher false-positive rate, reliably excludes the presence of significant CAD in women with negative results as well as it does in men.

MECHANISMS FOR GENDER-RELATED DIFFERENCES IN THE EXERCISE ELECTROCARDIOGRAM

The cited reasons for a lower sensitivity and specificity of exercise testing in women are (1) a lower prevalence of multivessel CAD, (2) a digitalis-like effect of estrogen, (3) a higher likelihood of an inadequate exercise response, (4) a higher incidence of underlying ECG repolarization abnormalities, and (5) altered hemodynamics. They are discussed in detail here.

Lower Prevalence of Multivessel Coronary Artery Disease

Coronary angiography studies have consistently demonstrated that women have a lower prevalence of multivessel disease.[35, 56, 57] This fact reduces the specificity of exercise testing. Single-vessel disease is more common in women, and multivessel and left main disease are more common in men.[56, 57] These characteristics lower the sensitivity of exercise testing. If the documented CAD in the population tested is more extensive, it follows that the probability of detecting disease is higher and the occurrence of a false-positive result lower. Stated simply, patients with more severe disease have a higher incidence of abnormal test results.[42, 43]

Digitalis-Like Effect of Estrogen

Jaffe[58, 59] reported that postexercise ST depression increased in the presence of oral estrogen and that administration of testosterone diminished the effect.[58, 59] A later study by Vaitkevicius and coworkers[60] has demonstrated a clear association between the hyperventilation-induced ST segment response and estrogen replacement in postmenopausal women.[60] In an elegant study, Marmor and associates[61] followed the ST segment response in a cohort of women with false-positive exercise test results who subsequently underwent oophorectomy. After surgery, not only did the ST segment response for these women normalize, but institution of estrogen replacement therapy resulted in return of exercise-induced ST depression. Estrogens and digitalis have similar chemical structures. The hypothesis is that estrogen may exert a selective coronary vasoconstrictive effect, similar to the postulated mechanism for digitalis-associated ST segment changes. The exact mechanisms, however, remain to be elucidated.

Inadequate Exercise Response

Compared with men of the same age, women are more likely to be deconditioned and are less capable of achieving an adequate heart rate response to exercise.[62] The normal physiologic responses to exercise also differ in men and women. In similarly conditioned populations, women demonstrated lower values for ejection fraction, peak workload, and oxygen consumption.[63] Moreover, women with heart disease generally present at a later age with a greater number of comorbidities. Both factors significantly alter exercise capacity and limit or prevent achievement of adequate exercise parameters.[2] During stress, women also have a higher documented incidence of vasospasm.[64, 65] These factors may influence the accuracy of the stress test.

Repolarization Abnormalities

Baseline repolarization abnormalities have traditionally limited the interpretation of the stress ECG. In addition to the limitations already cited, women are more likely to have baseline ST segment depression and ECG repolarization abnormalities in association with mitral valve prolapse, a different chest wall configuration, ventricular hypertrophy, concomitant pharmacologic therapy, motion, and hyperventilation.[62, 66] These features can significantly limit the accuracy and predictive value of the stress test.

Altered Hemodynamics

Kusumi and associates,[67] examining hemodynamic variables in middle-aged women with false-positive treadmill test results, found an association between ST segment depression and increases in oxygen demand, arterial blood pressure, and peripheral vascular resistance. Their hypothesis was that greater subendocardial oxygen demand may explain the occurrence of false-positive test results. Reasons for the greater vasoreactivity were not offered.

In order to further clarify the variables that may influence the sensitivity and specificity of exercise testing, Hlatky and coworkers[43] performed a multivariate logistic regression analysis of 3094 patients who underwent both exercise testing and coronary angiography. The overall sensitivity of exercise testing was lower for women. The variables that independently affected sensitivity were the maximal heart rate achieved, the number of vessels diseased, the presence of typical angina, age, and female sex. The only variable found to independently affect specificity was the maximal heart rate achieved during exercise.

In summary, the results of exercise stress testing in women are less accurate because the currently measured test variables are affected by factors other than the mere presence of CAD.

STRATEGIES TO IMPROVE THE DIAGNOSTIC VALUE OF EXERCISE TESTING

Exercise testing provokes the physiologic sequelae of myocardial ischemia that are not limited to the electrical consequences manifested by ST segment change, the limitations of which have been eloquently summarized by Gianrossi and colleagues.[37] Strategies designed to improve the diagnostic yield of exercise testing have thus incorporated alternative stress test criteria using non-ECG variables (such as heart rate, angina, and exercise duration) or have combined exercise testing with another modality, such as nuclear myocardial perfusion imaging or echocardiography. In addition, there is a provocative report of the improvement of stress ECG sensitivity with the simple addition of right precordial leads.[68] Among the strategies utilizing alternate stress criteria, the ST segment/heart rate (ST/HR) index and slope, the Duke Treadmill Score (DTS), the multivariate approach, and the probabilistic approach appear the most promising.

The ST Segment/Heart Rate Slope and Index

In 1980, Elamin and associates[69] proposed HR adjustment of ST segment depression as a predictor of severity of CAD. This rate-related change in exercise-induced ST segment depression, or the ST/HR slope, attempts to adjust the extent of ST depression for the HR and to serve as an index of exercise-induced augmentation of myocardial oxygen demand. The ST/HR slope is based on linear regressions of the ST segment on HR during the various exercise stages. The calculations are already incorporated in the software of many stress testing systems.

Kligfield and colleagues[70] reported that setting an ST/HR slope value of 1.1 μV/beat/min as the upper limit of normal improved test sensitivity from 57% to 91% while preserving a specificity of more than 90%. An ST/HR slope of 6.0 or more was found to distinguish patients with three-vessel CAD with a sensitivity of 78%, a specificity of 97%, a positive predictive value of 93%, and an overall accuracy of 90%. These data suggested that the ST/HR slope could significantly improve the evaluation of patients with suspected CAD.

Later, Kligfield and colleagues[71] proposed a simpler approach to HR adjustment, the ST/HR index.[71] The ST/HR index is the ratio between the maximal exercise-induced ST segment change from rest and the maximal exercise-induced HR change from rest. An ST/HR index of 1.6 μV/beat/min improved the exercise test sensitivity from 68% to 91%. Lachterman and coworkers[72] attempted to reproduce these findings in 328 men who underwent exercise treadmill testing and confirmatory coronary angiography. These researchers reported no significant difference in the sensitivity between standard visual interpretation and the ST/HR index in terms of discriminating the presence or absence of CAD and three-vessel disease.

Okin and Kligfield[73] compared the diagnostic value of these methods in both men and women. Sensitivities were evaluated in a group of patients with angina and without angiographic confirmation of CAD who were pooled with a group of patients with angiographically proven CAD. Specificities were evaluated in clinically normal patients referred for checkup. The sensitivities for the standard criteria were 67% in men and 60% in women; the specificities for the standard criteria were 99% in men and 93% in women. The sensitivities for the ST/HR index were 93% in men and 82% in women, and for the ST/HR slope, 95% in men and 93% in women. The specificity for the ST/HR index was 97% for both men and women, and for the ST/HR slope, 98% in men and 97% in women. This study has been criticized as overestimating the sensitivity because of the inclusion of patients with typical clinical angina in the sensitivity calculation as well a high rate of beta blocker use, which affects the ability to achieve higher heart rates and can affect the ST/HR criteria. Although these data are encouraging, controversy still exists in the literature concerning the ST/HR indexes. Nonetheless, it seems obvious today that ST depression cannot be used by itself to evaluate for the presence and extent of disease without adjustment for the corresponding myocardial workload.

The Duke Treadmill Score

The DTS is a weighted index combining the ST segment deviation, the treadmill time, and the presence or absence of exercise-induced angina. The formula for the DTS is as follows:

$$\begin{aligned}\text{DTS} = {} & \text{exercise time in minutes} - \\ & 5 \times \text{ST deviation, in mm} - \\ & 4 \times \text{treadmill angina index.}\end{aligned}$$

(For the treadmill angina index, a score of 0 indicates no angina; a score of 1, the presence of nonlimiting angina; and a score of 2, the presence of exercise-limiting angina.)

Low risk was defined as a DTS greater than 5; moderate risk as a DTS between 5 and −10; and high risk as a DTS of −11 or less.

The DTS diagnostic and prognostic values were initially developed and validated in predominantly male populations.[74, 75] In 1998, Alexander and coworkers[76] examined the diagnostic and prognostic value of the DTS in 976 women and 2249 men who underwent both treadmill testing and coronary angiography. At every DTS risk level, women had less CAD than their male counterparts. At low risk scores, 81% of women had no significant CAD at angiography, compared with 53% of men. Of women with moderate risk scores, 65% had no significant CAD, 35% had significant CAD, and 12% had severe CAD. In contrast, few men with a moderate DTS had no significant CAD (18%); significant disease (82%) or severe disease (39%) was more common. Patients with high risk scores frequently had severe CAD (men, 72%, and women, 46%). The 2-year mortality rates for women with low, moderate, and high risk scores were 1.0%, 2.2%, and 3.5%, respectively; for men, the 2-year mortality rates were 1.7%, 5.8%, and 16.6%, respectively.

Because of differences in disease prevalence, women had a better survival at all values of the DTS in this study. Risk categories were essentially shifted down one level of severity in women. Because of a lower prevalence in women, a low-risk DTS was actually better at excluding CAD in women than in men. The conclusion of the study was that the DTS accurately stratified diagnostic and prognostic risk in women and that routine initial use of the treadmill in suitable candidates of both genders was acceptable.

The Multivariate Approach

The multivariate approach is also based on the premise that multiple variables other than the ST segment are of diagnostic and prognostic value. It utilizes computer-assisted stress ECG analysis, which incorporates the ST/HR approach previously described and factors such as peak HR, ST segment shifts, angina, and workload into a multivariate model, and then generates a multivariate score. The score reflects the global probability of CAD and enhances the reliability and diagnostic value of exercise treadmill testing in both men and women. Examples that have integrated this approach or portions thereof are the Barolsky score, the Deckers score, and the Robert score.

The Barolsky score is an offspring of the ST/HR relationship. In 1979, Barolsky and associates[39] observed that in patients with similar CAD prevalence, the positive predictive value of ST segment depression was higher in men than in women. These researchers introduced an exercise score with varying ST segment weights for men and for women. At the same peak heart rate, the same amount of ST segment deviation confers a lower likelihood of CAD for a woman.

Deckers and colleagues[77] studied 189 women and derived a discriminant score for women. This score was then compared with the diagnostic performance of the ST/HR index, the Barolsky score, and standard ST segment depression. The sensitivities of these indexes were 73%, 77%, 60%, and 48%, respectively, at a specificity of 90%; the sensitivities were 90%, 83%, 76%, and 60%, respectively, at a specificity of 80%. Decker and colleagues[77] concluded that the diagnostic yield of exercise testing in females could be improved by the use of more sophisticated ECG and exercise variables.

Robert and coworkers[48] assessed whether the diagnostic value of exercise testing could be enhanced in women by using multivariate analysis of exercise data, which included workload, heart rate, and ST segment deviation, to build a diagnostic model. They compared their multivariate model with conventional ST analysis, with and without adjustment for heart rate, and the Deckers score. In a group of 115 women undergoing cardiac catheterization and 76 volunteers, the sensitivity of the model was better than that of conventional ST analysis (70% vs. 59%) without a loss of specificity (85% vs. 93%). Receiver operator characteristic curves also showed a better diagnostic accuracy with the model (Fig. 8–1). These researchers concluded that in women, logistic analysis of exercise variables improves the diagnostic value of exercise testing.

Williams and associates[78] compared the diagnostic accu-

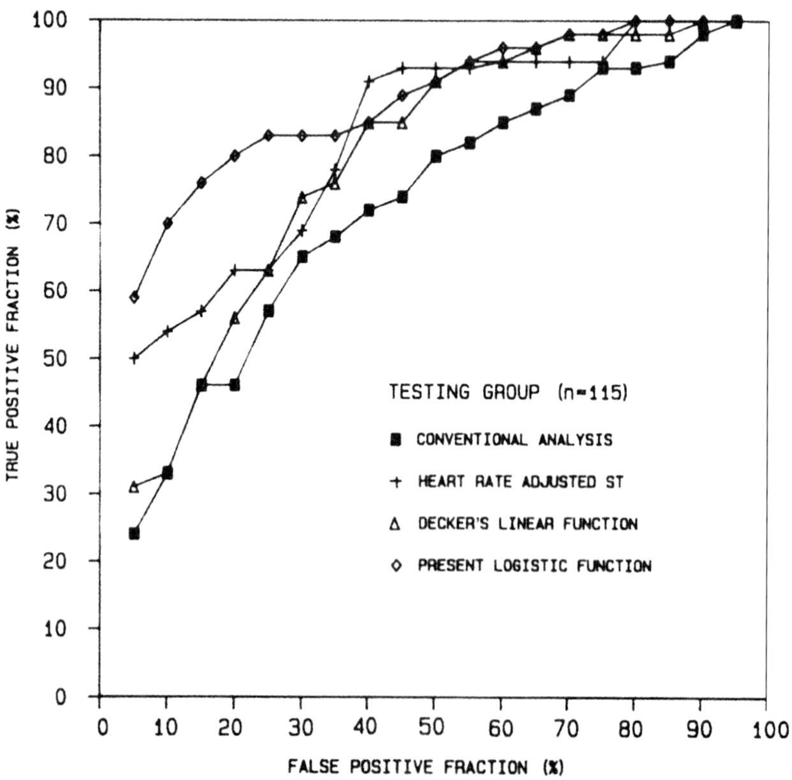

FIGURE 8–1. Plot of sensitivities at a fixed specificity for the prediction of CAD for conventional ST depression, heart rate–adjusted ST, Decker's score, and the Robert logistic function. The area under the Robert logistic analysis is significantly higher than that of the three other analyses and had the best diagnostic accuracy. (Modified from Robert AR, Melin JA, Detry JM: Logistic discriminant analysis improves diagnostic accuracy of exercise testing for coronary artery disease in women. Circulation 83:1202, 1991.)

racy of routine treadmill testing, a female-specific multivariate exercise score, and exercise echocardiography in 70 women who also underwent confirmatory coronary angiography. The reported sensitivities were 67%, 61%, and 88%, respectively, with specificities of 51%, 73%, and 84%, respectively. The accuracy of exercise echocardiography (86%) exceeded that of the exercise score (67%) and conventional ST analysis (59%). In comparison with conventional ST analysis, the exercise score yielded a better specificity without loss of sensitivity, although it was less accurate than stress echocardiography (Fig. 8–2).

Although these data are appealing, several areas of controversy remain. There is still disagreement as to (1) whether computerized ST analysis improves diagnostic accuracy, (2) which location of the ST segment is the optimal point of measurement, and (3) whether upsloping ST segments should be considered normal.[79–81] Clearly, further refinement and validation must occur before these techniques can take center stage.

The Probabilistic Approach

The probabilistic approach utilizes clinical and exercise test information in a sequential diagnostic strategy to arrive at the probability of a patient's having CAD.[82] A pretest probability (or prior risk ratio) is first obtained from the patient's age and symptomatology. A stress test is then performed, from which a likelihood ratio and then post-test probability of CAD are calculated. Depending on the value obtained, further imaging, or coronary angiography can be performed, or diagnostic workup ceases. If further imaging is performed, the prior post-test probability can be used as the pretest value for the subsequent test. As one would expect, such an approach could lead to a referral bias for coronary angiography. However, there are encouraging reports on the efficiency and cost effectiveness of this approach.[83] Furthermore, realistically, current practice and physician referral are already based on this principle.

Exercise Testing Combined with Myocardial Perfusion Imaging

Exercise myocardial perfusion imaging studies using thallium-201, technetium 99m (Tc-99m) sestamibi, or Tc-99m teboroxime have the advantage of directly imaging the myocardium and not depending on the ECG for diagnosis of ischemia. As with exercise ECG, reported sensitivities and specificities vary widely, ranging from 71% to 95% and 61% to 91%, respectively.[66] In a meta-analysis of five studies of exercise, thallium-201 perfusion imaging the weighted mean sensitivity was 78%, and the specificity was 64%.[36]

In a later study, Taillefer and associates[84] compared the sensitivity and specificity of either treadmill (n = 75) or dipyridamole (n = 37) thallium-201 perfusion, Tc-99m sestamibi perfusion, and Tc-99m sestamibi ECG-gated single photon emission tomography (SPECT) for the detection of CAD in women.[84] The overall sensitivities for detecting 50% or greater and 70% or greater stenoses were 75% and 84%, respectively, for thallium-201 perfusion imaging and 72% and 80%, respectively, for Tc-99m sestamibi perfusion studies (Fig. 8–3*A* and *B*). The specificity of Tc-99m sestamibi imaging was better for lesions 50% or greater (86% vs. 62% with thallium-201) and for lesions 70% or greater (82% vs. 59% for thallium-201) (Fig. 8–3*C*). The study demonstrates that thallium-201 and Tc-99m sestamibi studies have similar sensitivity levels for the detection of CAD in women, but that Tc-99m sestamibi has significantly better specificity.

Exercise Testing Combined with Echocardiography

Exercise echocardiography also has the advantage of directly imaging the myocardium and not relying on conventional ST

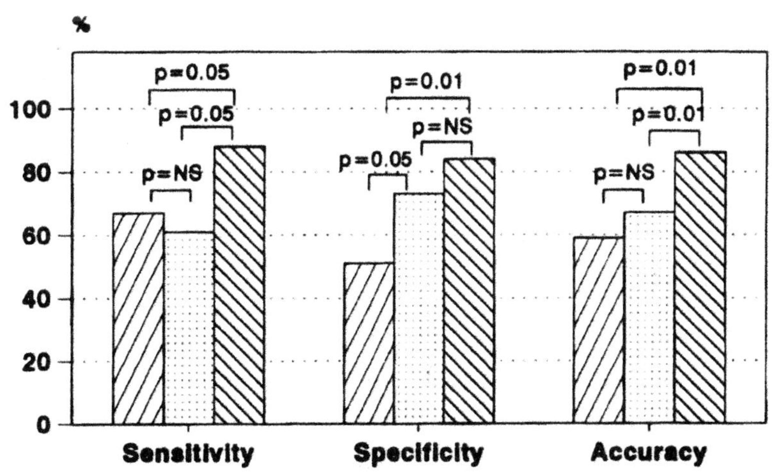

	Sensitivity	Specificity	Accuracy
ST analysis	67	51	59
Multivariate score	61	73	67
Exercise echo	88	84	86

ST analysis / Multivariate score / Exercise echo

FIGURE 8–2. Sensitivity, specificity, and accuracy of ST analysis, multivariate exercise score, and exercise echo in 70 women investigated for chest pain. Compared to conventional ST analysis, the exercise score yielded a better specificity without loss of sensitivity, although it was less accurate than stress echo. (From Williams MJ, Marwick TH, O'Gorman D, Foale RA: Comparison of exercise echocardiography with an exercise score to diagnose coronary artery disease in women. Am J Cardiol 74:435, 1994.)

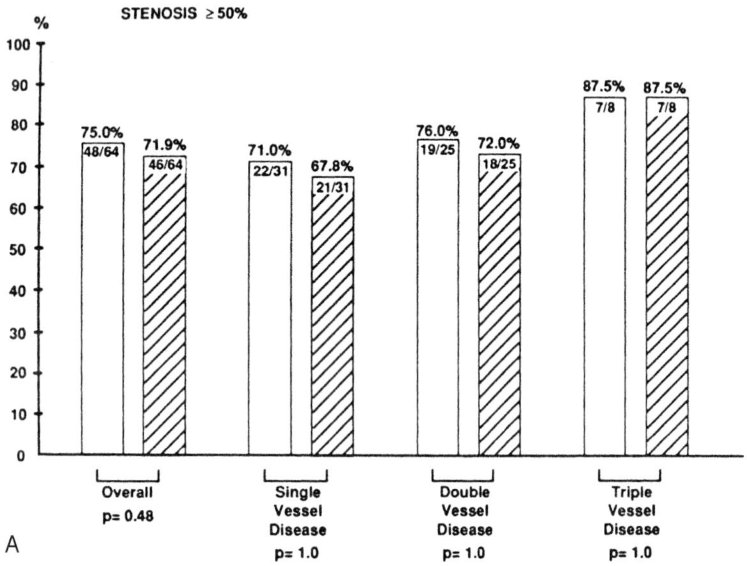

A

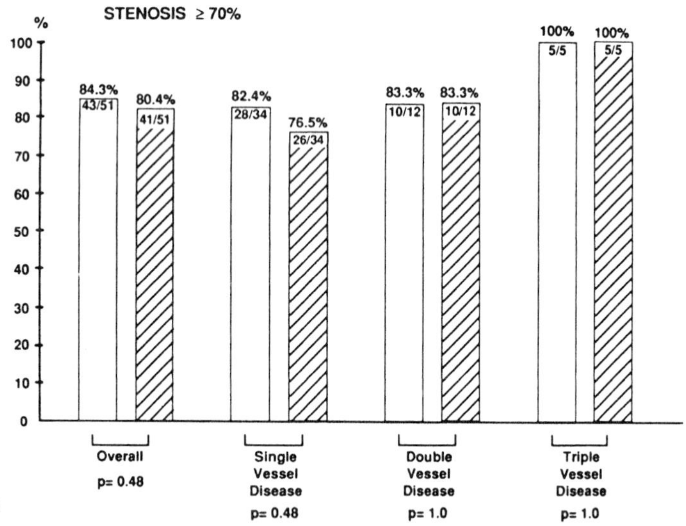

B

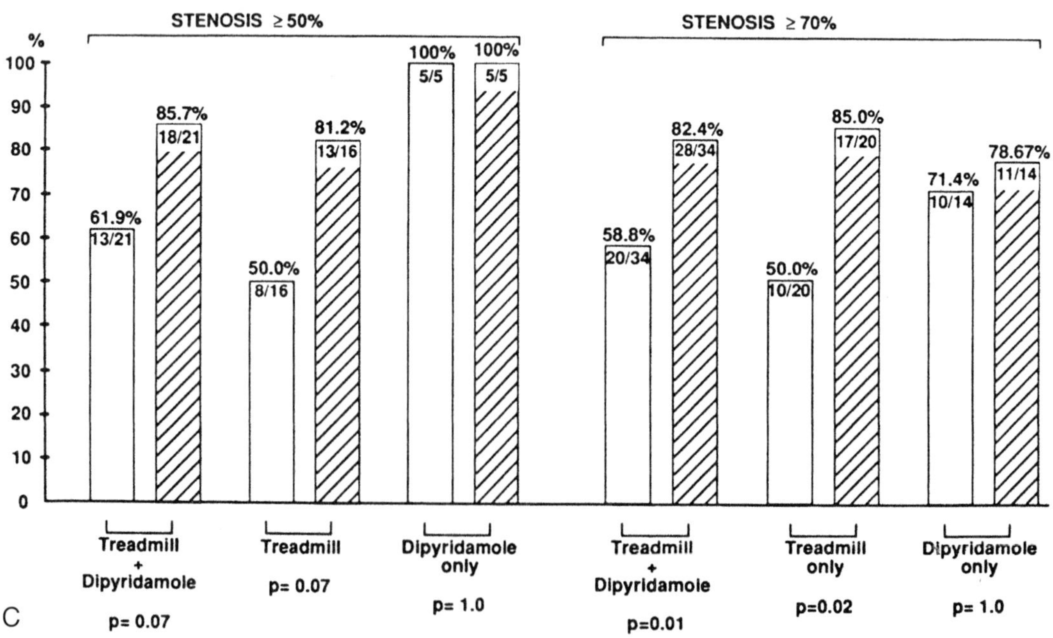

C

FIGURE 8–3. *A* and *B*, Sensitivity of thallium-201 *(open bars)* and Tc-99m sestamibi perfusion *(striped bars)* studies for the detection of single-, double-, and triple-vessel CAD in patients with 50% or more *(A)* and 70% or more *(B)* stenosis. *C*, Specificity of thallium-201 *(open bars)* and Tc-99m sestamibi *(striped bars)* studies for the detection of CAD in patients undergoing either treadmill testing or dipyridamole, or both. (From Taillefer R, DePuey EG, Udelson JE, et al: Comparative diagnostic accuracy of thallium-201 and Tc-99m sestamibi SPECT imaging [perfusion and ECG-gated SPECT] in detecting coronary artery disease in women. J Am Coll Cardiol 29:69, 1997.)

analysis for the diagnosis of ischemia. Furthermore, visualization of cardiac structures permits identification of disease that may explain the chest pain syndrome (i.e., mitral valve prolapse). Conversely, this technique is limited by local expertise and the ability to obtain a good "window." Chronic obstructive pulmonary disease, obesity, and other body habitus abnormalities may hinder the acquisition of good images. The available studies of exercise echocardiography have focused mostly on men, but the few available for women are very encouraging. Sawada and colleagues[46] studied 57 women subjected to either treadmill or bicycle echocardiography and coronary angiography. The sensitivity and specificity of exercise echocardiography were both 86%. In a meta-analysis of exercise echocardiography studies (total 296 women), the weighted mean sensitivity and specificity were 86% and 79%, respectively (Table 8–2).[36]

Right Precordial Leads

Michaelides and associates[68] compared the sensitivity and specificity of the standard 12-lead ECG, exercise ECG with right precordial leads (V_3R, V_4R, and V_5R), and thallium-201 scintigraphy in 218 men and 27 women, all of whom underwent confirmatory coronary angiography. Overall, the sensitivities of the three methods were 66%, 92%, and 93%, respectively, for the detection of any CAD, and the specificities were 88%, 88%, and 82%, respectively. A subset analysis of the women showed that use of the right precordial leads improved the sensitivity of exercise ECG from 71% to 88% without affecting specificity, which remained at 80%. However, we have tested this finding at our institution in a larger cohort of women (n = 40) and found no significant improvement in sensitivity (unpublished data).

CONCLUSIONS

Conventional ST segment analysis in conjunction with exercise treadmill testing is less accurate for the diagnosis of CAD in women than in men. However, a negative test result is a powerful tool for excluding the presence of CAD. Alternative strategies that incorporate various stress ECG and non-ECG variables improve the sensitivity and specificity of the conventional exercise treadmill test. Of these, the ST/HR indexes, DTS, and the multivariate approaches appear the most promising but require further refinement and validation. The sensitivity and specificity of the exercise test for the detection of CAD are also improved when the method is combined with myocardial perfusion imaging and echocardiography. Finally, the effect of the addition of right precordial leads is intriguing and deserves further study.

Table 8–2. SUMMARY OF EXERCISE ECHOCARDIOGRAPHY STUDIES

AUTHORS	YEAR	n	SENSITIVITY	SPECIFICITY
Sawada et al[46]	1989	57	0.86	0.86
Ryan et al[85]	1993	78	0.91	0.78
Marwick et al[55]	1995	161	0.80	0.81
All studies		296	0.86 (0.75–0.96)*	0.79 (0.72–0.86)*

*Weighted mean (95% confidence intervals).

Modified from Kwok Y, Kim C, Grady D, et al: Meta-analysis of exercise testing to detect coronary artery disease in women [see comments]. Am J Cardiol 83: 660, 1999.

References

1. American Heart Association: 2000 Heart and Stroke Statistical Update. American Heart Association, Dallas, TX, 1999.
2. Lerner DJ, Kannel WB: Patterns of coronary heart disease morbidity and mortality in the sexes. A 26-year follow-up of the Framingham population. Am Heart J 111:383, 1986.
3. Castelli WP: Cardiovascular disease in women. Am J Obstet Gynecol 158(6 Pt 2):1553, 1988.
4. Douglas PS, Ginsburg GS: The evaluation of chest pain in women [see comments]. N Engl J Med 334:1311, 1996.
5. Wenger NK, Speroff L, Packard B: Cardiovascular health and disease in women [see comments]. N Engl J Med 329:247, 1993.
6. Kennedy JW, Killip T, Fisher LD, et al: The clinical spectrum of coronary artery disease and its surgical and medical management, 1974–1979. The Coronary Artery Surgery study. Circulation 66(5 Pt 2): III16, 1982.
7. Kudenchuk PJ, Maynard C, Martin JS, et al: Comparison of presentation, treatment, and outcome of acute myocardial infarction in men versus women (the Myocardial Infarction Triage and Intervention Registry) [see comments]. Am J Cardiol 78:9, 1996.
8. Becker RC, Terrin M, Ross R, et al: Comparison of clinical outcomes for women and men after acute myocardial infarction. The Thrombolysis in Myocardial Infarction Investigators [see comments]. Ann Intern Med 120:638, 1994.
9. Kober L, Torp-Pedersen C, Ottesen M, et al: Influence of gender on short- and long-term mortality after acute myocardial infarction. TRACE study group. Am J Cardiol 77:1052, 1996.
10. Kostis JB, Wilson AC, O'Dowd K, et al: Sex differences in the management and long-term outcome of acute myocardial infarction: A statewide study. MIDAS Study Group. Myocardial Infarction Data Acquisition System. Circulation 90:1715, 1994.
11. Vaccarino V, Parsons L, Every NR, et al: Sex-based differences in early mortality after myocardial infarction. National Registry of Myocardial Infarction 2 Participants [see comments]. N Engl J Med 341:217, 1999.
12. Weitzman S, Cooper L, Chambless L, et al: Gender, racial, and geographic differences in the performance of cardiac diagnostic and therapeutic procedures for hospitalized acute myocardial infarction in four states. Am J Cardiol 79:722, 1997.
13. Wenger NK: Coronary heart disease in women: Gender differences in diagnostic evaluation. J Am Med Womens Assoc 49:181, 1994.
14. Shaw LJ, Miller DD, Romeis JC, et al: Gender differences in the noninvasive evaluation and management of patients with suspected coronary artery disease. Ann Intern Med 12:559, 1994.
15. Tobin JN, Wassertheil-Smoller S, Wexler JP, et al: Sex bias in considering coronary bypass surgery. Ann Intern Med 107:19, 1987.
16. Ayanian JZ, Epstein AM: Differences in the use of procedures between women and men hospitalized for coronary heart disease [see comments]. N Engl J Med 325:221, 1991.
17. Bell MR, Berger PB, Holmes DR Jr, et al: Referral for coronary artery revascularization procedures after diagnostic coronary angiography: Evidence for gender bias? J Am Coll Cardiol 25:1650, 1995.
18. Krumholz HM, Douglas PS, Lauer MS, Pasternak RC: Selection of patients for coronary angiography and coronary revascularization early after myocardial infarction: Is there evidence for a gender bias? [see comments]. Ann Intern Med 116:785, 1992.
19. Maynard C, Litwin PE, Martin JS, Weaver WD: Gender differences in the treatment and outcome of acute myocardial infarction: Results from the Myocardial Infarction Triage and Intervention Registry. Arch Intern Med 152:972, 1992.
20. Steingart RM, Packer M, Hamm P, et al: Sex differences in the management of coronary artery disease: Survival and Ventricular Enlargement Investigators [see comments]. N Engl J Med 325:226, 1991.
21. Khan SS, Nessim S, Gray R, et al: Increased mortality of women in coronary artery bypass surgery: Evidence for referral bias. Ann Intern Med 112:561, 1990.
22. Moen EK, Asher CR, Miller DP, et al: Long-term follow-up of gender-specific outcomes after thrombolytic therapy for acute myocardial infarction from the GUSTO-I trial: Global Utilization of Streptokinase

and Tissue Plasminogen Activator for Occluded Coronary Arteries. J Womens Health 6:285, 1997.
23. Fisher LD, Kennedy JW, Davis KB, et al: Association of sex, physical size, and operative mortality after coronary artery bypass in the Coronary Artery Surgery Study (CASS). J Thorac Cardiovasc Surg 84:334, 1982.
24. Kelsey SF, James M, Holubkov AL, et al: Results of percutaneous transluminal coronary angioplasty in women. 1985–1986 National Heart, Lung, and Blood Institute's Coronary Angioplasty Registry [see comments]. Circulation 87:720, 1993.
25. Bell MR, Holmes DR Jr, Berger PB, et al: The changing in-hospital mortality of women undergoing percutaneous transluminal coronary angioplasty. JAMA 269:2091, 1993.
26. Bell MR, Grill DE, Garratt KN, et al: Long-term outcome of women compared with men after successful coronary angioplasty. Circulation 91:2876, 1995.
27. Keelan ET, Nunez BD, Grill DE, et al: Comparison of immediate and long-term outcome of coronary angioplasty performed for unstable angina and rest pain in men and women [see comments]. Mayo Clin Proc 72:5, 1997.
28. Stone GW, Grines CL, Browne KF, et al: Comparison of in-hospital outcome in men versus women treated by either thrombolytic therapy or primary coronary angioplasty for acute myocardial infarction. Am J Cardiol 75:987, 1995.
29. Profant GR, Early RG, Nilson KL, et al: Responses to maximal exercise in healthy middle-aged women. J Appl Physiol 33:595, 1972.
30. Wu SC, Secchi MB, Radice M, et al: Sex differences in the prevalence of ischemic heart disease and in the response to a stress test in a working population. Eur Heart J 2:461, 1981.
31. Sketch MH, Mohiuddin SM, Lynch JD, et al: Significant sex differences in the correlation of electrocardiographic exercise testing and coronary arteriograms. Am J Cardiol 36:169, 1975.
32. Koppes G, McKiernan T, Bassan M, Froelicher VF: Treadmill exercise testing, part II. Curr Probl Cardiol 7:1, 1997.
33. Koppes G, McKiernman T, Bassan M, Froelicher VF: Treadmill exercise testing. Part I. Curr Probl Cardiol 7:1, 1977.
34. Amsterdam EA, Price JE, Chin R: Exercise stress testing in patients with angiographically normal coronary arteries: Similar frequency of false positive ischemic responses in males and females. Am J Cardiol 41:378, 1978.
35. Weiner DA, Ryan TJ, McCabe CH, et al: Exercise stress testing: Correlations among history of angina, ST-segment response and prevalence of coronary-artery disease in the Coronary Artery Aurgery Study (CASS). N Engl J Med 301:230, 1979.
36. Kwok Y, Kim C, Grady D, et al: Meta-analysis of exercise testing to detect coronary artery disease in women [see comments]. Am J Cardiol 83:660, 1999.
37. Gianrossi R, Detrano R, Mulvihill D, et al: Exercise-induced ST depression in the diagnosis of coronary artery disease: A meta-analysis. Circulation 80:87, 1989.
38. Detry JM, Kapita BM, Cosyns J, et al: Diagnostic value of history and maximal exercise electrocardiography in men and women suspected of coronary heart disease. Circulation 56:756, 1977.
39. Barolsky SM, Gilbert CA, Faruqui A, et al: Differences in electrocardiographic response to exercise of women and men: A non-Bayesian factor. Circulation 60:1021, 1979.
40. Guiteras P, Chaitman BR, Waters DD, et al: Diagnostic accuracy of exercise ECG lead systems in clinical subsets of women. Circulation 65:1465, 1982.
41. Friedman TD, Greene AC, Iskandrian AS, et al: Exercise thallium-201 myocardial scintigraphy in women: Correlation with coronary arteriography. Am J Cardiol 49:1632, 1982.
42. Hung J, Chaitman BR, Lam J, et al. Noninvasive diagnostic test choices for the evaluation of coronary artery disease in women: A multivariate comparison of cardiac fluoroscopy, exercise electrocardiography and exercise thallium myocardial perfusion scintigraphy. J Am Coll Cardiol 4:8, 1984.
43. Hlatky MA, Pryor DB, Harrell FE Jr, et al: Factors affecting sensitivity and specificity of exercise electrocardiography: Multivariable analysis. Am J Med 77:64, 1984.
44. Weiner DA: Accuracy of cardiomyography during exercise testing: Results of a multicenter study. J Am Coll Cardiol 6:502, 1985.
45. Masini M, Picano E, Lattanzi F, et al: High dose dipyridamole-echocardiography test in women: Correlation with exercise-electrocardiography test and coronary arteriography. J Am Coll Cardiol 12:682, 1988.
46. Sawada SG, Ryan T, Fineberg NS, et al: Exercise echocardiographic detection of coronary artery disease in women [see comments]. J Am Coll Cardiol 14:1440, 1989.
47. Pratt CM, Francis MJ, Divine GW, Young JB: Exercise testing in women with chest pain: Are there additional exercise characteristics that predict true positive test results? Chest 95:139, 1989.
48. Robert AR, Melin JA, Detry JM: Logistic discriminant analysis improves diagnostic accuracy of exercise testing for coronary artery disease in women. Circulation 83:1202, 1991.
49. Chae SC, Heo J, Iskandrian AS, et al: Identification of extensive coronary artery disease in women by exercise single-photon emission computed tomographic (SPECT) thallium imaging. J Am Coll Cardiol 21:1305, 1993.
50. Richardson MT, Holly RG, Amsterdam EA, Wang MQ: The value of ten common exercise tolerance test measures in predicting coronary disease in symptomatic females. Cardiology 86:243, 1995.
51. Severi S, Picano E, Michelassi C, et al: Diagnostic and prognostic value of dipyridamole echocardiography in patients with suspected coronary artery disease: Comparison with exercise electrocardiography. Circulation 89:1160, 1994.
52. Chikamori T, Hirakawa K, Seo H, et al: Diagnostic significance of exercise-induced ST-segment depression in the lateral limb leads in patients with suspected coronary artery disease. Am J Cardiol 76: 513, 1995.
53. Lee JH, Crump R, Ellestad MH: Significance of precordial T-wave increase during treadmill stress testing. Am J Cardiol 76:1297, 1995.
54. Morise AP, Diamond GA: Comparison of the sensitivity and specificity of exercise electrocardiography in biased and unbiased populations of men and women. Am Heart J 130:741, 1995.
55. Marwick TH, Anderson T, Williams MJ, et al: Exercise echocardiography is an accurate and cost-efficient technique for detection of coronary artery disease in women. J Am Coll Cardiol 26:335, 1995.
56. Chaitman BR, Bourassa MG, Davis K, et al: Angiographic prevalence of high-risk coronary artery disease in patient subsets (CASS). Circulation 64:360, 1981.
57. Welch CC, Proudfit WL, Sheldon WC: Coronary arteriographic findings in 1,000 women under age 50. Am J Cardiol 35:211, 1975.
58. Jaffe MD: Effect of oestrogens on postexercise electrocardiogram. Br Heart J 38:1299, 1976.
59. Jaffe MD: Effect of testosterone cypionate on postexercise ST segment depression. Br Heart J 39:1217, 1977.
60. Vaitkevicius P, Wright JG, Fleg JL: Effect of estrogen replacement therapy on the ST-segment response to postural and hyperventilation stimuli. Am J Cardiol 64:1076, 1989.
61. Marmor A, Zeira M, Zohar S: Effects of bilateral hystero-salpingo-oophorectomy on exercise-induced ST-segment abnormalities in young women. Am J Cardiol 71:1118, 1993.
62. Cerqueira MD: Diagnostic testing strategies for coronary artery disease: Special issues related to gender. Am J Cardiol 75:52D, 1995.
63. Gibbons RJ, Lee KL, Cobb F, Jones RH: Ejection fraction response to exercise in patients with chest pain and normal coronary arteriograms. Circulation 64:952, 1981.
64. Sullivan AK, Holdright DR, Wright CA, et al: Chest pain in women: Clinical, investigative, and prognostic features. BMJ 308:883, 1994.
65. Cannon RO, Camici PG, Epstein SE: Pathophysiological dilemma of syndrome X. Circulation 85:883, 1992.
66. Redberg RF: Diagnostic testing for coronary artery disease in women and gender differences in referral for revascularization. Cardiol Clin 16:67, 1998.
67. Kusumi F, Bruce RA, Ross MA, et al: Elevated arterial pressure and postexertional ST-segment depression in middle-aged women. Am Heart J 92:576, 1976.
68. Michaelides AP, Psomadaki ZD, Dilaveris PE, et al: Improved detection of coronary artery disease by exercise electrocardiography with the use of right precordial leads [see comments]. N Engl J Med 340:340, 1999.
69. Elamin MS, Mary DA, Smith DR, Linden RJ: Prediction of severity of coronary artery disease using slope of submaximal ST segment/heart rate relationship. Cardiovasc Res 14:681, 1980.
70. Kligfield P, Okin PM, Ameisen O, Borer JS: Evaluation of coronary artery disease by an improved method of exercise electrocardiography: The ST segment/heart rate slope. Am Heart J 112:589, 1986.
71. Kligfield P, Ameisen O, Okin PM: Heart rate adjustment of ST segment depression for improved detection of coronary artery disease. Circulation 79:245, 1989.
72. Lachterman B, Lehmann KG, Detrano R, et al: Comparison of ST

segment/heart rate index to standard ST criteria for analysis of exercise electrocardiogram [see comments]. Circulation 82:44, 1990.
73. Okin PM, Kligfield P: Identifying coronary artery disease in women by heart rate adjustment of ST-segment depression and improved performance of linear regression over simple averaging method with comparison to standard criteria. Am J Cardiol 69:297, 1992.
74. Mark DB, Shaw L, Harrell FE Jr, et al: Prognostic value of a treadmill exercise score in outpatients with suspected coronary artery disease [see comments]. N Engl J Med 325:849, 1991.
75. Mark DB, Shaw LK, DeLong ER, et al: Absence of sex bias in the referral of patients for cardiac catheterization [see comments]. N Engl J Med 330:1101, 1994.
76. Alexander KP, Shaw LJ, Shaw LK, et al: Value of exercise treadmill testing in women [published erratum appears in J Am Coll Cardiol 33: 289, 1999]. J Am Coll Cardiol 32:1657, 1998.
77. Deckers JW, Rensing BJ, Simoons ML, Roelandt JR: Diagnostic merits of exercise testing in females. Eur Heart J 10:543, 1989.
78. Williams MJ, Marwick TH, O'Gorman D, Foale RA: Comparison of exercise echocardiography with an exercise score to diagnose coronary artery disease in women. Am J Cardiol 74:435, 1994.
79. Detrano R, Salcedo E, Leatherman J, Day K: Computer-assisted versus unassisted analysis of the exercise electrocardiogram in patients without myocardial infarction. J Am Coll Cardiol 10:794, 1987.
80. Okin PM, Kligfield P: Effect of precision of ST-segment measurement on identification and quantification of coronary artery disease by the ST/HR index. J Electrocardiol 24(Suppl):62, 1992.
81. Froelicher V, Myers J, Follansbee W, Labovitz A: Special Methods: Computerized Exercise ECG Analysis, 3rd ed. Mosby, St. Louis, 1993.
82. Diamond GA, Forrester JS: Analysis of probability as an aid in the clinical diagnosis of coronary-artery disease. N Engl J Med 300:1350, 1979.
83. Melin JA, Wijns W, Vanbutsele RJ, et al: Alternative diagnostic strategies for coronary artery disease in women: Demonstration of the usefulness and efficiency of probability analysis. Circulation 71:535, 1985.
84. Taillefer R, DePuey EG, Udelson JE, et al: Comparative diagnostic accuracy of Tl-201 and Tc-99m sestamibi SPECT imaging (perfusion and ECG-gated SPECT) in detecting coronary artery disease in women. J Am Coll Cardiol 29:69, 1997.
85. Ryan T, Segar DS, Sawada SG, et al: Detection of coronary artery disease with upright bicycle exercise echocardiography. J Am Soc Echocardiogr 6:186, 1993.

8.2 Nuclear Imaging

A. Iain McGhie, Marcy Lim, and James T. Willerson

The early detection of coronary artery disease (CAD) in women is critical, because 40% of all coronary events in women are fatal. Moreover, 67% of all sudden coronary deaths occur in women who have no history of CAD.[1] Although women are more likely than men to present with angina, the reliability of chest pain as a predictor of underlying CAD is lower in women. Only about 50% of women have angiographic evidence of CAD when they present with angina.[2, 3] Therefore, noninvasive testing is important in the evaluation of women in whom CAD is suspected.

EXERCISE TESTING

Exercise testing is widely used either as a diagnostic aid in patients with suspected CAD or as a technique to provide information on prognosis and heart function in patients known to have CAD. The role of exercise testing in women is controversial, however, because exercise testing has a lower accuracy in women than in men. The existing literature is divided as to the reason for this lower accuracy in women; lower specificity and lower sensitivity have been cited.

The largest study of the predictive accuracy of exercise electrocardiography (ECG) testing in women and men is the CASS.[4] In that study, the false-positive rate was 12% for men (n = 1465) and 54% for women (n = 580). However, the prevalence rate of CAD was higher in men (70%) than in women (29%). Moreover, after matching for age, prevalence, and severity of CAD, investigators found no significant differences in test sensitivity between men (76%) and women (78%), but lower specificity in women (64%) than in men (73%). When only patients with a normal resting ECG were analyzed, no significant difference in test specificity was noted between men and women. These findings were similar to those reported by Barolsky and associates,[5] who found similar sensitivity values in men and women but a lower specificity value in women than in men (68% vs. 89%). However, when patients taking digoxin were excluded from analysis, the specificity was 95% in men and in women, but the sensitivity was lower in women than in men (50% vs. 64%).

Several studies have shown that using the ST/HR index and slope in the interpretation of the test impoves the diagnostic accuracy of exercise ECG testing. Okin and Kligfield[6] found that using standard ST segment criteria (0.1 mV of horizontal or downward depression 60 msec after the J point) yielded a similar specificity of 96% in both sexes, but a lower sensitivity in women than in men (Fig. 8–4). Although these investigators found no significant differences in the ST segment during exercise in normal women, women with CAD had significantly less ST segment depression. Applying gender-specific ST/HR slope criteria significantly improved sensitivity in both men and women with respect to the standard criteria, but the improvement in sensitivity was greater in women.

The explanation for lower sensitivity of exercise ECG testing in women is unclear but probably relates to less ST segment depression in women. The reason for this gender difference is also unclear but is likely multifactorial. For example, the difference may be related in part to lower exercise tolerance in women, which leads to lower maximal heart rates and systolic blood pressures at peak exercise. In addition, studies have shown that estrogen affects coronary vasomotor tone. Evidence suggests that estrogen may influence the response of the ST segment during exercise.[7, 8] In a double-blind crossover study of woman with CAD, Rosano and colleagues[8] reported that sublingual administration of estradiol lengthened the time to ST segment depression and the total duration of treadmill exercise testing.

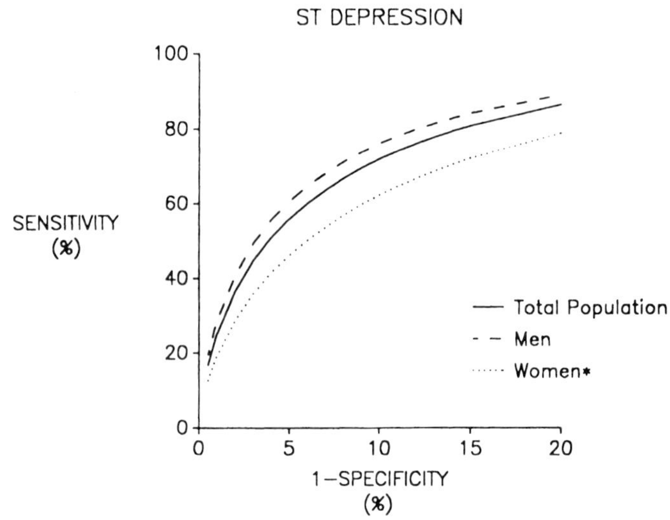

FIGURE 8–4. Receiver operating characteristic curves comparing the overall performance of the simple magnitude of ST depression for the identification of coronary artery disease in the total population and in men and women ($p < .05$). (From Okin PM, Kligfield P: Gender-specific criteria and performance of the exercise electrocardiogram. Circulation 92:1209, 1995.)

The use of exercise ECG testing in women with suspected or known CAD requires careful consideration and should be individualized for each patient. The low specificity of exercise testing in women relates in part to the lower prevalence of CAD in younger age groups and to the higher prevalence of baseline abnormalities in resting ECG. In addition to chest pain, these patients often have an abnormal resting ECG and a false-positive or inconclusive exercise ECG test result. In this situation, stress myocardial perfusion imaging may be useful in determining whether the chest pain is caused by underlying CAD.[9, 10]

In summary, if the pretest likelihood of CAD is low, the clinical examination is normal without evidence of mitral valve prolapse, the resting ECG is normal, and the woman can exercise adequately, an exercise ECG may be a reasonable initial diagnostic test. Otherwise, a stress test should be combined with an imaging procedure in a woman with suspected CAD.

EXERCISE RADIONUCLIDE VENTRICULOGRAPHY

Exercise radionuclide ventriculography, either a first-pass or gated equilibrium technique, is used as both a diagnostic and a prognostic tool in patients with suspected or known CAD.[11–15] In initial studies, the technique had a high level of accuracy for detecting CAD. For a variety of reasons, however, the specificity of radionuclide ventriculography declined once it became more widely applied to patients with suspected CAD.[16]

In exercise radionuclide ventriculography, the subject usually exercises with a bicycle ergometer, either in the upright position if the first-pass technique is employed or in the supine position if the gated equilibrium technique is used. Although significant hemodynamic differences are observed in the responses to upright and supine exercise,[17, 18] these differences do not appear to influence the accuracy of the technique.[19] Whether the patient's gender is of importance in the left ventricular response to exercise has been an area of contention. Several studies have suggested that there are significant gender-related differences in the left ventricular response to exercise.[20–25] In general, these studies have shown that the left ventricular ejection fraction increases less in women and that the incidence of an abnormal ejection fraction response is higher in women without apparent cardiac disease. For example, in a study from the Mayo Clinic, Hanley and associates[24] evaluated 192 men and 67 women with a low pretest likelihood of CAD who were undergoing supine exercise radionuclide ventriculography (Table 8–3). These researchers found that (1) men had lower ejection fractions at rest than women, (2) the ejection fraction increased more with exercise in men than in women, and (3) the left ventricular ejection fraction fell in 30% of women but in 16% of men. In addition, they found that the end-diastolic volume index at rest was lower and that it increased more with exercise in women than in men. In contrast, other studies of upright exercise ventriculography

Table 8–3. RADIONUCLIDE ANGIOGRAPHIC VARIABLES AT REST AND DURING EXERCISE

	MEN (n = 192) (mean ± SEM)	WOMEN (n = 67) (mean ± SEM)	*p* VALUE
EF			
Rest	0.63 (±0.01)	0.66 (±0.01)	<.05
Peak exercise	0.71 (±0.01)	0.68 (±0.01)	<.05
ΔEF			
Mean	0.08 (±0.01)	0.02 (±0.01)	<.0001
25th percentile	0.03	−0.02	
75th percentile	0.13	0.09	
EDVI			
Rest (ml/m^2)	97 (±2)	87 (±3)	<.005
Peak exercise (ml/m^2)	95 (±2)	93 (±4)	NS
ΔEDVI (ml/m^2)	−2 (±1)	6 (±2)	<.005

EDVI, end-diastolic volume index; ΔEDVI, exercise EDVI − rest EDVI; EF, ejection fraction; ΔEF, exercise EF − rest EF; SEM, standard error of the mean.

Adapted from Hanley PC, Zinsmeister AR, Clements IP: Gender-related differences in cardiac response to supine exercise assessed by radionuclide angiography. J Am Coll Cardiol 13:624, 1989.

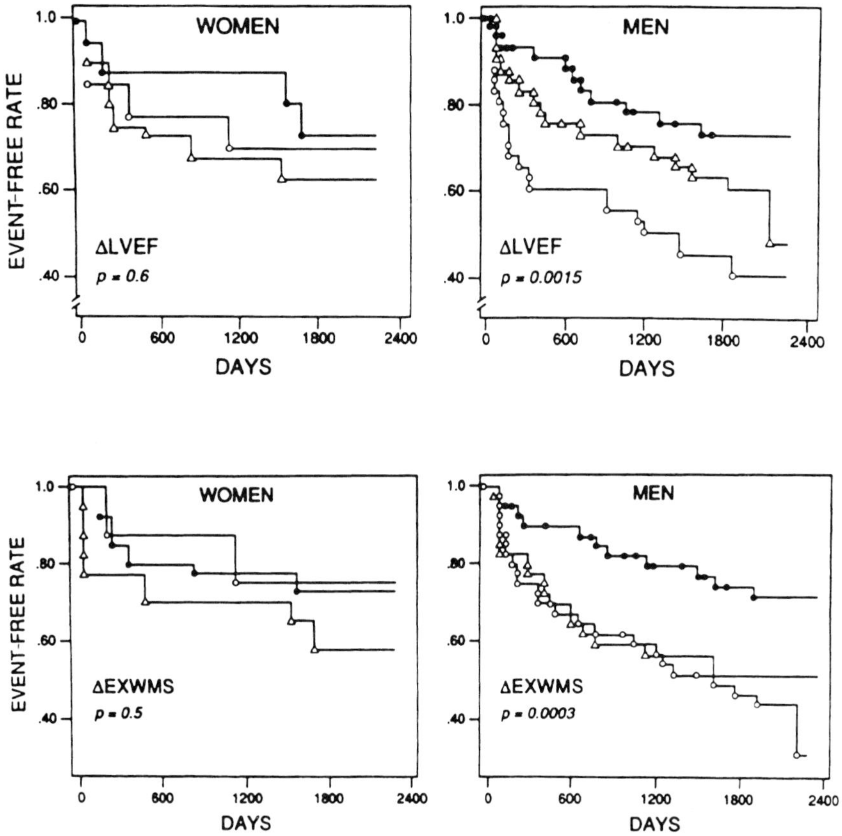

FIGURE 8–5. Kaplan-Meier survival curves for women and men with greater than 1 luminal diameter stenosis of 50% or more in a major coronary artery. *Upper Panels*, According to change in left ventricular ejection fraction (LVEF), expressed as change from rest to peak exercise in absolute %. Symbol key: *closed circles,* LVEF change ≥ 5%; *open triangles,* LVEF change −5% to +5%; *open circles,* LVEF change ≥ −5%. *Lower Panels*, According to worsening exercise wall motion score (△ EXWMS), calculated as (sum of the 5 left ventricular segmental scores at rest) − (sum of the 5 segmental scores at peak exercise). Symbol key: *closed circles,* worsening exercise wall motion score less than 1; *open triangles,* worsening exercise wall motion score 2 to 3; *open circles,* worsening exercise wall motion score of 4 or more. (From Moriel M, Rozanski A, Klein J, et al: The limited efficacy of exercise radionuclide ventriculography in assessing prognosis in women with coronary artery disease. Am J Cardiol 76:1030, 1995.)

have shown no gender-based differences in the left ventricular response to exercise.[26–27]

Exercise radionuclide ventriculography has been used to stratify patients with CAD by risk. Jones and colleagues[13] reported that patients with an abnormal exercise ejection fraction had a 20% higher mortality after 3 years than patients with a normal response. Bonow and coworkers[14] monitored a group of patients with triple-vessel coronary disease; the 18-month survival was less than 80% in patients who had a decrease in ejection fraction, an ST segment depression, and a limited capacity for exercise, whereas the remaining patients had an excellent prognosis. Similar results have been reported in patients with single- and double-vessel disease.[15] None of these studies specifically examined the influence of gender on their results. However, in a 5-year study, Moriel and associates[28] evaluated the influence of gender on the use of radionuclide ventriculography for establishing prognosis in 419 patients (74 women and 345 men) with CAD.[28] During the study, 96 patients (23%) experienced cardiac events. Although the left ventricular response to exercise (i.e., the change in left ventricular ejection fraction and wall motion score) provided prognostic information in both the combined population and men, it yielded no useful prognostic information in women (Fig. 8–5).

In summary, exercise radionuclide ventriculography appears to have limited application in the management of women with suspected or known CAD. This limit on usefulness may result from gender differences in the left ventricular response to exercise. Stress myocardial perfusion imaging, which has not been associated with gender differences, may be more useful than exercise radionuclide ventriculography in women with known or suspected CAD.

STRESS MYOCARDIAL PERFUSION IMAGING

Diagnostic Accuracy

Stress myocardial perfusion imaging is the most widely used nuclear technique for evaluating patients with suspected or known CAD. The widespread application of this technique is a consequence of its proven diagnostic accuracy, prognostic power, and widespread availability. In a meta-analysis of 122 studies of patients with suspected or known CAD, the mean sensitivity for planar exercise thallium-201 imaging was 84% (1775/2118), and the mean specificity was 87% (990/1140).[29] In a review of 13 studies of thallium-201 SPECT imaging, the mean sensitivity was 88% and the mean specificity was, 87%.[30]

Limited data are available on the accuracy of stress myocardial perfusion imaging in women (Table 8–4).[31–36] Friedman and colleagues[31] studied exercise-redistribution planar thallium-201 imaging in 60 women with suspected CAD. They reported a sensitivity of 75% and a specificity of 97% when only abnormal results induced by exercise were considered. When both fixed and reversible defects were considered, the sensitivity was 79% and the specificity was 88%. Sensitivity and specificity for exercise ECG were much lower (32% and 41%, respectively). In a similar study of exercise-redistribution planar thallium-201 imaging, Hung and associ-

Table 8–4. SENSITIVITY AND SPECIFICITY OF STRESS MYOCARDIAL PERFUSION IMAGING IN WOMEN

SOURCE	TECHNIQUE	STRESS	NO. OF WOMEN	SENSITIVITY (%)	SPECIFICITY (%)
Freidman et al[31]	Planar	Exercise	60	75	97
Hung et al[32]	Planar	Exercise	92	75	91
Melin et al[33]	Planar	Exercise	93	58	80
Kong et al[35]	Planar	Dipyridamole	43	87	58
Chae et al[36]	SPECT	Exercise	243	71	65
Ficaro et al[42]	SPECT	Exercise/pharmacologic	59	86	87
Ficaro et al[42]	AC-SPECT	Exercise/pharmacologic	59	93	98

AC-SPECT, attenuation-corrected single photon emission computed tomography; SPECT, single photon emission computed tomography.

ates[32] reported that in 92 symptomatic women without prior MI, the exercise ECG had a sensitivity of 73% and a specificity of 59%. The sensitivity of exercise ECG alone (75%) was not statistically different, but the specificity was significantly higher (91%). In a later study of exercise thallium-201 SPECT imaging in 243 women, Chae and colleagues[36] reported that the method had a sensitivity of 71% and a specificity of 65% for the detection of CAD. The exercise ECG had a sensitivity of 66% and a specificity of 60% after the exclusion of patients who did not attain 85% of predicted heart rate or who had baseline ECG abnormalities.

In a comparison of the diagnostic accuracies of planar and thallium-201 SPECT imaging methods, Fintel and coworkers[34] found that at a specificity of 90%, SPECT imaging had a sensitivity of 94% in men and of 86% in women. At the same specificity, planar imaging had a sensitivity of 82% in men and of 84% in women. Kong and associates[35] studied the effect of gender on the diagnostic accuracy of dipyridamole planar thallium-201 imaging in 114 patients. In this study, the overall sensitivity for detection of CAD was 87% for women and 94% for men, and the specificity was 58% in women and 63% in men; these differences did not reach statistical significance.

Tc-99m sestamibi imaging offers potential benefits over thallium-201 imaging in women because of the more favorable dosimetry and higher-energy photons associated with Tc-99m. Taillefer and colleagues[37] compared the diagnostic accuracy of Tc-99m sestamibi and thallium-201 perfusion imaging methods in 115 women (85 patients and 30 controls). All patients underwent stress perfusion imaging with both radiopharmaceuticals. These researchers reported no difference in sensitivity between the two techniques, with a value of 71.9% for Tc-99m sestamibi and 80.4% for thallium-201. However, the specificity of Tc-99m sestamibi was significantly lower than that for thallium-201 (58.8% versus 82.4%; $p = .01$).

Gender does not appear to have a significant effect on the clinical usefulness of preoperative dipyridamole thallium-201 imaging. Hendel and coworkers[38] found that preoperative thallium-201 imaging was equally useful for predicting short- and long-term events in both men and women undergoing vascular surgery. Interestingly, these researchers observed gender-specific differences in the predictive value of several clinical risk factors. The presence of Q waves on the electrocardiogram and a history of cardiac failure were predictors of both perioperative and late events in men but not in women. Similarly, dipyridamole-induced ST segment depression was strongly predictive of perioperative events in men but not in women.

Gender Differences in Myocardial Distribution of Activity

The normal distribution of activity of tracer uptake has certain characteristic patterns in cardiac SPECT imaging. Typically, the lateral wall–septal wall activity ratio is greater than 1. The activity at the base of the septum is diminished because of the reductions in thickness of the membranous septum and left ventricular outflow tract. The apex, which is a thin region, has reduced activity. In addition, the myocardial distribution of activity differs in men and women.[39, 40] In women, the activity of the anterior wall of the left ventricle is usually reduced because of breast attenuation (Color Plate 8–1). Depending on the size, shape, and location of the breasts, the attenuation can result in diminished activity of the anterolateral wall. Typically, the apex is not affected by breast attenuation, a fact that can be helpful in differentiating breast attenuation from left anterior descending CAD. If care is not taken to ensure that the position of the breasts does not change between acquisition of stress and rest images, varying degrees of attenuation can result in reversible or partial perfusion abnormalities, which can be incorrectly interpreted as ischemia. In men, the normal myocardial distribution of activity is characterized by reduced activity along the inferior aspects of the left ventricle, which is especially prominent toward the base (Color Plate 8–1).

Related Technical Developments

Because of important technical advances in nuclear cardiology, the diagnostic accuracy of myocardial perfusion imaging is likely to improve. The first of these advances has been the application of attenuation correction to conventional SPECT images. As discussed previously, attenuation, which is often gender related, can alter the activity distribution in SPECT images. Comparing polar-map displays of patients' perfusion studies with those of gender-matched, normal control subjects can help correct the attenuation. However, use of polar maps is only partially successful because of individual variability in body size and shape. Positron emission tomography (PET) uses attenuation correction that is individualized for each patient, eliminating attenuation artifacts and enhancing diagnostic accuracy.

Attenuation correction has also been applied to conventional SPECT images. Ficaro and associates[41] used simultaneous emission-transmission imaging with a multidetector system to produce attenuation-corrected images, which have significantly enhanced the diagnostic accuracy of myocardial

SPECT imaging. Figure 8–6 shows stress Tc-99m sestamibi tracer distribution in patients with less than 5% pretest likelihood of CAD. Tracer distribution in the posterior and lateral walls was 7% to 9% higher in women than in men ($p < .001$); after attenuation correction, there were no significant differences between the sexes. Also after attenuation correction, the sensitivity rose from 78% to 84%, and the specificity from 46% to 82%, in all patients. The same research group has presented data in women showing that the use of attenuation correction improves sensitivity from 86% to 93% with both visual and quantitative analyses and improves specificity from 87% to 98% with visual analysis and from 68% to 88% with quantitative analysis.[42]

With the advent of Tc-99m–labeled perfusion agents, the use of gated-SPECT myocardial perfusion imaging has increased.[37, 43–45] In addition to providing functional information and greater sensitivity and specificity, gated studies help to discriminate fixed defects caused by scar from attenuation artifacts and improve the accuracy of SPECT imaging in both sexes. For example, in women with a mild fixed anterior perfusion defect with normal wall thickening and wall motion, the abnormality most likely represents breast attenuation rather than scar, particularly if there is no ECG evidence of prior MI. In the future, these improvements in cardiac SPECT imaging will increase its use and thus its predictive accuracy.

NUCLEAR CARDIOLOGY TECHNIQUES IN WOMEN WITH KNOWN OR SUSPECTED HEART DISEASE

Several studies have examined the influence of gender on referral for cardiac catheterization after noninvasive testing.[45–49] In an early study by Tobin and associates,[45] only 4% of women were referred for cardiac catheterization after abnormal results on a stress nuclear procedure, compared with 40% of men. Even after results were controlled for age, previous MI, symptoms, and abnormal test results, men were 6.5 times more likely than women to be referred for cardiac catheterization. Mark and colleagues[48] also found a higher referral rate for men than women (27% versus 18%).

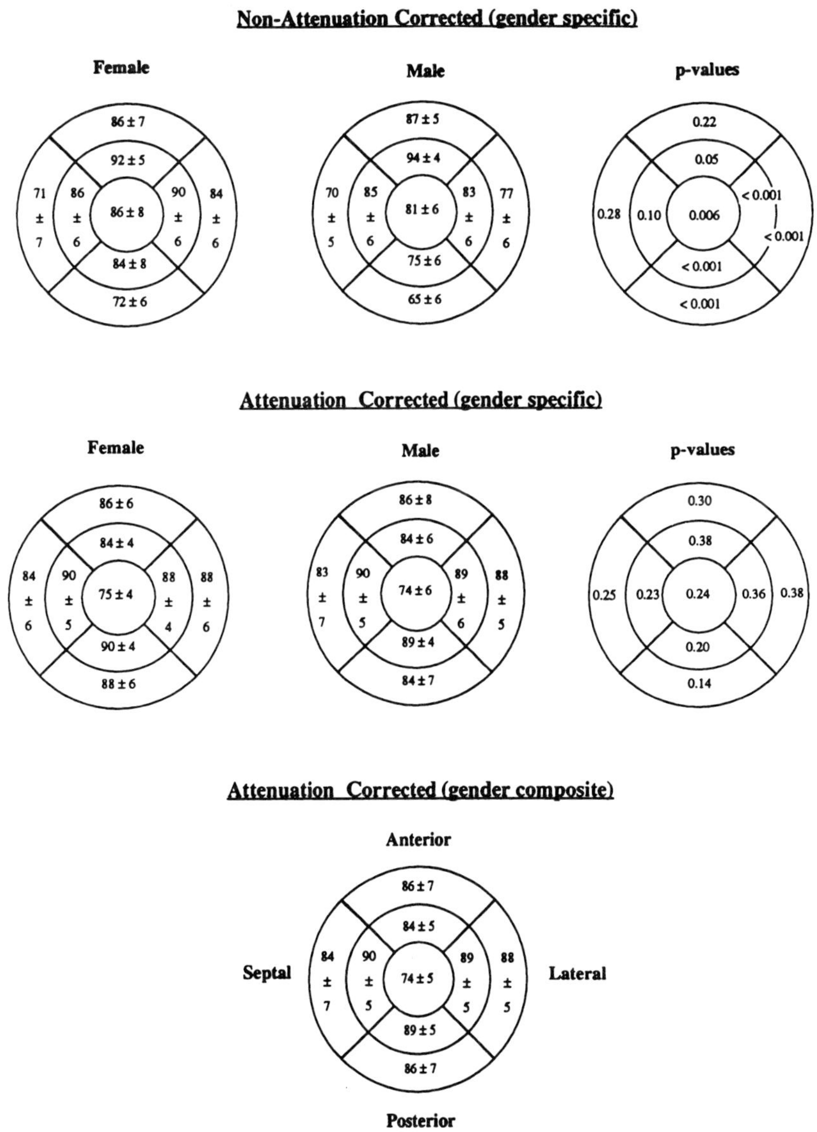

FIGURE 8–6. Stress Tc-99m sestamibi tracer distribution in the myocardium of patients with 5% or less pretest likelihood of coronary artery disease. Normal, gender-specific polar map distributions (n = 20) are presented for nonattenuated corrected and attenuated corrected images. Significant differences (p values) between the gender maps are displayed on the right. Based on the nonsignificant differences in the attenuated distributions for each gender, a single distribution is shown at the bottom for 10 women and 10 men. (From Chua T, Kiat H, Germano G, et al: Gated technetium-99m sestamibi for stimultaneous assessment of stress myocardial perfusion, postexercise regional ventricular function and myocardial viability. Correlation with echocardiography and rest thallium-201 scintigraphy. J Am Coll Cardiol 23:1107, 1994.)

Table 8–5. PROBABILITY OF CORONARY ARTERY DISEASE IN SYMPTOMATIC PATIENTS ACCORDING TO AGE AND GENDER*

AGE (yr)	NONANGINAL CHEST PAIN		ATYPICAL CHEST PAIN		TYPICAL CHEST PAIN	
	Men	Women	Men	Women	Men	Women
30–39	5.2±0.8	0.8±0.3	21.8±2.4	4.2±1.3	69.7±3.2	25.8±6.6
40–49	14.1±1.3	2.8±0.7	46.1±1.8	13.3±2.9	87.3±1.0	55.2±6.5
50–59	21.5±1.7	8.4±1.2	58.9±1.5	32.4±3.0	92.0±0.6	79.4±2.4
60–69	28.1±1.9	18.6±1.9	67.1±1.3	54.4±2.4	94.3±0.4	90.6±1.0

*Chest pain characteristics: substernal location, relief <10 min with rest or nitroglycerin, and precipitation by exertion. Nonanginal pain, two characteristics; atypical angina, two of three characteristics; typical angina, all three characteristics.

Adapted from Diamond GA, Forrester JS: Analysis of probability as an aid in the clinical diagnosis of coronary-artery disease. N Engl J Med 300:1350, 1979.

However, after adjustment for lower pretest probability and lower rate of positive exercise test results, these researchers found that patient gender was not an independent predictor of cardiac catheterization. In another study, gender was an independent predictor of cardiac catheterization following an abnormal stress test; 38% of women and 62% of men underwent cardiac catheterization.[47] In this study, the coronary revascularization rate was 4.9% in men and 2.0% in women and was associated with 2-year cardiac death or MI rates of 2.4% for men and 6.9% for women.

In a similar study, Hachamovitch and coworkers[49] noted a significantly lower referral rate for cardiac catheterization in women than in men (7.1% versus 10.6%). However, after results were controlled for the extent of the perfusion abnormality on the stress Tc-99m sestamibi SPECT study, these researchers found no gender-based difference in referral for catheterization or revascularization. Also in this study, the presence of severe abnormalities on the nuclear scan was associated with a significantly higher event rate in women than in men (17.5% vs. 6.3%). In a large multicenter study, the prognostic value of stress myocardial perfusion imaging was evaluated in 2084 women.[50] Predictors of death were the number of abnormal vascular areas on perfusion imaging ($\chi^2 = 44.7$, $p = .00001$), the clinical index ($\chi^2 = 29.7$; $p = .00001$), and the number of ischemic areas on perfusion imaging ($\chi^2 = 21.5$; $p = .0001$). Gender was not a predictor of death. In women, the strongest correlate of death after adjustments were made for exercise variables was the number of abnormal vascular areas demonstrated on perfusion imaging.

When evaluating either a man or a woman with suspected CAD, the physician should consider the likelihood of CAD in the particular patient. Table 8–5 is a modification of data collected by Diamond and Forrester[51] that relates the prevalence of CAD to patients' symptoms, gender, and age. This has been further refined using the Duke Databank for Cardiovascular Disease, which also takes into consideration findings on the ECG and risk factors.[52] The use of clinical variables to diagnose CAD in women younger than 50 years has a very low specificity (see Table 8–5). Therefore, unless the likelihood of CAD is very low, some form of noninvasive testing is usually required in this group.

Melin and colleagues[33] evaluated different diagnostic strategies in women with chest pain. Exercise ECG, thallium-201 imaging, and coronary arteriography were used to evaluate 135 women. The researchers found that performing an exercise ECG was no more helpful in diagnosis than the clinical evaluation. However, exercise thallium-201 imaging improved the diagnostic accuracy of stress testing in patients in whom the pretest likelihood of CAD was less than 10% or greater than 90%. Hung and associates[32] also found that the addition of thallium-201 imaging to exercise ECG testing increased diagnostic accuracy in different clinical subsets of women.

Stress echocardiography in women has been studied less than comparable nuclear imaging techniques. However, preliminary data suggest that stress echocardiography is significantly more accurate than exercise ECG in women with suspected CAD.[53, 54] In the absence of data favoring nuclear imaging over echocardiography, the choice of technique should depend on the expertise and quality of the local exercise laboratory.

CONCLUSION

The initial assessment of a woman with suspected CAD should consist of a careful history and physical examination, an evaluation for coronary risk factors, and a resting 12-lead ECG. The assessment should also include an estimate of the pretest likelihood of CAD. If the pretest likelihood exceeds 10% to 20%, exercise myocardial perfusion imaging should provide important diagnostic and prognostic information, which will be helpful in determining optimal management of the patient. If a patient would be unable to complete an exercise stress test, a pharmacologic stress test, usually with either adenosine or dipyridamole, should be considered if a nuclear imaging technique is to be performed.

References

1. Kannel WB, Abbott RD: Incidence and prognosis of myocardial infarction in women: The Framingham Study. In Eaker ED, Packard B, Wenger NK (eds): Coronary Heart Disease in Women. National Heart, Lung, and Blood Institute, National Institutes of Health, Bethesda, MD, 1987, p 47.
2. Kennedy JW, Killip T, Fisher LD, et al: The clinical spectrum of coronary artery disease and its surgical and medical management, 1974–1979. The Coronary Artery Surgery Study. Circulation 66:III16, 1982.
3. Waters DD, Halphen C, Theroux P, et al: Coronary artery disease in young women: Clinical and angiographic features and correlation with risk factors. Am J Cardiol 42:41, 1978.
4. Weiner DA, Ryan TJ, McCabe CH, et al: Correlations among history of angina, ST-segment response and prevalence of coronary-artery dis-

ease in the Coronary Artery Surgery Study (CASS). N Engl J Med 301: 230, 1979.

5. Barolsky SM, Gilbert CA, Faruqui A, et al: Differences in electrocardiographic response to exercise of women and men: A non-Bayesian factor. Circulation 60:1021, 1979.
6. Okin PM, Kligfield P: Gender-specific criteria and performance of the exercise electrocardiogram. Circulation 92:1209, 1995.
7. Morise AP, Dalal JN, Duval RD: Value of a simple measure of estrogen status for improving the diagnosis of coronary artery disease in women. Am J Med 94:491, 1993.
8. Rosano GM, Sarrel PM, Poole-Wilson PA, Collins P: Beneficial effect of oestrogen on exercise-induced myocardial ischaemia in women with coronary artery disease. Lancet 342:133, 1993.
9. Greenspan M, Iskandrian AS, Mintz GS, et al: Exercise myocardial scintigraphy with 201-thallium: Use in patients with mitral valve prolapse without associated coronary artery disease. Chest 77:47, 1980.
10. Klein GJ, Kostuk WJ, Boughner DR, Chamberlain MJ: Stress myocardial imaging in mitral leaflet prolapse syndrome. Am J Cardiol 42: 746, 1978.
11. Borer JS, Kent KM, Bacharach SL, et al: Sensitivity, specificity and predictive accuracy of radionuclide cineangiography during exercise in patients with coronary artery disease: Comparison with exercise electrocardiography. Circulation 60:572, 1979.
12. Jones RH, McEwan P, Newman GE, et al: Accuracy of diagnosis of coronary artery disease by radionuclide measurement of left ventricular function during rest and exercise. Circulation 64:586, 1981.
13. Jones RH, Floyd RD, Austin EH, Sabiston DC Jr: The role of radionuclide angiocardiography in the preoperative prediction of pain relief and prolonged survival following coronary artery bypass grafting. Ann Surg 197:743, 1983.
14. Bonow RO, Kent KM, Rosing DR, et al: Exercise-induced ischemia in mildly symptomatic patients with coronary-artery disease and preserved left ventricular function: Identification of subgroups at risk of death during medical therapy. N Engl J Med 311:1339, 1984.
15. Miller TD, Taliercio CP, Zinsmeister AR, Gibbons RJ: Risk stratification of single or double vessel coronary artery disease and impaired left ventricular function using exercise radionuclide angiography. Am J Cardio 165:1317, 1990.
16. Rozanski A, Diamond GA, Berman D, et al: The declining specificity of exercise radionuclide ventriculography. N Engl J Med 309:518, 1983.
17. Poliner LR, Dehmer GJ, Lewis SE, et al: Left ventricular performance in normal subjects: A comparison of the responses to exercise in the upright and supine positions. Circulation 62:528, 1980.
18. Manyari DE, Kostuk WJ: Left and right ventricular function at rest and during bicycle exercise in the supine and sitting positions in normal subjects and patients with coronary artery disease: Assessment by radionuclide ventriculography. Am J Cardiol 51:36, 1983.
19. Freeman MR, Berman DS, Staniloff H, et al: Comparison of upright and supine bicycle exercise in the detection and evaluation of extent of coronary artery disease by equilibrium radionuclide ventriculography. Am Heart J 102:182, 1981.
20. Greenberg PS, Berge RD, Johnson KD, et al: The value and limitation of radionuclide angiocardiography with stress in women. Clin Cardiol 6:312, 1983.
21. Gibbons RJ, Lee KL, Cobb F, Jones RH: Ejection fraction response to exercise in patients with chest pain and normal coronary arteriograms. Circulation 64:952, 1981.
22. Adams KF, Vincent LM, McAllister SM, et al: The influence of age and gender on left ventricular response to supine exercise in asymptomatic normal subjects. Am Heart J 113:732, 1987.
23. Higgenbotham MB, Morris KG, Coleman RE, Cobb FR: Sex-related differences in the normal cardiac response to upright exercise. Circulation 70:357, 1984.
24. Hanley PC, Zinsmeister AR, Clements IP: Gender-related differences in cardiac response to supine exercise assessed by radionuclide angiography. J Am Coll Cardiol 13:624, 1989.
25. Younis LT, Melin JA, Robert AR, Detry JM: Influence of age and sex on left ventricular volumes and ejection fraction during upright exercise in normal subjects. Eur Heart J 11:916, 1990.
26. Hakki AH, Iskandrian AS: Effect of gender on left ventricular function during exercise in patients with coronary artery disease. Am Heart J 111:543, 1986.
27. Sullivan MJ, Cobb FR, Higginbotham MB: Stroke volume increases by similar mechanisms during upright exercise in normal men and women. Am J Cardiol 67:1405, 1991.
28. Moriel M, Rozanski A, Klein J, et al: The limited efficacy of exercise radionuclide ventriculography in assessing prognosis in women with coronary artery disease. Am J Cardiol 76:1030, 1995.
29. Kotler TS, Diamond GA: Exercise thallium-201 scintigraphy in the diagnosis and prognosis of coronary artery disease. Ann Intern Med 113:684, 1990.
30. McGhie AI, Gould KL, Schelbert HR, Willerson JT: Coronary artery disease—nuclear cardiology. In Willerson JT, Cohn JN (eds): Cardiovascular Medicine. Churchill Livingstone, New York, 1995, p 475.
31. Friedman TD, Greene AC, Iskandrian AS, et al: Exercise thallium-201 myocardial scintigraphy in women: Correlation with coronary arteriography. Am J Cardiol 49:1632, 1982.
32. Hung J, Chaitman BR, Lam J, et al: Noninvasive diagnostic test choices for the evaluation of coronary artery disease in women: A multivariate comparison of cardiac fluoroscopy, exercise electrocardiography and exercise thallium myocardial perfusion scintigraphy. J Am Coll Cardiol 4:8, 1984.
33. Melin JA, Wijns W, Vanbutsele RJ, et al: Alternative diagnostic strategies for coronary artery disease in women: Demonstration of the usefulness and efficiency of probability analysis. Circulation 71:535, 1985.
34. Fintel DJ, Links JM, Brinker JA, et al: Improved diagnostic performance of exercise thallium-201 single photon emission computed tomography over planar imaging in the diagnosis of coronary artery disease: A receiver operating characteristic analysis. J Am Coll Cardiol 13:600, 1989.
35. Kong BA, Shaw L, Miller DD, Chaitman BR: Comparison of accuracy for detecting coronary artery disease and side-effect profile of dipyridamole thallium-201 myocardial perfusion imaging in women versus men. Am J Cardiol 70:168, 1992.
36. Chae SC, Heo J, Iskandrian AS, et al: Identification of extensive coronary artery disease in women by exercise single photon emission computed tomographic (SPECT) thallium imaging. J Am Coll Cardiol 21:1305, 1993.
37. Taillefer R, DePuey EG, Udelson JE, et al: Comparative diagnostic accuracy of Tl-201 and Tc-99m sestamibi SPECT imaging (perfusion and ECG-gated SPECT) in detecting coronary artery disease in woman. J Am Coll Cardiol 29:69, 1997.
38. Hendel RC, Chen MH, L'Italien GJ, et al: Sex differences in perioperative and long-term cardiac event-free survival in vascular surgery patients: An analysis of clinical and scintigraphic variables. Circulation 91: 1044, 1995.
39. Maddahi J, Van Train K, Prigent F, et al: Quantitative single photon emission computed thallium-201 tomography for detection and localization of coronary artery disease: Optimization and prospective validation of a new technique. J Am Coll Cardiol 14:1689, 1989.
40. Van Train KF, Maddahi J, Berman DS, et al: Quantitative analysis of tomographic stress thallium-201 myocardial scintigrams: A multicenter trail. J Nucl Med 31:1168, 1990.
41. Ficaro EP, Fessler JA, Shreve PD, et al: Simultaneous transmission/emission myocardial perfusion tomography: Diagnostic accuracy of attenuation-corrected 99mTc-sestamibi single-photon emission tomography. Circulation 93:463, 1996.
42. Ficaro EP, Shreve PD, Kritzman JN, et al: Evaluation of attenuation corrected cardiac SPECT perfusion imaging in women [abstract]. Circulation 94(Suppl):I13, 1996.
43. DePuey EG, Rozanski A: Using gated technetium-99m-sestamibi SPECT to characterize fixed myocardial defects as infarct or artifact. J Nucl Med 36:952, 1995.
44. Chua T, Kiat H, Germano G, et al: Gated technetium-99m sestamibi for simultaneous assessment of stress myocardial perfusion, postexercise regional ventricular function and myocardial viability: Correlation with echocardiography and rest thallium-201 scintigraphy. J Am Coll Cardiol 23:1107, 1994.
45. Tobin JN, Wassertheil-Smoller S, Wexler JP, et al: Sex bias in considering coronary bypass surgery. Ann Intern Med 107:19, 1987.
46. Shaw LJ, Miller DD, Romeis JC, et al: Gender differences in the noninvasive evaluation and management of patients with suspected coronary artery disease. Ann Intern Med 120:559, 1994.
47. Bickell NA, Pieper KS, Lee KL, et al: Referral patterns for coronary artery disease treatment: Gender bias or good clinical judgment? Ann Intern Med 116:791, 1992.
48. Mark DB, Shaw LK, DeLong ER, et al: Absence of sex bias in the referral of patients for cardiac catheterization. N Engl J Med 330: 1101, 1994.
49. Hachamovitch R, Berman DS, Kiat H, et al: Gender-related differences

in clinical management after exercise nuclear testing. J Am Coll Cardiol 26:1457, 1995.
50. Marwick TH, Lauer MS, Shaw LJ, et al: Myocardial perfusion imaging predicts cardiac mortality in women—multicenter study of 4753 patients followed-up over 2 years [abstract]. Circulation 94(Suppl):I13, 1996.
51. Diamond GA, Forrester JS: Analysis of probability as an aid in the clinical diagnosis of coronary-artery disease. N Engl J Med 300:1350, 1979.
52. Pryor DB, Harrell FE, Lee KL, et al: Estimating the likelihood of significant coronary artery disease. Am J Med 75:771, 1983.
53. Sawada SG, Ryan T, Fineberg NS, et al: Exercise echocardiographic detection of coronary artery disease in women. J Am Coll Cardiol 14: 1440, 1989.
54. Marwick TH, Anderson T, Williams MJ, et al: Exercise echocardiography is an accurate and cost-efficient technique for the detection of coronary artery disease in women. J Am Coll Cardiol 26:335, 1995.

8.3 Echocardiography

Eddy Barasch

Few data are available regarding the noninvasive evaluation of CAD in women. Most information on CAD has been derived from studies predominantly or exclusively involving middle-aged men.[1] Several hypotheses have been proposed to explain the lack of data for women: the low prevalence of CAD in premenopausal women, comorbidities present at an advanced age, the low specificity of exercise ECG tests in women, and the general perception that angina pectoris is a benign problem in women.[2]

Chest pain, the clinical hallmark of CAD, is less predictive for the presence of significant disease in women. Furthermore, predicting CAD from the history and physical examination in women is difficult.[3] Data from several studies have shown that abnormal results on coronary angiogram are seen in 60% to 75% of women with typical angina, in contrast to 30% to 40% of those with probable angina, and in 2% to 7% of those with atypical chest pain.[1] According to CASS data, 93% of men with anginal pain have CAD, and 66% of men with anginal pain have evidence of this disease.[4]

Exercise ECG, the primary noninvasive test for assessing CAD, has a similar level of sensitivity in women and men, but its specificity and positive and negative predictive value are lower in women.[5] The relatively high numbers of false-positive results in women may be explained by the following factors:[6, 7]

- Lower prevalence of CAD in women,
- Digoxin-like effect of estrogens,
- Lower hematocrit in women,
- Higher prevalence of mitral valve prolapse in women,
- Autonomic and hormonal influences,
- Decreased myocardial potassium levels,
- Higher pulmonary vascular resistance,
- Higher prevalence of changes in the resting ECG.

Myocardial nuclear perfusion techniques in conjunction with exercise or pharmacologic stress agents are often used in women with suspected CAD. However, the limitations of both exercise ECG and nuclear myocardial perfusion tests have prompted the search for other diagnostic techniques.

The echocardiographic detection of CAD is based primarily on the presence of regional wall motion abnormalities (WMAs) at rest[8] and on the propensity of provocative tests to induce WMAs. These provocative tests induce WMAs by raising the myocardial oxygen demand, by producing heterogeneity in myocardial perfusion, or both.[9] Echocardiography has also been used to assess changes in left ventricular systolic volumes,[9] to evaluate the left ventricular diastolic filling pattern,[10] and to assess the anatomy and the vascular reserve of coronary arteries.[11, 12]

In addition to detecting and possibly localizing CAD, stress echocardiography can assess the extent and functional significance of coronary stenosis. Furthermore, this technique is used to evaluate myocardial viability and functional recovery after revascularization procedures. Patients often undergo stress echocardiography after an acute MI or as a preoperative evaluation, especially before major vascular surgery or organ transplantation.

The myocardial stress modalities used in conjunction with transthoracic or transesophageal echocardiography are physical exercise (isotonic or isometric), atrial pacing, and administration of different pharmacologic agents, such as dobutamine, adenosine, and dipyridamole. Echocardiography can identify WMAs induced by hyperventilation, intravenous administration of ergonovine, or application of the cold pressor test, all of which produce coronary artery spasms.[13] The usefulness of echocardiography in evaluating CAD has been improved by digital image acquisition and technologic advances such as acoustic quantification, color kinesis, Doppler tissue imaging, and the use of myocardial contrast agents. However, high-quality images are not obtained in approximately 10% of patients because of poor echocardiographic windows.

EXERCISE ECHOCARDIOGRAPHY

Described by Wann and colleagues[14] in 1979, exercise echocardiography is based on the principle proposed by Galagher and associates,[15] which states that during stress-induced ischemia, the decrease in myocardial contractile function is directly related to the reduction in regional subendocardial blood flow.

A normal stress echocardiogram is characterized by a uniform increase in wall motion and a thickening of the systolic wall with a concomitant decrease in end-systolic volume. An abnormal test result is defined by baseline, new, or worsening regional asynergy, tardokinesia, or a failure to augment endocardial motion with stress.[16]

The most common means of physical exercise used in exercise echocardiography are the treadmill and the upright or supine bicycle.[17] Different exercise protocols are used.[17] A wall motion score index (WMSI) is derived to assess results. The left ventricular walls are divided into 16 segments, and in most laboratories, WMSI is computed by dividing the overall score of the analyzed segments by the number of the visualized segments.[18] The individual segment score usually ranges from 1 (normal) to 4 (dyskinetic). A higher WMSI implies a higher degree of wall motion abnormalities.

An exercise test, considered the most physiologic investigation, is preferred over a pharmacologic test. However, exercise echocardiography has two major disadvantages: (1) Accurate results depend on the patient's motivation to exercise at an expected level of stress and (2) the sonographer must acquire images within the first minute of exercise termination. Adding atropine (0.5 mg) 10 minutes before starting the exercise may increase the duration of the maximal heart rate and therefore prolong the scanning time.[19] Imaging at peak exercise is more sensitive than imaging after exercise in patients undergoing bicycle exercise.[20] Images should be obtained at rest and at peak stress and should be digitized and displayed in a cineloop format for analysis.

The use of the upright bicycle for exercise in exercise echocardiography has the same accuracy as that of treadmill exercise.[21, 22] The supine bicycle allows for continuous scanning during exercise, which is an advantage because rapid recovery may occur in approximately 20% of cases.[20] Pain experienced during exercise echocardiography has been associated with greater myocardial dysfunction.[23]

Women have a higher resting left ventricular ejection fraction (LVEF) than men, and the LVEF in women increases less with exercise. The routine treadmill exercise may be a "supermaximal stress" for women, which yields a relative lower LVEF. In addition, the mechanisms for increasing cardiac output may differ in men and women. Women increase cardiac output by increasing the end-diastolic volume index without significantly raising LVEF. In contrast, men increase cardiac output by decreasing the end-systolic volume index and raising LVEF.[24] LVEF does not rise during exercise radionuclide ventriculography in about 30% of women, a finding that may explain the poor specificity of this test in women.

A few studies have assessed the value of exercise echocardiography in women. In a study of 57 women presenting with chest pain (mean age, 57 years; range, 33 to 75 years), the sensitivity and specificity of exercise echocardiography were 86%; the sensitivity of stress ECG was 29% to 53% and the specificity was 65% to 83%. Exercise echocardiography was diagnostic in 82% of women with ST segment abnormalities at rest. Moreover, exercise echocardiography predicted the presence or absence of CAD in 84% of women with atypical chest pain and in 89% of those with typical chest pain. The correct diagnosis was made by echocardiography in 82% of patients for whom exercise ECG was nondiagnostic.[25]

In a study of 70 women (mean age, 60 ± 9 years) with chest pain, Williams and associates[26] compared the accuracy of exercise ECG, exercise score, and exercise echocardiography. Significant coronary stenosis was defined as 50% or greater. They found that exercise echocardiography had a sensitivity of 88%, a specificity of 84%, and an overall accuracy of 86%. The sensitivity of exercise echocardiography for detecting one-vessel CAD was 89%.[26] In a study of 161 women (mean age, 60 ± 8 years) without a prior Q-wave MI, Marwick and colleagues[7] reported that the sensitivity of exercise echocardiography for detecting one-vessel disease was 75 ± 2%, and for detecting multivessel CAD, 85 ± 2%. The overall sensitivity of exercise echocardiography was similar to that of exercise ECG (Table 8–6). However, the specificity and accuracy of exercise echocardiography were greater than those of exercise ECG. Although the positive predictive value was higher for exercise echocardiography, the negative predictive values were similar for the two tests.

In a study conducted with 228 patients (mean age, 62 years), of whom 75 were women, Crouse and associates[27, 28] found that exercise echocardiography had higher sensitivity, specificity, and negative predictive value than exercise ECG. In a retrospective analysis comparing results in men and women, these researchers did not find significant differences between the two sexes.[27, 28]

The prognostic value of post-treadmill exercise echocardiography was assessed in a study of 77 men and 71 women (mean age, 52.5 years) who had an intermediate probability of development of CAD. Only 4.1% of patients with a normal exercise echocardiogram had a cardiac event during follow-up at 28.4 ± 8.5 months. More than 40% of patients had an abnormal exercise ECG. Only 2 of 71 women (2.8%) had a cardiac event in this study; both were asymptomatic and had no ischemic changes on ECG. Neither woman had an abnormal exercise ECG or recurrent atypical chest pain even if she did not achieve 6 metabolic equivalents.[6]

In a study of 118 patients (93 men, 25 women) with a mean age of 57 years ± 12 years who underwent exercise echocardiography and coronary angiography, 23 patients had false-positive or false-negative results. Age, sex, weight, and image quality did not significantly affect the rate of false-negative or false-positive results. The following factors correlated with false-negative findings: submaximal exercise, one-vessel CAD, and moderate (50% to 70%) coronary stenosis.[29]

No studies comparing exercise echocardiography with nuclear myocardial perfusion tests have been conducted exclusively in women. However, studies in both sexes have shown that the sensitivity of exercise echocardiography (80%) is similar to that of thallium-201 SPECT (89%), and the specificity of exercise echocardiography (80%) is higher than that

Table 8–6. COMPARISON OF EXERCISE ECHOCARDIOGRAPHY AND EXERCISE ELECTROCARDIOGRAPHY IN 161 WOMEN

	EXERCISE ECHOCARDIOGRAPHY	EXERCISE ELECTROCARDIOGRAPHY
Sensitivity (%)	80 ± 3	77 ± 3
Specificity (%)	80 ± 3	56 ± 4*
Accuracy (%)	81 ± 5	64 ± 6†
Positive predictive value (%)	74 ± 4	54 ± 4‡
Negative predictive value (%)	86 ± 3	78 ± 3

*$p < .0004$; †$p < .0005$; ‡$p < .005$.

From Marwick TH, Anderson T, Williams MJ, et al: Exercise echocardiography is an accurate and cost-efficient technique for detection of coronary artery disease in women. J Am Coll Cardiol 26:335, 1995.

of thallium-201 imaging (65%). The specificity of gated Tc-99m sestamibi SPECT imaging (90%) is comparable to that of exercise echocardiography.[30, 31] The concordance between exercise echocardiography and thallium-201 SPECT was 82% in one study, and reversible perfusion defects on thallium-201 SPECT occurred in more than a third of the regions with fixed WMAs, suggesting the presence of viable myocardium.[32]

In summary, exercise echocardiography is superior to exercise ECG for detecting CAD in women. The specificity, positive predictive value, and accuracy are higher with exercise echocardiography than with exercise ECG; however, the sensitivity and negative predictive value are similar for the two techniques.

DIPYRIDAMOLE ECHOCARDIOGRAPHY

Intravenous administration of dipyridamole may induce WMAs by vertical coronary flow steal, horizontal steal, passive coronary collapse, and systemic steal "luxury perfusion."[33] Dipyridamole is usually administered intravenously at a concentration of 0.56 mg/kg (low dose) over 4 minutes, followed by a pause of 4 minutes, and then administration of another 0.28 mg/kg within 2 minutes (high dose).[34] Two-dimensional echocardiograms are obtained before the drug is given and continuously during and up to 10 minutes after its administration.

In one study, high-dose dipyridamole echocardiography and an upright bicycle exercise test were used to evaluate 83 women (mean age, 55 years ± 8 years) with chest pain; significant coronary disease was defined as 70% or greater luminal reduction. False-positive results with exercise ECG were recorded in 48% of patients. In 68 women without a previous MI, the sensitivities and negative predictive values of dipyridamole echocardiography and exercise ECG were similar; however, the specificity, accuracy, and positive predictive value were higher for dipyridamole echocardiography than for exercise ECG (Table 8–7).[35]

The prognostic value of dipyridamole echocardiography was clearly demonstrated in the Echo Persantine International Cooperative Study. Dipyridamole echocardiography was performed in 925 patients (mean age, 56 ± 9 years) 10 ± 5 days after a first uncomplicated MI, and patients were monitored for a mean of 14 months. Of the 925 patients,

Table 8–7. COMPARISON OF DIPYRIDAMOLE ECHOCARDIOGRAPHY AND EXERCISE ELECTROCARDIOGRAPHY IN 83 WOMEN

	DIPYRIDAMOLE ECHOCARDIOGRAPHY	EXERCISE ELECTROCARDIOGRAPHY
Sensitivity (%)	79	72
Specificity (%)	93	52*
Accuracy (%)	87	47*
Positive predictive value (%)	87	47†
Negative predictive value (%)	84	68

*$p < .001$; †$p < .01$.

From Masini M, Picano E, Lattanzi F, et al: High dose dipyridamole-echocardiography test in women: Correlation with exercise-electrocardiography test and coronary angiography. J Am Coll Cardiol 12:682, 1988.

133 were women. For all the spontaneous events (angina, reinfarction, death), Cox analysis showed a positive dipyridamole echocardiography result, age, and male sex to have an independent and additive value. Age was the most important predictor of survival, followed by WMSI during dipyridamole administration. Two percent of patients who had negative results on dipyridamole echocardiography died, 4% of patients with positive dipyridamole echocardiography high-dose results died, and 7% of patients with positive low-dose results died.[36] Considered safe, dipyridamole echocardiography has been performed more than 10,000 times, with no serious side effects seen within 10 minutes of the test.[37]

DOBUTAMINE STRESS ECHOCARDIOGRAPHY

Dobutamine is the most commonly used pharmacologic agent for stress echocardiography in the United States. With a complex mode of action, dobutamine stimulates $beta_1$, $beta_2$, and $alpha_1$ adrenoceptors, resulting in positive inotropic, lusitropic, and chronotropic actions on the myocardium. In addition, dobutamine alters left ventricular loading secondary to its action on vascular smooth muscle.

The central and peripheral hemodynamic responses to dobutamine stress at a peak dose of 33 μg/kg/min were studied with Doppler echocardiography and venous occlusion plethysmography in 18 healthy women, aged 54 to 73 years. Heart rate increased by 49% and cardiac output by 59%, whereas total vascular resistance decreased by 44% and leg peripheral vascular resistance by 26% ($p < .001$). Total peripheral vascular resistance (PVR) decreased more in patients who demonstrated hypotension, but similar changes in leg PVR were seen in patients with and without hypotension.[38]

Studying the normal myocardial response to dobutamine stress, Carstensen and coworkers[39] reported that the maximal increases in wall motion and thickening occur between baseline and administration of low-dose dobutamine; from low dose to peak dose, the mean absolute motion decreases by 13.1% and the relative thickening by 21.4% regardless of age, sex, and addition of atropine.[39] The magnitude of the ischemic response was 242% greater with dobutamine than with dipyridamole. In another study performed in pigs, dobutamine decreased blood flow in the ischemic zone, whereas dipyridamole had no effect; thus, dobutamine may contribute to the induction of myocardial ischemia.[40]

Protocols for dobutamine stress echocardiography (DSE) are described in detail elsewhere.[41–43] Following is a brief description. A complete Doppler echocardiographic study is performed at rest. Then, an infusion of dobutamine is started at a rate of 5 μg/kg/min and is increased after 3 minutes to 10 μg/kg/min. Incremental additions of 10 μg/kg/min are made every 3 minutes until a maximal dose (40 or 50 μg/kg/min) is achieved, an endpoint is reached, or a serious side effect occurs. The addition of atropine (usually no more than 1 mg) augments both the chronotropic and inotropic effects of dobutamine. If the heart rate does not reach more than 60% of the maximal predicted heart rate at 20 μg/kg/min, atropine may be administered to shorten the duration of the study.[44] The increase of stage duration from 3 to 5 minutes improves the sensitivity for detecting CAD, especially in patients with a moderate pretest probability of CAD or in those taking beta blockers.[45]

Digitally acquired images are displayed in a quad-screen format for analysis. Four different types of response can be elicited with dobutamine administration: (1) normal, consisting of progressive augmentation of wall motion and thickening; (2) fixed, in which the akinetic segment remains akinetic; (3) biphasic or ischemic increase in myocardial contraction at low dose followed by a decrease at a higher dose; and (4) progressive worsening, which suggests severe coronary stenosis.

Panza and colleagues[46] determined the DSE ischemic threshold to be 25.4 ± 11.2 μg/kg/min for one-vessel disease, 14.4 ± 7.9 μg/kg/min for two-vessel disease, and 9.1 ± 7.9 μg/kg/min for three-vessel disease.

Safety of DSE

A retrospective analysis of 3020 DSE studies conducted at a single institution showed that major side effects occurred in 0.2% of patients.[44] DSE was terminated prematurely because of side effects in 7% of patients; ventricular tachycardia (VT) occurred in 0.8% of cases, and supraventricular tachycardia in 0.5%. Sustained VT occurred in five patients, and one patient had an acute MI. Suboptimal stress was seen more often in women and in patients with diabetes and in those taking beta blockers or calcium channel blockers.

Mertes and associates[47] analyzed more than 118 DSE studies performed at one institution (488 in women) and found that patients with a recent MI more frequently had dobutamine-induced angina than patients without a recent MI, but the incidences of arrhythmias were similar in the two groups. No deaths, acute MIs, or sustained VT occurred. The frequency of noncardiac side effects (nausea, anxiety, headache, tremor, urgency) was 26%, but major side effects occurred in just 3% of patients. The most common side effects were arrhythmias, hypotension, nausea, and dyspnea.[47]

Acute MI during DSE, which rarely occurs, has been attributed to platelet activation secondary to dobutamine administration.[48] Hypotension (20 mm Hg or greater decrease in systolic blood pressure) during DSE, which relates to the development of dynamic left ventricular outflow tract (LVOT) obstruction or an increase in vagal stimulation, is seen in about 10% to 20% of patients and does not have the same grave prognosis as that in exercise tests. The incidences of hypotension, arrhythmias, and chest pain are similar in men and women.[49] However, in some studies, LVOT obstruction was more common in women, and hypotension was more common in elderly women with small ventricles who were not receiving beta-blocker therapy.[50, 51]

Only a few studies have separately analyzed the responses of men and women to DSE. In one such study, 342 DSEs were performed within 6 weeks of coronary angiography in patients with chest pain. False-positive results were seen in 39 patients (11.4%), more than 70% of whom were women. The incidence of false-positive results was 20.9% in women but only 5.3% in men. Approximately two thirds of the false-positive results were in the posterobasal and inferobasal segments, sections of the endocardium that are often poorly visualized. In addition, the tethering effect of the fibrous skeleton of the heart to these segments may contribute to inaccurate results.[52]

The rate of agreement between results of stress echocardiography and those of perfusion scintigraphy was lower in patients who had WMAs at rest.[32] A biphasic response to dobutamine increased the detection of CAD to 98% in a study of 50 men and 4 women in whom radionuclide perfusion imaging tests were positive for ischemia. The agreement of stress echocardiography results with Tc-99m sestamibi or Tc-99m tetrofosmin perfusion results was 89% for the biphasic response and only 56% at peak dose.[53]

The correlation between reversible perfusion defects detected on dobutamine sestamibi SPECT and transient WMAs detected on DSE was studied in 38 men and 16 women. More women than men had ischemia on dobutamine sestamibi SPECT but did not have transient WMAs on DSE. In addition, these women had a lower rate-pressure product. Because the predicted maximal heart rate with exercise is higher in men than in women at any age, a similar calculation of maximal heart rate during DSE may not be appropriate in women undergoing DSE, in which the detection of ischemia depends on an increase in heart rate.[54]

In patients with left ventricular hypertrophy or complete left bundle branch block who have not had an MI, DSE is more accurate than Tc-99m sestamibi perfusion. In women, the incidence of false-negative results was higher with both techniques because of the low grade of coronary stenosis. In accuracy, the two techniques are comparable.[55]

In 80 patients (mean age, 53 ± 8 years; 13 women) who underwent DSE, dipyridamole echocardiography (dosage, 0.84 mg/kg) over 10 minutes), and bicycle exercise echocardiography, DSE and exercise echocardiography had a higher sensitivity than dipyridamole echocardiography in patients with one-vessel CAD, whereas the three tests had similar levels of sensitivity in patients with multivessel disease. DSE and dipyridamole echocardiography had a higher specificity than exercise echocardiography, and DSE was more accurate than exercise echocardiography.[56]

Using a combination of dipyridamole and dobutamine in echocardiographic studies may be possible in some patients and may improve the sensitivity of DSE. In a study of 55 patients (45 men, 10 women) with CAD (most of whom had one-vessel disease and were receiving antianginal therapy), the addition of dobutamine to dipyridamole was feasible in 96% of patients and increased the sensitivity of the test from 71% to 92% without affecting specificity.[57]

In the two studies comparing exercise echocardiography, DSE, and dipyridamole echocardiography, the sensitivity of both exercise echocardiography and DSE was higher than that of dipyridamole echocardiography, but the specificity levels of the three tests were similar.[58, 59]

Evaluation of Myocardial Viability

DSE is used to evaluate myocardial viability; however, no studies have enrolled only women. Viable myocardium can be detected with low-dose dobutamine (5 to 10 μg/kg/min). A biphasic response is required to predict functionally recoverable myocardium after revascularization procedures.[60] The sensitivity level and positive and negative predictive values for detecting viable myocardium are comparable for DSE and thallium-201 reinjection imaging, but DSE has a higher specificity than thallium-201 reinjection.[61] The ability of DSE to detect viable myocardium is comparable to that of 18 fluorodeoxyglucose PET.[62–64]

OTHER, NONPHARMACOLOGIC MODALITIES OF STRESS TESTING

Atrial Pacing

Atrial pacing is used mainly in conjunction with transesophageal echocardiography. In a study of 70 patients (46 men, 24 women) in which 50% or greater arterial narrowing indicated the presence of CAD, atrial pacing had a sensitivity of 69% for detection of one-vessel CAD and 90% for three-vessel disease. The specificity for multivessel disease and the positive predictive value were both 100%, but the negative predictive value was only 44%.[65]

Hyperventilation Echocardiography Test

Hyperventilation at a rate of 30 respirations/min for 5 minutes induced WMAs in 104 hospitalized patients (27 women) within 30 to 300 seconds after hyperventilation. Only ST segment elevation corresponded to the site of asynergy. Hyperventilation echocardiography showed a specificity of 100%, a sensitivity of 84%, a positive predictive value of 100%, and a negative predictive value of 92%.[13]

CONCLUSION

Regardless of the chosen test, the evaluation of CAD in both men and women relies on the pretest likelihood of disease. If the probability of disease and the sensitivity and specificity of a particular diagnostic tool are known, the post-test likelihood can be quantified. The benefit of a noninvasive test is greatest when the pretest likelihood is in the intermediate range (20% to 80%).[66] A nomogram for estimating the likelihood of significant CAD in women has been published.[67]

Physical exercise should be the first choice for use as a stress agent in combination with echocardiography or nuclear scintigraphy for detection of CAD. Physical exercise has a higher sensitivity than dobutamine and dipyridamole and may provide additional information regarding functional capacity. If the patient will not or cannot exercise, dobutamine or dipyridamole can be chosen as a stress-inducing agent. DSE has a higher sensitivity than dipyridamole echocardiography for evaluation of CAD. Low-dose dobutamine is the agent of choice for assessing viability of cardiac tissue. Myocardial contraction of the inferior and posterobasal walls should be analyzed carefully, especially in women, because of the high rate of false-positive results related to interpretation of WMAs in these myocardial segments.[55]

Stress echocardiographic studies should be analyzed by a physician trained to interpret such studies to optimize test reliability and accuracy. Highly accurate results may not be obtained at institutions with a low volume of studies. Performed by trained sonographers and physicians and validated by other diagnostic techniques, stress echocardiography may be a powerful and reliable diagnostic tool. In fact, stress echocardiography may be preferable to other noninvasive diagnostic techniques for evaluating CAD in women because of the lack of radiation exposure, the ease with which it can be performed, and its ability to detect noncoronary causes of chest pain.

References

1. Wenger NK: Coronary heart disease in women: Gender differences in diagnostic evaluation. J Am Med Womens Assoc 49:181, 1994.
2. Lerner DJ, Kannel WB: Patterns of coronary heart disease morbidity and mortality in the sexes: A 26-year follow-up of the Framingham population. Am Heart J 111:383, 1986.
3. Fetters JK, Peterson ED, Shaw LI, et al: Sex-specific differences in coronary artery disease risk factors, evaluation and treatment; have they been adequately evaluated? Am Heart J 131:796, 1996.
4. Chaitman BR, Bourassa MG, Davis K, et al: Angiographic prevalence of high-risk coronary artery disease in patient subsets (CASS). Circulation 64:360, 1981.
5. Zhao D, Freeman DH, de Fillippi CR: A meta-analysis of gender differences in exercise stress testing. Circulation 94:1497, 1996.
6. Sawada SG, Ryan T, Conley MJ, et al: Prognostic value of a normal exercise echocardiogram. Am Heart J 120:49, 1990.
7. Marwick TH, Anderson T, Williams MJ, et al: Exercise echocardiography is an accurate and cost-efficient technique for detection of coronary artery disease in women. J Am Coll Cardiol 26:335, 1995.
8. Dec GW, Fuster V: Idiopathic dilated cardiomyopathy. N Engl J Med 331:1564, 1994.
9. Olson CE, Porter TR, Deligonul U, et al: Left ventricular volume changes during dobutamine stress echocardiography identify patients with more extensive coronary artery disease. J Am Coll Cardiol 24: 1268, 1994.
10. el-Said ES, Roelandt JR, Fioretti PM, et al: Abnormal left ventricular early diastolic filling during dobutamine stress Doppler echocardiography is a sensitive indicator of significant coronary artery disease. J Am Coll Cardiol 24:1618, 1994.
11. Stoddard MF, Prince CR, Morris GT: Coronary flow reserve assessment by dobutamine transesophageal Doppler echocardiogrphy. J Am Coll Cardiol 25:325, 1995.
12. Tardif LC, Vannan MA, Taylor K, et al: Delineation of extended lengths of coronary arteries by multiplane transesophageal echocardiography. Am J Cardiol 24:909, 1994.
13. Morales MA, Reisenhofer B, Rovai D, et al: Hyperventilation-echocardiography test for the diagnosis of myocardial ischaemia at rest. European Heart J 14:1088, 1993.
14. Wann LS, Faris JV, Childress RH, et al: Exercise cross-sectional echocardiography in ischemic heart disease. Circulation 60:1300, 1979.
15. Gallagher KP, Matsuzaki M, Osakada G, et al: Effect of exercise on the relationship between myocardial blood flow and systolic wall thickening in dogs with acute coronary stenosis. Circ Res 52:716, 1983.
16. Mazeika PK, Nihoyannopoulos P, Oakley CM: Stress echocardiography: Time for critical reappraisal. Br Heart J 70:208, 1993.
17. Roger VL, Pellikka PA, Oh JK, et al: Stress echocardiography. Part I: Exercise echocardiography: Techniques, implementation, clinical applications, and correlations. Mayo Clin Proc 70:1, 1995.
18. Segar DS, Brown SE, Sawada SG, et al: Dobutamine stress echocardiography: Correlation with coronary lesion severity as determined by quantitative angiography. J Am Coll Cardiol 19:1197, 1992.
19. Attenhofer C, Capps MA, Roger VL, et al: Does atropine injection prior to exercise echocardiography increase the heart rate during image acquisition? A randomized trial. J Am Soc Echocardiogr 9:398, 1996
20. Presti CF, Armstrong WF, Feigenbaum H: Comparison of echocardiography at peak exercise and after bicycle exercise in evaluation of patients with known or suspected coronary artery disease. J Am Soc Echocardiogr 1:119, 1988.
21. Ryan T, Segar DS, Sawada SG, et al: Detection of coronary artery disease with upright bicycle exercise echocardiography. J Am Soc Echocardiogr 6:186, 1993.
22. Hecht HS, DeBord L, Shaw R, et al: Digital supine bicycle stress

echocardiography: A new technique for evaluating coronary artery disease. J Am Coll Cardiol 21:950, 1993.
23. Nihoyannopoulos P, Marsoni A, Joshi J, et al: Magnitude of myocardial dysfunction is greater in painful than in painless myocardial ischemia: An exercise echocardiographic study. J Am Coll Cardiol 25:1507, 1995.
24. Merz CN, Moriel M, Rozanski A, et al: Gender-related differences in exercise ventricular function among healthy subjects and patients. Am Heart J 131:704, 1996.
25. Sawada SG, Ryan T, Fineberg NS, et al: Exercise echocardiographic detection of coronary artery disease in women. J Am Coll Cardiol 14: 1440, 1989.
26. Williams MJ, Marwick TH, O'Gorman D, Foale RA: Comparison of exercise echocardiography with an exercise score to diagnose coronary artery disease in women. Am J Cardiol 74:435, 1994.
27. Crouse LJ, Harbrecht JJ, Vacek JL, et al: Exercise echocardiography as a screening test for coronary artery disease and correlation with coronary arteriography. Am J Cardiol 67:1213, 1991.
28. Crouse LJ, Kramer PH: Are there gender differences related to stress or pharmacological echocardiography? Am J Card Imaging 10:65, 1996.
29. Marwick TH, Nemec JJ, Pashkow FI, et al: Accuracy and limitations of exercise echocardiography in a routine clinical setting. J Am Coll Cardiol 19:74, 1992.
30. Hecht HS, DeBord L, Shaw R: Supine bicycle stress echocardiography versus tomographic thallium-201 exercise imaging for the detection of coronary artery disease. J Am Soc Echocardiogr 6:177, 1993.
31. Nagueh SF, Zoghbi WA: Stress echocardiography for the assessment of myocardial ischemia and viability. Curr Probl Cardiol 21:445, 1996.
32. Quinones MA, Verani MS, Haichin RM, et al: Exercise echocardiography versus 201 Tl single-photon emission computed tomography in evaluation of coronary artery disease: Analysis of 292 patients. Circulation 85:1026, 1992.
33. Picano E, Lattanzi F: Dipyridamole echocardiography: A new diagnostic window on coronary artery disease. Circulation 83(suppl III):III19, 1991.
34. Picano E, Lattanzi F, Masini M, et al: High dose dipyridamole echocardiography test in effort angina pectoris. J Am Coll Cardiol 8:848, 1986.
35. Masini M, Picano E, Lattanzi F, et al: High dose dipyridamole-echocardiography test in women: Correlation with exercise-electrocardiography test and coronary angiography. J Am Coll Cardiol 12:682, 1988.
36. Picano E, Landi P, Bolognese L, et al: Prognostic value of dipyridamole echocardiography early after uncomplicated myocardial infarction: A large-scale, multicenter trial. The EPIC Study Group. Am J Med 95: 608, 1993.
37. Picano E, Marinin C, Pirreli S, et al: Safety of intravenous high dose dipyridamole echocardiography. The Echo-Persantine International Cooperative Study Group. Am J Cardiol 70:252, 1992.
38. Blomstrand P, Engvall J, Swahn E, et al: Cardiovascular effects of dobutamine stress testing in women with suspected coronary artery disease. Heart 75:436, 1996.
39. Cartensen S, Ali SM, Stensgaard-Habsen FV, et al: Dobutamine-atropine stress echocardiography in asymptomatic individuals: The relativity of stress-induced hyperkinesia. Circulation 92:3453, 1995.
40. Segar DS, Ryan T, Sawada SG, et al: Pharmacologically induced myocardial ischemia: A comparison of dobutamine and dipyridamole. J Am Soc Echocardiogr 8:9, 1995.
41. Pellika PA, Roger VL, Oh JK, et al: Stress echocardiography. Part II: Dobutamine stress echocardiography: Techniques, implementation, clinical applications, and correlations. Mayo Clin Proc 70:16, 1995.
42. Barasch E, Wilansky S: Dobutamine stress echocardiography in clinical practice with a review of the recent literature. Tex Heart Inst J 21: 202, 1994.
43. Marcovitz PA, Armstrong WF: Accuracy of dobutamine stress echocardiography in detecting coronary artery disease. Am J Cardiol 169: 1269, 1992.
44. Secknus MA, Marwick TH: Safety and efficacy of dobutamine-atropine stress: Prediction of submaximal stress in 3020 patients studied at a single center. Circulation 94:I-383, 1996.
45. Weissman NJ, Nidorf SM, Guerrero JL, et al: Optimal stage duration in dobutamine stress echocardiography. J Am Coll Cardiol 25;605, 1995.
46. Panza JA, Curiel RV, Laurenzo JM, et al: Relation between ischemic threshold measured during dobutamine stress echocardiography and known indices of poor prognosis in patients with coronary artery disease. Circulation 92:2095, 1995.
47. Mertes H, Sawada SG, Ryan T, et al: Symptoms, adverse effects, and complications associated with dobutamine stress echocardiography: Experience in 1118 patients. Circulation 88:15, 1993.
48. Galloway MT, Paglioroni T, Wun T, et al: Platelet activation during dobutamine stress echocardiography. Am Heart J 135:88, 1998.
49. Hiro J, Hiro T, Reid CL, et al: Safety and results of dobutamine stress echocardiography in women versus men and in patients older and younger than 75 years of age. Am J Cardiol 80:1014, 1997.
50. Gaos CM, Grosz S, Hernandez A, et al: Complications and risk factors for the development of an intracavitary gradient during dobutamine echocardiography. Circulation 92(suppl 1):1, 1995.
51. Marcovitz A, Bach DS, Mathias W, et al: Paradoxic hypotension during dobutamine stress echocardiography: Clinical and diagnostic implications. J Am Coll Cardiol 21:1080, 1993.
52. Bach D, Muller DW, Gross BJ, et al: False positive dobutamine stress echocardiograms: Characterization of clinical, echocardiographic and angiographic findings. J Am Coll Cardiol 24:928, 1994.
53. Senior R, Lahiri A: Enhanced detection of myocardial ischemia by stress dobutamine echocardiography utilizing the "biphasic" response of wall thickening during low and high dose dobutamine infusion. J Am Coll Cardiol 26:26, 1995.
54. Elhendy A, Geleijnse ML, Roelandt JR, et al: Dobutamine-induced hypoperfusion without transient wall motion abnormalities: Less severe ischemia or less severe stress? J Am Coll Cardiol 27:323, 1996.
55. Marwick T, D'Hondt A-M, Baudhuin T, et al: Optimal use of dobutamine stress for the detection and evaluation of coronary artery disease: Combination with echocardiography or scintigraphy, or both? J Am Coll Cardiol 22:159, 1993.
56. Previtali M, Lanzarini L, Fetiveau R, et al: Comparison of dobutamine stress echocardiography, dipyridamole stress echocardiography and exercise stress testing for diagnosis of coronary artery disease. Am J Cardiol 72:865, 1993.
57. Ostojic M, Picano E, Beleslin B, et al: Dipyridamole-dobutamine echocardiography: A novel test for the detection of milder forms of coronary artery disease. J Am Coll Cardiol 23:1115, 1994.
58. Beleslin BD, Ostojic M, Stepanovic J, et al: Stress echocardiography in the detection of myocardial ischemia. Head-to-head comparison of exercise, dobutamine, and dipyridamole tests. Circulation 90:1168, 1994.
59. Dagianti A, Penco M, Agati L, et al: Stress echocardiography: Comparison of exercise, dipyridamole, and dobutamine in detecting and predicting the extent of coronary artery disease. J Am Coll Cardiol 26: 18, 1995.
60. Afridi I, Kleiman NS, Raizner AE, Zoghbi WA: Dobutamine echocardiography in myocardial hibernation: Optimal dose and accuracy in predicting recovery of ventricular function after coronary angioplasty. Circulation 91:663, 1995.
61. Haque T, Furukawa T, Takahashi M, Kinoshita M: Identification of hybernating myocardium by dobutamine stress echocardiography: Comparison with thallium-201 reinjection imaging. Am Heart J 130:553, 1995.
62. Baer FM, Voth E, Deutsch HJ, et al: Assessment of viable myocardium by dobutamine transesophageal echocardiography and comparison with fluorine-18 fluorodeoxyglucose positron emission tomography. J Am Coll Cardiol 24:343, 1994.
63. Pierard LA, De Landsheere CM, Berthe C, et al: Identification of viable myocardium by echocardiography during dobutamine infusion in patients with myocardial infarction after thrombolytic therapy: Comparison with positron emission tomography. J Am Coll Cardiol 15:1021, 1990.
64. Barasch E, Kadipasaoglu K, Moore WH, et al: Low dose dobutamine echocardiography, 201 thallium scintigraphy and 18-fluorodeoxyglucose positron emission tomography for detection of myocardial viability in coronary artery disease. J Am Soc Echocardiogr 8:408, 1995.
65. Kamp O, De Cock CC, Kupper AJ, et al: Simultaneous transesophageal two-dimensional echocardiography and atrial pacing for detecting coronary artery disease. Am J Cardiol 69:1412, 1992.
66. Diamond GA, Forrester JS: Analysis of probability as an aid in the clinical diagnosis of coronary-artery disease. N Engl J Med 300;1350, 1979.
67. Pryor DB, Shaw L, Harrell FE Jr, et al: Estimating the likelihood of severe coronary artery disease. Am J Med 90:553, 1991.

8.4 Positron Emission Tomography

K. Lance Gould

The diagnosis and management of CAD in women remains suboptimal. The diagnostic accuracy of conventional noninvasive stress testing is particularly limited in women, being even lower than in men.[1–10] False-negative electrocardiographic or stress perfusion images are more common in women because of the lower workloads achieved, the inability to reach the target heart rate, and the presence of relatively diffuse disease that does not cause regional perfusion abnormalities. Moreover, women commonly have mitral valve prolapse, hyperventilation-induced ST segment changes, exertional vasoconstriction, and breast-related attenuation artifacts, which are known to cause false-positive electrocardiographic or stress perfusion images.

With standard SPECT stress perfusion imaging, there are significant sex-related differences in the test results, their prognostic value, and subsequent clinical management.[5, 6, 8–15] This method has significant benefits with respect to clinical management and cost effectiveness in women.[16] However, its diagnostic accuracy, particularly its specificity, remains suboptimal, even for severe CAD in women,[5, 17–19] and is not improved by electrocardiographic gating, SPECT attenuation correction, use of a size-based normal database, or Wiener filtering.[20–22] Consequently, PET has a greater specificity then SPECT.[23]

This section discusses the role of high-quality, attenuation-corrected myocardial perfusion imaging—PET and ultrafast computed tomography (CT)—in managing CAD in women. It also explains how such imaging has led to a new paradigm that, instead of relying primarily on revascularization procedures, emphasizes vigorous treatment of risk factors.

POSITRON EMISSION TOMOGRAPHY

Diagnostic Uses

For noninvasive diagnosis, cardiac PET accurately detects both localized and diffuse CAD and assesses its severity, providing a basis for the optimal, comprehensive, principally noninvasive management of CAD, including lifelong reversal treatment, as documented in reviews of the substantial literature.[24–26] PET identifies the coronary arteries involved and determines the quantitative severity of disease with comparable accuracy in asymptomafic and symptomatic patients of both sexes. Moreover, several new concepts in PET perfusion imaging provide additional clinical insights into diffuse atherosclerosis, endothelial dysfunction, and stabilization-reversal treatment of CAD.[24–28] This information is not obtainable with any other technology.

New Concepts in Positron Emission Tomography Perfusion Imaging

Graded, Longitudinal, Base-to-Apex Perfusion Gradient

The first new concept in perfusion imaging is that diffuse coronary atherosclerosis causes a graded, longitudinal, base-to-apex perfusion gradient (Color Plates 8–2 and 8–3). Relative perfusion is best at the base of the heart, poorer in the middle sections, and worst at the apex, in a continuous graded change. This pattern of abnormal perfusion contrasts with the circumscribed, localized perfusion defects that characterize segmental coronary artery stenoses. The fluid-dynamic basis for the base-to-apex perfusion gradient is a branch steal, in which relatively nonstenotic coronary branches shunt flow away from diffusely narrowed major coronary arteries after dipyridamole or adenosine stress.

Resting Perfusion Defects Related to Endothelial Dysfunction

The second new concept in perfusion imaging is that atherosclerosis-induced endothelial dysfunction of the coronary microcirculation may cause abnormal, inhomogeneous resting perfusion that improves after dipyridamole or adenosine stress.[24] Endothelium produces a variety of vasoactive substances, particularly nitric oxide, that are important for maintaining resting vasomotor tone and resting coronary blood flow. Endothelial function is impaired by many vascular insults, including smoking, hypercholesterolemia, hypertension, low levels of high-density lipoprotein cholesterol, and coronary atherosclerosis. The endothelial dysfunction may cause heterogeneous, altered vasomotor tone under resting conditions, with greater vasoconstriction at rest and vasoconstrictive responses to a variety of stimuli, such as acetylcholine and exercise, which normally cause vasodilation.

One manifestation of endothelial dysfunction on the resting PET image may be heterogeneously decreased perfusion with a "moth-eaten" appearance, or discrete resting perfusion defects that improve, resulting in more homogeneous perfusion, after dipyridamole or adenosine stress (Color Plate 8–4). In addition to perfusion heterogeneity at rest, severe endothelial dysfunction may reduce the coronary flow reserve after adenosine or dipyridamole stress because the component of increased flow related to flow-sensitive, endothelium-mediated vasodilation is lost or reduced.[28, 29]

Endothelial dysfunction associated with atherosclerosis may improve with vigorous risk factor management before anatomic disease regression occurs.[24, 28, 30–40] After vigorous lipid treatment is initiated, endothelial healing begins within weeks to months, improving the vasomotor tone and coronary flow reserve.[28, 37] Endothelial healing may also result in improved PET perfusion abnormalities at rest that are independent of improved perfusion defects during stress, reflecting anatomic regression of stenoses.[28]

Follow-Up of Coronary Artery Disease

The third new concept in perfusion imaging is that PET is comparable to or better than quantitative coronary arteriography for following up the progression or regression of CAD.[24, 29] Changes in coronary flow are a function of the luminal radius raised to the fourth power. Therefore, small changes in the radii of severe stenoses that are hard to measure accurately on an arteriogram cause definite, readily apparent effects on PET perfusion images. These images also reflect changes in multiple stenoses and in luminal size along the length of the artery. Furthermore, PET perfusion images reflect the endothelium-mediated vasomotor function of both the epicardial arteries and the microcirculation. Therefore, in contrast to arteriography, which yields only limited information concerning the anatomic luminal narrowing of one small segment, PET perfusion imaging shows the cumulative anatomic and functional changes that accompany disease progression or regression in the entire coronary vasculature.

On the basis of automated, objective quantitative analysis, PET images obtained after dipyridamole stress have shown that myocardial perfusion abnormalities decrease in size or severity in patients who make intense lifestyle changes, undergo cholesterol-lowering drug therapy, or both (Color Plate 8–5), but increase or worsen in patients who receive standard antianginal therapy alone.[24, 28, 29] The improved perfusion on PET images after vigorous cholesterol-lowering therapy shows the functional changes that occur in the atherosclerotic coronary artery tree after lipid-lowering treatment that are associated with modest regression of anatomic disease on arteriography and a markedly reduced risk of adverse coronary events.

Vigorous cholesterol-lowering therapy by means of strict dietary restriction or drug treatment over the relatively short time of 40 to 90 days improves myocardial perfusion in patients with CAD before anatomic regression occurs.[24, 28, 30–40] Within 60 days after lipid-lowering treatment is discontinued, the size and severity of perfusion abnormalities on PET return to baseline status.[28] These rapid alterations in perfusion appear to be due to changing vasomotor function rather than to anatomic regression or progression of stenoses during such short periods.

Maximum myocardial perfusion (ml/min/g) and the absolute coronary flow reserve, as measured by PET, improve in direct proportion to the decrease in serum cholesterol levels seen during 6 weeks of physical training and ingestion of low-fat food.[37] Similar changes are observed on SPECT images (see next section).

Substitution of Single Photon Emission Computed Tomography for Positron Emission Tomography

Because PET is not widely available, the same concepts can be applied to SPECT imaging, although use of this less definitive perfusion imaging technique necessitates more frequent confirmatory coronary arteriography. Such arteriography commonly leads to more revascularization procedures, because of frequent visual overestimations of stenosis severity.

Whereas the accuracy of SPECT in detecting mild to moderate perfusion defects may be questionable because of attenuation artifacts, the absence of severe large perfusion defects on SPECT images indicates a good prognosis and a low risk of coronary events during 1 to 3 years of follow-up observation. In addition, objective determination of stenosis severity by means of quantitative arteriography, Doppler examination, or pressure-wire studies may help the physician decide about the necessity of a revascularization procedure, but these methods are not widely used. If PET is not available, SPECT stress perfusion imaging should be used as a guide to invasive evaluation, despite the presence of attenuation artifacts, which may be "read through" to a limited extent on the basis of a thorough knowledge of coronary anatomy.

Short-term (12-week) lowering of cholesterol levels with fluvastatin is reported to decrease the severity of perfusion abnormalities on SPECT perfusion images obtained during exercise.[31] Because these improvements occur over such a brief period, they implicate altered vasomotor function rather than anatomic changes in the coronary arteries.[28, 30, 31, 37, 41] SPECT imaging during exercise also shows a decreased severity of perfusion defects after lipid-active drug therapy or exercise training and use of a low-fat diet.[31, 41]

ULTRAFAST COMPUTED TOMOGRAPHY FOR CORONARY CALCIFICATION

Ultrafast CT identifies coronary calcification as a marker of coronary atherosclerosis and quantifies the density, amount, or both, of calcium as an indirect indicator of CAD.[42–50] In older men the sensitivity of ultrafast CT for identifying coronary atherosclerosis is high, but its specificity for identifying focal coronary artery stenosis is low (40% to 55%) because many men older than 50 years have coronary calcification without stenosis. The sensitivity of ultrafast CT for identifying coronary artery stenosis may also be low in younger people—as low as 50% in women younger than 60 years, owing to the presence of newer, less calcified plaque. If calcium score criteria are used for diagnosing coronary stenosis, the specificity of ultrafast CT is increased to 95% but the sensitivity falls to 46%; if calcium score criteria are used that increase the specificity for diagnosing significant coronary artery stenosis to 90%, the sensitivity falls to 70%. Many older patients have high calcium scores but widely patent arteries. Younger patients may have extensive CAD, even angina or an MI, without having significantly abnormal calcium levels. Therefore, in clinical practice, calcium scores do not reliably predict the presence or severity of stenosis, and such scores may not be optimally reproducible. However, when Achenbach and coworkers[48] excluded 25% of their images (involving 37% of patients) because they did not conform to strict technical criteria for adequacy, the predictive accuracy of ultrafast CT for detecting high-grade stenosis improved to more than 90%.

In cases of coronary calcification, the great strength of ultrafast CT is its high sensitivity for detecting atherosclerosis manifested as calcified plaque. The importance of this fact is often lost because of an inappropriate preoccupation, on the part of both critics and supporters, with the technique's low specificity for significant stenoses. Like high cholesterol levels, a family history, or other risk factors, high coronary calcium scores on ultrafast CT indicate a higher, more specific risk of disease.[46] Compared with intracoronary ultrasonography for the detection of calcium, ultrafast CT is less sensitive for identifying noncalcified plaque,[49] which may occur in younger people. With respect to cardiovascular risk, ultrafast CT has a promising predictive value[50] but necessitates long-term follow-up owing to the relative stability of chronic calcified disease (compared to young, friable, lipid-rich plaques, which are prone to rupture and cause unstable coronary syndromes).

The value of ultrafast CT depends on one's orientation toward CAD. For a cardiologist focused on "significant" stenosis and on binary decision making with respect to revascularization procedures, ultrafast CT is of little value except to increase the number of diagnostic arteriograms, many of which show little obstructive disease. However, according to a new paradigm for the primarily noninvasive management of coronary atherosclerosis (see next section), there is substantial merit to screening for coronary calcification by means of ultrafast CT. Patients with a high calcium score would then be evaluated with definitive PET to assess the effects of endothelial dysfunction, diffuse CAD, or regional flow-limiting stenosis on myocardial perfusion. Evaluation of the severity and size of regional perfusion defects or of a longitudinal perfusion gradient provides a noninvasive basis for either instituting lifelong intense treatment of risk factors or proceeding to arteriography. In the latter case, revascularization would be highly likely in patients with large, life-threatening perfusion defects that objectively indicate severe stenosis of a major proximal coronary artery.

PARADIGM SHIFT IN THE TREATMENT OF CORONARY ARTERY DISEASE

High-quality perfusion imaging has led to a paradigm shift in the management of CAD—from relying primarily on revascularization procedures to emphasizing vigorous treatment of risk factors as the first step in therapy. Traditional diagnosis and management of CAD are characterized by binary thinking that relies on yes-or-no decisions about "significant disease" and the patient's suitability for coronary angioplasty or bypass surgery. Reflecting this binary mindset, the accuracy of a noninvasive diagnostic test is traditionally described in terms of sensitivity and specificity, compared with the standard of coronary arteriography. According to this viewpoint, the arteriogram is interpreted as either showing a significant segmental stenosis or not, although visual estimates are notoriously inaccurate. However, the pathophysiology of coronary atherosclerosis, as well as coronary events and their treatment, necessitates that cardiovascular medicine adopt an entirely different paradigm,[24–26, 51] on the basis of the following observations:

1. Eighty-five percent of MIs develop at coronary artery sites of less severely narrowed, lipid-rich plaques that rupture because of thrombosis and spasm.
2. Coronary atherosclerosis is diffuse and subject to plaque rupture throughout the length of all the epicardial arteries.
3. Coronary atherosclerosis alters the endothelial and vasomotor function of the microvasculature, causing altered rest/stress perfusion patterns as a sign of early CAD.
4. With diffuse coronary atherosclerosis, the diagnostic accuracy of coronary arteriography is poor (as low as 10%) compared with intracoronary ultrasonography, rendering arteriography suboptimal for identifying and quantifying the diffuse disease that is responsible for most clinical cardiac events.
5. Vigorous cholesterol-lowering strategies reduce the cardiac event rate and mortality much more than invasive procedures, which improve neither the cardiac event rate nor long-term survival.
6. Compared with coronary arteriography, new techniques for interpreting noninvasive PET perfusion images or absolute flow measurements better reflect the presence of diffuse coronary atherosclerosis, endothelial dysfunction, and the changes produced by vigorous cholesterol-lowering strategies.

These observations and their associated therapeutic options are not compatible with traditional binary, procedure-based decision making, in which diagnosis and treatment are focused on segmental stenoses and localized mechanical procedures. Coronary atherosclerosis is diffuse, not discrete. Its progression and outcome arise from diffuse, continuous processes that occur throughout the coronary tree. Quantifying the severity of CAD necessitates graded, multifaceted, continuous measurement with the use of both invasive and noninvasive methods. Treatment also necessitates a graded, multifaceted therapeutic approach, revascularization based on objective criteria being only one option. Therefore, it is time for diagnosis and treatment to be reoriented toward the new paradigm and for greater emphasis to be placed on intense risk factor treatment, which improves survival better than revascularization procedures.

CONCLUSIONS

Treatment regimens designed to partially reverse or to stop the progression of coronary atherosclerosis ideally require a lifelong commitment to a low-fat diet, a lean body habitus, moderate exercise, cessation of smoking, control of blood pressure, and cardiovascular and cholesterol-lowering drug therapy. A firm diagnosis of CAD is essential as the basis for such a reversal regimen. In clinical practice and cholesterol-lowering trials, CAD documented by quantitative coronary arteriography has traditionally been the basis both for definitive diagnosis and for following up changes in the severity of the disease. However, reliance on an invasive diagnostic test for noninvasive reversal treatment precludes a principally noninvasive approach to managing CAD.

It is time, in women's cardiovascular medicine, to acknowledge that the presence of attenuation artifacts in myocardial perfusion imaging is an unacceptable limitation that undermines diagnostic accuracy and becomes the reason for performing "definitive" coronary arteriograms. Coronary arteriography (with its reliance on visual interpretation) can now be replaced by PET imaging, which is just as accurate (or even more so for assessing diffuse disease). For moderate to severe stenoses, small changes in luminal size that are hard to measure reliably with coronary arteriography are quite apparent on PET images after administration of dipyridamole. Equally important, PET shows the cumulative hemodynamic effects of multiple stenoses or diffuse disease and of atherosclerotic endothelial dysfunction of both the arterial circulation and microcirculation, even in the absence of arteriographic stenosis.

The principally noninvasive management of CAD, based on PET and reversal treatment, is a valid, safe, effective alternative to invasive procedures.[24–26, 51] It is not antithetical to revascularization but may offer a better outcome, at lower risk and cost, for many women with CAD. Most patients pursue an effective reversal regimen if it is presented and managed appropriately, with strong support from a knowledgeable physician.[51] Nevertheless, some patients do not show response to vigorous medical treatment or will not alter their risk factors despite predictable future morbidity and mortality. For such patients, coronary arteriography, intravascular Doppler or pressure studies, and revascularization procedures may be appropriate, with reversal treatment playing a secondary role. In these cases, essential coronary arteriograms should be performed (by a physician with a thorough understanding of diffuse disease) and should be integrated with intracoronary flow-velocity and pressure measurements or quantitative arteriographic analyses of the entire coronary tree; by clearly defining the physiologic severity of stenoses and of diffuse disease, these studies can serve as the basis for revascularization in the relatively few cases that do not respond to vigorous management of risk factors.

References

1. Guiteras VP, Chaitman BR, Waters DD, et al: Diagnostic accuracy of exercise ECG lead systems in clinical subsets of women. Circulation 65:1465, 1982.
2. Hung J, Chairman BR, Lam J, et al: Noninvasive diagnostic test choices for the evaluation of coronary artery disease in women—a multivariate comparison of cardiac fluoroscopy, exercise electrocardiography and exercise thallium myocardial perfusion scintigraphy. J Am Coll Cardiol 4:8, 1984.
3. Sketch MH, Mohiuddin SM, Lynch JD, et al: Significant sex differences in the correlation of electrocardiographic exercise testing and coronary arteriograms. Am J Cardiol 36:169, 1975.
4. Waters DD, Szlachcic J, Bonan R, et al: Comparative sensitivity of exercise, cold pressor and ergonovine testing in provoking attacks of variant angina in patient with active disease. Circulation 67:310, 1983.
5. Wackers FJTH: Artifacts in planar and SPECT myocardial perfusion imaging. Am J Card Imaging 6:42, 1992.
6. Wenger NK: Symposium—gender differences in cardiac imaging. Am J Card Imaging 10:42, 1996.
7. Okin PM, Kligfield P: Gender-specific criteria and performance of the exercise electrocardiogram. Circulation 92:1209, 1995.
8. Chae SC, Heo J, Iskandrian AS, et al. Identification of extensive CAD in women by exercise single-photon emission computed tomographic (SPECT) thallium imaging. J Am Coll Cardiol 21:1305, 1993.
9. Pancholy S, Gioia G, Russell J, et al: Detection of CAD in women. Circulation 92:I130, 1995.
10. Hlatky MA, Pryor DB, Harrell FE, et al: Factors affecting sensitivity and specificity of exercise electrocardiography—multivariable analysis. Am J Med 77:64, 1984.
11. Hachamovitch R, Berman DS, Kiat H, et al: Gender-related differences in clinical management after exercise nuclear testing. J Am Coll Cardiol 26:1457, 1995.
12. Travin MI, Duca MD, Kline GM, et al: Relation of gender to physician use of test results and to the prognostic value of stress technetium 99m sestamibi myocardial single-photon emission computed tomography scintigraphy. Am Heart J 134:73, 1997.
13. Marwick TH, Shaw LJ, Lauer MS, et al: The noninvasive prediction of cardiac mortality in men and women with known or suspected coronary artery disease. Economics of Noninvasive Diagnosis (END) Study Group. Am J Med 106:172, 1999.
14. Ababneh AA, Sciacca RR, Kim B, Bergmann SR: Normal limits for left ventricular ejection fraction and volumes estimated with gated myocardial perfusion imaging in patients with normal exercise test results: Influence of tracer, gender, and acquisition camera. J Nucl Cardiol 7:661, 2000.
15. Toft J, Hesse B, Rabol A: The occurrence of false-positive technetium-99m sestamibi bull's eye defects in different reference databases: A study of an age- and gender-stratified healthy population. Eur J Nucl Med 24:179, 1997.
16. Shaw LJ, Heller GV, Travin MI, et al: Cost analysis of diagnostic testing for coronary artery disease in women with stable chest pain. Economics of Noninvasive Diagnosis (END) Study Group. J Nucl Cardiol 6: 559, 1999.
17. Hansen CL, Crabbe D, Rubin S: Lower diagnostic accuracy of thallium-201 SPECT myocardial perfusion imaging in women: An effect of smaller chamber size. J Am Coll Cardiol 28:1214, 1996.
18. Amanullah AM, Berman DS, Hachamovitch R, et al: Identification of severe or extensive coronary artery disease in women by adenosine technetium-99m sestamibi SPECT. Am J Cardiol 80:132, 1997.
19. Travin MI, Katz MS, Moulton AW, et al: Accuracy of dipyridamole SPECT imaging in identifying individual coronary stenoses and multivessel disease in women versus men. J Nucl Cardiol 7:213, 2000.
20. Chatziioannou SN, Moore WH, Dhekne RD, Ford PV: Gating of myocardial perfusion imaging for the identification of artifacts: Is it useful for experienced physicians? Tex Heart Inst J 27:14, 2000.
21. Lee DS, So Y, Cheon GJ, et al: Limited incremental diagnostic values of attenuation-noncorrected gating and ungated attenuation correction to rest/stress myocardial perfusion SPECT in patients with an intermediate likelihood of coronary artery disease. J Nucl Med 41:852, 2000.
22. Hansen CL, Kramer M, Rastogi A: Lower accuracy of TI-201 SPECT in women is not improved by size-based normal databases or Wiener filtering. J Nucl Cardiol 6:177, 1999.
23. Freedman N, Schechter D, Klein M, et al: SPECT attenuation artifacts in normal and overweight persons—insights from a retrospective comparison of Rb-82 positron emission tomography and TI-201 SPECT myocardial perfusion imaging. Clin Nucl Med 25:1019, 2000.
24. Gould KL: Coronary Artery Stenosis, 2nd ed. Arnold Publishers, London, 1999.
25. Gould KL: Focus for the new millennium—Diffuse coronary artery disease and new paradigms in cardiovascular medicine. ACC Curr J Review, January/February 2000.
26. Gould KL: New concepts and paradigms in cardiovascular medicine. The non-invasive management of coronary artery disease. Am J Med 104:25, 1998.
27. Gould KL, Nakagawa Y, Nakagawa N, et al: Frequency and clinical implications of fluid dynamically significant diffuse coronary artery disease manifest as graded, longitudinal, base-to-apex myocardial perfusion abnormalities by noninvasive positron emission tomography. Circulation 101:1931, 2000.
28. Gould KL, Martucci JP, Goldberg DI, et al: Short-term cholesterol lowering decreases size and severity of perfusion abnormalities by positron emission tomography after dipyridamole in patients with coronary artery disease: A positive noninvasive marker of healing coronary endothelium. Circulation 89:1530, 1994.
29. Gould K, Ornish D, Scherwitz L, et al: Changes in myocardial perfusion abnormalities by positron emission tomography after long-term, intense risk factor modification. JAMA 274:894, 1995.
30. Baller D, Notohamiprodjo G, Gleichmann U, et al: Improvement in coronary flow reserve determined by positron emission tomography after 6 months of cholesterol-lowering therapy in patients with early stages of coronary atherosclerosis. Circulation 99:2871, 1999.
31. Eichstadt HW, Eskotter H, Hoffman I, et al: Improvement of myocardial perfusion by short term fluvastatin therapy in coronary artery disease. Am J Cardiol 76:122A, 1995.
32. Tamai O, Matsuoka H, Itabe H, et al: Single LDL apheresis improves endothelium-dependent vasodilation in hypercholesterolemic humans. Circulation 95:76, 1997.
33. O'Driscoll G, Green D, Taylor RR: Simvastatin, an HMG-coenzyme A reductase inhibitor, improves endothelial function within 1 month. Circulation 95:1126, 1997.
34. De Divitiis M, Rubba P, DiSomma S, et al: Effects of short term reduction in serum cholesterol with simvastatin in patients with stable angina pectoris and mild to moderate hypercholesterolemia. Am J Cardiol 78:763, 1996.
35. Vogel A, Corretti MC, Plotnick GD: Effect of a single high-fat meal on endothelial function in healthy subjects. Am J Cardiol 79:350, 1997.

36. Plotnick GD, Corretti MC, Vogel RA: Effect of antioxidant vitamins on the transient impairment of endothelium-dependent brachial artery vasoactivity following a single high-fat meal. JAMA 278:1682, 1997.
37. Czernin J, Barnard J, Sun KT, et al: Effect of short-term cardiovascular conditioning and low-fat diet on myocardial blood flow and flow reserve. Circulation 92:197, 1995.
38. Armstrong ML, Heistad DD, Marcus ML, et al: Hemodynamic sequelae of regression in experimental atherosclerosis. J Clin Invest 71: 104, 1983.
39. Benzuly KH, Padgett RC, Kaul S, et al: Functional improvement precedes structural regression of atherosclerosis. Circulation 89:1810, 1994.
40. Reddy KG, Nair RV, Sheehan HM, Hodgson JM: Evidence that selective endothelial dysfunction may occur in the absence of angiographic or ultrasound atherosclerosis in patients with risk factors for atherosclerosis. J Am Coll Cardiol 23:833, 1994.
41. Schuler G, Hambrecht R, Schlierf G, et al: Myocardial perfusion and regression of coronary artery disease in patients on a regimen of intensive physical exercise and low fat diet. J Am Coll Cardiol 19: 34, 1992.
42. O'Rourke RA, Brundage BH, Froelicher VF, et al: American College of Cardiology/American Heart Association expert consensus document on electron-beam computed tomography for the diagnosis and prognosis of coronary artery disease. J Am Coll Cardiol 36:326, 2000.
43. Devries S, Wolfkiel C, Fusman B, et al: Influence of age and gender on the presence of coronary calcium detected by ultrafast computed tomography. J Am Coll Cardiol 25:76, 1995.
44. Kajinami K, Seki H, Takekoshi N, Mabuchi H: Noninvasive prediction of coronary atherosclerosis by quantification of coronary artery calcification using electron beam computed tomography: Comparison with electrocardiographic and thallium exercise stress test results. J Am Coll Cardiol 26:1209, 1995.
45. Rumberger JA, Behrenbeck T, Breen JF, Sheedy PF: Coronary calcification by electron beam computed tomography and obstructive coronary artery disease: A model for costs and effectiveness of diagnosis as compared with conventional cardiac testing methods. J Am Coll Cardiol 33:453, 1999.
46. Schmermund A, Baumgart D, Görge G, et al: Measuring the effect of risk factors on coronary atherosclerosis: Coronary calcium score versus angiographic disease severity. J Am Coll Cardiol 31:1267, 1998.
47. Fiorino AS: Electron-beam computed tomography, coronary artery calcium and evaluation of patients with coronary artery disease. Ann Intern Med 128:839, 1998.
48. Achenbach S, Moshage W, Ropers D, et al: Value of electron beam computed tomography for the noninvasive detection of high-grade coronary-artery stenoses and occlusions. N Engl J Med 339:1964, 1998.
49. Baumgart D, Schmermund, Goerge G, et al: Comparison of electron beam computed tomography with intracoronary ultrasound and coronary angiography for detection of coronary atherosclerosis. J Am Coll Cardiol 30:57, 1997.
50. Arad Y, Spadaro L, Goodman K, et al: Predictive value of electron beam computed tomography of the coronary arteries: 19 month follow-up of 1173 asymptomatic subjects. Circulation 93:1951, 1996.
51. Gould KL: Heal Your Heart: How You Can Prevent or Reverse Heart Disease. Rutgers University Press, New Brunswick, NJ, 1998.

CHAPTER 9

Invasive Diagnostic Testing

Carina M. Alfaro-Franco, Richard W. Smalling, and H. Vernon Anderson

Coronary artery disease is the leading cause of death among both women and men in the United States.[1] As public attention has focused on women's health care, recent studies have questioned whether gender bias exists in the diagnosis of coronary artery disease, especially in the use of invasive diagnostic procedures.[2–8]

TECHNICAL FEATURES AND RISKS

Cardiac catheterization is used to confirm the presence of clinically suspected heart disease, to define its anatomic and physiologic severity, and to determine the presence of associated conditions.[9] The same technical procedure is used to perform cardiac catheterization in women and men, but the smaller size of the coronary arteries and peripheral vessels in women[10] increases the technical difficulty of inserting the catheter, which may prolong the procedure. Longer procedures may require more contrast dye, which can lead to contrast-induced renal dysfunction in patients with underlying azotemia or diabetes mellitus.[11] Furthermore, a Foley catheter is often used in women during prolonged procedures and during the immobilization period after catheterization, whereas an external (condom) urinary catheter is commonly used in men.

The overall major complication rate is less than 1% in patients undergoing diagnostic cardiac catheterization.[12, 13] Shorter procedure times are associated with a decreased risk of adverse events.[14] The major complications of cardiac catheterization are death, acute myocardial infarction, pulmonary embolus, perforation or dissection of a major vessel or chamber, life-threatening dysrhythmias (ventricular tachycardia, ventricular fibrillation, or asystole), and neurologic damage lasting more than 24 hours after the procedure. Minor complications include thrombus or hemorrhage requiring surgical correction, hypotension, prolonged angina, pyrogenic reaction, and transient neurologic damage lasting less than 24 hours.[15, 16] Female gender is an independent predictor for developing an acute neurologic complication (e.g., visual disturbance, facial droop, hemiparesis) after cardiac catheterization and is associated with more than a threefold increase in risk for neurologic events.[17, 18] Visual disturbances occur more often in women than in men, but these disturbances are usually transient and benign, and resolve within 24 hours.[19] Women may be at higher risk for developing neurologic events because of having a small body area or because of presenting for cardiac evaluation at a more advanced age, which may correlate with more extensive generalized atherosclerosis.[17]

In a prospective review of unplanned admissions after outpatient cardiac catheterizations during a 1-year period at a large community-based tertiary care hospital, Clark and Dolce[12] found that women were more likely than men to be admitted with complications of hemodynamic instability after catheterization.

VASCULAR APPROACH

The femoral approach is preferred over the formerly used transbrachial approach in high-risk or unstable patients regardless of gender. The femoral approach allows for faster introduction of the catheter and for the use of larger sheaths, which provide the potential for performing a broad range of interventional procedures (e.g., angioplasty, stent placement, atherectomy) and the possibility of providing circulatory assist (e.g., intra-aortic balloon). Because of smaller-sized peripheral vessels, smaller sheaths and catheters are used in women to decrease the likelihood of peripheral vascular complications,[20] including obstruction of antegrade flow in the femoral artery. This type of obstruction causes leg ischemia, especially when the catheter dwell time is long[14] or when several catheters are exchanged.[21] In addition, the common femoral artery should be accurately punctured and initial bleeding after sheath removal should be controlled to avoid pseudoaneurysm formation.[14] Lilly and colleagues[22] found that in transfemoral arteriography, complications requiring surgical correction are more common when the arterial puncture site is outside the common femoral artery; age, gender, body type, and anticoagulation had less effect on patient risk. Furthermore, Lilly and colleagues[22] reported that the risk of complications was slightly higher in women and in patients over 65 years of age; however, these differences did not reach statistical significance.

The transbrachial approach is associated with a higher risk of local vascular complications requiring surgical repair.[13, 23–25] Recurrent thrombosis after initial thrombectomy and local brachial artery revision occurs more often in women than in men[13]; however, segmental arterial resection and overnight heparin anticoagulation reduce the risk for early post-thrombectomy failure in women.[26]

CLINICAL FEATURES

The presentation and manifestation of clinical heart disease differ in women and men. Although women are usually smaller in physical stature than men, gender alone does not completely determine the size of the coronary vessels. Roberts and Roberts[10] measured at autopsy the proximal portion of the coronary arteries in patients with cardiac disease. They found that patients with angina pectoris had smaller hearts with smaller coronary arteries, regardless of gender. The mean cross-sectional size of proximal coronary arteries was smaller in women (5.9 mm^2) than in men (7.7 mm^2). This difference, however, was attributed to lower heart weights in women. Small coronary arteries have a higher prevalence of atherogenesis than larger arteries, possibly because variables that suppress atherogenesis (e.g., volume flow rate, flow velocity, and shear stress) increase with vessel radius.[27]

Coronary artery disease in women develops approximately 6 to 10 years later than in men.[28] This difference has been attributed, in part, to the protective effects of estrogen before menopause.[29] After menopause, circulating levels of high-density lipoprotein (HDL) cholesterol decrease slightly, and levels of low-density lipoprotein (LDL) cholesterol increase. Both of these changes increase the risk of coronary heart disease.[30, 31] Women hospitalized with acute myocardial infarction are usually older than men and are more likely to have the risk factors of hypertension, diabetes mellitus, previous angina, peripheral or cerebrovascular disease, obesity, and congestive heart failure. However, women with acute myocardial infarction are less likely than men to have a history of smoking or chronic obstructive lung disease.[7, 29, 32–36] Therefore, women present in a later stage of cardiac disease than do men,[37] with more atypical symptoms and with more severe comorbidities.[8, 38]

For any risk factor, women have a lower rate of developing heart disease than do men.[7, 39, 40] Despite having worse symptoms, women have less severe and less extensive coronary disease on angiography than men.[5, 33, 34, 41] In the Coronary Artery Surgical Study (CASS),[42] 20,391 patients underwent cardiac catheterization from 1975 to 1979. Of the 401 women in the study who had definite angina, only 72% had significant obstructive coronary artery disease compared with 93% of 1919 men with definite angina. Of the men who were more than 50 years old, 50% had three-vessel or left main coronary artery disease. The prevalence of left main coronary artery disease among the 1012 women with probable angina did not exceed 5% regardless of age, and three-vessel or left main coronary artery disease was uncommon in women younger than 70. Of the 1397 women with nonspecific chest pain, the prevalence of left main coronary artery disease was less than 1% regardless of age. Of the 1282 men with nonspecific chest pain, three-vessel or left main coronary artery disease was uncommon in patients younger than 70 years of age and was seen in five (23%) of the 22 men older than 70 years of age.

FUNCTIONAL STATUS

Women usually have greater functional disability related to heart disease and may be less aggressively treated than men with similar symptoms[3, 43]; thus outcome is less favorable in women.[36, 44] Although small body size independently increases perioperative mortality of patients undergoing aortocoronary bypass surgery,[45, 46] Khan and associates[47] found that women had a higher perioperative mortality than did men because they were referred for surgery at a more advanced stage of the disease. Moreover, Tobin and coworkers[2] found that men were 10 times as likely as women to be referred for coronary angiography after an abnormal nuclear exercise stress test. In a review of enrollment for the Survival and Ventricular Enlargement study, Steingart and colleagues[3] reported that men were referred twice as often as women for coronary angiography and bypass surgery after admission to the hospital for myocardial infarction. Ayanian and Epstein[4] reported similar findings in a large study of patients hospitalized for coronary heart disease in Maryland and Massachusetts; women were one third less likely than men to have coronary angiography or coronary revascularization after admission for myocardial infarction, stable or unstable angina, chronic ischemic heart disease, or chest pain.[4]

Mark and colleagues[6] conducted a prospective study on the ability of physicians to make accurate predictions regarding diagnosis and outcome for outpatients referred to the exercise laboratory for evaluation of suspected coronary artery disease. They found that women were referred for cardiac catheterization significantly less often than men, but women had a significantly lower pretest probability of coronary disease (as estimated by their physicians) and a lower rate of positive exercise test results. Those findings suggest that gender is not an independent predictor of referral for catheterization and that physicians were not underestimating the risk of coronary disease in women.

Hachamovitch and coworkers[5] reported that women with severe ischemia on perfusion scan were referred more often for catheterization than were men, and that both men and women with normal scans and a low risk for coronary events were appropriately referred at a low rate. However, women with severe perfusion abnormalities (the high-risk subgroup) had a greater rate of cardiac death and myocardial infarction than did men; therefore, these authors suggested that women are underreferred for catheterization. Lauer and associates[48] studied 2351 men and 1318 women with no history of invasive cardiac procedures who were referred for treadmill thallium testing at the Cleveland Clinic Foundation. They reported that women were less likely to undergo coronary angiography but were also less likely to have an abnormal thallium scan. After adjusting for thallium results and age, the authors showed that women were as likely as men to be referred for coronary angiography, although women were less likely to have severe coronary disease on angiography. They concluded that gender-related differences in referral for coronary angiography after treadmill thallium testing can be explained by a higher rate of abnormal tests in men.

In other recent studies after adjusting for age, severity of disease, number of comorbidities, and other confounding factors, investigators have found no significant gender-related differences in the rate of referral for cardiac catheterization.[5, 7–8, 35, 49]

CONCLUSIONS

The issue of gender bias in the diagnosis of cardiovascular disease is debated. Whether cardiac catheterization is underused in women or overused in men is unresolved.[4] Furthermore, whether awareness of gender-related differences in the manifestation of heart disease has led physicians to treat men and women with cardiac symptoms differently is unknown.[50] Diagnostic cardiac catheterization is a valuable tool for assessing the presence and severity of heart disease in women and men, and the method should be used in all patients with suspected heart disease.

References

1. Eaker ED, Cheseboro JH, Sacks FM, et al: Cardiovascular disease in women. Circulation 88:1999, 1993.
2. Tobin JN, Wassertheil-Smoller S, Wexler JP, et al: Sex bias in considering coronary bypass surgery. Ann Intern Med 107:19, 1987.
3. Steingart RM, Packer M, Hamm P, et al: Sex differences in the management of coronary artery disease. Survival and Ventricular Enlargement Investigators. N Engl J Med 325:226, 1991.
4. Ayanian JZ, Epstein AM: Differences in the use of procedures between women and men hospitalized for coronary heart disease. N Engl J Med 325:221, 1991.
5. Krumholz HM, Douglas PS, Lauer MS, et al: Selection of patients for coronary angiography and coronary revascularization early after myocardial infarction: Is there evidence for a gender bias? Ann Intern Med 116:785, 1992.
6. Mark DB, Shaw LK, DeLong ER, et al: Absence of sex bias in the referral of patients for cardiac catheterization. N Engl J Med 330: 1101, 1994.
7. Bernstein SJ, Hilborne LH, Leape LL, et al: The appropriateness of use of cardiovascular procedures in women and men. Ann Intern Med 154:2759, 1994.
8. Hachamovitch R, Berman DS, Kiat H, et al: Gender-related differences in clinical management after exercise nuclear testing. J Am Coll Cardiol 26:1457, 1995.
9. Grossman W: Current practice standards. In Baim DS, Grossman W (eds): Cardiac Catheterization, Angiography, and Intervention. Williams & Wilkins, Baltimore, 1996, p 9.
10. Roberts CS, Roberts WC: Cross-sectional area of the proximal portions of the three major epicardial coronary arteries in 98 necropsy patients with different coronary events. Relationship to heart weight, age and sex. Circulation 62:953, 1980.
11. Cigarroa RG, Lange RA, Williams RH, et al: Dosing of contrast material to prevent contrast nephropathy in patients with renal disease. Am J Med 86:649, 1989.
12. Clark VL, Dolce J: Unplanned admissions after outpatient cardiac catheterization. Clin Cardiol 16:823, 1993.
13. Davis K, Kennedy JW, Kemp HG Jr, et al: Complications of coronary arteriography from the Collaborative Study of Coronary Artery Surgery (CASS). Circulation 59:1105, 1979.
14. Baim DS, Grossman W: Complications of cardiac catheterization. In Baim DS, Grossman W (eds): Cardiac catheterization, angiography, and intervention. Williams & Wilkins, Baltimore, 1996, p 17.
15. Fighali S, Krajcer Z, Gonzales-Camid F, et al: Safety of outpatient cardiac catheterization. Chest 88:349, 1985.
16. Gillinov AM, Davis EA, Alberg AJ, et al: Pulmonary embolism in the cardiac surgical patient. Ann Thorac Surg 53:988, 1992.
17. Lazar JM, Uretsky BF, Denys BG, et al: Predisposing risk factors and natural history of acute neurological complications of left-sided cardiac catheterization. Am J Cardiol 75:1056, 1995.
18. Brown DL, Topol EJ: Stroke complicating percutaneous coronary revascularization. Am J Cardiol 72:1207, 1993.
19. Vik-Mo H, Todnem K, Folling M, et al: Transient visual disturbance during cardiac catheterization with angiography. Cathet Cardiovasc Diagn 12:1, 1986.
20. Talley JD, Mauldin PD, Kupersmith J: Economic and angiographic factors in determining optimal catheter size in performing outpatient left-sided heart and coronary angiography. Am J Cardiol 77:374, 1996.
21. Kido DK, King PD, Manzione J, et al: The role of catheters and guidewires in the production of angiographic thromboembolic complications. Invest Radiol 23:S359, 1988.
22. Lilly MP, Reichman W, Sarazen AA Jr, et al: Anatomic and clinical factors associated with complications of transfemoral arteriography. Ann Vasc Surg 4:264, 1990.
23. Kitzmiller JW, Hertzer NR, Beven EG: Routine surgical management of brachial artery occlusion after cardiac catheterization. Arch Surg 117:1066, 1982.
24. Adams DF, Abrams HL: Complications of coronary arteriography: a follow-up report. Cardiovasc Radiol 2:89, 1979.
25. Kennedy JW, Baxley WA, Bunnel IL, et al: Mortality related to cardiac catheterization and angiography. Cathet Cardiovasc Diagn 8:323, 1982.
26. Kline RM, Hertzer NR, Beven EG, et al: Surgical treatment of brachial artery injuries after cardiac catheterization. J Vasc Surg 12:20, 1990.
27. Nwasokwa ON, Weiss M, Gladstone C, et al: Effect of coronary artery size on the prevalence of atherosclerosis. Am J Cardiol 78:741, 1996.
28. Castelli WP: Cardiovascular disease in women. Am J Obstet Gynecol 158:1553, 1988.
29. Wenger NK: Coronary disease in women. Annu Rev Med 36:285, 1985.
30. Lobo RA: Hormones, hormone replacement therapy, and heart disease. In Douglas PS (ed): Cardiovascular Health and Disease in Women. W.B. Saunders, Philadelphia, 1993, p 227.
31. Matthews KA, Meilahn E, Kuller LH, et al: Menopause and risk factors for coronary heart disease. N Engl J Med 321:641, 1989.
32. Lincoff AM, Califf RM, Ellis SG, et al: Thrombolytic therapy for women with myocardial infarction: Is there a gender gap? Thrombolysis and Angioplasty in Myocardial Infarction Study Group. J Am Coll Cardiol 22:1780, 1993.
33. Stone PH, Thompson B, Anderson HV, et al: Influence of race, sex, and age on management of unstable angina and non-Q-wave myocardial infarction: The TIMI III Registry. JAMA 275:1104, 1996.
34. Bell MR, Berger PB, Holmes DR Jr, et al: Referral for coronary artery revascularization procedures after diagnostic coronary angiography: Evidence for gender bias? J Am Coll Cardiol 25:1650, 1995.
35. Weintraub WS, Wenger NK, Jones EL, et al: Changing clinical characteristics of coronary surgery patients. Circulation 88(Pt II):79, 1993.
36. Kostis JB, Wilson AC, O'Dowd K, et al: Sex differences in the management and long-term outcome of acute myocardial infarction. A statewide study. MIDAS study group. Myocardial Infarction Data Acquisition System. Circulation 90:1715, 1994.
37. Lerner DJ, Kannel WB: Patterns of coronary heart disease morbidity and mortality in the sexes: A 26-year follow-up of the Framingham population. Am Heart J 111:383, 1986.
38. Jenkins JS, Flaker GC, Nolte B, et al: Causes of higher in-hospital mortality in women than in men after acute myocardial infarction. Am J Cardiol 73:319, 1994.
39. Robinson K, Conroy RM, Mulcahy R, et al: Risk factors and in-hospital course of first episode of myocardial infarction or acute coronary insufficiency in women. J Am Coll Cardiol 11:932, 1988.
40. Dittrich H, Gilpin E, Nicod P, et al: Acute myocardial infarction in women: Influence of gender on mortality and prognostic variables. Am J Cardiol 62:1, 1988.
41. He ZX, Dakik HA, Vaduganathan P, et al: Clinical and angiographic significance of a normal thallium-201 tomographic study in patients with a strongly positive exercise electrocardiogram. Am J Cardiol 78: 638, 1996.
42. Chaitman BR, Bourassa MG, Davis K, et al: Angiographic prevalence of high risk coronary artery disease in patient subsets (CASS). Circulation 64:360, 1981.
43. Wenger NK, Speroff L, Packard B: Cardiovascular health and disease in women. N Engl J Med 329:247, 1993.
44. Kudenchuck PJ, Maynard C, Martin JS, et al: Comparison of presentation, treatment, and outcome of acute myocardial infarction in men versus women. Am J Cardiol 78:9, 1996.
45. Fisher LD, Kennedy JW, Davis KB, et al: Association of sex, physical size, and operative mortality after coronary artery bypass in the Coronary Artery Surgery Study (CASS). J Thorac Cardiovasc Surg 84:334, 1982.
46. Loop FD, Golding LR, MacMillan JP, et al: Coronary artery surgery in women compared with men: Analyses of risks and long-term results. J Am Coll Cardiol 1:383, 1983.
47. Khan SS, Nessim S, Gray R, et al: Increased mortality of women in coronary artery bypass surgery: Evidence for referral bias. Ann Intern Med 112:561, 1990.
48. Lauer MS, Pashkow FJ, Snader CE, et al: Gender and referral for coronary angiography after treadmill thallium testing. Am J Cardiol 78: 278, 1996.
49. Vacek JL, Handlin LR, Rosamond TL, et al: Gender-related differences in reperfusion treatment allocation and outcome for acute myocardial infarction. Am J Cardiol 76:226, 1995.
50. Vaitkus PT: Gender differences in the utilization of cardiac catheterization for the diagnosis of chest pain. Am J Cardiol 75:79, 1995.

CHAPTER 10 Clinical Consequences

10.1 Access to Treatment

Judith K. Mickelson and Jane M. Geraci

As defined in the early 1990s by the National Academy of Science's Access Monitoring Project, access to personal health care services is "the timely use of [those] services to achieve the best possible health outcomes."[1] These services include the prevention, diagnosis, and treatment of disease as well as the recovery and rehabilitation of the patient.[1] Perfect health care can be defined as health care that is available to all and is the result of a process that provides the best possible outcomes at the least expense (Fig. 10–1).

There are, however, a number of potential barriers to access that may affect women and minority groups more than men.[1] These barriers fall into two broad categories: those related to the patient and those related to the structure of the health-care delivery system (Fig. 10–2). The first type of barrier includes the patient's age, race, sex, language, cultural background, social support system, insurance status, socioeconomic status (e.g., education and income), and medical profile (i.e., presence of comorbid diseases and the severity of each).

The second type of barrier includes the availability of services and specialists, coordination of those services, transportation to and from places of service, and third-party payment mechanisms. Not all services may be available at one location. Travel may be difficult for some patients. Many insurance providers and health maintenance organizations impose high deductibles, numerous exclusions, and copay-

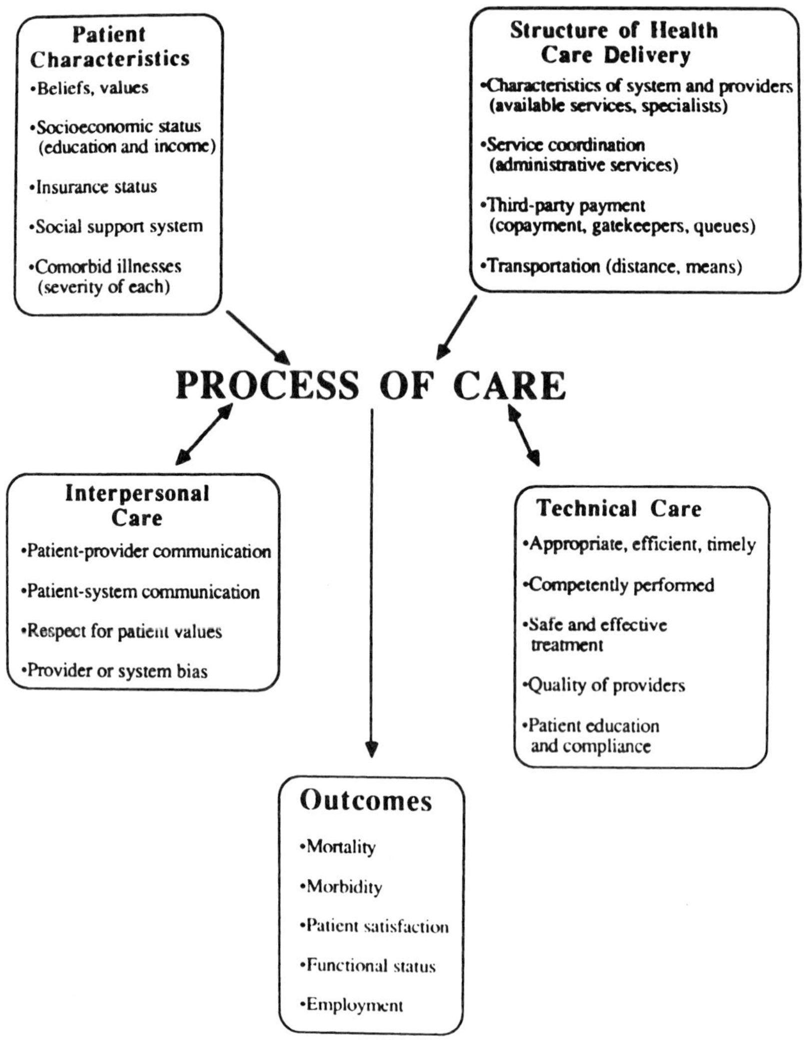

FIGURE 10–1. Access to and quality of health care. This schematic provides an overview of components of the overall process of providing health care for individuals.

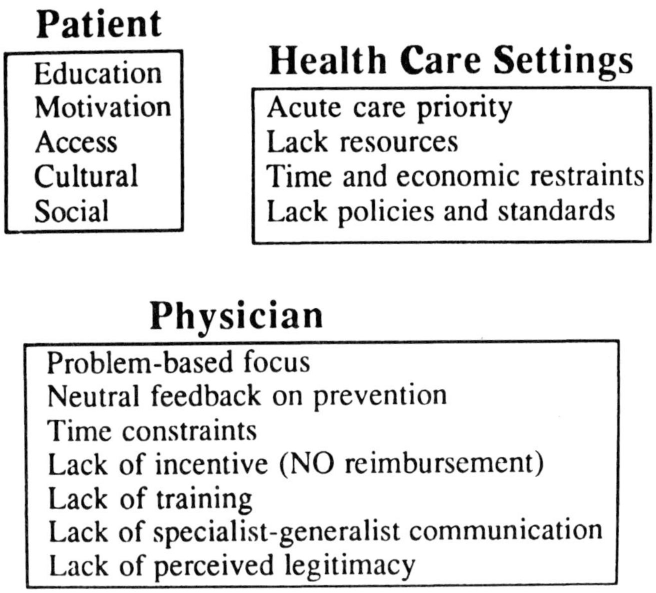

FIGURE 10–2. Barriers to preventive health care.

ments and require coordination of services through gatekeepers in order to control the use of office-based, specialty, and emergency room services.[2,3]

Access may also be affected by the technical aspects of care. These aspects include the appropriateness, efficiency, and safety of diagnostic or therapeutic modalities provided and may be monitored in several ways. The use of practice guidelines can be monitored to determine whether procedures or treatments are overutilized or underutilized by a provider or for a specific subgroup within the general population. The promptness or timeliness of care delivery can be monitored for its contribution to patient satisfaction and its influence on morbidity and mortality in emergent situations. The overall decision making of health-care providers can be monitored for its direct impact upon patient outcome, utilization of resources, and cost effectiveness. Patient outcomes can be analyzed in terms of morbidity, mortality, satisfaction, functional status, and employment status. By such monitoring, areas of health care that need improvement and specific subgroups in the population that deserve attention can be identified in order to provide more equal access to health care.

Ideally, access to health care would not differ by sex, age, race, ethnic origin, income, geographic location, or insurance status[4–7]; any differences in outcomes or utilization would be due only to patient preferences. However, this is not true in practice. This chapter specifically discusses differences in access to health care for women and men with heart disease.

HEART DISEASE MORTALITY RATE

Between 1960 and 1998, the overall age-adjusted mortality rate (per 100,000 people) for heart disease declined steadily (Table 10–1).[8] When analyzed by sex, the age-adjusted death rate for heart disease in 1998 was higher for men than women (167 versus 93, respectively). When analyzed by race among women exclusively, the death rate was over three

Table 10–1. MORTALITY RATES FOR HEART DISEASE (PER 100,000 PEOPLE), 1960 VERSUS 1998

	WHITE MEN		BLACK MEN		WHITE WOMEN		BLACK WOMEN	
	1960	1998	1960	1998	1960	1998	1960	1998
Age adjusted	375	162	381	232	197	88	293	147
Crude	455	283	331	231	306	287	269	225
45–54 years	413	140	514	283	103	43	361	133
55–64 years	1056	388	1236	700	383	154	952	362
65–74 years	2298	981	2281	1313	1229	494	1681	859
75–84 years	4840	2382	3533	2649	3630	1556	2927	2045
≥85 years	10136	6479	6037	5447	9281	5971	5650	5373

Source: Health, United States, 2000. Hyattsville, MD: U.S. Department of Health and Human Services, Public Health Service, Centers for Disease Control and Prevention, National Center for Health Statistics, 2000 [DHHS Publication No. (PHS) 00–1232].

times higher in black women than in white women aged 35 to 54 years and almost 1.5 times higher in black women than in white women aged 55 to 84 years.[9]

HEALTH CARE UTILIZATION

Sex-related differences in heart disease mortality rates may be related to how men and women use the health care system.[8] In 1993, the age-adjusted number of physician contacts was 5.2 for men versus 6.7 for women (Table 10–2). Women were also more likely to have seen a physician in the last year (84% versus 74%) (Table 10–2). Men and women differed slightly in their point of contact with the health care system: Men more often used a hospital, and women more often used the telephone (Table 10–3). For both sexes, the number of visits to physicians increased with age (Table 10–4).

WOMEN'S CONTACT WITH HEALTH CARE SERVICES

Women are more likely than men to have a usual source of health care and to consume more health services.[4,8] These

Table 10–2. PHYSICIAN CONTACTS, 1993

AGE (Years)	NO. VISITS (% <1 y, % >2 y)*			
	Men	Women	Whites	Blacks
All	5.2 (74, 15)	6.7 (84, 8)	6.0 (79, 11)	6.0 (79, 10)
15–44	3.6 (64, 23)	6.4 (83, 8)	5.1 (73, 15)	4.7 (74, 13)
45–64	6.1 (72, 18)	8.1 (83, 9)	7.0 (78, 14)	8.7 (80, 11)
65–74	9.3 (85, 10)	10.4 (88, 8)	9.7 (87, 9)	11.5 (86, 7)
≥75	11.7 (90, 6)	12.8 (91, 6)	12.2 (91, 6)	13.7 (89, 8)

*The numbers in parentheses represent, respectively, the percentages of patients who had seen a physician within the last year (<1 y) and the percentages of those who had not (>2 y).

Source: Health, United States, 1994. Hyattsville, MD: U.S. Department of Health and Human Services, Public Health Service, Centers for Disease Control and Prevention, National Center for Health Statistics, 1995 [DHHS Publication No. (PHS) 95–1232].

Table 10–3. POINT OF CONTACT WITH HEALTH CARE SYSTEM, 1993

	MEN (%)	WOMEN (%)	WHITE (%)	BLACK (%)
Office	56.7	56.5	58.4	47.7
Hospital department	14.6	12.6	11.8	21.2
Telephone	12.1	13.4	13.7	8.3
Other	16.6	17.5	16.0	22.8

Source: Health, United States, 1994. Hyattsville, MD: U.S. Department of Health and Human Services, Public Health Service, Centers for Disease Control and Prevention, National Center for Health Statistics, 1995 [DHHS Publication No. (PHS) 95-1232].

differences extend beyond the reproductive years and include differences in the number of office visits, hospitalization, and prescription medications. Whether this reflects appropriate use and positive outcomes of care has not been established. Several explanations for the difference in utilization between the sexes have been proposed: (1) women may have poorer health and more chronic disease processes than men (e.g., arthritis, diabetes, hypertension); (2) women may acknowledge symptoms or perceive the need for health care more readily than men; and (3) health-care services for women may be less coordinated among their providers (e.g., among internist, surgeon, and obstetrician-gynecologist).

For routine preventive care (i.e., physical examination, blood pressure testing, cholesterol testing, clinical breast examination, mammography, pelvic examination, and Pap smear), women receive better care from obstetrician-gynecologists than from general practitioners, family practitioners, or internists. Increasing income, education, and insurance are associated with increasing preventive health care for women.[5–7] Does this translate into a benefit for women who receive such care? Cancer screening studies indicate that early detection clearly improves survival and that abnormal screening results are seldom ignored.[5] When hypertension and hyperlipidemia are detected, are they appropriately treated? Even though modification of these two risk factors decreases the incidence of stroke, peripheral vascular disease, and heart attack, preventive care for hypertension and hyperlipidemia is limited by lack of time, resources, and insurance reimbursement. Nevertheless, women have a lower rate of death due to heart disease than do men. This difference may be related to women having less worrisome cardiac risk factor profiles or more physician contacts. It might also suggest that women do benefit from the preventive or therapeutic interventions provided by their physicians. Nevertheless, over the past three decades, the death rate for heart disease has steadily declined for both sexes.

Table 10–4. DISTRIBUTION OF VISITS TO COMMONLY USED PHYSICIANS, 1992

	No. Visits	PHYSICIAN TYPE (%)		
		GP/FP	IM	Ob/Gyn
Sex				
Men				
15–44 years	1.6	38	14	—
45–64 years	2.6	28	20	—
>65 years	5.3	21	20	—
Women				
15–44 years	3.2	32	9	31
45–64 years	3.7	29	18	9
>65 years	5.6	25	23	2
Race				
White	3.1	29	13	9
Black	2.6	29	16	9

GP/FP = General practice or family practice; IM = internal medicine; Ob/Gyn = obstetrics/gynecology.

Source: Health, United States, 1994. Hyattsville, MD: U.S. Department of Health and Human Services, Public Health Service, Centers for Disease Control and Prevention, National Center for Health Statistics, 1995 [DHHS Publication No. (PHS) 95-1232].

WOMEN AND HEART DISEASE

Do women have equal access to all the components of health care for heart disease? In terms of prevention (i.e., assessing and, if possible, modifying risk factors), it is common knowledge that men over 40 years old are at high risk for coronary artery disease; yet, it is often forgotten that postmenopausal women who are not receiving hormone replacement therapy are also at high risk.[10, 11] Premenopause is, in general, a very coronary-protective state, but once menopause has occurred, the risk of disease in women becomes similar to that in men. Most women who develop coronary artery disease are at least 10 years older than men with such disease. Women live longer than men, and the risk of developing or dying from coronary artery disease increases with age.

In general, death due to cardiovascular disease accounts for 58% of deaths in persons 85 years and older. There are several apparent reasons for this. Optimal use of medical therapy (e.g., aspirin, beta blockers, thrombolytic therapy) or interventional therapy for coronary artery disease seems to decline with age, along with appropriate and high-quality care.[12–15] Failure to treat is thought to contribute to the increased mortality rate among elderly patients with heart disease.[15, 16] Increased thrombolytic use and interventions after myocardial infarction have been associated with lower mortality rates in patients 65 years and older.[16] Thus, aging is a confounding factor that influences access to health care and final outcomes for women with heart disease.

Clinical evidence suggests that "the timely use of personal health services to achieve the best possible health outcomes" may not apply to women with coronary artery disease. Diagnosis is often made late in the disease process. Acute myocardial infarction has a worse outcome in women than in men.[17] This is thought to be related to advanced age and more unfavorable risk factors (hypertension and diabetes) in women. Women come to the hospital later and are less likely to receive thrombolytic therapy than men.[18–20] Even with thrombolytic therapy, the mortality rate is higher for women.[19, 21] Women are more likely to develop heart failure and to suffer reinfarction in the year following an index infarction. Even in cases of greater cardiac disability after myocardial infarction, women are managed less aggressively than men.[22–25] After myocardial infarction, women are referred for cardiac catheterization less often and receive fewer cardiovascular medications than men. One study of Medicare patients treated for myocardial infarction found that those treated by a cardiologist had a better 1-year survival rate than those treated by a primary care physician and that the cardiologists used more cardiac procedures and medications; the study also found that women were more likely to be treated by a primary care physician.[26] Although they are beneficial to both sexes, revascularization procedures carry higher morbidity and mortality rates for women.[27–30] This is presumably true because women are referred for such procedures later in the disease process when unstable or postinfarction angina is present and ejection fractions are low. One frustrating aspect of coronary artery disease in women is failure to diagnose it early in the disease process when interventions (nonpharmacologic, pharmacologic, or interventional) might be safer and simpler and thus might improve the long-term outcome.

EARLY DIAGNOSIS OF HEART DISEASE IN WOMEN

Women with chest pain syndromes are usually not seen by a cardiologist initially but instead present to the office of a primary care physician or an emergency room. In the emergency room setting, men with chest pain are more often admitted to the hospital than women.[31, 32] In several studies, women admitted to the hospital with angina pectoris were less likely to undergo cardiac catheterization than men.[33, 34] However, it is not clear whether women admitted to coronary care units undergo cardiac catheterization as frequently as men[33, 35]; the uncertainty is due to regional differences and small sample sizes in studies conducted so far.

Women who are not admitted to the hospital for evaluation of chest pain syndrome may be referred for stress testing. Again, the data are conflicting with respect to stress test results and referral for cardiac catheterization. Early data from Shaw and colleagues suggested that women were less often referred for additional diagnostic tests after a positive stress test and had higher cardiac morbidity and mortality rates at 2 years.[36] Several other investigators found that, after adjusting for age and the magnitude of myocardial ischemia (as determined by radionuclide perfusion imaging or radionuclide angiography), women were less likely than men to be referred for cardiac catheterization.[37–39] This difference may be related to whether a cardiologist was involved in determining the need for subsequent cardiac catheterization.[40] In the study by Shaw and associates,[36] a retrospective cohort study in a university medical center, it was not clear whether a cardiologist was involved in the decision for catheterization; in the other three studies, however, a cardiologist was clearly involved.[37–39] This same question of cardiologist as primary decision maker arose in the Systolic Hypertension in the Elderly Program (SHEP), which found that elderly patients and women with coronary heart disease were less often referred for invasive procedures.[41] Once catheterization is performed, gender does not appear to influence subsequent utilization of indicated revascularization procedures (and especially coronary angioplasty).[22, 33, 42, 43] However, women who suffer myocardial infarction or undergo revascularization procedures are referred for cardiac rehabilitation less often than men.[44]

CONCLUSIONS

It is well established that the decline in death rates for all heart diseases since 1960 has been most impressive for white men. However, the available literature suggests that women undergo cardiac procedures less often and later in the course of coronary heart disease than do men. Recent data also suggest that coronary disease risk factors are less well controlled in black women than in white women, resulting in a higher death rate from coronary heart disease in black women. Women patients and the physicians who care for them need to be educated about the importance of controlling risk factors (particularly in postmenopausal women) and of providing timely care for coronary heart disease. As managed care becomes more prevalent, it will be important to monitor the use of gatekeepers, copayments, and other mechanisms that can limit patient access to and utilization of needed specialty care. Further studies are needed to determine whether women and men have different preferences for their care, which might explain some differences in procedure rates.

References

1. A model for monitoring access. In Millman M (ed): Access to Health Care in America. National Academy Press, Washington, DC, 1993, pp 31–45.
2. The Medicaid Access Study Group: Access of Medicaid recipients to outpatient care. N Engl J Med 330:1426–1430, 1994.
3. Hurley RE, Freund DA, Gage BJ: Gatekeeper effects on patterns of physician use. J Fam Pract 32:167–174, 1991.
4. Weisman CS: Women's use of health care. In Falik MM, Collins KS (eds): Women's Health—The Commonwealth Fund Survey. Johns Hopkins University Press, Baltimore, 1996, pp 19–48.
5. Wyn R, Brown ER, Yu H: Women's use of preventive health services. In Falik MM, Collins KS (eds): Women's Health—The Commonwealth Fund Survey. Johns Hopkins University Press, Baltimore, 1996, pp 49–75.
6. Lyons B, Salganicoff A, Rowland D: Poverty, access to health care, and Medicaid's critical role for women. In Falik MM, Collins KS (eds): Women's Health—The Commonwealth Fund Survey. Johns Hopkins University Press, Baltimore, 1996, pp 273–295.
7. Reising AL: Health insurance and women's access to health care. In Falik MM, Collins KS (eds): Women's Health—The Commonwealth Fund Survey. Johns Hopkins University Press, Baltimore, 1996, pp 324–344.
8. Health, United States, 2000. Hyattsville, MD, US Department of Health and Human Services, Public Health Service, Centers for Disease Control and Prevention, National Center for Health Statistics, 2000 [DHHS Publication No. (PHS) 00–1232].
9. Gillum RF, Mussolino ME, Madans JH: Coronary heart disease incidence and survival in African-American women and men: The NHANES I epidemiologic follow-up study. Ann Intern Med 127:111–118, 1997.
10. Grodstein F, Sampfer MJ, Colditz GA, et al: Postmenopausal hormone therapy and mortality. N Engl J Med 336:1769–1775, 1997.
11. Grodstein F, Stampfer MJ, Manson JE, et al: Postmenopausal estrogen and progestin use and the risk of cardiovascular disease. N Engl J Med 335:453–461, 1996.
12. Gurwitz JH, Gore JM, Goldberg RJ, et al: Recent age-related trends in the use of thrombolytic therapy in patients who have had acute myocardial infarction. Ann Intern Med 124:283–291, 1996.
13. Gurwitz JH, Goldberg RJ, Chen Z, et al: Beta-blocker therapy in acute myocardial infarction: Evidence for underutilization in the elderly. Am J Med 93:605–609, 1992.
14. Krumholz HM, Radford MJ, Ellerbeck EF, et al: Aspirin in the treatment of acute myocardial infarction in elderly Medicare beneficiaries. Circulation 92:2841–2847, 1995.
15. Lindsay J, Reddy VM, Pinnow EE, et al: Morbidity and mortality rates in elderly patients undergoing percutaneous coronary transluminal angioplasty. Am Heart J 128:697–702, 1994.
16. Pashos C, Newhouse JP, McNeil BJ: Temporal changes in the care and outcomes of elderly patients with acute myocardial infarction, 1987 through 1990. JAMA 270:1832–1836, 1993.

17. Vaccarino V, Krumholz HM, Berkman LF, Horwitz RI: Sex differences in mortality after myocardial infarction. Circulation 91:1861–1871, 1995.
18. European Secondary Prevention Study Group: Translation of clinical trials into practice: A European population-based study of the use of thrombolysis for acute myocardial infarction. Lancet 347:1203–1207, 1996.
19. Weaver WD, White HD, Wilcox RG, et al: Comparisons of characteristics and outcomes among women and men with acute myocardial infarction treated with thrombolytic therapy. JAMA 275:777–782, 1996.
20. Dellborg M, Swedberg K: Acute myocardial infarction: Difference in the treatment between men and women. Qual Assur Health Care 5: 261–265, 1993.
21. Eysmann SB, Douglas PS: Reperfusion and revascularization strategies for coronary artery disease in women [review]. JAMA 268:1903–1907, 1992.
22. Steingart RM, Packer M, Hamm P, et al: Sex differences in the management of coronary artery disease. Survival and Ventricular Enlargement Investigators. N Engl J Med 325:226–230, 1991.
23. Iezzoni LI, Ash AS, Schwartz M, Mackiernan YD: Differences in procedure use, in-hospital mortality, and illness severity by gender for acute myocardial infarction patients: Are answers affected by data source and severity measure? Med Care 35:158–171, 1997.
24. Herholz H, Goff DC, Ramsey DJ, et al: Women and Mexican Americans receive fewer cardiovascular drugs following myocardial infarction than men and non-Hispanic whites: The Corpus Christi Heart Project, 1988–1990. J Clin Epidemiol 49:279-287, 1996.
25. Schwartz LM, Fisher ES, Tosteson ANA, et al: Treatment and health outcomes of women and men in a cohort with coronary artery disease. Arch Intern Med 157:1545–1551, 1997.
26. Jollis JG, DeLong ER, Peterson ED, et al: Outcome of acute myocardial infarction according to the specialty of the admitting physician. N Engl J Med 335:1880–1887, 1996.
27. Kelsey SF, James M, Holubkov AL, et al: Results of percutaneous transluminal coronary angioplasty in women: 1985–1986 National Heart, Lung, and Blood Institute's Coronary Angioplasty Registry. Circulation 87:720–727, 1993.
28. Malenka DJ, O'Connor GT, Quinton H, et al: Differences in outcomes between women and men associated with percutaneous transluminal coronary angioplasty. Circulation 94(Suppl II):II99–II104, 1996.
29. Weintraub WS, Wenger NK, Jones EL, et al: Changing clinical characteristics of coronary surgery patients: Differences between men and women. Circulation 88:II79–II86, 1993.
30. Christakis GT, Weisel RD, Buth KJ, et al: Is body size the cause of poor outcomes of coronary artery bypass operations in women? J Thorac Cardiovasc Surg 110:1344–1356, 1995.
31. Silbergleit R, McNamara RM: Effect of gender on the emergency department evaluation of patients with chest pain. Acad Emerg Med 2:115–119, 1995.
32. Johnson PA, Goldman L, Orav EJ, et al: Gender differences in the management of acute chest pain. J Gen Intern Med 11:209–217, 1996.
33. Bergelson BA, Tommaso CL: Gender differences in clinical evaluation and triage in coronary artery disease. Chest 108:1510–1513, 1995.
34. Maynard C, Beshansky JR, Griffith JL, Selker HP: Influence of sex on the use of cardiac procedures in patients presenting to the emergency department: A prospective multicenter study. Circulation 94(Suppl II): II93–II98, 1996.
35. Schecter AD, Goldschmidt-Clermont PJ, McKee G, et al: Influence of gender, race, and education on patient preferences and receipt of cardiac catheterizations among coronary care unit patients. Am J Cardiol 78:996–1001, 1996.
36. Shaw LJ, Miller DD, Romeis JC, et al: Gender differences in the noninvasive evaluation and management of patients with suspected coronary artery disease. Ann Intern Med 120:559–566, 1994.
37. Hachamovitch R, Berman DS, Kiat H, et al: Gender-related differences in clinical management after exercise nuclear testing. J Am Coll Cardiol 26:1457–1464, 1995.
38. Lauer MS, Pashkow FJ, Snader CE, et al: Gender and referral for coronary angiography after treadmill thallium testing. Am J Cardiol 78: 278–283, 1996.
39. Mark DB, Shaw LK, DeLong ER, et al: Absence of sex bias in the referral of patients for cardiac catheterization. N Engl J Med 330: 1101–1106, 1994.
40. Borowsky SJ, Kravitz RL, Laouri M, et al: Effect of physician specialty on use of necessary coronary angiography. J Am Coll Cardiol 26: 1484–1491, 1995.
41. Bearden D, Allman R, McDonald R, et al: Age, race, and gender variation in the utilization of coronary artery bypass surgery and angioplasty in SHEP. SHEP Cooperative Research Group. Systolic Hypertension in the Elderly Program. J Am Geriatr Soc 42:1143–1149, 1994.
42. Bell MR, Berger PB, Holmes DR, et al: Referral for coronary artery revascularization procedures after diagnostic coronary angiography: Evidence for gender bias? J Am Coll Cardiol 25:650–655, 1995.
43. Laouri M, Kravitz RL, French WJ, et al: Underuse of coronary revascularization procedures: Application of a clinical method. J Am Coll Cardiol 29:891–897, 1997.
44. Thomas RJ, Miller NH, Lamendola C, et al: National survey on gender differences in cardiac rehabilitation programs: Patient characteristics and enrollment patterns. J Cardiopulm Rehab 16:402–412, 1996.

10.2 Psychiatric Aspects of Coronary Artery Disease

Priscilla Ray

For 'tis the mind that makes the body rich.

William Shakespeare

To see the intertwining of the mind and the heart, one need look no further than our language: phrases such as "a broken heart," "a gift from the heart," and "heart-to-heart talks" demonstrate this close connection. The relationship also holds true for women with coronary artery disease; psychiatric factors play vital roles in a patient's development of, treatment for, and attitude toward an illness. A doctor's understanding of these factors may mean the difference between compliance and noncompliance and—at times—between life and death.

PSYCHIATRIC FACTORS IN THE DEVELOPMENT OF CORONARY ARTERY DISEASE

One of the most widely cited associations between emotions and physical health is that of stress as a cause of heart disease. However, most studies have defined "stress" loosely and do not often consider differences between men and women. The increased incidence of myocardial infarction in persons with "type A" personality characteristics (aggression, competitiveness, work-orientation, and sense of urgency) was reported years ago and has been widely publicized.[1, 2] How-

Table 10–5. FACTORS TO CONSIDER BEFORE DIAGNOSIS OF CORONARY ARTERY DISEASE

Assess for depression
Counsel patient on role of psychiatric factors
Invite communication on psychiatric symptoms

ever, the significance of this association is unclear, especially in women. Likewise, the roles of hostility, cynicism, and aggression in the development of coronary artery disease are not well defined. This is a difficult area for study, as coronary artery disease may progress slowly and silently over years, making the causal relationship with a particular stressor more difficult to detect.

However, recognition of the effect of psychiatric factors on the development of heart disease is receiving increased attention. In a recent prospective study of 1551 people, 8.2% of those with a history of clinical depression had a myocardial infarction (MI), whereas 3.3% of those without a history of clinical depression had one. This difference was even greater when other risk factors, such as hypertension or tobacco use, were excluded. The risk of MI was twice the baseline risk for those who suffered prolonged periods of sadness that fell below threshold criteria for depression. Depressed patients taking antidepressants lowered their risk of MI[1] (Table 10–5).

PSYCHIATRIC FACTORS FOLLOWING DIAGNOSIS OF CORONARY ARTERY DISEASE

After a patient has been diagnosed with coronary artery disease, she often seeks direction with regard to prevention and treatment. A discussion of these processes can easily include a discussion of the psychiatric factors that are involved, and the physician can assess the patient's psychiatric profile at this time.

Stress

In patients with coronary artery disease, mental stress may contribute to silent ischemia by causing frequent wall motion abnormalities[3] or coronary artery spasms.[4] Stress may also aggravate coronary heart disease by activation of blood platelets and associated coronary artery occlusion or constriction.[5]

Depression

Although not all the effects of depression on the heart are known, mean heart rate in patients with coronary artery disease was found to be increased in those who were depressed.[6]

Inhibition of Expression

The combination of two "type D" personality factors (the tendency to experience negative emotions and the tendency to inhibit self-expression) significantly predicted the rate of death within 5 years in patients with coronary heart disease.[7]

Table 10–6. FACTORS TO CONSIDER FOLLOWING DIAGNOSIS OF CORONARY ARTERY DISEASE

Assess tendency toward "negative" emotions and inhibition of self-expression—counsel and refer if needed
Assess "type A" traits, remembering uncertainty about their significance
Assess for depression—treat or refer
Assess for anxiety about diagnosis—reassure patient
Assess mental "stress"—counsel and refer if needed
Remind patient of willingness to discuss psychiatric factors

Adjustment

Feelings of anxiety may, understandably, follow a new diagnosis of coronary artery disease. Communication of this fact to the patient often reassures her and helps limit fears about how her new anxiety affects her heart (Table 10–6).

PSYCHIATRIC FACTORS FOLLOWING MYOCARDIAL INFARCTION: HOSPITALIZATION

The period of hospitalization following an acute MI may be the first opportunity to address a patient's coping style and abilities, her psychiatric symptoms, her attitudes and beliefs about cardiac disease, and factors that might limit her compliance with necessary treatment (Table 10–7). The most common psychiatric symptoms during this period are anxiety and, often a day or two later, depression.[8] These symptoms are not uncommon, though they may go unrecognized at this time.

Factors contributing to post-MI anxiety include fear of death or disability, apprehension about inability to detect an impending recurrence, concern about how the illness will affect family members, negative experiences of the patient or others with similar illnesses, and the patient's beliefs about the illness. For patients unfamiliar with hospitals, treatments that seem commonplace to physicians may inspire fear; for example, some patients view oxygen administered by nasal cannula as "life-support." Some will not mention feelings of hopelessness or fear to avoid "bothering" the doctor.

Depression is more common in women than in men, and it may be a danger sign following an acute MI. Prompt

Table 10–7. FACTORS TO CONSIDER FOLLOWING MYOCARDIAL INFARCTION: HOSPITALIZATION

Assess for anxiety, especially first few days, and treat or refer
Assess for acute depression, especially next several days; treat or refer
Assess for cognitive deficits, investigate cause, and treat or refer
Ask about feelings of fear or discouragement
Explore patient's expectations about future disability and activities
Communicate expectations about resuming activities (work, sex, and exercise)
Invite and solicit questions

treatment may prevent serious future morbidity and even death. In the first 8 to 10 days after acute MI, 18% of the patients in one study developed major depression and an additional 23% developed minor depression. These symptoms were not correlated with the severity of the cardiac disease. Those patients who developed major depression during this period were more likely to be depressed 3 to 4 months later and less likely to have returned to work.[9] Depression occurring during hospitalization after an acute MI is a significant predictor of cardiac death within 18 months, especially in patients with 10 or more premature ventricular contractions (PVCs) per hour.[10] Depression was the most significant of only two predictors of poor post-MI outcome in a New York study.[11]

The hospitalization period is a good time to discuss the patient's feelings with her openly, to solicit questions and concerns, and, specifically, to inquire about feelings of anxiety, depression, or discouragement. It also provides an opportunity to investigate the possibility of mild or moderate cognitive deficits for a baseline measurement and, if deficits are present, to investigate the cause or causes. Expectations about recovery and the resumption of usual activities, including sexual activity, can be communicated at this time. The patient's attitudes during her hospitalization about recovery and about future ability and disability may significantly influence future functioning, including return to work.

PSYCHIATRIC FACTORS FOLLOWING MYOCARDIAL INFARCTION: RECOVERY

Psychiatric factors may be even more important than nonpsychiatric factors in predicting recovery from MI (Table 10–8). Following discharge from the hospital after an MI, many patients suffer from psychological alterations such as impaired self-esteem, perceptions of poor health, subjective emotional distress, and increased interpersonal dependency. A patient's beliefs about her illness, such as whether she feels she can control or cure it, may significantly influence compliance with the recommended treatment and promptness in returning to work.[12]

Support Systems

Following acute MI, overall emotional distress, anxiety, and depression in women declined. Women may activate social support systems more effectively than men, which may aid in their adjustment to illness; these support systems may not be as significantly relevant to illness adjustment in men.[13]

Table 10–8. FACTORS TO CONSIDER FOLLOWING MYOCARDIAL INFARCTION: RECOVERY

Assess self-esteem and feelings about illness
Assess support system and assist in activation of it
Make recommendations for return to work
Assess for depression and treat or refer
Assess level of perceived control over illness
Assess for anxiety and tension symptoms and treat or refer
Counsel about sexual activity matter-of-factly, invite questions, reassure
Stress treatment compliance

This ability to mobilize social support systems may be important not only in women's adjustment to illness but also in recovery from MI. Decreased emotional support was associated with a significant increase in mortality rate in elderly patients in the first 6 months following an acute MI.[14]

Employment

Women who returned to their former employment status had higher levels of social support, self-esteem, and subjective quality of life.[15] Early clarification of the physician's recommendations regarding if and when the patient may return to work allows the patient to plan accordingly while also reassuring her about expectations for her recovery.

Personality

Several studies with mostly male patients have suggested the value of reducing type A behaviors, such as time-urgency and expressed hostility, in decreasing cardiac morbidity and mortality rates.[2, 16] However, other studies contradict this, and many researchers question whether findings for men can be generalized to women, who often express emotions such as anger in ways different from men.[17] Some studies have shown hostility to be predictive of all diseases and mortality rate in general.[18]

Long-term, stable type D personality factors, including negative affectivity (worry, pessimism, unhappiness, irritability, depression, tension, impaired sense of well-being) and social inhibition (inhibition of expression of feelings, tendency to keep others at a distance, subjectively low levels of social support) significantly predicted longer-term survival (at least 5 years) in men and women with coronary artery disease. This may occur because of the direct effects of suppressing emotions on disease promotion and the effects of associated factors, such as social alienation or depression, on increased mortality rate.[7]

Perceived Control

Subjectively high levels of control related to MI or coronary artery bypass have been correlated with lower rates of anxiety, depression, and hostility and improved psychosocial adjustment 6 months after the cardiac event.[19]

Anxiety and Tension

One year after acute MI, women had a higher incidence of cardiac, psychosomatic, and psychological symptoms, including headache, sweating, difficulty relaxing, anxiety, initial insomnia, and restless sleep, as well as difficulties in social life.[20] These factors are significant in that anxiety and tension, as well as infrequent vacations, predict coronary-related deaths and MI in women.[21]

Five years after MI, anxiety, along with physical factors such as angina and dyspnea, correlated with impaired quality of life. Myocardial infarction patients who suffered from anxiety at this point in their recovery reported decreases in sleep, energy, sex life, mobility, and hobby- and holiday-related activity compared with the healthy population.[22]

Depression

A patient may believe that her depression following an MI is "normal" and may not report symptoms such as insomnia, appetite change, fatigue, or decreased interest unless the physician specifically inquires about them. Patients frequently feel guilty about continuing risk behaviors, such as smoking, eating foods with too much cholesterol, and exercising too little, as well as the effects on their family members.

Sex

Patients, both male and female, frequently fear that resumption of sexual activity may worsen or even cause an MI, but they are often embarrassed about broaching the subject, especially in the presence of other people. It is often helpful for the physician to address this issue with the same matter-of-fact tone used for discussing diet and medications, and to include sex with the other "activities" permitted. It is also helpful to mention some concerns that many patients have; for example, they may need to change the position of either partner during intercourse. Reassure her that more than 80% of patients are able to engage in their previous levels of sexual functioning within 3 months after MI.[23] A successful return to normal sexual functioning often reassures the patient and her spouse or partner that her recovery is progressing well.

Treatment Compliance

The importance of treatment compliance should also be stressed after an MI. In one study, patients who did not adhere well to their treatment regimen were 2.6 times more likely to die within the first year after an MI.[24]

PSYCHIATRIC FACTORS BEFORE CORONARY ARTERY BYPASS SURGERY

Psychiatric variables present before coronary artery bypass surgery may help in the prediction of future psychosocial adjustment to illness, functioning, and even postoperative cognitive dysfunction.

Depression and Anxiety

Several studies have identified a more frequent occurrence of depression and anxiety before cardiac surgery in women than in men.[25] In a 1995 study, 66% of women, compared with 38% of men, reported depression the day before coronary bypass surgery; women also tended to have greater anxiety and less social support. On the day before discharge from the hospital, 75% of women and 54% of men reported depression.[26]

Table 10–9. FACTORS TO CONSIDER BEFORE CORONARY ARTERY BYPASS SURGERY

Assess for anxiety and irritability; treat or refer
Assess for depression and treat or refer
Assess social support system; encourage its activation

Predictive Variables

Preoperative psychiatric symptoms may predict poorer postoperative adjustment. In the 25% of patients with new or persistent psychiatric symptoms 1 year after coronary artery bypass surgery, over two thirds had had significant preoperative distress. The variables predicting poorer psychosocial adjustment included higher hypochondriasis, irritability, high anxiety, and depression (Table 10–9).[27]

PSYCHIATRIC FACTORS FOLLOWING CORONARY ARTERY BYPASS SURGERY

Adjustment

Several studies done following coronary artery bypass surgery have found few or no gender differences in psychiatric complications either acutely[28] or at a year[27]; although many women had more severe cardiac impairment at the time of surgery, their physical and psychosocial functioning 6 months later equaled that of men.[29] The psychological effects of coronary artery bypass surgery itself may benefit patients; some studies have found reduction in levels of somatization, depression, anxiety, obsessive-compulsive behavior, and sleep disturbance. However, as mentioned earlier, 25% of bypass patients who were studied 1 year postoperatively suffered new or persistent psychological distress.[27]

Denial

Denial may serve as an adaptive mechanism immediately following coronary artery bypass surgery. Higher levels of denial may actually predict better functioning for up to 6 months after surgery.[30] However, denial can also be problematic if it interferes with treatment compliance. Denial or minimization of the patient's illness and their effects on her and her family should be investigated; they may be underreported by patients and families who want to believe that the patient is "well" as long as she appears to be compliant with treatment.

Psychosis

The incidence of psychosis immediately after coronary artery bypass surgery may vary depending on the method of assessment; one early study found a much higher incidence of "postcardiotomy psychosis" in patients who were interviewed (70%) than the incidence obtained via chart review (27%).[31] Especially in a patient with no prior psychotic history, any appearance of psychosis in the postoperative period should prompt an investigation for underlying delirium.

Delirium

Postcardiotomy delirium has been reported in 32% of patients with no correlation to gender.[32] The delirium can be caused by medications, such as anesthetics, metabolic abnormalities, infection, or sensory deprivation. In her confusion, the patient may develop paranoid ideation and believe that treatment team personnel are trying to harm her, leading to agitation, fear, and the pulling out of tubes, lines, and other necessary medical equipment. The delirium usually subsides when the underlying causes are corrected, but the confusion (even without paranoia) may be terrifying to the patient and her family.

Cognitive Dysfunction

Compared with preoperative scores, cognitive dysfunction measured 4 days after coronary artery bypass correlated positively with higher levels of preoperative depression.[33] Decreased regional cerebral blood flow was not related.[34]

Recovery

During the period following bypass surgery, the patient may feel considerable relief and believe that the "new" blood supply to the heart has "fixed" the problem; the danger here is that denial or minimization may contribute to noncompliance with treatment recommendations. However, depression may also lead to noncompliance, especially when accompanied by hopelessness, worthlessness, guilt, or feelings of being a burden to one's family. The recovery period is a good opportunity to assess the patient's attitude about her illness; to discuss her expectations about returning to her role in employment, family, leisure activities, and sexual relations; and to open lines of communication regarding any psychiatric symptoms that may arise (Table 10–10).

PSYCHIATRIC FACTORS ASSOCIATED WITH CORONARY ANGIOPLASTY

Symptoms of vital exhaustion (fatigue, irritability, and demoralization) present 2 weeks after hospital discharge predicted cardiac events in the first 18 months after successful percutaneous transluminal coronary angioplasty (PTCA)[35]; however, the relationship of vital exhaustion and anger were not as significant in predicting mortality in women.[36]

Table 10–10. FACTORS TO CONSIDER FOLLOWING CORONARY ARTERY BYPASS SURGERY

Assess denial; address if interfering with treatment
Assess for psychosis and treat or refer
Assess delirium, dementia, or cognitive dysfunction; look for causes and treat or refer
Assess for depression, including hopelessness, worthlessness, or being a burden, and treat or refer
Clarify expectations about recovery, including work, exercise, sex, hobbies
Stress treatment compliance even when "feeling good"

PSYCHIATRIC FACTORS ASSOCIATED WITH CARDIAC TRANSPLANTATION

Predictive Variables

About half of heart transplant patients were preoperatively diagnosed with a psychiatric problem, although many of these were "minor"; the number dropped to about one fifth of patients 1 year after transplant. There was a significant correlation between a preoperative psychiatric diagnosis and treatment noncompliance.[37]

Anxiety and Depression

Preoperative anxiety may be related to fears of disability or death, the wait for a donor organ, and uncertainty about the effects of medication and surgery. Anxiety symptoms are often similar to those experienced with angina (chest discomfort, shortness of breath, lightheadedness, diaphoresis, and nausea). Depression may be aggravated by these same factors, as well as by feelings of guilt about wishing for a donor organ and by the effects of the illness and treatment on the patient's family and support system. Additionally, patients with cardiomyopathies may have a higher frequency (83%) of definite or probable panic disorder.[38] Postoperative anxiety may be related to fears of organ rejection and infection. This is a complex topic, because acute graft rejection may cause anxiety.[39] The manifestations of anxiety after cardiac transplantation may differ from pretransplant symptoms because of less rate variability in the denervated heart.

Delirium and Dementia

Mild and sometimes moderate dementia preceding transplantation may be due to a variety of factors, including medications, previous cardiac surgery, and inadequate cerebral perfusion due to heart failure or cardiopulmonary arrest. Delirium and psychotic features newly occurring in the immediate post-transplant period are often reversible and may be related to medications, electrolyte abnormalities, impairment in liver or kidney function, infection (in immunosuppressed patients), transplant rejection, and cerebral emboli. Later cognitive impairment is more likely to be due to rejection, infection, or medications such as steroids and immunosuppressants.

Adjustment

Adjustment issues in cardiac transplant patients may include the re-evaluation of priorities, re-examination of relationships, acceptance of the ongoing nature of treatment, apprehension about the possibility of rejection or infection, and conscious and unconscious concerns about the meaning of the transplant. This last issue is especially relevant, because the heart often symbolizes the "life" of a person and the locus of emotions.

Table 10–11. FACTORS TO CONSIDER BEFORE CARDIAC TRANSPLANTATION

Assess for panic disorder and treat or refer
Assess anxiety symptoms, differentiate from angina and treat or refer
Assess for dementia, investigate causes, treat or refer
Assess emotional coping with and adjustment to transplant
Clarify patient's and family's expectations about recovery
Collaborate with transplant team on patient's psychiatric needs

Recovery

Psychosocial evaluations are frequently performed preoperatively, but the predictive value of these is not entirely clear. These evaluations do provide an opportunity, as do post-transplantation evaluations, to screen for the presence of a psychiatric illness while simultaneously exploring the patient's beliefs, expectations, and attitudes about recovery and her ability to live with a chronic illness. Postoperative cognitive functioning should be assessed, and each physician's role on the treatment team should be clarified. The patient's feelings about functioning with "someone else's heart" inside her can be explored, and the physician can communicate willingness to hear concerns and fears and can clarify expectations about recovery (Tables 10–11 and 10–12).

COPING WITH ILLNESS

The ability of patients to cope successfully with coronary artery disease can be assessed using characteristics common to coping with other chronic diseases. Some of these are listed here:

1. Unexpectedness/acuteness: A shorter interval between initial symptom development and the diagnosis of a major illness limits the time available for adapting to the diagnosis.
2. Denial: Some denial may actually improve coping by reducing anxiety; however, too much may interfere with treatment compliance or reduction of modifiable risk factors or lead to excessive work or exercise.
3. Meaning of the illness for the patient: The patient's experiences in her life, those of family members with the illness, how the illness affects her image of herself, and how she believes others will perceive her differently may affect her ability to cope with her illness. As an example, a woman whose mother was severely limited for years after an acute MI and subsequently died of congestive heart failure had very different expectations of herself after a diagnosis of coronary artery disease than another patient, similarly diagnosed, whose mother, still alive, played golf, swam, and worked full time.
4. Personality: Patients with certain personality types, for example, dependent-demanding, orderly-controlling, dramatic-histrionic, self-sacrificing and masochistic, guarded-suspicious, narcissistic, schizoid, or impulsive, may have very different ways of coping with illness.[40] As an example, a dependent patient may focus on the disabling characteristics of her illness or abandonment, an obsessional patient on control, and a narcissistic patient on loss of autonomy and perfection.
5. Patterns of coping: Patients who cope with stressors with optimism, flexibility, resourcefulness, practicality, and openness to advice generally cope better with illnesses.
6. Meaning of illness within family: How her family interprets her illness and any resulting disability, as well as whether it is perceived to affect her roles (e.g., employment or childbearing), may significantly affect the patient's response to her illness.
7. Degree of emotional support.
8. Age and maturity: The patient's developmental and psychological state at the time of diagnosis may play a significant role in how she comes to understand and integrate her illness into her self-perception.
9. Stage of emotional healing: Coping with illness is a process marked by the following stages, which, of course, are affected by many of the variables listed here.
   - "Surviving": feelings of inner chaos, isolation, re-examination of beliefs, search for meaning, redefinition of relationships, heightened awareness of time.
   - "Originating": redefinition of priorities, more appreciation of life, search for necessary support, identification of new emotional and physical abilities, creation of beneficial relationships.
   - "Patterning balance": refinement of personal goals, consideration of opportunities, acceptance of uncertainty, reaching out to others.[41]

Table 10–12. FACTORS TO CONSIDER FOLLOWING CARDIAC TRANSPLANTATION

Assess for delirium or psychotic symptoms, investigate possible causes, treat or refer
Assess for anxiety (symptoms may differ); differentiate from graft rejection and treat or refer
Assess for depression and/or guilt, treat or refer
Assess adjustment, degree of denial, and patient's evaluation of priorities
Explore expectations about recovery and disability
Clarify roles of treatment team members

TREATMENT AND PREVENTION

In addition to appropriate treatment for the physical aspects of coronary artery disease, a patient needs attention for the psychiatric factors that may affect recovery, a number of which have been previously discussed.

Cardiac Rehabilitation

Male patients who participated in comprehensive cardiac rehabilitation experienced a decrease in tranquilizer use and depression and an improved activity profile; they improved more and deteriorated less than patients who did not undergo such rehabilitation.[42]

Prevention of Emotional Stress

Complete prevention of stress is, of course, impossible, but in the face of ongoing or severe stress, strategies for coping may need to be explored.

Clarification of Expectations

Patients, their families, and support system members may have unrealistic expectations about physical recovery, the effort involved in everyday activities, reactions to emotional stress, changes in self-image, and feelings of anxiety, uncertainty, and depression. The expression and clarification of these issues should contribute to a stable social support system and an avoidance of frustration, disappointment, and increased emotional stress because of unachievable expectations.

Expression of Feelings

Because the psychological factors usually studied have been stable, long-term personality traits, the effects of encouraging appropriate, open expression of feelings are unclear, but this openness may lead to improved communication with the physician and family members. This may contribute to more realistic expectations by the patient and her social support system.

Activation of Support System

Activation of a support system may be an essential element of the female patient's recovery, because women's socialization focuses on these systems as priorities.

Psychotherapy

Many of these factors, such as clarification of expectations, learning of coping skills, constructive and appropriate expression of feelings, and exploration of ways of activating a social support system, may be responsive to psychotherapy if encouragement is ineffective. Psychotherapy is also useful for treating depression, anxiety, and other psychiatric illnesses. Brief psychotherapy for disturbances of emotion (anger, depression, anxiety) focuses on identifying the source of the emotion and helping the patient regain control over the intensity and expression of the emotion.

Different personality styles may respond to somewhat different ways of interaction; for example, an obsessional patient, with anxiety and need for control, may respond better to scientific explanations, details, and repetition. A dependent patient with fears of abandonment, however, may need a nurturing approach, fewer details, and encouragement toward independence. A caring, supportive approach encouraging the ventilation of feelings may work well with a histrionic personality but stimulate feelings of threat and fear in a paranoid or schizoid patient.

Pharmacotherapy

Anxiety may be successfully treated by explanation and reassurance or by psychotherapy alone, depending on the psychological causes. When adjunctive medication is required, benzodiazepines, especially fast-acting ones such as alprazolam, are often the first choice; lorazepam may be administered parenterally. On a cautionary note, these medications do have a potential for increased tolerance, withdrawal effects, and respiratory depression.

Depression also may respond to supportive psychotherapy but may require other modalities. Pharmacologic treatment should be tailored to the specific patient with consideration of the effects of medications on her cardiac disease and specific symptoms of depression. Her family history, previous response to treatment, medication side effects and their cardiac and psychiatric significance, and potential interaction with other medications should also be considered. Lithium is difficult to use in patients with cardiac failure and during the acute postoperative period. Levels may also be affected by a number of medications, including cyclosporine.

Psychosis usually requires the administration of antipsychotics with, again, an emphasis on individualized therapy; the higher-potency antipsychotics are usually preferred because they are less likely to cause hypotension.

References

1. Friedman M, Manwaring JH, Rosenman RH: Instantaneous and sudden deaths: Clinical and pathological differentiation in coronary artery disease. JAMA 225:1319, 1973.
2. Rosenman RH: Role of type A behavior pattern in the pathogenesis of ischemic heart disease and modification for prevention. Adv Cardiol 25:35, 1978.
3. Rozanski A, Bairey CN, Krantz DS, et al: Mental stress and the induction of silent myocardial ischemia in patients with coronary artery disease. N Engl J Med 318:1005, 1988.
4. Yeung AC, Vekshtein VI, Krantz DS, et al: The effect of atherosclerosis on the vasomotor response of coronary arteries to mental stress. N Engl J Med 325:1551, 1991.
5. Malkoff SB, Muldoon MF, Zeigler ZR, et al: Blood platelet responsivity to acute mental stress. Psychosom Med 55:477, 1993.
6. Carney RM, Rich MW, teVelde A, et al: The relationship between heart rate, heart rate variability and depression in patients with coronary artery disease. J Psychosom Res 32:159, 1988.
7. Denollet J, Sys SU, Stroobant N, et al: Personality as independent predictor of long-term mortality in patients with coronary heart disease. Lancet 347:417, 1996.
8. Cassem NH, Hackett TP: Psychiatric consultation in a coronary care unit. Ann Intern Med 75:9, 1971.
9. Schleifer SJ, Macari-Hinson MM, Coyl D, et al: The nature and course of depression following myocardial infarction. Arch Intern Med 149:1785, 1989.
10. Frasure-Smith N, Lesperance F, Talajic M: Depression and 18-month prognosis after myocardial infarction. Circulation 91:999, 1995.
11. Kennedy GJ, Hofer M, Cohen D, et al: Significance of depression and cognitive impairment in patients undergoing programmed stimulation of cardiac arrhythmias. Psychosom Med 49:410, 1987.
12. Petrie KJ, Weinman J, Sharpe N, et al: Role of patients' view of their illness in predicting return to work and functioning after myocardial infarction: Longitudinal study. BMJ 312:1191, 1996.
13. Riegel B, Gocka I: Gender differences in adjustment to acute myocardial infarction. Heart Lung 24:457, 1995.
14. Berkman LF, Leo-Summers L, Horwitz RI: Emotional support and survival after myocardial infarction: A prospective, population-based study of the elderly. Ann Intern Med 117:1003, 1992.
15. Wingate S: Quality of life for women after a myocardial infarction. Heart Lung 24:467, 1995.
16. Friedman M, Thoresen CE, Gill JJ, et al: Alteration of type A behavior and its effect on cardiac recurrences in post myocardial infarction patients: Summary results of the recurrence coronary prevention project. Am Heart J 112:653, 1986.
17. Powell LH, Shaker LA, Jones BA, et al: Psychosocial predictors of mortality in 83 women with premature acute myocardial infarction. Psychosom Med 55:426, 1993.

18. Barefoot JC, Dahlstrom WG, Williams RB Jr: Hostility, CHD incidence and total mortality: A 25-year follow-up study of 225 physicians. Psychosom Med 45:59, 1983.
19. Moser DK, Drakup K: Psychosocial recovery from a cardiac event: The influence of perceived control. Heart Lung 24:273, 1995.
20. Wiklund I, Herlitz J, Johansson S, et al: Subjective symptoms and well-being differ in women and men after myocardial infarction. Eur Heart J 14:1315, 1993.
21. Eaker ED, Pinsky J, Castelli WP: Myocardial infarction and coronary death among women: Psychosocial predictors from a 20-year follow-up of women in the Framingham Study. Am J Epidemiol 135:854, 1992.
22. Wiklund I, Herlitz J, Hjalmarson A: Quality of life five years after myocardial infarction. Eur Heart J 10:464, 1989.
23. Khan MIG: Complications of myocardial infarction and postinfarction care. In Khan MIG (ed): Heart Disease Diagnosis and Therapy: A Practical Approach. Williams & Wilkins, Baltimore, 1996, p 61.
24. Horwitz RI, Viscoli CM, Berkman L, et al: Treatment adherence and risk of death after a myocardial infarction. Lancet 336:542, 1990.
25. Sokol RS, Folks DG, Herrick RW, et al: Psychiatric outcome in men and women after coronary bypass surgery. Psychosomatics 28:11, 1987.
26. Burker EJ, Blumenthal JA, Feldman M, et al: Depression in male and female patients undergoing cardiac surgery. Br J Clin Psychol 34: 119, 1995.
27. Magni G, Unger HP, Valfre C, et al: Psychosocial outcome one year after heart surgery: A prospective study. Arch Intern Med 147:473, 1987.
28. Rabiner CJ, Willner AE, Fishman J: Psychiatric complications following coronary bypass surgery. J Nerv Ment Dis 160:342, 1975.
29. Ayanian JZ, Guadagnoli E, Cleary PD: Physical and psychosocial functioning of women and men after coronary artery bypass surgery. JAMA 274:1767, 1995.
30. Folks DG, Freeman AM 3d, Sokol RS, et al: Denial: Predictor of outcome following coronary bypass surgery. Int J Psychiatry Med 18: 57, 1988.
31. Kornfeld DS, Zimberg S, Malm JR: Psychiatric complications of open heart surgery. N Engl J Med 273:287, 1965.
32. Smith LW, Dimsdale JE: Postcardiotomy delirium: Conclusions after 25 years? Am J Psychiatry 146:452, 1989.
33. Folks DG, Freeman AM 3d, Sokol RS, et al: Cognitive dysfunction after coronary artery bypass surgery: A case-controlled study. South Med J 81:202, 1988.
34. Freeman AM 3d, Folks DG, Sokol RS, et al: Cognitive function after coronary bypass surgery: Effect of decreased cerebral blood flow. Am J Psychiatry 142:110, 1985.
35. Kop WJ, Appels AP, Mendes de Leon CF, et al: Vital exhaustion predicts new cardiac events after successful coronary angioplasty. Psychosom Med 56:281, 1994.
36. Mendes de Leon CF, Kop WJ, de Swart HB, et al: Psychosocial characteristics and recurrent events after percutaneous transluminal coronary angioplasty. Am J Cardiol 77:252, 1996.
37. Mai FM, McKenzie FN, Kostuk WJ: Psychosocial adjustment and quality of life following heart transplantation. Can J Psychiatry 35: 223, 1990.
38. Kahn JP, Drusin RE, Klein DF: Idiopathic cardiomyopathy and panic disorder: Clinical association in cardiac transplant candidates. Am J Psychiatry 144:1327, 1987.
39. Levenson JL, Olsbrich ME: Psychiatric aspects of heart transplantation. Psychosomatics 34:114, 1993.
40. Kahana RJ, Bibring GL: Personality types and medical management. In Zinberg N (ed): Psychiatry and Medical Practice in a General Hospital. International Universities Press, New York, 1964.
41. Fleury J, Kimbrell LC, Kruszewski MA: Life after a cardiac event: Women's experiences in healing. Heart Lung 24:474, 1995.
42. Denollet J, Brutsaert DL: Enhancing emotional well-being by comprehensive rehabilitation in patients with coronary heart disease. Eur Heart J 16:1070, 1995.

CHAPTER

11 Therapy

11.1 Pharmacologic Therapy for Stable Angina

Susan Wilansky and James T. Willerson

Patients with stable angina have symptoms usually after physical activity or during periods of emotional stress. Angina can also be triggered by a dream, by eating a large meal, and by exposure to cold. Any increase in heart rate, blood pressure, contractile state, or ventricular wall tension can raise myocardial oxygen demand. When supply lags behind demand, angina results. When stable angina is diagnosed, pharmacologic therapy can be prescribed to reduce myocardial oxygen demand and to increase blood flow to ischemic areas of the myocardium. However, a patient's risk factors and the extent of underlying disease must be determined before a specific treatment decision is made.

Treatment usually comprises pharmacologic agents from three classes, alone or in combination: nitrates, beta-adrenergic antagonists (beta blockers), and calcium channel blockers.[1] There is growing evidence that angiotensin-converting enzyme (ACE) inhibitors may also be beneficial, especially in reducing future risks of coronary events.[2] Because of their positive effects on morbidity and mortality, beta blockers should be strongly considered as initial therapy for chronic stable angina. Although they improve symptoms, nitrates have not been shown to reduce mortality or the future development of myocardial infarction (MI) in patients with coronary artery disease (CAD). Immediate-release or short-acting dihydropyridine calcium antagonists have been reported to increase the risk of adverse cardiac events, although these reports remain controversial.[1] Long-acting or slow-release dihydropyridines, or nondihydropyridines, have the potential to relieve symptoms without increasing the risk of adverse events.[1]

We were unable to find any reports that unequivocally proved significant gender differences in the treatment of stable angina. We do know, however, that women are less likely than men to receive appropriate treatment for their disease, including treatment with the staples of therapy—aspirin, beta blockers, and calcium antagonists,[3, 4] with a resultant increase in mortality. Regardless of the mechanism and extent of effects that sex differences have on approaches to cardiovascular disease, the outcomes of pharmacologic therapy are at least as beneficial for women as they are for men.[4, 5]

All of the pharmacologic agents used to treat stable angina are associated with some adverse effects, drug-drug interactions, and drug-food interactions. These effects and interactions are too complex and varied to describe here. Therefore, we suggest that before making decisions about therapy, physicians consult a source such as Micromedex (Micromedex Inc. 1974–2001, Healthcare Series), which is available online in many institutions.

NITRATES

Nitrates increase the availability of nitric oxide in the vasculature and reduce platelet aggregation and, possibly, inflammation at the site of endothelial injury. Of the nitrates, nitroglycerin is most often prescribed (Table 11–1). Nitro-

Table 11–1. MOST COMMONLY PRESCRIBED NITRATE PREPARATIONS USED IN THE TREATMENT OF ANGINA PECTORIS

PREPARATION	DOSAGE	DURATION OF EFFECT	FREQUENCY OF ADMINISTRATION
Sublingual nitroglycerin	0.3–0.5 mg	15–30 min	For individual episodes
Sublingual or chewable isosorbide dinitrate	2.5–10 mg	30 min–1 h	May be used instead of nitroglycerin
Oral isosorbide mononitrate (Ismo)	10–20 mg	24 h	Daily
Oral isosorbide mononitrate (Imdur)	30–90 mg	24 h	Daily
Oral isosorbide dinitrate (Tembid), longer-acting preparation	40 mg	6–8 h	Every 6–8 h
Pentaerythritol tetranitrate (Peritrate)			
Oral	10–40 mg	3–4 h	4 times a day
Sustained	80 mg (maximum of 240 mg)	8–10 h	2 times a day
Sustained-release oral nitroglycerin (Nitro-Bid)	2.5–6.5 mg	6 h	Every 6 h
Nitroglycerin ointment	Thin film on 1–2 inches over small area of anterior chest	4–6 h	Every 4–6 h
Nitroglycerin patches (sustained-release)	0.1 mg/h, 0.2 mg/h, 0.4 mg/h	Approximately 12 h	Every 12–24 h Nitrate-free period for 8 h
Nitroglycerin spray (Nitrolingual Pumpspray)	1 puff prn	Few minutes	Prn for chest pain

With permission from Willerson JT, Cohn JN (eds): Cardiovascular Medicine, 2nd ed., Churchill Livingstone, Philadelphia, 2000; adapted from Willerson JT, Hillis LD, Buja LM (eds): Ischemic Heart Disease: Clinical and Pathophysiological Aspects. Raven, New York, 1982.

glycerin is a potent smooth muscle vasodilator that can relieve angina within minutes of use. This agent acts on the peripheral vascular system, causing dilatation of systemic veins and decreased venous return to the right side of the heart and a subsequent reduction in myocardial wall tension and myocardial oxygen demand. Its effect on vascular resistance in arteries lowers systolic blood pressure. The vasodilator effect carries over to the medium-sized and large coronary arteries, thereby increasing blood flow to areas of the subendocardium being supplied by a narrowed or occluded coronary artery. Because they help balance myocardial oxygen demand and supply, nitroglycerin and the nitrates are different from most other coronary vasodilators, which increase blood flow and oxygen delivery to the epicardium or middle myocardium but do not affect oxygen supply in the endocardium.

For an acute anginal episode or for preventive care before exercise, 0.3 to. 0.6 mg of sublingual nitroglycerin is prescribed. Pain relief occurs in 7 minutes (often much sooner) and will last up to 30 minutes. If pain does not subside, the patient can repeat the dose 3 times at 5-minute intervals. Quickly relieving ischemic episodes is extremely important, so patients should be advised to carry their nitroglycerin (tablets or aerosol) with them at all times. Women, who experience typical angina pain less frequently, may be less likely to keep their medication with them. All women should be counseled about the importance of (1) recognizing their particular anginal symptoms and (2) quickly relieving an anginal episode.

Long-acting nitrates, which improve exercise tolerance for several hours for patients with angina, are available in oral and cutaneous preparations (see Table 11–1). Isosorbide mononitrate, which appears to be effective without causing drug tolerance, is now available in extended-release tablets (30 or 60 mg/day, which can be increased up to 240 mg/day, if needed). Cutaneous nitroglycerin paste or patches exert a prolonged therapeutic effect through a sustained, slow release of the drug. Nitroglycerin paste is readily absorbed into the skin, especially in a moist environment. Prescribed in a 2% preparation, the paste must be removed for about 8 hours each day to avoid tolerance, which is caused by continuous administration of the same nitrate preparation.[6] Tolerance is caused, at least partially, by sulfhydryl depletion in the smooth muscle, which decreases activation of cyclic guanosine monophosphate (GMP).

Because the incidence of acute MI is highest in the early morning hours, we generally tell patients to remove the nitroglycerin paste or patch in the late morning and replace it in the early evening or at bedtime, if possible. This approach provides the optimal use of the "nitrate effect" while avoiding the tolerance caused by continuous administration of the same preparation.[7, 8] Some investigators have suggested that the antioxidant vitamins C and E may reduce tolerance to nitrates, although this effect has not been rigorously proven.[9]

Some researchers believe that tolerance to nitroglycerin is clinically unimportant.[10] Although the nitrates are considered relatively safe drugs, side effects can occur; they include blueness of lips or fingernails, dyspnea, easy fatigability, headache, blurred vision, upset stomach, and skin rash. Nitroglycerin and nitrates are relatively contraindicated in patients with hypertrophic obstructive cardiomyopathy and severe aortic valve stenosis. In addition to the recommendations of nitrate use mentioned previously, we recommend that long-acting nitrates be added to patients' regimens when a beta blocker does not provide sufficient prevention of angina to allow them to be as physically active and productive as they wish to be or when they have angina at rest.

BETA-ADRENERGIC ANTAGONISTS (BETA BLOCKERS)

Beta-adrenergic antagonists (beta blockers) completely block sympathetic stimulation of the heart and reduce heart rate, systolic blood pressure, contractility, and cardiac output at rest and during exercise. When patients take a beta blocker, more oxygen is extracted from capillary blood, thus improving the systemic arteriovenous oxygen difference. The decrease in myocardial oxygen demand and the resultant increase in exercise tolerance may allow patients to resume previous activities without the threat of angina. Beta blockers can also be prescribed to control exercise-induced ventricular arrhythmias and arterial hypertension.

Beta-adrenergic antagonists are classified as nonspecific or $beta_1$-specific (Table 11–2). Nonspecific beta blockers may interfere with bronchial smooth muscle dilatation and exacerbate bronchospasm. At higher doses, the $beta_1$-specific blockers, such as metoprolol, may do the same. However, at reduced dosages, $beta_1$-specific blockers can be prescribed with careful monitoring for patients who have chronic obstructive pulmonary disease and reactive airway disease. The $beta_1$-specific blockers may also be better for treating patients with diabetes, because they decrease insulin release less than the nonspecific beta blockers. Beta blockers are available today in sustained-release formulations, which allow patients to receive an even distribution of response from the drug on a 24-hour basis. In general, we have found that beta blockers, in all of their preparations, should be started at lower dosages in women (i.e., half the usual starting dose to minimize side effects). For patients with exercise or stress-related angina, combining a beta blocker with nitrates often controls anginal symptoms.

As with all potent medications, beta blockers are associated with side effects. Besides bronchospasm, they can cause bradycardia, atrioventricular (AV) block, and hypotension. They may also decrease myocardial contractility and increase the severity and incidence of coronary artery spasm, so beta blockers should never be prescribed for patients with these conditions. Because of these side effects, these agents must be used cautiously in patients who have severe heart failure or peripheral vascular disease and insulin-dependent diabetes mellitus, especially if their blood glucose levels have been difficult to control. Beta blockers may also cause easy fatigability, insomnia, dizziness or syncope, dyspnea with effort, and sexual impotence, in addition to other side effects.

Side effects of beta blockers may be more common and more pronounced in women with the usual starting dosages. They are definitely contraindicated for patients with (1) severe bradycardia, (2) preexisting high degree of AV block, (3) sick sinus syndrome in the absence of a pacemaker, or (4) severe, unstable left ventricular failure. Beta blockers are used in the treatment of some patients with severe heart

Table 11–2. SELECTED BETA-ADRENERGIC ANTAGONISTS

NAME	BETA-BLOCKADE POTENCY RATIO (PROPRANOLOL = 1.0)	CARDIOSELECTIVE	USUAL THERAPEUTIC DOSE RANGE (mg/day)	ELIMINATION HALF-LIFE (h)	ROUTE OF EXCRETION
Propranolol (nonspecific)	1.0	0	40–480	3.5–6.0	Urine
Timolol	6.0	0	5–60	4–5	Urine
Sotalol	0.3	0	160–320	5–13	Urine
Metoprolol ($beta_1$)	1.0	+	Given IV at 5 mg in each of 3 doses at 2-min intervals, given orally at 100–800	3–4	Urine
Pindolol	6.0	0	20–60	3–4	Urine
Atenolol ($beta_1$)	1.0	+	25–100	6–9	Approximately 40% of unchanged drug in urine
Acebutolol ($beta_1$)	0.3	+	400–800	8	Uncertain
Nadolol	0.5–1.0	0	40–320	20–24	Urine
Sotalol*	1	0	80–640	12	Urine
Esmolol† ($beta_1$)	0.025	+	Given IV at 25–300 mg/kg/min	12	Hydrolysis by plasma
Labetalol	0.3	Selective alpha and nonselective beta blockers	Given IV 0.25 mg/kg over 2 min and additional 40–80 mg at 1-h intervals, given orally at 200–2400	8–10	Urine and bile
Toprol XL	—	Selective long-acting metoprolol	50–200	24	—

IV, intravenously.
*Seen only at low dosage.
†Given intravenously for immediate control of supraventricular tachycardia or systemic arterial hypertension.
With permission from Willerson JT, Cohn JN (eds): Cardiovascular Medicine, 2nd ed., Churchill Livingstone, Philadelphia, 2000; adapted from Hillis LD, Firth BG, Willerson JT: Manual of Clinical Problems in Cardiology, 2nd ed. Little, Brown, Boston, 1984.

failure; however, these agents should be started in very low doses, which should be increased very gradually in patients with relatively stable, albeit severe, heart failure. Asthma and bronchospastic disease, severe depression, and peripheral vascular disease are relative contraindications.

CALCIUM ANTAGONISTS (CALCIUM CHANNEL BLOCKERS)

Calcium antagonists are the third arm of the pharmacologic treatment of angina and CAD (Table 11–3). These agents cause vasodilatation of vascular smooth muscle and increase coronary blood flow by altering slow calcium channel transport into the cells. Like beta blockers, the calcium channel blockers verapamil and diltiazem reduce myocardial oxygen demand at rest and exercise by decreasing heart rate and contractility. They work by decreasing the formation of sinus node impulses and AV conduction. These agents also increase blood flow to ischemic regions of the epicardium.

In contrast to verapamil and diltiazem, the dihydropyridine calcium antagonist nifedipine raises heart rate and does not slow impulse formation in the sinus node delay AV conduction (Fig. 11–1). It is a potent vasodilator. Thus, like verapamil and diltiazem, it increases blood flow to ischemic regions of the epicardium. Nifedipine can be given to patients with severe congestive heart failure, because its negative inotropic effect is abrogated by its ability to reduce systemic vascular resistance and afterload, thus allowing the heart to contract more effectively. Although it has been

Table 11–3. SELECTED PROTOTYPE SLOW CALCIUM CHANNEL BLOCKERS

	DOSAGE		ONSET OF ACTION		THERAPEUTIC PLASMA CONCENTRATION	METABOLISM	EXCRETION
	Oral	IV	Oral	IV			
Diltiazem	120–140 mg/d	75–150 μg/kg (10–20 mg)	>30 min	>10 min	50–200 ng/ml	Deacetylation *N*-Demethylation *O*-Demethylation	60% fecal
Nifedipine SR (dihydropyridine calcium antagonist)	30–90 mg/d q 6–8 h	5–15 μg/kg*	>20 min	>5 min (3 min SL)	25–100 ng/ml	Alpha-hydroxycarboxylic acid and alpha-lactone with no known activity	20%–40% fecal 50%–80% renal
Verapamil	80–120 mg q 6–12 h	150 μg/kg (2.5–10 mg)	>30 min	>5 min	<100 ng/ml	*N*-Dealkylation *N*-Demethylation Major hepatic first-pass effect	15% fecal 70% renal

IV, intravenous; SL, sublingual.
*Not available in U.S.
With permission from Willerson JT, Cohn JN (eds): Cardiovascular Medicine, 2nd ed. Churchill Livingstone, Philadelphia, 2000; adapted from Packer M, Frishman WH: Calcium Channel Antagonists in Cardiovascular Disease. Appleton-Century-Crofts, East Norwalk, CT, 1984.

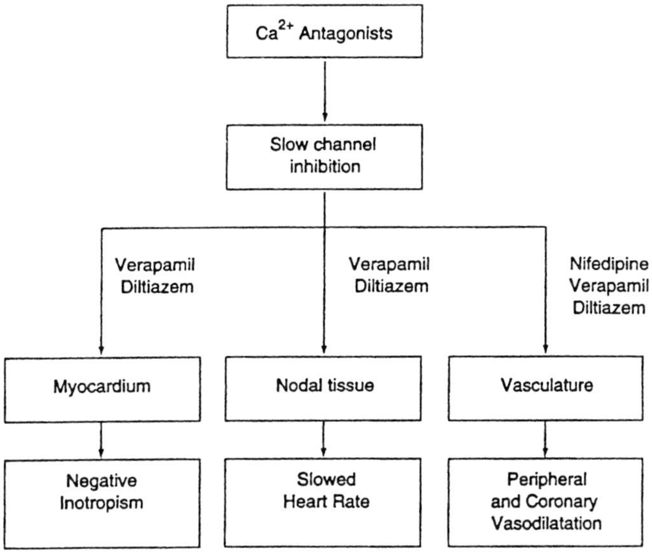

FIGURE 11–1. Effects produced by slow calcium channel antagonists. (From Willerson JT, Cohn JN [eds]: Cardiovascular Medicine, 2nd ed., Churchill Livingstone, Philadelphia, 2000.)

suggested that the blood pressure responses to nifedipine may be different in women and men, a study of matched (but very small) groups found no such difference.[11]

Calcium antagonists are indicated for patients who experience chest pain at relatively low levels of exercise or stress (Tables 11–3 and 11–4) and can be used alone or in combination with nitrates, beta blockers, or both. Calcium antagonists should be used in combination with beta blockers when initial treatment with beta blockers is not successful or as a substitute for a beta blocker when initial treatment leads to unacceptable side effects or the beta blocker is contraindicated. Calcium antagonists may also be indicated for treating stable angina in patients who have systemic arterial hypertension, atrial arrhythmias, and exercise-induced ventricular tachycardia. We generally prescribe calcium antagonists at half the recommended starting dose in women (e.g., amlodipine, 2.5 mg qd; or verapamil SR, 120 mg qd).

Varied side effects are associated with calcium channel blockers. With verapamil or diltiazem, patients and their physicians must be wary of marked bradycardia, hypotension, constipation, congestive heart failure, skin rash, and heart block. Of the calcium channel blockers, diltiazem usually causes the fewest side effects.

The combination of a beta blocker with verapamil is likely to lead to bradycardia and depression of cardiac contractility or AV block. Thus, it should be used only for patients who have atrial arrhythmias or angina that is very difficult to control, and even then, very carefully and with close monitoring for side effects. The safest clinical combination of a calcium antagonist with a beta blocker is with a dihydropyridine calcium antagonist, such as nifedipine. With nifedipine (and other dihydropyridine calcium antagonists), patients may experience a flushing sensation, dizziness, hypotension, peripheral edema, tachycardia, and rash. Physicians must take care when prescribing these medications in large dosages to patients with CAD and especially when prescribing them for patients with unstable angina or history of MI, to avoid tachycardia and hypotension in such patients.

Overt decompensated heart failure is a contraindication for the use of calcium antagonists, although newer-generation vasoselective dihydropyridines, like amlodipine and felodipine, are tolerated by patients with poorer ejection fractions. Bradycardia, sinus node dysfunction, and AV nodal block are contraindications for the use of heart rate–modulating calcium antagonists. A long QT interval is a contraindication to the use of mibefradil and bepridil.[1]

COMBINATION THERAPY

Patients who experience angina pain at very low levels of effort or whose symptoms are not easily controlled with one agent can be prescribed a combination of nitrates, beta blockers, and calcium channel blockers. However, a combination regimen must be prescribed cautiously and monitored regularly. The combination of nitrates and beta blockers has additive effects in the treatment of angina, because nitrates primarily cause peripheral and coronary vasodilation, and beta blockers reduce heart rate and myocardial contractility. In addition, the chronotropic effect of beta blockers may reduce any reflex tachycardia caused by the nitrates, and the vasodilation of the nitrates may counter the increase in peripheral vascular resistance caused by beta blockers.

Because both nitrates and rapid-acting dihydropyridine calcium antagonists can produce reflex tachycardia, a slower-onset calcium antagonist such as amlodipine or, alternatively,

Table 11–4. ADDITIONAL SLOW CHANNEL CALCIUM ANTAGONISTS

ANTAGONIST (TYPE)	DOSAGE	SPECIAL USES	EXCRETION
Nisoldipine (dihydropyridine)	10 mg PO q 12 h	Treat systemic arterial hypertension and angina	Renal
Felodipine (dihydropyridine)	5–10 mg PO q 24 h	Treat systemic arterial hypertension and angina	Renal
Nicardipine (dihydropyridine)	20–40 mg PO tid	Treat systemic arterial hypertension and angina	Renal
Nimodipine (dihydropyridine)	60 mg q 4 h PO for 21 days	Reduce cerebral vascular ischemia after subarachnoid hemorrhage	Renal
Isradipine (dihydropyridine)	2.5 mg PO bid increasing up to 20 mg PO qd	Hypertension	Renal
Amlodipine (dihydropyridine)	5–10 mg PO qd	Systemic arterial hypertension and angina	Bile and renal
Bepridil (sodium and calcium channel blocker)	200 mg PO qd increasing to 400 mg PO qd	Angina	Renal and fecal

With permission from Willerson JT, Cohn JN (eds): Cardiovascular Medicine, 2nd ed. Churchill Livingstone, Philadelphia, 2000; modified from Packer M, Frishman WH: Calcium Channel Antagonists in Cardiovascular Disease. Appleton-Century-Crofts, East Norwalk, CT, 1984.

diltiazem may be an appropriate choice. However, the combination of a beta blocker with nifedipine may prevent the increase in heart rate associated with nifedipine therapy, and the combination of an agent that reduces systemic vascular resistance and increases coronary blood flow (nifedipine) with one that reduces myocardial oxygen demand (beta blocker) can relieve angina.

When beta blockers are combined with calcium antagonists, the safest choice of calcium antagonist is one of the dihydropyridine type. When any calcium channel blocker is prescribed in combination with a beta blocker, the calcium antagonist should be prescribed first in small doses, which may be increased for clinical response only after the safety of the regimen has been reevaluated. In some cases, especially with verapamil but also with diltiazem, the added catecholamine-blocking action may produce an excessive reduction of resting sympathetic nervous system activity, which may result in marked bradycardia, hypotension, vertigo, syncopal attacks, or orthostatic hypotension. Therefore, verapamil and diltiazem must be prescribed very cautiously when a patient has already been prescribed a beta blocker.

PLATELET ANTAGONISTS

Platelet antagonists have been shown to reduce the risk of MI and mortality for patients with chronic stable angina.[1] These drugs combat platelet aggregation, which occurs after endothelial injury. Endothelial injury exposes the subendothelial collagen and other matrix proteins, allowing platelets to attach and aggregate. Platelet aggregation begins a cascade of events, including the accumulation of the mediators thromboxane A_2, serotonin, platelet-activating factor, thrombin, adenosine diphosphate, oxygen-derived free radicals, tissue factor, and endothelin,[6] which can lead to unstable angina and MI.

Fibrinogen levels vary directly with age and inversely with high-density lipoprotein (HDL) levels,[12] and age-adjusted fibrinogen levels are higher in women than in men, especially in the perimenopausal years. Increased fibrinogen levels are associated with a higher risk of coronary disease and stroke.[13–16] In addition, higher levels of factors VII and VIII and increased clotting activity are also more prevalent in elderly women, as are greater reactivity of circulating platelets and lower responsiveness of the fibrinolytic system.[17] All of these differences raise the risk for thromboembolism and vascular disease in women.

Aspirin has clearly been shown to reduce the rate of cardiac events, stroke, and acute myocardial syndromes.[18–21] In the Antiplatelet Trialists' Collaborative Study, aspirin was shown to statistically reduce the rate of nonfatal infarctions or strokes by 30% and the total vascular mortality rate by 15%.[19] When the daily dose of aspirin was 300 to 325 mg, the risk for total vascular events was reduced by 24%. Another meta-analysis that included a significant number of women with chronic stable angina reached the same conclusion.[22] In this study, aspirin dosages of 75 mg per day reduced the odds of a vascular event by 29%, which was not substantially different from the percentage reduction achieved with prescription of higher dosages. The Nurses' Health Study reported a reduction in risk for the first MI associated with the use of 1 to 6 aspirin tablets per week in women older than 50 years; however, this was not a randomized study, and the risk of cardiovascular death, stroke, or important vascular events was not altered.[23]

Aspirin inhibits platelet and endothelial cyclooxygenase (COX-1 and COX-2), thereby decreasing the formation of platelet thromboxane and endothelial cell prostacyclin. Because aspirin inhibits COX-2 activity, it may also reduce inflammation of vulnerable atherosclerotic plaques, thus reducing the risk of death from acute MI or from recurrent infarction, especially for patients who have sustained non–Q wave infarctions.[19]

Generally, we prescribe 1 aspirin (81 or 325 mg) every other day to 1 aspirin per day for women we believe to be at increased risk for future coronary events and for whom there is no contraindication. Aspirin use is associated with risk, however. Potential side effects include gastritis, stomach or gastrointestinal ulceration, gastrointestinal bleeding, easy bruising and bleeding with minor trauma, asthma, decreased renal function, and thrombocytopenia. Therefore, the risks and benefits must be weighed for each patient, and as with all pharmacologic therapy, follow-up is mandatory.

Although aspirin has been documented to be effective in treating and preventing complications of atherosclerotic disease, it only partially inhibits platelet aggregation, and some patients appear to be immune to its effects, even in large doses.[24] In some cases, especially patients at high risk for transient ischemic attack, stroke, ischemic heart disease, and peripheral artery occlusion, aspirin may be combined with clopidogrel (Plavix)—an analogue of ticoplidine that inhibits adenosine diphosphate activation of platelets—to produce an additional protective effect.[25] In the Clopidogrel versus Aspirin in Patients at Risk for Ischemic Events (CAPRIE) Study, aspirin (325 mg/day) was compared with clopidogrel (75 mg/day) for reducing the combined incidence of ischemic stroke, MI, or vascular death in 19,185 patients who had had a recent stroke or MI or who had symptomatic peripheral arterial disease.[26] After an average of 2 years of follow-up, clopidogrel showed a significant 8.7% benefit in efficacy over aspirin (5.32% vs. 5.83%, $p = .043$). Adverse events were similar, and neutropenia, which has been noted with ticlopidine therapy, was rare. Follow-up is also mandatory for patients taking clopidogrel.

ANGIOTENSIN-CONVERTING ENZYME INHIBITORS

Angiotensin-converting enzyme inhibitors block activation of the renin-angiotensin system. Experimental and epidemiologic data have suggested that activation of this system may play an important role in increasing the rate of cardiovascular events. Use of ACE inhibitors has been investigated for treatment of stable angina, but until recently, the efficacy of these agents had not been documented.

In the large multicenter Heart Outcomes Prevention Evaluation (HOPE) trial, ACE inhibitor therapy with ramipril was found to significantly affect the primary outcome composite of cardiovascular death, MI, or stroke (14.0% for ramipril vs. 17.8% for placebo; $p < .001$; relative risk [RR], .78; 95% confidence interval [CI], .70 to .86) in patients at high risk for cardiovascular events.[2] Significant benefits were also noted for the individual endpoints of cardiovascular death (6.1% vs. 8.1%; $p < .001$; RR, .74; 95% CI, .64 to .87), MI (9.9% vs. 12.3%; $p < .001$; RR, .80; 95% CI, .70 to .90), stroke (3.4% vs. 4.9%; $p < .001$; RR, .68; 95% CI, .56 to .84), and total mortality (10.4% vs. 12.2%; $p < .005$; RR, .84; 95% CI, .75 to .95). Stable angina was present in 5162 of the 9297 patients enrolled in the study (56%). The clinical benefit was also significant for patients with normal left ventricular ejection fractions and for patients in almost all of the major subgroups of the study, including those with and without cerebrovascular disease, diabetes, hypertension, CAD, and peripheral vascular disease; men and women; and young and old patients. In fact, the investigators observed a marked decrease in the incidence of complications of diabetes and of new cases of diabetes with the use of ramipril. In addition, the drug was well-tolerated in the treatment group.

The Brachial Artery Normalization of Forearm Function (BANFF) study examined the effects of quinapril, enalapril, losartan, and amlodipine on flow-mediated vasodilatation of the brachial artery in 80 patients with documented CAD and found quinapril to be the superior drug.[27] The reason may be the agent's higher affinity for tissue ACE, which would seem reasonable in consideration of the HOPE study, in which the high-affinity ramipril significantly improved cardiovascular endpoints.

Whereas ACE inhibitors are not currently initial or routine therapy for patients with stable angina, they may have a role in the future in the treatment of patients with atherosclerotic disease. These agents can also be considered for patients at higher risk, whose angina is difficult to manage with the standard medications. Adverse effects of ACE inhibitors include cough, rash, angioneurotic edema, hyperkalemia, and acute respiratory failure. Although fewer than 1% of men experience cough as a side effect of ACE inhibitors, at least 3% of women do so.

POTASSIUM CHANNEL BLOCKERS AND OPENERS

Another new class of potential anti-ischemic, vasodilator drugs consists of the bradycardic potassium channel blockers and openers. More studies are needed before efficacy can be established, but in one study, tedisamil exerted favorable hemodynamic, neurohumoral, and anti-ischemic effects in patients with coronary disease. This agent induced a dose-dependent decrease in both heart rate and the index of myocardial oxygen consumption and was associated with an improvement in ST segment depression. These effects compared favorably with those of the beta blockers esmolol and atenolol.[28]

INFECTION AND INFLAMMATION

Infection with certain bacteria (*Chlamydia pneumoniae, Helicobacter pylori*) and viruses (cytomegalovirus and herpes simplex virus 1) has also been implicated in the development of CAD.[29] In addition, inflammatory reactions in coronary plaques play an important role in the pathogenesis of acute atherothrombotic events. Inflammation elsewhere in the body may be associated with atherogenesis and thrombosis, and studies have found that an elevated level of C-reactive protein is associated with a higher risk of coronary events.[30, 31] In a meta-analysis, other inflammatory markers found to be associated with CAD were higher fibrinogen level, lower albumin level, and increased leukocyte count.[31]

The roles of antibiotics, antiviral agents, anti-inflammatory agents, and immunization in the treatment of CAD have not been established. Gender implications remain unknown as well. However, a better understanding of the role of infectious agents and the inflammatory process in general may provide additional avenues for earlier prevention of this disease. Whether chronic or acute infections increase the risk of CAD still remains to be established.

DRUG-DRUG INTERACTIONS

As in prescribing any medication, the physician must consider the potential drug-drug interactions when prescribing pharmacologic therapy for CAD. Of the lipid-lowering agents (discussed in Chapter 5.3), some statins may interact with other cardiovascular therapeutic agents, especially drugs metabolized by the cytochrome P450 enzyme pathway, such as the calcium channel blockers verapamil, nifedipine, and diltiazem; analgesics such as ibuprofen; antiarrhythmics such as amiodarone; anticoagulants such as warfarin; and antidepressants such as fluoxetine and amitriptyline, among others.[32] Predicting which patients will have side effects from drug-drug interactions can be difficult, so caution must always be taken in prescription of drugs to patients with coronary disease.

A number of factors may be responsible for the unpredictability of patient reactions, including a genetic polymorphism in the cytochrome P450 enzymes that may result in large differences in drug clearance rates among individuals[32–34] as well as in the incidence of side effects, such as myopathy and rhabdomyolysis. Drug-drug interactions should always be considered in the prescription of medications for patients with stable angina, and we suggest consultation of a pharmacologic database (such as Micromedex) for current information.

CONCLUSION

Women with stable angina can benefit from treatment with nitrates, beta blockers, calcium antagonists, antiplatelet agents (aspirin either alone or in combination with clopidogrel), and, possibly, ACE inhibitors. In prescribing these medications, we follow the protocol outlined in Figure 11–2. For patients with noncrescendo angina at low levels of activity, we prescribe nitrates, aspirin, a beta blocker, a calcium antagonist, or a combination of such agents, and we correct all probable risk factors, including abnormal serum lipid profiles. For patients whose angina resolves or occurs with only high levels of activity, we continue the prescribed therapy, with appropriate follow-up (see Table 11–2). Patients in whom significant ischemia is demonstrated by noninvasive testing or in whom functional alterations occur at low or moderate levels of stress are referred for coronary arteriography, as are patients who continue to have angina at low levels of effort.

Patients who have angina only with moderate activity or

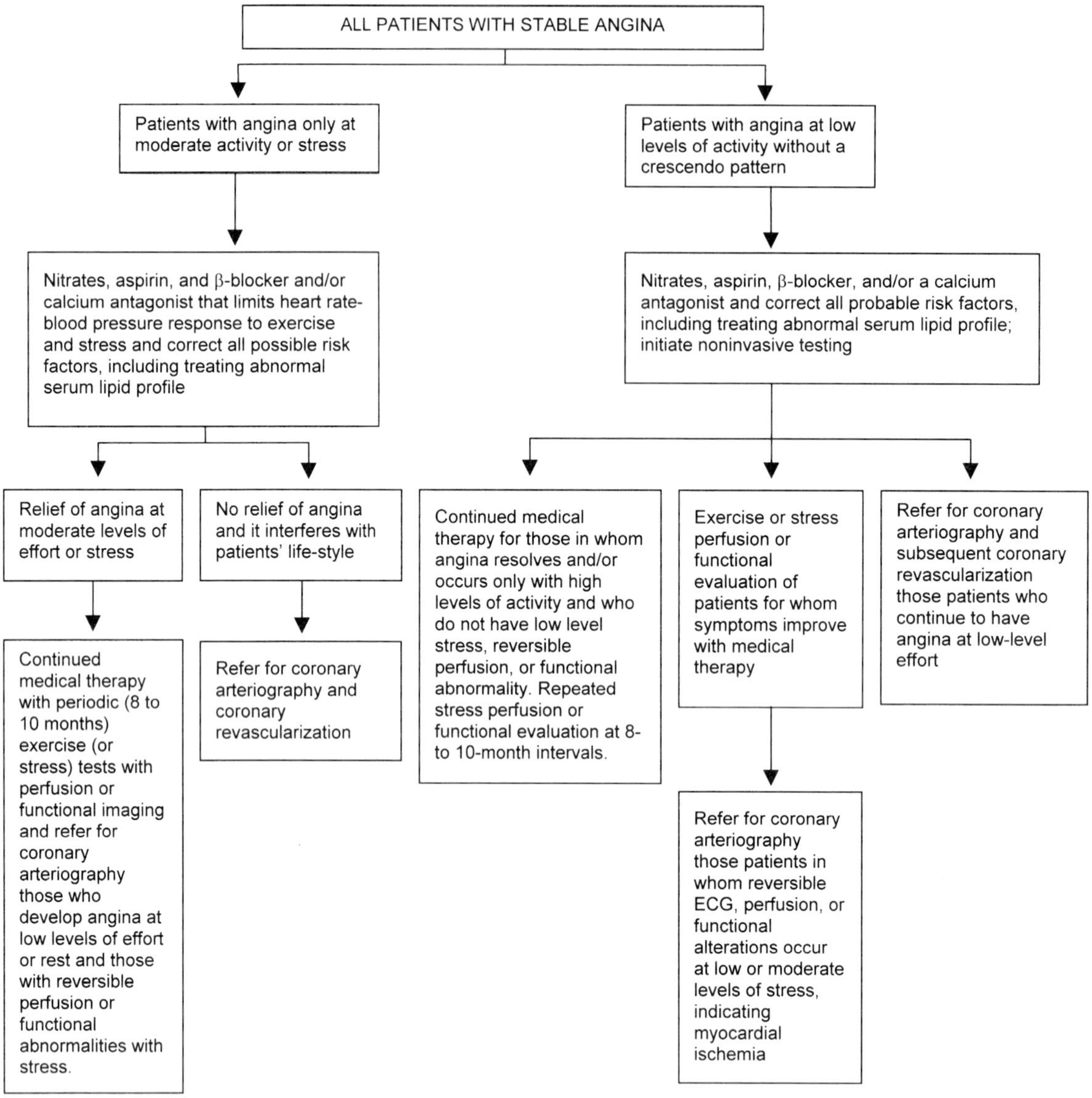

FIGURE 11–2. Treatment options for patients with stable angina. (From Willerson JT, Cohn JN [eds]: Cardiovascular Medicine, 2nd ed., Churchill Livingstone, Philadelphia, 2000.)

stress are prescribed nitrates, aspirin, a beta blocker, a calcium antagonist, or a combination of these agents. When serum lipid levels are abnormal, this condition is treated as well (see Chapter 5.3). When angina is relieved, medical therapy is continued, with appropriate follow-up (see Table 11–1). When angina is not relieved and it interferes with the patient's lifestyle, the patient is referred for coronary arteriography and possible coronary revascularization.

References

1. ACC/AHA/ACP-ASIM guidelines for the management of patients with chronic stable angina [erratum published in J Am Coll Cardiol 34:314, 1999]. J Am Coll Cardiol 33:2092, 1999.
2. The Heart Outcomes Prevention Evaluation Study Investigators: Effects of an angiotensin-converting enzyme inhibitor, ramipril, on cardiovascular events in high-risk patients. N Engl J Med 342:145, 2000.
3. Chandra NC, Ziegelstein RC, Rogers WJ, et al: Observations of the treatment of women in the United States with myocardial infarction: A report from the National Registry of Myocardial Infarction—I. Arch Intern Med 158:981, 1998.
4. Tsang TSM, Barnes ME, Gersh BJ, et al: Risks of coronary heart disease in women: Current understanding and evolving concepts. Mayo Clin Proc 75:1289, 2000.
5. Bernstein SJ, Hilborne LH, Leape LL, et al: The appropriateness of use of cardiovascular procedures in women and men. Arch Intern Med 154:2759, 1994.
6. Willerson JT: Medical treatment of stable angina. In Willerson JT, Cohn JN (eds): Cardiovascular Medicine, 2nd ed. Churchill Livingstone, New York, 2000, p 709.
7. Needleman P, Johnson EM Jr: Mechanism of tolerance development to organic nitrates. J Pharmacol Exp Ther 184:709, 1973.
8. Abrams J: Nitrate tolerance and dependence. Am Heart J 99:113, 1980.
9. Aronow WS, Chesluk HM: Evaluation of nitroglycerin in angina in patients on isosorbide dinitrate. Circulation 42:61, 1970.
10. Elkayam U, Aronow WS: Glyceryl trinitrate (nitroglycerin) ointment and isosorbide dinitrate: A review of their pharmacological properties and therapeutic uses. Drugs 23:165, 1982.
11. Klassen GA, Yeung PK, Barclay KD, et al: Effect of diltiazem on intraarterial blood pressure and heart rate during stress testing in patients with angina: A gender comparison study. J Clin Pharmacol 37:297, 1997.

12. Barash E, Benderly M, Graff E, et al: Plasma fibrinogen levels and their correlates in 6457 coronary heart disease patients: The Bezafibrate Infarction Prevention (BIP) Study. J Clin Epidemiol 48:757, 1995.
13. Meade TW, Mellows S, Brozovic M, et al: Haemostatic function and ischaemic heart disease: Principal results of the Northwick Park Heart Study. Lancet 2:533, 1986.
14. Wilhelmsen L, Svardsudd K, Korsan-Bengtsen K, et al: Fibrinogen as a risk factor for stroke and myocardial infarction. N Engl J Med 311: 501, 1984.
15. Kannel WB, Wolf PA, Castelli WP, et al: Fibrinogen and risk of cardiovascular disease: The Framingham Study. JAMA 258:1183, 1987.
16. Folsom AR, Wu KK, Rosamond WD, et al: Prospective study of hemostatic factors and incidence of coronary heart disease: The Atherosclerosis Risk in Communities (ARIC) Study. Circulation 96:1102, 1997.
17. Abbate R, Prisco D, Rostagno C, et al: Age-related changes in the hemostatic system. Int J Clin Lab Res 23:1, 1993.
18. Steering Committee of the Physicians' Health Study Research Group: Final report on the aspirin component of the ongoing Physicians' Health Study. N Engl J Med 321:129, 1989.
19. Secondary prevention of vascular disease by prolonged antiplatelet treatment: Antiplatelet Trialists' Collaboration. Br Med J (Clin Res Ed) 296:320, 1988.
20. Klimt CR, Knatterud GL, Stamler J, et al: Persantine-aspirin reinfarction study. Part II: Secondary coronary prevention with Persantine and aspirin. J Am Coll Cardiol 7:251, 1986.
21. Zanger DR, Solomon AJ, Gersh BJ: Contemporary management of angina. Part II: Medical management of chronic stable angina. Am Fam Physician 61:129, 2000.
22. Collaborative overview of randomised trials of antiplatelet therapy—I: Prevention of death, myocardial infarction, and stroke by prolonged antiplatelet therapy in various categories of patients. Antiplatelet Trialists' Collaboration [erratum published in BMJ 308:1540, 1994]. BMJ 308:81, 1994.
23. Manson JE, Stampfer MJ, Colditz GA, et al: A prospective study of aspirin use and primary prevention of cardiovascular disease in women. JAMA 266:521, 1991.
24. Helgason CM, Tortorice KL, Winkler SR, et al: Aspirin response and failure in cerebral infarction. Stroke 24:345, 1993.
25. Anand SS, Salim Y: Oral anticoagulant therapy in patients with coronary artery disease: A meta-analysis. JAMA 282:2058, 1999.
26. CAPRIE Steering Committee: A randomised, blinded, trial of clopidogrel versus aspirin in patients at risk of ischaemic events (CAPRIE). Lancet 348:1329, 1996.
27. Anderson TJ, Elstein E, Haber H, et al: Comparative study of ACE-inhibition, angiotensin II antagonism, and calcium channel blockade on flow-mediated vasodilation in patients with coronary disease (BANFF study). J Am Coll Cardiol 34:60, 1999.
28. Mitrovic V, Oehm E, Thormann J, et al: Potassium channel openers and blockers in coronary artery disease. Herz 25:130, 2000.
29. Roivainen M, Viik-Kajander M, Palosuo T, et al: Infections, inflammation, and the risk of coronary heart disease. Circulation 101:252, 2000.
30. Koenig W, Sund M, Frolich M, et al: C-reactive protein, a sensitive marker of inflammation, predicts future risk of coronary heart disease in initially healthy middle-aged men: Results from the MONICA (Monitoring Trends and Determinants in Cardiovascular Disease) Augsburg Cohort Study, 1984 to 1992. Circulation 99:237, 1999.
31. Gram J, Bladbjerg EM, Moller L, et al: Tissue-type plasminogen activator and C-reactive protein in acute coronary heart disease: A nested case-control study. J Intern Med 247:205, 2000.
32. Danesh J, Muir J, Wong YK, et al: Risk factors for coronary heart disease and acute-phase proteins: A population-based study. Eur Heart J 20:954, 1999.
33. Bertz RJ, Granneman GR: Use of in vitro and in vivo data to estimate the likelihood of metabolic pharmacokinetic interactions. Clin Pharmacokinet 32:210, 1997.
34. Gonzalez FJ, Nebert DW: Evolution of the P450 gene superfamily: Animal-plant "warfare," molecular drive and human genetic differences in drug oxidation. Trends Genet 6:182, 1990.

11.2 Pharmacologic Therapy for Unstable Angina and Non–Q Wave Infarction

Susan Wilansky and James T. Willerson

Unstable angina is characterized by increased, progressive symptoms of angina (crescendo angina) or onset of prolonged angina, angina at rest, or nocturnal angina (decubitus)—Braunwald classification IIIB and C (Table 11–5). Compared with the pain of stable angina, the pain of unstable angina is often more intense, lasts longer, and occurs with less effort. Unstable angina is generally precipitated by acute coronary obstruction. The obstruction usually results from rupture of atherosclerotic plaque, an injury that causes a consequent cascade of platelet aggregation, thrombosis, and dynamic vasoconstriction. This cascade leads to ischemia and MI, often within 3 months of onset of the unstable angina.

Unstable angina usually occurs when periods of severe reduction in coronary blood flow persist for less than 30 minutes. The periods of angina are usually repetitive, resulting from transient thrombus or subtotal occlusion of the culprit artery. Non–Q wave MI occurs when the critical period of coronary occlusion lasts between 30 minutes and 2 or 3 hours.[1] In both conditions, the occlusive thrombus and dynamic vasoconstriction are usually transient. Expeditious treatment to dissolve the thrombus may prevent Q wave MI from occurring. However, patients with either unstable angina or non–Q wave MI are at substantially higher risk of another MI for about 12 weeks, or until the endothelial injury heals. Unstable angina must be considered a relative medical emergency. Patients who experience these symptoms should be hospitalized immediately in a cardiac care unit to rule out MI and to begin treatment to prevent MI.

All patients with unstable angina must be screened for non–Q wave infarction, as these two acute coronary syndromes are closely related. The signs of non–Q wave infarction are (1) prolonged, severe chest pain, (2) ST segment depression or flattening, inversion, or both of the T wave on electrocardiogram (ECG), and (3) elevated concentrations of serum creatine kinase (CK), the MB isoenzyme of CK, and troponin I or T. Patients with non–Q wave infarctions are treated similarly to patients with unstable angina (Fig. 11–3). The goals of treatment of these acute syndromes are to prevent sustained thrombus formation at the site of the unstable plaque and to relieve associated vasoconstriction.

Unstable angina and non–Q wave MI are serious health

Table 11–5. BRAUNWALD'S CLASSIFICATION OF UNSTABLE ANGINA*

SEVERITY	A: DEVELOPS IN PRESENCE OF EXTRACARDIAC CONDITION THAT INTENSIFIES MYOCARDIAL ISCHEMIA (SECONDARY UA)	B: DEVELOPS IN ABSENCE OF EXTRACARDIAC CONDITION (PRIMARY UA)	C: DEVELOPS WITHIN 2 WEEKS AFTER AMI (POSTINFARCTION UA)
I. New onset of severe angina or accelerated angina; no rest pain	IA	IB	IC
II. Angina at rest within past month but not within preceding 48 h (angina at rest, subacute)	IIA	IIB	IIC
III. Angina at rest within 48 h (angina at rest, acute)	IIIA	IIIB	IIIC

*Patients with UA may also be divided into three groups depending on whether UA occurs (1) in the absence of treatment for chronic stable angina, (2) during treatment for chronic stable angina, or (3) despite maximal anti-ischemic drug therapy. These three groups may be designated by subscript 1, 2, or 3, respectively. Patients with UA may be further divided into those with and without transient ST-T wave changes during pain.

AMI, acute myocardial infarction; UA, unstable angina.

From Braunwald E: Unstable angina: A classification. Circulation 80:410, 1989, with permission.

threats for women. Even though fewer women than men have coronary disease, more women than men have unstable angina, coronary vasospasm,[2] and thromboembolic events.[3] Once atherosclerotic plaques develop in women, the threat of thromboembolic complications seems to be much higher than in men.[4, 5] Even when thrombolytic agents are administered expeditiously, women do not fare as well. The reason may be the increased thrombogenicity of women's platelets, which thus requires stronger inhibitors of platelet aggregation to suppress ischemic events.[3]

The American College of Cardiology/American Heart Association (ACC/AHA) Guidelines for managing patients with unstable angina and non–Q wave infarction recommend that women be treated similarly to men.[2] Unfortunately, women tend to receive less intensive pharmacologic therapy than men, including therapy with the mainstays of treatment, aspirin and antithrombotic agents.[6–8] In the Thrombolysis in Myocardial Infarction IIIB (TIMI IIIB) trial, women were found to have had fewer MIs or cardiac procedures, but their symptoms (including duration of symptoms) and ST changes on ECG were similar to those of men (Fig. 11–4).[8] When they were treated, the outcome of medical therapy was the same for women as for men.

Investigators from the Global Use of Strategies to Open Occluded Coronary Arteries in Acute Coronary Syndromes IIB (GUSTO-IIB) study also found that women were more likely to have unstable angina and less likely to have had an acute MI.[9] These investigators found that the 30-day event rate (death/MI) was significantly lower in women than in men (events odds ratio, 0.65; $p = .003$) when women had appropriate treatement.[9]

Patients with unstable angina who are at highest risk for complicated courses and poor outcomes have higher serum levels of the inflammatory markers C-reactive protein,[10–14] troponins I and T (necrosis markers),[15–17] fibrinogen,[18–20] interleukins 1 and 6,[21] and serum amyloid–like protein.[22] C-reactive protein may also directly contribute to the inflammatory process. Patients with increased levels of inflammatory markers require close monitoring. They will likely need more intensive medical therapy, interventional therapy (angioplasty, stenting, or both), or surgical therapy (coronary artery bypass graft [CABG] procedures).

Pharmacologic therapy begins with nitrates; antithrombotic therapies, especially aspirin, which inhibit thromboxane A_2, platelets, white blood cells, and inflammation; and unfractionated or low-molecular-weight (LMW) heparin to inhibit thrombin. For patients whose angina is not relieved by this regimen, additional antithrombotic medications can be prescribed, including clopidogrel and platelet glycoprotein IIb/IIIa (GPIIb/IIIa) receptor antagonists. For patients who experience angina with limited effort, hypertension, anxiety, or increased heart rate, beta blockers should be added to the regimen; they should be given intravenously at first, followed by oral administration (see Chapter 11.1). If beta blockers are contraindicated, a nondihydropyridine calcium antagonist (e.g., verapamil or diltiazem) can be given, usually followed by an oral form of the agent.[2]

NITRATES

The use of nitroglycerin in treating unstable angina is based on pathophysiologic principles and clinical observations. Nitroglycerin reduces myocardial oxygen demand and increases myocardial oxygen delivery (see Chapter 11.1). Nitroglycerin dilates normal and atherosclerotic epicardial coronary arteries as well as smaller arteries that constrict with stress (e.g., cold temperatures, mental stress, physical exercise).[2] Nitroglycerin also promotes development of collateral flow, redistributes blood flow to ischemic areas of the myocardium, and inhibits platelet aggregation.[2]

Nitroglycerin is generally started with three 0.4-mg sublingual nitroglycerin tablets (or spray), taken at 5-minute intervals (and initiation of an intravenous beta blocker in the absence of contraindications). Whether or not symptoms are relieved, nitroglycerin is generally given intravenously (also in the absence of contraindications), because it is protective against recurrent thrombosis. Intravenous nitroglycerin is recommended to start at a rate of 10 μg/min through continuous infusion with nonabsorbent tubing; it is then increased

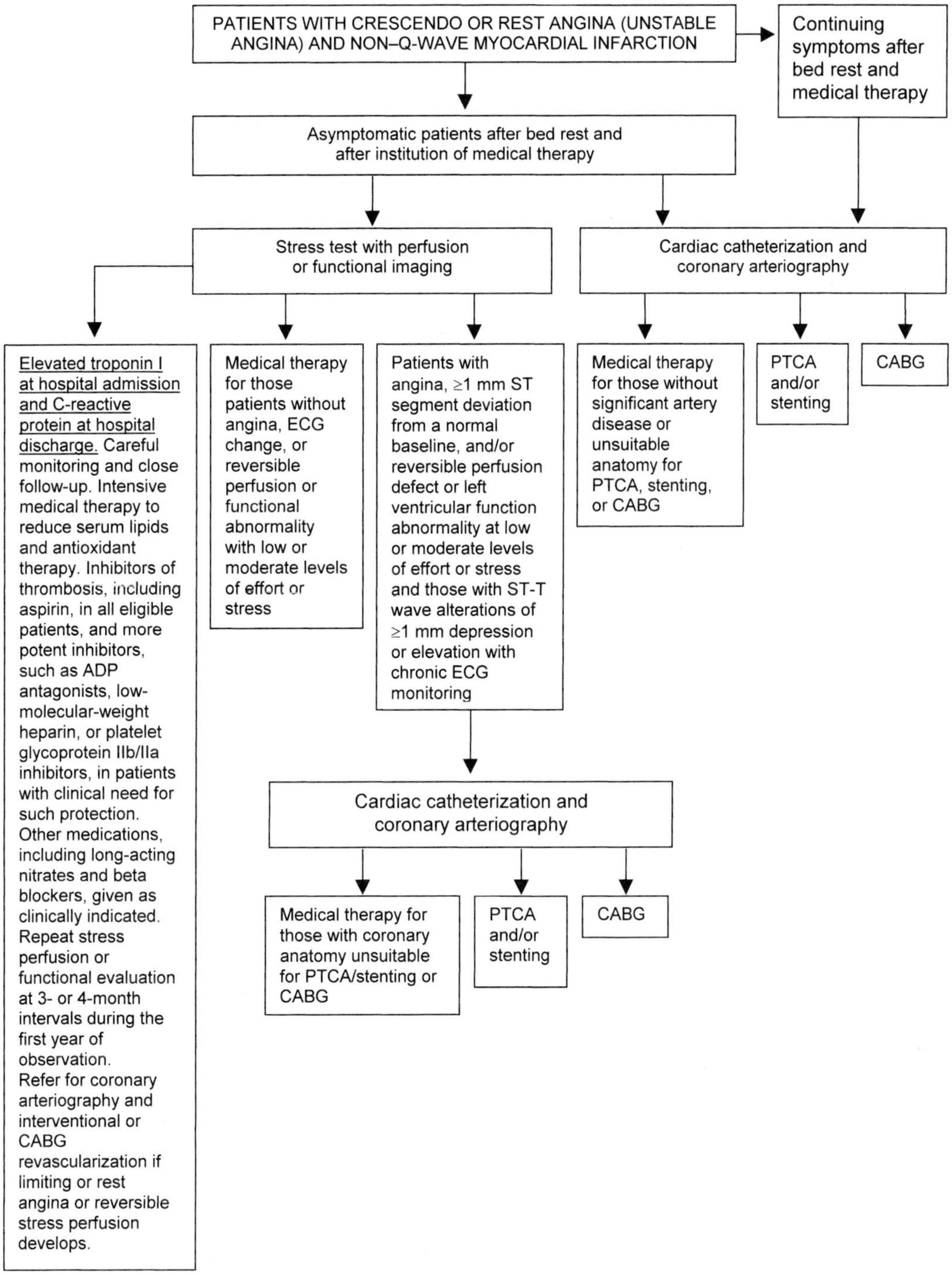

FIGURE 11–3. Therapeutic alternatives for patients with unstable angina and non–Q wave myocardial infarction. ADP, adenosine diphosphate; CABG, coronary artery bypass grafting; ECG, electrocardiogram; PTCA, percutaneous transluminal coronary angioplasty. (From Willerson JT: Medical treatment of unstable angina and non–Q wave myocardial infarction. In Willerson JT, Cohn JN [eds]: Cardiovascular Medicine, 2nd ed., Churchill Livingstone, Philadelphia, 2000, p 723. With permission from Churchill Livingstone.)

by 10 μg/min every 3 to 5 minutes until symptom or blood pressure response occurs.[2] Blood pressure response is not necessary if symptoms are relieved.

If symptoms are not relieved, the nitroglycerin dose should be increased until a blood pressure response occurs (usually a 10 mm Hg decrease in systolic blood pressure), at which point the dosage can be reduced and the interval lengthened. The maximum dose of nitroglycerin is as large an amount as is needed to relieve angina—up to the point that blood pressure decreases to unacceptably low levels or heart rate increases to 100 or more beats per minute. Later, when the situation is stable, a nonparenteral drug (orally administered long-acting nitrate) should be administered in a regimen that will not produce drug tolerance (see Chapter 11.1). Systolic blood pressure should not fall below 110 mm Hg in previously normotensive patients or decrease more than 25% in patients who were hypertensive before initiation of nitroglycerin therapy. If nitrates do not relieve symptoms

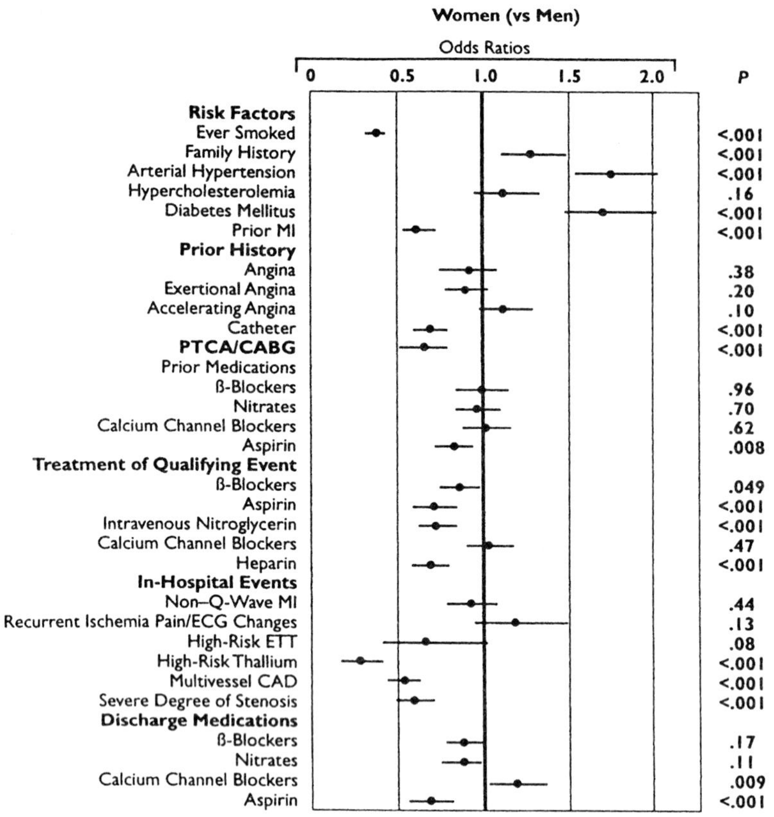

FIGURE 11–4. Odds ratios for selected characteristics comparing men versus women enrolled in the TIMI III registry. (From Stone PH, Thompson B, Anderson HV, et al: Influence of race, sex, and age on management of unstable angina and non-Q-wave myocardial infarction: The TIMI III registry. JAMA 275: 1104, 1996. Percentages indicate percentages of patients suffering a vascular event. With permission from the American Medical Association.)

after 3 sublingual tablets, morphine sulfate (1 to 5 mg) can be given intravenously.

ANTITHROMBOTIC THERAPIES

Antithrombotic therapy is necessary to prevent progression or recurrence of thrombus formation, first MI, or recurrent MI. Most typically, a combination of aspirin and unfractionated or LMW heparin (dalteparin or enoxaparin) is prescribed (Table 11–6). A platelet GPIIb/IIIa receptor antagonist (abciximab, eptifibatide, or tirofiban) is added for patients with continued chest pain despite this regimen and for those believed to be at high risk (i.e., those with elevations of C-reactive protein,[10–14] troponin I or T,[15–17] serum amyloid–like proteins,[22] interleukins 1 and 6,[21] or fibrinogen[18–20]) who are scheduled to undergo an interventional procedure (angioplasty or stent placement). Abciximab or, possibly, another GPIIb/IIIa antagonist is especially helpful for patients with diabetes.[23] Because both platelet activation and thrombin generation are involved in the thrombotic process, inhibitors of both platelet aggregation and coagulation are needed in treating patients with unstable angina or non–Q wave MI (and for patients with acute Q wave MI).

ORAL ANTIPLATELET THERAPY (ASPIRIN, TICLOPIDINE, CLOPIDOGREL)

Aspirin inhibits platelet aggregation and thromboxane A_2 synthesis and decreases inflammation and the interaction between platelets and white blood cells. When aspirin and heparin are combined, they work synergistically to inhibit thromboxane and thrombin, thereby improving myocardial blood flow and decreasing potential thrombus formation. In the patient with unstable angina, 162 to 325 mg aspirin per day reduces the risk of death and MI for women and men (see Table 11–6).[24–26] All trials of aspirin in unstable angina and non–Q wave MI have documented this benefit.[2] Similar efficacy for daily doses ranging from 75 to 325 mg has been shown.[27] However, it has been postulated that women's platelets are less responsive to aspirin therapy than men's,[2] possibly making aspirin therapy less effective for women.

For patients with unstable angina, the first dose of aspirin can be chewed to achieve blood levels rapidly. Thereafter, doses can be swallowed. If patients are already taking aspirin, it should be continued. Contraindications to aspirin therapy include (1) intolerance and allergy (development of asthma), (2) active bleeding, (3) hemophilia, (4) active retinal bleeding, (5) severe untreated hypertension, (6) an active peptic ulcer, and (7) gastrointestinal or genitourinary bleeding.[2]

Ticlopidine and clopidogrel (thienopyridines) are adenosine diphosphate (ADP) antagonists that have been approved as antiplatelet therapy[28] (see Chapter 11.1). These agents have a broad inhibitory effect on platelet-derived mediators, including thromboxane A_2 and serotonin. Aspirin and ADP inhibitors have different effects on platelets, so they can be used in combination for added antiplatelet effects. For patients with aspirin sensitivity, thienopyridines should be the first choice for therapy. Although ticlopidine has been used successfully in the treatment of MI,[29] it is associated with more adverse effects than clopidogrel. Side effects of ticlopidine are mainly gastrointestinal, although neutropenia has occurred in approximately 2.4% of patients;[30] thus, patients

Table 11–6. CLINICAL USE OF ANTITHROMBOTIC THERAPY

ORAL ANTIPLATELET THERAPY	
Aspirin	Initial dose of 162–325 mg nonenteric formulation followed by 75–160 mg/d of an enteric or a nonenteric formulation
Clopidogrel	75 mg/d; a loading dose of 4–8 tablets (300–600 mg) can be used when rapid onset of action is required
Ticlopidine	250 mg twice daily; a loading dose of 500 mg can be used when rapid onset of inhibition is required; monitoring of platelet and white cell counts during treatment is required
HEPARINS	
Dalteparin	120 IU/kg subcutaneously every 12 h (maximum 10,000 IU twice daily)
Enoxaprin	1 mg/kg subcutaneously every 12 h; the first dose may be preceded by a 30-mg IV bolus
Unfractionated heparin	Bolus 60–70 U/kg (maximum 5000 U) IV followed by infusion of 12–15 $U \cdot kg^{-1} \cdot h^{-1}$ (maximum 1000 U/h) titrated to aPTT 1.5–2.5 times control
INTRAVENOUS ANTIPLATELET THERAPY	
Abciximab	0.25 mg/kg bolus followed by infusion of 0.125 $\mu g \cdot kg^{-1} \cdot min^{-1}$ (maximum 10 μg/min) for 12 h
Eptifibatide	180 μg/kg bolus followed by infusion of 2.0 $\mu g \cdot kg^{-1} \cdot min^{-1}$ for 72 to 96 h*
Tirofiban	0.4 $\mu g \cdot kg^{-1} \cdot min^{-1}$ for 30 minutes followed by infusion of 0.1 $\mu g \cdot kg^{-1} \cdot min^{-1}$ for 48 to 96 h*

*Different dose regimens were tested in recent clinical trials before percutaneous interventions.

From ACC/AHA guidelines for the management of patients with unstable angina and non–ST-segment elevation myocardial infarction: A report of the American College of Cardiology/American Heart Association Task Force on Practice Guidelines (Committee on the Management of Patients with Unstable Angina). J Am Coll Cardiol 36:970, 2000. Copyright 2000 by the American College of Cardiology and American Heart Association, Inc.

taking ticlopidine must regularly be monitored with blood counts.

In contrast to ticlopidine, clopidogrel has not been associated with excess neutropenia (CAPRIE trial)[31] and has been found to be as effective as aspirin.[31] We prefer clopidogrel over ticlopidine for this reason and because of more rapid inhibition of platelets. Generally, we treat higher-risk patients with intravenous nitroglycerin, heparin, and clopidogrel (in addition to aspirin first), and with a GPIIb/IIIa antagonist started later, if necessary.

THROMBIN INHIBITORS

Patients with angina at rest should be given heparin along with aspirin, unless they have a contraindication (known hypersensitivity, active bleeding, blood dyscrasias, hemophilia, or other blood disorder). The combination of heparin and aspirin, however, raises the risk for bleeding complications.[24] When heparin (and other antithrombins) are withdrawn abruptly, heparin rebound can occur and cause worsening of angina and even MI.[32, 33] Thus, heparin must be withdrawn slowly over a period of several hours, and aspirin or other antiplatelet therapy must be administered concomitantly during the withdrawal period.

Under development are a variety of other thrombin inhibitors, including LMW heparins and direct thrombin antagonists (hirudin, bivalirudin, argatroban), which may be useful alternatives to unfractionated heparin in patients with unstable angina or non–Q wave MI. The direct thrombin antagonists may replace heparin for patients who experience thrombocytopenia, vascular thrombosis, or bleeding as an allergic reaction to heparin.

Low-Molecular-Weight Heparin

LMW heparin acts primarily through antithrombin III–mediated inhibition of factor Xa, but there is also some direct thrombin inhibition.[1] As is true of conventional heparin, LMW heparin promotes the release of tissue factor pathway inhibitor, a factor that may contribute to its antithrombotic effects[34, 35] and its lessened level of protein binding. LMW heparin is administered subcutaneously (usually 2 times per day) (see Table 11–6). The anticoagulant response to LMW heparin is predictable without the need for laboratory monitoring,[34, 35] and the patient receives a sustained anticoagulant and antithrombin effect.

Women were included in the Fragmin during Instability in Coronary Artery Disease (FRISC) Study.[35] In that study, dalteparin was given at 120 IU/kg body weight with a maximal dose of 10,000 IU given twice daily for 6 days, and then at 7500 IU once daily for the next 35 to 45 days. The patients given dalteparin, including the women in the study, showed a significant decrease in the composite endpoint of death, MI, revascularization, and need for intravenous heparin. A risk of reactivation and reinfarction occurred when the dose of dalteparin was decreased. The usefulness of LMW heparin was also shown in the TIMI 11B[36] trial as well as the Efficacy and Safety of Subcutaneous Enoxaparin in Non-Q-wave Coronary Events (ESSENCE) trial.[37] Results from all three of these trials suggest the superiority of LMW heparin over unfractionated heparin in reducing both the incidence of MI and death and the need for revascularization in patients with unstable angina and non–Q wave MI.

There is some higher risk of minor bleeding in the first week of therapy with LMW heparin, but the risk of heparin-induced thrombocytopenia is less than with unfractionated heparin.[38] When therapy is continued beyond a week, the risk of bleeding increases. Of the trials that evaluated prolonged treatment with LMW heparin, only the FRISC II study showed a benefit of prolonged administration beyond the acute phase.[39]

For patients who are not allergic to heparin, we now choose LMW heparin as therapy while patients are hospitalized. At this time, there have been no direct trials comparing the different LMW heparins, although dalteparin did outperform nadroparin and enoxaparin in comparisons with unfractionated heparin.

INTRAVENOUS ANTIPLATELET AGENTS

Platelet Glycoprotein IIb/IIIa Receptor Antagonists

In at least one study, a GPIIb/IIIa inhibitor was significantly more effective than aspirin in controlling ischemia in women with unstable angina.[3] Platelet activation causes changes in the shape of platelets and conformational changes in the GPIIb/IIIa receptors, transforming the receptors from a ligand-unreceptive to a ligand-receptive state. Ligand-receptive GPIIb/IIIa receptors bind fibrinogen molecules, which form bridges between adjacent platelets and facilitate platelet aggregation. Inhibitors of GPIIb/IIIa receptors bind to the receptors, thus blocking the binding of fibrinogen and thereby preventing platelet aggregation.[1]

GPIIb/IIIa is not expressed by resting platelets in a manner suitable for ligand binding, but upon platelet activation, a conformational change occurs that allows GPIIb/IIIa to bind to fibrinogen.[1, 40] Once activated, the original platelet monolayer recruits additional platelets, eventually forming a platelet thrombus through GPIIb/IIIa–fibrinogen–GPIIb/IIIa bridging.[1] This process repeats itself until platelet thrombus covers the denuded endothelium or area of ulceration in the atherosclerotic plaque.

The process can be attenuated somewhat if normal endothelium surrounds the area of injury. Normal endothelium secretes substances that inhibit thrombus formation, such as prostacyclin, nitric oxide, and tissue plasminogen activator.[41, 42] Because GPIIb/IIIa inhibitors interfere with platelet aggregation in the final common pathway of platelet aggregation, they are especially useful in the treatment of acute coronary syndromes, unstable angina, and non–Q wave MI.[43–45]

When given in conjunction with aspirin and heparin, the GPIIb/IIIa receptor antagonists, including the synthetic peptide eptifibatide, and the nonpeptide, LMW inhibitor tirofiban, decrease the risk of death, MI, and need for interventional therapy,[1, 46] although they do not provide complete protection. They should be administered to patients who have continuing ischemia or who are otherwise at high risk and to patients who are likely to undergo a percutaneous interventional procedure (abciximab) (see Table 11–6). The investigators of the Do Tirofiban and ReoPro Give Similar Efficacy Trial (TARGET) presented results of their study comparing tirofiban with abciximab for patients undergoing interventional procedures.[47] Tirofiban was associated with a significantly inferior primary endpoint compared with abciximab: 7.55% vs. 6.01% (odds ratio, 1.26; $p = .037$). Patients treated with a GPIIb/IIIa antagonists are at higher risk for bleeding, which is typically mucocutaneous or involves the access site of vascular intervention.[2]

BETA-ADRENERGIC BLOCKERS

At this time, use of beta blockers in the treatment of unstable angina and non–Q wave MI is based mostly on results in patients with acute MI, recent MI, or stable angina—all of which have shown significant reductions in rates of mortality and morbidity. In the absence of contraindications, beta blockers may be started early. For patients with unstable angina or non–Q wave MI who are hypertensive, have tachycardia, or have persistent rest angina, beta blockers should be given intravenously, followed by oral administration. Patients at low or intermediate risk can be started with oral preparations, however, unless they have contraindications (see Chapter 11.1).

Several regimens are recommended in the ACC/AHA Guidelines for Unstable Angina, including intravenous metoprolol, given in 5-mg increments by slow intravenous administration (5 mg over 1 to 2 min), repeated every 5 minutes for a total initial dose of 15 mg.[2] If patients tolerate the initial dose, oral therapy can be started (15 minutes after the last intravenous dose, 25 to 50 mg every 6 h for 48 h). After this dosage regimen is complete, a maintenance dose of 50 to 100 mg twice daily is prescribed. Atenolol can be prescribed to patients for whom a longer-acting agent is suitable. Atenolol is given starting with a 5-mg intravenous dose, followed 5 minutes later by a second 5-mg intravenous dose, after which oral therapy is started (25 to 100 mg/day begun 1 to 2 hours after the intravenous dose).[2]

LIPID-LOWERING THERAPY WITH HYDROXYMETHYLGLUTARYL COENZYME A REDUCTASE INHIBITORS

Treating patients with 3-hydroxy-3-methylglutaryl coenzyme A (HMG CoA) reductase inhibitors (statins) is another approach that may be useful for patients with acute coronary syndromes. These agents have proven benefits in lowering low-density lipoprotein (LDL) cholesterol and in reducing major coronary event rate and all-cause mortality for men and women with coronary disease.[48–52] Statins have also been shown to have pleiotropic effects on the mechanisms of atherosclerosis, including plaque thrombogenicity, cellular migration, endothelial function, and thrombotic tendency.[48, 53] In one study, improved endothelial function was seen in patients given pravastatin for 6 weeks.[54] Preoperative lipid control with simvastatin has been shown to decrease thrombocytosis and thrombotic complications after coronary artery bypass surgery.[55] Trials are under way that will evaluate the effects of lipid-lowering on early recurrent ischemic events in patients with unstable angina and non–Q wave MI.[48, 56]

For patients with CAD or other atherosclerotic disease, the National Cholesterol Education Program (NCEP) recommends an LDL value less than or equal to 100 mg/dl. For primary prevention, the NCEP recommends a minimal LDL goal of less than 160 mg/dl, and in patients with increased risk factors, the recommended LDL goal is less than 130 mg/dl.[57] The pharmacologic characteristics, including daily recommended dosages, of the different statin drugs differ and are listed in Table 11–7.

CORONARY ARTERY SPASM

Coronary artery spasm is probably more common in women than in men.[3] Treatment of patients with coronary artery spasm should begin with nitrates and a calcium antagonist.[1, 58, 59] (Beta blockers are not given because they may cause more frequent and severe episodes of spasm.) Patients normally show a good response to this regimen.

DRUG-DRUG INTERACTIONS

As with any medication, potential drug-drug interactions must be considered. Predicting which patients will have side effects from drug-drug interactions can be difficult, so caution must always be taken in the prescription of drugs to patients with coronary disease. In addition, clearance rates differ among individuals. We suggest consulting a pharmaco-

Table 11–7. PHARMACOLOGIC CHARACTERISTICS OF DIFFERENT HMG-CoA REDUCTASE INHIBITORS

DRUG	DAILY DOSE (mg)	ABSORPTION (%)	PLASMA PROTEIN BINDING (%)	RENAL EXCRETION (%)	HALF-LIFE (h)	SOLUBILITY
Lovastatin	20–80	31	95	30	2–3	Lipophilic
Simvastatin	10–80	60–85	98	13	2–3	Lipophilic
Pravastatin	20–40	35	40–50	60	1–3	Hydrophilic
Fluvastatin	20–80	98	99	6	0.5–1	Hydrophilic
Atorvastatin	5–80	NA	98	2	13–16	Lipophilic

From Vaughan CJ, Gotto AM, Basson CT. The evolving role of statins in the management of atherosclerosis. J Am Coll Cardiol 35:1, 2000.

logic database (such as Micromedex) for the current information. Many such databases are online in health-care institutions.

SUMMARY

Patients with unstable angina or non–Q wave MI are treated in a similar fashion because the two syndromes are closely related. Both usually result from platelet aggregation, thrombosis, and dynamic vasoconstriction at the site of a fissure or ulceration in an atherosclerotic plaque. In both unstable angina and non–Q wave MI, the occlusive thrombus and dynamic vasoconstriction are generally transient.

The treatment regimen for unstable angina or non–Q wave MI begins with nitrates (usually in the form of intravenous nitroglycerin) and antithrombotic agents (aspirin and unfractionated or LMW heparin). For patients who continue to have angina at rest, additional antithrombotic medications can be given. We usually choose clopidogrel and/or GPIIb/IIIa antagonists. We prescribe beta blockers for patients who have angina with limited effort, with elevated blood pressure or heart rate, or with anxiety. On the basis of results of the HOPE trial,[60] most patients with vascular disease who are older than 55 years could also benefit from an ACE inhibitor with tissue specificity for long-term prophylaxis (see Chapter 11.1). In addition, studies have also shown that HMG CoA reductase inhibitors, or statins, have proven beneficial effects on many components of atherosclerosis, including plaque thrombogenicity, cellular migration, endothelial function, and thrombotic tendency[53] (see Chapter 5.3). Under any circumstance, if medical therapy fails, the patient must be referred for cardiac catheterization and possible interventional or surgical therapy.

Determining which patients are likely to have MIs is more difficult. Patients who have elevations of troponin I or T with unstable angina or non–Q wave MI on admission are at higher risk for acute MI. Such patients may benefit from treatment with a GPIIb/IIIa antagonist in addition to interventional or surgical therapy. Similarly, patients with increased C-reactive protein on admission or at discharge are also more likely to have a future MI, as are patients with recurrent ST-T wave changes on ECG.[1, 10–14] These patients, as well as patients with reversible ischemia on stress imaging studies, should be scheduled for cardiac catheterization once their condition stabilizes. They most likely will require more intensive medical therapy, interventional therapy, or CABG.

References

1. Willerson JT: Medical treatment of unstable angina and non-Q-wave myocardial infarction. In Willerson JT, Cohn JN (eds): Cardiovascular Medicine. Churchill Livingstone, Philadelphia, 2000, p 723.
2. Braunwald E, Antman EM, Beasley, et al: ACC/AHA guidelines for the management of patients with unstable angina and non–ST-segment elevation myocardial infarction: A report of the American College of Cardiology/American Heart Association Task Force on Practice Guidelines (Committee on the Management of Patients with Unstable Angina). J Am Coll Cardiol 36:970, 2000.
3. Goldschmidt-Clermont PJ, Schulman SP, Bray PF, et al: Refining the treatment of women with unstable angina—a randomized, double-blind, comparative safety and efficacy evaluation of Integrelin™ versus aspirin in the management of unstable angina. Clin Cardiol 19:869, 1996.
4. Maynard C, Litwin PE, Martin JS, Weaver WD: Gender differences in the treatment and outcome of acute myocardial infarction: Results from the Myocardial Infarction Triage and Intervention Registry. Arch Intern Med 152:972, 1992.
5. Becker RC, Terrin M, Ross R, et al: Comparison of clinical outcomes for women and men after acute myocardial infarction. Ann Intern Med 120:638, 1994.
6. Stone PH, Thompson B, Anderson HV, et al: Influence of race, sex, and age on management of unstable angina and non–Q-wave myocardial infarction: The TIMI III registry. JAMA 275:1104, 1996.
7. Shaw LJ, Miller DD, Romeis JC, et al: Gender differences in the noninvasive evaluation and management of patients with suspected coronary artery disease. Ann Intern Med 120:559, 1994.
8. Hochman JS, McCabe CH, Stone PH, et al: Outcome and profile of women and men presenting with acute coronary syndromes: A report from TIMI IIIB. TIMI Investigators. Thrombolysis in Myocardial Infarction. J Am Coll Cardiol 30:141, 1997.
9. Hochman JS, Tamis JE, Thompson TD, et al: Sex, clinical presentation, and outcome in patients with acute coronary syndromes: Global Use of Strategies to Open Occluded Coronary Arteries in Acute Coronary Syndromes IIb Investigators. N Engl J Med 341:226, 1999.
10. Liuzzo G, Biasucci LM, Gallimore JR, et al: The prognostic value of C-reactive protein in severe angina. N Engl J Med 331:417, 1994.
11. Berk BC, Weintraub WS, Alexander RW: Evaluation of C-reactive protein in "active" coronary artery disease. Am J Cardiol 65:168, 1990.
12. Tomoda H, Aoki N: Instability of coronary lesions in unstable angina assessed by C-reactive protein values following coronary interventions. Am J Cardiol 87:221, 2001.
13. Haverkate F, Thompson SG, Pyke SD, et al: Production of C-reactive protein and risk of coronary events in stable and unstable angina: European Concerted Action on Thrombosis and Disabilities Angina Pectoris Study Group. Lancet 349:462, 1997.
14. Morrow DA, Rifai N, Antman EM, et al: C-reactive protein is a potent predictor of mortality independently of and in combination with troponin T in acute coronary syndromes: A TIMI 11A substudy. Thrombolysis In Myocardial Infarction. J Am Coll Cardiol 31:1460, 1998.
15. Zimmerman J, Fromm R, Meyer D, et al: Diagnostic Marker Cooperative Study for the diagnosis of myocardial infarction. Circulation 99: 1671, 1999.
16. Apple FS, Christenson RH, Valdes RJ, et al: Simultaneous rapid measurement of whole blood myoglobin, creatine kinase MB, and cardiac troponin I by the triage cardiac panel for detection of myocardial infarction. Clin Chem 45:199, 1999.
17. Antman EM, Tanasijevic MJ, Thompson B, et al: Cardiac-specific troponin 1 levels to predict the risk of mortality in patients with acute coronary syndromes. N Engl J Med 335:1342, 1996.
18. Kruskal JB, Commerford PJ, Franks JJ, Kirsch RE: Fibrin and fibrinogen-related antigens in patients with stable and unstable coronary artery disease. N Engl J Med 317:1361, 1987.

19. Ardissino D, Merlini PA, Gamba G, et al: Thrombin activity and early outcome in unstable angina pectoris. Circulation 93:1634, 1996.
20. Becker RC, Cannon CP, Bovill EG, et al: Prognostic value of plasma fibrinogen concentration in patients with unstable angina and non-Q-wave myocardial infarction (TIMI IIIB trial). Am J Cardiol 78: 142, 1996.
21. Biasucci LM, Liuzzo G, Fantuzzi G, et al: Increasing levels of interleukin (IL)-1Ra and IL-6 during the first 2 days of hospitalization in unstable angina are associated with increased risk of in-hospital coronary events. Circulation 99:2079, 1999.
22. Morrow DA, Rifai N, Antman EM, et al: Serum amyloid A predicts early mortality in acute coronary syndromes: A TIMI 11A substudy. J Am Coll Cardiol 35:358, 2000.
23. The EPISTENT Investigators: Randomised placebo-controlled and balloon-angioplasty-controlled trial to assess safety of coronary stenting with use of platelet glycoprotein IIb/IIIa blockage. Lancet 352:87, 1998.
24. Théroux P, Ouimet H, McCans J, et al: Aspirin, heparin, or both to treat acute unstable angina. N Engl J Med 319:1105, 1988.
25. Cairns JA, Gent M, Singer J, et al: Aspirin, sulfinpyrazone, or both in unstable angina: Results of a Canadian multicenter trial. N Engl J Med 313:1369, 1985.
26. De Caterina R, Giannessi D, Bernini W, et al: Low-dose aspirin in patients recovering from myocardial infarction: Evidence for selective inhibition of thromboxane-related platelet function. Eur Heart J 6: 409, 1985.
27. Antiplatelet Trialists' Collaboration: Collaborative overview of randomised trials of antiplatelet therapy–I: Prevention of death, myocardial infarction, and stroke by prolonged antiplatelet therapy in various categories of patients. BMJ 308:81, 1994.
28. Schror K: The basic pharmacology of ticlopidine and clopidogrel. Platelets 4:252, 1993.
29. Balsano F, Rizzon P, Violi F, et al: Antiplatelet treatment with ticlopidine in unstable angina: A controlled multicenter clinical trial. The Studio della Ticlopidina nell'Angina Instabile Group. Circulation 82: 17, 1990.
30. Love BB, Biller J, Gent M: Adverse haematological effects of ticlopidine: Prevention, recognition and management. Drug Saf 19:89, 1998.
31. CAPRIE Steering Committee: A randomised, blinded, trial of clopidogrel versus aspirin in patients at risk of ischemic events (CAPRIE). Lancet 348:1329, 1996.
32. Gold HK, Torres FW, Garabedian HD, et al: Evidence for a rebound coagulation phenomenon after cessation of a 4-hour infusion of a specific thrombin inhibitor in patients with unstable angina pectoris. J Am Coll Cardiol 21:1039, 1993.
33. Théroux P, Waters D, Lam J, et al: Reactivation of unstable angina after the discontinuation of heparin. N Engl J Med 327:141, 1992.
34. Hirsh J, Levine MN. Low-molecular-weight heparin. Blood 79:1, 1992.
35. Fragmin during Instability in Coronary Artery Disease (FRISC) Study Group: Low-molecular-weight heparin during instability in coronary artery disease. Lancet 347:561, 1996.
36. Antman EM, McCabe CH, Gurfinkel EP, et al: Enoxaparin prevents death and cardiac ischemic events in unstable angina/non-Q-wave myocardial infarction: Results of thrombolysis in myocardial infarction (TIMI) 11B trial. Circulation 100:1593, 1999.
37. Goodman SG, Cohen M, Bigonzi F, et al, for the Efficacy and Safety of Subcutaneous Enoxaparin in Non-Q-wave Coronary Events (ESSENCE) Study Group: Randomized trial of low molecular weight heparin (enoxaparin) versus unfractionated heparin for unstable coronary artery disease: one-year results of the ESSENCE Study. Efficacy and Safety of Subcutaneous Enoxaparin in Non-Q Wave Coronary Events. J Am Coll Cardiol 36:693, 2000.
38. Warkentin TE, Levine MN, Hirsh J, et al: Heparin-induced thrombocytopenia in patients treated with low-molecular-weight heparin or unfractionated heparin. N Engl J Med 332:1330, 1995.
39. FRagmin and Fast Revascularisation during InStability in Coronary artery disease Investigators: Long-term low-molecular-mass heparin in unstable coronary-artery disease: FRISC II prospective randomised multicentre study. Lancet 354:701, 1999.
40. Kroll MH, Harris TS, Moake JL, et al: Von Willebrand factor binding to platelet GpIB initiates signals for platelet activation. J Clin Invest 88:1568, 1991.
41. Shah PK: Pathophysiology of plaque rupture and the concept of plaque stabilization. Cardiol Clin 14:17, 1996.
42. Willerson JT, Golino P, Eidt J, et al: Specific platelet mediators and unstable coronary artery lesions: Experimental evidence and potential clinical implications. Circulation 80:198, 1989.
43. The Platelet Receptor Inhibition in Ischemic Syndrome Management (PRISM) Study Investigators: A comparison of aspirin plus tirofiban with aspirin plus heparin for unstable angina. N Engl J Med 338: 1498, 1998.
44. Platelet Receptor Inhibition in Ischemic Syndrome Management in Patients Limited by Unstable Signs and Symptoms (PRISM-PLUS) Study Investigators: Inhibition of the platelet glycoprotein IIb/IIIa receptor with tirofiban in unstable angina and non-Q-wave myocardial infarction. N Engl J Med 338:1488, 1998.
45. The PURSUIT Trial Investigators: Inhibition of platelet glycoprotein IIb/IIIa with eptifibatide in patients with acute coronary syndromes. N Engl J Med 339:436, 1998.
46. Lincoff AM, Topol EJ: Overview of the glycoprotein IIb/IIIa inhibitor trials. In: Platelet Glycoprotein IIb/IIIa Inhibitors In Cardiovascular Disease. Humana Press, Totowa, NJ, 1999.
47. Topol EJ, for the TARGET Investigators: TARGET. Do Tirofiban and ReoPro Give Similar Efficacy Trial. Abstracts, American Heart Association Scientific Sessions 2001. Available at: http://www.scientificsessions.org/archive/abstracts/latebreakingclinicaltrials@TARGET.pdf.
48. Cohen M: Calming the plaque to delay intervention for 24 hours in acute coronary syndromes. Am J Cardiol 86:18M, 2000.
49. Scandinavian Simvastatin Survival Group: Randomised trial of cholesterol lowering in 4444 patients with coronary heart disease: The Scandinavian Simvastatin Survival Study (4S). Lancet 344:1383, 1994.
50. Sacks FM, Pfeffer MA, Moye LA, et al, for the Cholesterol and Recurrent Events Trial Investigators: The effect of pravastatin on coronary events after myocardial infarction in patients with average cholesterol levels. N Engl J Med 337:1001, 1996.
51. Downs JR, Clearfield M, Weis W, et al, for the AFCAPS/TexCAPS Research Group: Primary prevention of acute coronary events with lovastatin in men and women with average cholesterol levels: Results of AFCAPS/TexCAPS. JAMA 279:1615, 1998.
52. The Long-Term Intervention with Pravastatin in Ischemic Disease (LIPID) Study Group: Prevention of cardiovascular events and death with pravastatin in patients with coronary heart disease and a broad range of initial cholesterol levels. N Engl J Med 339:1349, 1998.
53. Vaughan CJ, Gotto AM Jr, Basson CT: The evolving role of statins in the management of atherosclerosis. J Am Coll Cardiol 35:1, 2000.
54. Dupuis J, Tardif JC, Cernacek P, Theroux P: Cholesterol reduction rapidly improves endothelial function after acute coronary syndromes: The RECIFE (reduction of cholesterol in ischemic and function of the endothelium) trial. Circulation 99:3227, 1999.
55. Christenson JT: Preoperative lipid-control with simvastatin reduces the risk of postoperative thrombocytosis and thrombotic complications following CABG. Eur J Cardiothorac Surg 15:394, 1999.
56. Schwartz GG, Oliver MF, Ezekowitz MD, et al: Rationale and design of the Myocardial Ischemia Reduction with Aggressive Cholesterol Lowering (MIRACL) study that evaluates atorvastatin in unstable angina pectoris and in non-Q-wave myocardial infarction. Am J Cardiol 81:578, 1998.
57. National Cholesterol Education Program: Second report of the Expert Panel on Detection, Evaluation, and Treatment of High Blood Cholesterol in Adults (Adult Treatment Panel II). Circulation 89:1329, 1994.
58. Gunther S, Green L, Muller JE, et al: Prevention by nifedipine of abnormal coronary vasoconstriction in patients with coronary artery disease. Circulation 63:849, 1981.
59. Johnson SM, Mauritson DR, Willerson JT, Hillis LD: A controlled trial of verapamil for Prinzmetal's variant angina. N Engl J Med 304: 862, 1981.
60. The Heart Outcomes Prevention Evaluation Study Investigators: Effects of an angiotensin-converting-enzyme inhibitor, ramipril, on cardiovascular events in high-risk patients. N Engl J Med 342:145, 2000.

11.3 Thrombolytic Therapy

Jamie Doucet and James M. Wilson

The concept of pharmacologic thrombolysis arose in 1933, when a product of streptococcal cultures was observed to liquefy clotted human blood. Over a period of 20 years, study of this substance, which would become known as streptokinase, illuminated the hitherto poorly understood process of fibrinolysis or thrombolysis. Streptokinase associates with an inactive plasma protein, plasminogen, to form a plasminogen activator complex. Plasmin, the product of plasminogen activation, hydrolyzes bonds between fibrin monomers, thereby dissolving newly formed thrombi.

Streptokinase was the first of several activators of plasmin that were discovered and stimulated interest in the field of thrombolysis. Its potential for treating thrombotic diseases was clearly evident. Unfortunately, about the time that streptokinase became available to clinicians, the world of cardiology was mired in controversy as to the true relationship between thrombosis of the coronary vessels and MI. One school of thought was that coronary thrombosis was a secondary phenomenon resulting from sluggish blood flow in the artery supplying an infarcted territory. The second school, following the traditional interpretation of postmortem studies, argued that thrombosis within the coronary artery was the actual cause of infarction. While the debate raged, popular and financial support for a serious study of thrombolytic therapy for acute MI was hard to find.

In 1980, DeWood and coworkers[1] published their findings from coronary angiography performed during the first 24 hours after Q wave MI. Almost 90% of patients studied within 4 hours of symptom onset had complete occlusion of the infarct-related artery. Beyond 12 hours of symptom onset, the proportion of patients with complete occlusion fell to 65%. Fogarty catheter thrombectomy retrieved thrombus in a large proportion of patients, confirming the nature of the lesions. These observations clearly established that coronary thrombosis was an early event in MI that declined rather than increased as time passed from the event. Arguments about the cause-and-effect relationship between coronary thrombosis and MI were essentially laid to rest. Large-scale trials of thrombolytic therapy for MI soon followed.

Numerous trials of thrombolytic therapy have established that restoration of normal blood flow in an infarct-related artery improves the short- and long-term survival expectancy of both men and women with acute MI. The earlier that treatment is instituted after the onset of the event, the greater the benefit observed in terms of survival and prevention of complications such as congestive heart failure. The average reduction in 30-day mortality is about 20%, which works out to about 30 lives saved for every 1000 patients treated.[2] The introduction of thrombolytic therapy represents the most significant and widely applicable advance in the treatment of acute MI since the development of the defibrillator and the concept of the coronary care unit. However, general acceptance of thrombolytic therapy as safe and effective has not been rapid, resulting in a failure to treat some eligible patients, particularly women.

An amazing one third of women eligible for thrombolytic therapy are not treated.[3] Part of the reason for this unfortunate observation undoubtedly is lack of education about the benefits of thrombolytic therapy and fear of a rare but grave side effect of thrombolytic therapy, intracranial hemorrhage. Women suffering MI are older, are frequently hypertensive, and are smaller than their male counterparts. Each characteristic increases the risk for development of intracranial hemorrhage. Although this observation is widely publicized, rarely is mention made of the outcome of untreated MI in women. After MI, women are more likely to develop complications such as recurrent ischemia and reinfarction, and their mortality is roughly twice that of men. In spite of the fact that women have worse outcomes after MI than men and thus have great potential for enjoying the benefits of appropriate therapy, women are *less* likely to be treated with aspirin, heparin, beta blockers, ACE inhibitors, and thrombolytic therapy. Ironically, the group of people with the greatest risk of suffering complications from thrombolytic therapy actually has the most to gain from timely therapy. This section of the chapter provides an overview of MI in women and discusses the risks and benefits of thrombolytic therapy.

EPIDEMIOLOGY

Age

Cardiovascular disease is the leading cause of death in the United States and many industrialized countries. Each year, 500,000 American women die of cardiovascular disease, a death rate equal to that of men.[4] The impression that female gender affords nearly complete protection from the development of atherosclerosis is in part related to the exclusion of patients 75 years and older from most clinical trials. Female gender is associated with a delay in the time of onset of clinical atherosclerosis. At ages 25 through 49 years, men are more than six times more likely to experience an acute coronary event. The difference between genders narrows by age 60 to 64 years, so that men are only twice as likely as women to experience a clinical event.

The observed gender difference in the time of first presentation is believed to be due to a lower prevalence of risk factors for early-onset atherosclerosis in women and the vascular protection afforded by estrogens. On average, women presenting with symptomatic CAD are 7 to 10 years older than men. Therefore, a large fraction of women may be excluded from clinical studies that use age as an entry criterion.[5–7] An additional effect of the gender difference in the time of occurrence of a first event is overrepresentation of risk factors such as diabetes mellitus, hypertension, and cigarette smoking in women who gain entry into clinical trials (Table 11–8).[6–10]

Table 11–8. COMORBIDITIES AND MORTALITY OF WOMEN VS. MEN TREATED WITH THROMBOLYTIC DRUGS IN VARIOUS CLINICAL TRIALS

STUDY	MEN	WOMEN	*p* VALUE
MITI[8]			
N	246	851	
Age (yr)	57	65	.001
HTN (%)	35	49	.001
CHF (%)	5	9	.03
Mortality (%)	4.7	6.7	NS
SPRINT[6]			
N	4315	1524	
Age (yr)	61.4	67.3	<.0005
Diabetes (%)	18	29.1	<.0005
HTN (%)	35.5	50	<.0005
CHF (%)	24.4	26.8	.02
Mortality (%)	15.7	23.1	<.0005
MILIS[7]			
N	590	226	
Age (yr)	56	60	<.05
Diabetes (%)	15	28	<.05
HTN (%)	50	63	<.05
CHF (%)	7	12	<.05
Mortality (%)	7	13	<.05
Robinson et al[9]			
N	643	337	
Age (yr)	58.6	64.4	<.001
HTN (%)	28.5	42.7	<.001
Mortality (%)	6.6	12.6	.02
GUSTO[10]			
N	30706	10315	
Age (yr)	59	66	<.001
Diabetes (%)	13	21	<.001
HTN (%)	34	50	<.001
CHF (%)	14.3	17.6	<.001
Mortality (%)	5.5	11.3	<.001

CHF, congestive heart failure; N, total number of subjects; NS, not significant.

Diabetes Mellitus

Diabetes mellitus is a powerful risk factor for CAD in women, accelerating the atherosclerotic process more so than in men. This fact abolishes the gender difference in the age at the time of first MI that normally favors women.[11, 12] Mortality rates are threefold to sevenfold higher in women with diabetes. Mortality rates in men are less severely affected by diabetes.[11, 12] Diabetes mellitus is associated with hypertension, hyperlipidemia, and obesity. Each associated condition adds to the risk of cardiovascular morbidity. Hyperglycemia may impair estrogen binding in the vascular system, negating the protective effects that endogenous estrogens confer on premenopausal women.[13]

Cigarette Smoking

Cigarette smoking is a powerful predictor of MI and sudden cardiac death in women.[14] Smoking and oral contraceptive therapy in combination are particularly dangerous. The risk of MI in smokers taking oral contraceptives is approximately eight times that of nonsmokers. In women older than 35 years, this risk increases to 20 times that of nonsmokers.[15] Modern oral contraceptive therapy carries a very low risk of MI in women without other risk factors such as smoking, hypertension, and age more than 35 years. The higher likelihood of acute coronary events attributable to oral contraceptive use alone is 0.83 per 1 million woman-years treated.[16]

Men are more likely than women to be current smokers at the time of first MI.[9, 17, 18] Women are less likely to quit smoking.[9, 19, 20] Women are also more likely to smoke low-tar cigarettes than men, despite the fact that the risks of MI from high- and low-tar cigarettes are virtually identical. The risk of MI declines rapidly with smoking cessation, approaching that of nonsmokers after 2 to 3 years.[19]

Cholesterol

An unfavorable evolution of the lipoprotein profile in the absence of estrogens may be of central importance to the observed higher incidence of atherosclerotic events after menopause. Premenopausal women have lower total cholesterol and higher HDL cholesterol levels than men. Total cholesterol and LDL cholesterol concentrations rise following menopause.[21–23] HDL levels decrease[21] or remain the same.[23] Total cholesterol levels are actually higher in elderly women than in their male counterparts.[9, 22]

CLINICAL CHARACTERISTICS OF ACUTE MYOCARDIAL INFARCTION

Pathophysiology

Female gender is associated with certain unusual causes of MI, including severe and prolonged vasospasm and spontaneous dissection of the coronary arteries.[24–26] The reason for a higher rate of vasospastic disease in women is unknown. Spontaneous dissection of a coronary artery is a rare cause of MI that is seen most commonly during the peripartum period, perhaps in relation to the effects of progesterone. Although these entities are seen with greater frequency in women, they remain extraordinarily rare. In the vast majority of women, the cause of acute MI is rupture of an advanced, lipid-filled atherosclerotic plaque leading to coronary thrombosis. Critical reduction in myocardial blood flow results in acute myocardial dysfunction and, with time, myocardial cell death.[1, 27–30]

Delays in Diagnosis

Delays in seeking medical therapy are a serious problem in both women and men with acute MI. On average, women wait almost 20 minutes longer than men to seek medical attention.[5, 31, 32] Even after women seek medical attention, the diagnosis of acute MI is delayed.[32] Physicians, perhaps falsely comforted by reports of the vascular protection afforded by estrogens, are less likely to suspect that chest discomfort and shortness of breath in a woman have a cardiac etiology.

Symptoms

Classic angina pectoris is usually described as burning, boring, or pressure-like chest discomfort radiating to the back, neck, arms, or jaw (most often the arms) that is associated with nausea, diaphoresis, or breathlessness. Women with acute MI are just as likely as men to report chest discomfort[5, 8] but less likely to provide the classic description. Rather, they describe the discomfort as stabbing and epigastric in location.[8] Women more frequently report discomfort in the back, neck, and jaw. Women with MI are less likely (1) to experience radiation of discomfort to the upper arm, (2) to have diaphoresis as a presenting symptom,[8] and (3) to have ongoing pain at the time of initial evaluation.[31] Despite a more normal resting ejection fraction, women are more likely to present with paroxysmal nocturnal dyspnea, shortness of breath, and signs of congestive heart failure.[5, 8, 17, 31, 33]

Diagnostic Testing

After critical reduction in coronary blood flow, myocardial cell death becomes a time-dependent phenomenon. The majority of irreversible injury probably takes place within the first 2 hours of arterial closure. The event is essentially complete within 6 to 12 hours. Therefore, clinical evaluation, diagnosis, and the implementation of a therapeutic plan must take place within as short a time as possible. The time constraints placed on diagnostic evaluation make ECG the most powerful tool available. It may be performed rapidly and noninvasively, and when it reveals ST segment elevation in two or more contiguous leads of 0.1 mV or greater, ECG is very specific for the diagnosis of myocardial injury.

There is no reported difference in the ability of the ECG to recognize ongoing myocardial injury in women and men.[5, 7, 8] There is no difference in infarct distribution (anterior versus inferior or inferolateral).[5, 7, 8] The recognition of abnormal Q waves on the presenting ECG may be slightly less common in women.[8] This may be the result of a higher frequency of conduction abnormalities, although studies differ on this point.[5, 7, 8]

Cardiac isoenzymes do not usually play a role in the decision to give thrombolytic therapy. That decision is made on the basis of a compatible clinical history and ST segment elevation or new left bundle branch block on the 12-lead ECG. There is no gender difference in the utility of cardiac enzymes for the diagnosis of MI. The total CK elevation following MI is smaller in women. This probably reflects a difference in body and total heart mass rather than a real difference in infarct size.[5, 6, 9, 18, 34]

THROMBOLYTIC THERAPY

Thrombolytic agents act on plasminogen, producing the protease plasmin, which has the primary function of hydrolysis of new, fibrin-rich thrombi. The prototypic thrombolytic agent, streptokinase, is a member of the nonfibrin selective family that includes urokinase and anistreplase.[35] These agents act on both circulating and fibrin-bound plasminogen, producing a systemic fibrinolytic state. The concomitant reduction in circulating fibrinogen concentrations and the release of fibrinogen degradation products (FDPs) may have an additional anticoagulant effect.[36]

Fibrin-selective thrombolytic agents, including tissue-type plasminogen activator (tPA), recombinant tPA (r-tPA), reteplase, and single-chain urokinase (Scu-PA), have a much greater affinity for fibrin-bound plasminogen than for circulating plasminogen. They are 1000 times less potent than their nonselective counterparts in activating circulating plasminogen. The purported advantage of these agents is concentration of their activity at the site of interest without requiring systemic thrombolysis.

Attempts to uncover differences in the effectiveness of individual thrombolytic agents have involved comparisons of hard outcomes, such as death and intracranial hemorrhage, and other measures, such as the angiographic appearance of the culprit vessel, at different time points. Angiographic analysis from the large clinical trials directly comparing thrombolytic agents suggests that fibrin-selective agents produce significant intracoronary clot lysis more quickly than do nonselective agents. This difference translates to a marginally smaller mortality with the fibrin-selective agents, but only for patients treated within 2 hours of symptom onset. Surprisingly, intracranial hemorrhage may actually be more common when fibrin-selective agents are used.[10, 37]

Indications and General Considerations

Thrombolytic therapy is indicated for the treatment of acute ST segment elevation MI within 6 hours of symptom onset.[38] Acute ST segment elevation is defined as 0.1 mV or greater rises in two or more contiguous leads on a standard 12-lead ECG. Therapy is also indicated for patients who have a clinical history compatible with acute MI and now have left bundle branch block. New-onset left bundle branch block complicating acute MI is associated with higher mortality. The ST segment changes accompanying acute infarction may be obscured, and the duration of left bundle branch block is often difficult to document. This is a common reason for patients with acute MI to go untreated[3] despite strong evidence for benefit from thrombolysis.[2] The mortality reduction afforded by thrombolytic therapy is greatest when treatment is instituted within 2 hours of symptom onset. Measurable benefit falls drastically after 6 hours, although there is some evidence that treatment between 6 and 12 hours after symptom onset may be effective, particularly in those patients who present with stuttering symptoms.[39]

Ironically, thrombolytic agents that are given in an effort to dissolve new, fibrin-rich thrombi may actually increase platelet activation, leaving a prothrombotic state in their wake. Therefore, antiplatelet therapy with aspirin at a dose of 160 to 325 mg should be given immediately and continued indefinitely in all patients without a specific contraindication (e.g., angioedema).[38, 40]

The short half-life of fibrin-selective agents and their failure to routinely produce a systemic "lytic" state require adjunctive heparin administration. If heparin is not given as well, the risk of early vessel reocclusion is increased. Theoretically, the anticoagulant effect of fibrinogen depletion and fibrin degradation products produced by nonselective agents, such as streptokinase, obviates the need for heparin. In general, the body of evidence supports theoretical considerations.[37, 41] Therefore, the administration of heparin during therapy with a nonselective thrombolytic drug is not currently recommended.[38] New antithrombin drugs (desirudin, bivalirudin), which may be more effective than heparin during prothrombotic periods and may provide additional benefit when used with streptokinase, are currently under study.[42–44]

Contraindications

Thrombolytic therapy is contraindicated in patients with active bleeding or conditions that would expose them to life-threatening hemorrhage if such therapy were used (Table 11–9). Thrombolytic therapy has been given successfully in menstruating females and during pregnancy. Therefore, although caution is warranted, these conditions are not considered *absolute* contraindications to thrombolytic therapy. The notable exception in pregnant patients is reteplase. Animal studies have shown reteplase to be abortifacient in mammals; its use in pregnancy is contraindicated. Lastly, patients who have previously been treated with streptokinase or anisoylated plasminogen-streptokinase activator complex (APSAC; anistreplase) and have an active streptococcal infection should not be treated with streptokinase or its derivatives, owing to the possibility of the presence of neutralizing antibodies.

Many of the clinical trials of thrombolytic agents have excluded patients older than 75 years. This fact has produced a general reticence to provide a potential life-saving therapy to elderly patients. The elderly are at increased risk of suffering bleeding side effects after treatment with thrombolytic drugs. However, their risk of death after untreated MI is substantial, and the potential benefit of thrombolytic therapy is greater than the risk of intracranial hemorrhage. Therefore, although age greater than 75 years remains a consideration in the decision to apply thrombolytic therapy, it is not a contraindication.[45]

Table 11–9. CONTRAINDICATIONS TO THROMBOLYTIC THERAPY*

- Previous hemorrhagic stroke at any time; other strokes or cerebrovascular events within 1 year
- Known intracranial neoplasm
- Active internal bleeding (does not include menses)
- Suspected aortic dissection

Cautions/Relative Contraindications

- Severe uncontrolled hypertension on presentation (blood pressure >180/110 mm Hg)†
- History of prior cerebrovascular accident or known intracerebral pathology not covered in contraindications
- Current use of anticoagulants in therapeutic doses (INR ≥2–3); known bleeding diathesis
- Recent trauma (within 2–4 weeks), including head trauma or traumatic or prolonged (>10 min) CPR or major surgery (<3 weeks)
- Noncompressible vascular punctures
- Recent internal bleeding (within 2–4 weeks)
- For streptokinase/anistreplase: prior exposure (especially within 5 d to 2 y) or prior allergic reaction
- Pregnancy
- Active peptic ulcer
- History of chronic severe hypertension

*Viewed as advisory for clinical decision making and may not be all-inclusive or definitive.

†Could be an absolute contraindication in low-risk patients with myocardial infarction.

CPR, cardiopulmonary resuscitation; INR, International Normalized Ratio.

From Ryan TJ, Anderson JL, Antman EM, et al: ACC/AHA guidelines for the management of patients with acute myocardial infarction. A report of the American College of Cardiology/American Heart Association Task Force on Practice Guidelines (Committee on Management of Acute Myocardial Infarction). J Am Coll Cardiol 28: 1328, 1996. Copyright 2000 by the American College of Cardiology and American Heart Association.

Thrombolytic Agents

Streptokinase

Streptokinase is a sterile, purified protein extract produced by group C beta-hemolytic streptococci (Table 11–10).[46] It binds in a noncovalent fashion to plasminogen, forming an "activator complex" which then converts circulating plasminogen to plasmin. The activator complex has a half-life of approximately 23 minutes and is cleared by the liver. No active metabolites have been identified.

When given intravenously, streptokinase reduces total peripheral vascular resistance and systemic blood pressure. It may not be the fibrinolytic agent of choice in patients with preexisting hypotension or shock. Allergic reactions such as fever and shivering are seen in 1% to 4% of patients. Anaphylactic shock is very rare, occurring in 0.1% of patients treated. Streptokinase is considered a Pregnancy Category C agent (risk cannot be ruled out). No animal reproduction studies have been performed to date. It is not known whether streptokinase can cause fetal harm or affect reproduction capacity.

The first large-scale trial of streptokinase was the Gruppo Italiano per lo Studio della Streptokinasi Nell'infarcto Miocardio (GISSI) study.[47] It included 11,806 patients of all ages, 19.7% of whom were women. Although patients were eligible for inclusion in this trial if they were treated up to 12 hours after symptom onset, 80% of the patients enrolled were treated before 6 hours. The GISSI investigators reported a mortality benefit in treated women with acute MI. Mortality at 1 month was 18.5% in treated women, compared with 22.6% in women receiving placebo. These investigators also reported a gender difference in outcomes. Mortality rates in men were 8.8% in the treated group and 10.6% in the placebo group. The mortality benefit obtained by thrombolytic therapy is preserved for up to 10 years and is most prominent in patients treated within 2 hours of symptom onset.

Anistreplase

Anistreplase is a heat-treated Lys-plasminogen-streptokinase activator complex derived from human plasma (see Table 11–10). The complex is able to bind fibrin with high affinity but, like streptokinase, has a systemic fibrinolytic affect. The half-life of the fibrinolytic activity of the circulatory complex is 70 to 120 minutes. Anistreplase is a Pregnancy Category C agent (risk cannot be ruled out).

This agent was studied in the Anistreplase in Myocardial Infarction Study (AIMS) and the Third International Study of Infarct Survival (ISIS-3).[48] AIMS was a randomized placebo controlled trial of 1258 patients with symptoms suggesting acute MI accompanied by ST segment elevation. Women constituted 18% of study participants. Patients were randomly assigned to receive either 30 IU of anistreplase or placebo. Patients older than 70 years were excluded. Intravenous heparin was initiated 6 hours after anistreplase

Table 11–10. THROMBOLYTIC DRUG DOSING

AGENT	ROUTE	HEPARIN	DOSE
Streptokinase	IV	No	1,500,000 IU over 60 min
Anistreplase (APSAC)	IV	No	30 U over 2–3 min
Urokinase	IV	No	2,000 IU/lb bolus over 10 min, then 2000 IU/lb infused @ 15 ml/h for 12 h
Recombinant tissue plasminogen activator	IV	Yes	Weight ≥ 67 kg: 15 mg bolus, then 50 mg over 30 min, then 35 mg over 60 min Weight < 67 kg: 15 mg bolus, then 0.75 mg/kg not to exceed 50 mg over 30 min, then 0.50 mg/kg over 60 min
Reteplase	IV	Yes	10 IU bolus over 2 min, then 10 IU over 2 min 30 min later

APSAC, anisoylated plasminogen streptokinase activator complex; IU, international units; IV, intravenous.

or placebo was given. Oral anticoagulation using warfarin was continued for 3 months. Aspirin use was not recorded.

The mortality rates for women in AIMS at 30 days were 5.5% with anistreplase and 17.9% with placebo. Mortality rates for men were 6.6% and 10.9%, respectively. This lower mortality was preserved at 1 year. This finding represents the greatest reduction in mortality specific to women reported in any large placebo-controlled trial. Further study may be warranted to confirm this dramatic lowering of mortality specific to women.

ISIS-3 compared several thrombolytic regimens (streptokinase, anistreplase, and tPA) and also examined the independent effect of supplemental heparin administration. More than 40,000 patients were entered into the trial. No difference was apparent among the three thrombolytic regimens in terms of survival.

Urokinase

Urokinase is a nonselective activator of plasminogen that is produced by the kidney and excreted in the urine (see Table 11–10). Abbokinase (Abbott Laboratories) is a low-molecular-weight form of urokinase that is produced in a tissue culture from human kidney cells. The use of intravenous urokinase for acute MI has not been studied extensively in the United States. The largest international experience is from Italy.[49] Urokinase deserves mention because it is the only thrombolytic agent that has been studied in pregnancy. It is a Pregnancy Category B drug (no evidence of risk in humans). Reproduction studies in mice and rats have been performed with up to 1000 times the human dose without causing harm to the fetus or impairing fertility.

Recombinant Tissue Plasminogen Activator

The r-tPA alteplase (Activase) is a purified glycoprotein of 527 amino acids (see Table 11–10). It is made using complementary DNA (cDNA) from a human melanoma cell line, which is genetically inserted into a line of hamster ovary cells in tissue culture. It has the property of fibrin-enhanced conversion of plasminogen to plasmin. It has an initial half-life of approximately 5 minutes. Because of its short half-life and fibrin selectivity, concomitant therapy with heparin is considered mandatory. Like urokinase, tPA occurs naturally in humans. Therefore, allergic reactions do not occur. It is considered a Pregnancy Category C drug (risk cannot be ruled out), although there are case reports of its use in the peripartum period without fetal harm or uncontrolled maternal hemorrhage.

The Anglo Scandinavian Study of Early Thrombolysis (ASSET) trial[50] compared r-tPA (dose) with placebo in 5005 patients with acute MI and ST segment elevation. Women constituted 23% of study participants. The mortality rates in women at 1 month were 8.6% for r-tPA and 10.9% for placebo. Mortality rates in men were 6.8% and 9.4%, respectively. This lower mortality was preserved for up to 6 months.

The TIMI II trial was a randomized trial of invasive and conservative treatment strategies in men and women treated with thrombolytic drugs for acute MI.[51] The total dosage of r-tPA used in the first 520 patients was 150 mg IV over a period of 6 hours. An unacceptably high rate of intracranial hemorrhage was observed, prompting a reduction in dosage to 100 mg IV and centering attention upon thrombolytic drug dose and the risk of hemorrhage. The dosing regimen for r-tPA was modified as experience grew. In an attempt to speed the onset of thrombolysis, a large initial bolus dose was administered with a stepwise tapering in subsequent doses. This regimen—the accelerated, front-loaded r-tPA dose regimen—proved to be superior to standard dosing regimens. Questions were soon raised about the superiority of this agent over streptokinase.

The GUSTO trial studied 41,021 patients to compare the efficacy of tPA and streptokinase.[10] Women constituted 25% of study participants. A 1% absolute risk reduction favoring tPA was found, primarily in patients treated less than 2 hours from symptom onset. Once again, women were observed to have a twofold higher mortality in comparison with men (11.3% vs. 5.5%, $p < .001$). This difference was maintained after adjustment for baseline characteristics (RR = 1.15; 95% confidence interval, 1.0 to 1.31).

Reteplase

Reteplase is a nonglycosylated modified form of tPA, produced through the use of recombinant DNA technology (see Table 11–10). Reteplase has a half-life of 13 to 16 minutes in plasma and is cleared by the kidneys and the liver. Like tPA, reteplase must be given concomitantly with aspirin and intravenous heparin. Reteplase has been studied in pregnancy. It is a known abortifacient in rabbits when given at three times the human dose. No data currently exist on the use of this drug in pregnant humans. Reteplase is therefore a Pregnancy Category C drug (risk cannot be ruled out).

The International Joint Efficacy Comparison of Thrombolytics (INJECT) trial was a randomized, double-blind trial of 6010 patients who had a clinical history of and ECG criteria for acute MI.[52] The patients were randomly assigned to receive either 10 units of reteplase, given as a double bolus, or 1.5 million units of streptokinase as a 1-hour infusion. The 35-day mortality rates were 8.90% in the reteplase arm and 9.43% in the streptokinase arm (p = NS). Although almost 30% of the study population was female, no post-hoc analysis of gender differences in outcome has been reported.

Complications

The two complications common to all forms of thrombolytic therapy are stroke and bleeding. Stroke is more common in women than men after thrombolytic therapy. In the GUSTO study, women had a twofold higher risk of stroke (2.1% vs. 1.2%, $p < .0001$). Similar findings have been reported from other thrombolytic trials, including the Fibrinolytic Therapy Trialists' (FTT) Collaborative Group.[2]

Bleeding also occurs with greater frequency in women. Minor bleeding, such as leaking from intravenous catheter sites and gingival bleeding associated with dental caries, is not uncommon and does not warrant cessation of thrombolytic therapy. Bleeding complications may be minimized by attention to blood pressure control, avoidance of arterial puncture, and minimal use of venipuncture for laboratory testing.[53] Major bleeding complications include intracranial hemorrhage, retroperitoneal hemorrhage, and a requirement for transfusion of more than 2 units of packed red blood cells. Risk factors for severe bleeding complications are greater age, female gender, and small body size. Major bleeding complications are seen in 43% of women older than 65 years, compared with only 17% of all other patients.

The most feared bleeding complication of thrombolytic therapy is hemorrhagic stroke, which occurs in almost 1% of patients treated with tPA or reteplase. The mortality of intracranial hemorrhage as a complication of thrombolytic therapy is greater than 50%. Risk factors for intracranial hemorrhage include older age, female sex, black ethnicity, hypertension, history of stroke, tPA dose exceeding 1.5 mg/kg, and low body weight.[54] The lowest incidence of intracranial hemorrhage was reported in ISIS-2, a study of streptokinase in acute MI.[40] Only 7 of 12,884 patients (0.05%) had confirmed intracranial hemorrhage. A further 20 patients (0.15%) suffered a new neurologic event during the early treatment period that may have been due to intracranial hemorrhage. Ultimately, the risk of stroke was not increased by thrombolytic therapy with streptokinase. The overall risk of stroke was 0.7% with streptokinase compared with 0.8% in the control group. The observation that new neurologic events are less common with streptokinase than with tPA has led some investigators to recommend that streptokinase become the treatment of choice for patients with a higher risk of neurologic events who present with acute MI.

In the event of a major bleeding complication, thrombolytic infusions should be ceased immediately. If thrombolytic therapy is ongoing or has been recently given at the time an event is recognized, treatment with aprotinin, tranexamic acid, or epsilon-aminocaproic acid should be considered.[55, 56] Adjunctive heparin therapy should be reversed with intravenous protamine. The effect of antiplatelet drugs may be overcome with platelet transfusion.

Future

Although thrombolytic therapy has enjoyed remarkable success in the treatment of acute MI, a substantial proportion of patients experience incomplete recanalization and late reocclusion of the infarcted artery. Experience has shown that the effectiveness of thrombolytic therapy partly depends on additional antithrombotic therapy, such as with aspirin and heparin. Therefore, improving adjuvant therapy has become a central issue in ongoing research.

The search is under way for the safest and most effective antithrombin drug regimen for use with thrombolytic drugs. Candidates include low-molecular-weight heparins and specific antithrombin agents. The most exciting work is the use of normal or low-dose thrombolytic drug regimens with the potent antiplatelet drug family GPIIb/IIIa antagonists. The addition of eptifibatide (Integrelin) or abciximab to tPA is reported to restore patency and normal flow to about 70% of treated patient compared with 30% to 50% of patients receiving thrombolytic drug with placebo or standard thrombolytic regimens. The risk of intracranial hemorrhage does not appear to be markedly increased.[57, 58] This regimen will probably become the standard of care for treatment of acute MI.

CONCLUSION

Female gender is associated with several well-publicized differences in the incidence and outcome of atherosclerotic disease. The onset of clinically evident disease is delayed 7 to 10 years in women compared with men. Symptoms of myocardial ischemia may be atypical, and physicians have a lower index of suspicion for the presence of CAD when evaluating women. As a result, women with acute MI are treated later in the course of the event, are older, and typically have other comorbidities that negatively influence their likelihood of survival. Even when the same comorbidities exist and treatments are identical, women do not have the same prognosis for survival as men. The reason for the gender difference in survival after MI is unexplained but serves to emphasize the importance of interrupting acute ischemic events and salvaging myocardium.

The most successful and widely available method of aborting acute MI is thrombolytic therapy. Women are at higher risk than men of experiencing severe side effects from currently available thrombolytic drug regimens. The most feared side effect is intracranial hemorrhage. The risk associated with female gender is, in part, due to a relatively smaller body size, greater age at the time of the event, and higher prevalence of hypertension.

Despite the risk of therapy, there is clear evidence that the survival of women with acute MI is favorably influenced by treatment with thrombolytic drugs. Potential improvements in thrombolytic therapy that are on the horizon include combination therapy with GPIIb/IIIa antagonists and, perhaps, the new antithrombin drugs. Future studies with greater attention to outcome in women with acute MI may uncover the reasons for worse outcome and allow the application of gender-specific therapy.

References

1. DeWood MA, Spores J, Notske R, et al: Prevalence of total coronary occlusion during the early hours of transmural myocardial infarction. N Engl J Med 303:897, 1980.
2. Indications for fibrinolytic therapy in suspected acute myocardial infarction: Collaborative overview of early mortality and major morbidity results from all randomised trials of more than 1000 patients. Fibrinolytic Therapy Trialists' (FTT) Collaborative Group [see comments] [erratum appears in Lancet 343:742, 1994]. Lancet 343:311, 1994.
3. Barron HV, Bowlby LJ, Breen T, et al: Use of reperfusion therapy for acute myocardial infarction in the United States: Data from the National Registry of Myocardial Infarction 2. Circulation 97:1150, 1998.
4. Silent epidemic: The truth about women and heart disease. In: American Heart Association, Dallas, 1988.
5. Weaver WD, White HD, Wilcox RG, et al: Comparisons of characteristics and outcomes among women and men with acute myocardial infarction treated with thrombolytic therapy. GUSTO-I investigators [see comments]. JAMA 275:777, 1996.
6. Greenland P, Reicher-Reiss H, Goldbourt U, Behar S: In-hospital and 1-year mortality in 1,524 women after myocardial infarction: Comparison with 4,315 men [see comments]. Circulation 83:484, 1991.
7. Tofler GH, Stone PH, Muller JE, et al: Effects of gender and race on prognosis after myocardial infarction: Adverse prognosis for women, particularly black women. J Am Coll Cardiol 9:473, 1987.
8. Kudenchuk PJ, Maynard C, Martin JS, et al: Comparison of presentation, treatment, and outcome of acute myocardial infarction in men versus women (the Myocardial Infarction Triage and Intervention Registry) [see comments]. Am J Cardiol 78:9, 1996.
9. Robinson K, Conroy RM, Mulcahy R, Hickey N: Risk factors and in-hospital course of first episode of myocardial infarction or acute coronary insufficiency in women. J Am Coll Cardiol 11:932, 1988.
10. An international randomized trial comparing four thrombolytic strategies for acute myocardial infarction. The GUSTO investigators [see comments]. N Engl J Med 329:673, 1993.
11. Abbott RD, Donahue RP, Kannel WB, Wilson PW: The impact of diabetes on survival following myocardial infarction in men vs women: The Framingham Study [see comments] [erratum in JAMA 261:1884, 1989]. JAMA 260:3456, 1988.
12. Kannel WB: Metabolic risk factors for coronary heart disease in women: Perspective from the Framingham Study. Am Heart J 114:413, 1987.
13. Ruderman NB, Haudenschild C: Diabetes as an atherogenic factor. Prog Cardiovasc Dis 26:373, 1984.
14. Oparil S: Pathophysiology of sudden coronary death in women: Implications for prevention [editorial; comment]. Circulation 97:2103, 1998.
15. Croft P, Hannaford PC: Risk factors for acute myocardial infarction in women: Evidence from the Royal College of General Practitioners' oral contraception study [see comments]. BMJ 298:165, 1989.
16. Acute myocardial infarction and combined oral contraceptives: Results of an international multicentre case-control study. WHO Collaborative Study of Cardiovascular Disease and Steroid Hormone Contraception. Lancet 349:1202, 1997.
17. White HD, Barbash GI, Modan M, et al: After correcting for worse baseline characteristics, women treated with thrombolytic therapy for acute myocardial infarction have the same mortality and morbidity as men except for a higher incidence of hemorrhagic stroke. The Investigators of the International Tissue Plasminogen Activator/Streptokinase Mortality Study. Circulation. 88:2097, 1993.
18. Karlson BW, Herlitz J, Hartford M: Prognosis in myocardial infarction in relation to gender. Am Heart J 128:477, 1994.
19. Rosenberg L, Palmer JR, Shapiro S: Decline in the risk of myocardial infarction among women who stop smoking. N Engl J Med. 322: 213, 1990.
20. Fiore MC, Novotny TE, Pierce JP, et al: Trends in cigarette smoking in the United States: The changing influence of gender and race. JAMA 261:49, 1989.
21. Hjortland MC, McNamara PM, Kannel WB: Some atherogenic concomitants of menopause: The Framingham Study. Am J Epidemiol 103: 304, 1976.
22. Brunner EJ, Marmot MG, White IR, et al: Gender and employment grade differences in blood cholesterol, apolipoproteins and haemostatic factors in the Whitehall II study. Atherosclerosis 102:195, 1993.
23. Bonithon-Kopp C, Scarabin PY, Darne B, et al: Menopause-related changes in lipoproteins and some other cardiovascular risk factors. Int J Epidemiol 19:42, 1990.
24. Kovacs KA, Burggraf GW, Dewar CL: Reversible cardiogenic shock in an angry woman—case report and review of the literature. Can J Cardiol 12:689, 1996.
25. Jang IK: Images in clinical medicine: Acute myocardial infarction and coronary spasm. N Engl J Med 330:1420, 1994.
26. Fujiwara Y, Yamanaka O, Nakamura T, Yamaguchi H: Coronary spasm in two sisters. Jpn Circ J 57:472, 1993.
27. Buja LM, Willerson JT: Clinicopathologic correlates of acute ischemic heart disease syndromes. Am J Cardiol 47:343, 1981.
28. Gibson RS, Beller GA, Gheorghiade M, et al: The prevalence and clinical significance of residual myocardial ischemia 2 weeks after uncomplicated non-Q wave infarction: A prospective natural history study. Circulation 73:1186, 1986.
29. Falk E: Plaque rupture with severe pre-existing stenosis precipitating coronary thrombosis: Characteristics of coronary atherosclerotic plaques underlying fatal occlusive thrombi. Br Heart J 50:127, 1983.
30. Davies MJ, Thomas AC: Plaque fissuring—the cause of acute myocardial infarction, sudden ischaemic death, and crescendo angina. Br Heart J 53:363, 1985.
31. Becker RC, Terrin M, Ross R, et al: Comparison of clinical outcomes for women and men after acute myocardial infarction. The Thrombolysis in Myocardial Infarction Investigators [see comments]. Ann Intern Med 120:638, 1994.
32. Moser DK, Dracup K: Gender differences in treatment-seeking delay in acute myocardial infarction. Prog Cardiovasc Nurs 8:6, 1993.
33. Kimmelstiel C, Goldberg RJ: Congestive heart failure in women: Focus on heart failure due to coronary artery disease and diabetes. Cardiology 77:71, 1990.
34. Collinson PO, Stubbs PJ: Early 'rule-in' diagnosis of acute myocardial infarction 4 h post admission for rapid risk stratification by creatine kinase increment (creatine kinase change). Ann Clin Biochem 33: 308, 1996.
35. Willerson JT: Cardiovascular Medicine. Churchill Livingstone, New York, 1995.
36. Collen D, Lijnen HR, Verstraete M: Thrombolysis: Biological and Therapeutic Properties of New Thrombolytic Agents. Churchill Livingstone, New York, 1985.
37. ISIS-3: A randomised comparison of streptokinase vs tissue plasminogen activator vs anistreplase and of aspirin plus heparin vs aspirin alone among 41,299 cases of suspected acute myocardial infarction. ISIS-3 (Third International Study of Infarct Survival) Collaborative Group [see comments]. Lancet 339:753, 1992.
38. Ryan TJ, Anderson JL, Antman EM, et al: ACC/AHA guidelines for the management of patients with acute myocardial infarction: Executive summary. A report of the American College of Cardiology/American Heart Association Task Force on Practice Guidelines (Committee on Management of Acute Myocardial Infarction). Circulation 94:2341, 1996.
39. Yusuf S, Collins R, Peto R, et al: Intravenous and intracoronary fibrinolytic therapy in acute myocardial infarction: Overview of results on mortality, reinfarction and side-effects from 33 randomized controlled trials. Eur Heart J 6:556, 1985.
40. Randomized trial of intravenous streptokinase, oral aspirin, both, or neither among 17,187 cases of suspected acute myocardial infarction: ISIS-2. ISIS-2 (Second International Study of Infarct Survival) Collaborative Group. J Am Coll Cardiol 12(6 Suppl A):3A, 1988.
41. GISSI-2: A factorial randomised trial of alteplase versus streptokinase and heparin versus no heparin among 12,490 patients with acute myocardial infarction. Gruppo Italiano per lo Studio della Sopravvivenza nell'Infarto Miocardico [see comments]. Lancet 336:65, 1990.
42. White HD: Direct thrombin inhibition and thrombolytic therapy: Rationale for the Hirulog and Early Reperfusion/Occlusion (HERO-2) trial. Am J Cardiol 82:57P, 1998.
43. White HD, Ellis CJ, French JK, Aylward P: Hirudin (desirudin) and

Hirulog (bivalirudin) in acute ischaemic syndromes and the rationale for the Hirulog/Early Reperfusion Occlusion (HERO-2) Study. Aust N Z J Med 28:551, 1998.
44. White HD, Aylward PE, Frey MJ, et al: Randomized, double-blind comparison of Hirulog versus heparin in patients receiving streptokinase and aspirin for acute myocardial infarction (HERO). Hirulog Early Reperfusion/Occlusion (HERO) Trial Investigators [see comments]. Circulation 96:2155, 1997.
45. Woods KL, Ketley D: Utilisation of thrombolytic therapy in older patients with myocardial infarction. Drugs Aging 13:435, 1998.
46. Physician's Desk Reference, 53rd ed. Medical Economics, Montvale, NJ, 1999, p 576.
47. Effectiveness of intravenous thrombolytic treatment in acute myocardial infarction. Gruppo Italiano per lo Studio della Streptochinasi nell'Infarto Miocardico (GISSI). Lancet 1:397, 1986.
48. Effect of intravenous APSAC on mortality after acute myocardial infarction: Preliminary report of a placebo-controlled clinical trial. AIMS Trial Study Group. Lancet 1:545, 1988.
49. Rossi P, Bolognese L: Comparison of intravenous urokinase plus heparin versus heparin alone in acute myocardial infarction. Urochinasi per via Sistemica nell'Infarto Miocardico (USIM) Collaborative Group [see comments]. Am J Cardiol 68:585, 1991.
50. Wilcox RG, von der Lippe G, Olsson CG, et al: Trial of tissue plasminogen activator for mortality reduction in acute myocardial infarction. Anglo-Scandinavian Study of Early Thrombolysis (ASSET). Lancet 2: 525, 1988.
51. Comparison of invasive and conservative strategies after treatment with intravenous tissue plasminogen activator in acute myocardial infarction: Results of the thrombolysis in myocardial infarction (TIMI) phase II trial. The TIMI Study Group [see comments]. N Engl J Med 320: 618, 1989.
52. Smalling RW, Bode C, Kalbfleisch J, et al: More rapid, complete, and stable coronary thrombolysis with bolus administration of reteplase compared with alteplase infusion in acute myocardial infarction. RAPID Investigators. Circulation 91:2725, 1995.
53. Rao AK, Pratt C, Berke A, et al: Thrombolysis in Myocardial Infarction (TIMI) Trial–phase I: Hemorrhagic manifestations and changes in plasma fibrinogen and the fibrinolytic system in patients treated with recombinant tissue plasminogen activator and streptokinase. J Am Coll Cardiol 11:1, 1988.
54. Gurwitz JH, Gore JM, Goldberg RJ, et al: Risk for intracranial hemorrhage after tissue plasminogen activator treatment for acute myocardial infarction. Participants in the National Registry of Myocardial Infarction 2. Ann Intern Med 129:597, 1998.
55. Gulba DC, Dechend R: Thrombolysis in thromboembolic diseases. Ann Hematol 69:S41, 1994.
56. Efstratiadis T, Munsch C, Crossman D, Taylor K: Aprotinin used in emergency coronary operation after streptokinase treatment [see comments]. Ann Thorac Surg 52:1320, 1991.
57. Ohman EM, Kleiman NS, Gacioch G, et al: Combined accelerated tissue-plasminogen activator and platelet glycoprotein IIb/IIIa integrin receptor blockade with Integrilin in acute myocardial infarction: Results of a randomized, placebo-controlled, dose-ranging trial. IMPACT-AMI Investigators [see comments]. Circulation 95:846, 1997.
58. Ferguson JJ: Meeting highlights: Highlights of the 70th Scientific Sessions of the American Heart Association [news]. Circulation 97:1217, 1998.

11.4 Percutaneous Transluminal Coronary Angioplasty

Paolo Angelini

Introduced in 1977 by Andreas Gruentzig and colleagues,[1] percutaneous transluminal coronary angioplasty (PTCA)* has been the most commonly used intervention for CAD since the early 1990s.[2, 3] With the introduction of coronary stents into clinical practice,[4–6] the use of angioplasty has increased even further. The literature contains abundant general information about PTCA as well as details of specific angioplasty techniques.[7–9] This discussion examines the differences between men and women in the context of PTCA of any type. The sex of the patient can affect the presentation of CAD, technical aspects of PTCA, and early and late outcomes of intervention.

PRESENTATION OF CORONARY ARTERY DISEASE

CAD is essentially an aging process, as it manifests mainly in older individuals and progresses with time. The significance of statistical data regarding the frequency of CAD is limited by the variable strength of the diagnostic parameters used, such as angina, a history of MI, coronary revascularization, or both, or autopsy evidence. Despite these limitations, epidemiologic studies have substantiated the following basic findings, which are discussed more extensively in Chapter 3.

1. Premenopausal women have a lower incidence of CAD than men of the same age. Before menopause (or age 50 years), only women with severely increased risk factors (family history of CAD, hypercholesterolemia, severe hypertension, cigarette smoking, diabetes, previous arteritis) experience coronary obstructive disease.[10]
2. After menopause (or age 50 years), the incidence of CAD in women progressively rises with age in comparison with men, until around 70 years, when incidences are equal.[2, 11, 12]
3. Women live longer than men, so by age 70 years, the absolute number of women with CAD exceeds that of men.[2]
4. In contrast to men, women more frequently present with atypical angina[13] or unstable coronary syndromes (resting angina, MI, or sudden coronary death).[10, 14, 15] Women do not have effort angina as often, possibly because they engage in a lower level of physical activity,[16] especially at the advanced age at which they develop CAD.

*In this chapter, the term percutaneous transluminal coronary angioplasty and its abbreviation, PTCA, are used as generic names for any type of catheter-based angioplasty (modification of a vessel). Specific types of angioplasty are identified by qualifying terms, such as "stent-PTCA" and "balloon-PTCA."

5. According to the AHA, a higher absolute number of women (502,938) than of men (450,172) died of cardiovascular causes in 1997.[17] This mortality trend has changed substantially since 1979 (when about 470,000 women died of cardiovascular disease, versus 500,000 men).[2] In different age groups, the incidence of cardiovascular death varies dramatically: The male-to-female ratio is 2.0:1 in persons younger than 65 years, 1.0–1.1:1 in people 65 to 84 years old, and 0.8–1.0:1 in people 85 years and older.[2, 12]

In summary, the postmenopausal state seems to be as important a risk factor for CAD as male sex. This finding may be based not only on the natural history of the disease in humans but also on complex interactions among natural factors, lifestyles, environment, and clinical interventions in westernized nations.

Regarding sex-related differences in anatomic features and clinical manifestations of CAD, pertinent findings can be summarized with the following five points:

First, the coronary arteries tend to be smaller in women,[18–20] probably because of their lower body weight and lower level of physical training. The patterns of dominance in the branching of the coronary arteries are identical in women and men (in more than 90% of humans, the right coronary artery is dominant).[5, 12, 21] In older women, the coronary arteries tend to be curly and tightly bent as seen on angiography, but specific comprehensive studies of this phenomenon have not been carried out. The fact that coronary artery sinuosity progresses with age and that women undergo angiography at an older age than men may contribute to the popular notion that female coronary arteries are curly.[22] In some instances, a small luminal size may at least partially be due to diffuse CAD, especially in older women with diabetes.[23]

Second, coronary atherosclerosis manifests the same spectrum of multiple anatomic,[24] physiologic, and clinical forms[25] in both sexes. The only difference is the relative frequency of the individual forms.[5, 12, 14, 26] In contrast to men, female candidates for revascularization are generally older and have more associated risk factors,[5, 12, 14, 26, 27] especially diabetes,[28] so they tend to have more calcific, diffuse disease.[22, 23]

It is possible that women more commonly have a reduced coronary vasodilatory capacity in the absence of obstructive disease[29]; this reduced capacity might or might not contribute to the greater frequency of chest pain with "normal coronary arteries" observed in women.[29, 30]

Consistent with the fact that resting angina (as opposed to effort-related angina) is seen more frequently in women, the angiographic incidence of clot-complicated, ulcerated plaques may be higher in women than in men. As has been widely discussed in the literature, clinical and angiographic descriptors of the forms of CAD subjected to angioplasty are of variable relevance with respect to prognostic and procedural implications.[31] In contrast to stable, effort-related angina, unstable angina—especially in its prolonged, resting, recent-onset, or de novo form—is a clinical marker that predicts a more severe prognosis with medical treatment; nevertheless, unstable angina has been a poor predictor of the immediate risk and late prognosis associated with coronary intervention, especially since the introduction of coronary stenting[5] as a bailout procedure or even as a generalized treatment "when feasible."[32]

A history of a recent MI, with or without the use of thrombolytics,[33] is a strong predictor of the outcome of medical treatment or angioplasty.[34–36] The following angiographic descriptors seem to have important procedural and prognostic implications[31, 37]:

- Diffuse versus localized ("segmental") CAD
- The presence of coronary calcifications
- Lesion length of 1.5 cm or more
- Lesion location at a curve of more than 45 or 90 degrees, at a bifurcation, in a proximal versus a distal artery, in a large (greater than 3 mm) rather than small vessel, or in a vein graft rather than a native artery
- Intrinsic lesion-related characteristics, such as eccentricity, ulceration, and clot burden

A limited number of investigators have presented initial studies concerning the incidence of different angiographic features in men and women, both in general and specifically in the context of PTCA. Sex-related differences in this regard probably do exist in the general population as well as in patients selected for angioplasty. In female angioplasty candidates, the following extracardiac conditions may be relevant: (1) coagulation state,[38, 39] (2) capillary fragility, (3) diameter of the entry vessel (brachial, radial, or femoral), (4) extent of coexisting peripheral vascular disease (iliofemoral, ilioaortic, aortic wall), (5) renal function, and (6) age by itself. Specific, exhaustive sex-related studies regarding most of these variables have not yet been conducted.

Third, when the population-based cardiovascular mortality is compared with the coronary angiography and revascularization rates in male and female patients, the result may reveal an important referral bias.[40] Consistent with the reported higher incidence of CAD in older women, the male-female ratio in populations selected for angioplasty is reported to decrease slightly (from 3.0–5.7:1 before age 65 years to 2.3–3.0:1 after age 65 years).[4, 41–44] Justifiably or not, there is a clear, universal propensity towards prescribing medical treatment rather than surgical intervention for older women; this fact probably accounts for the difference between the rates of diagnostic angiography and revascularization procedures carried out in women and men. With the realization that CAD is a leading cause of death in women as well as in men came the suspicion that, in women, this condition is less aggressively treated by physicians, who are predominantly male.[12, 36, 40, 45–54] The perceived underrepresentation of women in interventional studies for CAD is called the "Yentl syndome."[55] However, global population data concerning United States health care expenses show that, compared with men, women spend more money on cardiovascular care (58% versus 42% of total health expenses).[56, 57] Whereas the cost efficiency of medical interventions in women could be improved, any supposed prejudice on the part of male physicians can be substantially dismissed.[58] Differences in the observed use of treatment modalities do exist,[12] but they are mainly due to a different incidence of comorbid states and atypical clinical presentations.

Fourth, during the diagnostic workup, major sex-related differences are observed.[59] The clinical history of women with or without CAD is less predictable than that of men.[13] A pathognomonic correlation between chest pain and physical activity is less frequently seen in women, probably because of their less active lifestyles and advanced age at presentation.[14, 60] Because CAD-related chest pain in women tends to be atypical[13] and to occur at rest,[15] the cardiac workup has a much lower predictive value than in men, and it more often yields false-positive or false-negative results.[14] Provocative tests (involving exercise and pharmacologic, ECG, or nuclear studies) are also persistently less reliable in female patients.[14, 61–63] Indeed, stress echocardiography may be the most accurate test in women.[14, 64]

These problems lead to higher rates of missed diagnosis (a major cause of the apparent discrepancy between the incidence of cardiovascular death and of revascularization procedures in female and male patients)[65] and of negative coronary angiographic findings in women than in men studied for suspected CAD.[66] For example, when coronary angiography is performed because of chest pain, "normal" coronary arteries are diagnosed in 41% of women versus 8% of men ($p < .001$).[67] Similarly, if coronary angiography is done because of an abnormal nuclear stress test result, women have a doubled incidence of the finding of "normal" coronary arteries.[40, 63] Weiner and colleagues[60] reported that the probability of finding significant coronary obstructions in female patients at diagnostic angiography is 62% for typical angina, 40% for probable angina, and 4% for atypical angina. Prospective, comprehensive population studies, such as the Monitoring Trends and Determinants of Cardiovascular Disease (MONICA) Project organized by the World Health Organization (WHO), have confirmed that women admitted to the hospital for acute MI have a 56% higher incidence of atypical chest pain than is seen in men.[68] Women probably have a higher incidence of "primary" coronary thrombosis in previously unobstructed arteries (as assessed by angiography after thrombolytic therapy)[69] and of mitral valve prolapse and hypercoagulopathy of any kind. Similarly, because of their more advanced age at presentation, women more often have occlusion resulting from a large clot burden.

Fifth, in PTCA series, there tends to be a noticeable but not consistent sex-related difference in the indications for intervention.[12] Whereas effort-related angina is a frequent indication for intervention in men (especially if they are younger, active, employed, and responsible for the financial support of a family), prevention of coronary occlusion and MI is a more common indication for intervention in women. Women, especially older women, tend to be advised not to have complex (multivessel) angioplasty, and they also frequently refuse intervention for a variety of reasons, such as living alone, fear of intervention, lack of functional limitations, and lack of motivation to improve their life expectancy while taking a substantial procedural risk.

In recent years, female patients and their physicians have gradually become more aggressive about pursuing coronary interventions, so that their attitudes currently seem to match those seen in cases involving men; nevertheless, one must consider a referral bias when retrospectively evaluating classic concepts regarding sex-related differences at PTCA based on the results of procedures performed during the early years of angioplasty (mainly the 1980s).

TECHNICAL ASPECTS OF CORONARY ANGIOPLASTY

Over the years, PTCA techniques have increased in variety, complexity, and safety. In most institutions, these techniques currently consist of balloon angioplasty, rotablation, directional atherectomy, and stenting. Because the general features of these procedures have been reviewed in several excellent textbooks,[7–9] this discussion deals only with sex-related technical issues.

From the previous discussion of the presentation of CAD, it is clear that PTCA involves no essential sex-related differences: In female and male patients, a substantially identical disease process is treated through the use of the same instruments and techniques. With respect to outcomes and technical modifications in individual cases, however, a few sex-related differences may be noted.

Indications for Intervention

Catheter revascularization is generally indicated by one or more of the following criteria, which are the same in men and women[37]:

1. The patient has a stenotic lesion that causes more than 70% narrowing of the luminal diameter in one or more coronary arteries (or bypass grafts) that have a reference inner diameter of 2 mm or more.
2. The lesion is reachable by the selected angioplasty catheter.
3. The planned procedure is likely to reduce the degree of stenosis to less than 50% (or better, to less than 30% since the introduction of stents).
4. The dependent myocardium is substantially viable.
5. The patient has related symptoms (angina or dyspnea).
6. There is objective evidence of ischemia (as documented by ECG, echocardiography, or nuclear myocardial scintigraphy).
7. The patient is at risk for significant lesion-related angina or its equivalents, MI, or death.
8. The immediate, or procedure-related, risks are lower than the risk of surgical revascularization.

The current tendency has been to evaluate the results of PTCA with respect to the 6- or 12-month incidence of major adverse cardiac events (MACEs), namely, acute MI, "redo" revascularization, and death.

The indications for intervention should be carefully individualized. Specifically, compared with men, older women are less interested in recovering a theoretical maximal cardiovascular exercise capacity. Also, the risks of surgical revascularization are usually higher in older women than in men of the same age,[70] especially when the procedure is carried out during an emergency bailout procedure after failed angioplasty.[71–75]

Preparation for Angioplasty

Before undergoing angioplasty, women (even more than men) should have an adequate preliminary visit with the operator or a responsible member of the team, who will explain the procedure, reassure the patient, and answer any questions.[8]

For routine procedures (lasting less than 90 minutes), minimal preliminary sedation is required. It should be administered orally at least 2 hours before the procedure (not on an on-call basis), because anxiety tends to mount during this period and may complicate the procedure by inducing coronary spasm and vagal hypertonicity. Further sedation is induced during the procedure as needed. Maximal epicardial coronary arterial vasodilatation is particularly important in women, in whom superimposed spasm in small arteries may complicate the procedure and significantly worsen the results, especially since the advent of coronary stents, which require optimal sizing of the reference arterial diameter.

Bladder catheterization is not usually necessary unless the procedure is expected to take more than 90 minutes, deep sedation is required, or the patient is unable to void in a bedpan. One of the advantages of prompt bladder emptying may be the diminished systemic toxicity of the contrast medium, which tends to be reabsorbed when left in the bladder; this fact may be important in the patient with renal failure.

Monitoring of the coagulation status has become more relevant, especially since the widespread adoption of combined antiplatelet and antithrombin therapy. The coagulation status is particularly important in women, in whom bleeding complications at the catheter entry site and the angioplasty site (with intramural or subadventitial hematoma formation) are more common than in men. Patients are generally advised to discontinue dicumarol, ticlopidine, and clopidogrel therapy at least 3 days before an elective procedure, because these drugs increase the bleeding risk, both at the entry site and, more importantly, during bailout surgery if it becomes necessary. On the other hand, discontinuation of acetylsalicylic acid therapy is not generally necessary or advisable. Since the introduction of coronary stents, the incidence of emergency surgery has decreased significantly,[32] and physicians have realized the advantage of decreased platelet aggregability during the early postoperative period. This realization has tilted the balance in favor of aggressive use of antiplatelet agents before routine stent-PTCA.

When a high-risk, prolonged, or uncomfortable procedure is anticipated, general anesthesia with endotracheal intubation is indicated from the start. The definition of high-risk PTCA continues to change with improvements in angioplasty technique and expansion of the indications for intervention, mainly with respect to the introduction of stents. Because female sex is indeed a risk factor for increases in the number and severity of perioperative complications,[76] supportive and preventive measures should be used more aggressively in women, especially frail, older patients with large myocardial areas at risk. Preservation of myocardial function during balloon inflation may be achieved by means of either active or passive coronary perfusion techniques.[8] Consideration should be given to the use of intra-aortic balloon counterpulsation for patients who undergo PTCA during an acute MI or who undergo a PTCA of crucial vessels. The extensive utilization of intra-aortic balloon counterpulsation in women is counterbalanced by the higher risk of vascular complications related to clotting at the accessed iliofemoral artery. Although temporary electronic pacing was considered necessary in the past, it is no longer routinely used. Nevertheless, a femoral venous sheath should be routinely inserted to allow quick placement of a temporary pacing catheter if it becomes necessary; this sheath also permits expeditious, reliable blood sampling for monitoring of the coagulation status. Continuous ECG, hemodynamic, and respiratory monitoring is routinely required, particularly if the patient is deeply sedated.

Entry Site

Because the female body is generally smaller than the male body, a woman's peripheral arteries are also smaller. Consequently, particularly in women, prolonged use of a sheath or catheter larger than 7F in the brachial or radial arteries tends to cause ischemic pain, local arterial spasm, and clotting. Because most new catheter devices generally require 7F or larger sheaths,[5] the brachial approach has been almost completely abandoned, even in men. With the femoral approach, the size of the vessel is not usually a limiting factor, even in women, because a 2- to 3-mm (6F to 9F) guiding catheter can be easily passed through the iliofemoral arteries, whose luminal diameter (in both women and men) generally exceeds 5 mm.

In women, it is particularly important to detect any obstructive disease at the site of vascular entry, owing to the frequent presence of specific risk factors, such as advanced age, smoking, and diabetes.[77] A history of claudication, uneven pulses or absence of pulses in the lower extremities, and the presence of femoral bruits are all indicators of vascular disease. The physician is justified in ordering a duplex Doppler scan before selecting the procedural approach, especially when these factors are present.

Angioplasty Procedure

The angioplasty procedure is basically conducted by means of the same techniques in both sexes. A careful review of the pretreatment angiogram should clearly suggest the objectives of the procedure (i.e., which lesions to address), the sequence of treatment, and the equipment to be used (guiding catheters, guidewires, balloon catheters, and/or other catheter devices). Such a preliminary review should also establish the minimal (versus ideal) objectives and should determine what adverse intraprocedural events will indicate the need for bailout surgery, if this is an available option.[78]

In both women and men, the angiographic anatomy is the main element that guides procedural choices and provides operative feedback. Intravascular ultrasound imaging has been extensively used in the development and research of new PTCA procedures; occasionally, this modality is required during routine clinical intervention, especially in the small vessels of female patients. In women who weigh less than 125 lb (56 kg), particular attention should be paid to estimating the coronary ostial and aortic root anatomy in order to choose an appropriate guiding catheter (with respect to size, degree of curvature, presence or absence of sideholes, etc.).

EARLY AND LATE OUTCOMES OF ANGIOPLASTY

Classic reports concerning the results of PTCA refer mainly to the era of stand-alone balloon-PTCA, as performed in the 1980s.[7] Since that time, the procedure's indications, techniques, and outcome have undergone dramatic changes, mainly because of the advent of coronary stents.[4, 6] The introduction of GPIIb/IIIa platelet receptor antagonists has also substantially lowered the incidence of perioperative complications, if not improved the angiographic success rate.

Stand-Alone Balloon Angioplasty

Early Outcome

Most investigators consistently report that early success rates for stand-alone balloon angioplasty are similar in men and women[12, 26, 34, 42, 44, 71, 72, 79, 80] but also that complication and mortality rates are higher in women.[12, 26, 41, 42, 44, 71, 72, 76, 80, 81] Moreover, women may have an equal or a slightly lower postprocedural restenosis rate.[12, 26, 42, 44, 71, 73, 74, 79, 80, 82]

Most researchers who have studied the specific influence of risk factors have concluded that sex, by itself, is a weak independent predictor of immediate success[37] but a clear predictor of morbidity and mortality in case of sudden reclosure (which entails a worse prognosis in women).[71–75] Women undergoing balloon angioplasty have more risk factors,[42, 83, 84] such as unstable angina, hypertension, hyperlipidemia, diabetes mellitus,[83] advanced age,[83] diffuse disease,[83] smaller vessels,[83] and calcification. In addition, women more commonly undergo treatment at a single coronary site.[85]

As in coronary artery bypass surgery, the smaller body size and stature of women seem to be mild independent variables associated with a higher risk during PTCA.[41, 44, 72] Currently, despite a probable sex-related selection bias in choice of the treatment for CAD, the following three specific procedural risks are higher in women:

- Dissection after balloon angioplasty[10, 37, 76, 86, 87]
- Bleeding at the entry site[86, 87]
- Mortality in the event of emergency bailout surgery[22, 73, 86–89]

The increased dissection rate is probably related to smaller coronary diameter, advanced age, more diffuse nature of the disease, and more frequent presence of adverse metabolic conditions (especially diabetes and coronary calcifications).[10, 22, 51, 66, 75] Post-PTCA bleeding or clotting at the entry site is more common in women.[42, 84, 87] Local factors, such as calcification of the femoral artery and exceptional smallness of the brachial artery, may play a role, along with the coagulation status, but these factors have not been specifically studied. Interestingly, the rate of intracranial bleeding after intravenous administration of tissue plasminogen activator for acute MI is almost eight times higher in women than in men.[90]

A retrospective analysis of the catheterization database at St. Luke's Episcopal Hospital, in Houston, showed that from 1993 through 1995, some form of PTCA was performed in 5663 patients, 1469 (25.9%) of whom were women (Angelini P, Vaughn WK: Incidence of postoperative complications in PTCA during the years 1993–1995. Data on file at St. Luke's Episcopal Hospital/Texas Heart Institute, Houston). The likelihood of development of "any complication" ("redo" revascularization, perioperative MI, bleeding, restenosis, or death) was higher for women than for men (13.8% versus 10.8%; $p = .004$). Specifically, the incidences of shock (0.9% versus 0.4%; $p = .01$) and of bleeding at the entry site requiring blood transfusion or surgical repair (13.3% versus 2.3%; $p = .001$) were higher in women. When the 768 procedures that involved coronary stenting (with an early protocol of aggressive anticoagulation) were considered, the incidence of bleeding at the entry site was higher (but not significantly more so) in women than in men (13.8% and 8.9%, respectively). It is not clear whether this greater bleeding tendency in women is caused by local factors at the entry site[72] or by an abnormal coagulation status.[91]

In most published series, a higher mortality was observed in women than in men in the subset of patients who required urgent surgery after failed PTCA.[81, 86, 89] Sex-related factors that may be important in this regard are advanced age, a frail constitution (a parameter that is real, but hard to quantitate), small coronary vessels, and extensive dissections.[87] Indeed, even in elective coronary artery bypass operations, women have a higher risk than men (more than double).[57, 92–96] Similarly, with the use of thrombolytics, the mortality related to the treatment of an acute MI is higher in women.[57, 68, 97–100]

Analysis of the subset of patients undergoing primary angioplasty for an acute MI (as selected de facto) does not implicate female sex as an independent risk factor.[34, 98] It may be relevant to recall that the degree of ST segment elevation during an acute MI and also during balloon inflation at PTCA is lower in women than in men,[101] probably because of the smaller absolute myocardial mass at risk in women, despite an involved territory equivalent in percentage of the total to that in men. On the other hand, in a continuous series of 75 patients,[72] the incidence of hemodynamic collapse during sudden reclosure was 38% in women versus 20% in men. Also relevant (but contradictory) in this regard are data from the MONICA Project's Scottish study, in which the mortality rate 1 hour after the onset of an acute MI was 32.8% in men and 24.9% in women.[68] Furthermore, 74.3% of the men who died during an acute MI (versus 67.8% of the women) did so outside the hospital. These results are probably related to the more extensive pathophysiologic impairment caused by sudden coronary occlusion in men.

As indirect evidence of the additional complexity of PTCA in women,[86, 102] hospital stays averaged about 1.5 days longer for women than men in the series described by Fortin and coworkers,[10] which involved 591 treated patients.

Female sex does not seem to be an independent risk factor for restenosis 3 to 6 months after PTCA, but the following clinical and angiographic risk factors entail a higher restenosis rate in both sexes[34, 37, 72, 74, 103, 104]:

- Unstable angina
- Recent MI
- Diabetes
- Small vessel diameter
- Lesions longer than 1.5 cm
- Lesions that are calcific, eccentric, ulcerated, or complicated by a clot

Other important risk factors for restenosis are postprocedural angiographic filling defects, dissections (type C, D, or E), and residual stenosis involving more than 30% luminal narrowing.[67, 75] Many of these factors may be more common in women than in men.[102]

Long-Term Outcome

When corrected for risk factors, long-term post-PTCA follow-up studies have documented similar survival rates in men and women[10, 26, 71, 103–105] but a higher incidence of chest pain (especially severe angina) and a lower incidence of bypass grafting in women.[10, 26, 71, 103, 106] Later studies regarding the angiographic incidence of restenosis have not identified male sex as an independent correlate of higher risk,[107] even though earlier reports suggested that it was.[71] Adequately large and detailed studies (including assessments of comorbidity parameters, disease state, and early postoperative results) have not yet been carried out.

Some reports have suggested that estrogen replacement therapy in postmenopausal patients may inhibit the restenotic process.[108–112] Another preliminary finding is that eptifibatide (Integrilin), a more potent platelet aggregation inhibitor than aspirin, has a more protective influence in women than in men.[113]

The Bypass Angioplasty Revascularization Investigation (BARI),[114] which randomized 1829 patients to undergo PTCA (mostly balloon) or bypass surgery, showed that women have the same 5-year mortality as men (12.8% versus 12.0%) despite a higher risk profile. This finding led the investigators to conclude that female sex has a favorable influence on long-term results.

Newer Devices

Initial reports (published in 1990 to 1995) suggested that women are more often treated with stand-alone balloon angioplasty than with newer interventional devices, probably because these devices generally require larger guiding catheters and larger target coronary arteries.[5, 115–118] Coronary spasticity may be more common and more intense in women who undergo rotablation angioplasty. Directional atherectomy and stenting were initially recommended only for vessels with an inner diameter of more than 3 mm, which are most often encountered in men. Otherwise, no sex-related differences have been observed with these methods.[5, 115] Because of the higher level of anticoagulation and the need for larger catheter devices, the incidence of bleeding complications at the entry site (as reflected by the need for blood transfusion and surgical repair) is generally greater in women who undergo angioplasty with the newer devices.[5, 41, 81, 115–117] The importance of the reference luminal diameter in causing adverse events (specifically restenosis) has been well recognized, and this factor may account for some of the negative implications associated with female sex after PTCA.[118–123]

Experience with coronary stents initially suggested that, in women, use of stents leads to higher rates of bleeding and vascular complications as well as of perioperative non–Q wave MIs and a lower early success rate.[124, 125] For example, Fishman and associates[124] reported an early success rate of 89% in women versus 96% in men (p = .005). In contrast, most later investigators have observed that the rate of late restenosis, infarction, and mortality was unaffected by sex.[5, 124]

Over the last few years, the angiographic success and MACE rates after coronary stenting have consistently improved in women, approximating the results achieved in men; unfortunately, the same is not true of individual event rates such as mortality (and possibly the incidence of non–Q wave MI).[126] The advanced age and smallness of the treated coronary segments are the most likely reasons for the excess mortality in women.[30, 127, 128] Similar risk factors common to the female sex have been associated with a persistently higher mortality rate after CABG.[129]

In an observational study conducted from 1992 to 1998 at a large cardiovascular center in Germany, indications for and results of PTCA in women and men were reassessed with respect to the use of coronary stents.[130] Of a total of 6532 cases of PTCA, 4264 cases involved stent use, the incidence being the same in men and women (about 65%). Women were significantly older (69 versus 63 years) and more frequently had hypertension (75% versus 68%), diabetes (27% versus 19%), and hypercholesterolemia (57% versus 47%). The left anterior descending artery was more frequently treated in women than in men (46% versus 40%). The angiographic success rates were identical (98.2%). The incidence of acute MI and death was higher in women (3.1% versus 1.8%) at 30 days but the incidences were essentially equal (6.0% versus 5.8%) at 1 year. The incidence of revascularization at 1 year was lower in women (14.5% versus 17.5%), but no data were available concerning angiographic restenosis.

Since stents became available for bailout procedures, the clinical consequences of dissection after balloon-PTCA have been reevaluated, specifically with respect to comparing the results in women and men. The incidence of angiographic dissection has been confirmed to be significantly higher in women (37.9% vs. 21.7%; p =.001), leading to a higher incidence of stent deployment as a bailout procedure (70.4% vs. 52.2%).[131]

With respect to the use of platelet GPIIb/IIIa inhibitors during PTCA,[132–134] similar advantages have been seen in the two sexes, although women have had a slightly higher rate of bleeding events. The Evaluation of Platelet IIb/IIIa Inhibitor for Stenting (EPISTENT) trial revealed that abciximab (ReoPro) seems to be more advantageous in men than in women subjected to stent-PTCA.[135, 136] Specifically, the rate of primary adverse events at 30 days was reduced from 10.5% to 4.2% in men but only from 11.7% to 8.7% in women.[135] Furthermore, the lowest 30-day event rates in women were achieved after balloon-PTCA with abciximab versus stent-PTCA with abciximab (5.1% and 8.7%, respectively).[135] The reported data do not clarify whether vessel size had an important influence on the women's results.

Apparently, the use of newer platelet inhibitors during coronary stenting mainly prevents small infarctions,[133, 135] not mortality per se, and the data concerning women in the EPISTENT trial confirm the (previously unsubstantiated) suspicion that the basic mechanism for the early protection achieved by such drugs is related to the prevention of side branch occlusion.[135, 136] This complication is more frequently seen after stent utilization, but it has only minor clinical implications in the general population treated with PTCA. Despite a lack of specific studies in women, there is no evidence to suggest that the rates of subacute stent thrombosis or 6-month restenosis are significantly affected by platelet inhibitors.

The hypothesis that estrogens may have a protective effect after PTCA[111, 112, 137] has been retested since the introduction of coronary stents, and the preliminary results have been promising.

CONCLUSION

PTCA has similar indications in the two sexes, but clinical recognition of CAD may be more difficult in women, because (1) the disease tends to have an atypical clinical presentation and (2) the results of noninvasive testing are less accurate. In themselves, the technical aspects of PTCA are not different in women and men; nevertheless, because post-PTCA complications are more common and more severe in women, emphasis should be placed on the prudent use of optimal techniques, more aggressive use of support devices, and optimization of postoperative entry-site care in order to prevent bleeding complications. In both sexes, the risk of restenosis depends more on the specific risk factors involved in individual cases than on sex itself. Especially since the introduction of coronary stents, PTCA has become a more reliable and more attractive revascularization modality than CABG, specifically for older, fragile women.

The higher incidence of dissection after balloon-PTCA[131] and of early (less than 24 hours) recoil after stand-alone balloon-PTCA[40] in women might be construed to support an even more definite policy of routine "stenting when feasible"[32] in women than in men.

References

1. Gruentzig AR, Senning A, Sieganthaler WE, et al: Percutaneous transluminal coronary angioplasty in women compared with men. J Am Coll Cardiol 24:81, 1994.
2. Heart and Stroke Facts (Suppl). American Heart Association, Dallas, 1996, p 3.
3. Weintraub WS, Jones EL, King SB, et al: Changing use of coronary angioplasty and coronary bypass surgery in the treatment of chronic coronary artery disease. Am J Cardiol 65:183, 1990.
4. Serruys PW, De Jaegere P, Kiemeneij F: A comparison of balloon-expandable-stent implantation with balloon angioplasty in patients with coronary artery disease. N Engl J Med 331:489, 1994.
5. Robertson T, Kennard ED, Mathis S, et al: Influence of gender on in-hospital clinical and angiographic outcomes and one-year follow-up in the new approaches to coronary intervention (NACI) Registry. Am J Cardiol 80:26K, 1997.
6. Fischman DL, Leon MB, Baim DS, et al: A randomized comparison of coronary stent placement and balloon angioplasty in the treatment of coronary artery disease. N Engl J Med 331:496, 1994.
7. Ellis S: Elective coronary angioplasty: Techniques and complications. In Topol E (ed): Textbook of Interventional Cardiology, 3rd ed. WB Saunders, Philadelphia, 1999, p 147.
8. Angelini P: Balloon Catheter Coronary Angioplasty. Futura, Mount Kisco, NY, 1987, p 30.
9. Meier B: Balloon angioplasty. In Topol E (ed): Textbook in Cardiovascular Medicine, Lippincott Raven, Philadelphia, 1998, p 1977.
10. Fortin DF, Roubin GS: Epidemiology of restenosis. In Roubin GS, Califf RM, O'Neill WW, et al (eds): Interventional Cardiovascular Medicine: Principles and Practice, Churchill Livingstone, New York, 1994, p 187.
11. Gillum RF: Trends in acute MI and CHD death in the U.S. J Am Coll Cardiol 23:1273, 1994.
12. Houssain KMA, Estrada AQ, Kogan A, et al: Trends in success rate after percutaneous transluminal coronary angioplasty in men and women with coronary artery disease. Am Heart J 134:719, 1997.
13. Milner KA, Funk M, Richards S, et al: Gender differences in symptom presentation associated with coronary heart disease. Am J Cardiol 84:396, 1999.
14. Douglas PS, Ginsburg GS: The evaluation of chest pain in women. N Engl J Med 334:1311, 1996.
15. Scirica BM, Moliterno DJ, Every NR, et al: Differences between men and women in the management of unstable angina pectoris (the GUARANTEE Registry). Am J Cardiol 84:1145, 1999.
16. Chandra NC, Zeigelstein RC, Rogers WJ, et al: Observations of the treatment of women in the United States with myocardial infarction. Arch Intern Med 158:981, 1998.
17. 2000 Heart and Stroke Statistical Update. American Heart Association, Dallas, 2000, p 3.
18. Roberts C, Roberts W: Cross-sectional area of the proximal portions of the three major epicardial coronary arteries in 98 necropsy patients with different coronary events: Relationship to heart weight, age and sex. Circulation 62:953, 1980.
19. O'Connor NJ, Morton JR, Birkmeyer JD, et al: Effect of coronary artery diameter in patients undergoing coronary bypass surgery. Circulation 93:652, 1996.
20. Dodge JT Jr, Brown BG, Bolson EL, et al: Lumen diameter of normal human coronary arteries: Influence of age, sex, anatomic variation, and left ventricular hypertrophy or dilation. Circulation 86:232, 1992.
21. Angelini P: Normal and anomalous coronary arteries in humans. In Angelini P (ed): Coronary Artery Anomalies. Lippincott Williams & Wilkins, Philadelphia, 1999, p 27.
22. Tan K, Sulke N, Taub N, et al: Clinical and lesion morphologic determinants of coronary angioplasty success and complications: Current experience. J Am Coll Cardiol 25:855, 1995.
23. Mintz GS, Painter JA, Pichard AD, et al: Atherosclerosis in angiographically "normal" coronary artery reference segments: An intravascular ultrasound study with clinical correlations. J Am Coll Cardiol 25:1479, 1995.
24. Mautner SL, Lin F, Mautner GC, et al: Comparison in women versus men of composition of atherosclerotic plaques in native coronary arteries and in saphenous veins used as aortocoronary conduits. J Am Coll Cardiol 21:1312, 1993.
25. Lerner DJ, Kannel WB: Patterns of CHD morbidity and mortality in the sexes: A 26-year follow-up of the Framingham population. Am Heart J 111:383, 1986.
26. Cowley MJ, Mullin SM, Kelsey SF, et al: Sex differences in early and long-term results of coronary angioplasty in the NHLBI PTCA registry. Circulation 71:90, 1985.
27. Findlay IN: Coronary bypass surgery in women. Curr Opin Cardiol 9:650, 1994.
28. Barrett-Connor E, Cohn BA, Wingard DL, et al: Why is diabetes mellitus a stronger risk factor for fatal ischemic heart disease in women than in men? JAMA 265:627, 1991.
29. Reis SE, Holubkov R, Lee JS, et al: Coronary flow velocity response to adenosine characterizes coronary microvascular function in women with chest pain and no obstructive coronary disease: Results from the pilot phase of the Women's Ischemia Syndrome Evaluation (WISE) Study. J Am Coll Cardiol 33:1469, 1999.
30. Murabito JM, Evans JC, Larson MG, et al: Prognosis after the onset of coronary heart disease: An investigation of differences in outcome between the sexes according to initial coronary disease presentation. Circulation 88:2548, 1993.
31. Kastrati A, Schomig A, Elezi S, et al: Prognostic value of the modified American College of Cardiology/American Heart Association stenosis morphology classification for long-term angiographic and clinical outcome after coronary stent placement. Circulation 100:1285, 1999.
32. Angelini P, Vaughn WK, Zaqqa M, et al: Impact of the "stent when feasible" policy on in-hospital and 6-month success and complication rates after coronary angioplasty: Single-center experience with 17,956 revascularization procedures (1993–1997). Tex Heart Inst J 27:337, 2000.
33. Maynard C, Litwin PE, Martin JS, et al: Gender differences in the treatment and outcome of acute myocardial infarction: Results from the Myocardial Infarction Triage and Intervention registry. Arch Intern Med 152:972, 1992.
34. Welty FK, Mittleman MA, Healy RW, et al: Similar results of percutaneous transluminal coronary angioplasty for women and men with postmyocardial infarction ischemia. J Am Coll Cardiol 23:35, 1994.

35. Tofler GH, Stone PH, Muller JE, et al: Effects of gender and race on prognosis after myocardial infarction: Adverse prognosis for women, particularly black women. J Am Coll Cardiol 9:473, 1987.
36. Krumholz HM, Douglas PS, Lauer MS, et al: Selection of patients for coronary angiography and coronary revascularization early after myocardial infarction: Is there evidence for a gender bias? Ann Intern Med 116:785, 1992.
37. Ryan TJ, Bauman WB, Kennedy JW, et al: Guidelines for percutaneous transluminal coronary angioplasty. Circulation 88:2987, 1993.
38. Bray PF, Becker LC, Goldschmidt-Clermont PJ: Differences in platelet fibrinogen binding relate to recurrent myocardial ischemic events and are dependent upon gender, age and hormonal status [abstract]. Blood 86:88, 1995.
39. Roberts JW, Goldschmidt-Clermont PJ, Bray PF, et al: Effect of gender on thrombogenic factors in asymptomatic people at high risk for coronary artery disease [abstract]. Circulation 90:I-283, 1994.
40. Ayanian JZ, Epstein AM: Differences in the use of procedures between women and men hospitalized for coronary heart disease. N Engl J Med 325:221, 1991.
41. Karrillon GJ, Morice MC, Benveniste E, et al: Intracoronary stent implantation without ultrasound guidance and with replacement of conventional anticoagulation by antiplatelet therapy: 30-day clinical outcome of the French Multicenter Registry. Circulation 94:1519, 1996.
42. Keelan ET, Nunez BD, Grill DE, et al: Comparison of immediate and long-term outcome of coronary angioplasty performed for unstable angina and rest pain in men and women. Mayo Clin Proc 72: 5, 1997.
43. Ruygrok PN, de Jaegere PPT, van Domburg RT, et al: Clinical outcome 10 years after attempted percutaneous transluminal coronary angioplasty in 856 patients. J Am Coll Cardiol 27:1669, 1996.
44. Weintraub WS, Wenger NK, Kosinski AS, et al: Percutaneous transluminal coronary angioplasty in women compared with men. J Am Coll Cardiol 24:81, 1994.
45. Clarke KW, Gray D, Keating NA, et al: Do women with acute myocardial infarction receive the same treatment as men? BMJ 309:563, 1994.
46. Weintraub WS, Kosinski AS, Wenger NK: Is there a bias against performing coronary revascularization in women? Am J Cardiol 78: 1154, 1996.
47. Pettigrew M, McKee M, Jones J: Coronary artery surgery: Are women discriminated against? BMJ 306:1164, 1993.
48. Bearden D, Allman R, McDonald R, et al: Age, race, and gender variation in the utilization of coronary artery bypass surgery and angioplasty in SHEP. Am J Geriatr Soc 42:1143, 1994.
49. Mark DB, Shaw LK, DeLong ER, et al: Absence of sex bias in the referral of patients for cardiac catheterization. N Engl J Med 330: 1101, 1994.
50. Shaw LJ, Miller DD, Romeis JC, et al: Gender differences in the noninvasive evaluation and management of patients with suspected coronary artery disease. Ann Intern Med 120:559, 1994.
51. Odes PA, Waldmann ML, Polk DM, et al: Referral patterns and exercise response in the rehabilitation of female patients aged >62 years. Am J Cardiol 69:1422, 1992.
52. Gillum RF: Coronary artery bypass surgery and coronary angiography in the United States, 1979–1983. Am Heart J 113:1255, 1987.
53. Steingart RM, Packer M, Hamm P, et al: Sex differences in the management of coronary artery disease. N Engl J Med 325:226, 1991.
54. Cole PL: Coronary artery disease in women: Differences in diagnosis, therapy, and treatment. Coron Artery Dis 4:595, 1993.
55. Healy B: The Yentl syndrome. N Engl J Med 3:274, 1991.
56. Eaker ED, Castelli WP: Coronary heart disease and its risk factors among women in the Framingham study. In Eaker ED, Packard B, Wenger NK, et al (eds): Coronary Heart Disease in Women. Haymarket Doyma, New York, 1987, p 122.
57. Taylor AL, Mueller SD: Coronary artery disease in women. In Willerson JW (ed): Cardiovascular Medicine. Churchill Livingstone, Philadelphia, 1995, p 1715.
58. Bernstein SJ, Hilborne LH, Leape LL, et al: The appropriateness of use of cardiovascular procedures in women and men. Arch Intern Med 154:2759, 1994.
59. Wenger N: Coronary disease in women. Ann Rev Med 36:285, 1985.
60. Weiner DA, Ryan TJ, McCabe CH, et al: Exercise stress testing: Correlations among history of angina, ST-segment response and prevalence of coronary-artery disease in the Coronary Artery Surgery Study. N Engl J Med 301:230, 1979.
61. Sawada SG, Ryan T, Fineberg NS, et al: Exercise echocardiographic detection of coronary artery disease in women. J Am Coll Cardiol 14: 1440, 1989.
62. Taillefer R, DePuey EG, Udelson JE: Comparative diagnostic accuracy of Tl-201 and Tc-99m sestamibi SPECT imaging (perfusion and ECG-gated SPECT) in detecting coronary artery disease in women. J Am Coll Cardiol 29:69, 1997.
63. Iskandrian AE, Heo J, Nallamothu N: Perfusion imaging for the diagnosis and risk assessment of coronary artery disease in women. In Marwick TH (ed): Cardiac Stress Testing and Imaging: A Clinician's Guide. Churchill Livingstone, Philadelphia, 1996, p 177.
64. Marwick TH, Anderson T, Williams MJ, et al: Exercise echocardiography is an accurate and cost-efficient technique for the detection of coronary artery disease in women. J Am Coll Cardiol 26:335, 1995.
65. Eysmann SB, Douglas PS: Reperfusion and revascularization strategies for coronary artery disease in women. JAMA 268:1903, 1992.
66. Ellis SG, Roubin GS, King S III, et al: In hospital cardiac mortality after acute closure after coronary angioplasty: Analysis of risk factors from 8,207 patients. J Am Coll Cardiol 11:211, 1988.
67. Sullivan AK, Holdright DR, Wright CA, et al: Chest pain in women: Clinical, investigative, and prognostic features. Br Med J 308:883, 1994.
68. Tunstall-Pedoe H, Morrison C, Woodward M, et al: Sex differences in myocardial infarction and coronary deaths in the Scottish MONICA population of Glasgow 1985 to 1991. Circulation 93:1981, 1996.
69. Llevadot J, Giugliano RP, McCabe CH, et al: Degree of residual stenosis in the culprit coronary artery after thrombolytic administration (Thrombolysis in Myocardial Infarction [TIMI] Trials). Am J Cardiol 85:1409, 2000.
70. Khan SS, Nessim S, Gray R, et al: Increased mortality of women in coronary artery bypass surgery: Evidence for referral bias. Ann Intern Med 112:561, 1990.
71. Kelsey SF, James M, Holubkov AL, et al: Results of PTCA in women: 1985–1986 NHLBI coronary angioplasty registry. Circulation 87:720, 1993.
72. Malenka DJ, O'Connor GT, Quinton H, et al: Differences in outcomes between women and men associated with percutaneous transluminal coronary angioplasty: A regional prospective study of 13061 procedures. Circulation 94(Suppl):II99, 1996.
73. Bell MR, Holmes DR Jr, Berger PB, et al: The changing in-hospital mortality of women undergoing percutaneous transluminal coronary angioplasty. JAMA 269:2091, 1993.
74. Ruygrok PN, de Jaegere PT, van Domburg RT, et al: Women fare no worse than men 10 years after attempted coronary angioplasty. Cathet Cardiovasc Diagn 39:9, 1996.
75. Ellis SG, Roubin GS, King S III, et al: Angiographic and clinical predictors of acute closure after native vessel coronary angioplasty. Circulation 77:372, 1988.
76. Ilia R, Bigham H, Brennan J, et al: Predictors of coronary dissection following percutaneous transluminal coronary balloon angioplasty. Cardiology 85:229, 1994.
77. Omoigui NA, Califf RM, Pieper K, et al: Peripheral vascular complications in the Coronary Angioplasty versus Excisional Atherectomy Trial. J Am Coll Cardiol 26:922, 1995.
78. Angelini P: Guidelines for surgical standby for coronary angioplasty: Should they be changed? J Am Coll Cardiol 33:1266, 1999.
79. Fetters JK, Peterson ED, Shaw IJ, et al: Sex-specific differences in coronary artery disease risk factors, evaluation, and treatment: Have they been adequately evaluated? Am Heart J 131:796, 1996.
80. Williams DO, Thompson B, Braunwald E, et al: Contemporary PTCA for acute coronary ischemia: Results in women match those of men. J Am Coll Cardiol 25:138A, 1995.
81. Greenberg MA, Mueller HS: Why the excess mortality in women after PTCA? Circulation 87:1032, 1993.
82. Mich WJ, Piedmonte MR, Arnold AM, et al: Risk stratification for long-term outcome after elective coronary angioplasty: A multivariate analysis of 5,000 patients. J Am Coll Cardiol 24:74, 1994.
83. Faxon DP: Effect of high dose angiotensin-converting enzyme inhibition on restenosis: Final results of the MARCATOR study, a multicenter, double-blind, placebo-controlled trial of cilazapril. J Am Coll Cardiol 25:362, 1995.
84. Arnold AM, Mick MJ, Piedmonte MR, et al: Gender differences for coronary angioplasty. Am J Cardiol 74:18, 1994.
85. Alexander KP, Mark DB: Effect of gender on angioplasty outcome: Are we closer to the answer? Mayo Clin Proc 72:89, 1997.

86. Wolfe MW, Roubin GS, Schweiger M, et al: Length of hospital stay and complications after percutaneous transluminal coronary angioplasty. Circulation 92:311, 1995.
87. Jacobs AK, Kelsey SF, Yeh W, et al: Documentation of decline in morbidity in women undergoing coronary angioplasty (a report from the 1993–94 NHLBI Percutaneous Transluminal Coronary Angioplasty Registry). Am J Cardiol 80:979, 1997.
88. Vacek JL, Rosamond TL, Kramer PH, et al: Sex-related differences in patients undergoing direct angioplasty for acute myocardial infarction. Am Heart J 126(3 Pt 1):521, 1993.
89. Carey JA, Davies SW, Balcon R, et al: Emergency surgical revascularization for coronary angioplasty complications. Br Heart J 72:428, 1994.
90. Stone GW, Grines CL, Browne KF, et al: Comparison of in-hospital outcome in men versus women treated by either thrombolytic therapy or primary coronary angioplasty for acute myocardial infarction. Am J Cardiol 75:987, 1995.
91. Conlan MG, Folsom AR, Finch A, et al: Associations of factor VIII and von Willebrand factor with age, race, sex, and risk factors for atherosclerosis. Semin Thromb Hemost 70:380, 1993.
92. He G, Acuff TE, Ryan WH, et al: Influence of old age, gender, and internal mammary artery grafting on operative morality and morbidity in coronary artery bypass grafting. Am J Geriatr Cardiol 5:10, 1996.
93. Fisher LD, Kennedy JW, Davis KB, et al: Association of sex, physical size, and operative mortality after coronary bypass surgery in the Coronary Artery Surgery Study. J Thorac Cardiovasc Surg 84:334, 1982.
94. Kouchoukos NT, Oberman A, Kirklin JW, et al: Coronary bypass surgery: Analysis of factors affecting hospital mortality. Circulation 62(Suppl 1):84, 1980.
95. Cosgrove DM, Loop FD, Lytle BW, et al: Primary myocardial revascularization: Trends in surgical mortality. J Thorac Cardiovasc Surg 88: 673, 1984.
96. Loop FD, Golding LR, MacMillan JP, et al: Coronary artery surgery in women compared with men: Analyses of risks and long-term results. J Am Coll Cardiol 1:383, 1983.
97. White HD, Barbash GI, Modan M, et al: After correcting for worse baseline characteristics, women treated with thrombolytic therapy for acute myocardial infarction have the same mortality and morbidity as men except for a higher incidence of hemorrhagic stroke. Circulation 88:2097, 1993.
98. Chandra NC, Ziegelstein RC, Rogers WJ, et al: Observations of the treatment of women in the United States with myocardial infarction. Arch Intern Med 158:981, 1998.
99. Becker RC, Terrin M, Ross R, et al: Comparison of clinical outcomes for women and men after acute myocardial infarction. Ann Intern Med 120:638, 1994.
100. Lincoff AM, Califf RM, Ellis SG, et al: Thrombolytic therapy for women with myocardial infarction: Is there a gender gap? Thrombolysis and Angioplasty in Myocardial Infarction Study Group. J Am Coll Cardiol 22:1780, 1993.
101. Dellborg M, Herlitz J, Emanuelsson H, et al: ECG changes during myocardial ischemia: Differences between men and women. J Electrocardiol 27(Suppl):42, 1994.
102. Kahn JK, Rutherford BD, McConahay DR, et al: Comparison of procedural results and risks of coronary angioplasty in men and women for conditions other than acute myocardial infarction. Am J Cardiol 69:1241, 1992.
103. Bell MR, Grill DE, Garratt KN, et al: Long-term outcome of women compared with men after successful coronary angioplasty. Circulation 91:2876, 1995.
104. Califf RM, Ohman EM, Frid D: Restenosis: The clinical issues. In Topol E (ed): Textbook of Interventional Cardiology. WB Saunders Co, Philadelphia, 1990, p 363.
105. Arora RR, Konard K, Badhwar K, et al: Restenosis after transluminal coronary angioplasty: A risk factor analysis. Cathet Cardiovasc Diagn 19:17, 1990.
106. McEniery PT, Hollman J, Knezinek V, et al: Comparative safety and efficacy of percutaneous transluminal coronary angioplasty in men and in women. Cathet Cardiovasc Diagn 13:364, 1987.
107. Forrester JS, Fishbein M, Helfant R, et al: A paradigm for restenosis based on cell biology: Clues for the development of new preventive therapies. J Am Coll Cardiol 17:758, 1991.
108. O'Brien JE, Peterson ED, Keeler GP, et al: Relation between estrogen replacement therapy and restenosis after percutaneous coronary interventions. J Am Coll Cardiol 28:111, 1996.
109. O'Keefe JH, Kim SC, Hall RR, et al: Estrogen replacement therapy after coronary angioplasty in women. J Am Coll Cardiol 29:1, 1997.
110. Abu-Halawa SA, Thompson K, Kirkeeide RL, et al: Estrogen replacement therapy and outcome of coronary balloon angioplasty in postmenopausal women. Am J Cardiol 82:409, 1998.
111. Moraghan TJ, Grenert JP, Johnson CM, et al: Gender related differences in smooth muscle cell proliferation in response to estradiol and dihydrotestosterone [abstract]. J Am Coll Cardiol 25:14A, 1995.
112. Foegh ML, Asotra S, Howell MH, et al: Estradiol inhibition of arterial neointimal hyperplasia after balloon injury. J Vasc Surg 19:722, 1994.
113. Goldschmidt-Clermont PJ, Schulman SP, Bray PF, et al: Refining the treatment of women with unstable angina—a randomized, double-blind, comparative safety and efficacy evaluation of Integrelin versus aspirin in the management of unstable angina. Clin Cardiol 19:869, 1996.
114. Jacobs AK, Kelsey SF, Brooks MM, et al: Better outcome for women compared with men undergoing coronary revascularization: A report from the Bypass Angioplasty Revascularization Investigation (BARI). Circulation 98:1279, 1998.
115. Bell MR, Garratt KN, Bresnahan JF, et al: Immediate and long-term outcome after directional coronary atherectomy: Analysis of gender differences. Mayo Clin Proc 69:723, 1994.
116. Casale PN, Whitlow PL, Franco L, et al: Comparison of major complication rates with atherectomy devices for percutaneous coronary intervention in women versus men. Am J Cardiol 71:1221, 1993.
117. Moscucci M, Mansour KA, Kent C, et al: Peripheral vascular complications of directional coronary atherectomy and stenting: Predictors, management and outcome. Am J Cardiol 74:448, 1994.
118. Kuntz RE, Safian RD, Carrozza JP, et al: The importance of acute luminal diameter in determining restenosis after coronary atherectomy or stenting. Circulation 86:1827, 1992.
119. Brodie BR, Stuckey TD, Hansen C, et al: Influence of vessel size on early and late outcomes after primary angioplasty for acute myocardial infarction. J Invasive Cardiol 12:13, 2000.
120. Diaz L, Fajadet J, Cassagneau B, et al: The short term results and angiographic predictors of subacute thrombosis in the coronary implantation of the Palmaz-Schatz endoprosthesis. Rev Esp Cardiol 47: 747, 1994.
121. Akiyama T, Moussa I, Reimers B, et al: Angiographic and clinical outcome following coronary stenting of small vessels: A comparison with coronary stenting of large vessels. J Am Coll Cardiol 32:1610, 1998.
122. Miketic S, Carlsson J, Tebbe U: Clinical and angiographic outcomes of NIR stent implantation in small vessels with unfavorable lesion morphology. J Invasive Cardiol 11:269, 1999.
123. Elezi S, Kastrati A, Neuman FJ: Vessel size and long term outcome after coronary stent placement. Circulation 98:1875, 1998.
124. Fishman RF, Kuntz RE, Carrozza JP Jr, et al: Acute and long-term results of coronary stents and atherectomy in women and the elderly. Coron Artery Dis 6:159, 1995.
125. Mak KH, Belli G, Ellis SG, et al: Subacute stent thrombosis: Evolving issues and current concepts. J Am Coll Cardiol 27:494, 1996.
126. Gowda MS, Vacek JL, Hallas D: Gender-related risk factors and outcomes for non-Q wave myocardial infarction patients receiving in-hospital PTCA. J Invasive Cardiol 11:121, 1999.
127. Brodie BR: Why is mortality rate after percutaneous transluminal coronary angioplasty higher in women? Am Heart J 137:582, 1999.
128. Malenka DJ, O'Rourke D, Miller MA, et al: Cause of in-hospital death in 12,232 consecutive patients undergoing percutaneous transluminal coronary angioplasty. Am Heart J 137:632, 1999.
129. Abramov D, Tamariz MG, Sever JY, et al: The influence of gender on the outcome of coronary bypass surgery. Ann Thorac Surg 70: 800, 2000.
130. Mehilli J, Kastrati A, Dirschinger J, et al: Differences in prognostic factors and outcomes between women and men undergoing coronary artery stenting. JAMA 284:1799, 2000.
131. Carcagni A, Camellini M, Maiello L, et al: Percutaneous transluminal coronary revascularization in women: Higher risk of dissection and need for stenting. Ital Heart J 8:536, 2000.
132. EPILOG Investigators: Effect of the platelet glycoprotein IIb/IIIa receptor inhibitor abciximab with lower heparin dosages on ischemic complications of percutaneous coronary revascularization. N Engl J Med 336:1689, 1997.
133. Califf RM, Abdelmeguid AE, Kuntz RE, et al: Myonecrosis after revascularization procedures. J Am Coll Cardiol 31:241, 1998.
134. Kereiakes DJ, Lincoff AM, Miller DP, et al, for the EPILOG Trial

Investigators: Abciximab therapy and unplanned coronary stent deployment: Favorable effects on stent utilization, clinical outcomes and bleeding complications. Circulation 97:857, 1998.
135. The EPISTENT Investigators: Randomised placebo-controlled and balloon-angioplasty-controlled trial to assess safety of coronary stenting with use of platelet glycoprotein-IIb/IIIa blockade. Lancet 352:87, 1998.
136. Topol EJ, Mark DB, Lincoff AM, et al, for the EPISTENT Investigators: Evaluation of platelet IIb/IIIa inhibitor for stenting: Outcomes at 1 year and economic implications of platelet glycoprotein IIb/IIIa blockade in patients undergoing coronary stenting: Results from a multicentre randomised trial. Lancet 354:2019, 1999.
137. Khan MA, Liu MW, Singh D, et al: Long-term (three years) effect of estrogen replacement therapy on major adverse cardiac events in postmenopausal women after intracoronary stenting. Am J Cardiol 86: 330, 2000.

11.5 Surgical Therapy

O. H. Frazier and Nancy A. Nussmeier

Cardiovascular disease continues to be the leading health threat to women in the Western world, being the cause of one of every two female deaths.[1] In the United States, in 1997, CABG operations were performed in 116,000 women,[2] accounting for 32% of all CABG procedures. Although a growing number of women are being referred for such operations, men remain the predominant recipients of cardiac catheterization and CABG surgery. Some researchers have suggested that this disparity represents a referral bias (the "Yentl syndrome"),[3–7] but others have found no evidence for such a bias.[8, 9] Multiple published reports suggest that CABG yields a higher operative mortality and poorer overall outcome in women than in men.[10–21] Nevertheless, emerging evidence suggests that this gender gap is narrower than previously believed and that female sex, per se, is not necessarily an independent risk factor.[22–24]

This discussion briefly reviews the comparative results of CABG in women and men and suggests methods for improving the surgical outcome. Because the two sexes present with significantly different preoperative characteristics and risk profiles, comparison is not always straightforward.

PREOPERATIVE PRESENTATION

Compared with men, women are shorter, weigh less, and have a smaller body surface area (BSA) and smaller coronary arteries.[24, 25] Because natural estrogen has a protective effect against CAD, this condition rarely affects women before menopause (or age 50 years). The Framingham Heart Study is the most extensive source of epidemiologic data concerning CAD in women.[26–28] This longitudinal study found that (1) women manifest symptoms of CAD an average of 10 years later than men do, (2) in women, the primary presenting symptoms are consistent with unstable angina (compared with frank MI in men), and (3) angiography reveals obstructive CAD in more than 90% of men with unstable angina but in only 60% of women. Therefore, women receive fewer aggressive procedures, including PTCA and CABG, until a later age.

After age 50, the incidence of CAD begins to increase in women, but not until age 70 does it equal the incidence in men. Likewise, MI is relatively rare in women younger than 55 years, but after age 75, the frequency of infarction in women equals that in men. These observations led to the hypothesis that premenopausal women have a lower relative risk of CAD compared with postmenopausal women and that the most likely protective factor is estrogen. The other inference is that, when referred for evaluation of CAD, women tend to be older than men and in worse overall condition.

Women are more likely than men to have comorbid conditions that predict a poor outcome after CABG surgery, including diabetes mellitus,[11, 12, 22, 24, 25] hypertension,[11, 22, 24] congestive heart failure,[11, 12, 24] and peripheral vascular disease.[11, 12] With respect to the extent and distribution of CAD, women have basically the same patterns as men.[8, 22, 29, 30] Nevertheless, they have a higher incidence of Canadian Cardiovascular Society class 3 or 4 angina,[23, 25] and their angina tends to be acute and unstable rather than effort-related.[14, 22] Women have higher rates of preoperative intra-aortic balloon pump support and of previous PTCA, and they are more likely to require urgent CABG.[23]

CORONARY ARTERY BYPASS GRAFTING

Studies concerning the outcome of surgical revascularization in women have had conflicting results. Traditionally, most reports have shown that women fare worse than men with respect to operative mortality and morbidity as well as postoperative outcome.[10–12, 14–19, 31, 32] On the basis of these findings, female sex, per se, would appear to be an independent risk factor in patients undergoing CABG. Nevertheless, when the population is adjusted for BSA,[13, 33] coronary artery size,[34, 35] or risk-factor profile,[23, 24, 36, 37] the male-female difference in mortality and morbidity tends to lose its significance, and the poor results appear to be related mainly to those confounding variables.

In fact, even in men, smaller body size is associated with an overall poorer outcome.[11, 38] With small coronary arteries, the creation of suitable anastomoses may be technically more difficult, and fewer distal anastomoses are attempted.[24] Therefore, women are less likely to undergo complete revascularization than men. Moreover, internal mammary artery (IMA) grafts, which are known to offer superior patency and to increase postoperative survival, may be used less often in women.[23]

Operative Mortality

Since the early days of CABG, reporters have cited operative mortality rates up to twice as high for women (1.3% to 8.8%) as for men (0.9% to 3.0%).[12, 14, 15, 20, 21, 39–44] However, after adjusting for risk factor profile in 1743 patients who underwent primary CABG from 1994 to 1997, Aldea and colleagues[24] found no significant difference between women and men with respect to perioperative mortality. Likewise, after allowing for risk-factor profile in 4823 patients undergoing CABG, Abramov and coworkers[23] concluded that female sex is not an independent predictor of early mortality and is only a weak independent predictor for the combined endpoint of early mortality and cardiovascular morbidity. Furthermore, in 347 women and 2098 men undergoing isolated CABG from 1992 to 1997, Nardi and associates[25] observed no significant intergroup difference in operative mortality. Finally, in the Bypass Angioplasty Revascularization Investigation (BARI),[22] which evaluated 1829 patients undergoing PTCA or CABG for multivessel disease, the in-hospital mortality rates were similar for the two sexes once the investigators allowed for the higher baseline risk status of women. In fact, in a review of the literature concerning referral patterns and outcomes for male versus female patients undergoing CABG, Hussain and coauthors[12] concluded that once other variables are taken into account, female sex is no longer a statistically significant predictor of operative mortality.

On the other hand, Edwards and colleagues[11] evaluated 97,153 women and 247,760 men registered in the Society of Thoracic Surgeons (STS) National Cardiac Surgery Database, all of whom underwent isolated CABG between 1994 and 1996. These investigators showed that, even when confounding risk factors were taken into account, women still had a significantly higher operative mortality (4.5% versus 2.6%).[11, 14] Only among the patients at highest risk did the significance of sex tend to disappear.

Hormone Replacement Therapy

At the Texas Heart Institute from 1993 through 1999, women receiving hormone replacement therapy (HRT) had a significantly lower mortality after CABG than those not receiving HRT; this result was confirmed by multivariate analysis, essentially establishing a parity between HRT recipients and men (Table 11–11).[45] The patients consisted of 4265 women and men aged 55 years or more. Of the 1133 postmenopausal women, 222 (19.6%) were taking HRT at the time of admission to the hospital for CABG. The rate of HRT in our study was similar to the 20% rate of estrogen use reported by the National Center for Health Statistics.[46] Because differences in baseline characteristics might have affected the outcomes for estrogen users, a multivariate analysis was performed, with mortality as the dependent variable. Considering all 4265 patients (including those at high risk because of emergency status, performance of "redo" CABG, or the need for a concomitant surgical procedure such as valve replacement), multivariate analysis confirmed that female sex without HRT was an independent predictor of a higher CABG mortality (p = .0001; see Table 11–11). Similarly, in the subset of patients having an elective, primary, isolated CABG (n = 2910) (excluding those undergoing "redo" surgery, emergency surgery, or a concomitant procedure), multivariate analysis again confirmed that female sex without HRT was an independent predictor of a higher CABG mortality ($p < .0001$; see Table 11–11).

The effect of HRT on the cardiovascular system is not clear.[47–49] A large number of observational studies have suggested that HRT offers substantial cardiovascular benefit for primary and secondary prevention of cardiovascular disease.[50–60] However, observational data may be subject to bias by the following factors: (1) *selection:* a healthy cohort of women is typically prescribed estrogen; (2) *self-selection:* women who use estrogen beyond the period of perimenopausal symptoms both tend to be free of disease and to demonstrate compliance and healthy lifestyle patterns; (3) *limited population:* women who use estrogen appear to be better educated and to have better access to health care; and (4) *limited power:* many studies are conducted in relatively few subjects. Women taking HRT tend to be younger, wealthier, more educated, and healthier than untreated women.[61] Thus, some of estrogen's putative benefits might be spurious, in that women who are less likely to develop severe coronary artery disease are more likely to take estrogen.

In fact, the results of large randomized, controlled clinical trials designed to study the effects of HRT in women with or without known coronary artery disease, the Heart and Estrogen/Progestin Replacement (HERS) study,[47] the Estrogen Replacement and Atherosclerosis (ERA) trial,[62] and preliminary trends in the Women's Health Initiative (WHI) study[63] have shown no significant benefit and have raised the possibility of short-term increases in risk. Specifically, in

Table 11–11. MORTALITY AFTER CORONARY ARTERY BYPASS GRAFTING (CABG) IN MEN, WOMEN RECEIVING HORMONE REPLACEMENT THERAPY (HRT), AND WOMEN NOT RECEIVING HORMONE REPLACEMENT THERAPY, 55 YEARS AND OLDER

PATIENT GROUP	ALL PATIENTS UNDERGOING CABG* (n = 4265)		PATIENTS UNDERGOING ELECTIVE PRIMARY ISOLATED CABG (n = 2910)	
	Number	Mortality (%)	Number	Mortality (%)
Men	3132	7.5	2108	2.6
Women				
With HRT	222	5.8	165	2.4
Without HRT	911	11.8†	632	7.1

*Includes redo, emergency, and concomitant procedures, e.g., valve replacement.
†$p < .0005$ versus both other groups.

the HERS trial of HRT for secondary prevention, there was no overall effect of 4.1 years of treatment with conjugated estrogen plus medroxyprogesterone acetate on the risk of nonfatal myocardial infarction and death from coronary heart disease among women with established coronary atherosclerosis.[47] These results were complicated by an early increase, but a late reduction, in risk within the overall null effect. Therefore, there may be an initial acceleration of the rate of cardiovascular events in women taking HRT, leaving a lower-risk group for continued follow-up.[62, 64] For secondary prevention of cardiovascular events, the latest American Heart Association recommendations state that HRT should not be initiated for this purpose.[65] Definitive evidence regarding the benefits and risks of HRT for primary prevention of cardiovascular disease should emerge from the ongoing, large-scale WHI trial, which should be completed in 2005.[63]

Perhaps the benefits of HRT are most evident in the presence of a vascular injury, as noted in numerous laboratory studies.[66–80] It has been clearly shown that endothelial cells and vascular smooth-muscle cells possess estrogen receptors, and thus are physiologic targets for estrogen action.[67, 68] Evidence from animal models suggests that, in normal blood vessels, estrogen inhibits hyperproliferation after acute injury.[66] Apparently, the response to endoluminal injury involves the activation of adventitial cells and their migration toward the lumen.[69–72] Using a rat model with a balloon-injured common carotid artery, Oparil and colleagues[66, 73–75] showed that estrogen inhibited neointima formation by affecting all three layers of the vascular wall—inhibiting medial smooth-muscle-cell migration and proliferation, stimulating regrowth of the endothelium, and inhibiting adventitial-cell migration into neointima. In responding to vascular injury, this rat model exhibited a sexual dimorphism, with intact males developing a more robust hyperproliferative response than intact females.[75, 76] Apparently, estrogen modulates the expression of vascular smooth-muscle cells and the secretion of a factor or factors that promote the migration of adventitial fibroblasts, by means of a mechanism that depends on intact estrogen receptors.[77, 78] Current laboratory investigations are directed toward identifying the soluble factor(s) involved in this process.[79, 80] Our data suggest that chronic HRT is somehow beneficial in the presence of the vascular injury that occurs to each of the grafted coronary arteries during the surgical anastomoses. It is not clear which aspect of estrogen action might mediate this beneficial effect.

Some clinical data support this beneficial effect. O'Keefe and coauthors[81] retrospectively studied 337 postmenopausal women undergoing elective percutaneous transluminal coronary angioplasty (PTCA). The treatment groups consisted of 137 consecutive women receiving long-term estrogen therapy at the time of PTCA, and the control group comprised 200 nonusers of estrogen who were computer-matched with the estrogen group. All the women were followed up for 65 ± 5 months. Actuarial survival was superior in the estrogen group. Even at 7 years, the cardiovascular event rate was significantly lower in the estrogen group.[81] Also, Khan and associates[82] studied 129 women who underwent stenting of a single coronary artery. Estrogen treatment significantly reduced the need for repeat revascularization. The mean duration of HRT was 8.2 ± 7.9 years. Sullivan and coworkers[83] studied 1098 postmenopausal women undergoing CABG. Although only 92 women (8.4%) were receiving HRT at the time of CABG, they had a 5-year survival rate of 98.8%, compared with 82.3% in estrogen nonusers. The 10-year survival rates were 81.4% and 65.1%, respectively. In a multivariate analysis of long-term survival after CABG, HRT remained significantly beneficial. More recently, Shackelford and colleagues[84] retrospectively studied 734 consecutive postmenopausal women undergoing isolated CABG from 1992 to 1997, of whom 102 (13.9%) received estrogen. Univariate analysis showed that the perioperative mortality was significantly lower in the women receiving HRT (2.7% versus 7.4% [odds ratio = .38; confidence interval = .07–1.2]), although stepwise logistic regression failed to confirm that HRT was a significant predictor of lower mortality. Our data are strikingly similar in a larger patient group. Female sex with HRT was a significant independent predictor of lower in-hospital mortality after isolated or complicated CABG.

Prospective clinical trials designed to confirm our institution's evidence of lower mortality in women who took HRT before admission (see Table 11–11) and to clarify the importance of the duration of postmenopausal status and of HRT administration would be extremely important in predicting the true risk of women undergoing CABG. The resulting knowledge could affect decisions regarding the risk-benefit ratio in individual women considering CABG.

Perioperative Morbidity

With respect to perioperative morbidity, women traditionally have a lower postoperative cardiac output[15, 23] and higher rates of MI[12, 15, 23] and congestive heart failure.[22] Also, one single-institution study[15] and one large multi-institution study examining the STS National Cardiac Surgery Database[85] have shown that female sex is an independent risk factor for perioperative stroke.

Women tend to have shorter cardiopulmonary bypass and aortic cross-clamp times, probably because fewer vessels are bypassed.[23, 32] Compared with men, however, women have a higher transfusion requirement after CABG. Transfusion is known to be a risk factor for mortality and morbidity in women undergoing this operation.[23, 31, 86–89] It is possible that estrogen administration may exert some of its beneficial effect by reducing the transfusion requirements.[90, 91]

Women also tend to have a longer period of mechanical ventilation,[23, 86] longer time in the intensive care unit,[24, 92, 93] and longer hospitalization.[23] Again, this increased morbidity may be related to male-female differences in body size and risk factor profiles rather than to female sex per se.

POSTOPERATIVE OUTCOME

Compared with men, women traditionally have a poorer CABG outcome with respect to relief from angina[12, 94] (85.0% vs. 91.7% at 1 year[94]), improvement in cardiac function,[95, 96] and benefit from rehabilitation programs.[97, 98] These results may reflect the fact that women have a higher degree of preoperative cardiac compromise. They also have a higher rate of early and late graft occlusion.[12, 94] This high occlusion rate is no doubt related to difficulty of anastomosis, lack of complete revascularization, and less frequent use of IMA grafts in women.

Nevertheless, after allowing for different risk profiles, Aldea and associates[24] found no statistical differences between men and women with respect to the incidence of postoperative death, MI, or cerebrovascular accident or transient ischemic attack. These researchers concluded that women are as likely as men to have relief from angina and are less likely to require subsequent reintervention, especially if the IMA was used. Likewise, at 1-year follow-up evaluation of 910 patients undergoing CABG, Tan and coauthors[94] found that women had similar graft patency but a worse clinical outcome because of excess risk factors.

With respect to late (5-year) survival, women appear to equal or even surpass men. In a large Swedish study reported by Herlitz and colleagues,[99] the adjusted relative risks of death during the 5 years after CABG were equal in the two sexes, but the women had more angina. Furthermore, in the BARI series,[22] the unadjusted rates for mortality and for mortality plus MI were similar in the two sexes. The investigators in this study concluded that because women have a higher baseline risk status, female sex is an independent predictor of *better* 5-year survival. Likewise, in the CABG series reported by Abramov and coworkers,[23] involving 4823 patients, actuarial survival at 60 months was greater in women than men (93.1% + 1.7% vs. 90.0% + 1.0%). After adjustment for other risk factors, female sex was found to be protective for long-term survival.

Other studies of late survival after CABG have shown no difference between men and women.[16, 18, 20, 39, 43, 100–103] This lack of difference in mortality persists, holding firm even at 10 years.[18, 20] Therefore, women are most vulnerable during the operative and early postoperative periods, after which their survival rate begins to improve, eventually approaching or surpassing that of men.

COMMENTS

Until recently, CAD was viewed as a "man's disease," and research was focused almost exclusively on men. Even now, clinical decision making continues to be widely influenced by the results of major trials from which women were excluded. In fact, unless a woman has already had an MI, she may be less likely than a man to undergo coronary catheterization or cardiac revascularization.[4, 6, 7]

Investigators in the Fragmin and fast Revascularization during Instability in Coronary artery disease (FRISC II) trial have recently noted that an early invasive strategy did not reduce the risk of future events among women.[103] This study further emphasizes the need for additional research to identify the most appropriate treatment strategy in women with unstable CAD.

Although the outcome of CABG has traditionally been believed to be poorer in women than in men, this disparity tends to disappear when confounding variables are taken into account. Unfortunately, we do not know the extent to which female sex, per se, influences the outcome of CABG. What we do know is that physicians are not justified in withholding this operation from female patients for fear that the results will be less than optimal. Indeed, emerging evidence suggests that women can benefit from CABG at least as much as men. Therefore, public awareness of CAD in women should be promoted so that the disease is diagnosed early, before comorbid conditions supervene. Any gaps in male-female referral rates for coronary diagnosis or treatment should be acknowledged and eliminated, along with any controllable factors that place women at unnecessary risk. If CABG is necessary, revascularization should be complete, with the use of IMA grafts wherever appropriate. Because intraoperative blood transfusion is a major risk factor, it should be minimized with use of techniques to conserve blood. These strategies can optimize the results of CABG in women, allowing similar excellent results to be obtained in both sexes.

Future studies addressing the long-term follow-up of female survivors of CABG in the presence or absence of estrogen would yield valuable information. It is possible that estrogen protection against neointimal formation during and after coronary artery injury (trauma during grafting) maintains graft patency, thus reducing early and late mortality.[45, 81–83] In addition, further studies are needed to evaluate sex-related differences in autonomic responses to acute coronary occlusion, complications related to cardiopulmonary bypass, susceptibility to abnormalities in coagulation (coagulopathy versus thromboembolism), and other factors that might account for discrepant outcomes in men and women undergoing CABG.[92]

References

1. Mosca L, Jones WK, King KB: Awareness, perception, and knowledge of heart disease risk and prevention among women in the United States. American Heart Association Women's Heart Disease and Stroke Campaign Task Force. Arch Fam Med 9:506, 2000.
2. American Heart Association: Estimated Inpatient Cardiovascular Operations, Procedure and Patient Data by Sex, Age and Region. 2000 Heart and Stroke Statistical Update. American Heart Association, Dallas, 1999, p 27.
3. Johnson PA, Goldman L, Orav EJ, et al: Gender differences in the management of acute chest pain: Support for the "Yentl syndrome." J Gen Intern Med 11:209, 1996.
4. Healy B: The Yentl syndrome. N Engl J Med 325:2714, 1991.
5. Tobin JN, Wassertheil-Smoller S, Wexler JP, et al: Sex bias in considering coronary bypass surgery. Ann Intern Med 107:19, 1987.
6. Steingart RM, Packer M, Hamm P, et al: Sex differences in the management of coronary artery disease. Survival and Ventricular Enlargement Investigators. N Engl J Med 325:226, 1991.
7. Ayanian JZ, Epstein AM: Differences in the use of procedures between women and men hospitalized for coronary heart disease. N Engl J Med 325:221, 1991.
8. Roeters van Lennep JE, Zwinderman AH, Roeters van Lennep HW: Gender differences in diagnosis and treatment of coronary artery disease from 1981 to 1997: No evidence for the Yentl syndrome. Eur Heart J 21:911, 2000.
9. Orth-Gormer K: New light on the Yentl syndrome. Eur Heart J 21: 874, 2000.
10. Kennedy JW, Kaiser GC, Fisher LD: Multivariate discriminant and angiographic predictors of operative mortality from the Collaborative Study in Coronary Artery Surgery (CASS). J Thorac Cardiovasc Surg 80:876, 1980.
11. Edwards FH, Carey JS, Grover FL, et al: Impact of gender on coronary bypass operative mortality. Ann Thorac Surg 66:125, 1998.
12. Hussain KMA, Kogan A, Estrada AQ: Referral pattern and outcome in men and women undergoing coronary artery bypass surgery: A critical review. Angiology 49:243, 1998.
13. O'Connor GT, Morton JR, Diehl MJ, et al: Differences between men and women in in-hospital mortality associated with coronary artery bypass graft surgery. The Northern New England Cardiovascular Disease Study Group. Circulation 88(5 Part 1):2104, 1993.

14. Wenger NK: Women, myocardial infarction, and coronary revascularization: Concordant and discordant clinical trial and registry data. Cardiol Rev 7:117, 1999.
15. Hogue CW, Murphy SF, Schechtman KB, et al: Risk factors for early or delayed stroke after cardiac surgery. Circulation 100:642, 1999.
16. Davis KB, Chaitman B, Ryan T, et al: Comparison of 15-year survival of men and women after initial medical or surgical treatment for coronary artery disease: A CASS Registry study. J Am Coll Cardiol 25: 1000, 1995.
17. Krumholz HM, Douglas PS, Lauer MS, et al: Selection of patients for coronary angiography and coronary revascularization early after myocardial infarction: Is there evidence for a gender bias? Ann Intern Med 116:785, 1992.
18. Eaker ED, Kronmal R, Kennedy JW, et al: Comparison of the long-term, postsurgical survival of women and men in the Coronary Artery Surgery Study (CASS). Am Heart J 117:71, 1989.
19. Adler DS, Goldman L, O'Neil A, et al: Long-term survival of more than 2,000 patients after coronary artery bypass grafting. Am J Cardiol 58:195, 1986.
20. Loop FD, Golding LR, Macmillan JP, et al: Coronary artery surgery in women compared with men: Analyses of risks and long-term results. J Am Coll Cardiol 1:383, 1983.
21. Killen DA, Reed WA, Arnold M, et al: Coronary artery bypass in women: Long-term survival. Ann Thorac Surg 34:559, 1982.
22. Jacobs AK, Kelsey SF, Brooks MM, et al: Better outcome for women compared with men undergoing coronary revascularization: A report from the bypass angioplasty revascularization investigation. Circulation 98:1279, 1998.
23. Abramov D, Tamariz MG, Sever JY, et al: The influence of gender on the outcome of coronary artery bypass surgery. Ann Thorac Surg 70: 800, 2000.
24. Aldea GS, Gaudiani JM, Shapira OM, et al: Effect of gender on postoperative outcomes and hospital stays after coronary artery bypass grafting. Ann Thorac Surg 67:1097, 1999.
25. Nardi P, Pellegrino A, De Paulis R, et al: Coronary heart surgery in women: The risk factors and short-term results. Ital Heart J 1(4 Suppl):537, 2000.
26. Stokes J III, Kannel WB, Wolf PA, et al: The relative importance of selected risk factors for various manifestations of cardiovascular disease among women and men from 35–64 years: 30 years of follow-up in the Framingham Study. Circulation 75(suppl V):V65, 1987.
27. Lerner DJ, Kannel WB: Patterns of coronary heart disease morbidity and mortality in the sexes: A 26 year follow-up of the Framingham population. Am Heart J 111:383, 1986.
28. Castelli WP: Epidemiology of coronary heart disease: The Framingham study. Am J Med 76:4, 1984.
29. Leaf DA, Sanmarco ME, Bahl RA: Gender differences in coronary angiographic findings from 1972 through 1981 in Los Angeles, California. Angiology 41:609, 1990.
30. Kyriakidis J, Petropoulakis P, Androulakis A, et al: Sex differences in anatomy of coronary artery disease. J Clin Epidemiol 48:723, 1995.
31. Utley JR, Wilde EF, Leyland SA, et al: Intraoperative blood transfusion is a major risk factor for coronary artery bypass grafting in women. Ann Thorac Surg 60:570, 1995.
32. Williams MR, Choudhri AF, Morales DLS: Gender differences in patients undergoing coronary artery bypass surgery, from a mandatory statewide database. Journal of Gender-Specific Medicine 3:41, 2000.
33. Hannan EL, Bernard HR, Kilburn JR, et al: Gender differences in mortality rates for coronary bypass surgery. Am Heart J 123:866, 1992.
34. Davis KB: Coronary artery bypass graft surgery in women. In Eaker ED, Packard B, Wenger NK, et al (eds): Coronary Artery Disease in Women, New York, Haymarket-Doyma, 1987, p 247.
35. Weintraub WS, Wenger NK, Jones EL, et al: Changing clinical characteristics of coronary surgery patients: Differences between men and women. Circulation 88(Part 2):79, 1993.
36. Khan SS, Nessim S, Gray R, et al: Increased mortality of women in coronary artery bypass surgery: Evidence for referral bias. Ann Intern Med 112:561, 1990.
37. Koch CG, Higgins TL, Capdeville M, et al: The risk of coronary artery surgery in women: A matched comparison using preoperative severity of illness scoring. J Cardiothorac Vasc Anesth 10:839, 1996.
38. Yap AG, Baladi N, Allman G, et al: Coronary artery bypass surgery on small patients. J Invasive Cardiol 12:542, 2000.
39. Douglas JS Jr, King SB III, Jones EL, et al: Reduced efficacy of coronary bypass surgery in women. Circulation 64(Suppl II):II11, 1981.
40. Bolooki H, Vargas A, Green R, et al: Results of direct coronary artery surgery in women. J Thorac Cardiovasc Surg 69:271, 1975.
41. Tyras DH, Barner HB, Kaiser GC, et al: Myocardial revascularization in women. Ann Thorac Surg 25:449, 1978.
42. Kennedy JW, Kaiser GC, Fisher LD, et al: Clinical and angiographic predictors of operative mortality for the Collaborative Study in Coronary Artery Surgery Study (CASS). Circulation 63:793, 1981.
43. Hall RJ, Elayda MA, Gray, et al: Coronary artery bypass: Long-term follow-up of 22,284 consecutive patients. Circulation 68:II20, 1983.
44. Laird-Meeter K, Penn OCKM, Haalebos MMP, et al: Survival in 1041 patients with consecutive aortocoronary bypass operations. Eur Heart J 5:35, 1984.
45. Nussmeier NA, Marino MR, Vaughn WK: Women undergoing coronary artery surgery: Hormone replacement therapy improves survival. Anesth Analg 90:SCA5, 2000.
46. Brett KM, Makans JH: Use of postmenopausal hormone replacement. Am J Epidemiol 145:56, 1997.
47. Hulley S, Grady D, Bush T, et al: Randomized trial of estrogen plus progestin for secondary prevention of coronary heart disease in postmenopausal women. JAMA 280:605, 1998.
48. Bush TL: Lessons from HERS: The null and beyond. J Womens Health 7:781, 1998.
49. Herrington DM: The HERS trial results: Paradigms lost? Ann Intern Med 131:463, 1999.
50. Stampfer MJ, Colditz GA, Willett WC, et al: Postmenopausal estrogen therapy and cardiovascular disease: Ten-year follow-up from the Nurses' Health Study. N Engl J Med 325:756, 1991.
51. Grodstein F, Stampfer MJ, Manson JE, et al: Postmenopausal estrogen and progestin use and the risk of cardiovascular disease. N Engl J Med 335:453, 1996.
52. Henderson BE, Paganini-Hill A, Ross RK: Decreased mortality in users of estrogen replacement therapy. Arch Intern Med 151:75, 1991.
53. Grodstein F, Stampfer M: The epidemiology of coronary heart disease and estrogen replacement in postmenopausal women. Prog Cardiovasc Dis 38:199, 1995.
54. Grodstein F, Stampfer MJ, Colditz GA, et al: Postmenopausal hormone therapy and mortality. N Engl J Med 336:1769, 1997.
55. Ettinger B, Friedman GD, Bush T, et al: Reduced mortality associated with long-term postmenopausal estrogen therapy. Obstet Gynecol 87: 6, 1996.
56. Gruchow HW, Anderson AJ, Barboriak JJ, et al: Postmenopausal use of estrogen and occlusion of coronary arteries. Am Heart J 154: 954, 1988.
57. Hong MK, Romm PA, Reagan K, et al: Effects of estrogen replacement therapy on serum lipid values and angiographically defined coronary artery disease in postmenopausal women. Am J Cardiol 69: 176, 1992.
58. Sullivan JM, Vander Zwagg R, Lemp GF, et al: Estrogen replacement and coronary artery disease: Effect on survival in postmenopausal women. Arch Intern Med 150:2557, 1990.
59. Stampfer MJ, Colditz GA: Estrogen replacement therapy and coronary heart disease: A quantitative assessment of the epidemiologic evidence. Prev Med 20:47, 1991.
60. Writing Group for the PEPI Trial: Effects of estrogen or estrogen/progestin regimens on heart disease risk factors in postmenopausal women: The Postmenopausal Estrogen/Progestin Interventions (PEPI) Trial. JAMA 273:199, 1995.
61. Matthews KA, Kuller LH, Wing RR, et al: Prior to the use of estrogen replacement therapy, are users healthier than non-users? Am J Epidemiol 143:971, 1996.
62. Herrington DM, Reboussin DM, Brosnihan B, et al: Effects of estrogen replacement on the progression of coronary-artery atherosclerosis. N Engl J Med 343:522, 2000.
63. Lenfant C: Preliminary trends in the Women's Health Initiative. National Heart, Lung, and Blood Institute Communications Office, Bethesda, MD, April 3, 2000.
64. Manson JE, Martin KA: Postmenopausal hormone replacement therapy. N Engl J Med 345:34, 2001.
65. Mosca L, Collins P, Herrington DM, et al: Hormone replacement therapy and cardiovascular disease. A statement for healthcare professionals from the American Heart Association, 2001.
66. Oparil S, Chen SJ, Chen YF, et al: Estrogen attenuates the adventitial contribution to neointima formation in injured rat carotid arteries. Cardiovasc Res 44:608, 1999.
67. Orimo A, Inoue S, Ouchi Y, et al: Vascular smooth muscle cells possess estrogen receptors and respond to estrogen. Ann N Y Acad Sci 748: 592, 1995.

68. Farhat MY, Abi-Younes S, Ramwell PW: Non-genomic effects of estrogen and the vessel wall. Biochem Pharmacol 51:571, 1996.
69. Shi Y, O'Brien JE Jr, Fard A, et al: Adventitial myofibroblasts contribute to neointimal formation in injured porcine coronary arteries. Circulation 94:1655, 1996.
70. Shi Y, O'Brian JE Jr, Ala-Kokko L, et al: Origin of extracellular matrix synthesis during coronary repair. Circulation 95:997, 1997.
71. Shi Y, Pienick M, Fard A, et al: Adventitial remodeling after coronary arterial injury. Circulation 93:340, 1996.
72. Scott NA, Cipolla GD, Ross CE, et al: Identification of a potential role for the adventitia in vascular lesion formation after balloon overstretch injury of porcine coronary arteries. Circulation 93:2178, 1996.
73. White CR, Shelton J, Chen SJ, et al: Estrogen restores endothelial cell function in an experimental model of vascular injury. Circulation 96:1624, 1997.
74. Mori T, Durand J, Chen YF, et al: Effects of short-term estrogen treatment on the neointimal response to balloon injury of rat carotid artery. Am J Cardiol 85:1276, 2000.
75. Chen SJ, Li H, Durand J, et al: Estrogen reduces myointimal proliferation after balloon injury of the rat carotid artery. Circulation 93: 577, 1996.
76. Oparil S, Levine RL, Chen SJ, et al: Sexually dimorphic response of the balloon-injured rat carotid artery to hormone treatment. Circulation 95:1301, 1997.
77. Li G, Chen YF, Greene GL, et al: Estrogen inhibits vascular smooth muscle cell-dependent adventitial fibroblast migration in vitro. Circulation 100:1639, 1999.
78. Bakir S, Mori T, Durand J, et al: Estrogen-induced vasoprotection is estrogen-receptor dependent: Evidence from the balloon-injured rat carotid artery model. Circulation 101;2342, 2000.
79. Li G, Chen YF, Kelpke SS, et al: Estrogen attenuates integrin-B3-dependent adventitial fibroblast migration after inhibition of osteopontin production in vascular smooth muscle cells. Circulation 101:2949, 2000.
80. Srivatsa SS, Fitzpatrick LA, Tsao PW, et al: Selective avB3 integrin blockade potently limits neointimal hyperplasia and lumen stenosis following deep coronary arterial stent injury: Evidence for the functional importance of integrin avB3 and osteopontin expression during neointima formation. Cardiovasc Res 36:408, 1997.
81. O'Keefe JH, Kim SC, Hall RR, et al: Estrogen replacement therapy after coronary angioplasty in women. J Am Coll Cardiol 29:1, 1997.
82. Khan MA, Liu MW, Singh D, et al: Long-term (three years) effect of estrogen therapy on major adverse cardiac events in postmenopausal women after intracoronary stenting. Am J Cardiol 86:330, 2000.
83. Sullivan JM, El-Zeky F, Vander Zwaag R, et al: Effect on survival of estrogen replacement therapy after coronary artery bypass grafting. Am J Cardiol 79:847, 1997.
84. Shackelford DP, Daniels S, Hoffman MK, et al: Estrogen therapy in women undergoing coronary artery bypass grafting: Effect on surgical complications. Obstet Gynecol 95:732, 2000.
85. Hogue CW, Barzilai B, Pieper KS, et al: Sex differences in neurological outcomes and mortality after cardiac surgery. Circulation 103:2133, 2001.
86. Women CABG patients require more blood, ventilator time. Qual Lett Healthc Lead 10:10, 1998.
87. Ramani R, Pagala M, Tyagaraj C, et al: Characteristics of female and male patients who require blood transfusion during coronary artery bypass graft surgery [abstract A-121]. Abstracts of the 2000 Meeting of the American Society of Anesthesiologists, San Francisco, October 14–18, 2000. Available at: http://lww.anesthesiology.org. Accessed October 20, 2000.
88. Punjala M, Udeh C, Pagala M, et al: Blood volume and blood transfusion for female and male patients undergoing coronary artery bypass graft surgery [abstract A-310]. Abstracts of the 2000 Meeting of the American Society of Anesthesiologists, San Francisco, October 14–18, 2000. Available at: http://lww.anesthesiology.org. Accessed October 20, 2000.
89. Shevde K, Pagala M, Kashikar A, et al: Gender is an essential determinant of blood transfusion in patients undergoing coronary artery bypass graft procedure. J Clin Anesth 12:109, 2000.
90. Boyd G, Diethelm G, Gelman S: Correcting prolonged bleeding during renal transplantation with estrogen or plasma. Arch Surg 131: 160, 1996.
91. Frenette L, Cox J, McArdle P, et al: Conjugated estrogen reduces transfusion and coagulation factor requirements in orthotopic liver transplantation. Anesth Analg 86:1183, 1998.
92. Butterworth J, James R, Prielipp R, et al: Female gender associates with increased duration of intubation and length of stay after coronary artery surgery. CABG Clinical Benchmarking Database Participants. Anesthesiology 92:414, 2000.
93. Rankin SH: Differences in recovery from cardiac surgery: A profile of male and female patients. Heart Lung 19:481, 1990.
94. Tan ES, van der Meer J, Jan de Kam P, et al: Worse clinical outcome but similar graft patency in women versus men one year after coronary artery bypass graft surgery owing to an excess of exposed risk factors in women. CABADAS. Research Group of the Interuniversity Cardiology Institute of The Netherlands. Coronary Artery Bypass Graft Occlusion by Aspirin, Dipyridamole and Acenocoumarol/phenoprocoumon Study. J Am Coll Cardiol 34:1760, 1999.
95. Gardner TJ, Horneffer PJ, Gott VL, et al: Coronary artery bypass surgery in women: A ten-year prospective. Ann Surg 201:780, 1985.
96. Jeffery DL, Vijayanagar RR, Bognolo DA, et al: Results of coronary bypass surgery in elderly women. Ann Thorac Surg 42:550, 1986.
97. Ades PA, Waldmann ML, Polk DM, et al: Referral patterns and exercise response in the rehabilitation of female coronary patients aged >62 years. Am J Cardiol 69:1422, 1992.
98. Murdaugh C: Coronary heart disease in women. Prog Cardiovasc Nurs 1:2, 1986.
99. Herlitz J, Brandrup-Wognsen G, Karlson BW, et al: Mortality, risk indicators of death, mode of death and symptoms of angina pectoris during 5 years after coronary artery bypass grafting in men and women. J Intern Med 247:500, 2000.
100. Council on Ethical and Judicial Affairs, American Medical Association: Gender disparities in clinical decision making. JAMA 266:559, 1991.
101. Lindenau KF, Olthoff D, Adam H, et al: Coronary surgery in females. Herz 12:296, 1987.
102. Rahimtoola SH, Bennett AJ, Grunkemeier GL, et al: Survival at 15 to 18 years after coronary bypass surgery for angina in women. Circulation 88(Part 2):II71, 1993.
103. Lagerqvist B, Säfström K, Ståhle E, et al: Is early invasive treatment of unstable coronary artery disease equally effective for both women and men? J Am Coll Cardiol 38:41, 2001.

11.6 Rehabilitation

Susan Wilansky

At each stage in the diagnosis and treatment of heart disease, women appear to be at a disadvantage with respect to referral patterns and resource utilization. In the long term, women benefit from cardiac diagnosis and treatment at least as much as men[1–3] but are less likely to receive optimal therapy.[4, 5] Moreover, once the diagnosis has been established and they have received treatment, women are less likely to be referred to a cardiac rehabilitation program. In fact, comprehensive cardiac rehabilitation is generally directed toward young or middle-aged white men who have had a first, uncomplicated MI. These patients are easy to treat but may have the least to gain from rehabilitation.[6] Relatively few data are available concerning the rehabilitation of other groups, including women, the elderly, and racial minorities.

This discussion examines the goals and benefits of cardiac rehabilitation, the types of currently available programs, and sex-related differences in such programs. It also points out ways in which women can be encouraged to participate in rehabilitation.

GOALS AND BENEFITS OF CARDIAC REHABILITATION

Cardiac rehabilitation originated during the 1950s as an exercise-based response to treatment regimens involving prolonged bed rest.[7, 8] Over the years, it has evolved into a multidisciplinary effort that involves baseline patient assessment, nutritional counseling, risk factor modification (lipids, hypertension, weight, diabetes, and smoking), psychosocial management, physical activity counseling, and exercise training.[9] The goals of rehabilitation are to (1) limit the impact of heart disease, (2) minimize mortality, (3) prevent further cardiac events, and (4) enhance the patient's quality of life. Specifically, rehabilitation lowers the cardiovascular death rate,[10, 11] improves exercise tolerance (by 30%[12–15]), reduces ischemia,[16, 17] decreases stress,[18] improves blood lipid levels,[18] decreases cigarette smoking,[18] and slows the progress of CAD.[19–21] Rehabilitation also reduces depression, promotes emotional well-being, and enhances psychosocial function.[18, 22–24] These benefits may be at least as great in women as in men.[12, 15, 22, 25]

Most patients are referred for cardiac rehabilitation because they have undergone MI, CABG, or PTCA. Other indications are heart transplantation, valve surgery, angina, heart failure, and conduction disturbances. Of the patients who could benefit from a rehabilitation program, as few as 11%[26] actually enroll in such a program.

TYPE AND DURATION OF REHABILITATION

The traditional cardiac rehabilitation program is initiated 3 to 6 weeks after a cardiac event and lasts for 12 weeks. The program is usually held on the hospital premises but may also take place in a university, a community center, or some other private facility. Program personnel include cardiologists, physiotherapists, nurses, occupational therapists, psychologists, social workers, and dietitians.

Traditional cardiac rehabilitation programs have been criticized because of suboptimal participation, poor facilitation of independent exercise, use of expensive ECG monitoring, and lack of insurance reimbursement.[27] As a result, some centers have adopted a home-based exercise protocol for low- to moderate-risk patients. This protocol is implemented with the aid of educational support meetings, telephone follow-up, and transtelephonic monitoring if necessary.[28] Compared with traditional programs, the home-based protocol is equally effective at improving physiologic outcomes while costing considerably less and being more attractive to patients.[27, 28]

Exercise conditioning alone, without modification of dietary intake, may be insufficient for attaining the desired risk factor goals.[29] Cardiac rehabilitation exercise programs burn surprisingly few calories, and, in the short term (3 months), have little effect on obesity and dyslipidemia.[30] Even aggressive cardiac rehabilitation may fail to alter the postoperative weight or risk profile of severely obese patients undergoing CABG,[31] leaving them at risk for further disease progression and further CABG procedures. To maximize caloric expenditure and modify obesity and lipid risk factors, alternative training programs should be considered.[30]

Programs that last for longer than 12 weeks may confer an even greater level of benefit. In fact, in CABG recipients, the effects of rehabilitation may not be fully realized even within the first 12 months after surgery.[32] Morrin and colleagues[33] found that physical activity and physical function peaked at 3 months and were maintained at 6 months; with respect to mental health recovery, however, a significant improvement was not achieved until between 3 and 6 months. This finding is important for the 20% of coronary patients who have symptoms of depression.[34] If not treated, depression tends to persist, raising the risk of major adverse coronary events and of death as much as fourfold at 6 months and 1 year.[24, 35]

Cardiac rehabilitation is not necessarily limited to the period after hospital admission or surgery. Some experts believe that, for low-risk patients awaiting elective cardiovascular procedures, preoperative exercise training can improve functional capacity and quality of life, allowing such patients to recover more quickly from surgery.[36] Such training can be continued during the hospital stay and after the patient returns home.

Minimization of Risk

Although cardiac rehabilitation programs are normally quite safe, they must be designed to minimize risk. For cardiac patients undergoing a brisk unsupervised workout, the risk of sudden death is 1 in 60,000 to 65,000 person-hours of exercise.[37] In a supervised cardiac rehabilitation program, that risk decreases to 1 in 763,972 person-hours of exercise.[38] When exercise-related cardiac arrest does occur, it is usually caused by ventricular fibrillation or tachycardia; in a supervised situation, rapid defibrillation is possible, so the event is rarely fatal. Arrhythmias are recorded in a third of program participants (33.5%) but preclude rehabilitation in only 5%.[39]

Before embarking upon any exercise program, patients should be in stable condition and receiving an optimal regimen of medication. They should undergo an exercise test while taking their customary medication.

High-risk patients include those with large or multiple infarcts, an ejection fraction of less than 30%, a low exercise tolerance, and residual ischemia or ventricular arrhythmias.[6] These patients should be enrolled in a formal, supervised program that includes ECG monitoring if necessary.

Medium-risk patients have medium-sized infarcts and a moderately reduced exercise tolerance, possibly with residual ischemia.[6] These patients should begin rehabilitation in a supervised setting; if no problems develop, the patients may be transferred to a home-based program.

In contrast, low-risk patients have small infarcts, a satisfactory exercise tolerance, and no residual ischemia or ventricular arrhythmias. These patients can safely follow a home-based exercise plan from the start.[6, 40, 41]

SEX-RELATED DIFFERENCES IN CARDIAC REHABILITATION

Participation Patterns

Although women have 40% of all adverse coronary events,[42] they account for only 20% of all participants in structured cardiac rehabilitation programs.[43–45] Enrollment in such programs is particularly low among minority populations and patients older than 65 years.[46] In fact, increased age and female sex are independently associated with not being invited to attend cardiac rehabilitation.[47] The greatest sex-related disparity in enrollment occurs among post-MI patients, followed by post-CABG patients; in contrast, the disparity is minimal among post-PTCA patients.[46] Up to 70% of these patients undergoing cardiac procedures could probably benefit from a supervised exercise program.[46] The most important factors that influence a patient's decision to participate in rehabilitation are physician recommendation and encouragement from family members.[48]

Patient Profiles

Upon becoming eligible for cardiac rehabilitation, women tend to be older and sicker than men and to have a lower exercise tolerance.[12, 13, 46] Women have more cardiac risk factors[15, 49] than men but are less likely to have undergone an invasive cardiac procedure.[50] In at least one study, severity of disease was positively related to functional impairment in women but not in men.[23] Women are more likely to be unemployed or retired[12]; if employed, they have significantly lower return-to-work rates than men.[22] Women are also more likely to be nonwhite,[12] to be depressed,[23] to live alone,[46] to be socially inhibited,[51] and to lack adequate psychosocial support.[22] On quality of life surveys, they have a significantly lower score than men do.[50, 52]

Because women have a greater degree of dysfunction, they stand to gain a greater benefit from cardiac rehabilitation. Unfortunately, they are also less likely to participate in this intervention. Even when they do enroll, they have poorer adherence rates and significantly higher dropout rates than men.[22] Moreover, despite a greater prevalence of coronary risk factors and a higher mortality after MI, black women are less likely than white women to complete a 12-week rehabilitation program.[53]

Barriers to female participation in cardiac rehabilitation include advanced age, concomitant illness, lack of transportation, insufficient insurance, inconvenient timing, work conflicts, family responsibilities, and language difficulties.[26, 48, 54] Also, many eligible women are simply not encouraged by their primary care physician to attend such programs.

Patient Preferences

In old-style rehabilitation programs, all patients tended to receive the same type of therapy. Because most of these programs were designed for middle-aged men, they were unappealing and unsatisfying to women. For women older than 60 years, the most important self-defined issues are (1) maintaining their functional capacity, (2) promoting resiliency, and (3) dealing with memory problems; for younger women, emotional concerns are paramount.[55] In general, women want to feel safe and to exercise without having symptoms or feeling tired.[51, 56–58] They want peer group support, social bonding with other patients, and pleasant interaction with staff members.[25, 57]

Ideally, women should be presented with a personalized regimen that gradually builds in intensity and duration. High-impact activities should be avoided because they place older women at risk for injury.[57] Exercise programs must adopt a flexible approach: A good outcome is more desirable than rigid adherence to a formal protocol.[7] During treadmill exercise, elevation may be more important than speed in achieving the desired intensity of activity.[25] During home-based exercise, the entire activity need not be accomplished during a single session but, rather, may be divided into intermittent short sessions.[25]

Rather than promoting physical fitness per se, rehabilitation programs should emphasize health benefits and quality of life.[59, 60] For instance, early sessions might focus on the activities of daily living.[61] Women prefer to have more options besides cycling and treadmill exercise. Additional options should include resistance training and recreational games.[57, 58] Pleasant surroundings and background music can make these activities more enjoyable. Also, the patient's family or spouse may be invited to attend rehabilitation sessions.

Women prefer to engage in joint goal-setting and periodic discussion of progress with staff members.[56] Participants who achieve their stated goals should receive positive reinforcement, including some type of award or other recognition.

Unfortunately, without a long-term commitment to the maintenance of healthy habits, the benefits of cardiac rehabilitation disappear. In assessing women's patterns of exercise after cardiac rehabilitation, Moore and coauthors[62] found that, during the first month, 83% of the subjects participated in exercise; after the first month, one third of the subjects stopped exercising, and by the end of the 3-month study period, only 50% of the women were still exercising. Therefore, one of the most important goals of rehabilitation is to promote a permanently healthy lifestyle, including a long-term commitment to exercise. By empowering women to take responsibility for their own physical and emotional well-being, cardiac rehabilitation can have the maximal benefit.

CONCLUSION

When indicated, rehabilitation should be standard practice for both men and women with cardiac disease. Because women generally enter these programs with a greater functional deficit, they may benefit even more than men. Nevertheless, women tend to be underrepresented in rehabilitation programs. As the main gatekeepers for such programs, primary care physicians must be made more aware of the importance of rehabilitation. In the future, the growing average age of westernized populations and the increasing longevity of patients with cardiovascular disease will lead to an even greater emphasis on cardiac rehabilitation services.

References

1. Jacobs AK, Kelsey SF, Brooks MM, et al: Better outcome for women compared with men undergoing coronary revascularization: A report from the Bypass Angioplasty Revascularization Investigation. Circulation 98:1279, 1998.
2. Abramov D, Tamariz MG, Sever JY, et al: The influence of gender on the outcome of coronary artery bypass surgery. Ann Thorac Surg 70: 800, 2000.
3. Aldea GS, Gaudiani JM, Shapira OM, et al: Effect of gender on postoperative outcomes and hospital stays after coronary artery bypass grafting. Ann Thorac Surg 67:1097, 1999.
4. Johnson PA, Goldman L, Orav EJ, et al: Gender differences in the management of acute chest pain: Support for the "Yentl syndrome." J Gen Intern Med 11:209, 1996.
5. Hussain KMA, Kogan A, Estrada AQ: Referral pattern and outcome in men and women undergoing coronary artery bypass surgery: A critical review. Angiology 49:243, 1998.
6. Bethell HJ: Cardiac rehabilitation: From Hellerstein to the millennium. Int J Clin Pract 54:92, 2000.
7. Thompson DR, De Bono DP: How valuable is cardiac rehabilitation and who should get it? Heart 82:545, 1999.
8. Hellerstein HK, Hornsten E: Rehabilitation of patients with heart disease. Postgrad Med 15:265, 1954.
9. Balady GJ, Ades PA, Comoss P, et al: Core components of cardiac rehabilitation/secondary prevention programs: A statement for healthcare professionals from the American Heart Association and the American Association of Cardiovascular and Pulmonary Rehabilitation. Circulation 102:1069, 2000.
10. Oldridge NB, Guyatt GH, Fischer ME, et al: Cardiac rehabilitation after myocardial infarction: Combined experience of randomized trials. JAMA 260:945, 1988.
11. O'Connor GT, Buring JE, Yusuf S, et al: An overview of randomized trials of rehabilitation with exercise after myocardial infarction. Circulation 80:234, 1989.
12. Cannistra LB, Balady GJ, O'Malley CJ, et al: Comparison of the clinical profile and outcome of women and men in cardiac rehabilitation. Am J Cardiol 69:1274, 1992.
13. Ades PA, Waldmann ML, Polk DM, et al: Referral patterns and exercise response in the rehabilitation of female coronary patients aged greater than or equal to 62 years. Am J Cardiol 69:1422, 1992.
14. Kavanaugh T, Mertens DJ, Kennedy J: Can women benefit from cardiac rehabilitation programmes? Circulation 94:I419, 1996.
15. Lavie CJ, Milani RV: Effects of cardiac rehabilitation and exercise training on exercise capacity, coronary risk factors, behavioral characteristics, and quality of life in women. Am J Cardiol 75:340, 1995.
16. Ehsani AA, Health GW, Hagberg JM, et al: Effects of 12 months of intense exercise training on ischemic ST-segment depression in patients with coronary artery disease. Circulation 64:1116, 1981.
17. Todd IC, Ballantyne D: Antianginal efficacy of exercise training: A comparison with beta blockade. Br Heart J 64:14, 1990.
18. Cardiac Rehabilitation Guideline Panel, Wenger NK, co-chair, Froelicher ES, co-chair: Cardiac Rehabilitation. (Clinical Practice Guideline No. 17; DHHS publication No. PHS 88-3427.) U.S. Department of Health and Human Services, Public Health Service, National Center for Health Services Research and Health Care Technology Assessment, Rockville, MD, 1995.
19. Hambrecht R, Niebauer J, Marburger C, et al: Various intensities of leisure time physical activity in patients with coronary artery disease: Effects of cardiorespiratory fitness and progression of coronary atherosclerotic lesions. J Am Coll Cardiol 22:468, 1993.
20. Schuler G, Hambrecht R, Schlierf G, et al: Regular physical exercise and low-fat diet: Effects on progression of coronary artery disease. Circulation 86:1, 1992.
21. Schuler G, Hambrecht R, Schlierf G, et al: Myocardial perfusion and regression of coronary artery disease in patients on a regimen of intensive physical exercise and low fat diet. J Am Coll Cardiol 19: 34, 1992.
22. Brezinka V, Kittel F: Psychosocial factors of coronary heart disease in women: A review. Soc Sci Med 42:1351, 1996.
23. Con AH, Linden W, Thompson JM, et al: The psychology of men and women recovering from coronary artery bypass surgery. J Cardiopulm Rehabil 19:152, 1999.
24. Lavie CJ, Milani RV, Cassidy MM, et al: Effects of cardiac rehabilitation and exercise training programs in women with depression. Am J Cardiol 83:1480, 1999.
25. Limacher MC: Exercise and cardiac rehabilitation in women. Cardiol Rev 6:240, 1998.
26. Blackburn GG, Foody JM, Sprecher DL, et al: Cardiac rehabilitation participation patterns in a large, tertiary care center: Evidence for selection bias. J Cardiopulm Rehabil 20:189, 2000.
27. Carlson JJ, Johnson JA, Franklin BA, et al: Program participation, exercise adherence, cardiovascular outcomes, and program cost of traditional versus modified cardiac rehabilitation. Am J Cardiol 86:17, 2000.
28. Ades PA, Pashkow FJ, Fletcher G, et al: A controlled trial of cardiac rehabilitation in the home setting using electrocardiographic and voice transtelephonic monitoring. Am Heart J 139:543, 2000.
29. Brochu M, Poehlman ET, Savage P, et al: Modest effects of exercise training alone on coronary risk factors and body composition in coronary patients. J Cardiopulm Rehabil 20:180, 2000.
30. Savage PD, Brochu M, Scott P, et al: Low caloric expenditure in cardiac rehabilitation. Am Heart J 140:527, 2000.
31. Rohs T Jr, Polanski P, Just SC, et al: Early complications and long-term survival in severely obese coronary bypass patients. Am Surg 61: 949, 1995.
32. Ashton KC, Saccucci MS: A follow-up study of ethnic and gender differences in cardiac rehabilitation. Rehabil Nurs 21:187, 1996.
33. Morrin L, Black S, Reid R: Impact of duration in a cardiac rehabilitation program on coronary risk profile and health-related quality of life outcomes. J Cardiopulm Rehabil 20:115, 2000.
34. Lavie CJ, Milani RV: Benefits of cardiac rehabilitation and exercise training. Chest 117:5, 2000.
35. Milani RV, Lavie CJ: Prevalence and effects of cardiac rehabilitation on depression in the elderly with coronary artery disease. Am J Cardiol 81:1233, 1998.
36. Arthur HM, Daniels C, McKelvie R, et al: Effect of a preoperative intervention on preoperative and postoperative outcomes in low-risk patients awaiting elective coronary artery bypass graft surgery: A randomized, controlled trial. Ann Intern Med 133:253, 2000.
37. Fletcher GF, Froelicher VF, Hartley LH, et al: Exercise standards: A statement for health professionals from the American Heart Association. Circulation 82:2286, 1990.
38. Van Camp SP, Peterson RA: Cardiovascular complications of outpatient cardiac rehabilitation programs. JAMA 256:1160, 1986.
39. Galante A, Pietroiusti A, Cavazzini C, et al: Incidence and risk factors associated with cardiac arrhythmias during rehabilitation after coronary artery bypass surgery. Arch Phys Med Rehabil 81:947, 2000.

40. Lewin B, Robertson IH, Casy EL, et al: Effects of self-help myocardial infarction rehabilitation on psychological adjustment and use of health services. Lancet 339:1036, 1992.
41. Thompson DR, Bowman DS, Kitson AL, et al: Cardiac rehabilitation services in England and Wales: A national survey. Int J Cardiol 59: 299, 1997.
42. Lerner DJ, Kannel WB: Patterns of coronary heart disease morbidity and mortality in the sexes: A 26-year follow-up of the Framingham population. Am Heart J 111:383, 1986.
43. Schuster P, Waldron J: Gender differences in cardiac rehabilitation patients. Rehabil Nursing 16:248, 1991.
44. Ades PA, Waldmann ML, McCann WJ, et al: Predictors of cardiac rehabilitation participation in older coronary patients. Arch Intern Med 52:1033, 1992.
45. Evenson KR, Rosamond WD, Luepker RV: Predictors of outpatient cardiac rehabilitation utilization. The Minnesota Heart Surgery Registry. J Cardiopulm Rehabil 18:192, 1998.
46. Thomas RJ, Miller NJ, Lamendola C, et al: National survey on gender differences in cardiac rehabilitation programs. J Cardiopulm Rehabil 16:402, 1996.
47. Pell J, Pell A, Morrison C, et al: Retrospective study of influence of deprivation on uptake of cardiac rehabilitation. BMJ 313:267, 1996.
48. Lieberman L, Meana M, Stewart D: Cardiac rehabilitation: Gender differences in factors influencing participation. J Womens Health 7: 717, 1998.
49. O'Farrel P, Murray J, Huston P, et al: Sex differences in cardiac rehabilitation. Can J Cardiol 16:319, 2000.
50. Deshotels A, Planchock N, Dech Z, et al: Gender differences in perceptions of quality of life in cardiac rehabilitation patients. J Cardiopulm Rehabil 15:143, 1995.
51. Brezinka V, Dusseldorp E, Maes S: Gender differences in psychosocial profile at entry into cardiac rehabilitation. J Cardiopulm Rehabil 18: 445, 1998.
52. Loose MS, Fernhall B: Differences in quality of life among male and female cardiac rehabilitation participants. J Cardiopulm Rehabil 15: 225, 1995.
53. Cannistra LB, O'Malley CJ, Balady GJ: Comparison of outcome of cardiac rehabilitation in black women and white women. Am J Cardiol 75:890, 1995.
54. King KM, Humen DP, Teo KK: Cardiac rehabilitation: The forgotten intervention. Can J Cardiol 15:979, 1999.
55. Murray JC, O'Farrell P, Huston P: The experiences of women with heart disease: What are their needs? Can J Public Health 91:98, 2000.
56. Moore SM, Kramer FM: Women's and men's preferences for cardiac rehabilitation program features. J Cardiopulm Rehabil 16:163, 1996.
57. Limacher MC: Exercise and rehabilitation in women: Indications and outcomes. Cardiol Clin 16:27, 1998.
58. Carhart RL Jr, Ades PA: Gender differences in cardiac rehabilitation. Cardiol Clin 16:37, 1998.
59. Richardson LA, Buckenmeyer PJ, Bauman BD, et al: Contemporary cardiac rehabilitation: Patient characteristics and temporal trends over the past decade. J Cardiopulm Rehabil 20:57, 2000.
60. Froelicher VF: Cardiac rehabilitation. In Willerson JT, Cohn JN (eds): Cardiovascular Medicine. Churchill Livingstone, New York, 2000, p 906.
61. Halm M, Penque S, Doll N, et al: Women and cardiac rehabilitation: referral and compliance patterns. J Cardiovasc Nurs 13:83, 1999.
62. Moore SM, Ruland CM, Pashkow FJ, et al: Women's patterns of exercise following cardiac rehabilitation. Nurs Res 47:318, 1998.

11.7 Secondary Prevention

John C. LaRosa

Coronary atherosclerosis in women, as in men, is the most common cause of death in Western society. In large populations, coronary disease can be prevented by eating a diet low in animal fat, exercising regularly, avoiding tobacco use, preventing weight gain, and detecting and treating hypertension and hypercholesterolemia. Indeed, in societies where the diets are low in animal fat, coronary disease is uncommon despite high rates of cigarette smoking, hypertension, diabetes, and other risk factors for coronary disease.[1, 2]

Until recently, the treatment of established coronary atherosclerosis has focused on interventional procedures such as coronary angioplasty and bypass surgery. These procedures do not address the diffuse nature of atherosclerosis, which spreads throughout the arterial wall and is not an isolated lesion. Moreover, if present in one area, such as the coronary arteries, atherosclerosis may likely be found throughout the arterial tree. Thus, patients with evidence of carotid atherosclerosis or peripheral vascular disease often have coronary disease even if it is not clinically demonstrable.[3] In addition, the atherosclerotic lesions that are most active (those most likely to cause organ damage as a result of sudden occlusion) are not necessarily those that appear the most severe on angiography. Almost 70% of coronary occlusions occur in arteries with lesions that have less than 50% stenosis.[4] As a result, the procedures directed to the most severe lesions as noted on angiograms may not effectively prevent recurrent coronary events.[5, 6] Even in patients with clinically documented atherosclerosis, nonanatomic, medical interventions must be considered to prevent recurrence of coronary events.

CURRENT GUIDELINES FOR COMPREHENSIVE RISK REDUCTION IN PATIENTS WITH CORONARY OR OTHER ATHEROSCLEROTIC VASCULAR DISEASE

In 1995, the AHA released a Consensus Panel Statement outlining specific recommendations for the prevention of heart attack and death in patients with coronary disease (Table 11–12).[7] These recommendations are based on a large number of studies that link major risk factors to coronary disease and on clinical trials that show the benefit of risk factor intervention in patients with established coronary disease. The recommendations emphasize hygienic interventions, such as quitting smoking, increasing physical activity, reducing weight, and lowering intake of animal fat. In addition, the guidelines recommend that cholesterol levels be lowered with diet and, if necessary, with cholesterol-lowering drugs.[7]

Most of the data that support these recommendations came from studies of middle-aged white men. Less is known

Table 11–12. AMERICAN HEART ASSOCIATION CONSENSUS PANEL STATEMENT: GUIDE TO COMPREHENSIVE RISK REDUCTION FOR PATIENTS WITH CORONARY AND OTHER VASCULAR DISEASE

<table>
<tr><th>RISK INTERVENTION</th><th colspan="5">RECOMMENDATIONS</th></tr>
<tr><td>Smoking:
Goal
complete cessation</td><td colspan="5">Strongly encourage patient and family to stop smoking.
Provide counseling, nicotine replacement, and formal cessation programs as appropriate.</td></tr>
<tr><td rowspan="6">Lipid management:
Primary goal
LDL <100 mg/dl
Secondary goals
HDL >35 mg/dl;
TG <200 mg/dl</td><td colspan="5">Start AHA Step II Diet in all patients: ≤30% fat, <7% saturated fat, <200 mg/d cholesterol.
Assess fasting lipid profile. In post-MI patients, lipid profile may take 4 to 6 weeks to stabilize. Add drug therapy according to the following guide:</td></tr>
<tr><td rowspan="5">LDL <100 mg/dl
No drug therapy</td><td colspan="2">LDL 100 to 130 mg/dl
Consider adding drug therapy to diet, as follows:</td><td>LDL >130 mg/dl
Add drug therapy to diet, as follows:</td><td rowspan="5">HDL <35 mg/dl
Emphasize weight management and physical activity.
Advise smoking cessation.

If needed to achieve LDL goals, consider niacin, statin, fibrate.</td></tr>
<tr><td colspan="3">↘ Suggested drug therapy ↙</td></tr>
<tr><td>TG <200 mg/dl</td><td>TG 200 to 400 mg/dl</td><td>TG >400 mg/dl</td></tr>
<tr><td>Statin
Resin
Niacin</td><td>Statin
Niacin</td><td>Consider combined drug therapy (niacin, fibrate, statin)</td></tr>
<tr><td colspan="3">If LDL goal not achieved, consider combination therapy.</td></tr>
<tr><td>Physical activity:
Minimum goal
30 minutes 3 to 4 times per week</td><td colspan="5">Assess risk, preferably with exercise test, to guide prescription.
Encourage minimum of 30 to 60 minutes of moderate-intensity activity 3 or 4 times weekly (walking, jogging, cycling, or other aerobic activity) supplemented by an increase in daily lifestyle activities (e.g., walking breaks at work, using stairs, gardening, household work). Maximum benefit 5 to 6 hours a week.
Advise medically supervised programs for moderate- to high-risk patients.</td></tr>
<tr><td>Weight management:</td><td colspan="5">Start intensive diet and appropriate physical intervention, as outlined above, in patients >120% of ideal weight for height.
Particularly emphasize need for weight loss in patients with hypertension, elevated triglycerides, or elevated glucose levels.</td></tr>
<tr><td>Antiplatelet agents/
anticoagulants:</td><td colspan="5">Start aspirin 80 to 325 mg/d if not contraindicated.
Manage warfarin to international normalized ratio = 2 to 3.5 in post-MI patients not able to take aspirin.</td></tr>
<tr><td>ACE inhibitors post-MI:</td><td colspan="5">Start early post-MI in stable high-risk patients (anterior MI, previous MI, Killip class II [S_3 gallop, rales, radiographic CHF]).
Continue indefinitely for all with LV dysfunction (ejection fraction ≤40%) or symptoms of failure.
Use as needed to manage blood pressure or symptoms in all other patients.</td></tr>
<tr><td>Beta-blockers:</td><td colspan="5">Start in high-risk post-MI patients (arrhythmia, LV dysfunction, inducible ischemia) at 5 to 28 days. Continue 6 months minimum. Observe usual contraindications.
Use as needed to manage angina, rhythm, or blood pressure in all other patients.</td></tr>
<tr><td>Estrogens:</td><td colspan="5">Consider estrogen replacement in all postmenopausal women.
Individualize recommendation consistent with other health risks.</td></tr>
<tr><td>Blood pressure control:
Goal
≤140/90 mm Hg</td><td colspan="5">Initiate lifestyle modification—weight control, physical activity, alcohol moderation, and moderate sodium restriction—in all patients with blood pressure >140 mm Hg systolic or 90 mm Hg diastolic.
Add blood pressure medication, individualized to other patient requirements and characteristics (i.e., age, race, need for drugs with specific benefits) if blood pressure is not less than 140 mm Hg systolic or 90 mm Hg diastolic in 3 months or if initial blood pressure is >160 mm Hg systolic or >100 mm Hg diastolic.</td></tr>
</table>

ACE, angiotension-converting enzyme; CHF, congestive heart failure; MI, myocardial infarction; TG, triglycerides; LV, left ventricular.

about the risk factors in racial and ethnic minority groups, and almost nothing is known about the efficacy of risk factor reduction in these populations. More is known about risk factors for coronary disease in women; however, the data are incomplete. This discussion briefly reviews how coronary risk factors and interventions affect the onset and progression of coronary atherosclerosis in women.

CORONARY RISK FACTORS IN WOMEN

The same risk factors that predict coronary disease in men apply to women. Hypercholesterolemia, hypertension, and cigarette smoking are all significant antecedents of coronary disease in both sexes, and they predict important coronary events after coronary disease is clinically manifest.[8] However, some aspects of coronary risk factors are unique in women. Total and LDL cholesterol levels predict coronary disease less strongly in women than in men.[9] This finding may be related in part to the larger contribution that HDL makes to total cholesterol levels in women. Furthermore, LDL is less easily oxidized and therefore less likely to be taken up by the vascular wall in the presence of estrogen.[10] In both men and women, levels of total LDL and HDL cholesterol are less predictive of the relative risk of coronary disease in older patients[11]; this is of particular interest in women, who usually do not demonstrate clinical coronary disease until the sixth or seventh decade of life.

Some investigators have suggested that modulation of total cholesterol levels in older patients may not be useful.[12]

However, the severity of atherosclerosis is related not only to the level of cholesterol at any given time but also to the lifetime exposure to cholesterol.[13] Moreover, in older people, the relative risk of coronary disease is less important than the absolute risk. Coronary disease is more prevalent in older patients, and the absolute number of coronary events relates directly to cholesterol levels in older men[14] and, presumably, in older women. Finally, the protective effects of estrogen progressively diminish as women age and pass through menopause. Estrogen decreases oxidation and uptake of LDL by the intima and reduces vasospasm and clotting in the area of atherosclerotic plaque.[10] Thus, older estrogen-deficient women are at particular risk for the progression of atherogenesis.

Other risk factors are of unique importance in women. Diabetes is a particularly important risk factor in women. In fact, diabetic men and women have almost the same risk of coronary disease.[15] The 5- to 10-year delay in the onset of coronary disease in nondiabetic women compared with nondiabetic men is lost in the presence of diabetes. Both hypertriglyceridemia and low HDL levels, which are present in both diabetic men and women, are much stronger predictors of coronary risk in diabetic women. This predictive capability indicates that these factors play a more important role in atherogenesis in diabetic women than in diabetic men.[16] Even in the absence of diabetes, hypertriglyceridemia and low HDL levels are stronger predictors of coronary risk in women than in men.[17, 18]

Other risk factors are common to both men and women. For both groups, coronary risk directly relates to cigarette smoking and, more specifically, to the number of cigarettes smoked per day.[19] Even moderate obesity (as indicated by a body mass index of 25 to 29) raises the risk of coronary heart disease, and that risk increases further with weight gain.[20] The distribution of weight may affect the risk of coronary disease. A larger waist-hip ratio is independently associated with higher risk of coronary disease in both women and men.[21] Both greater body mass index and higher waist-to-hip ratio may indirectly raise risk by promoting hypertension, diabetes, and dyslipidemia.

In both men and women, regular physical activity, particularly over several years, decreases the risk of coronary disease.[22] Many of the benefits of physical activity may result from its effect on blood pressure and lipid levels. Another benefit of exercise is the inverse association seen between physical activity and smoking.

A strong association exists between high blood pressure and coronary disease in both men and women.[8] The degree of association does not appear to be gender-specific. However, systolic hypertension, which is more prevalent among older women than older men, may be of particular importance in the higher incidence of coronary disease in older women.[23]

Finally, a larger intake of alcohol decreases the risk of coronary disease in both women and men. Like estrogen, alcohol has many protective effects, including elevation of HDL levels and reduction of levels of certain clotting factors, that may help stabilize atherosclerotic plaques and make them less likely to occlude arteries. Unlike estrogen, however, increased alcohol consumption has also been shown to raise blood pressure and, in more extreme cases, to induce cardiomyopathies. Alcohol should be considered beneficial only when used in moderation and only if its intake is controllable.[24]

MEDICAL INTERVENTIONS IN WOMEN WITH ATHEROSCLEROSIS

The AHA Guidelines recommend a series of risk interventions for people with coronary disease (see Table 11–12).[7] In fact, these interventions may be useful in patients without clinically apparent coronary disease who have evidence of atherosclerosis in other vascular beds. No distinction between men and women is made in the AHA guidelines in applying these risk interventions.

Progression of atherosclerosis is the most common cause of disability and death in both men and women with coronary disease. However, participants in interventional trials for the prevention of coronary disease are usually men.

Although the rate of onset of new coronary disease is lower in women than in men at any age, the consequences of *recurrent* coronary disease are greater in women than in men. Women of all ages are more likely than men to die of coronary disease. This means that the prognosis for women who have had a previous coronary event is worse than that for men. Moreover, women are more likely than men to suffer from prolonged disability after a coronary event as well as to have complications after bypass surgery.[25] Although a more conservative approach to primary prevention of coronary disease in women may be justified by the lower risk of a first event in women, the severity of this disease in women once it is established dictates that secondary prevention be applied as aggressively in women as in men.

SPECIFIC INTERVENTIONS

Smoking

There is a linear relationship between the number of cigarettes smoked and the risk of coronary disease in women.[19] Moreover, when women stop smoking, their risk of MI decreases almost immediately and reaches that of a nonsmoker after approximately 2 years.[26] Specific studies of smoking cessation in women with coronary disease have not been conducted. Nevertheless, it is reasonable to assume that smoking cessation is an important means of lowering the risk of coronary disease. Although it is beyond the scope of this discussion to review all interventions for smoking cessation, several issues should be addressed.

First, more men than women have quit smoking.[27] Whether this difference is related to fear of weight gain or to some other gender-related difference is unclear. Although women who quit smoking may gain an average of 3 to 5 pounds, women who smoke actually have a *higher* waist-to-hip ratio. This higher ratio may relate to greater estrogen catabolism in smoking women.[28, 29] Weight gain may be minimized by the use of nicotine replacement patches or gum[30]; however, the use of nicotine replacement without behavioral interventions is less likely to be successful.

Second, although formal programs are worth trying, most men and women who quit smoking do so on their own. Some evidence indicates that women may have more success

Table 11–13. EARLY SECONDARY PREVENTION TRIALS IN WOMEN WITH CORONARY DISEASE

TRIAL	NO. OF WOMEN (TOTAL NO. OF PATIENTS)	TYPES OF CHD	INTERVENTION	% REDUCTION IN TOTAL CHOLESTEROL	RR (95% CI) FOR WOMEN	
					CHD Mortality	Total Mortality
Stockholm Ischaemic Heart Disease Study[35]	103 (555)	MI survivors	Clofibrate and nicotinic acid	13	NA	NA
Scottish Society of Physicians[36]	124 (717)	Recent MI and/ or angina	Clofibrate	16	0.17 (0.02, 1.37)	NA
Newcastle upon Tyne[37]	97 (497)	MI or angina (MI not recent)	Clofibrate	NA	0.29 (0.19, 1.37)	NA
Scandinavian Simvastatin Survival Study[31]	827 (4444)	MI or angina	Simvastatin	28	0.79 (0.37, 1.6)	1.12 (0.65, 1.93)

Abbreviations: CHD, coronary heart disease; MI, myocardial infarction; NA, not applicable; RR, risk reduction.

in settings in which there is strong social support; however, in general, no unique interventions are more successful for women than for men.

Finally, any successful intervention must involve clear and unambiguous advice from a physician that smoking is dangerous for women with coronary disease. Despite the variable success rate, quitting smoking is a very important intervention for the prevention of coronary disease.

Lipid Management

Elevated cholesterol levels are essential for atherogenesis. In societies in which average cholesterol levels are less than 160 mg/dl (4 mmol/l), coronary disease is uncommon even in the presence of other risk factors, such as smoking and hypertension.[1, 2] Lowering cholesterol levels in patients with coronary disease has been studied more commonly in clinical trials than any other medical intervention. Evidence from both older and newer trials has shown unequivocally that lowering LDL cholesterol can reduce morbidity and mortality from subsequent coronary disease by 25% to 40%.[31–34] Most patients in these studies were men. No clinical trial of the effects of lowering cholesterol levels has been conducted exclusively in women.

Women with coronary disease, however, were included in four older secondary prevention trials (Table 11–13).[31, 35–37] These four studies included women and used coronary disease endpoints as indices of benefit. A significant beneficial effect of cholesterol lowering on mortality from coronary heart disease was found only in the Stockholm Ischemic Heart Disease Study (in which the data from women were not analyzed separately). No studies yet completed have involved a sufficient number of women to allow conclusions to be drawn about total mortality.

In other interventional trials, serial coronary angiography or carotid sonography has been used to examine atherosclerotic vessels before and after cholesterol lowering. Women were included in three of these trials. In one study in which men and women with familial hypercholesterolemia were treated with bile acid sequestrants and niacin to lower LDL and raise HDL levels, women had twice the level of atherosclerotic regression as men. In fact, the regression was statistically significant only in women.[38] Similarly, in a study of lovastatin, both progression of established lesions and appearance of new lesions were significantly less in treated women than in treated men and in women receiving placebo.[39] In a study of cholesterol lowering induced by ileal bypass surgery, cholesterol levels of women in the surgical group were reduced 24%, and significantly less progression of disease was seen on coronary angiography in women 5 years later.[40]

In the Cholesterol and Recurrent Events (CARE) study, in which cholesterol lowering was examined in patients with average cholesterol levels of 209 mg/dl (5.3 mmol/l, approximating the U.S. mean), women had twice the reduction of subsequent coronary events seen in men (Table 11–14).[41] Although fewer data are available for women than for men, all evidence indicates that lowering cholesterol in women with coronary disease is likely to prevent events from recurring. Reduction in overall mortality has not been assessed because of the small numbers of women in these studies; however, it is reasonable to assume that if the rate of recurring events is decreased, then the risk of subsequent death also will be reduced.

None of these clinical trials has addressed the issue of lowering triglyceride levels or increasing HDL levels in women with coronary disease. Because triglyceride and HDL levels are better predictors of coronary risk in women than in men, this issue is of particular importance in women. Unfortunately, the data indicating that lowering triglyceride levels is beneficial either in men or in women are incomplete.[42] No clinical trial has enrolled patients primarily on the basis of triglyceride levels. Indeed, patients with triglyceride levels exceeding 300 or 400 mg/dl (3.4 to 4.5 mmol/l) have

Table 11–14. REDUCTION IN OCCURRENCE OF CORONARY EVENTS IN THE CHOLESTEROL AND RECURRENT EVENTS (CARE) STUDY

ENDPOINT	DECREASE IN OCCURRENCE (%)
Primary	
Fatal CHD or nonfatal MI	
All patients (N = 4076)	24
Women only (n = 576)	45
Others	
Angioplasty	22
Bypass surgery	26
Stroke	28

CHD, coronary heart disease; MI, myocardial infarction.

LaRosa JC: Triglycerides and coronary risk in women and the elderly. Arch Intern Med 157:961, 1997.

usually been excluded from cholesterol-lowering trials. Nevertheless, two studies have provided some help. First, in the Stockholm Study, the extent of triglyceride lowering, but not the change in total cholesterol, correlated with a reduction in mortality from coronary events.[35] Second, in the Bezafibrate Coronary Artery Intervention Trial (BECAIT), triglyceride levels were lowered with relatively little change in LDL levels and only modest increases in HDL levels.[43] However, as demonstrated by serial coronary angiograms, the benefit was comparable to that seen in LDL-lowering trials in which the reduction in triglyceride levels was minimal.

The AHA guidelines focus on lowering LDL levels because of the lack of definitive evidence for other lipid interventions.[7] These guidelines recommend that all patients with coronary atherosclerosis be started on the AHA Step 2 Diet, in which fewer than 7% of calories come from saturated fat and patients consume less than 200 mg per day of cholesterol. Debate continues as to the length of time that diet intervention alone is appropriate before cholesterol-lowering drugs are introduced in patients after an acute coronary event.

The goal of lipid intervention is to reduce LDL levels to less than 100 mg/dl (2.5 mmol/l). To achieve that goal, most patients require more than diet intervention. The drug of choice is usually one of the HMG-CoA inhibitors, which are potent agents for lowering LDL cholesterol. In patients whose triglyceride levels are higher than 400 mg/dl (4.5 mmol/l), drugs such as niacin or one of the fibric acid derivatives (including gemfibrozil and clofibrate in the United States) may be selected first. However, the addition of a statin is often necessary to sufficiently lower LDL levels. In patients with high triglyceride and low HDL levels, weight reduction and greater physical activity are especially important, because these lipids are particularly sensitive to such interventions. Again, it is important to emphasize that there are no gender differences in these recommendations because the risk of recurrent disease is very high in both men and women.

Physical Activity and Weight Management

Lack of physical activity and obesity are predictive factors of coronary disease in women and men. However, the benefits of greater physical activity and lower body weight have not been studied in clinical trials either in men or in women. Nevertheless, the beneficial effects that exercise and fitness have on lipid levels and blood pressure justify this type of intervention. Patients with coronary disease must, of course, undergo formal exercise testing to ensure an appropriate exercise level. Only moderate regular exercise is required to achieve the desired benefits. Appropriate moderate activities include walking, jogging, and cycling. Many patients are discouraged by the misguided notion that benefit is derived only from vigorous exercise.

Regular exercise is also an indispensable ingredient in any weight reduction program. Weight reduction should be prescribed for any patient with a body weight greater than 120% of the ideal level. Weight loss can be frustrating for both patient and physician, especially if the patient has been a smoker. As with smoking cessation, different patients respond to different regimens for weight loss, which may range from office counseling to more formalized group programs. The importance of exercise and weight reduction cannot be overemphasized.

Antiplatelet Agents

Treatment with aspirin or other antiplatelet agents reduces the rate of recurrent coronary disease by approximately 25%. Meta-analysis of interventional trials of these agents (two thirds of which have used aspirin) has shown that men and women benefit equally from the use of aspirin and antiplatelet agents (Fig. 11–5).[44] Clinical trials in men and observational studies in women have shown that regular use of aspirin is beneficial; however, no clinical trials of the effect of aspirin on primary prevention of coronary disease in women have been completed.[45] Aspirin use is indicated in both women and men who have documented coronary disease. For those women who cannot take aspirin, low-dose warfarin may be considered as an alternative.

Angiotensin-Converting Enzyme Inhibitors

In two large clinical trials, ACE inhibitors reduced both the risk of recurrent coronary disease and associated mortality.[46, 47] Because patients in these studies had left ventricular dysfunction and congestive heart failure, we do not know whether the results can be extrapolated to patients without heart failure. Furthermore, the effects on women in these studies were mixed. In the Studies of Left Ventricular Dysfunction (SOLVD) trials, which composed a large study of enalapril, the reduction of recurrent coronary disease was more substantial in women (35%) than in men (19%) (Table 11–15).[47] However, in the Survival and Ventricular Enlargement (SAVE) trial, which was a study of captopril, only men had a significant reduction in recurrent coronary risk with

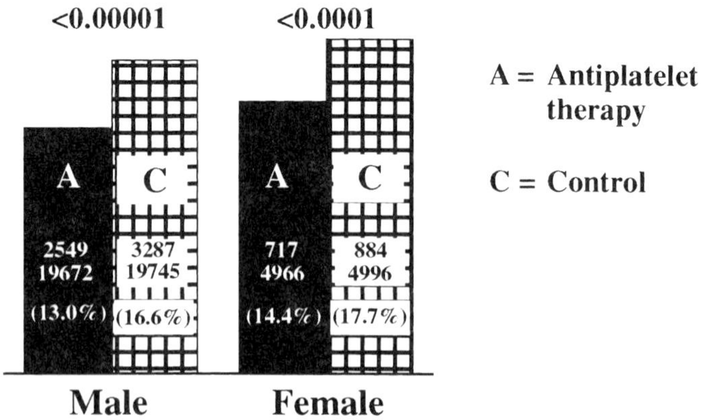

FIGURE 11–5. Results of meta-analysis showing the effect of antiplatelet therapy on vascular events in men and women with occlusive vascular disease. (Two thirds of subjects treated on aspirin.) Percentages indicate percentages of patients suffering a vascular event. (From Antiplatelets Trialists' Collaboration: Collaborative overview of randomised trials of antiplatelet therapy–I: Prevention of death, myocardial infarction, and stroke by prolonged antiplatelet therapy in various categories of patients. BMJ 308:81, 1994.)

Table 11–15. EFFECT OF ANGIOTENSIN-CONVERTING ENZYME INHIBITORS ON CORONARY HEART DISEASE (CHD) BY GENDER

TRIAL	CHD EVENTS (%) Placebo	Drug	REDUCTION IN RISK (%)
SOLVD[48] (enalapril)			
Women	28.8 (n = 496)	19.6 (n = 484)	35
Men	24.6 (n = 2905)	21.1 (n = 2911)	19
SAVE[49] (captopril)			
Women	20.1 (n = 204)	19.9 (n = 186)	2
Men	25.7 (n = 912)	20.6 (n = 929)	22

therapy. No benefits of captopril were seen in women.[46] The discrepancy in results between the SOLVD and SAVE trials may be attributed to the smaller number of patients in the SAVE trial. Nevertheless, because of the significant findings in the SOLVD Study, the AHA recommends that all patients with coronary disease who are at high risk of congestive failure be started on an ACE inhibitor. In patients who have ejection fractions less than 40% or symptoms of heart failure, ACE inhibitors should be continued indefinitely.

Beta-Adrenergic Blockade

Meta-analyses have shown that regular use of beta blockers reduces the rate of subsequent coronary events by 20% to 25%, especially in patients with a history of previous coronary event who have arrhythmias, left ventricular dysfunction, or recurrent ischemia.[48] Although both men and women have been included in beta blocker trials, analyses by gender have not been reported. Nevertheless, it has been assumed that both women and men benefit from this intervention. The use of beta blockers is most beneficial in the first year after MI. Therefore, the AHA guidelines recommend routine use of beta blockers only for the first 6 months after MI, except for patients with other indications, including recurrent angina, arrhythmias, and hypertension, who may continue taking beta blockers.

Estrogen

Several observational prospective cohort studies have indicated that women who have taken estrogen at any time during the first 10 years after menopause have half the mortality rates (both coronary and total mortality rates) of women who have not taken estrogen.[49] Some reports have shown that estrogen, even when supplemented with progesterone, has a beneficial effect on coronary morbidity; however, effects on mortality have not been reported because of insufficient data.[50–52] These benefits in observational studies are apparent in women with and without coronary disease. No clinical trials can corroborate results from these observational studies. Nevertheless, many physicians believe that estrogen replacement therapy is useful, especially in women with established coronary disease, because the results of observational studies have been consistent and significant.

Estrogen exerts its benefit not only by modulating lipoprotein levels but also by acting directly on the vascular wall. Estrogen therapy decreases LDL levels by an average of 15% and similarly increases HDL levels. These beneficial effects, however, are often accompanied by a small increase in triglyceride levels.[53] Estrogen also reduces levels of fibrinogen and the lipoprotein particle Lp(a).[53, 54] Adding progestin does not affect the estrogen-induced decrease in LDL levels; however, depending on the dose, progestin can prevent the increase in HDL levels. Progestin does not alter the estrogen-induced decrease in fibrinogen but may diminish estrogen's effect on Lp(a).

Estrogen can directly affect the vascular wall by preventing the oxidation of LDL and its uptake by the vascular wall and by inhibiting platelet adhesiveness, clotting, and vasospasm in the area of the atheroma. How progestin affects these estrogen-induced changes is unknown. The clinical observational studies previously mentioned indicate that the addition of progestin to an estrogen regimen does not reduce the benefit of estrogen alone. In addition, animal studies indicate that the inhibition of atherogenesis by estrogen is effective even when HDL levels are lowered.[55] These studies imply that the vascular effects of estrogen on atherogenesis are very important and that these effects are relatively uninhibited by progestins.

Pending the completion of ongoing clinical trials, it seems prudent to consider the use of estrogen replacement therapy in women with coronary disease. Contraindications to starting such therapy include a recent history of thrombophlebitis or breast cancer. There are no recommendations about the use of estrogen-progestin combinations because the data are incomplete. Relatively few data concerning estrogen use in older women are available, even though this group has a high incidence of coronary disease. More definitive recommendations about estrogen use await the completion of clinical trials of estrogen in women with and without coronary disease.

Blood Pressure

Reducing high blood pressure, both systolic and diastolic, substantially lowers the risk of stroke, especially in older women with systolic hypertension.[56] The beneficial effects of lowering blood pressure on coronary disease predicted by observational studies have not, however, been completely supported by clinical trial results. In a meta-analysis of 17 trials, drug treatment to lower blood pressure in patients with hypertension reduced the risk of coronary heart disease.[56] In this meta-analysis, the 16% reduction in the risk of coronary heart disease was less than that observed in lipid-lowering trials, in trials of beta blockade, and in studies of ACE inhibitors. Nevertheless, these benefits are great enough to justify lowering blood pressure to prevent coronary heart disease.

Lifestyle interventions, such as weight reduction, salt and alcohol restriction, and regular exercise, may in many cases be sufficient to reduce blood pressure to acceptable levels without drug intervention. It is important to remember that approximately 30% of women older than 65 years have isolated systolic hypertension. The Systolic Hypertension in the Elderly Program (SHEP)[57] has shown that treatment of elevated systolic blood pressure can reduce the incidence of stroke by 36% and the incidence of coronary heart disease by 25%. Because most coronary heart disease occurs in women older than 65 years, reducing blood pressure is a useful and important intervention.

Diabetes Mellitus

Diabetes is an important risk factor for the development of coronary heart disease. However, diabetes is less important in populations in which the intake of dietary animal fat and blood cholesterol are lower than in Western populations.[58] Diabetes is a more important risk factor in women than in men. Unfortunately, controlled trials of lowering blood glucose levels or controlling diabetes have not been conducted. These trials would be useful for establishing recommendations for the prevention of coronary disease in women with non–insulin-dependent diabetes mellitus. Clearly, lifestyle changes such as weight loss and exercise reduce hyperglycemia, but whether these changes would decrease the risk of coronary disease in diabetics is unknown. Furthermore, clinical trials of lipid lowering in diabetics have not been reported. Whether strict control of blood glucose levels, independent of any other risk factor modifications, prevents expression or progression of recurrent coronary disease is also unknown. Nevertheless, the risk of atherosclerosis in diabetics is so high that controlling lipid and glucose levels seems prudent.

Alcohol

Alcohol protects against the development and expression of coronary atherosclerosis. However, alcohol is also a metabolic poison capable of causing cardiomyopathy, aggravating diabetes, and raising blood pressure. Moreover, alcohol is highly addictive. For these reasons, regular use of alcohol for the prevention of coronary disease cannot be endorsed, although patients who are able to limit their intake to very modest amounts may derive some benefit.

Antioxidant Drugs

Observational studies in both men and women have indicated that diets high in antioxidants such as vitamin E and beta-carotene may reduce the risk of coronary disease. In a study limited to men, beta-carotene ingestion protected against coronary disease.[59] That finding was not supported by results of other, larger clinical trials. Once thought harmless, beta-carotene ingestion may be associated with a higher rate of lung cancer in smokers.[60] Another study indicated that vitamin E supplementation may raise the risk of hemorrhagic stroke.[61] Results of observational studies have not been confirmed by clinical trials of antioxidant supplementation; therefore, physicians should recommend diets naturally high in antioxidant vitamins rather than antioxidant supplements.

SUMMARY

Coronary disease is the most common cause of death in women and men in the United States. Because atherosclerosis is a diffuse disease of arteries, it cannot be treated definitively by focused anatomic procedures such as bypass surgery and angioplasty. The only definitive treatments for atherosclerosis are medical. In women and men with coronary disease, medical treatments include interventions such as the following:

- Quitting smoking
- Lowering lipid levels and blood pressure
- Restricting intake of calories, fat, and salt
- Increasing physical activity
- Reducing weight
- Therapy with beta blockers for the first 6 to 12 months after an infarction
- Use of ACE inhibitors for patients with congestive heart failure

Specific guidelines for the use of these interventions have been released by a Consensus Panel of the AHA. These guidelines apply to both women and men with coronary disease, even though most of the evidence on which the guidelines are based has been derived from interventional trials that included mostly men. The application of these guidelines cannot guarantee that coronary disease will not recur. Unlike anatomic procedures, however, these interventions attack the underlying process of atherogenesis. Failure to include these interventions in the care of men and women with established coronary disease is a serious and potentially life-threatening omission.

References

1. Roberts WC: Atherosclerotic risk factors: Are there ten or is there only one? Am J Cardiol 64:552, 1989.
2. Alexander RW: Theodore Cooper Memorial Lecture: Hypertension and the pathogenesis of atherosclerosis: Oxidative stress and the mediation of arterial inflammatory responses: A new perspective. Hypertension 25:155, 1995.
3. Wilt TJ, Rubins HB, Collins D, et al: Correlates and consequences of diffuse atherosclerosis in men with coronary heart disease. Veterans Affairs High-Density Lipoprotein Intervention Trial Study Group. Arch Intern Med 156:1181, 1996.
4. Falk E, Shah PK, Fuster V: Coronary plaque disruption. Circulation 92:657, 1995.
5. Yusuf S, Zucker D, Peduzzi P, et al: Effect of coronary artery bypass graft surgery on survival: Overview of 10-year results from randomised trials by the Coronary Artery Bypass Graft Surgery Trialists Collaboration. Lancet 344:563, 1994.
6. Eichner JE, Moore WE, McKee PA, et al: Fibrinogen levels in women having coronary angiography. Am J Cardiol 78:15, 1996.
7. Smith SC Jr, Blair SN, Criqui MH, et al: Preventing heart attack and deaths in patients with coronary disease. Circulation 92:2, 1995.
8. Wolf PA: Risk factors for stroke: How they differ from those for coronary artery disease. In Perspectives in Lipid Disorders. Postgraduate Medicine: Custom Communications, Morris Plains, NJ, 1986, p 16.
9. Bass KM, Newschaffer CJ, Klag MJ, et al: Plasma lipoprotein levels as predictors of cardiovascular death in women. Arch Intern Med 153: 2209, 1993.
10. LaRosa JC: Metabolic effects of estrogen and progestins. Fertil Steril 62(Suppl):140S, 1994.
11. Manolio TA, Pearson TA, Wenger NK, et al: Cholesterol and heart disease in older persons and women: Review of an NHLBI workshop. Ann Epidemiol 2:161, 1992.
12. Garber AM, Browner WS, Hulley SB: Cholesterol screening in asymptomatic adults, revisited. Part 2. Ann Intern Med 124:518, 1996.
13. Davenport J, Whittaker K: Secondary prevention in elderly survivors of heart attacks. Am Fam Physician 38:216, 1988.
14. Rubin S, Sidney S, Black DM et al: High blood cholesterol in elderly

men and the excess risk for coronary heart disease. Ann Intern Med 113:916, 1990.
15. Krolewski AS, Warram JH, Valsania P, et al: Evolving natural history of coronary artery disease in diabetes mellitus. Am J Med 90(Suppl 2A): 56S, 1991.
16. Goldschmid MG, Barrett-Conner E, Edelstein SL, et al: Dyslipidemia and ischemic heart disease mortality among men and women with diabetes. Circulation 89:991, 1994.
17. Gordon DJ, Probstifield JL, Garrison RJ, et al: High-density lipoprotein cholesterol and cardiovascular disease: Four prospective American studies. Circulation 79:8, 1989.
18. Castelli WP: The triglyceride issue: A view from Framingham. Am Heart J 112:432, 1986.
19. Palmer JR, Rosenberg L, Shapiro S: "Low yield" cigarettes and the risk of nonfatal myocardial infarction in women. N Engl J Med 320; 1569, 1989.
20. Manson JE, Colditz GA, Stampfer MJ, et al: A prospective study of obesity and risk of coronary heart disease in women. N Engl J Med 322:882, 1990.
21. Folsom AR, Kaye SA, Sellers TA, et al: Body fat distribution and 5 year risk of death in older women. JAMA 269:483, 1993.
22. Scragg R, Stewart A, Jackson R, et al: Alcohol and exercise in myocardial infarction and sudden coronary death in men and women. Am J Epidemiol 126:77, 1987.
23. Saltzberg S, Stroh JA, Frishman WH: Isolated systolic hypertension in the elderly: Pathophysiology and treatment. Med Clin North Am 72: 523, 1988.
24. Stampfer MJ, Colditz GR, Willett WC, et al: A prospective study of moderate alcohol consumption and the risk of coronary disease and stroke in women. N Engl J Med 319:267, 1988.
25. Wenger NK: Coronary heart disease: Diagnostic decision making. In Douglas PS (ed): Cardiovascular Health and Disease in Women. WB Saunders, Philadelphia, 1993, p 25.
26. Rosenberg L, Palmer JR, Shapiro S: Decline in the risk of myocardial infarction among women who stop smoking. N Engl J Med 322:213, 1990.
27. Schoenborn CA, Boyd G: Smoking and other tobacco use. Vital Health Stat 169:1, 1989.
28. Schwartz JL: Review and evaluation of smoking cessation methods: The United States and Canada 1978–1985 (NIH Publication No. 87-2940). U.S. Department of Health and Human Services, Bethesda, MD, 1987.
29. Hall SM, McGee R, Tunstall C et al: Changes in food intake and activity after quitting smoking. J Consult Clin Psychol 57:81, 1989.
30. Gross J, Stitzer ML, Maldonado J: Nicotine replacement: Effects of postcessation weight gain. J Consult Clin Psychol 57:87, 1989.
31. Scandinavian Simvastatin Survival Study Group: Randomised trial of cholesterol lowering in 4444 patients with coronary heart disease: The Scandinavian Simvastatin Survival Study (4S). Lancet 344:1383, 1994.
32. Shepherd J, Cobbe SM, Ford I, et al: Prevention of coronary heart disease with pravastatin in men with hypercholesterolemia. West of Scotland Coronary Prevention Study Group. N Engl J Med 333:1301, 1995.
33. Sacks FM, Pfeffer MA, Moye LA et al: The effect of pravastatin on coronary events after myocardial infarction in patients with average cholesterol levels. Cholesterol and Recurrent Events Trial Investigators. N Engl J Med 335:1001, 1996.
34. The Post Coronary Artery Bypass Graft Trial Investigators: The effect of aggressive lowering of low-density lipoprotein cholesterol levels and low-dose anticoagulation on obstructive changes in saphenous-vein coronary-artery bypass grafts. N Engl J Med 336:153, 1997.
35. Carlson LA, Rosenhamer G: Reduction of mortality in the Stockholm Ischaemic Heart Disease Secondary Prevention Study by combined treatment with clofibrate and nicotinic acid. Acta Med Scand 223: 405, 1988.
36. Research Committee of the Scottish Society of Physicians: Ischemic heart disease: A secondary prevention trial using clofibrate. Br Med J 4:775, 1971.
37. Group of Physicians of the Newcastle upon Tyne Region: Trial of clofibrate in the treatment of ischemic heart disease. Br Med J 4: 767, 1971.
38. Kane JP, Malloy MJ, Ports TA, et al: Regression of coronary atherosclerosis during treatment of familial hypercholesterolemia with combined drug regimens. JAMA 264:3007, 1990.
39. Waters D, Higginson L, Gladstone P, et al: Effects of cholesterol lowering on the progression of coronary atherosclerosis in women: A Canadian Coronary Atherosclerosis Intervention Trial (CCAIT) substudy. Circulation 92:2404, 1995.
40. Buchwald H, Vargo RL, Matts JP, et al: Effect of partial ileal bypass surgery on mortality and morbidity from coronary heart disease in patients with hypercholesterolemia. Report of the Program on the Surgical Control of the Hyperlipidemias. N Engl J Med 323:946, 1990.
41. Braunwald E, Pfeffer M, Sacks F: CARE trial results. Reported at the American College of Cardiology 45th Annual Scientific Session, Orlando, Florida, March 24–26, 1996.
42. LaRosa JC: Triglycerides and coronary risk in women and the elderly. Arch Intern Med 157:961, 1997.
43. Ericsson CG, Hamsten A, Nilsson J, et al: Angiographic assessment of effects of bezafibrate on progression of coronary artery disease in young male postinfarction patients. Lancet 347:849, 1996.
44. Antiplatelets Trialists' Collaboration: Collaborative overview of randomised trials of antiplatelet therapy–I: Prevention of death, myocardial infarction, and stroke by prolonged antiplatelet therapy in various categories of patients. BMJ 308:81, 1994.
45. Manson JE, Stampfer MJ, Colditz GA, et al: A prospective study of aspirin use and primary prevention of cardiovascular disease in women. JAMA 266:521, 1991.
46. Pfeffer MA, Braunwald E, Moye LA, et al: Effect of captopril on mortality and morbidity in patients with left ventricular dysfunction after myocardial infarction: Results of the survival and ventricular enlargement trial. The SAVE Investigators. N Engl J Med, 327:669, 1992
47. Yusuf S, Pepine CJ, Garces C, et al: Effect of enalapril on myocardial infarction and unstable angina in patients with low ejection fractions. Lancet 340:1173, 1992.
48. Yusuf S, Peto R, Lewis J, et al: Beta blockade during and after myocardial infarction: An overview of randomized trials. Prog Cardiovasc Dis 27:335, 1985.
49. Henderson BE, Paganini-Hill A, Ross RK: Decreased mortality in users of estrogen replacement therapy. Arch Intern Med 151:75, 1991.
50. Falkeborn M, Persson I, Adami HO: The risk of acute myocardial infarction after oestrogen and oestrogen-progestogen replacement. Br J Obstet Gynecol 99:821, 1992.
51. Psaty BM, Heckbert SR, Atkins D, et al: The risk of myocardial infarction associated with the combination use of estrogens and progestins in postmenopausal women. Arch Intern Med 154:1333, 1994.
52. Grodstein F, Stampfer M, Manson JE, et al: Postmenopausal estrogen and progestin use and the risk of cardiovascular disease. N Engl J Med 335:453, 1996.
53. Writing Group for the PEPI Trial: Effects of estrogen or estrogen/progestin regimens on heart disease risk factors in postmenopausal women: The Postmenopausal Estrogen/Progestin Interventions (PEPI) Trial. JAMA 273:199, 1995.
54. Kim CJ, Min YK, Ryu WS, et al: Effect of hormone replacement therapy on lipoprotein(a) and lipid levels in postmenopausal women: Influence of various progestogens and duration of therapy. Arch Intern Med 156:1693, 1996.
55. Adams MR, Clarkson TB, Koritnik DR, et al: Contraceptive steroids and coronary artery atherosclerosis in cynomolgus macaques. Fertil Steril 47:1010, 1987.
56. Hebert PR, Moser M, Mayer J, et al: Recent evidence on drug therapy of mild to moderate hypertension and decreased risk of cardiovascular heart disease. Arch Intern Med 153:578, 1993.
57. SHEP Cooperative Research Group: Prevention of stroke by antihypertensive drug treatment in older persons with isolated systolic hypertension: Final results of the Systolic Hypertension in the Elderly Program (SHEP). JAMA 265:3255, 1991.
58. Ruderman NB, Schneider SH: Diabetes, exercise, and atherosclerosis. Diabetes Care 15:1787, 1992.
59. Gaziano JM, Manson JE, Branch LG, et al: Dietary beta carotene and decreased cardiovascular mortality in an elderly cohort [abstract]. J Am Coll Cardiol 19(Suppl A):377A, 1992.
60. Hennekens CH, Buring JE, Peto R: Antioxidant vitamins—benefits not yet proved. N Engl J Med 330:1080, 1994.
61. The Alpha-Tocopherol, Beta Carotene Cancer Prevention Study Group: The effect of vitamin E and beta carotene on the incidence of lung cancer and other cancers in male smokers. N Engl J Med 330:1029, 1994.

SECTION

III

VALVULAR HEART DISEASE

CHAPTER 12

Aortic Valve Disease

William A. Zoghbi and Sherif F. Nagueh

Diseases of the aortic valve are prevalent in the general population, particularly in older persons. Aortic valve disease causes a significant morbidity and mortality. Several underlying conditions may affect the structure of the aortic valve and may restrict cusp mobility, which causes aortic stenosis. Or, underlying conditions may disturb coaptation of the valve, which leads to aortic insufficiency or regurgitation. In this chapter, we discuss aortic stenosis and aortic regurgitation, and address possible gender differences in the presentation and outcome of both conditions. Although we discuss aortic stenosis and regurgitation separately, they frequently coexist, particularly when the underlying disease is aortic stenosis. When they coexist, pressure and volume overload of the left ventricle may cause symptoms to develop earlier than in patients with isolated aortic stenosis or regurgitation; consequently, intervention may be required earlier.

ANATOMY OF THE AORTIC VALVE

The normal aortic valve has three cusps: the left, right, and noncoronary (posterior) cusps (Fig. 12–1). The corresponding sinuses of Valsalva are located above the cusps. The left sinus gives rise to the left coronary artery, and the right sinus gives rise to the right coronary artery. The right and noncoronary sinuses are located close to the right ventricular outflow tract and the right atrium, whereas the left coronary sinus is close to the left atrium. The cuspal markings become more prominent with age.[1] The sinotubular junction marks the beginning of the tubular portion of the ascending aorta.

AORTIC STENOSIS

Aortic stenosis can be at the valvular, subvalvular, or supravalvular level. The increased afterload associated with aortic stenosis results in compensatory left ventricular hypertrophy. However, as the stenosis increases, left ventricular systolic dysfunction gradually ensues, and symptoms develop. Aortic stenosis is readily diagnosed by physical examination and Doppler echocardiography. In this chapter, we focus on valvular aortic stenosis.

Etiology

Aortic stenosis may be congenital, degenerative, or rheumatic. Congenital aortic stenosis may exist in isolation or as part of complex cardiac malformations. Obstruction may occur at the valvular, subvalvular, or supravalvular level. Supravalvular aortic stenosis has been linked to the elastin gene on chromosome 7q.[2] Deletion of the terminal segment of the long arm of chromosome 4 has also been described in children with aortic stenosis.[3] In a population-based study, aortic stenosis was more frequent in boys than in girls (ratio of 1.95:1).[4]

Congenital aortic stenosis usually results from a bicuspid aortic valve (see Fig. 12–1) with commissures that are fused to varying degrees. Unicuspid or unicommissural valves may occasionally be seen. Malformed valves undergo dystrophic calcification and are at risk of infection during episodes of bacteremia. The most frequently associated lesion with congenital aortic stenosis is coarctation of the aorta.

In adults, aortic valvular stenosis is most frequently caused by degenerative calcific aortic stenosis (51%), followed by the presence of bicuspid valves (36%), and finally by postinflammatory stenosis (9%).[5] In developing countries, rheumatic fever is a significant underlying cause of aortic valvular stenosis and is almost always associated with mitral valve involvement. The inflammation associated with rheumatic fever causes the commissures to fuse and the cusps to subsequently retract (see Fig. 12–1). Consequently, the valve is often regurgitant. Systemic lupus erythematosus and alkaptonuric ochronosis with homogentisic acid oxidase deficiency are rare causes of aortic stenosis.[6]

Calcific deposits on the aortic valve are microcrystalline products with various amounts of sodium, magnesium, carbonate, fluoride, and organic fraction. The deposits have a high calcium-to-phosphorus ratio and low solubility.[7] In degenerative calcific aortic stenosis, valvular fibroblasts have been shown to express HLA-DR antigen and smooth muscle cell markers in vitro, which suggests that the fibroblasts are chronically activated.[8]

Pathophysiology

In the presence of a stenotic aortic valve, the resistance to left ventricular ejection is greater. Thus, left ventricular systolic pressure and stroke work increase. The result is left ventricular hypertrophy, which tends to normalize wall stress. In addition, coronary flow reserve is affected in patients with aortic stenosis even in the absence of coronary artery disease. The effect on coronary flow is associated with left ventricular hypertrophy. In severe aortic stenosis, reversal of coronary systolic flow and abnormal diastolic flow are observed. The severity of coronary flow abnormalities relates to the transvalvular pressure gradient.[9]

In patients with aortic stenosis who have a hypertrophied left ventricle, the degree of diastolic dysfunction varies, even in the early stages of preserved systolic performance. The pressure-volume relation usually shifts to the left and the chamber stiffness increases because of a low volume-to-mass ratio.[10] Furthermore, subendocardial fibrosis, which

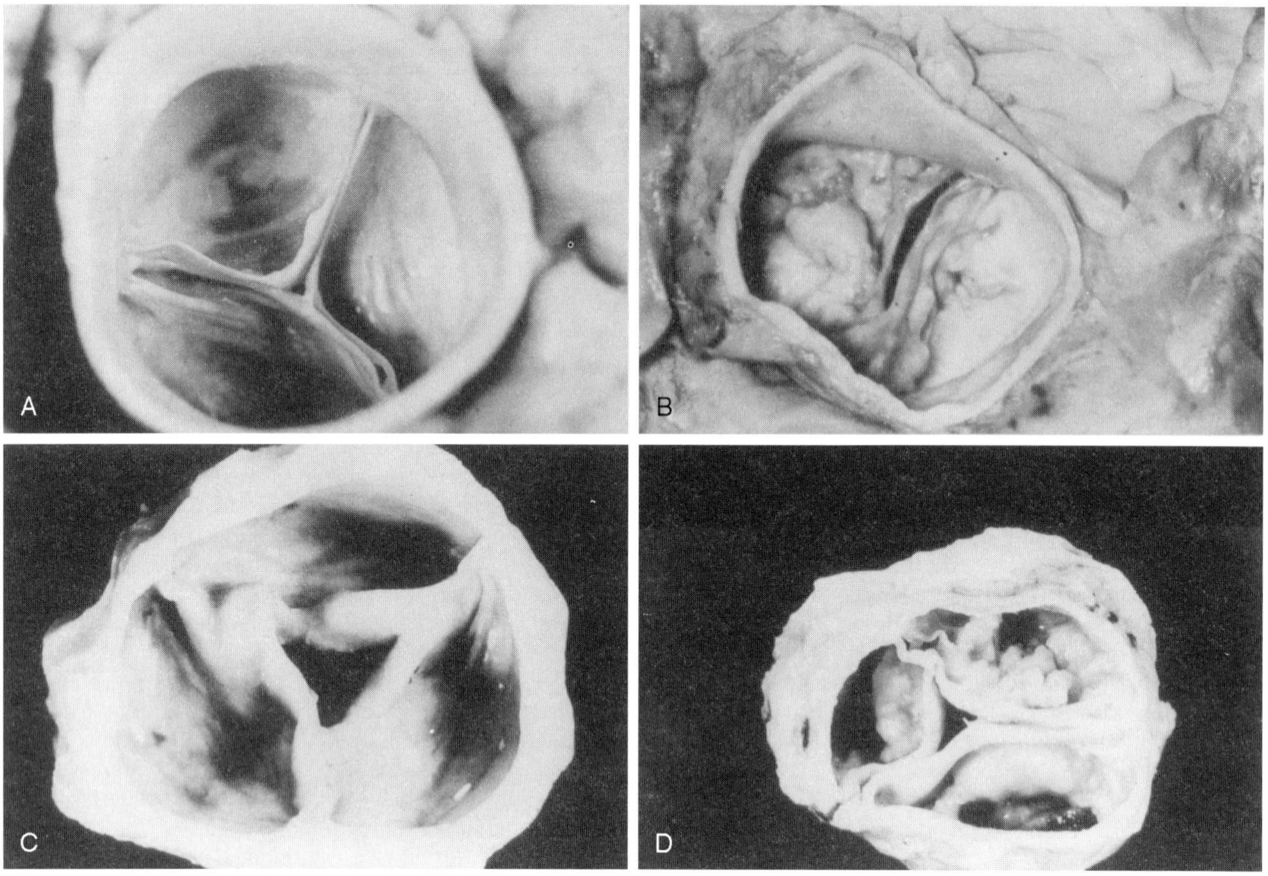

FIGURE 12–1. Pathologic specimen of a normal aortic valve *(upper left)*. Calcific bicuspid aortic stenosis *(upper right)* shows a transverse slit across the aortic root with masses of calcium bulging from each cusp. Rheumatic aortic stenosis *(lower left)* shows fusion of all three commissures and a triangular aortic valve aperture. Calcific aortic stenosis *(lower right)* shows extreme degenerative changes and calcification in the cusps. (From Sutton GC, Fox KM: Valve disease. In Sutton GC, Fox KM [eds]: A Color Atlas of Heart Disease. Pathological, Clinical and Investigatory Aspects. Current Medical Literature Ltd, London, 1990, p 105.)

increases intrinsic myocardial stiffness, is often present in hypertrophied hearts.[11] The reduced uptake of calcium by the sarcoplasmic reticulum during diastole prolongs myocardial relaxation.[12] In addition, elevated intracardiac levels of angiotensin II and angiotensin-converting enzyme contribute to diastolic dysfunction in these patients.[13] The result is an increase in left ventricular end-diastolic pressure. During later stages of the disease, left atrial pressure increases, which allows for adequate ventricular filling in the presence of impaired myocardial relaxation. Later in the course of aortic stenosis, with the prolonged duration of afterload mismatch, left ventricular systolic dysfunction develops. Left ventricular dimensions and volumes increase, and the ejection fraction decreases.

Surgical correction of aortic valve stenosis invariably leads to improvement. Systolic function frequently returns to normal after aortic valve replacement.[14, 15] Many diastolic abnormalities can be improved or reversed. After aortic valve replacement, the myocardial stiffness constant decreases, and left ventricular relaxation returns to normal with the concomitant decrease in left ventricular mass, muscle fiber diameter, and interstitial fibrosis.[16]

Gender Differences

Left ventricular function at rest and during exercise differs in men and women who have the same severity of aortic stenosis. Women have a smaller end-diastolic volume, end-systolic volume, and left ventricular mass, and they have a higher frequency of functional impairment.[17, 18] Furthermore, women have a higher shortening fraction, generate more ventricular pressure with a greater maximum positive dp/dt, and therefore sustain higher transvalvular gradients than men with the same degree of valvular stenosis (Fig. 12–2).[17–19] In a recent study on exercise testing, women with aortic stenosis exercised for a shorter time (4.5 ± 4.1 min versus 8 ± 3.9 min; $p < .0001$) and had a smaller increase in cardiac output (5.4 ± 3.5 L/min versus 8 ± 4.3 L/min, $p < .01$) than men, even though peak heart rate and blood pressure were similar.[17] After adjusting for age, fractional shortening, left ventricular systolic pressure, and functional status, left ventricular hypertrophy was independently associated with gender.[19]

Diagnosis

History

Valvular aortic stenosis can be asymptomatic in children or can occasionally cause a medical emergency in the first year of life. In preschool children with severe stenosis, growth retardation may occur. Similarly, the presentation of the

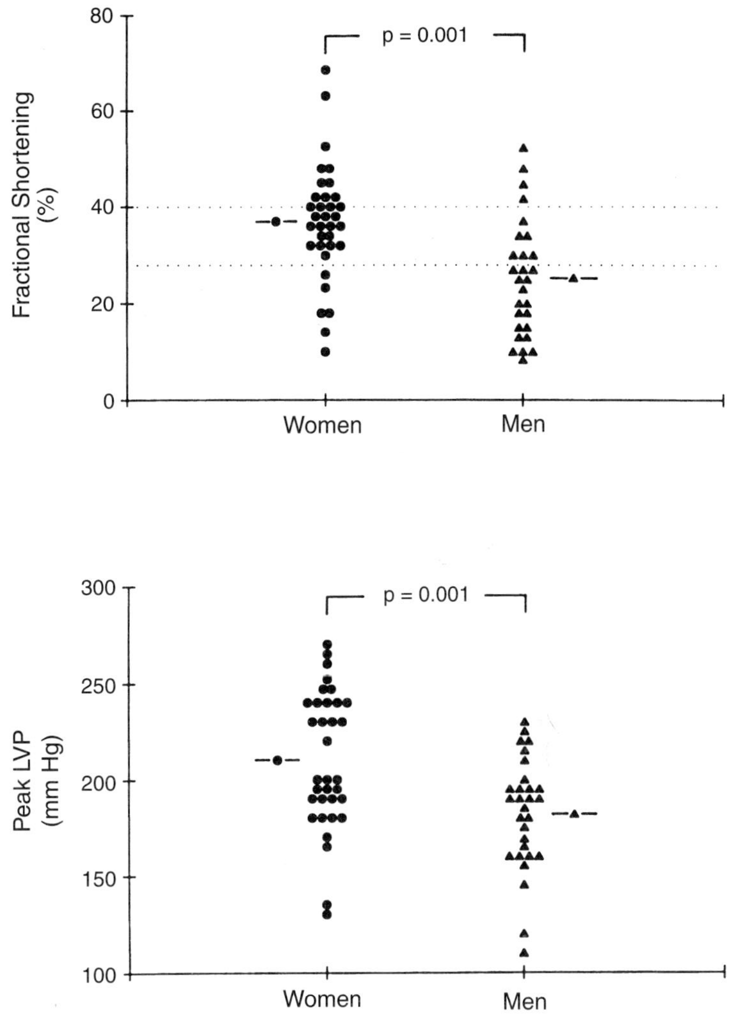

FIGURE 12–2. Fractional shortening and peak left ventricular pressure in women and men with similar degrees of aortic stenosis. (LVP, left ventricular pressure.) (From Carroll JD, Carroll EP, Feldman T, et al: Sex-associated differences in left ventricular function in aortic stenosis of the elderly. Circulation 86:1099, 1992.)

older child or adult with aortic stenosis may range from asymptomatic to development of congestive heart failure. Symptoms usually include dyspnea, fatigue, chest pain, and syncope. The development of symptoms significantly reduces life span.[20] Angina may be related to epicardial coronary disease or to reduction of coronary flow reserve secondary to ventricular hypertrophy. Calcific coronary embolism in patients with normal coronary arteries may rarely cause angina.[21, 22]

Syncope, a typical symptom in patients with aortic stenosis, may result during peripheral vasodilation, which can lead to increased transvalvular gradient and decreased perfusion pressure. This scenario is usually related to physical exertion. However, syncope may result from tachyarrhythmias, bradyarrhythmias, and even transient ischemic attacks from aortic or carotid emboli. Symptoms of pulmonary congestion in patients with aortic stenosis usually result from systolic and diastolic ventricular dysfunction, which leads to increased left atrial pressure. During pregnancy, the reduction in afterload and coronary perfusion pressure, along with the increase in left ventricular stroke volume, can cause asymptomatic patients with aortic stenosis to develop clinically serious disease. However, the outcome in pregnant patients with congenital lesions has been satisfactory in retrospective studies.[23] Sudden cardiac death, a rare presentation of aortic stenosis, is probably related to dysrhythmias or acute ischemia.[24]

Physical Examination

The arterial pulse in severe aortic stenosis typically increases slowly to a small amplitude and then follows a prolonged downslope. These findings, however, may not be present in patients with associated regurgitation or in elderly patients, in whom an increased pulse pressure is observed. The forceful, sustained cardiac impulse in significant aortic stenosis becomes weak and diffuse with the onset of left ventricular failure.

On auscultation, the first heart sound is usually normal. The aortic component of the second heart sound is present at first, becomes soft, and finally disappears with gradual immobility of the aortic cusps. The prominent fourth heart sound reflects the forceful atrial contribution to left ventricular filling. With the onset of left ventricular dysfunction, an S_3 gallop may be heard, and the pulmonic component of the second heart sound becomes accentuated. An ejection click, often present with preserved leaflet mobility, is best heard along the left sternal border. The click is usually heard in patients with bicuspid aortic valves and disappears with advanced valvular calcifications.

The murmur of aortic stenosis is systolic. Best heard at the cardiac base, the murmur radiates to the carotids and is crescendo-decrescendo, starting after the first heart sound and ending before the second sound. Its intensity is diminished when transvalvular flow is reduced and is barely audible when severe heart failure is present. The murmur is accentuated by the inhalation of amyl nitrite and is reduced on standing and on performing the Valsalva maneuver. In contrast, the Valsalva maneuver intensifies the murmur of hypertrophic cardiomyopathy.

Noninvasive Tests

Chest Radiography and Electrocardiography

In the early stages of aortic stenosis, the chest radiograph shows a normal cardiac silhouette or left ventricular prominence. Later in the course of the disease, left ventricular and left atrial enlargement and pulmonary congestion may be seen. The ascending aorta may have poststenotic dilatation. In patients with severe degenerative changes, calcifications of the aortic valve are observed.

Electrocardiography may show evidence of left ventricular hypertrophy with or without a ventricular strain pattern. Left atrial enlargement may also be present. Various degrees of atrioventricular block may be observed, and calcifications may extend into the conduction system.

Echocardiography

Echocardiography is the technique of choice for the noninvasive evaluation of aortic valve stenosis and for assessment of the heart's adaptation to the pressure overload state. Leaflet separation and calcification can be seen with M-mode and two-dimensional echocardiography. Furthermore, the site of obstruction can be determined, and subvalvular, valvular, and supravalvular stenosis can be differentiated. The dimensions, volumes, and systolic and diastolic function of the left ventricle are readily evaluated with echocardiography. In technically difficult studies, transesophageal echocardiography can improve the definition of the aortic valve and surrounding structures.

Differentiating between moderate and severe aortic stenosis with imaging alone is often difficult because of heavy calcification of the valve and because of the small areas involved. Doppler echocardiography, which provides a hemodynamic evaluation of the stenotic valve, has significantly improved the assessment of aortic stenosis by allowing for the derivation of gradient through the valve and valve area. By estimating the velocity of the stenotic jet, the transvalvular gradient can be derived with a modification of the Bernoulli equation as follows:

$$\text{Gradient} = 4V^2$$

where gradient is in mm Hg and V is the velocity of the stenotic jet in m/s. Data obtained with this equation have correlated well with simultaneously acquired data from cardiac catheterization (Fig. 12–3).[25, 26] Gradients depend on transvalvular flow; therefore, the valve area must be assessed.

Aortic valve area, which depends less on flow, can be derived with Doppler echocardiography based on the continuity equation (Fig. 12–4). Flow through a given area is calculated as the product of area and velocity. With conservation of mass, velocity through a stenotic orifice is higher than that before stenosis (see Fig. 12–4). The site of flow

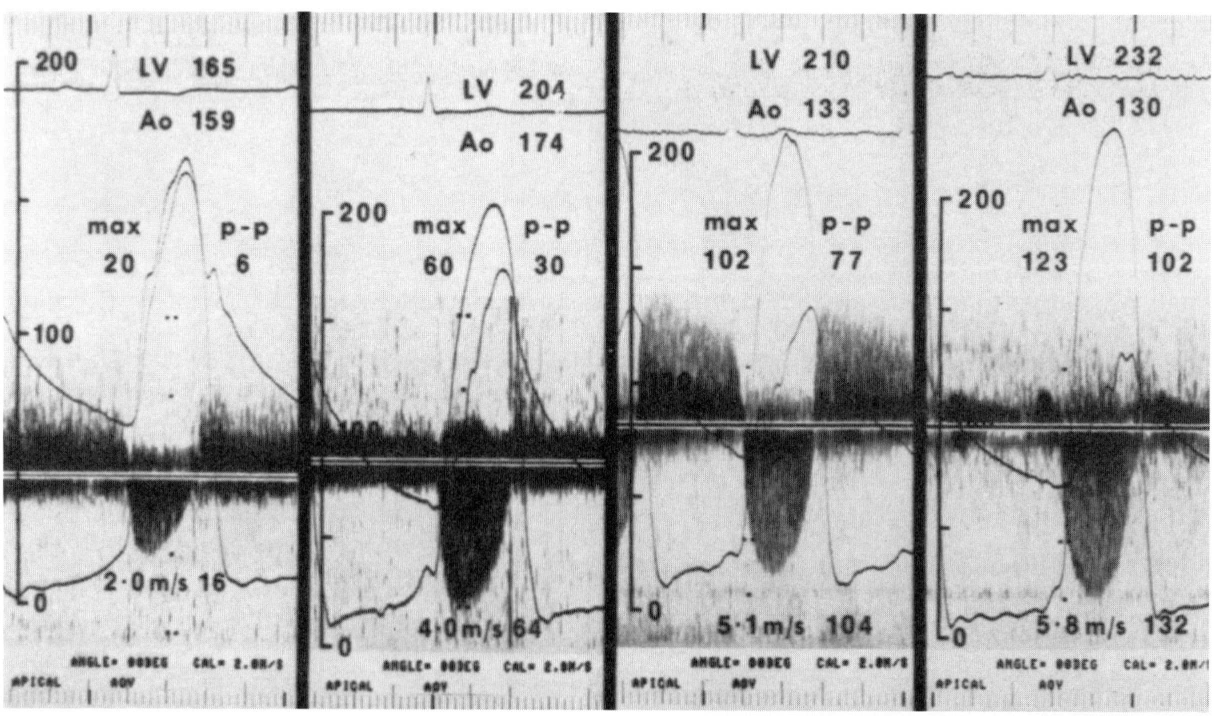

FIGURE 12–3. Simultaneous pressure recordings in the aorta and left ventricle and Doppler recordings of aortic stenosis jet velocity in four patients with increasing severity of aortic stenosis. The maximum and peak-to-peak (p-p) catheter gradients are shown with the corresponding velocities and calculated gradient using the modified Bernoulli equation. (From Currie PJ, Seward JB, Reeder GS, et al: Continuous-wave Doppler echocardiographic assessment of severity of calcific aortic stenosis: A simultaneous Doppler-catheter correlative study in 100 adult patients. Circulation 71:1162, 1985.)

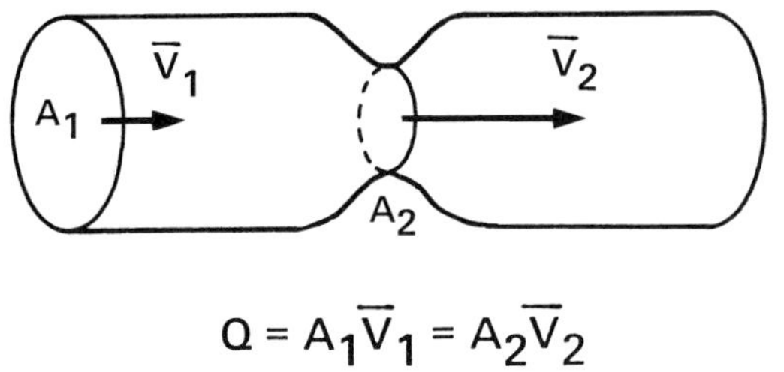

FIGURE 12–4. Schematic representation of the continuity equation. A1 and A2 are the corresponding areas at sites 1 and 2, and V1 and V2 are the corresponding mean velocities. (Q, flow.) (From Zoghbi WA: Echocardiographic and Doppler ultrasonic evaluation of valvular aortic stenosis. Echocardiography 5:23, 1988.)

calculation is usually the left ventricular outflow tract, just proximal to the aortic stenosis. Accordingly, the aortic valve area is derived as follows:

$$AVA = \frac{A_1 \times V_1}{V_2} = \frac{CSA_{(AoA)} \times Velocity_{(LVO)}}{Velocity_{(jet)}}$$

where A_1 and V_1 refer to the area and velocity proximal to the stenosis; $CSA_{(AoA)}$ is the cross-sectional area of the aortic annulus; and $Velocity_{(LVO)}$ and $Velocity_{(jet)}$ are the blood velocities in the left ventricular outflow and aortic jet, respectively (Fig. 12–5).[27–29]

The normal aortic valve area in adults is approximately 3 to 4 cm^2. In mild aortic stenosis, the valve area is usually larger than 1 cm^2; in moderate stenosis, between 1 and 0.75 cm^2; and in severe stenosis, less than 0.75 cm^2. These values are clinical guidelines, not rigid criteria for intervention. The physician's decision to replace a valve should be based on valvular hemodynamics, the patient's clinical status, and myocardial adaptations to the pressure overload state. Most patients who require valve replacement have severely stenotic valves; however, some patients may become symptomatic with moderate stenosis and require intervention.[30]

In some patients with severely depressed ventricular systolic function, the aortic valve area may be underestimated because of the low-flow state. This underestimation possibly results from poor leaflet separation caused by low flow and has been described for both the hydraulic Gorlin equation at cardiac catheterization[31] and the continuity equation.[32] In these situations, the severity of stenosis should be reassessed under conditions that augment flow, such as exercising or administering pharmacologic agents (e.g., dobutamine). In addition to the transvalvular gradient and valve area, valve resistance (mean transvalvular gradient/mean flow rate) and stroke work loss (mean transvalvular gradient/left ventricular systolic pressure) can be calculated and used as indices of stenotic severity. These indices depend to a certain extent on transvalvular flow.[33, 34] Because of its accuracy and noninvasive approach, Doppler echocardiography is ideally suited for evaluating the progression and prognosis of aortic stenosis.[35, 36]

Radionuclide Studies

Radionuclide studies are used only to assess ventricular function and myocardial perfusion. Adenosine scintigraphy has been shown to be safe and accurate in the noninvasive evaluation of coronary artery disease in patients with aortic stenosis.[37]

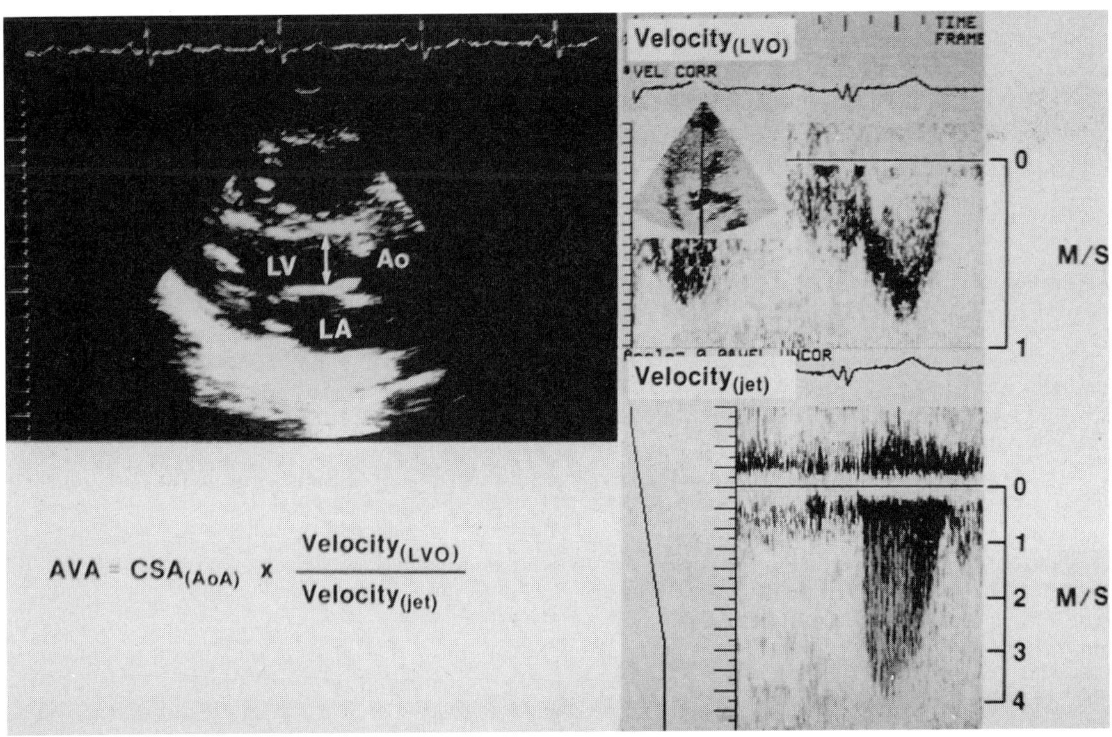

FIGURE 12–5. Example of the derivation of aortic valve area using Doppler echocardiography. Imaging of the calcific aortic valve and surrounding structures is obtained from the apical window. (AVA, aortic valve area; $CSA_{(AoA)}$, cross-sectional area of the aortic annulus; LVO, left ventricular outflow.) (From Zoghbi WA: Echocardiographic and Doppler ultrasonic evaluation of valvular aortic stenosis. Echocardiography 5:23, 1988.)

Cardiac Catheterization

Before the advent of Doppler echocardiography, cardiac catheterization was the only way to accurately assess the severity of aortic valve stenosis. The site and magnitude of the transvalvular gradient can be determined, and the valve area can be calculated with the Gorlin equation. Moreover, filling pressures are accurately recorded. The aortic valve area (AVA) is calculated using the Gorlin equation:

$$\text{AVA} = \frac{\text{CO/SEP} \times \text{HR}}{44.3 \times \sqrt{\text{mean gradient}}}$$

where CO is cardiac output, HR is heart rate, and SEP is systolic ejection period. The cardiac output is typically measured with the thermodilution technique, whereas the mean gradient is obtained by recording pressures in the left ventricle and the ascending aorta.

Valve resistance is another measure of stenosis severity and is calculated as follows:

$$\text{valve resistance} = \frac{\text{mean gradient} \times \text{HR} \times \text{SEP} \times 1.33}{\text{CO}}$$

where resistance is expressed in dynes·sec·cm^{-5}, CO is cardiac output in liters per minute, and SEP is systolic ejection period in seconds. Valve resistance of greater than 250 dynes·sec·cm^{-5} usually indicates severe aortic stenosis. As mentioned earlier, exercise or dobutamine infusion can be used in the catheterization laboratory to augment flow and to reassess valve severity in patients with low-flow state and apparent severe aortic stenosis.

The most common indication for left-sided heart catheterization in adults with aortic stenosis is epicardial coronary artery disease. The incidence of coronary artery disease in adults with aortic stenosis ranges between 33% and 50%.[38, 39] Left-sided heart catheterization is also indicated in patients in whom clinical and Doppler estimates of valvular severity differ or in patients with inadequate Doppler studies.

Natural History

Congenital aortic valve stenosis is usually mild at presentation and gradually worsens over time. Fewer than 20% of patients are likely to have only mild stenosis after 30 years.[40] Adults with calcific aortic stenosis can be asymptomatic for long periods; however, the time to progression of symptoms varies.[41, 42] Echocardiographic studies have shown variable rates of progression. The mean gradient increased by an average of 6 to 8 mmHg/yr.[42–44] Valve area decreased by an average of 0.1 to 0.14 cm^2/yr.[42, 43] Left ventricular hypertrophy developed as an adaptive response to the pressure overload, and progressive mitral regurgitation developed as left ventricular systolic function deteriorated and transvalvular gradients increased.[42] Once symptoms of aortic stenosis develop, mortality is high in the absence of surgery. The average survival rate is 2 years after the onset of heart failure and 5 years after development of angina.[20]

Treatment

Patients with asymptomatic aortic stenosis can be monitored with serial clinical and echocardiographic examinations.[45] Once symptoms develop, patients with significant stenosis should undergo valve replacement given the high mortality rate without surgery.[46]

Medical Therapy

Patients with aortic stenosis, particularly those with rheumatic or bicuspid valves, should receive prophylaxis for endocarditis before undergoing dental or other surgical procedures. In addition, patients with rheumatic aortic stenosis should receive prophylaxis for rheumatic fever, possibly until the fourth decade of life. Because of increased ventricular stiffness and impaired relaxation, left ventricular filling depends heavily on atrial contraction. Thus, these patients tolerate atrial fibrillation poorly and should be converted to and maintained in sinus rhythm. Vasodilators should be used with extreme caution. Stroke volume and cardiac output are not likely to increase in the presence of severe obstruction; therefore, vasodilators may induce hypotension, which can be detrimental to peripheral and myocardial circulation. In patients with congestive heart failure secondary to aortic stenosis, treatment with digoxin and diuretics is only a temporary measure until the stenosis can be surgically corrected.

Balloon Valvuloplasty

Percutaneous balloon valvuloplasty is a therapeutic option for adults with severe valvular stenosis who are not good candidates for surgery. Valvuloplasty increases the valve area by fracturing the calcified nodules, splitting fused commissures, and possibly dilating the valve ring. The procedural mortality rate is 3%; the complication rate is 30%; and the 30-day mortality rate is 14%.[47] Otto and colleagues[48] reported on the 3-year outcome of 674 patients who underwent balloon aortic valvuloplasty as part of the National Heart, Lung and Blood Institute Balloon Valvuloplasty Registry. The mean age of the group was 78 ± 9 years, and 56% were women. Early after the procedure, the aortic valve area increased from 0.5 ± 0.2 cm^2 to 0.8 ± 0.3 cm^2, and the mean gradient decreased from 55 ± 21 mm Hg to 29 ± 13 mm Hg.[47] In 187 patients who underwent echocardiography 6 months after the procedure, values for the area and the gradient were midway between the baseline and postvalvuloplasty measurements, and the severity of aortic regurgitation had slightly increased. Overall survival was 55% at 1 year, 35% at 2 years, and 23% at 3 years; 70% of the deaths had a cardiac etiology. Predictors of outcome were systolic ventricular function, valve gradient, and concomitant mitral regurgitation. Clinical predictors were functional status, cachexia, renal function, and female gender. Although survival rates were higher in women than in men, gender was a univariate predictor of survival only in the subgroup with cardiac output less than 3 L/min. Balloon valvuloplasty does not significantly alter the natural history of the disease because the outcome of unoperated, severe symptomatic aortic stenosis is similar to that of valvuloplasty-treated disease.

Surgical Treatment

In children, valvotomy is usually performed before valve replacement surgery and can be a life-saving procedure in critically ill neonates.[49] Pulmonary autografts have been used,[50, 51] and cryopreserved allografts have produced favorable clinical results.[52]

The use of a bioprosthesis to replace the aortic valve does not require anticoagulation; therefore, bleeding complications are avoided. However, bioprosthetic valves begin to degenerate and calcify a few years after implantation; 20% to 30% of patients undergo repeat surgery in 10 years.[53] The failure rate is higher in patients younger than 35 years of age and in patients with renal failure. Anticoagulation is recommended for the first 3 months after operation because of an increased risk of embolism. Preliminary results with a stentless porcine bioprosthesis have been promising.[54, 55]

In contrast to bioprosthetic valves, mechanical valves have the advantage of durability (except for the Bjork-Shiley 60-degree convex-concave valve, which has a 10-year fracture rate of 10.5% for 29- to 33-mm valves) and the disadvantage of thromboembolic and hemorrhagic risks. Anticoagulation decreases the risk of thromboembolism but increases the risk of hemorrhage. An International Normalized Ratio (INR) of 2.5 to 3.5 is recommended in patients with mechanical valves. Older patients have an increased risk of bleeding (usually gastrointestinal).

In addition to valve type, valve size is an important consideration in patients undergoing aortic valve replacement. To achieve a good exercise capacity postoperatively, a valve area index greater than 1.5 cm²/m² is desirable.[56] Furthermore, a greater reduction in left ventricular mass is seen when the size of the prosthesis exceeds 21 mm[57]; therefore, aortic root reconstruction may be necessary in patients with small aortic roots.

Several factors affect surgical and long-term mortality: age, left ventricular systolic function, rhythm, and emergency status. Surgical mortality varies between 6.2% and 12.4%.[58–60] The presence of coronary artery disease and the need for bypass surgery increase early mortality (10.4% mortality rate in combined procedures versus 4.9% in valve replacement only). Actuarial survival at 9 years is higher in patients who undergo aortic valve replacement only (78.9% versus 66%).[39]

Early (14%) and late mortality rates associated with aortic valve replacement are high in patients who have had previous coronary artery bypass surgery. Risk factors for early mortality include the number of diseased vessels, renal failure, and prior myocardial infarction. Risk factors for late mortality are preoperative diabetes mellitus, postoperative acute respiratory distress syndrome, and ventricular arrhythmias.[61]

Gender Differences in the Response to Valve Replacement

In a study of 1012 patients (329 women) undergoing aortic valve replacement, women were older than men and had a

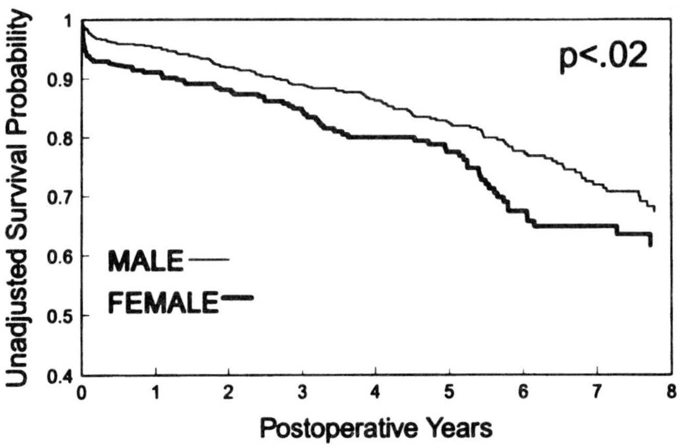

FIGURE 12–6. Unadjusted survival probability in men and women after aortic valve replacement relative to gender. (From Morris JJ, Schaff HV, Mullany CJ, et al: Gender differences in left ventricular functional response to aortic valve replacement. Circulation 90:II183, 1994.)

higher preoperative left ventricular ejection fraction.[62] Furthermore, isolated aortic stenosis was more frequent in women. Women with coronary disease were as likely as men to undergo complete revascularization. After a mean follow-up of 1.4 years, ejection fraction increased more in women (from 33 ± 8% to 48 ± 15%) than in men (from 32 ± 9% to 42 ± 15%). Female gender was an independent predictor of early improvement in ejection fraction and conferred a survival benefit (Fig. 12–6).[62] Men and women who underwent aortic valve replacement in addition to coronary artery bypass surgery had higher operative mortality rates (10.3%) than those who underwent valve replacement only (2.9%). Coronary artery bypass surgery and New York Heart Association class IV were significant predictors of operative mortality in older women (mean age, 77 years).[63]

AORTIC REGURGITATION

Prevalence

Most adults with aortic regurgitation are men; however, the combination of aortic regurgitation with mitral valve prolapse is more common in women. Studies of Doppler echocardiography have shown that trivial to mild aortic regurgitation, although not usually audible, is common in the normal population. The prevalence of aortic regurgitation increases with age. Although aortic regurgitation is not usually detected in normal children and adolescents, the incidence increases to 14% in patients in their sixties and to 33% in patients older than 70 years of age.[64, 65] In a prospective study of the evaluation of regurgitation by Doppler echocardiography during pregnancy, aortic regurgitation was not detected in any stage of pregnancy, but the prevalence of mitral, tricuspid, and pulmonic regurgitation increased in later stages of pregnancy.[66]

Etiology

Aortic regurgitation can result from abnormalities of the aortic cusp or the aortic root or from an increased afterload

Table 12–1. CAUSES OF AORTIC REGURGITATION

AORTIC CUSP ABNORMALITIES	
Infectious: Bacterial endocarditis, rheumatic fever	
Congenital: Bicuspid aortic valve, Marfan's syndrome	
Inflammatory: systemic lupus erythematosus, rheumatoid arthritis, Behçet's syndrome, Reiter's syndrome	
Degenerative: myxomatous (floppy) valve, calcific aortic valve	
Trauma	
Postaortic valvuloplasty	
AORTIC ROOT ABNORMALITIES	
Aortic root dilatation: Marfan's syndrome, syphilis, ankylosing spondylitis, relapsing polychondritis, idiopathic aortitis, annuloaortic ectasia, cystic medial necrosis, Ehlers-Danlos syndrome, osteogenesis imperfecta, mucopolysaccharidosis	
Loss of commissural support: Aortic dissection, trauma, ventricular septal defect	
INCREASED AFTERLOAD	
Systemic hypertension	
Supravalvular aortic stenosis	

(Table 12–1). Congenital aortic regurgitation is seen in patients with fenestrations of the aortic valve and prolapse of an aortic cusp, usually the right cusp in the presence of a supracristal ventricular septal defect. An aortic-left ventricular tunnel, which is rare, can lead to diastolic volume overload of the left ventricle and can be associated with aortic regurgitation and a bicuspid aortic valve.

In adults, regurgitation resulting from abnormalities of the aortic cusps can be caused by inflammatory, infectious, and degenerative diseases and by trauma. In patients with rheumatic fever, thickening, fibrosis, and fusion of aortic valve cusps may be seen. Aortic regurgitation results from improper coaptation, with a variable degree of valvular stenosis. Infective endocarditis, which is an important cause of life-threatening, acute aortic regurgitation, can cause cusp perforation and perivalvular leaks.

Marfan's syndrome and other diseases of the aorta that lead to root dilatation are important causes of valvular insufficiency associated with the aortic root. Type A aortic dissection can lead to acute massive regurgitation by disturbing the annular support of the aortic cusp and causing subsequent prolapse.[67] Although the condition is infrequent, syphilis can lead to dilatation of the aortic root and the ascending aorta. In rare metabolic diseases such as Ehlers-Danlos syndrome, osteogenesis imperfecta, and mucopolysaccharidoses (MPS), the prevalence of aortic insufficiency may be as high as 40%.[68] The incidence is highest in MPS VI (100%) and lowest in MPS IV (33%). Hypertension that leads to aortic dilatation at the commissural attachment may predispose patients to aortic regurgitation. However, in a recent study of healthy, asymptomatic individuals with hypertension, the diameter of the supra-aortic ridge and proximal ascending aorta was only slightly increased, and the incidence of aortic regurgitation was not increased.[69]

Pathophysiology

Aortic insufficiency results in a volume overload of the left ventricle. Although it is usually a diastolic phenomenon, aortic regurgitation can occasionally be observed during systole, when premature beats cause the left ventricular systolic pressure to be lower than the aortic pressure.[70, 71] In patients with chronic insufficiency, left ventricular dilatation and eccentric hypertrophy occur, and left ventricular compliance increases. Initially, the ejection fraction is preserved and forward stroke volume is maintained. With compensatory hypertrophy, the larger left ventricular stroke volume increases the myocardial oxygen demand. As the disease progresses, left ventricular compliance decreases and left ventricular diastolic pressure increases. The inotropic state of the myocardium eventually weakens; ejection fraction and forward stroke volume fall.

The size of the regurgitant orifice and the aortic left ventricular pressure gradient help determine the regurgitant volume. An increase in either factor will lead to a larger regurgitant volume. In addition, the distensibility of the aorta is an important determinant of diastolic regurgitation and ventricular function. Aortic distensibility decreases with age, which imposes a higher afterload on the left ventricle and may lead to further deterioration in ventricular function.[72]

In contrast to chronic aortic regurgitation, acute regurgitation forces a large regurgitant volume on a normal-sized left ventricle. Thus, left ventricular diastolic pressure markedly increases and often exceeds left atrial pressure, which causes premature closure of the mitral valve. To maintain forward stroke volume, left atrial pressure increases and acute pulmonary edema ensues. Moreover, acute aortic regurgitation affects coronary blood flow reserve. Phasic epicardial coronary blood flow becomes predominantly systolic with retrograde diastolic flow.[73]

History

Patients with aortic regurgitation can remain asymptomatic for years when the left ventricle adequately compensates for the chronic volume overload. Some patients may have palpitations possibly related to the large stroke volume or to ectopic beats. Later, patients present with symptoms of pulmonary congestion, including dyspnea, orthopnea, and paroxysmal nocturnal dyspnea. Chest pain may be related to epicardial coronary atherosclerosis or to disease of the aortic root involving the coronary ostia (e.g., chronic dissection or syphilis). However, nocturnal angina can occur in the absence of coronary artery disease and may be related to increased regurgitation and reduced coronary perfusion with slower heart rates. In patients with a history of congenital heart disease, the etiology of aortic insufficiency may also be congenital. Fever and chills may indicate infective endocarditis. Family history is important in patients with hereditary diseases such as Marfan's syndrome.

In contrast to the insidious onset of symptoms in chronic aortic insufficiency, patients with acute regurgitation often present with a sudden onset of symptoms that can rapidly progress to severe dyspnea and hemodynamic collapse.

Physical Examination

The peripheral signs of significant chronic aortic regurgitation are related to the large pulse pressure and include

Table 12–2. PERIPHERAL SIGNS OF AORTIC REGURGITATION

Corrigan's sign:	Rapid and forceful distention of arterial pulse with quick collapse
de Musset's sign:	Up-and-down head bobbing
Müller's sign:	Visible pulsation of uvula
Quincke's sign:	Capillary pulsations seen on light compression of nail bed
Traube's sign:	Systolic and diastolic sounds (so-called pistol shots) over the femoral artery
Duroziez's sign:	Bruit heard over femoral artery on light compression by stethoscope
Hill's sign:	Popliteal cuff systolic blood pressure exceeding brachial pressure by 60 mm Hg or more

prominent carotid pulsations, head-bobbing, and prominent pulsations of the uvula and the nail beds (Table 12–2). So-called pistol-shot sounds can be heard over the peripheral arteries, and a to-and-fro bruit is heard over the femoral artery when it is lightly compressed with a stethoscope. A reduction of left ventricular systolic function and stroke volume decreases the incidence of these signs.

On cardiac examination, the apex is often displaced caudally and laterally. The first heart sound is usually of normal intensity. With severe regurgitation, the intensity of the aortic component of the second heart sound is diminished, and a third heart sound is heard in approximately 28% of patients. This third heart sound is not necessarily related to left ventricular failure.[74] The classic valvular murmur of aortic regurgitation is a soft, high-pitched, early diastolic, decrescendo murmur heard along the left sternal border; maximum intensity is heard at the third left intercostal space. The murmur, which begins with the aortic second sound, is earlier than a pulmonic regurgitation murmur. When aortic root pathology is the cause of the regurgitation, the murmur is loudest at the right sternal border. The murmur is typically accentuated when patients sit up, lean forward, and hold their breath at end-expiration. A systolic murmur of variable intensity can be heard in the aortic area in the absence of valvular stenosis and is related to the large forward systolic flow. Another diastolic murmur (Austin-Flint murmur) that mimics mitral stenosis can be heard over the apex and is probably related to the displacement of the anterior mitral leaflet by the aortic regurgitant jet.[75] The diastolic murmur, which usually indicates significant aortic insufficiency, can be differentiated from mitral stenosis by inhalation of amyl nitrite. In patients with aortic insufficiency, amyl nitrite reduces the intensity of the diastolic murmur because of a decrease in aortic diastolic pressure, whereas amyl nitrite increases the murmur in mitral stenosis because of an increase in left atrial pressure during tachycardia.

In patients with acute aortic regurgitation, the decrease in the intensity of the first heart sound is related to the premature closure of the mitral valve. The diastolic murmur of aortic insufficiency is usually soft, early, and of short duration. The murmur may be difficult to hear, especially in hemodynamically unstable patients. Occasionally, the murmur may have a musical quality, suggesting leaflet laceration or separation from the annulus.[76] Signs of increased pulse pressure or left ventricular enlargement are not usually detected, even though a third heart sound is often heard.

Joint deformities (connective tissue disease), blue sclera (osteogenesis imperfecta), ectopia lentis, skeletal deformities, and arachnodactyly (Marfan's syndrome) can indicate the underlying etiology.

Noninvasive Diagnosis

Chest Radiography

In chronic aortic regurgitation, left ventricular enlargement is present. Aneurysmal dilatation of the ascending aorta may be noted. In acute aortic regurgitation, pulmonary congestion and pulmonary edema occur with a normal-sized heart.

Electrocardiography

The electrocardiogram does not provide specific signs of aortic regurgitation. Changes of left ventricular hypertrophy with secondary ST-T wave changes are the most common findings. Ventricular ectopy may be present in advanced disease.[77] When the atrioventricular (AV) node is inflamed, the P-R interval may be prolonged and AV block may be observed.

Echocardiography and Doppler Techniques

Echocardiographic and Doppler techniques, which are the most common noninvasive tests for assessing the severity and etiology of aortic regurgitation, provide imaging of the aortic valve structure and the aortic root. M-mode and two-dimensional echocardiograms provide indirect clues for detecting the presence or severity of the lesion. These clues include diastolic fluttering of the anterior mitral leaflet or the septum and a ventricle with a volume overload pattern. In the case of severe acute regurgitation, the mitral valve closes prematurely. Aortic regurgitation can be detected and the severity quantified with the use of pulsed, continuous wave, and color-flow Doppler techniques; thus, Doppler techniques are the techniques of choice for the primary evaluation of patients with aortic regurgitation. Most patients can be evaluated with transthoracic imaging; however, transesophageal echocardiography may be needed in selected cases to define the etiology of the regurgitation and to determine its severity.

Color-flow Doppler provides a semiquantitative measure of the severity of aortic regurgitation by imaging the aortic regurgitation jet (Color Plate 12–1). The size of the regurgitant jet at its origin provides a good assessment of the severity of the regurgitation.[78] However, color-flow mapping depends on many factors including machine settings and gains. Furthermore, color Doppler may underestimate the severity of the lesion in patients with eccentric regurgitant jets. Another index used to determine the severity of regurgitation is the pressure half-time obtained by continuous-wave Doppler. This index represents the time required for the maximal diastolic pressure gradient between aorta and left ventricle to decrease by 50%. As aortic regurgitation worsens, this pressure gradient decreases rapidly during diastole,

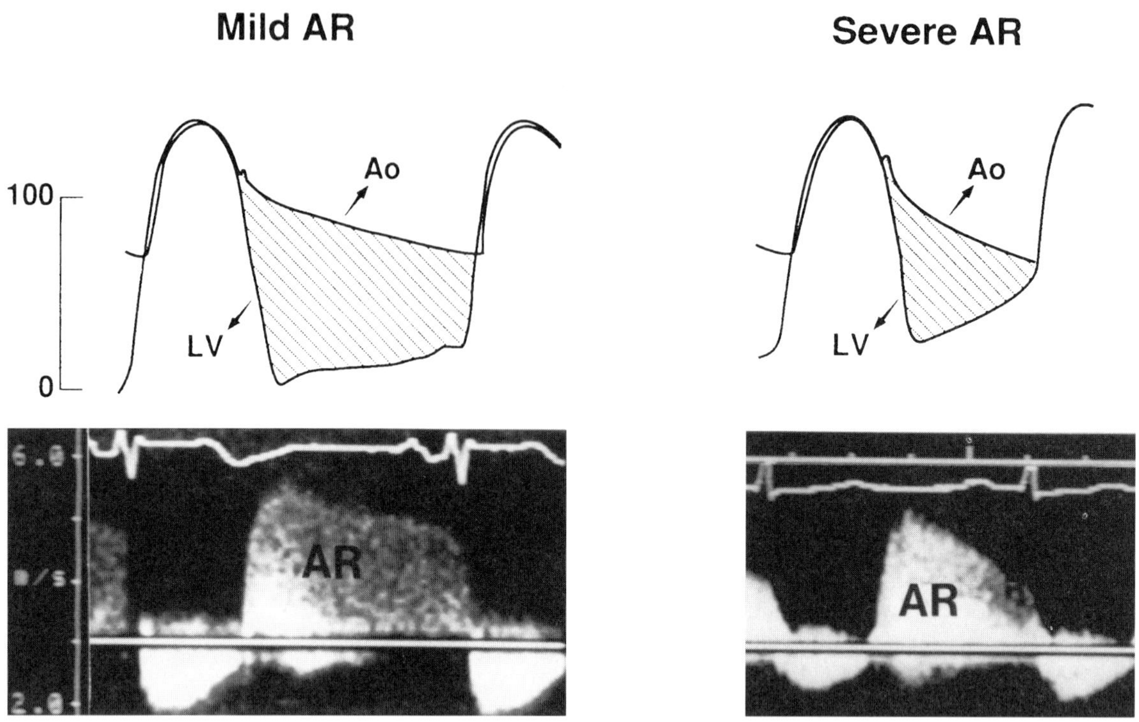

FIGURE 12–7. Schematic of aortic and left ventricular pressure tracings in patients with mild and severe aortic regurgitation with corresponding examples of continuous wave Doppler recording of aortic jet velocity. (AR, aortic regurgitation; Ao, aorta; LV, left ventricle.) (From Zoghbi WA, Afridi I: Aortic regurgitation. In Crawford MH [ed]: Current Diagnosis and Treatment in Cardiology. Appleton & Lange, Norwalk, Conn, 1995, p 99.)

thus shortening the pressure half-time (Fig. 12–7).[79] In patients with high left ventricular diastolic pressures, the pressure half-time overestimates the severity of aortic regurgitation. Finally, pulsed Doppler allows for the evaluation of regurgitant volume and regurgitant fraction.[80] Table 12–3 summarizes a grading system that uses Doppler and echocardiographic techniques.

The effect of aortic regurgitation on hemodynamic function can be assessed by changes in left ventricular size (volume and mass) and function. Simple two-dimensional measurements of end-diastolic and end-systolic dimensions can predict disease progression[81] and can help establish the best time for surgical intervention.

Radionuclide Studies

Left ventricular function at rest and during exercise can be evaluated with radionuclide angiography; a decrease in ejection fraction may herald myocardial impairment. A reduction in ejection fraction during exercise, however, does not necessarily indicate a bad outcome when the resting left ventricular systolic function is normal.[81] The decrease in ejection fraction during exercise is partly accounted for by the reduction in aortic regurgitant volume and left ventricular preload during the tachycardic state. Thus, determination of ejection fraction during exercise is not recommended in patients with aortic regurgitation. Regurgitant volume and regurgitant fraction can be calculated with radionuclide angiography by using differences in stroke volume between the left and right ventricles. However, these differences in stroke volumes are not specific for aortic regurgitation and can be seen in other regurgitant lesions and in shunts.

Magnetic Resonance Imaging

Left ventricular volumes and mass can be accurately measured with magnetic resonance imaging (MRI). Furthermore, MRI can be used to measure regurgitant volume and

Table 12–3. GRADING THE SEVERITY OF AORTIC REGURGITATION USING DOPPLER AND ECHOCARDIOGRAPHIC TECHNIQUES

SEVERITY	COLOR-FLOW DOPPLER JH/LVOH (%)	CONTINUOUS-WAVE DOPPLER Pressure Half-time (msec)	PULSED DOPPLER Regurgitant Fraction (%)
Mild	<24	>500	<20
Moderate	25–45	500–350	20–35
Moderately severe	46–64	350–200	35–50
Severe	≥65	<200	>50

JH/LVOH, ratio of aortic regurgitant jet height to left ventricular outflow height in the parasternal long-axis view.
From Zoghbi WA, Afridi I: Aortic regurgitation. In Crawford MH (ed): Current Diagnosis and Treatment in Cardiology. Appleton & Lange, Norwalk, Conn, 1995, p 99.

orifice. Disadvantages of MRI include limited availability and expense. In addition, MRI cannot be performed in patients with metallic objects such as defibrillators and pacemakers.

Cardiac Catheterization

The severity of aortic regurgitation can be determined during cardiac catheterization by aortography. A semiquantitative grading system can be used with this method (Table 12–4). However, this assessment depends not only on the size of the regurgitant orifice but also on the size of the left ventricle and the position of the catheter in relation to the aortic valve. In addition, the severity of aortic regurgitation can be quantified by determining the regurgitant volume and fraction at catheterization. Because of improved noninvasive tests, routine cardiac catheterization is not recommended in most patients. Cardiac catheterization should be used to assess the severity of aortic insufficiency when results from noninvasive tests are equivocal or discordant with the clinical presentation and, more commonly, when coronary artery disease is assessed before aortic valve surgery.

Prognosis and Natural History

Left ventricular systolic function is an important determinant of long-term outcome in patients with chronic aortic regurgitation. Asymptomatic patients with normal systolic function have an excellent prognosis with an annual mortality less than 0.5%. Fewer than 4% of patients per year require valve replacement because of symptoms or because of left ventricular dysfunction at rest. Serial follow-up studies allow for the detection of patients with left ventricular dysfunction before the development of symptoms.[82, 83] In one study, a baseline end-systolic ventricular diameter greater than 50 mm and an ejection fraction less than 60% were predictors of cardiac symptoms or left ventricular dysfunction where the risk of surgery was 12% at 5 years and 24% at 10 years.[83] Bonow and associates[81] noted that patients with extreme left ventricular dilatation (end-diastolic dimension greater than 80 mm; end-systolic dimension greater than 55 mm) had a higher risk of sudden cardiac death before surgery. Extreme left ventricular dilatation, seen mostly in men, is frequently associated with a reduced ejection fraction but, by itself, is not a marker of irreversible left ventricular dysfunction.[84] Accordingly, extreme dilatation is not a contraindication to surgery but involves an excess late mortality.[84] Valve replacement surgery should still be considered in patients with aortic regurgitation and severe left ventricular dysfunction, but mortality is higher and postoperative ejection fraction is lower in these patients.[84, 85]

Treatment

Medical Treatment

Prophylaxis for endocarditis and rheumatic fever in patients with aortic regurgitation is the same as that described for patients with aortic stenosis. Patients with syphilis should receive a full course of penicillin therapy. Surgery should be considered in patients with symptoms or with evidence of left ventricular dysfunction. Asymptomatic patients can be followed clinically and with serial echocardiography to determine the timing of valve replacement before irreversible left ventricular dysfunction. Vasodilators may improve hemodynamic status and may help postpone valve replacement in asymptomatic patients; however, some differences have been noted between the various classes of vasodilators.[86, 87] After 1 year of treatment, quinapril (10 to 20 mg/day) significantly reduced left ventricular volumes, left ventricular mass, and regurgitant fraction in patients with moderate to severe aortic regurgitation.[88] In a study of 143 patients with isolated asymptomatic severe aortic regurgitation and normal left ventricular systolic function, Scognamiglio and coworkers[89] found that after 6 years of therapy, only 15% of patients treated with nifedipine (20 mg twice a day) underwent aortic valve replacement compared with 34% of those treated with digoxin. After a 1-year follow-up, in a study comparing enalapril with hydralazine in asymptomatic, nonrheumatic patients with mild to severe chronic aortic regurgitation, Lin and colleagues[86] showed that only enalapril significantly reduced left ventricular volume indices and mass index, even though both drugs decreased left ventricular mean wall stress.

Patients with acute severe aortic regurgitation require aggressive supportive therapy. Vasodilator therapy with intravenous sodium nitroprusside decreases preload and afterload, and thus optimizes forward output and wedge pressure. Dobutamine can be added to the regimen in patients with associated hypotension and low output. The definitive therapy is urgent, early surgical correction.

Surgical Treatment

A schematic diagram for management of patients with significant aortic regurgitation is presented in Figure 12–8. Symptomatic patients do poorly with medical therapy only. Surgery is clearly indicated to relieve symptoms and to try

Table 12–4. ANGIOGRAPHIC GRADING OF THE SEVERITY OF AORTIC REGURGITATION

GRADE	DEGREE OF LV OPACIFICATION	INTENSITY OF DYE	CLEARANCE OF DYE FROM LV
I (mild)	Incomplete	Ao>LV	Complete on each beat
II (moderate)	Complete but faint	Ao>LV	Incomplete
III (moderately severe)	Complete in several beats	Ao=LV	Slow
IV (severe)	Complete on first beat	Ao<LV	Slow

Ao, aorta; LV, left ventricle.

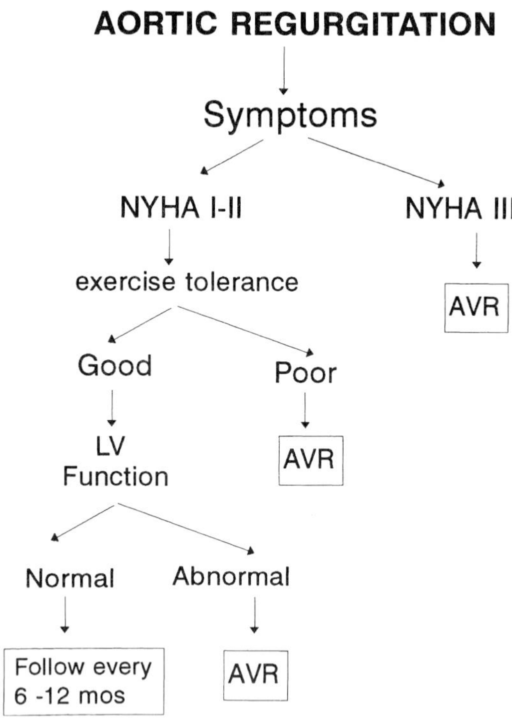

FIGURE 12–8. Schematic for management of patients with chronic aortic regurgitation. (AVR, aortic valve replacement; LV, left ventricle.) (From Zoghbi WA, Afridi I: Aortic regurgitation. In Crawford MH [ed]: Current Diagnosis and Treatment in Cardiology. Appleton & Lange, Norwalk, Conn, 1995, p 99.)

to prevent irreversible left ventricular dysfunction. Postoperative left ventricular function can be predicted by several preoperative parameters including end-diastolic dimension (greater than 70 mm) and volume (greater than 150 ml/m^2). However, both of these measurements depend on preload. End-systolic dimension (greater than 55 mm) and volume (greater than 55 to 60 ml/m^2), also powerful predictors, do not depend on preload but are strongly influenced by afterload. Finally, the ejection fraction (less than 50%) can be used to predict postoperative function, but it depends on both preload and afterload. Thus, the relationship between end-systolic stress and ejection fraction more accurately reflects the myocardial inotropic state. However, this relationship is difficult to calculate and is not routinely used. Moreover, serial acquisition of such data is valuable for the detection of relative deterioration of ventricular systolic function.

Surgery is essential for patients with acute aortic regurgitation. The native valve is usually replaced with a mechanical or bioprosthetic valve. An aortic homograft may be preferred in cases of acute infective endocarditis with severe aortic regurgitation. In selected patients with normal aortic leaflets who are undergoing repair of an ascending aortic aneurysm, the ascending aorta can be replaced and the native valve resuspended within the vascular prosthesis along with reimplantation of the coronary ostia. The intermediate results of this approach are good, but long-term durability has not been determined.[90] Half of patients with type A dissection who are either treated medically or untreated die within 48 hours of onset of symptoms; therefore the need for surgery is urgent. The ascending aorta is replaced with a Dacron prosthesis after resection of the entry site of the dissection flap, reconstruction of the aortic root, and resuspension of the aortic valve.[67] With aortic annular ectasia, the aorta and the valve are usually replaced with a composite graft according to the Bentall technique and its modifications.[91–93]

Early mortality for aortic valve replacement for aortic regurgitation is 2% to 3%.[94, 95] Risk factors for mortality are previous myocardial infarction, coronary artery disease, heart failure, and atrial fibrillation. Late mortality is valve related in 22% of patients, including sudden death in 7% and cerebral vascular accidents in another 7%. In patients with aortic regurgitation and preoperative heart failure, heart failure accounts for 44% of deaths.[95] Postoperative care and the use of anticoagulants are similar to those in patients with aortic stenosis who undergo valve replacement. Doppler echocardiography can be used postoperatively to assess left ventricular function and prosthetic valve performance. A baseline evaluation of prosthetic valve function should be performed in the few months after valve replacement to facilitate interpretation of subsequent studies.

References

1. Waller BF, Roberts WC: Cardiovascular disease in the very elderly. Analysis of 40 necropsy patients aged 90 years or over. Am J Cardiol 51:403, 1983.
2. Kumar A, Olson TM, Thibodeau SN, et al: Confirmation of linkage of supravalvular aortic stenosis to the elastin gene on chromosome 7q. Am J Cardiol 74:1281, 1994.
3. Ho NK, Ng IS: Deletion of the terminal segment of the long arm of chromosome 4 with aortic stenosis. J Paediatr Child Health 29: 473, 1993.
4. Samanek M: Boy:girl ratio in children born with different forms of cardiac malformation: A population-based study. Pediatr Cardiol 15: 53, 1994.
5. Dare AJ, Veinot JP, Edwards WD, et al: New observations on the etiology of aortic valve disease: A surgical pathologic study of 236 cases from 1990. Hum Pathol 24:1330, 1993.
6. Cortina R, Moris C, Astudillo A, et al: Familial ochronosis. Eur Heart J 16:285, 1995.
7. Tomazic BB, Edwards WO, Schoen FJ: Physicochemical characterization of natural and bioprosthetic heart valve calcific deposits: Implications for prevention. Ann Thorac Surg 60(Suppl 2):S322, 1995.
8. Olsson M, Rosenqvist M, Nilsson J: Expression of HLA-DR antigen and smooth muscle cell differentiation markers by valvular fibroblasts in degenerative aortic stenosis. J Am Coll Cardiol 24:1664, 1994.
9. Yoshikawa J, Akasaka T, Yoshida K, Takagi T: Systolic coronary flow reversal and abnormal diastolic flow patterns in patients with aortic stenosis: Assessment with an intracoronary Doppler catheter. J Am Soc Echocardiogr 6:516, 1993.
10. Glantz SA, Parmley WW: Factors which affect the diastolic pressure-volume curve. Circ Res 42:171, 1978.
11. Gaasch WH, Bing OH, Mirsky I: Chamber compliance and myocardial stiffness in left ventricular hypertrophy. Eur Heart J 3(Suppl A):139, 1982.
12. Lorell BH, Grossman W: Cardiac hypertrophy: The consequences for diastole. J Am Coll Cardiol 9:1189, 1987.
13. Friedrich SP, Lorell BH, Rousseau MF, et al: Intracardiac angiotensin-converting enzyme inhibition improves diastolic function in patients with left ventricular hypertrophy due to aortic stenosis. Circulation 90: 2761, 1994.
14. Robiolio PA, Rigolin VH, Hearne SE, et al: Left ventricular performance improves late after aortic valve replacement in patients with aortic stenosis and reduced ejection fraction. Am J Cardiol 76:612, 1995.
15. Uwabe K, Kitamura M, Hachida M, et al: Long-term outcome of left ventricular dysfunction after surgery for severe aortic stenosis. J Heart Valve Dis 4:503, 1995.
16. Villari B, Vassalli G, Monrad ES, et al: Normalization of diastolic

dysfunction in aortic stenosis late after valve replacement. Circulation 91:2353, 1995.
17. Legget ME, Kuusisto J, Healy NL, et al: Gender differences in left ventricular function at rest and with exercise in asymptomatic aortic stenosis. Am Heart J 131:94, 1996.
18. Carroll JD, Carroll EP, Feldman T, et al: Sex-associated differences in left ventricular function in aortic stenosis of the elderly. Circulation 86: 1099, 1992.
19. Douglas PS, Otto CM, Mickel MC, et al: Gender differences in left ventricle geometry and function in patients undergoing balloon dilatation of the aortic valve for isolated aortic stenosis. NHLBI Balloon Valvuloplasty Registry. Br Heart J 73:548, 1995.
20. Ross J Jr, Braunwald E: Aortic stenosis. Circulation 38(Suppl 1):61, 1968.
21. Jondeau G, Dubourg O, Partovian C, et al: Acute myocardial infarction in a patient with severe aortic stenosis and normal coronary arteries. Eur Heart J 15:715, 1994.
22. Brockmeier LB, Adolph RJ, Gustin BW, et al: Calcium emboli to the retinal artery in calcific aortic stenosis. Am Heart J 101:32, 1981.
23. Lao TT, Sermer M, MaGee L, et al: Congenital aortic stenosis and pregnancy—a reappraisal. Am J Obstet Gynecol 169:540, 1993.
24. Frank S, Johnson A, Ross J Jr: Natural history of valvular aortic stenosis. Br Heart J 35:41, 1973.
25. Oh JK, Taliercio CP, Holmes DR Jr, et al: Prediction of the severity of aortic stenosis by Doppler aortic valve area determination: Prospective Doppler-catheterization correlation in 100 patients. J Am Coll Cardiol 11:1227, 1988.
26. Currie PJ, Seward JB, Reeder GS, et al: Continuous-wave Doppler echocardiographic assessment of severity of calcific aortic stenosis: A simultaneous Doppler-catheter correlative study in 100 adult patients. Circulation 71:1162, 1985.
27. Skjaerpe T, Hegrenaes L, Hatle L: Noninvasive estimation of valve area in patients with aortic stenosis by Doppler ultrasound and two-dimensional echocardiography. Circulation 72:810, 1985.
28. Zoghbi WA, Farmer KL, Soto JG, et al: Accurate noninvasive quantification of stenotic aortic valve area by Doppler echocardiography. Circulation 73:452, 1986.
29. Otto CM, Pearlman AS, Comess KA, et al: Determination of the stenotic aortic valve area in adults using Doppler echocardiography. J Am Coll Cardiol 7:509, 1986.
30. Galan A, Zoghbi WA, Quinones MA: Determination of severity of valvular aortic stenosis by Doppler echocardiography and relation of findings to clinical outcome and agreement to hemodynamics determined at cardiac catheterization. Am J Cardiol 67:1007, 1991.
31. Casale PN, Palacios IF, Abascal VM, et al: Effects of dobutamine on Gorlin and continuity equation valve areas and valve resistance in valvular aortic stenosis. Am J Cardiol 70:1175, 1992.
32. deFilippi CR, Willett DL, Brickner ME, et al: Usefulness of dobutamine echocardiography in distinguishing severe from nonsevere valvular aortic stenosis in patients with depressed left ventricular function and low transvalvular gradients. Am J Cardiol 75:191, 1995.
33. Voelker W, Reul H, Nienhaus G, et al: Comparison of valvular resistance, stroke work loss, and Gorlin valve area for quantification of aortic stenosis. An in vitro study in a pulsatile aortic flow model. Circulation 91:1196, 1995.
34. Burwash IG, Pearlman AS, Kraft CD, et al: Flow dependence of measures of aortic stenosis severity during exercise. J Am Coll Cardiol 24:1342, 1994.
35. Roger VL, Tajik AJ: Progression of aortic stenosis in adults: New insights provided by Doppler echocardiography. J Heart Valve Dis 2: 114, 1993.
36. Aronow WS: Usefulness of M-mode, 2-dimensional, and Doppler echocardiography in the diagnosis, prognosis, and management of valvular aortic stenosis, aortic regurgitation, and mitral annular calcium in older patients. J Am Geriatr Soc 43:295, 1995.
37. Samuels B, Kiat H, Friedman JD, Berman OS: Adenosine pharmacologic stress myocardial perfusion tomographic imaging in patients with significant aortic stenosis. Diagnostic efficacy and comparison of clinical, hemodynamic and electrocardiographic variables with 100 age-matched control subjects. J Am Coll Cardiol 25:99, 1995.
38. Moraski RE, Russell RO Jr, Mantle JA, Rackley CE: Aortic stenosis, angina pectoris, coronary artery disease. Cathet Cardiovasc Diagn 2: 157, 1976.
39. Iung B, Drissi MF, Michel PL, et al: Prognosis of valve replacement for aortic stenosis with or without coexisting coronary heart disease: a comparative study. J Heart Valve Dis 2:430, 1993.
40. Kitchiner D, Jackson M, Walsh K, et al: The progression of mild congenital aortic valve stenosis from childhood into adult life. Int J Cardiol 42:217, 1993.
41. Kelly TA, Rothbart RM, Cooper CM, et al: Comparison of outcome of asymptomatic to symptomatic patients older than 20 years of age with valvular aortic stenosis. Am J Cardiol 61:123, 1988.
42. Brener SJ, Duffy CI, Thomas JD, Stewart WJ: Progression of aortic stenosis in 394 patients: relation to changes in myocardial and mitral valve dysfunction. J Am Coll Cardiol 25:305, 1995.
43. Otto CM, Pearlman AS, Gardner CL: Hemodynamic progression of aortic stenosis in adults assessed by Doppler echocardiography. J Am Coll Cardiol 13:545, 1989.
44. Peter M, Hoffmann A, Parker C, et al: Progression of aortic stenosis. Role of age and concomitant coronary artery disease. Chest 103:1715, 1993.
45. Pellikka PA, Nishimura RA, Bailey KR, Tajik AJ: The natural history of adults with asymptomatic, hemodynamically significant aortic stenosis. J Am Coll Cardiol 15:1012, 1990.
46. Stone PH: Management of the patient with asymptomatic aortic stenosis. J Card Surg 9:139, 1994.
47. Percutaneous balloon aortic valvuloplasty. Acute and 30-day follow-up results in 674 patients from the NHLBI Balloon Valvuloplasty Registry. Circulation 84:2383, 1991.
48. Otto CM, Mickel MC, Kennedy JW, et al: Three-year outcome after balloon aortic valvuloplasty. Insights into prognosis of valvular aortic stenosis. Circulation 89:642, 1994.
49. Hosokawa Y, Chibana M, Nakama T et al: [A case report of successful open valvotomy in neonate with critical aortic stenosis]. [Japanese]. Nippon Kyobu Geka Gakkai Zasshi 42:126, 1994.
50. Ross D: Pulmonary valve autotransplantation (the Ross operation). J Card Surg 3:313, 1988.
51. Fabiani JN, Dreyfus GD, Marchand M, et al: The autologous tissue cardiac valve: A new paradigm for heart valve replacement. Ann Thorac Surg 60(Suppl 2):S189, 1995.
52. Shapira OM, Shemin RJ: Aortic valve replacement with cryopreserved allografts: Mid-term results. J Cardiac Surg 9:292, 1994.
53. Hammermeister KE, Sethi GK, Henderson WG, et al: A comparison of outcomes in men 11 years after heart-valve replacement with a mechanical valve or bioprosthesis. Veterans Affairs Cooperative Study on Valvular Heart Disease. N Engl J Med 328:1289, 1993.
54. Del Rizzo DF, Goldman BS, David TE: Aortic valve replacement with a stentless porcine bioprosthesis: Multicentre trial. Canadian Investigators of the Toronto SPV Valve Trial. Can J Cardiol 11:597, 1995.
55. David TE, Feindel CM, Bos J, et al: Aortic valve replacement with a stentless porcine aortic valve. A six-year experience. J Thorac Cardiovasc Surg 108:1030, 1994.
56. Hirooka K, Kawazoe K, Kosakai Y, et al: Prediction of postoperative exercise tolerance after aortic valve replacement. Ann Thorac Surg 58: 1626, 1994.
57. Sim EK, Orszulak TA, Schaff HV, Shub C: Influence of prosthesis size on change in left ventricular mass following aortic valve replacement. Eur J Cardiothorac Surg 8:293, 1994.
58. Chocron S, Etievent JP, Viel JF, et al: Aortic valve replacement in the elderly: A comparative assay of potential risk factor modification. J Heart Valve Dis 4:268, 1995.
59. Obadia JF, Eker A, Rescigno G, et al: Valvular replacement for aortic stenosis on patients in NYHA class III and IV. Early and long term results. J Cardiovasc Surg (Torino) 36:251, 1995.
60. Logeais Y, Langanay T, Roussin R, et al: Surgery for aortic stenosis in elderly patients. A study of surgical risk and predictive factors. Circulation 90:2891, 1994.
61. Fighali SF, Avendano A, Elayda MA, et al: Early and late mortality of patients undergoing aortic valve replacement after previous coronary artery bypass graft surgery. Circulation 92(Suppl 9):II163, 1995.
62. Morris JJ, Schaff HV, Mullany CJ, et al: Gender differences in left ventricular functional response to aortic valve replacement. Circulation 90:II183, 1994.
63. Aranki SF, Rizzo RJ, Couper GS, et al: Aortic valve replacement in the elderly. Effect of gender and coronary artery disease on operative mortality. Circulation 88:II17, 1993.
64. Brand A, Dollberg S, Keren A: The prevalence of valvular regurgitation in children with structurally normal hearts: A color Doppler echocardiographic study. Am Heart J 123:177, 1992.
65. Klein AL, Burstow DJ, Tajik AJ, et al: Age-related prevalence of valvular regurgitation in normal subjects: A comprehensive color flow examination of 118 volunteers. J Am Soc Echocardiogr 3:54, 1990.

66. Campos O, Andrade JL, Bocanegra J, et al: Physiologic multivalvular regurgitation during pregnancy: A longitudinal Doppler echocardiographic study. Int J Cardiol 40:265, 1993.
67. Guilmet D, Bachet J, Goudot B, et al: Aortic dissection: Anatomic types and surgical approaches. J Cardiovasc Surg (Torino) 34:23, 1993.
68. Wippermann CF, Beck M, Schranz D, et al: Mitral and aortic regurgitation in 84 patients with mucopolysaccharidoses. Eur J Pediatr 154: 98, 1995.
69. Kim M, Roman MJ, Cavallini MC, et al: Effect of hypertension on aortic root size and prevalence of aortic regurgitation. Hypertension 28:47, 1996.
70. Kronzon I, Konecky N, Tunick PA: Systolic aortic regurgitation: A hemodynamic challenge for the clinician. J Am Soc Echocardiogr 8: 941, 1995.
71. Unger P, Vandenbossche JL: Doppler demonstration of systolic aortic regurgitation. Am Heart J 123:805, 1992.
72. Wilson RA, McDonald RW, Bristow JD, et al: Correlates of aortic distensibility in chronic aortic regurgitation and relation to progression to surgery. J Am Coll Cardiol 19:733, 1992.
73. Ardehali A, Segal J, Cheitlin MD: Coronary blood flow reserve in acute aortic regurgitation. J Am Col Cardiol 25:1387, 1995.
74. Folland ED, Kriegel BJ, Henderson WG, et al: Implications of third heart sounds in patients with valvular heart disease. The Veterans Affairs Cooperative Study on Valvular Heart Disease. N Engl J Med 327:458, 1992.
75. Landzberg JS, Pflugfelder PW, Cassidy MM, et al: Etiology of the Austin Flint murmur. J Am Coll Cardiol 20:408, 1992.
76. Wigle ED, Labross CJ: Sudden, severe aortic insufficiency. Circulation 32:705, 1965.
77. Martinez-Useros C, Tomos P, Montoyo J, et al: Ventricular arrhythmias in aortic valve disease: A further marker of impaired left ventricular function. Int J Cardiol 34:49, 1992.
78. Perry GJ, Helmcke F, Nanda NC, et al: Evaluation of aortic insufficiency by Doppler color flow mapping. J Am Coll Cardiol 9:952, 1987.
79. Teague SM, Heinsimer JA, Anderson JL, et al: Quantification of aortic regurgitation utilizing continuous wave Doppler ultrasound. J Am Coll Cardiol 8:592, 1986.
80. Rokey R, Sterling LL, Zoghbi WA, et al: Determination of regurgitant fraction in isolated mitral or aortic regurgitation by pulsed Doppler two-dimensional echocardiography. J Am Coll Cardiol 7:1273, 1986.
81. Bonow RO, Lakatos E, Maron BJ, Epstein SE: Serial long-term assessment of the natural history of asymptomatic patients with chronic aortic regurgitation and normal left ventricular systolic function. Circulation 84:1625,1991.
82. Bonow RO: Asymptomatic aortic regurgitation: Indications for operation. J Card Surg 9(Suppl 2):170, 1994.
83. Tornos MP, Olona M, Permanyer-Miralda G, et al: Clinical outcome of severe asymptomatic chronic aortic regurgitation: A long-term prospective follow-up study. Am Heart J 130:333, 1995.
84. Klodas E, Enriquez-Sarano M, Tajik AJ, et al: Aortic regurgitation complicated by extreme left ventricular dilation: Long-term outcome after surgical correction. J Am Coll Cardiol 27:670, 1996.
85. Bonow RO, Nikas D, Elefteriades JA: Valve replacement for regurgitant lesions of the aortic or mitral valve in advanced left ventricular dysfunction. Cardiol Clin 13:73, 1995.
86. Lin M, Chiang HT, Lin SL, et al: Vasodilator therapy in chronic asymptomatic aortic regurgitation: Enalapril versus hydralazine therapy. J Am Coll Cardiol 24:1046, 1994.
87. Rothlisberger C, Sareli P, Wisenbaugh T: Comparison of single-dose nifedipine and captopril for chronic severe aortic regurgitation. Am J Cardiol 72:799, 1993.
88. Schon HR: Hemodynamic and morphologic changes after long-term angiotensin converting enzyme inhibition in patients with chronic valvular regurgitation. J Hypertens Suppl 12:S95, 1994.
89. Scognamiglio R, Rahimtoola SH, Fasoli G, et al: Nifedipine in asymptomatic patients with severe aortic regurgitation and normal left ventricular function. N Engl J Med 331:689, 1994.
90. Simon P, Mortiz A, Moidl R, et al: Aortic valve resuspension in ascending aortic aneurysm repair with aortic insufficiency. Ann Thorac Surg 60:176, 1995.
91. Bentall H, De Bono A: A technique for complete replacement of the ascending aorta. Thorax 23:338, 1968.
92. Cabrol C, Gandjbakhch I, Cham B: Aneurismes de l'aorte ascendante: Remplacement total avec reimplantation des arteres coronaires. [Aneurysms of the ascending aorta: total replacement with reimplantation of the coronary arteries.] Nouv Presse Med 7:363, 1978.
93. Kawazoe K, Eishi K, Kawashima Y: New modified Bentall procedure: Carrel patch and inclusion technique. Ann Thorac Surg 55:1578, 1993.
94. Henry WL, Bonow RO, Borer JS, et al: Observations on the optimum time for operative intervention for aortic regurgitation. I. Evaluation of the results of aortic valve replacement in symptomatic patients. Circulation 61:471, 1980.
95. Verheul HA, van den Brink RB, Bouma BJ, et al: Analysis of risk factors for excess mortality after aortic valve replacement. J Am Coll Cardiol 26:1280, 1995.
96. Zoghbi WA, Afridi I: Aortic regurgitation. In Crawford MH (ed): Current Diagnosis and Treatment in Cardiology. Appleton & Lange, Norwalk, Conn, 1995, p 99.
97. Sutton GC, Fox KM: Valve disease. In Sutton GC, Fox KM (eds): A Color Atlas of Heart Disease. Pathological, Clinical and Investigatory Aspects. Current Medical Literature Ltd, London, 1990, p 105.
98. Zoghbi WA: Echocardiographic and Doppler ultrasonic evaluation of valvular aortic stenosis. Echocardiography 5:23, 1988.

CHAPTER

13 Mitral Valve Disease

Charles Pollick

ANATOMY

Embryology

By the third week of gestation, an embryo can no longer be adequately nourished by diffusion alone; therefore, the vascular system develops.[1] At approximately 30 days, the atrioventricular endocardial cushions develop at either end of the atrioventricular canal, and by 35 days, they divide the canal into right and left atrioventricular orifices. The ventricular surface of the tissue in each canal becomes hollow, and the atrioventricular valves are formed. The valves remain attached to the ventricular wall by muscular cords, which eventually degenerate and are replaced by dense connective tissue. Composed of connective tissue covered by endocardium, the valves are connected to papillary muscles in the wall of the ventricle by means of the chordae tendineae. In the left atrioventricular canal, two valve leaflets form the mitral valve; on the right side, three leaflets form the tricuspid valve. Abnormalities of the atrioventricular canal include not only atrial and ventricular septal defects but also mitral and tricuspid valvular defects.

Morphology

In addition to leaflet tissue, the valve apparatus consists of supporting structures, which include the chordae tendineae and papillary muscles, the left ventricular myocardium subjacent to the papillary muscles, and the fibromuscular annulus. To work properly, the valve needs each of these parts. The mitral valve leaflets comprise an anterior mitral leaflet and a posterior mitral leaflet. The anterior leaflet is relatively long and semicircular, whereas the posterior leaflet is shorter with a larger area of attachment to the mitral annulus. The distal third of both leaflets is rough, whereas the proximal two thirds is smooth. The anterior and posterior mitral leaflets are separated by the anterolateral and posteromedial mitral commissures. The chordae tendineae insert into the rough area on the ventricular surface of the mitral leaflets. The leaflets coapt at the superior margin of this rough area. The posteromedial papillary muscle chordae attach to the medial half of both the anterior and posterior mitral leaflets, and the anterolateral papillary muscle chordae attach to the lateral half of both leaflets.

PATHOPHYSIOLOGY

The thin, pliable mitral leaflets move in concert with the flow of blood through the valve orifice and are restrained by supporting structures. At the onset of diastole, the leaflet tips suddenly and rapidly open until they near the endocardial surfaces of the ventricle. At the maximum point of peak leaflet separation, the distance between the leaflets exceeds the diameter of the mitral annulus, and the annulus automatically limits left ventricular inflow.[2] After opening, the leaflets start to reclose, possibly because of the eddy currents swirling around the leaflets. After atrial systole, the leaflets reopen. Coaptation of the leaflets is initiated by atrial relaxation and completed by ventricular systole.

Different factors can influence the timing and degree of mitral leaflet motion. When flow is slow or reduced through the mitral orifice, or when initial diastolic left ventricular pressure is high, then initial opening of the leaflets is slow, which reduces the rate of initial diastolic closure (EF slope) of the mitral valve and increases E-point septal separation. Closure of the mitral valve may be delayed by first-degree atrioventricular block with a prolonged PR interval and poor inotropy, which prolongs the pre-ejection period. In patients with severe aortic regurgitation, the rapid rise in left ventricular diastolic pressure may reverse the atrioventricular pressure gradient and cause premature closure of the mitral valve leaflets.

Congenital Valvular Pathology

Mitral atresia is characterized by the embryologic absence of a mitral valve. Instead, the fetus has a dimple in the floor of the left atrium; a patent ductus arteriosus or ventricular septal defect is necessary for survival.

Mitral Stenosis

The following are anatomic varieties of congenital mitral stenosis: parachute mitral valve, supravalvular mitral ring, mitral arcade, malformed leaflets and chordae, accessory mitral valve tissue, and obstructing papillary muscle or anomalous left ventricular muscle bundles. In patients with a parachute mitral valve, leaflets and commissures may be relatively normal, but chordae tendineae from both leaflets converge to insert into a single left ventricular papillary muscle. Thus, flow through the mitral valve is both interleaflet and interchordal. Stenosis occurs because the only access to the left ventricle is through the slitlike interchordal spaces; circulation between the leaflets is impossible because the two leaflets cannot separate. In addition, short, thick chordae tendineae limit the movement of the leaflets.[3] In patients with parachute mitral valve in whom the chordae are elongated and are not fused, the valve becomes regurgitant. Parachute mitral valve is often associated with three other obstructive anomalies: supravalvular stenosing ring, subvalvular aortic stenosis, and coarctation of the aorta. Rarely, congenital mitral valve stenosis may result from a mitral arcade, which is a rigid tissue of the free edge of the valve that obstructs the mitral valve orifice.

Double orifice of the mitral valve is another anomaly that may lead to mitral stenosis.[4] In this condition, a band extends across part of the left component of the mitral valve, producing two small annuli, valve leaves, and support apparatus. The lesion may be a true extra valve orifice or just a fibrous strand of tissue.

Mitral Regurgitation

Many different congenital conditions can lead to mitral valve regurgitation. In corrected transposition, the left-sided atrioventricular valve may be an anatomic tricuspid valve with Ebstein's malformation, and "mitral" regurgitation may be produced. Although this condition is called left-sided atrioventricular valve regurgitation, it is really tricuspid regurgitation.

Cleft mitral valve, often with a cleft in the anterior mitral leaflet, may be associated with an endocardial cushion defect or may be an isolated lesion. The anterior leaflet may be partially or entirely cleft. Extra chordae arise from the interventricular septum and attach to the margins of the cleft. The chordae, which are inadequate, do not allow the valve to close properly in systole, and mitral regurgitation results.

Coarctation of the aorta is associated with congenital anomalies of the mitral valve. The leaflets, chordae, papillary muscles, and the left ventricular wall are commonly involved. Clefts, perforations, and myxomatous changes may be present in the mitral valve leaflets, and leaflet tissue may be deficient. In addition, abnormally long or short chordae with poorly developed interchordal spaces may be seen. Furthermore, abnormalities of papillary muscle and endocardial fibroelastosis of the left ventricular wall are also sometimes present. These abnormalities frequently produce a murmur of mitral regurgitation.

The severity of mitral valve prolapse ranges from mildly thickened and myxomatous valve leaflets with mild superior displacement of the valve to severely thickened, grossly abnormal, and redundant mitral valve leaflets. Similarly, the degree of regurgitation with mitral valve prolapse varies. Myxomatous degeneration may affect the cusps of the mitral valve, the chordae tendineae, and the annulus. Chordal rupture may result from degeneration of collagen within the central core of the chordae tendineae. Myxomatous changes in the annulus may cause annular dilatation and calcification. Mitral valve prolapse is sometimes inherited as an autosomal dominant trait but may be associated with Marfan's syndrome, Ehlers-Danlos syndrome, osteogenesis imperfecta, pseudoxanthoma elasticum, muscular dystrophy, and polycystic kidney disease. Congenital thoracic deformities, including a straight back, pectus excavatum, or a shallow chest, are often found in patients with mitral valve prolapse.

Acquired Valvular Pathology

Mitral Stenosis

Rheumatic endocarditis is the most common cause of mitral stenosis in the United States. Almost half of patients with mitral stenosis have a history of rheumatic fever. The acute stage of rheumatic fever does not cause mitral stenosis; rather, mitral regurgitation develops as the valve leaflets become shortened and diseased. Slow, progressive changes occur over several years; leaflet thickening, commissural fusion, shortening, and fusion of the chordae tendineae produce stenosis of the valve. Although rheumatic fever occurs more frequently in men than in women, mitral stenosis is four times more frequent in women.

The stenosed mitral valve limits inflow into the left ventricle with three major consequences: (1) increased left atrial pressure with subsequent pulmonary venous hypertension and pulmonary congestion, (2) right ventricular hypertension, and (3) a possible decrease in left ventricular function. As pulmonary venous hypertension develops and capillary pressures rise above 25 mm Hg, fluid accumulates in the pulmonary alveolar space. This fluid accumulation can lead to pulmonary congestion and pulmonary edema with symptoms of dyspnea on exertion, orthopnea, and paroxysmal nocturnal dyspnea. Pulmonary hypertension can cause right ventricular pressure overload with increased pulmonary vascular resistance, which can lead to right heart failure. Some patients with mitral stenosis have abnormal left ventricular systolic function, which may be related to the reduced preload and underfilled left ventricle associated with mitral stenosis, or which may be caused by a "myocardial factor" related to the rheumatic process.

Mitral Regurgitation

Mitral regurgitation can develop for many reasons that are not primarily based on congenital abnormalities of the mitral valve apparatus.[5] The most common cause of severe mitral regurgitation requiring mitral valve replacement is ischemic heart disease and papillary muscle dysfunction. Ischemia of the papillary muscle may be reversible and may cause reversible mitral regurgitation. However, papillary ischemia may lead to infarction and fibrosis of the papillary muscles, which causes varying degrees of chronic mitral regurgitation. Occasionally, acute myocardial infarction may cause necrosis of papillary muscle and may lead to frank rupture of papillary muscle. Total rupture of a papillary muscle, usually fatal, produces extremely severe mitral regurgitation. However, patients may survive subtotal rupture of one or two of the apical heads of a muscle, which produces milder mitral regurgitation.

Left ventricular dilatation of any cause, including ischemia, can enlarge the mitral annulus and alter the spatial relationships between the papillary muscles in the chordae tendineae, thereby producing mitral regurgitation.

The mitral annulus, normally a flexible structure, contracts in systole and dilates in diastole. When the mitral annulus becomes calcified, it can no longer change shape during the cardiac cycle. This calcification can lead to significant and sometimes severe mitral regurgitation. Mitral annular calcification, which is an important cause of mitral regurgitation in the elderly, is more common in women than in men. Mitral annular calcification is associated with systemic hypertension, aortic stenosis, hypertrophic cardiomyopathy, diabetes, renal failure, and Marfan's and Hurler's syndromes. In addition, patients with an elevated calcium phosphorus product such as hyperparathyroidism may have mitral annular calcification.

Mitral regurgitation may be associated with abnormalities of the mitral valve leaflets seen in inflammatory conditions other than rheumatic fever, such as systemic lupus erythematosus, infective endocarditis, and trauma.

In hypertrophic obstructive cardiomyopathy, the mitral valve leaflets are often elongated and are located in an abnormal anterior position in the left ventricle. In some patients, the anterior mitral leaflet and sometimes the posterior mitral leaflet may move anteriorly in systole and partially or completely obstruct the left ventricular outflow tract. This process can cause significant and sometimes severe mitral regurgitation.

CLINICAL RECOGNITION AND DIAGNOSIS

Physical Examination

Mitral Valve Prolapse

Patients with mitral valve prolapse often have a slender physique with a variety of congenital thoracic deformities including a straight back, a pectus excavatum, or a shallow chest. On auscultation, the characteristic abnormality in mitral valve prolapse is the presence of one or more systolic nonejection clicks. The click occurs at least 140 milliseconds after the first heart sound and can be differentiated from a systolic ejection click because the nonejection click is heard after the beginning of the upstroke of the carotid pulse. Sometimes several mid and late systolic clicks can be heard, particularly along the lower left sternal border. The click occurs as the elongated chordae tendineae snap and the mitral valve prolapses into or toward the left atrium in systole. The click may or may not be accompanied by a mid- to late systolic murmur. The murmur results from mitral regurgitation produced by the abnormal coaptation of the valve leaflets. The click and murmur may vary in intensity and position within the cardiac cycle, both with different phases of respiration and with different positions of the patient. When the ventricle gets smaller, such as when the patient is standing or dehydrated, or when the Valsalva maneuver is performed, prolapse of the mitral valve occurs earlier and is more pronounced; the click occurs sooner in systole (and therefore closer to the first heart sound), and the murmur starts earlier in systole and increases in duration and sometimes in intensity. In some patients, the click and murmur may be absent in the recumbent position but prominent when the patient stands or performs a Valsalva maneuver (Table 13–1). The murmur is shorter than the classic pansystolic murmur of mitral regurgitation and may be confused with a systolic ejection pulmonary flow murmur sometimes heard in healthy individuals. The differentiating feature is that the pulmonary flow murmur is typically heard in the pulmonic area, but the murmur of mitral valve prolapse is best heard at the apex. Rarely, an opening snap may be associated with the mitral valve prolapse after the second heart sound. Other causes of midsystolic clicks include ventricular and atrial septal aneurysms, aortic and pulmonary valve disease, and aortic root dilatation.

Table 13–1. EFFECT OF MANEUVERS ON VARIOUS SYSTOLIC MURMURS

	VALSALVA	STANDING	HAND GRIP	SQUATTING
Mitral Prolapse	↑	↑	↓	↓
Mitral Regurgitation	↓	↓	↑	↑
HOCM	↑	↑	↓	↓
Aortic Stenosis	↓	↔	↔	↔

HOCM, hypertrophic obstructive cardiomyopathy; ↑, increases; ↓, decreases; ↔, usually does not change.

Mitral Stenosis

Chest palpation may reveal a "tapping" apex beat, which correlates with a loud first heart sound. The loud first heart sound reflects the transmitral gradient that keeps the mitral leaflets open throughout diastole so that they close with full momentum after ventricular systole. If the mitral valve becomes calcified or severely diseased, however, apposition of the mitral valve leaflets will not produce a loud sound. In addition, if leaflet mobility is reduced, the first heart sound may be soft. Usually, the second heart sound is physiologically split, but if pulmonary hypertension develops, the second component of the second heart sound (the pulmonic component) is increased in intensity. After the second heart sound, an opening snap is followed by the low-pitched diastolic rumble, which is the hallmark of mitral stenosis. In patients in sinus rhythm, presystolic accentuation of the murmur may be heard at the end of diastole resulting from left atrial contraction, which increases the transmitral gradient. The interval between the second heart sound and the opening snap is related to several variables, including the height of the aortic diastolic pressure, the height of the left atrial pressure, and the rate of fall of left ventricular diastolic pressure. In general, the shorter the interval the higher the left atrial pressure. As the stenosis increases, left atrial pressure increases, the mitral valve opens earlier in diastole, and the opening snap is heard closer to the second heart sound. A short S2–OS interval of 80 milliseconds suggests severe mitral stenosis, whereas an interval of greater than 120 milliseconds suggests mild mitral stenosis. Just as the first heart sound gets softer as the valve gets calcified, so the opening snap disappears when the valve becomes less pliable and calcified. When the patient is in atrial fibrillation, presystolic accentuation of the diastolic murmur is not heard. As the duration of the diastolic murmur increases, the severity of the mitral stenosis increases because the transmitral gradient remains significant throughout diastole to produce a long diastolic rumble. A short diastolic rumble suggests mild mitral stenosis. Physical examination may show signs of pulmonary hypertension including a right ventricular lift along the left sternal border or a prominent a-wave in the jugular venous pulse. Hepatomegaly, edema, and ascites may indicate late-stage pulmonary hypertension.

Mitral Regurgitation

Patients with mild mitral regurgitation may have no abnormal findings on physical examination; however, florid signs may be seen in severe cases. In patients with severe mitral regurgitation who have good left ventricular function, the carotid arterial upstroke may be quite sharp in contrast to the delayed arterial upstroke of aortic stenosis, which may produce a similar prominent precordial systolic murmur. In patients with severe mitral regurgitation and a dilated left ventricle, the apex beat is brisk, hyperdynamic, and displaced to the left. Rarely, a greatly enlarged left atrium can be felt in the third left intercostal space during systole. When mitral regurgitation is chronic and severe because of abnormal valve cusps, the first heart sound produced by valve closure is usually diminished. The second heart sound may be widely split because of the shortened left ventricular ejection time and an earlier aortic second sound, which results from reduced resistance to left ventricular outflow. With pulmonary hypertension, the pulmonary second sound is louder than the aortic second sound. The abnormal increase in flow rate across the mitral orifice during the rapid filling phase is usually associated with a third heart sound. The presence of a third heart sound excludes predominant mitral stenosis.

The systolic murmur is the most dramatic finding in mitral regurgitation. With mitral prolapse, the murmur may be midsystolic or late systolic. A pansystolic murmur radiating to the axilla is usually heard in other forms of mitral regurgitation. The murmur is usually constant in intensity, blowing and high pitched, and loudest at the apex. The murmur can radiate toward the sternum or aortic area in patients with an anteriorly directed mitral regurgitant jet, which is usually associated with severe prolapse of the posterior mitral leaflet or chordal rupture attached to the posterior mitral leaflet. The murmur may radiate to the left posterior chest when a defective anterior leaflet is present and when the regurgitant jet is directed posterolaterally.

The murmur of rheumatic mitral regurgitation varies little with the phases of respiration. However, standing suddenly or administering amyl nitrite usually diminishes the murmur, whereas squatting or administering phenylephrine enhances the murmur. The murmur is reduced during the straining phase of the Valsalva maneuver and returns 6 to 8 beats after release. These responses are different from the responses that would occur in patients with mitral regurgitation associated with mitral prolapse (in the absence of chordal rupture).

The differential diagnosis of the pansystolic murmur of mitral regurgitation includes ventricular septal defect, aortic stenosis, and pulmonary stenosis. The quality of the murmur, its radiation, and its response to various maneuvers help distinguish mitral regurgitation from other entities. In the beat after a long pause in atrial fibrillation, the murmur of aortic stenosis is usually louder (because of the increased stroke volume) than the softer murmur of mitral regurgitation (because aortic diastolic pressure and afterload will be less at the onset of systole).

Mitral regurgitation secondary to hypertrophic obstructive cardiomyopathy varies in a similar way to that of mitral valve prolapse. The murmur is enhanced by performing the Valsalva maneuver, by standing, and by administering amyl nitrite. The murmur is diminished by hand gripping, squatting, or placing the patient supine with the legs elevated.

Electrocardiography

Mitral Valve Prolapse

No specific electrocardiogram (ECG) abnormalities are associated with mitral valve prolapse. In fact, ECG is usually normal in asymptomatic patients. However, some patients have ST-segment and T-wave abnormalities, often in the inferior leads. Supraventricular arrhythmias are more common in patients with mitral valve prolapse. Some studies have reported that the incidence of supraventricular arrhythmias is 25% in patients with mitral valve prolapse as compared with 15% in controls. Ventricular tachycardia has been noted in patients with mitral valve prolapse. In one study, the incidence was 5%, whereas in other studies the incidence of ventricular tachycardia was not increased in patients with mitral valve prolapse.

Mitral Stenosis

Characteristic changes in the ECG are seen in moderate or severe mitral stenosis. When the patient is in sinus rhythm, the predominant finding is left atrial enlargement, as demonstrated by a terminal negative P wave in lead V_1 greater than 0.1 mV in height and 40 msec in duration. When atrial fibrillation develops, the fibrillatory waves may be coarse and greater than 0.1 mV in height in V_1, which suggests left atrial enlargement. Evidence of right ventricular enlargement on ECG is seen in about half of patients with pulmonary hypertension (pulmonary artery systolic pressure greater than 70 mm Hg). When right ventricular systolic pressures exceed 100 mm Hg, right ventricular hypertrophy is invariably found. In addition, the QRS axis correlates with the severity of stenosis and pulmonary vascular resistance. An axis measurement between 0 and +60 degrees correlates with a mitral valve area greater than 1.3 cm^2. An axis greater than 60 degrees generally indicates a valve area less than 1.3 cm^2. When pulmonary vascular resistance is greatly increased, the mean axis usually exceeds 110 degrees.

Mitral Regurgitation

The main ECG finding in patients with mitral regurgitation is left atrial enlargement. Left ventricular enlargement occurs when mitral regurgitation is severe and chronic. In patients with pulmonary hypertension, signs of right ventricular hypertrophy are seen on ECG.

Chest Radiography

The earliest sign of mitral stenosis on the chest radiograph is enlargement of the left atrial appendage. Left atrial enlargement is also evident on the lateral views. Right ventricular enlargement occurs with pulmonary hypertension. Calcification of the mitral valve is more often seen by fluoroscopy. Elevated capillary pressure is indicated by upper lobe venous distention and interstitial edema manifested as Kerley B lines, which are short horizontal lines seen at the costophrenic angles. Severe mitral stenosis may lead to Kerley A lines, which are vertical lines running toward the hilum. In longstanding mitral stenosis, evidence of pulmonary hemosiderosis may be seen.

Enlargement of the left ventricle and left atrium is seen in chronic, severe mitral regurgitation. Left atrial size and left atrial pressure do not usually correlate. Interstitial edema with Kerley B lines can be seen with left ventricular failure, and calcification of the mitral annulus may be seen.

Echocardiography

Mitral Valve Prolapse

On M-mode echocardiography, mitral valve prolapse is diagnosed by posterior displacement of the valve in systole (3 mm or more behind the line connecting the closure point with the opening point of the mitral valve). Holosystolic prolapse is associated with "hammocking" with posterior displacement throughout systole. Midsystolic prolapse is associated with a "? on its side," where the posterior displacement of the coapted leaflet does not occur until midsystole. Pansystolic bowing or hammocking is less specific than midsystolic bowing for mitral valve prolapse.

On two-dimensional echocardiography, the accepted criteria for mitral valve prolapse include superior displacement of either the anterior or the posterior leaflet in the parasternal long-axis view behind the imaginary plane of the mitral annulus. The posterior mitral leaflet is usually involved and can be seen to curl behind this imaginary line. Superior displacement of the anterior mitral leaflet in the apical four-chamber view is seen in up to 30% of healthy individuals.[6] However, any superior displacement of the posterior mitral leaflet on the apical four-chamber view usually indicates mitral valve prolapse. Other features are often seen on two-dimensional echocardiography. Thickening and typical myxomatous changes of the valve leaflets may be seen; the degree of thickening correlates with the risk of subsequent endocarditis and mitral regurgitation. Redundancy of the mitral valve leaflets can be seen in the short-axis view of the mitral valve, where the valve appears to be too large for the size of the mitral orifice. In addition, torn chordae, which indicate significant mitral regurgitation, can be seen.

The presence and degree of mitral regurgitation can be assessed with color-flow Doppler, which can demonstrate the direction of the jet. In patients with significant mitral regurgitation from posterior mitral leaflet prolapse, the jet is directed anteriorly under the aortic root. In anterior mitral leaflet prolapse, the jet is generally directed posteriorly and laterally. The size of the jet roughly correlates with the degree of regurgitation. When the jet area is greater than 8 cm^2, the regurgitation is often severe.[7]

Mitral valve prolapse may be diagnosed based on the presence of one major criterion or two minor criteria (Table 13–2). Diagnosis is made entirely by auscultation or echocardiography. In 80% of patients who have only isolated nonejection systolic clicks, midsystolic clicks, which are classic for mitral valve prolapse, are heard, but the echocardiogram is normal. When patients have a midsystolic click and murmur, the echocardiogram is usually concordant with the diagnosis of mitral valve prolapse. Occasionally, patients with classic echocardiographic signs of mitral valve prolapse have no auscultatory signs.

Mitral Stenosis

The classic triad of signs of mitral stenosis on M-mode echocardiography is thickening of the mitral valve echoes, anterior motion of the posterior mitral leaflet, and a reduced rate of closure of the diastolic EF slope. In addition, left atrial enlargement secondary to increased left atrial pressure or atrial fibrillation and right ventricular enlargement from pulmonary hypertension may be seen. On two-dimensional echocardiography, the valve leaflets have a domed appearance with restricted leaflet tips (Fig. 13–1). In the early stages, the bodies of both the anterior and posterior mitral leaflets are fairly mobile. Thus, the anterior mitral leaflet has a "hockey stick" appearance. Four aspects of mitral stenosis should be assessed from the two-dimensional echocardiogram when considering mitral valvuloplasty: (1) thickness, (2) mobility of the valve leaflets, (3) calcification of the valve leaflets, and (4) subvalvular involvement. The area of the mitral valve can be determined by planimetry in the short-axis view. This assessment is usually accurate except in patients who have had a commissurotomy. In patients with long-standing mitral stenosis, particularly atrial fibrillation, a thrombus may be present in the left atrial appendage. These patients should be assessed with transesophageal echocardiography.

With the use of spectral Doppler (Fig. 13–2), the transmitral gradient and valve area in mitral stenosis can be calculated using planimetry and the pressure half-time equation, which depends on the decrease in the transmitral gradient with time in diastole.

Mitral Regurgitation

M-mode echocardiography may show mitral prolapse, mitral annular calcification, or a rheumatic mitral valve as the

Table 13–2. DIAGNOSIS OF MITRAL VALVE PROLAPSE

	MAJOR CRITERIA (ONE ESTABLISHES DIAGNOSIS)	MINOR CRITERIA (TWO ESTABLISHES DIAGNOSIS)
Auscultation	Typical clicks and late systolic murmur, or "whoop" at cardiac apex	Loud first sound with apical pansystolic murmur
Two-dimensional echo/ Doppler	Marked superior displacement (SD) of mitral leaflets	Mild to moderate SD of posterior leaflet
	Mild to moderate SD with chordal rupture, MR	Moderate SD of both leaflets
Auscultation/History and two-dimensional echo	Mild to moderate SD on two-dimensional echo with either (i) typical clicks or (ii) late systolic murmur	One of the above two-dimensional echo findings plus either (i) focal neurologic attacks or (ii) first-degree relatives with minor criteria

MR, mitral regurgitation.

Reprinted from Perloff JK, Child JS, Dewards JE: New guidelines for the clinical diagnosis of mitral valve prolapse. Am J Cardiol 52:112, 1986, with permission from Excerpta Medica, Inc.

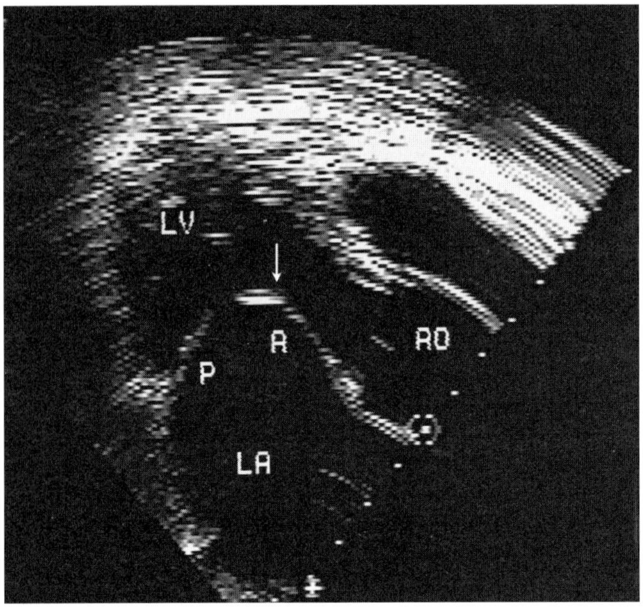

FIGURE 13–1. Two-dimensional echocardiogram from transesophageal window of mitral stenosis. Arrow points to the "hockey-stick" anterior leaflet. Both leaflets are "domed" in diastole. (A, anterior mitral leaflet; AO, aorta; LA, left atrium; LV, left ventricle; P, posterior mitral leaflet.)

cause of mitral regurgitation. In addition, left atrial and left ventricular enlargement may be seen. Moreover, right ventricular enlargement may be seen if pulmonary hypertension is present. When a cord ruptures, systolic fluttering of the mitral valve may be seen on the M-mode echocardiogram.

On two-dimensional echocardiography, mitral valve pathology may be seen with the diagnoses mentioned earlier. Other diagnoses for mitral valve pathology include hypertrophic cardiomyopathy, cleft mitral valve, endocarditis, and ruptured papillary muscle (Fig. 13–3).

Doppler flow study is useful for assessing the degree of valvular regurgitation. The most common method for assessing the degree of regurgitation is to quantify the color Doppler jet. The proximal isovelocity surface area (PISA) method is another way of assessing mitral regurgitation.[8]

Transesophageal echocardiography may be helpful in assessing patients with mitral regurgitation. However, the degree of regurgitation may be underestimated by transthoracic echocardiography, although sometimes the reverse may also occur. Transesophageal echocardiography can be used to assess pulmonary venous flow. Pulmonary venous systolic reversal is a fairly specific finding for severe mitral regurgitation (Fig. 13–4). In patients with a large compliant left atrium, severe mitral regurgitation may occur without reversal of pulmonary venous systolic flow.

Invasive Testing

Invasive testing is not frequently used in the diagnosis of mitral valve prolapse. In patients with mitral stenosis, hemodynamic information usually is obtained by a combination of echocardiography and Doppler analysis. Cardiac catheterization may be useful to calculate the pulmonary vascular resistance or to assess pulmonary artery pressure when Doppler analysis cannot be used. In mitral regurgitation, the left ventricular angiogram may be used to assess the degree of mitral regurgitation and to obtain information that supplements the Doppler and echocardiographic assessment. In most patients, mitral regurgitation can be assessed fully by noninvasive tests; however, if the mitral regurgitant jet is directed against one of the left atrial walls, an accurate assessment of the degree of mitral regurgitation by color Doppler is difficult.

TREATMENT

Medical Treatment

Mitral Valve Prolapse

Antibiotic prophylaxis for infective endocarditis is recommended for patients who have mitral valve prolapse and the murmur of mitral regurgitation. Patients who have a click and no murmur do not need antibiotic prophylaxis. Prophylaxis may be recommended for patients with mitral valve prolapse who have significant (more than physiologic) mitral regurgitation by color-flow Doppler imaging, even if they do

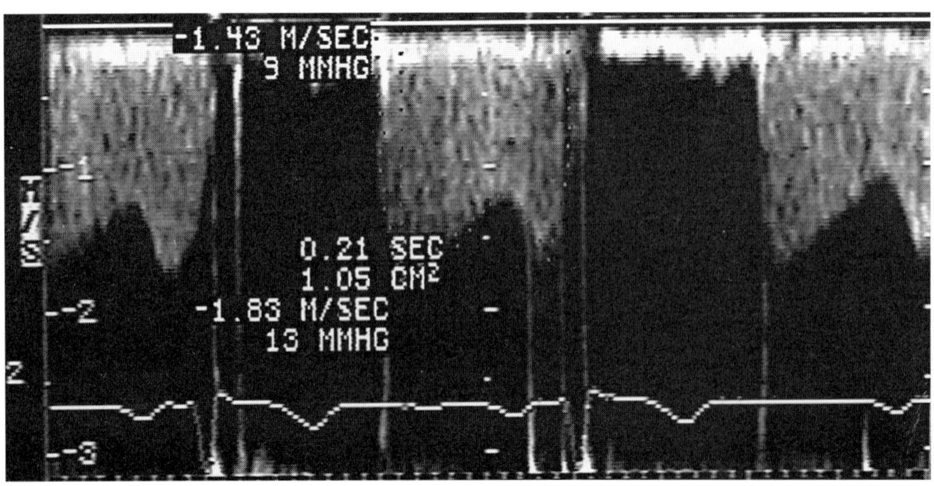

FIGURE 13–2. Spectral continuous-wave Doppler of mitral inflow of patient in Figure 13–3. Mean gradient, 9 mm Hg; peak gradient, 13 mm Hg; valve area, 1.05 cm^2.

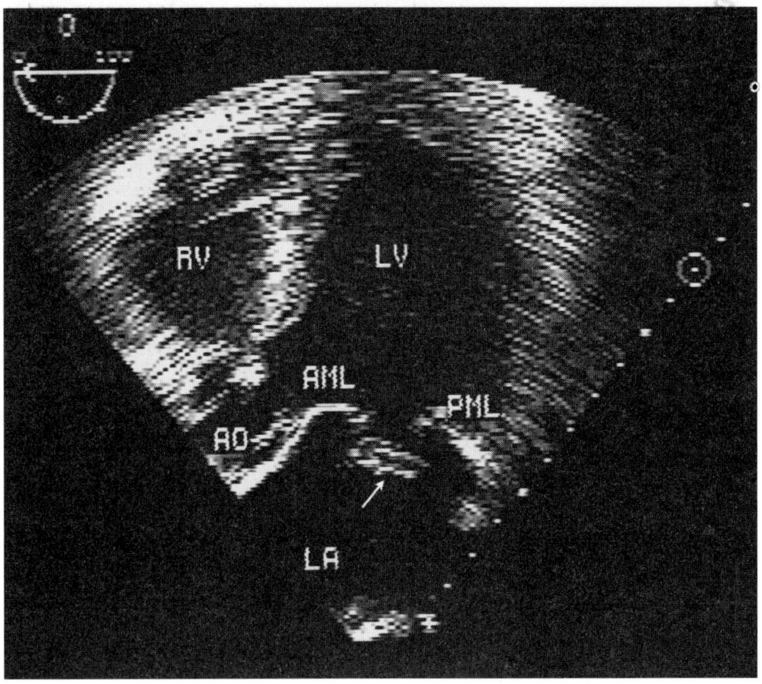

FIGURE 13–3. Transesophageal two-dimensional echocardiogram of ruptured papillary muscle *(arrow)*. (AML, anterior mitral leaflet; AO, aorta; LA, left atrium; LV, left ventricle; PML, posterior mitral leaflet; RV, right ventricle.)

not have the murmur of mitral regurgitation. In the past, physicians believed that patients with mitral valve prolapse who had atypical chest pain syndrome might benefit from beta blockers. More recent studies have shown that atypical chest pain is more common in patients with mitral valve prolapse than in the normal population. Furthermore, the use of beta blockers in the treatment of atypical chest pain has had mixed success.[6] Standard guidelines for antiarrhythmic therapy should be applied to patients with mitral valve prolapse who have cardiac arrhythmias. Beta blockers have traditionally been used for supraventricular arrhythmias, but no study has shown that beta blockers are more successful in treating arrhythmias associated with mitral valve prolapse than they are in other situations. Aspirin or warfarin (Coumadin) should be given to patients with mitral valve prolapse who have had a stroke.

Mitral Stenosis

The goal of pharmacologic therapy for mitral stenosis is to lower left atrial pressure. Diuretic therapy may help reduce left atrial pressure. Beta blockers and digoxin can be used

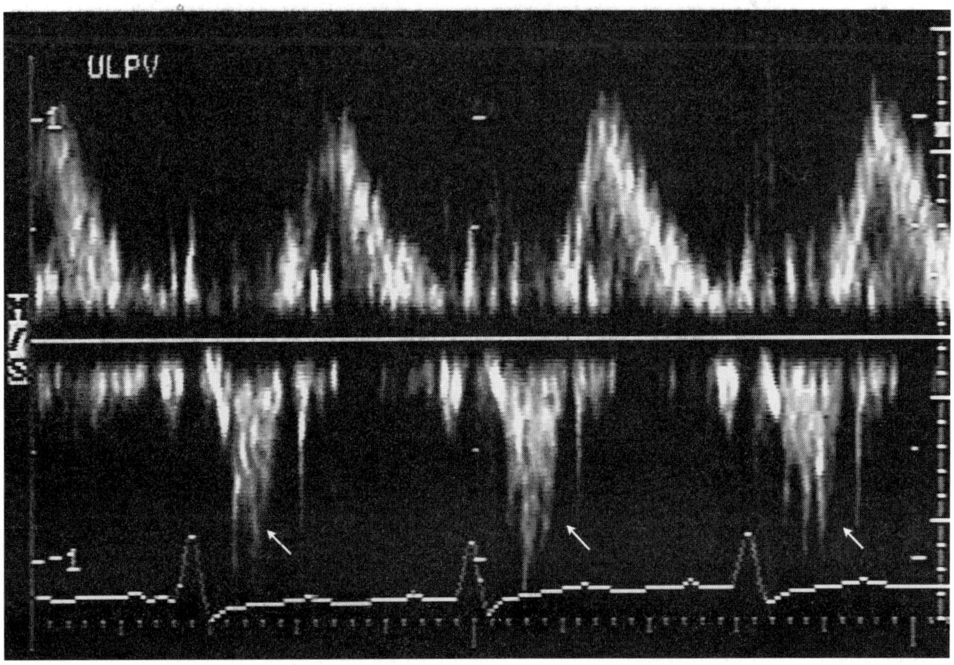

FIGURE 13–4. Spectral pulsed Doppler of pulmonary venous flow, demonstrating systolic reversal *(arrows)*. (ULPV, upper left pulmonary vein.) (Patient from Figure 13–3.)

Table 13–3. MANAGEMENT OF MITRAL REGURGITATION (IN THE ABSENCE OF CORONARY DISEASE, CONCOMITANT MITRAL STENOSIS, OR UNRELATED CARDIOMYOPATHY)

DEGREE OF MR	LV SIZE*	EF	SYMPTOMS	MEDICAL THERAPY	SURGICAL REPAIR/ REPLACEMENT
Mild	N	N	None	None	None
Moderate	N	N	None	√	None
Severe	N	N	None	√√	None
Severe	N	N	Any	√	√√
Severe	>60 ml/m³	N	None	√	√√
Severe	N	35%–50%	NR	√	√√
Severe	>60 ml/m³	20%	NR	√√	None

MR, mitral regurgitation; LV size*, end-systolic left ventricular volume; N, normal; EF, ejection fraction (N > 0.5); √, therapy indicated; √√, therapy of choice; NR, not relevant.

in patients with sinus rhythm to slow the heart rate and to increase the diastolic filling period.

Pharmacologic therapy should be used at the onset of atrial fibrillation to convert the patient back to sinus rhythm or to control the ventricular rate. No particular antiarrhythmic drug for atrial fibrillation has been more effective for atrial fibrillation in patients with mitral stenosis than for atrial fibrillation from other causes. Digoxin is the most effective drug for controlling the ventricular rate in patients with established atrial fibrillation. If digoxin alone is ineffective, then calcium channel blockers (such as verapamil or diltiazem) or beta blockers may be added to the regimen. Patients who develop paroxysmal or chronic atrial fibrillation require anticoagulation; 25% of patients with mitral stenosis who are not given anticoagulants in such a situation develop systemic emboli. Aspirin therapy is insufficient, and warfarin should be given to attain an International Normalized Ratio (INR) range between 2 and 2.5 times the control.

Once mitral stenosis impairs exercise tolerance to an unacceptable degree, then mechanical therapy such as balloon valvuloplasty or mitral valve repair or replacement is indicated. The decision to institute mechanical therapy often depends on the lifestyle of the patient. Younger patients with a greater exercise and activity level who have a valve area of 1.5 cm² may need mechanical therapy. As the patient gets older, the exercise demands of life decrease, and a patient with this degree of stenosis may not require mechanical therapy.

Balloon valvuloplasty performed in the cardiac catheterization laboratory is feasible when mitral regurgitation is less than moderate and when the valve is suitable for valvuloplasty. The valve is scored on the basis of thickness, calcification, mobility, and subvalvular involvement. Some studies have shown that the success of valvuloplasty decreases when the score exceeds 8 out of a possible 16. Heterogeneity of calcification improves the chances of successful balloon valvuloplasty. When mitral valve balloon valvuloplasty is not possible, then surgical repair or replacement may be necessary. In general, surgery is used in patients who have severe mitral stenosis with a valve area of 1.0 cm² or less and who have pulmonary hypertension. In pregnant patients with mitral stenosis, medical therapy with diuretics and beta blockers usually overcomes congestive heart failure that may be precipitated by the blood volume changes and increased heart rate associated with pregnancy. Balloon valvuloplasty can be successfully performed during pregnancy when medical therapy does not prevent or control the heart failure.

Mitral Regurgitation

Vasodilators and afterload reduction, which may delay or prevent the progression of mitral regurgitation, are usually indicated when mitral regurgitation is moderate or greater, especially when left atrial enlargement and pulmonary hypertension are present. The use of angiotensin-converting enzyme (ACE) inhibitors or other vasodilators (e.g., hydralazine) may be appropriate. Surgery for mitral valve replacement is usually indicated when the patient becomes symptomatic with mitral regurgitation. Treatment of asymptomatic patients with severe mitral regurgitation is controversial. Asymptomatic patients may develop dilated and hypokinetic left ventricles, which may not be reversible upon the onset of symptoms. Several studies have been performed to determine the optimal time for mitral valve surgery in patients with asymptomatic severe mitral regurgitation. The development of significant pulmonary hypertension is one potential indication for surgery because pulmonary hypertension may be irreversible and may cause right ventricular failure. An end-systolic dimension on the left ventricular minor axis of 4.5 cm or an end-systolic volume greater than 60 ml/m² have been recommended as indicators of surgery in asymptomatic patients (Table 13–3). Waiting until the ejection fraction reaches 35% or less might be too late; however, surgery for mitral valve replacement can produce significant clinical and ventricular improvement even in patients with a poor ejection fraction. Improvements in myocardial preservation over the last few years have allowed surgery to be performed in patients who previously would have done poorly with surgery.

References

1. Sadler TW: Langman's Medical Embryology, 6th ed. Williams & Wilkins, Baltimore, 1990.
2. Weyman AE: Principles and Practice of Echocardiography, 2nd ed. Lea & Febiger, Philadelphia, 1994, pp 91–480.
3. Perloff JK: The Clinical Recognition of Congenital Heart Disease. WB Saunders, Philadelphia, 1992.
4. Silverman NH: Pediatric Echocardiography. Williams & Wilkins, Baltimore, 1993.
5. Carabello BA: Mitral valve disease. Curr Probl Cardiol 18:423, 1993.
6. Pollick C, Wilansky S, Parker S: Mitral valve prolapse: Clinical and echocardiographic perspective. Can Med Assoc J 104:641, 1986.
7. Cujec B, Wilansky S, David TE, Pollick C: Colorflow imaging in severe mitral and aortic regurgitation. Can J Cardiol 4:341, 1988.
8. Feigenbaum H. Echocardiography, 5th ed. Lea & Febiger, Philadelphia, 1994.

CHAPTER 14

Tricuspid and Pulmonary Valve Disease

Raymond F. Stainback

TRICUSPID VALVE DISEASE

Anatomy and Normal Physiology

Embryology

The morphogenesis of the two atrioventricular (AV) valves is intimately related to atrial and ventricular septation of the primitive AV canal. This complex and miraculous series of directed developmental events is initiated around fetal day 28 (9-mm stage), with completion of AV valve formation (tricuspid and mitral) at about day 55.[1, 2] The right and left AV valve leaflets (tricuspid and mitral) begin as proliferations of the five endocardial cushions. The septal tricuspid leaflet and part of the anterior mitral leaflet are derived from the same (inferior) endocardial cushion. Thus, congenital AV septal defects (AV canal defects) result in both mitral and tricuspid valve abnormalities. Mesenchymal proliferations, which will become the free tricuspid valve leaflets and associated chordae tendineae, are continuous with the underlying ventricular myocardium. Connective tissue proliferation into this matrix proceeds alongside resorption of the underlying ventricular myocardium, allowing the free tricuspid (and mitral) leaflets and the fibrous chordae tendineae to take shape. The papillary muscles are residual ventricular muscular attachments. Errors in this "delamination" of the tricuspid leaflets from the ventricular myocardium result in congenital malformations.

Morphology

The tricuspid valve is a complex asymmetric structure with the same morphologic features as the mitral valve: annulus, leaflets, commissures, chordae tendineae, and papillary muscles. The tricuspid valve's basic function is to provide low resistance and unidirectional blood flow between the right atrium and right ventricle. In addition, the tricuspid annulus, along with the rest of the cardiac skeleton, ensures AV electrical isolation. Unlike the tough fibromuscular mitral annulus, the tricuspid annulus is composed of relatively loose connective tissue, which is more subject to dilatation and tricuspid regurgitation (TR) in response to right-sided pressure or volume overload. A four-chamber view of the heart (Fig. 14–1) reveals a slightly more apical location of the septal tricuspid leaflet annular attachment than that of the opposing anterior mitral leaflet. This relationship is important for determining ventricular situs in congenital malformations and for diagnosing Ebstein's anomaly.

The three leaflets (anterior, septal, and posterior) vary considerably in size and shape. The anterior leaflet is the largest and most mobile, hanging curtain-like between the right ventricular inflow and outflow tracts. The systolic tethering action of this tensor apparatus (papillary muscles and associated chordae tendineae) prevents systolic leaflet prolapse and regurgitation. Because each papillary muscle supplies chordae to each of two adjacent leaflets, shortening of the systolic papillary muscle tends to assist leaflet closure. The anterior papillary muscle, arising at least partially from the right ventricular moderator band, is the largest and most well defined.[3–6] A small degree of natural leaflet redundancy and a leaflet coaptation zone allow continued leaflet competency despite mild enlargement of the tricuspid annulus diameter.

Physiology

In the absence of shunt lesions, flow across the tricuspid and mitral valves is equal. The tricuspid valve area is larger, however, accounting for a lower diastolic tricuspid inflow velocity. Significant respiratory variation in tricuspid valve flow occurs—increased with inspiration (lowered intrathoracic pressure) and decreased with Valsalva's maneuver or

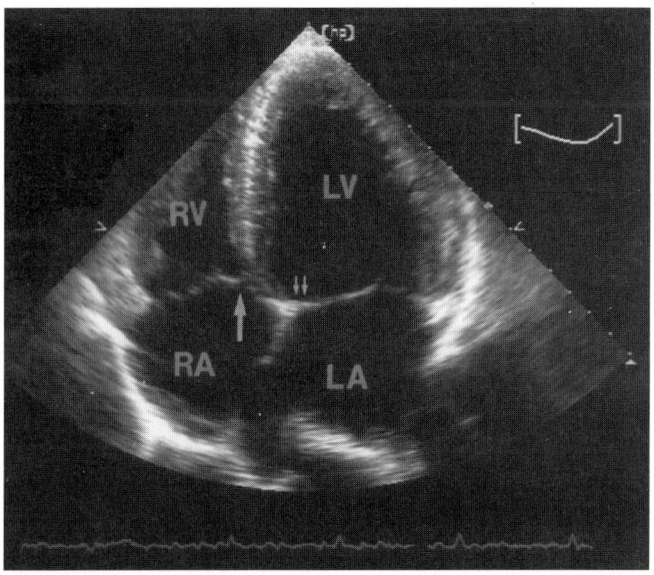

FIGURE 14–1. Apical four-chamber echocardiographic view in a patient with mild dilated cardiomyopathy but an otherwise morphologically normal heart. The tricuspid valve's septal leaflet (*single arrow*) is more apically located than the mitral valve's anterior leaflet-septal attachment (*double arrows*). RV, right ventricle; LV, left ventricle; RA, right atrium; LA, left atrium. (Photo courtesy of Todd Belcik, RDCS.)

positive pressure ventilation (raised intrathoracic pressure). Because the intensity of auscultated cardiac resistance murmurs increases with increased flow, respiratory maneuvers may, therefore, be valuable in distinguishing right-sided (tricuspid or pulmonary valve) pathology from left-sided (mitral or aortic valve) lesions at the bedside.

Under normal physiologic conditions, the tricuspid valve opposes no more than 20 to 30 mm Hg peak systolic right ventricular pressure. However, it is capable of much more. The structural integrity of the intact tricuspid valve is best illustrated by a case of congenitally corrected transposition of the great arteries, wherein the tricuspid valve serves as the systemic AV valve, functioning without failure under systemic arterial pressure for more than 2 or 3 decades.

Noninvasive Measurement of Systolic Pulmonary Artery Pressure. Normal or physiologic TR may be seen in the majority of normal individuals undergoing color-flow Doppler examination.[7] This small, usually inaudible regurgitant volume is measurable by continuous-wave Doppler echocardiography in more than 60% of subjects.[8–10] Application of the modified Bernoulli formula ($\Delta P = 4V^2$) to the peak TR velocity (V) yields an accurate peak systolic pressure difference (ΔP) in millimeters of mercury between the right ventricle and right atrium.[11] In the absence of right ventricular outflow obstruction, an accurate and reproducible estimate of peak systolic pulmonary artery pressure is obtained when the calculated transvalvular pressure gradient is added to an estimated right atrial pressure.[12] Thus, Doppler-measurable physiologic (and pathologic) TR enables accurate noninvasive estimates of peak systolic pulmonary artery pressure in most clinical situations (Fig. 14–2).[13]

Pathophysiology

Tricuspid Regurgitation

Tricuspid valve pathology may be divided according to whether the defects are acquired or congenital (Table 14–1). Asymptomatic TR, which may be mild to moderate in severity, is common. However, severe TR requiring medical or surgical management is not as common. A defect in any of the tricuspid valve components may result in TR.

ACQUIRED TRICUSPID VALVE REGURGITATION

Functional Tricuspid Valve Regurgitation

The most common cause of TR is not intrinsic tricuspid valve pathology but secondary or functional TR. Functional TR may complicate any condition, leading to right ventricular failure or dilatation because the relatively lax tricuspid annulus dilates along with the enlarging right ventricle. Right

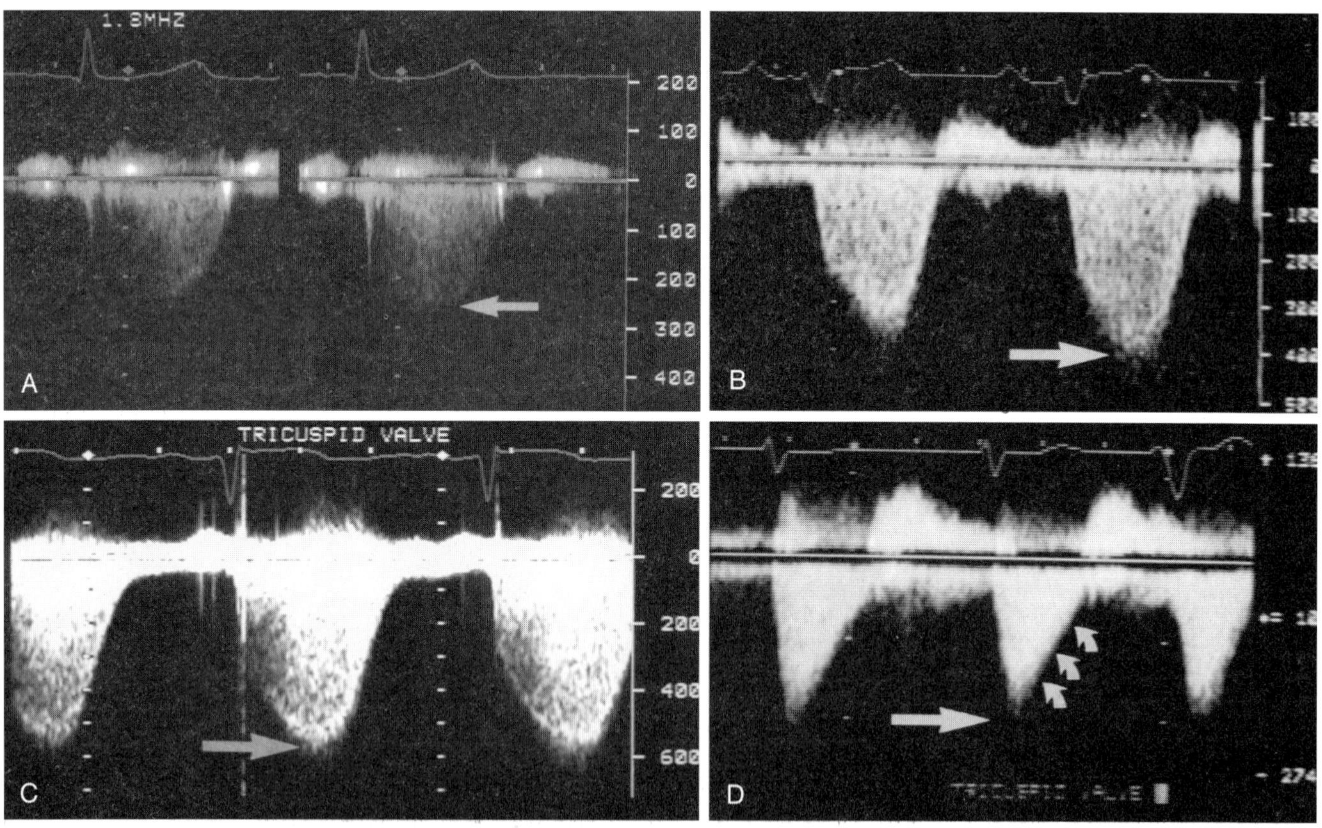

FIGURE 14–2. Four examples of tricuspid regurgitation (TR) velocity measurement and systolic pulmonary artery pressure (PAP) estimation by continuous-wave Doppler echocardiography ($PAP = 4V_{TR}^2 + P_{RA}$, see text). *A*, Mild "physiologic" TR and normal PAP. Peak TR velocity (*arrow*) = 2.5 m/s; estimated RA pressure = 5 mm Hg, systolic PAP = 30 mm Hg. *B*, Moderate functional TR (chronic obstructive lung disease). Peak TR velocity (*arrow*) = 4 m/s; estimated RA pressure = 15 mm Hg, systolic PAP = 79 mm Hg. *C*, Moderate functional TR (advanced primary pulmonary hypertension). Peak TR velocity (*arrow*) = 5.7 m/s; estimated RA pressure = 20 mm Hg, systolic PAP = 150 mm Hg. *D*, Severe "low-pressure" TR (torn tricuspid leaflet). "V-wave cutoff" (*triple arrows*) and a dense regurgitation velocity signal indicate a large regurgitation volume.

Table 14–1. ETIOLOGY OF TRICUSPID REGURGITATION

Acquired TR
Functional
RV pressure or volume overload
Rheumatic
Endocarditis
Myxomatous degeneration
Endomyocardial biopsy complication
Tricuspid prosthesis dysfunction
Rare causes
Carcinoid heart disease
Traumatic injury
Myocardial infarction (papillary muscle rupture)
Endomyocardial fibroelastosis
Methylsergide-induced valve disease
Systemic lupus erythematosuis
Radiation injury
Cardiac tumors (valve destruction or distortion)
Congenital TR
Ebstein's anomaly
Congenital non-Ebstein's anomaly

RV, right ventricular; TR, tricuspid regurgitation.

ventricular dilatation also leads to excessive tricuspid leaflet systolic tethering by the subvalvular tensor apparatus. Increased flow resistance at any site downstream (right ventricular outflow tract, pulmonary vasculature, mitral valve, left ventricle, aortic valve, peripheral vasculature) augments the tricuspid regurgitant volume and exacerbates clinical symptoms of severe TR. Functional TR and right ventricular failure may occur secondary to severe left-sided valve pathology; severe mitral valve disease (regurgitation or stenosis) is the leading cause. Less commonly, functional TR accompanies untreated or end-stage aortic stenosis or aortic insufficiency with left ventricular failure. Functional TR from low-pressure right ventricular failure is usually due to right-sided volume overload conditions, such as severe pulmonary insufficiency and large atrial septal defect (atrial level left-to-right shunting). Significant functional TR is common in patients with acute pulmonary embolus[14] because of sudden right ventricular dilatation from elevation of acute pulmonary artery pressure.

Under conditions of slowly progressive pulmonary hypertension (chronic pulmonary emboli, Eisenmenger's syndrome, primary pulmonary hypertension), right ventricular dilatation and severe functional TR occur as late complications (Fig. 14–3). At least moderate functional TR is not an uncommon complication of cor pulmonale due to chronic obstructive pulmonary disease. Tricuspid regurgitation from *any* cause imposes an added regurgitant volume load on the right ventricle. In a circular process, the ensuing compensatory right ventricular dilatation leads to increased annular dilatation and worsening functional TR.

Rheumatic Tricuspid Regurgitation

Important TR occurs in only 5% of patients with rheumatic heart disease, whereas the mitral and aortic valves are affected in 85% and 55% of patients, respectively. Rheumatic TR is twice as likely to occur in women and is almost always accompanied by significant mitral valve disease, usually mitral stenosis.[15–17] The pathologic changes that produce TR are the same as those that produce rheumatic mitral regurgitation. Acute and chronic inflammation produces fibrosis, thickening, and shortening of the tricuspid leaflets and chordae tendineae. TR results from retraction of the fibrosed leaflets and tethering due to chordal shortening. A degree of tricuspid stenosis may coexist or even be the predominant lesion. Some progression of disease is likely to occur from functional wear and tear on the morphologically abnormal

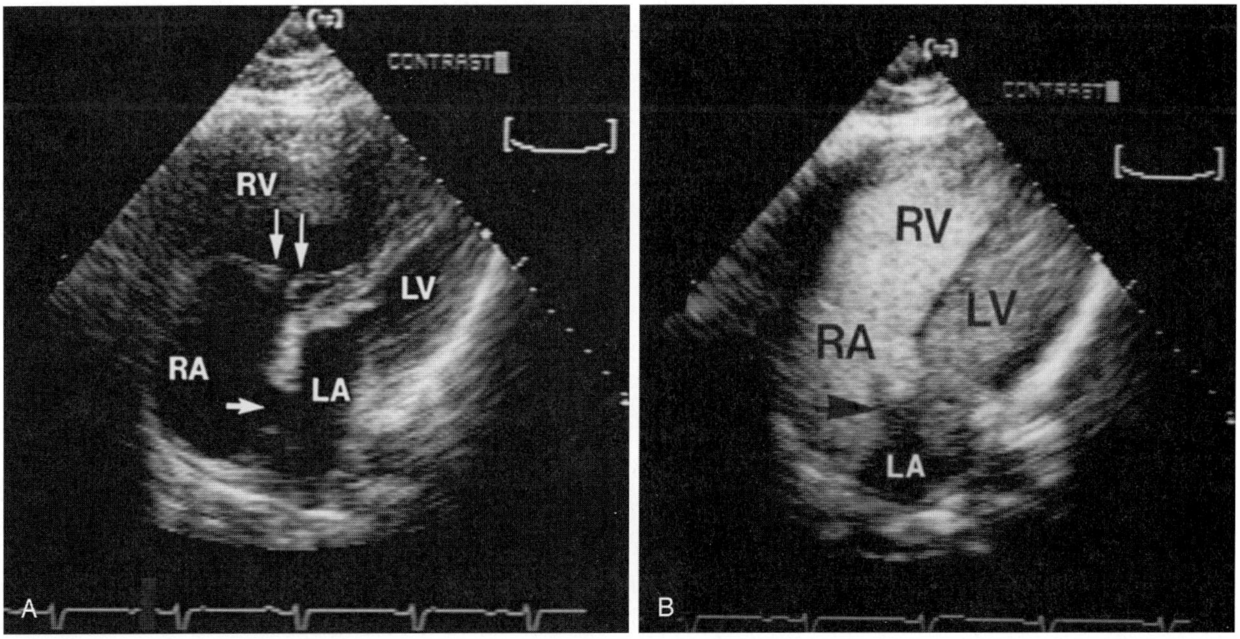

FIGURE 14–3. Severe functional TR secondary to a large atrial septal defect (ASD = *arrows*) and concomitant severe pulmonary hypertension. Severely dilated right ventricle (RV); small, underfilled left ventricle (LV). Cyanosis was present due to high right atrium (RA) pressure and right-to-left shunting across the atrial septal defect, demonstrated in *B* by complete left-sided opacification after intravenous agitated-saline "contrast" injection. A "negative contrast jet" (*black arrow*) from intermittent left-to-right shunting further demonstrates the ASD.

valve, even after rheumatic inflammation has become quiescent. Progression to severe TR is accelerated by pulmonary hypertension from concomitant mitral or aortic valve disease, or both, and occasionally, superimposed infective endocarditis. Rheumatic TR and right-sided failure may progress without echocardiographic evidence for progression of accompanying rheumatic mitral stenosis.[18]

Nonrheumatic Organic Tricuspid Regurgitation

Infective endocarditis may result in severe TR due to leaflet, annulus, or chordae tendineae destruction. Intravenous drug use is a major risk factor wherein highly virulent organisms (such as *Staphylococcus aureus*) can infect a morphologically normal tricuspid valve. Valvular abnormalities increase the risk of endocarditis. Infecting organisms that may involve the other heart valves directly or by local extension include *Staphylococcus* and *Streptococcus* species, gonococci, gram-negative rods, and mycotic organisms. In a reported series of illicit intravenous drug use–related bacterial endocarditis cases in Chicago, 32% of 125 cases occurred in women; the tricuspid valve was involved in 46% of cases. The causative organism was a *Staphylococcus* species in 66% and *Streptococcus* in 26%.[19] Other patients at risk for bacterial endocarditis include those with prior episodes of endocarditis, rheumatic heart disease, and congenital anomalies. Chronic and temporary indwelling right-sided catheters may traumatize the tricuspid valve (and pulmonary valve), providing both a nidus and an entry site for infectious organisms.[20–22]

Isolated tricuspid valve prolapse is rare but can occur in approximately 20% of patients with mitral valve prolapse due to myxomatous degeneration (floppy mitral valve) or Marfan's syndrome. A complication of percutaneous right ventricular biopsy is injury to the tricuspid leaflets or chordae. For this reason, severe TR, often due to a flail leaflet, may occur in cardiac transplant patients who must undergo periodic right ventricular diagnostic and surveillance biopsies.[23–25] Dysfunctional prosthetic tricuspid valves may produce regurgitation due to leaflet degeneration (bioprosthesis) or malfunctioning mechanical leaflets from obstructing thrombus or pannus (infiltrating fibrous tissue) formation.

Rare Causes of Tricuspid Regurgitation

Carcinoid Heart Disease. A complication of metastatic carcinoid tumors can be severe TR, which occurs via a complex mechanism.[26, 27] The primary lesion, a carcinoid tumor, is an uncommon (0.7 per 100,000) indolent malignancy of the midgut (>90%) or, occasionally, the foregut (3.5% bronchial). The carcinoid syndrome (e.g., episodic cutaneous flushing, diarrhea, bronchospasm, hypotension, tachycardia) occurs in 20% to 30% of patients who develop advanced, metastatic liver involvement. Approximately half of those with carcinoid syndrome go on to develop significant cardiac complications (cardiac carcinoid) due to tricuspid and pulmonary valve destruction. Carcinoid syndrome usually occurs in the 5th or 6th decade, during which there is no significant male or female predilection. However, evidence has shown that early carcinoids are rare in women during the reproductive years, suggesting a role for hormonal factors upon etiology.[26]

Carcinoid tumors (malignant chromaffin cells) are apudomas, exhibiting amino uptake and decarboxylation (APUD). The complex array of monoamine and peptide hormones (e.g., serotonin, bradykinin, histamine, catecholamines, prostaglandins) released into the portal circulation by these tumors is largely metabolized by the liver in a first-pass effect until late in the disease course, when hepatic metastasis occurs. At this stage, tumor products bypass the liver, enter the systemic venous circulation directly, and cause the peripheral manifestations of the carcinoid syndrome. Elevated right atrial and right ventricular serotonin (a smooth-muscle mitogen) and bradykinin (known to damage endothelium) levels are thought to stimulate formation of dense, superficial plaques on the tricuspid and pulmonary valves. Both serotonin and bradykinin undergo pulmonary metabolism, possibly explaining why the left-sided heart valves are spared in the absence of an intracardiac shunt lesion or in rare bronchial carcinoids. The classic tricuspid valve changes are easily recognized by echocardiography (Fig. 14–4). The leaflets and chordae tendineae appear severely thickened and partially frozen in a semiopen position. Varying degrees of pulmonary valve stenosis or insufficiency worsen the extent of TR. With metastatic carcinoid disease, long-term survival is poor.[28] Administration of parenteral octreotide (somatostatin analogue) inhibits the secretory activity of carcinoid tumors and may greatly improve the systemic symptoms.[29] The cardiac manifestations, however, are not reversed by this therapy.

Other Rare Causes of Tricuspid Valve Regurgitation. Deceleration injuries (chest striking the steering wheel or a fall from a ladder) or penetrating trauma may cause severe

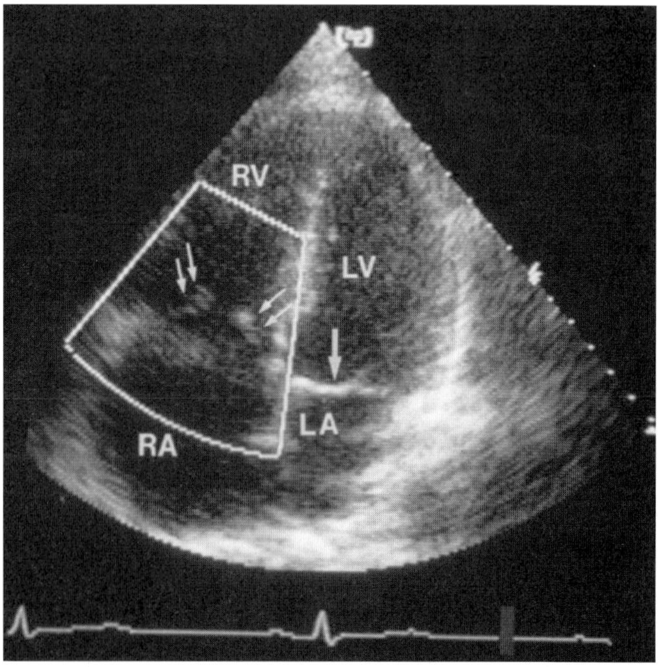

FIGURE 14–4. Carcinoid heart disease with RV and RA dilatation due to severe tricuspid regurgitation. The tricuspid valve leaflets (*double arrows*) are thickened and frozen in the open position during ventricular systole, while the mitral valve (*single arrow*) closes appropriately.

TR, usually due to anterior leaflet papillary muscle or chordal rupture.[30, 31] A history suggesting post-traumatic TR may be difficult to elicit because the onset of symptoms may be remote from the injury. Another unusual cause of severe TR that may result in cardiogenic shock is papillary muscle rupture after right ventricular infarction.[32] Degeneration and insufficiency may rarely be diagnosed in endomyocardial fibrosis, methysergide-induced valvular disease, or systemic lupus erythematosus, although, again, disease primarily affects the mitral valve. Infiltration, compression, or destruction of the valve apparatus by primary intracardiac or metastatic cardiac tumors may lead to TR. Significant TR from radiation injury may rarely occur.

Congenital Tricuspid Regurgitation

Ebstein's Anomaly

Ebstein's anomaly, although rare, is the most common congenital malformation of the tricuspid valve. Because of incomplete leaflet delamination during morphogenesis, the valve opening occurs at a distance from the true tricuspid annulus. The basal leaflet portions are adherent to the underlying myocardium with so-called apical displacement of the proximal tricuspid leaflet attachments.[33, 34] Cases usually occur spontaneously in both sexes, although familial occurrences have been described. A case-control study suggests an association between first-trimester maternal lithium ingestion and an increased risk of Ebstein's anomaly in the offspring.[35] However, this association was not demonstrated in a more recent prospective study.[36] Severe TR from poor leaflet coaptation is the predominant hemodynamic lesion in symptomatic patients. The right atrium is potentially massively enlarged, owing to severe TR and incorporation of an atrialized portion of the basal right ventricle into the chamber (Fig. 14–5). An interatrial communication (atrial septal defect or patent foramen ovale [PFO]) is present in 50% of patients and allows atrial level right-to-left shunting and cyanosis due to right atrial pressure elevation. Varying degrees of tricuspid valve malformation and the presence or absence of associated defects produce a wide range of severity and patient ages at presentation. Patients diagnosed in adolescence or adulthood generally have mild disease and an excellent prognosis. Although late hemodynamic compromise from right ventricular failure, development of cyanosis, left ventricular failure, or arrhythmia may occur, mild Ebstein's anomaly does not preclude a normal life expectancy.[37]

In Ebstein's anomaly, fertility is not affected, but pregnancy and its associated risks are important considerations. Clinical data for Ebstein's anomaly and pregnancy are limited. The largest series reports 44 women with 111 documented conceptions.[38] Maternal risk was low in this population despite a wide spectrum of disease severity, including documented cyanosis in 16 patients. Even though supervised pregnancy was well tolerated in these women, an increased risk of fetal loss, congenital cardiac defects, prematurity, and low birth weight (in cyanotic mothers) was observed. Although it is not precluded, pregnancy in women with Ebstein's anomaly should be considered high risk due to the number of potential complications. Prenatal evaluation and follow-up at a tertiary referral center is recommended.

Non-Ebstein's Congenital Tricuspid Regurgitation

Atrioventricular septal defects can produce TR, although the mitral valve is usually more insufficient in this condition. Localized adherence of tricuspid leaflet tissue is a recognized means of spontaneous closure of perimembranous ventricu-

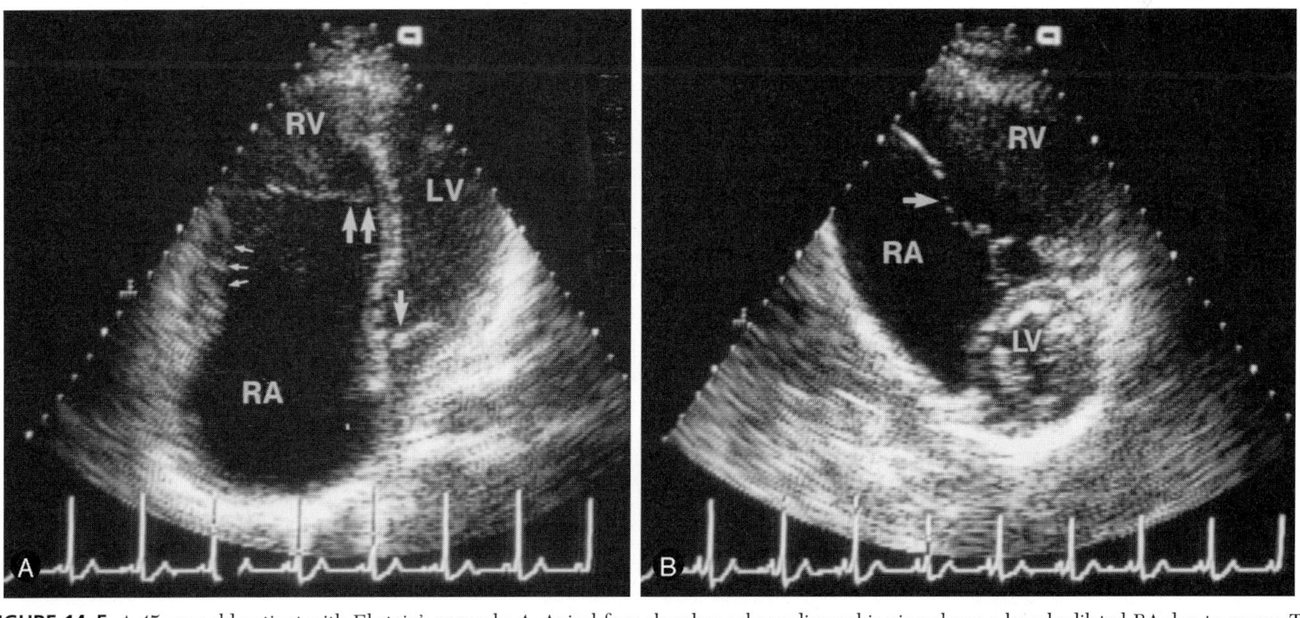

FIGURE 14–5. A 45-year-old patient with Ebstein's anomaly. *A*, Apical four-chamber echocardiographic view shows a hugely dilated RA due to severe TR and an "atrialized" RV component (*triple arrows*), along with marked apical displacement of the tricuspid valve's septal-leaflet attachment (*double arrows*) relative to the mitral valve's anterior leaflet (*single arrow*). *B*, Parasternal short-axis view: massive RA and RV dilatation and a small, underfilled LV in cross-section. The anterior tricuspid valve's leaflet (*single arrow*) is markedly elongated and "sail-like."

lar septal defects with development of a ventricular septal aneurysm. In this case, distortion of the tricuspid valve from septal leaflet adherence to a perimembranous ventricular septal defect may result in TR.[39] Other congenital cardiac defects may result in functional TR due to right ventricular pressure or volume overload. In congenitally corrected transposition of the great arteries, the morphologic right ventricle and its associated morphologic tricuspid valve may fail over time due to systemic arterial pressure.

Tricuspid Stenosis

Acquired Tricuspid Stenosis

Rheumatic Tricuspid Stenosis

Acquired tricuspid stenosis (TS) is unusual and is typically due to rheumatic heart disease. Although only 10% of patients with chronic rheumatic valvular disease develop hemodynamically significant TS, the overwhelming majority of cases occur in women.[40] On the Indian subcontinent, the prevalence of TS in chronic rheumatic heart disease is approximately 30%, according to autopsy studies. The reason rheumatic TS predominantly occurs in women is not known. Differing immunologic responses and a smaller valve orifice may be factors. Rheumatic TS is almost always accompanied by significant mitral stenosis, which tends to dominate the clinical picture. Pathologic changes of chronic rheumatic inflammation lead to insidious development of an AV membrane–like partition with a reduced, circular fish-mouthed orifice.

Nonrheumatic Tricuspid Stenosis

The rate of mechanical tricuspid valve thrombotic obstruction (clinical TS) is approximately 4%, compared with 0.5% for mechanical mitral or aortic valves.[41] Calcific degeneration of a bioprosthetic valve occasionally produces TS. Rarely, intracardiac or extracardiac tumors, which obstruct or compress the right ventricular inflow tract, may manifest as TS.

Congenital Tricuspid Stenosis

Tricuspid atresia is a complex cyanotic congenital heart defect characterized by complete agenesis of the tricuspid valve. Consequently, there is no direct right atrium–to–right ventricle communication. Tricuspid atresia is uncommon (identified in 1% to 3% of patients with congenital heart disease at autopsy) and is slightly more common in men (55%). An adequately sized interatrial communication (patent foramen ovale in 80% or a secundum or primum atrial septal defect) is essential for survival.

Clinical Recognition

Tricuspid Regurgitation

History and Physical Examination. Mild or moderate TR is difficult to detect clinically. In advanced severe TR with right-sided heart failure, fatigue, nausea, abdominal discomfort, early satiety, and bloating are prominent symptoms due to reduced forward blood flow, gut edema, and salt water retention. Reduced caloric intake, malabsorption, liver dysfunction, and increased circulating tumor necrosis factor (cachectin)[42, 43] conspire to produce malnutrition and cardiac cachexia in these patients. In patients with severe TR, massive jugular venous engorgement accompanied by large systolic waves may be forceful enough to produce a mild head bob. With severe right atrial hypertension, the superimposed systolic waves may even be visible in the superficial temporal or frontal scalp veins. Chest inspection and palpation in a patient with severe TR and relatively preserved right ventricular function may reveal apical systolic retraction (rapid emptying of a large right ventricle) accompanied by right parasternal lift (right atrial expansion). Subsequent brisk diastolic expansion of the cardiac apex (rapid right ventricular filling) should not be mistaken for an apical systolic impulse. If a PFO or other interatrial communication is present, the classic signs of central cyanosis due to right-to-left atrial-level shunting may be observed. Systolic flow reversal produces a "pulsatile" liver that may be tender to palpation.

Auscultation. The abnormal heart sounds of aortic, mitral, and pulmonary valve disease usually overshadow sounds produced by the tricuspid valve. The TR murmur is frequently heard best over the left lower sternal border. Organic TR with elevated right ventricular pressure produces a high-frequency holosystolic murmur that is mild to moderate in intensity. Except in end-stage disease, the TR murmur intensifies on inspiration (Carvallo's sign). In torrential TR, the systolic murmur may be soft or absent (due to nearly unobstructed flow) and accompanied by a soft, early diastolic rumble accentuated by inspiration and a right-sided S_3. Tricuspid stenosis should be suspected when a substantial right-sided diastolic rumble (varying with respiration) is appreciated. In Ebstein's anomaly, TR can range from inaudible (unusual) to extremely loud, with a palpable thrill. The first heart sound is widely split, owing to right bundle branch block and increased excursion of the oftentimes billowing, redundant anterior leaflet. An additional systolic clicking sound from early systolic tensing of the redundant anterior leaflet increases with inspiration and has been called the sail sound.

Laboratory. In severe TR with right-sided heart failure, modest elevations of the hepatic transaminases and both conjugated and unconjugated bilirubin may occur early on, whereas long-standing disease may produce marked hyperbilirubinemia, prothrombin time (PT) prolongation, and low albumin from impaired protein synthesis. Ultimately, cardiac cirrhosis occurs with a macroscopic "nutmeg liver" appearance (alternating areas of red congestion with pale centrilobular necrosis and fibrosis).

Tricuspid Stenosis

History and Physical Examination. When the mean tricuspid valve gradient exceeds 5 to 8 mm Hg, signs and symptoms commonly associated with right-sided heart failure—jugular venous distention, hepatomegaly, ascites, and anasarca—occur. Significant exertional fatigue, abdominal discomfort, and edema are usually present. Patients may complain of hepatic pain on exertion. If sinus rhythm is present, the hallmark physical finding is "giant *a* waves," jugular vein flow reversal from atrial contraction against an obstructed tricuspid orifice. The jugular vein *y* descent (early diastolic collapse) is prolonged, owing to impeded right atrial emptying. Chronic severe TS (usually rheumatic) can protect the pulmonary circuit from exercise-induced surges in venous return, thereby preventing exertional dyspnea and masking the presence of concomitant severe rheumatic mitral stenosis. Cyanosis in a patient with TS may be explained by a large atrial level right-to-left shunt through a PFO—which is present in 30% of normal individuals. Obstructive right ventricular inflow tract lesions (tumors or prosthetic valve malfunction) may progress more rapidly than organic tricuspid valve disease and should be suspected when concomitant aortic and mitral valve pathology is not present.

Auscultation. Distinguishing a TS murmur from mitral stenosis (usually also present) can be challenging. The diastolic murmur (rumble) of TS is usually best heard near the left lower sternal border. Mitral stenosis is typically louder at the apex; a dead zone may lie in between. Another of Carvallo's distinguishing signs is accentuation of the TS diastolic murmur with inspiration. In atrial fibrillation, the TS murmur is primarily mid-diastolic, distinguishing it from the early diastolic murmur of severe TR. In sinus rhythm, the diastolic murmur is loudest in late diastole, corresponding with atrial contraction. Because the right atrium contracts earlier than the left atrium, onset of the late diastolic TS murmur precedes its mitral counterpart. When TS is due to mechanical valve obstruction, the examination is remarkable for muffling or absence of the normally crisp prosthetic leaflet opening or closing sounds or a new systolic or diastolic murmur.

Noninvasive Testing

Electrocardiography

Right atrial enlargement from either TR or TS frequently produces large P waves (P-pulmonale). Suggestive findings include tall P waves (more than 2.5 mm) of normal duration (0.08–0.11 second) in leads II, III, and aVF or P waves more than 1.5 mm in leads V_1 and V_2. Unfortunately, these electrocardiographic (ECG) criteria are relatively insensitive and nonspecific for right atrial abnormalities caused by valvular disease.[44] Right ventricular volume or pressure overload produces right ventricular hypertrophy. Clues to right ventricular hypertrophy are listed in Table 14–2. In many patients, particularly asymptomatic patients, the ECG is less than diagnostic of right ventricular hypertrophy, although incomplete right bundle branch block is commonly seen. In Ebstein's anomaly, the ECG alone may lead to the diagnosis. Accessory bypass tracts (also from abnormal tricuspid annulus development) produce the Wolff-Parkinson-White (WPW) syndrome in some patients. Overt ventricular preexcitation with delta waves is evident in 10% to 20% of patients.[44, 45]

Table 14–2. ELECTROCARDIOGRAPHIC EVIDENCE FOR RIGHT VENTRICULAR HYPERTROPHY

Right axis deviation (≥ +90 degrees QRS axis)
$RV_1 \geq 7$ mm
$RV_1 + SV_5$ or $SV_6 \geq 10$ mm
R/S ratio in $V_1 \geq 1.0$
S/R ratio in $V_6 \geq 1.0$
Late intrisicoid deflection in V_1 (>0.035 sec)
Incomplete RBBB pattern
Repolarization abnormality ("strain" pattern) leads II, III, and aVF
Right atrial enlargement

RBBB, right bundle branch block.
Adapted from Marriott, HJL: Chamber enlargement. In Marriott, HJL, (ed): Practical Electrocardiography, 8th ed. Williams & Wilkins, Baltimore, 1988, p 57.

Echocardiography

Tricuspid Regurgitation

Echocardiography is the most important modality in the assessment of tricuspid valve pathology because transvalvular flow velocities are obtainable noninvasively by Doppler in most patients. A comprehensive examination addresses the severity of stenosis or regurgitation and the presence and severity of other cardiac pathology. Although transthoracic leaflet imaging may be challenging owing to asymmetric morphology, thinness, and retrosternal location, adjunctive transesophageal echocardiography can be helpful in guiding treatment when structural abnormalities (e.g., ruptured chord, flail leaflet, vegetation, or obstruction) are suspected.

Regardless of etiology, severe TR ultimately results in pronounced right ventricular and right atrial dilatation, which is immediately obvious on the apical four-chamber and subcostal views (see Figs. 14–3, 14–4, and 14–5). The right ventricle, instead of the left ventricle, appears to form the cardiac apex. Severe right ventricular volume overload (from TR, pulmonary insufficiency, or atrial septal defect) should be suspected when a paradoxical motion of the interventricular septum is observed (Fig. 14–6). A pressure overloaded right ventricle (primary pulmonary hypertension, severe pulmonary stenosis) should be suspected when continuous flattening of the interventricular septum is observed. A hemodynamically significant interatrial communication should be ruled out when an unexplained right ventricular enlargement and functional TR are discovered (see Fig. 14–3). With right-sided heart failure, the subcostal view (Fig. 14–7) reveals engorgement of the hepatic vein and inferior vena cava, confirming right atrial pressure elevation. In rheumatic TR, the morphologic appearance is similar to that seen with rheumatic mitral disease. Myxomatous tricuspid valve disease (often associated with a thickened, myxomatous, and prolapsing mitral valve) can be appreciated by virtue of a dilated annulus and prolapse of the leaflets past the annular plane. Carcinoid heart disease is generally evident by echocardiography (see Fig. 14–4). ECG is generally sufficient for establishing the diagnosis and severity of Ebstein's anomaly (see Fig. 14–5).[46]

Doppler echocardiography may be used to determine severity and to accurately estimate peak systolic pulmonary artery pressure noninvasively (see Tricuspid Valve Physiology, earlier). Continuous-wave Doppler signal density correlates directly with the regurgitant volume (see Fig. 14–2*B* to

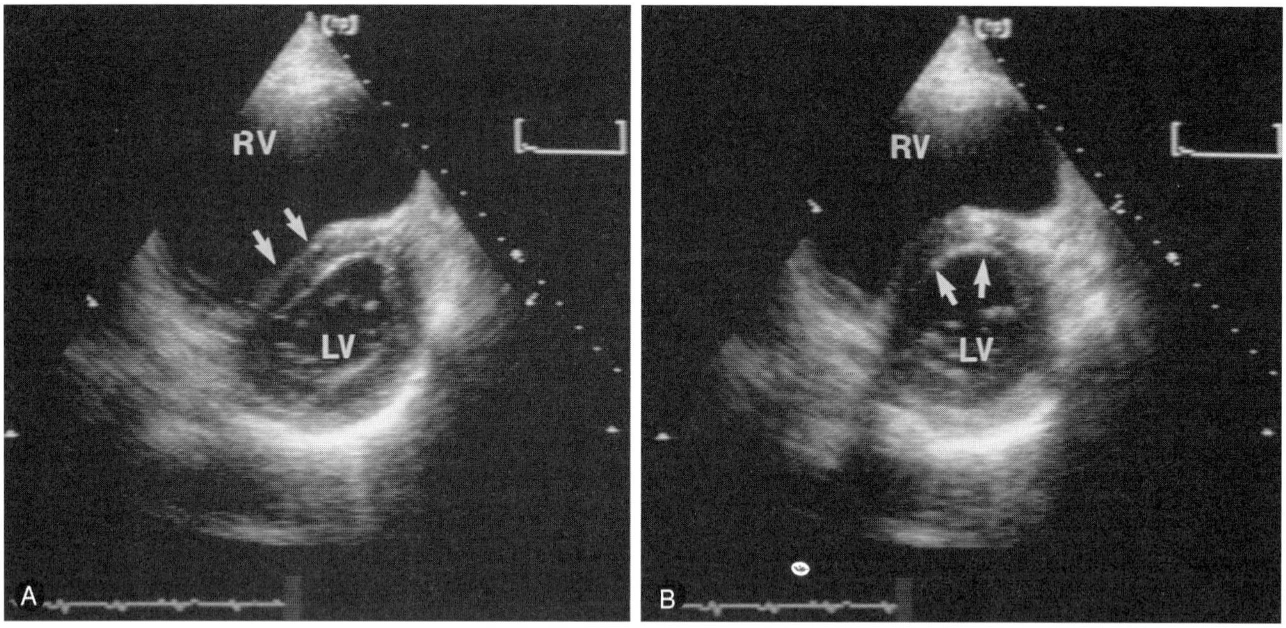

FIGURE 14–6. Paradoxical septal motion indicates severe right ventricular volume overload, due in this case to isolated severe TR. *A*, Diastole—the interventricular septum flattens toward the LV cavity. *B*, Systole—paradoxical bulging of the interventricular septum away from the LV cavity.

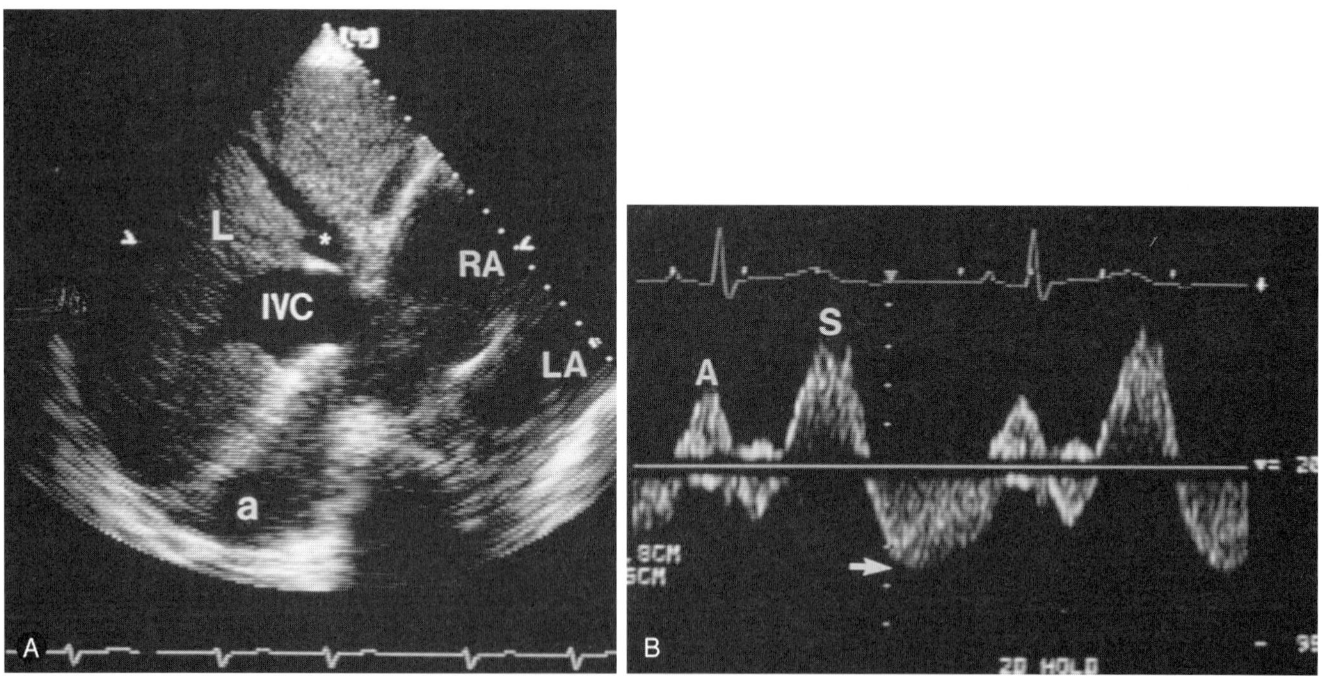

FIGURE 14–7. *A*, Subcostal echocardiographic view: severe right-sided heart failure is indicated by an engorged inferior vena cava (IVC) and hepatic vein (°), ascites (a) surrounding the liver (L), and a dilated right atrium (RA). *B*, In the same patient, pulsed Doppler blood-flow velocity measurement in the hepatic vein demonstrates two significant flow reversals: diastolic "A wave" (A) indicating high RV end-diastolic pressure and a large systolic "S wave" (S) indicating severe tricuspid regurgitation. (*Arrow*, early diastolic forward flow [prominent *y* descent of severe TR].)

D). A tricuspid inflow velocity of more than 1 cm/s usually accompanies severe TR and is due to increased transvalvular forward flow from the large regurgitant volume. Pulsed Doppler sampling in the hepatic vein demonstrates large systolic flow reversals in severe TR (see Fig. 14–7). Color-flow Doppler reveals an aliased regurgitant jet area occupying more than 30% of the right atrial area.[47]

Tricuspid Stenosis

The transvalvular peak, mean forward flow velocity, and pressure gradients are easily calculated using continuous-wave Doppler. Doppler echocardiography is invaluable for detecting thrombotic obstruction of prosthetic valves and for following response to thrombolytic therapy (Fig. 14–8).

Invasive Testing

With the advent of noninvasive Doppler and two-dimensional echocardiography, cardiac catheterization is generally not required for the assessment of tricuspid valve disease. When echocardiographic examination is technically inadequate, right-sided heart catheterization can be invaluable for confirming the diagnosis. With severe TR, significant whip of the catheter within the right atrium can be observed by fluoroscopy. Prominent right atrial and great vein V waves (systolic waves) are invariably present in association with high mean right atrial pressure. In tricuspid valve stenosis, the right atrial pressure is elevated, large *a* waves accompany a prolonged *y* descent, and the mean transvalvular gradient is greater than 5 mm Hg.

Prevention

In acquired tricuspid disease, prevention is the most effective but also the most difficult medical strategy to implement. From a global health perspective, organic tricuspid disease in women could largely be eliminated by the effective recognition and treatment of group A streptococcal pharyngitis—the prevention of acute rheumatic fever.[48] Rheumatic valvular disease is commonly diagnosed at institutions caring for large numbers of patients originating from developing countries where rheumatic fever continues to be prevalent.[49, 50] Prevention of recurrent streptococcal infection and superimposed bacterial endocarditis using antibiotic prophylaxis is necessary for lessening the sequelae of rheumatic heart disease in those already affected.[51] Reducing illicit intravenous drug use would reduce acquired TR due to bacterial endocarditis.

Treatment

Medical Management

Congestive Heart Failure. In most cases of functional TR, medical or surgical treatment of downstream valve abnormalities, shunt lesions, or left ventricular dysfunction generally improves valve function if the right ventricular volume regresses and the pulmonary artery pressure falls. Routine adjunctive therapy includes hypertension control, digitalis, diuretics, and pharmacologic afterload reduction for left-sided heart failure. For symptomatic patients who are not surgical candidates, treatment is aimed at reducing the systemic venous pressure. Oral sodium restriction and diuretics are mainstays of therapy. Decreased arterial perfusion, venous congestion, and bowel edema accompany right-sided heart failure and may reduce oral medication bioavailability. The patient or caretaker should maintain a daily log of body weight. When weight increases cannot be reversed by changes in oral medication, early institution of judicious intravenous loop diuretic therapy (inpatient or outpatient) and curtailment in physical activity generally enhances diuresis and improves symptoms. In selected patients with severe end-stage disease, inpatient infusion of low-dose intravenous dobutamine may be palliative.

Surgical Management

Because of a relatively high risk for tricuspid prosthesis dysfunction from structural deterioration (bioprosthesis) and thrombosis (mechanical prosthesis), a basic admonition is to avoid tricuspid valve replacement when possible. In fact, repair rather than replacement for severe TR is often possi-

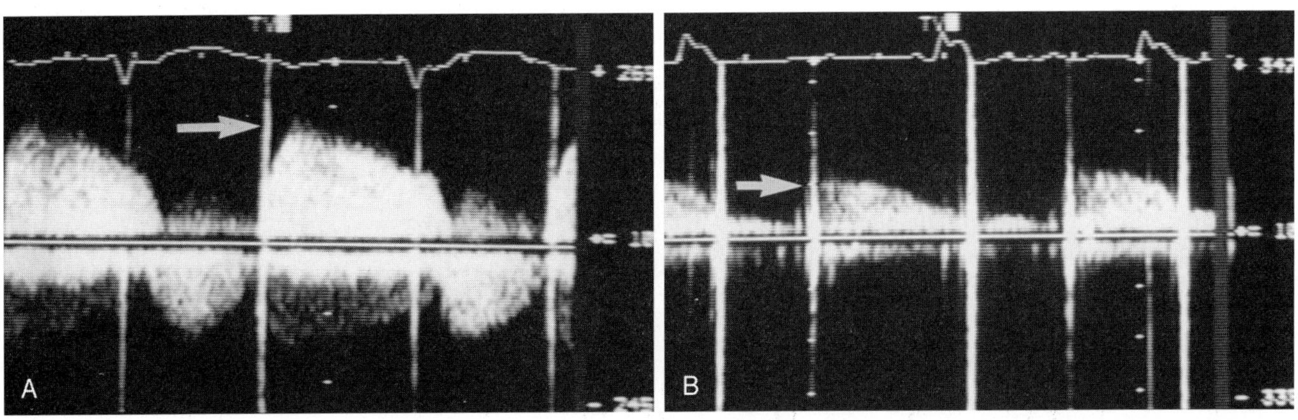

FIGURE 14–8. Tricuspid stenosis due to thrombosis of a bileaflet mechanical prosthesis before (*A*) and 36 hours after (*B*) continuous intravenous urokinase therapy. In *A*, the peak tricuspid inflow velocity (*arrow*) equals 1.8 m/s (13 mm Hg), with normalization of the inflow velocity to 1 m/s in *B*.

ble because the etiology is usually functional or due to myxomatous disease. Tricuspid repair is performed in approximately 10% of patients undergoing mitral or aortic valve operations. Reduction of the tricuspid annulus using a prosthetic ring or, more commonly, a De Vega[52, 53] or modified De Vega[54] purse-string suture repair generally produces valve competence. Tricuspid débridement and annuloplasty are also possible in acute endocarditis,[55] avoiding the need for prosthetic replacement or, in the case of intravenous drug addicts, complete tricuspid valvulectomy. When possible, tricuspid valve reconstruction is attempted for traumatic injury and Ebstein's anomaly.

Tricuspid Valve Prostheses. Fewer than 1.5% of all prosthetic cardiac valves are placed in the tricuspid position. The most common indication is rheumatic TS or TR; however, valve replacement may be required for any condition in which native valve morphologic derangement is severe. Because of rheumatic disease, the majority of tricuspid valve replacements occur in women. Combining the subjects from three recent and relatively large outcome studies reveals that 233 (77%) of 303 tricuspid valve replacements were performed in women.[56–58]

In the past, conventional wisdom has dictated that a bioprosthesis is desirable even when no contraindications for anticoagulation therapy exist and despite left-sided mechanical valves being placed concomitantly. The risk of thrombosis with mechanical tricuspid valve prostheses is high; however, recent evidence suggests that modern bileaflet devices have a lower risk than their ball-in-cage or single disk predecessors.[59] Tricuspid bioprostheses are subject to late structural failure (7 to 10 years) due to calcific degeneration and may necessitate reoperation, particularly in the young or in those with renal failure. Regardless of valve type, patients with prosthetic tricuspid valves are at significant risk for valve failure and should be followed closely by physical exam and echocardiography. For mechanical valves, high-risk periods include pregnancy and whenever anticoagulation therapy is relaxed for invasive procedures. Unless a PT international normalized ratio (INR) can be rigorously maintained in the range of 2.5 to 3.5,[60, 61] a mechanical prosthesis is best avoided. Intravenous heparinization is probably cost effective when oral warfarin therapy must be curtailed for any reason. The advent of thrombolytic therapy has enabled medical management of obstructed mechanical valves (low risk) rather than operative replacement (high risk).[41, 62–65] Thrombolysis (with no consensus on the most appropriate agent) for tricuspid prosthesis obstruction has an 86% success rate without the significant risk of peripheral embolization, which attends left-sided valve thrombolysis.[41] Thrombolytic infusion endpoints include the development of side effects (such as bleeding) or the demonstration of normal prosthetic leaflet motion by cinefluoroscopy and normalized valve flow velocities by Doppler echocardiography. If valve obstruction persists after 48 to 72 hours of therapy, it is likely that significant pannus formation is present. In such cases, the patient should be referred for surgical valve replacement.

Cardiac Carcinoid. Carcinoid heart disease can lead to progressive right-sided heart failure. Because medical palliation of right-sided heart failure has improved considerably in recent years, surgical palliation of carcinoid disease should be considered, even though the surgical risks are not well defined and recent data suggest a high perioperative mortality for valve replacement in this setting (35% to 68%).[66, 67] Younger patients with few comorbidities tend to fare better.

Ebstein's Anomaly. Surgical correction of Ebstein's anomaly is technically difficult and carries a significant perioperative risk. Furthermore, surgery has not been shown to reduce the incidence of arrhythmic death. Thus, patients who are in New York Heart Association (NYHA) functional classes I and II are probably best managed medically. When NYHA functional class III to IV symptoms are present, the prognosis is poor enough to warrant consideration of surgical repair. Prosthetic valve replacement is possible but difficult due to annular distortion.[68] When the anterior leaflet is large and redundant without free-edge tethering, successful surgical reconstruction is possible with echocardiography-guided patient selection.[69–71]

PULMONARY VALVE DISEASE

Anatomy and Normal Physiology

The pulmonary valve lies directly anterior, slightly superior, and to the left of the aortic valve. As opposed to the asymmetric and geometrically complex AV valves, hemodynamic integrity of the normal pulmonary valve (like the aortic valve) is derived from a simple but perfect symmetric relationship of three leaflets. During systole, the highly mobile leaflets open widely by straightening, allowing negligible flow resistance within a nearly circular orifice. With forward flow cessation, adjacent leaflets (one anterior and two posterior) fall back tightly on each other to support normal or even highly elevated diastolic pressures. Any variations from this leaflet arrangement may create systolic leaflet deformation and a propensity for fibrotic thickening or endocarditis. The pulmonary valve is the only major heart valve that is not part of the fibrous cardiac skeleton, arising completely from the muscular infundibulum of the right ventricular outflow tract. It is, therefore, relatively easily harvested along with a thin sleeve of infundibular muscle without damage to its vital structures. The size and tensile strength of the pulmonary and aortic valves are similar. Thus, the pulmonary valve can be used as a cryopreserved cadaveric homograft in the pulmonary or aortic position or as a fresh autograft in the aortic position (Ross procedure).[72, 73] The pulmonary valve's primary function is to provide low-resistance unidirectional flow from the right ventricle to the pulmonary arteries. In normal, young individuals, the pulmonary vascular resistance is so low that cardiac output is preserved in the absence of a pulmonary valve. As with the tricuspid valve, a very small degree of physiologic pulmonary insufficiency may be observed by color Doppler in a large percentage of normal subjects.[7]

Pathophysiology

Pulmonary Insufficiency. Acquired pulmonary valve disease is unusual and rarely of functional significance. In drug addicts or in patients with chronic indwelling right-sided central venous or pulmonary artery catheters, pulmonary valve endocarditis and pulmonary insufficiency (PI) can occur. In carcinoid heart disease, valve fibrotic plaque may cause varying degrees of PI or pulmonary stenosis (PS), complicating the predominant tricuspid valve lesions. High-pressure pulmonary regurgitation commonly occurs in patients with pulmonary artery hypertension (e.g., primary pulmonary hypertension, severe mitral stenosis, or mitral regurgitation) owing to annular dilatation. As with TR, severe PI may be tolerated for years as long as the pulmonary artery pressure remains normal. This explains the excellent short- and medium-term results achieved by complete pulmonary valvotomy in intravenous drug users with infectious endocarditis or in patients with congenital PS. However, the PI regurgitant volume gradually increases with aging (higher pulmonary vascular resistance and poorer left ventricular compliance) or with any disease process that leads to elevated pulmonary artery pressures. Compensatory right ventricular dilatation may ultimately produce worsening functional TR and right ventricular failure.

Pulmonary Stenosis. Isolated pulmonary valve stenosis is the most common congenital form of right ventricular outflow tract obstruction, with 50% of patients being women.[74] The congenitally stenotic pulmonary valve may be mobile and either bicuspid or tricuspid, with commissural fusion resulting in reduced valve area. Pulmonary valve dysplasia (severely deformed, immobile, thickened, or cartilaginous valve leaflets) is less common, being found in a significant minority of patients with tetralogy of Fallot and in association with Noonan's syndrome (autosomal dominant transmission). Pulmonary stenosis or pulmonary atresia may also occur as a component of other complex congenital heart diseases, such as transposition of the great arteries, tricuspid atresia, or Ebstein's anomaly. Along with right ventricular hypertrophy, ventricular septal defect, and overriding aorta, PS (right ventricular outflow obstruction) is one component of tetralogy of Fallot. In half of patients with tetralogy of Fallot, right ventricular outflow obstruction is due primarily to hypertrophied muscle bands (subpulmonic stenosis). Valvular and subpulmonic PS may coexist.

Clinical Recognition

History

Pulmonary Insufficiency. PI usually produces few symptoms unless it is accompanied by some degree of pulmonary hypertension, in which case severe right ventricular dilatation and functional TR ensue, producing symptoms of right-sided heart failure (see Tricuspid Valve Regurgitation, earlier). When PI is secondary to severe pulmonary hypertension, symptoms include fatigue, breathlessness due to reduced cardiac output, and arterial hypoxia.

Pulmonary Stenosis. Although severe congenital PS generally requires treatment in childhood because of heart failure symptoms and growth retardation, mild to moderately severe isolated PS is usually well tolerated. Presentation in early adulthood may occur because of progressive valvular stenosis and/or a progressive contributing gradient from infundibular subpulmonic stenosis. Severe stenosis limits cardiac output; thus, effort intolerance and fatigue are common complaints. However, the degree of stenosis frequently does not correlate well with symptoms. Some patients with relatively severe obstruction may remain essentially asymptomatic, and some with moderate obstruction easily tire or become breathless. Exertional chest pain analogous to angina pectoris may occur from transient subendocardial ischemia of the hypertrophied right ventricle. In severe PS, the right ventricular systolic pressure may exceed that of the left ventricle.

Physical Examination

Central cyanosis may occur in patients with advanced PI or PS when rising right atrial pressures allow right-to-left shunting across a PFO or atrial septal defect. Most patients with severe low-pressure PI appear well on examination, although a prominent pulmonary artery pulsation and diastolic thrill may be palpated in the pulmonary region (left upper sternal border, 2nd to 3rd interspace). The right ventricular hypertrophy of severe PS produces a forceful and sustained precordial right ventricular impulse that is accompanied by a palpable systolic thrill over the pulmonary region. Most patients with either PI or PS maintain sinus rhythm. Inspection of the jugular vein reveals a prominent *a* wave due to right ventricular diastolic hypertension. The jugular venous pulse becomes elevated and distended only if right ventricular failure becomes advanced.

Auscultation. In low-pressure PI, a variety of first and second heart sounds may be heard depending on the etiology of the defect (associated endocarditis, congenital abnormalities, or postvalvotomy). If the pulmonary valve is absent, S_2 is single. With congenital PI and low pulmonary artery pressure, a soft to moderate intensity early diastolic murmur is heard in the pulmonary region. In the setting of pulmonary hypertension, one may appreciate the characteristic high-pitched diastolic Graham Steell murmur of pulmonary insufficiency, which may be difficult to distinguish from aortic insufficiency. This blowing decrescendo murmur begins promptly with S_2 and either fades out in early to mid-diastole with severe pulmonary hypertension or extends throughout diastole in less severe pulmonary hypertension.

Severe PS produces a loud, high-pitched crescendo-decrescendo murmur in the pulmonary region. A mobile but morphologically abnormal valve whose excursion is arrested soon after opening produces a pulmonary ejection sound (click) soon after S_1. When an ejection click is not heard, this suggests a severely dysplastic valve with relatively thick and immobile leaflets. As PS becomes increasingly severe, the systolic murmur peaks later in systole. In addition, late systolic accentuation of the murmur may occur if there is subpulmonic dynamic obstruction from infundibular muscle hypertrophy. With severe PS, S_2 becomes increasingly split, with some widening on inspiration, and the late-peaking systolic murmur extends past and obscures the earlier aortic valve closure (A_2). With marked PS, a right-sided S_4 may be heard.[75] In patients with unrepaired tetralogy of Fallot, however, the duration and intensity of the PS murmur are *inversely* proportional to the severity of right ventricular outflow tract obstruction, because a ventricular septal defect allows decompression of the right ventricle. For similar reasons, prominent jugular vein *a* waves may be absent in tetralogy of Fallot patients despite severe PS.

Noninvasive Testing

Electrocardiography

The ECG can be normal in about half of patients with mild or moderate isolated PS (systolic pulmonary artery pressure less than 60 mm Hg). Sinus rhythm is generally found. In severe PS, however, large P waves and the findings of right ventricular hypertrophy (Table 14–2) are almost always present and often dramatic. Although the ECG alone cannot be used to predict the right ventricular pressure, a large monophasic R wave or a QR complex with T-wave inversion in ECG lead V_1 suggests severe disease.[76]

Echocardiography

Excellent long-axis pulmonary valve images in the parasternal window are routinely obtained and are ideal for guiding noninvasive transvalvular Doppler measurement of blood flow velocity. Bright, thickened, or doming leaflets by two-dimensional echocardiography suggest organic valve disease. Normal pulmonary valve flow is laminar, with mid-systolic peaking at less than 1 m/s in adults.

Pulmonary Insufficiency. Trivial to mild PI is generally detectable on echocardiography for normal and diseased valves. In mild PI, the velocity profile density recorded using continuous-wave Doppler is faint, and a significant residual regurgitation velocity persists at end diastole. With severe pulmonary incompetence, however, the diastolic continuous-wave Doppler signal is dense; the end-diastolic regurgitation velocity is small or zero, owing to end-diastolic right ventricular and pulmonary artery pressure equalization (Fig. 14–9). Severe PI produces a dilated, volume-overloaded right ventricle, which often exhibits significant functional TR (see Echocardiography, under Tricuspid Valve Regurgitation).

Pulmonary Stenosis. Poststenotic pulmonary artery dilatation may be dramatic but does not correlate with PS severity, which is best determined using continuous-wave Doppler. Application of the modified Bernoulli equation ($\Delta P = 4V^2$) to the peak transvalvular velocity (V) yields the peak instantaneous pressure drop across the valve (ΔP). The pulmonary valve flow velocity may have a superimposed dynamic, late-peaking obstructive velocity profile, owing to subpulmonic muscular hypertrophy. This muscular subpulmonic stenosis may persist but will gradually regress after balloon valvuloplasty or surgical correction. Doppler-derived instantaneous valve gradients may be somewhat higher than peak-to-peak measurements obtained by right-sided heart catheterization, but several clinical investigations have demonstrated a very high correlation between the two methods, with correlation coefficients generally exceeding 0.9.[77] A resting transvalvular gradient less than 40 mm Hg represents mild stenosis; 40 to 70 mm Hg, moderate stenosis; and greater than 70 mm Hg, severe stenosis.[78]

Treatment

Medical Management

Medical treatment of symptomatic isolated PS is seldom effective or indicated because percutaneous balloon valvuloplasty (see later) is generally a safe and effective therapy. As with other flow-limiting cardiac lesions, patients with either untreated or residual pulmonary stenosis require advice regarding the extent of physical activity that may be safely undertaken. For patients with a resting systolic right ventricular outflow gradient of less than 50 mm Hg, no symptoms, and no evidence of right ventricular systolic dysfunction, annual re-evaluation is recommended, with no specific limitations in competitive sports believed necessary. With a resting systolic gradient more than 50 mm Hg, balloon or operative valvuloplasty is recommended.[78] Others have advocated a more conservative approach, advising unrestricted physical activity only with resting systolic gradients

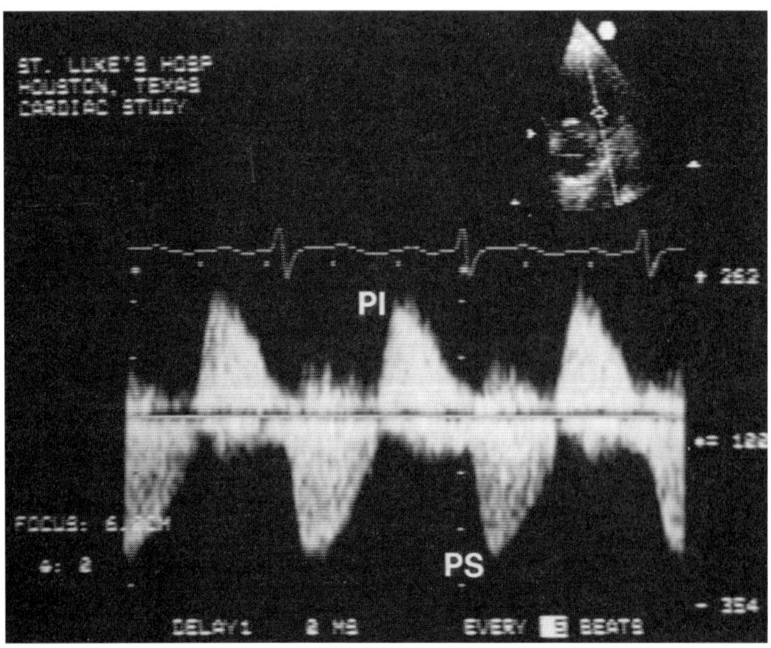

FIGURE 14–9. Continuous-wave Doppler pulmonary valve signal in a patient with carcinoid heart disease and severe pulmonary valve insufficiency (PI, reverse diastolic flow above the baseline) and mild pulmonary stenosis (PS, forward systolic flow below the baseline). The forward velocity equals 2.5 m/s (25 mm Hg peak transvalvular gradient).

less than 25 mm Hg and advising against intensive competitive sports with moderate obstruction in the range of 25 to 50 mm Hg because of unpredictable exercise flow–related increases in right ventricular systolic pressure.[79] Pregnancy is generally well tolerated in mild to moderate PS.[80]

Interventional Catheterization in Pulmonary Stenosis

If the pulmonary valve is crossed, a careful pullback through the right ventricular outflow tract is required to detect and measure the degree of subpulmonic stenosis. Balloon valvuloplasty of the congenitally stenosed pulmonary valve has been used since the early 1980s.[81–83] This procedure is now considered the treatment of choice for moderate or greater stenosis. In the absence of significant annular hypoplasia, balloon dilatation relieves the obstruction by tearing the leaflets or by separating the leaflet commissures. Despite the uncontrolled nature of leaflet splitting using balloon valvuloplasty, the degree of PI is generally no more than mild and recurrence of stenosis does not appear to be a significant problem.

Surgical Management

A cadaveric pulmonary homograft or valved prosthetic conduit may be placed in the pulmonary position when severe, symptomatic PI is present, when PS is not amenable to balloon valvuloplasty, and in certain cases of severe congenital right ventricular outflow tract anomalies. Although organic PS is a moderate risk factor for the development of endocarditis, prosthetic valve endocarditis is a potentially lethal complication. Prosthetic pulmonary valves can thrombose and may develop structural failure. Pulmonary homografts may be difficult to size, particularly if poststenotic dilatation is severe, and late structural failure can occur. Mechanical valves in the pulmonary position must be treated with lifelong oral anticoagulation therapy.

References

1. Langman J: Cardiovascular system. In Langman J (ed): Medical Embryology, 4th ed. Williams & Wilkins, Baltimore, 1981, pp 170–202.
2. Feldt RH, Porter CJ, Edwards WD, et al: Atrioventricular septal defects. In Emmanouilides GC, Reimenschneider TA, Allen HD, Gutgesell HP (eds): Moss and Adams' Heart Disease in Infants, Children, and Adolescents, 5th ed. Williams & Wilkins, Baltimore, 1995, pp 702–707.
3. Edwards WD: Cardiac anatomy and examination of cardiac specimens. In Emmanouilides GC, Reimenschneider TA, Allen HD, Gutgesell HP (eds): Moss and Adams' Heart Disease in Infants, Children, and Adolescents, 5th ed. Williams & Wilkins, Baltimore, 1995, pp 80–82.
4. Wilcox BR, Anderson RH: Surgical anatomy of the valves of the heart. In Wilcox BR, Anderson RH (eds): Surgical Anatomy of the Heart, 2nd ed. Gower Medical Publishing, London, 1992, pp 3.4–3.10.
5. Silver MD, Lam JH, Ranganathan N, Wigle ED: Morphology of the human tricuspid valve. Circulation 43:333–348, 1971.
6. Rosenquist GC, Sweeney LJ: Normal variations in tricuspid valve attachments to the membranous ventricular septum: A clue to the etiology of left ventricle–to–right atrial communication. Am Heart J 89: 186–188, 1975.
7. Yoshida K, Yoshikawa J, Shakudo M, et al. Color Doppler evaluation of valvular regurgitation in normal subjects. Circulation 78:840–847, 1988.
8. Yock PG, Popp RL: Noninvasive estimation of right ventricular systolic pressure by Doppler ultrasound in patients with tricuspid regurgitation. Circulation 70:657–662, 1984.
9. Beard JT, Byrd BF: Saline contrast enhancement of trivial Doppler tricuspid regurgitation signals for estimating pulmonary artery pressure. Am J Cardiol 62:486–488, 1988.
10. Himelman RB, Stulbarg MS, Lee E, et al: Noninvasive evaluation of pulmonary artery systolic pressures during dynamic exercise by saline-enhanced Doppler echocardiography. Am Heart J 119:685–688, 1990.
11. Feigenbaum H: Hemodynamic information derived from echocardiography. In Feigenbaum H (ed): Echocardiography, 5th ed. Lea & Febiger, Philadelphia, 1994, pp 195–197.
12. Kircher BJ, Himelman RB, Schiller NB: Noninvasive estimation of right atrial pressure from the inspiratory collapse of the inferior vena cava. Am J Cardiol 66:493–496, 1990.
13. Borgeson DD, Seward JB, Miller FAJ, et al: Frequency of Doppler measurable pulmonary artery pressures. J Am Soc Echocardiogr 9: 832–837, 1996.
14. Wolfe MW, Lee RT, Feldstein ML, et al: Prognostic significance of right ventricular hypokinesis and perfusion lung scan defects in pulmonary embolism. Am Heart J 127:1371–1375, 1994.
15. Sepulveda G, Lukas DS: The diagnosis of tricuspid insufficiency: Clinical features in 60 cases with associated mitral valve disease. Circulation 11:552, 1955.
16. Salazar E, Levine HD: Rheumatic tricuspid regurgitation: The clinical spectrum. Am J Med 33:111, 1962.
17. Chiang CW, Kuo CT, Chen WJ, et al: Comparisons between female and male patients with mitral stenosis. Br Heart J72:567–570, 1994.
18. Sagie A, Freitas N, Padial LR, et al: Doppler echocardiographic assessment of long-term progression of mitral stenosis in 103 patients: Valve area and right heart disease. J Am Coll Cardiol 28:472–479, 1996.
19. Mathew J, Addai T, Anand A, et al: Clinical features, site of involvement, bacteriologic findings, and outcome of infective endocarditis in intravenous drug users. Arch Intern Med 155:1641–1648, 1995.
20. Liepman MK, Jones PG, Kauffman CA: Endocarditis as a complication of indwelling right atrial catheters in leukemic patients. Cancer 54: 804–807, 1984.
21. Rowley KM, Clubb KS, Smith GJ, Cabin HS. Right-sided infective endocarditis as a consequence of flow-directed pulmonary-artery catheterization. A clinicopathological study of 55 autopsied patients. N Engl J Med 311:1152–1156, 1984.
22. Ford SE, Manley PN: Indwelling cardiac catheters. An autopsy study of associated endocardial lesions. Arch Pathol Lab Med 106:314–317, 1982.
23. Williams MJ, Lee MY, DiSalvo TG, et al: Biopsy-induced flail tricuspid leaflet and tricuspid regurgitation following orthotopic cardiac transplantation. Am J Cardiol 77:1339–1344, 1996.
24. Wiklund L, Suurkula MB, Kjellstrom C, Berglin E: Chordal tissue in endomyocardial biopsies. Scand J Thorac Cardiovasc Surg 28:13–18, 1994.
25. Tucker PA, Jin BS, Gaos CM, et al: Flail tricuspid leaflet after multiple biopsies following orthotopic heart transplantation: Echocardiographic and hemodynamic correlation [see comments]. J Heart Lung Transplant 13:466–472, 1994.
26. Neary PC, Redmond PH, Houghton T, et al: Carcinoid disease: Review of the literature. Dis Colon Rectum 40:349–362, 1997.
27. Anderson AS, Krauss D, Lang R: Cardiovascular complications of malignant carcinoid disease. Am Heart J 134:693–702, 1997.
28. Kaplan LM: Endocrine tumors of the gastrointestinal tract and pancreas. In Isselbacher KJ, Braunwald E, Wilson JD, et al (eds). Harrison's Principles of Internal Medicine, 13th ed. McGraw-Hill,New York, 1994, pp 1535–1542.
29. Kvols LK, Moertel CG, O'Connell MJ, et al: Treatment of the malignant carcinoid syndrome. Evaluation of a long-acting somatostatin analogue. N Engl J Med 315:663–666, 1986.
30. Maisano F, Lorusso R, Sandrelli L, et al: Valve repair for traumatic tricuspid regurgitation. Eur J Cardiothorac Surg 10:867–873, 1996.
31. Gayet C, Pierre B, Delahaye JP, et al: Traumatic tricuspid insufficiency. An underdiagnosed disease. Chest 92:429–432, 1987.
32. Bolinger BS, Winslow TM: Transesophageal echocardiographic diagnosis of a ruptured tricuspid valve chordae tendineae as the etiology for cardiogenic shock. Chest 105:1286–1288, 1994.
33. Anderson KR, Zuberbuhler JR, Anderson RH, et al: Morphologic spectrum of Ebstein's anomaly of the heart: A review. Mayo Clin Proc 54:174–180, 1979.

34. Celermajer DS, Bull C, Till JA, et al: Ebstein's anomaly: Presentation and outcome from fetus to adult. J Am Coll Cardiol 23:170–176, 1994.
35. Zalzstein E, Koren G, Einarson T, Freedom RM: A case-control study on the association between first trimester exposure to lithium and Ebstein's anomaly. Am J Cardiol 65:817–818, 1990.
36. Jacobson SJ, Jones K, Johnson K, et al: Prospective multicentre study of pregnancy outcome after lithium exposure during first trimester. Lancet 339:530–533, 1992.
37. Perloff JK: Ebstein's anomaly of the tricuspid valve. In Perloff JK, ed: The clinical recognition of congenital heart disease, 4th ed. W.B. Saunders, Philadelphia, 1994, pp 247–272.
38. Connolly HM, Warnes CA: Ebstein's anomaly: Outcome of pregnancy. J Am Coll Cardiol 23:1194–1198, 1994.
39. Winslow TM, Redberg RF, Foster E, Schiller NB. Transesophageal echocardiographic detection of abnormalities of the tricuspid valve in adults associated with spontaneous closure of perimembranous ventricular septal defect. Am J Cardiol 70:967–969, 1992.
40. Guyer DE, Gillam LD, Foale RA, et al: Comparison of the echocardiographic and hemodynamic diagnosis of rheumatic tricuspid stenosis. J Am Coll Cardiol 3:1135–1144, 1984.
41. Hurrell DG, Schaff HV, Tajik A. Thrombolytic therapy for obstruction of mechanical prosthetic valves. Mayo Clin Proc 71:605–613, 1996.
42. Levine B, Kalman J, Mayer L, et al: Elevated circulating levels of tumor necrosis factor in severe chronic heart failure. N Engl J Med 323:236–241, 1990.
43. Packer M: Is tumor necrosis factor an important neurohormonal mechanism in chronic heart failure? Circulation 92:1379–1382, 1995.
44. Chou T: Atrial abnormalities. In Chou T (ed): Electrocardiography in Clinical Practice, 2nd ed. W.B. Saunders, Philadelphia, 1986, pp 27–45.
45. Van Hare GF, Lesh MD, Stanger P: Radiofrequency catheter ablation of supraventricular arrhythmias in patients with congenital heart disease: Results and technical considerations. J Am Coll Cardiol 22:883–890, 1993.
46. Shiina A, Seward JB, Edwards WD, et al: Two-dimensional echocardiographic spectrum of Ebstein's anomaly: Detailed anatomic assessment. J Am Coll Cardiol 3:356–370, 1984.
47. Oh JK, Seward JB, Tajik AJ: Valvular heart disease. In Oh JK, Seward JB, Tajik AJ (eds): The Echo Manual. Little, Brown, Boston, 1994, pp 87–115.
48. Dajani AS, Bisno AL, Chung KJ, et al: Prevention of rheumatic fever: A statement for health professionals by the Committee on Rheumatic Fever, Endocarditis and Kawasaki Disease of the Council on Cardiovascular Disease in the Young, the American Heart Association. Pediatr Infect Dis J 8:263–266, 1989.
49. Ayoub EM: Acute rheumatic fever. In Emmanouilides GC, Reimenschneider TA, Allen HD, Gutgesell HP (eds): Moss and Adams' Heart Disease in Infants, Children, and Adolescents, 5th ed. Williams & Wilkins, Baltimore, 1995, pp 1400–1416.
50. Sanyal SK: Long-term sequelae of the first attack of acute rheumatic fever during childhood. In Emmanouilides GC, Reimenschneider TA, Allen HD, Gutgesell HP (eds): Moss and Adams' Heart Disease in Infants, Children, and Adolescents, 5th ed. Williams & Wilkins, Baltimore, 1995, pp 1416–1440.
51. Dajani AS, Taubert KA, Wilson W, et al: Prevention of bacterial endocarditis: Recommendations by the American Heart Association. JAMA 277:1794, 1997.
52. De Vega NG, De Rabago G, Castillon L, et al: A new tricuspid repair. Short-term clinical results in 23 cases. J Cardiovasc Surg, Spec No: 384–386, 1973;
53. De Vega NG: [Selective, adjustable and permanent annuloplasty. An original technique for the treatment of tricuspid insufficiency]. [Spanish]. Rev Esp Cardiol 25:555–556, 1972.
54. Antunes MJ, Girdwood RW: Tricuspid annuloplasty: A modified technique. Ann Thorac Surg 35:676–678, 1983.
55. Lange R, De Simone R, Bauernschmitt R, et al: Tricuspid valve reconstruction, a treatment option in acute endocarditis. Eur J Cardiothorac Surg 10:320–326, 1996.
56. Munro AI, Jamieson WR, Tyers GF, Germann E: Tricuspid valve replacement: Porcine bioprostheses and mechanical prostheses. Ann Thorac Surg 60:S470–S474, 1995.
57. Scully HE, Armstrong CS: Tricuspid valve replacement. Fifteen years of experience with mechanical prostheses and bioprostheses. J Thorac Cardiovasc Surg 109:1035–1041, 1995.
58. Van Nooten GJ, Caes F, Taeymans Y, et al: Tricuspid valve replacement: postoperative and long-term results. J Thorac Cardiovasc Surg 110: 672–679, 1995.
59. Singh AK, Feng WC, Sanofsky SJ: Long-term results of St. Jude Medical valve in the tricuspid position. Ann Thorac Surg 54:538–540 1992.
60. Hirsh J, Dalen JE, Deykin D, Poller L: Oral anticoagulants. Mechanism of action, clinical effectiveness, and optimal therapeutic range. Chest 102:312S–326S, 1992.
61. Litin SC, Gastineau DA: Current concepts in anticoagulant therapy. Mayo Clin Proc 70:266–272, 1995.
62. Luluaga IT, Carrera D, D'Oliveira J, et al: Successful thrombolytic therapy after acute tricuspid-valve obstruction. Lancet 1:1067–1068, 1971.
63. Roudaut R, Labbe T, Lorient-Roudaut MF, et al: Mechanical cardiac valve thrombosis. Is fibrinolysis justified? Circulation 86:II8–II15, 1992.
64. Silber H, Khan SS, Matloff JM, et al: The St. Jude valve: Thrombolysis as the first line of therapy for cardiac valve thrombosis. Circulation 87: 30–37, 1993.
65. Connolly HM, Miller FAJ, Taylor CL, et al: Doppler hemodynamic profiles of 82 clinically and echocardiographically normal tricuspid valve prostheses. Circulation 88:2722–2727, 1993.
66. Moertel CG: Treatment of the carcinoid tumor and the malignant carcinoid syndrome. J Clin Oncol 1:727–740, 1983.
67. Robiolio PA, Rigolin VH, Harrison JK, et al. Predictors of outcome of tricuspid valve replacement in carcinoid heart disease. Am J Cardiol 75:485–488, 1995.
68. Tasdemir O, Katircioglu SF, Tezcaner T, et al: Surgical treatment of Ebstein's anomaly: Valve replacement and reconstruction. J Cardiovasc Surg 30:740–743, 1989.
69. Carpentier A, Chauvaud S, Mace L, et al: A new reconstructive operation for Ebstein's anomaly of the tricuspid valve. J Thorac Cardiovasc Surg 96:92–101, 1988.
70. Mair DD: Ebstein's anomaly: Natural history and management [editorial; comment]. J Am Coll Cardiol 19:1047–1048; 1992.
71. Mair DD, Seward JB, Driscoll DJ, Danielson GK: Surgical repair of Ebstein's anomaly: Selection of patients and early and late operative results. Circulation 72:II70–II76, 1985.
72. Ross D, Jackson M, Davies J: Pulmonary autograft aortic valve replacement: Long-term results. J Card Surg 6:529–533, 1991.
73. Kouchoukos NT, Davila-Roman VG, Spray TL, et al: Replacement of the aortic root with a pulmonary autograft in children and young adults with aortic-valve disease. N Engl J Med 330:1–6, 1994.
74. Perloff JK: The Clinical Recognition of Congenital Heart Disease, 4th ed. W.B. Saunders, Philadelphia, 1994.
75. Stapleton JF: Clinical aspects of nonrheumatic valvular disease. In Chizner MA (ed): Classic Teachings in Clinical Cardiology: A Tribute to W. Proctor Harvey. Laennec Publishing, Cedar Grove, NJ, 1996, pp 1017–1048.
76. Chou T: Congenital heart disease in adults. In Chou T (ed): Electrocardiography in Clinical Practice, 2nd ed. W.B. Saunders, Philadelphia, 1986, pp 336–337.
77. Weyman AE: Right ventricular ouflow tract. In Weyman AE (ed): Principles and Practice of Echocardiography, 2nd ed. Lea & Febiger, Philadelphia, 1994, pp 863–900.
78. Graham TPJ, Bricker JT, James FW, Strong WB: 26th Bethesda Conference: Recommendations for determining eligibility for competition in athletes with cardiovascular abnormalities. Task Force 1: Congenital heart disease. J Am Coll Cardiol 24:867–873, 1994.
79. Perloff JK: Congenital heart disease in adults. In Braunwald E (ed): Heart Disease: A Textbook of Cardiovascular Medicine, 5th ed. W. B. Saunders, Philadelphia, 1997, pp 963–987.
80. Perloff JK, Koos BL: Pregnancy and congenital heart disease. In Perloff JK, Child JS (ed): Congenital Heart Disease in Adults, 2nd ed. W. B. Saunders, Philadelphia, 1998, pp 144–164.
81. Pepine CJ, Gessner IH, Feldman RL: Percutaneous balloon valvuloplasty for pulmonic valve stenosis in the adult. Am J Cardiol 50: 1442–1445, 1982.
82. Kan JS, White RIJ, Mitchell SE, Gardner TJ: Percutaneous balloon valvuloplasty: A new method for treating congenital pulmonary-valve stenosis. N Engl J Med 307:540–542, 1982.
83. Beekman RH, Thomas RL: Balloon valvuloplasty and stenting for congenital heart disease. In Topol EJ (ed): Textbook of Interventional Cardiology, 2nd ed. W. B. Saunders, Philadelphia, 1994, pp 1277–1297.

SECTION IV

ENDOCARDITIS

CHAPTER 15

Infective Endocarditis

Barry Zeluff

Infective endocarditis is an infection of the endocardial surface of the heart. Although endocarditis usually involves the heart valves, it may also affect the mural surface or septal defects. The older term *bacterial endocarditis* is no longer used because pathogens other than typical bacteria, such as fungi, *Rickettsia,* and *Chlamydia,* also can cause endocarditis. Furthermore, the terms *acute* and *subacute endocarditis* are no longer commonly used because they represent the clinical presentation and progression of endocarditis in the preantibiotic era. *Subacute endocarditis* was used when a pathogen such as viridans streptococcus was the cause, and *acute endocarditis* was usually used when *Staphylococcus aureus* or *Streptococcus pneumoniae* was the cause of infection. These terms, however, did not allow for the large overlap in clinical presentation of endocarditis, which can be caused by many pathogens. The current terminology is based on the causative agent, which has implications for the underlying abnormality of the heart, the clinical presentation of the disease, and therapy.

Infective endocarditis is less common in women than in men, occurring twice as often in men as in women according to Lerner and Weinstein.[1] This difference increases to 6.5:1 in patients 61 to 70 years old and to 9:1 in patients 50 to 60 years old. Seaworth and Durack[2] reported only 124 cases of infective endocarditis in obstetric or gynecologic patients over a 40-year period. Although infective endocarditis is uncommon in women, certain unique aspects seen in women warrant further discussion.

EPIDEMIOLOGY

The overall incidence of endocarditis has not changed dramatically over time[3, 4]; however, the age distribution of patients with endocarditis has changed over the last 50 years. Before the introduction of antibiotics, infective endocarditis mostly affected young adults. In fact, in 1926 the median age of patients with endocarditis was less than 30 years.[5] Now, more than 50% of cases occur in patients older than 50 years.[6] The increase in the age of these patients is even more significant when certain pathogens are involved; the age range of patients with endocarditis caused by group D streptococci is 61 to 67 years.[7] The reason for the increase in age is unclear. Durack and Petersdorf[8] have suggested several explanations for this trend: (1) the large number of atherosclerotic-resultant sites that may be infected during bacteremia, (2) the increase in the frequency of cardiac surgery and in the placement of intravascular lines in severely ill elderly patients, (3) the large number of elderly patients with nosocomial bacteremia, (4) the more common occurrence of rheumatic fever in the elderly, and (5) the increased life expectancy of patients with congenital heart disease, who are more likely to require a prosthesis.

An exception to the trend of increasing age among patients with endocarditis is infective endocarditis associated with intravenous drug abuse: The mean age of these patients is 27 years.[9] Women are also affected by endocarditis associated with drug use. In a study of three cases of endocarditis associated with drug use in pregnant women, Pastorek and associates reported a higher than previously stated rate of endocarditis in an urban, inner city population of women.[10] They attributed the high rate to the widespread problem of drug abuse.

PATHOGENESIS AND PATHOPHYSIOLOGY

Most cases of infective endocarditis are associated with the presence of an abnormal valve, which leads to hemodynamic changes that promote endothelial damage. In turn, the endothelial damage promotes platelet aggregation, and the deposition of fibrin results in sterile vegetation or nonbacterial thrombotic endocarditis. This type of endocarditis is seen in patients with other conditions such as cancer, chronic wasting disease, rheumatic or congenital heart disease, uremia, and connective tissue diseases.[11] This vegetative area is a favorable environment for colonization by circulating bacteria. The deposition of bacteria promotes further thrombus formation and the development of an infected thrombus or infective endocarditis. Not all patients with endocarditis have an abnormal valve. Certain bacteria such as *S. aureus, Neisseria gonorrhoeae,* and *S. pneumoniae*, however, have virulence factors that enable them to infect a normal valve. The incidence of endocarditis caused by *N. gonorrhoeae* and *S. pneumoniae* has decreased. *S. aureus,* however, remains a major cause of endocarditis and commonly infects both intact and abnormal valves.

Multiple factors influence the development of endocarditis. These factors include the amount of valvular trauma, the mean pressure across the valve, the number of circulating organisms, the duration of the bacteremia, and the virulence of the infecting organism. The left side of the heart has an increased risk of endothelial damage because of the higher pressure system. Thus, the aortic and mitral valves are infected more often than the tricuspid and pulmonic valves. The mitral valve is infected in 40% of cases, and the aortic valve is infected in 5% to 36% of cases. Involvement of both valves is less common.[12] Other sites of the endothelium may be damaged when a regurgitant jet of blood strikes the endothelial wall of a cardiac chamber. Endocarditis is more likely to develop in the presence of a small defect with a high relative pressure than when there is a large defect with low pressure. Turbulent flow also promotes the deposition of bacteria on endothelial surfaces, which may lead to development of an infected thrombus.

Many cardiac abnormalities are associated with endocarditis. The frequency of these abnormalities has changed over the years.[13] In the past, rheumatic heart disease was the most common cause of valvular abnormalities associated with infective endocarditis. Although it is still a common risk factor in many parts of the world, rheumatic heart disease has decreased significantly in the United States in the last 40 years because the incidence of rheumatic fever has decreased. Rheumatic heart disease usually affects the mitral valve; mitral stenosis develops in 90% of cases and mitral regurgitation in 6.6%. The aortic valve is less frequently involved; aortic regurgitation develops in 2.5% of cases and aortic stenosis in less than 1%.[14] Both valves may occasionally be involved. The tricuspid and pulmonary valves are rarely affected by rheumatic heart disease.

Congenital heart disease and degenerative valvular diseases have become important causes of endocarditis in the United States. Degenerative disease is the most common valvular lesion among the elderly, whereas congenital heart disease is more common in young and middle-aged patients.[8] Congenital lesions often seen in patients with endocarditis include patent ductus arteriosus, coarctation, tetralogy of Fallot, pulmonary stenosis, and a bicuspid aortic valve. Other common lesions are idiopathic hypertrophic subaortic stenosis, systemic to pulmonary artery shunts, and small ventricular septal defects (VSD). The high pressure and jet stream of a small VSD creates a higher risk for the development of endocarditis than do lesions such as a large VSD or an uncomplicated secundum atrial defect. Valves previously damaged from endocarditis are at a higher risk for subsequent episodes of endocarditis. Prosthetic valves, which create some turbulent flow, are always at increased risk for development of endocarditis.

The potential of mitral valve prolapse (MVP) to cause endocarditis has been controversial. Since its recognition as a clinical entity in 1963,[15] MVP has become one of the most common valvular abnormalities found on physical examination or echocardiographic study.[16, 17] MVP affects women more often than men; about 6% to 10% of women have MVP of varying severity.[18] The frequency and variable severity of MVP make it difficult to assess its potential as a risk factor for the development of endocarditis. Most clinicians believe that patients who have MVP with a regurgitant murmur or a significantly prolapsing valve are at greatest risk for developing endocarditis and should receive antibiotic prophylaxis. In fact, the risk for these patients may be 5 to 8 times greater than the risk for patients with normal valves. Although MVP is more common in women, men with MVP are at greater risk for developing complications such as endocarditis or stroke.[19, 20]

The diagnostic trend for endocarditis is to identify the pathogen rather than to label the disease as acute or subacute. The likelihood of an organism's causing endocarditis depends on the frequency and duration of bacteremia and the intrinsic virulence factors of the organism. Routine daily activities such as brushing or flossing teeth or eating hard candy can cause transient bacteremia.[21] The two most common sources of transient bacteremia are the oropharynx and the genitourinary system. The gastrointestinal tract also is a common source, but organisms from this site are usually filtered out by the reticuloendothelial system of the liver and spleen. Iatrogenic procedures such as dental surgery or bronchoscopy (with a rigid scope) may cause transient bacteremia, as may urologic procedures such as urethral dilatation, cytoscopy, and catheterization. Even diagnostic procedures such as transesophageal echocardiography have led to transient bacteremia and the subsequent development of endocarditis.[22–24]

Bacteremia can occur routinely in gynecologic or obstetric patients. Transient bacteremias have been reported after common gynecologic procedures such as endometrial biopsy.[25] Endocarditis has been noted after both vaginal and cesarean section deliveries.[2, 10, 26–28] Several studies have investigated the frequency of bacteremia and clinical outcome in these patients. In a retrospective study of indigent obstetric patients at a county hospital, Blanco and coworkers[29] reported that the incidence of bacteremia was 7.5 per 1000 hospital admissions, or 9.7% of patients sampled. These investigators found no deaths, no evidence of septic shock, and no cases of postinfectious endocarditis. They reported that the most frequently seen organisms were *Escherichia coli*, group B streptococcus, and *Bacteroides* sp. Other studies have indicated that endocarditis after vaginal delivery is rare. In a study in Scotland conducted between 1969 and 1972, Smith and associates[30] reported no cases of endocarditis in women after normal delivery. Cesarean sections pose a potentially greater risk for bacteremia; however, data supporting this assumption are scarce. In a prospective study, Boggess and colleagues[31] reported that the frequency of bacteremia was 11% in 119 women undergoing cesarean section. Furthermore, all 13 episodes of bacteremia occurred after labor or after rupture of the membranes. Although the follow-up period in their study was not long, Boggess and associates concluded that cesarean sections may pose a potential risk for endocarditis and that antibiotic prophylaxis should be considered.

MICROBIOLOGY

An understanding of the pathogens involved in endocarditis is important in prescribing effective empiric antibiotic therapy. Although many different organisms can cause endocarditis, only a few are responsible for most cases. In endocarditis of native valves, the gram-positive cocci cause about 80% of cases (Table 15–1). Of the gram-positive cocci, viridans streptococci are the most common and are found in the oropharynx, the gastrointestinal tract, and the female genital

Table 15–1. COMMON GRAM-POSITIVE ORGANISMS IN INFECTIVE ENDOCARDITIS

PATHOGEN	PERCENTAGE OF CASES	COMMENT
Viridans streptococci	25–30	Commonly associated with transient bacteremia
Group D streptococci	15–20	Seen in obstetric and gynecologic patients
Other streptococci	15–25	Group B streptococci are important in neonates and adults
Staphylococcus aureus	15–25	Often seen in drug users and prosthetic valve infections
Staphylococcus epidermidis	2–5	Common in prosthetic valve infections

tract. Because of their prevalence and location, viridans streptococci are often associated with transient bacteremia and thus may seed a sterile thrombus on the endocardium. These organisms have been associated with transient bacteremias caused by dental manipulations or oral infections. Group D streptococci are the second most common streptococcal isolates seen in endocarditis. Enterococci *(Enterococcus faecalis, E. faecium,* and *E. durans)* and nonenterococcus group D streptococci *(Streptococcus bovis)* may all cause endocarditis. Enterococcal endocarditis is increasing in frequency and accounts for 15% to 20% of all endocarditis cases.[8] Women who have undergone gynecologic or obstetric procedures are at risk for enterococcal endocarditis. Older men who have undergone gastrointestinal or genitourinary manipulations, those with prostatic hypertrophy, or those who have enterococcal urinary tract infections also are at risk. *S. bovis* is seen in 20% to 25% of cases and is common in patients with underlying gastrointestinal abnormalities such as cancer or polyps.

Group B streptococci *(Streptococcus agalactiae),* which are common flora of the gastrointestinal tract, the genitourinary tract, and the pharynx, are important pathogens in neonates and adults.[32, 33] Although originally recognized in the preantibiotic era as a cause of endocarditis in postpartum women, group B streptococci are now rare in this population and are more often seen in elderly patients and in patients with underlying cardiac disease, diabetes, alcoholism, drug abuse, and genitourinary disease. In a review of group B streptococcal endocarditis, Sexton and colleagues[34] noted a bimodal distribution of 19 previously reported cases, with one peak in young or middle-aged women undergoing obstetric or gynecologic procedures and the other peak in older patients with underlying conditions. In another review of 12 cases of endocarditis caused by *S. agalactiae*, none was associated with pregnancy, and all patients had serious underlying conditions.[35]

S. aureus, which can infect both normal and damaged valves, causes about 20% of all cases of endocarditis. In addition, *S. aureus* causes 50% of cases of acute endocarditis with a fulminant presentation and may also cause a subacute infection.[36] Endocarditis seen in intravenous drug users and in patients with prosthetic valves is often caused by *S. aureus.* Almost 20% of the population may carry *S. aureus,* usually in the anterior nares or on the skin. Patients with underlying skin conditions and those who receive frequent injections, such as diabetics, dialysis patients, and intravenous drug users, have a higher rate of colonization with *S. aureus* and thus may be at greater risk for bacteremia.[37–39] Often, *S. aureus* causes nosocomial bacteremia, and distinguishing between transient bacteremia and endocarditis may be difficult. The teichoic acid antibody test may be suggestive for making this determination, but it has a low sensitivity and specificity.[40]

Other organisms such as gram-negative bacilli, anaerobes, and fungi are less common causes of endocarditis on native valves. Although they cause less than 5% of cases of endocarditis, these organisms may be more common in such subgroups as patients who have endocarditis associated with prosthetic valve or intravenous drug use. One unusual cause of endocarditis deserves mention. *Listeria monocytogenes,* like *S. agalactiae,* has been associated with puerperal and neonatal sepsis. However, *L. monocytogenes*–induced endocarditis is infrequent, and women are not predisposed to infection with this organism. In a review of 34 cases of infective endocarditis caused by *L. monocytogenes*, the left side of the heart was most often involved, and the male-to-female ratio was 2:1.[41] Only two of the 34 cases involved pregnant women.

Culture-negative endocarditis is common and may involve organisms that are difficult to grow with routine blood culture techniques. Such organisms include fastidious or slow-growing organisms such as nutritionally deficient streptococci, *Brucella* sp., *Rickettsia*, and *Coxiella burnetii*. However, prior antibiotic use is the most common cause of culture-negative endocarditis.[42]

Endocarditis of prosthetic valves has a distinct microbiology. Prosthetic valve endocarditis (PVE) is usually categorized as either early or late; the pathogenesis and microbiology of the two periods differ. PVE that occurs within 60 days of surgery has traditionally been defined as early PVE. However, data suggest that the time line is less distinct and that the separation point between early and late PVE should be 12 months.[43, 44] The most common predisposing factor for early PVE is perioperative contamination of the valve, usually from the patient's own skin. However, contamination may come from operating room personnel, aerosolized droplets, the heart-lung bypass machine, intravascular catheters, and rarely, the prosthetic valve itself.[45, 46] The most common organisms seen in early prosthetic valve endocarditis are coagulase-negative staphylococci and *S. aureus.* Other frequent causes of early infection are gram-negative bacilli such as *Pseudomonas aeruginosa* and yeasts such as *Candida albicans*.[47, 48] Organisms that are common skin contaminants, such as *Bacillus* spp. or diphtheroids, also can cause endocarditis in this setting. All positive cultures from patients with prosthetic valves must be carefully analyzed to ensure that they are not clinically significant.

The characteristics and microbiology of late PVE are more similar to those of native valve endocarditis. Viridans streptococci are the most common cause of late infection in PVE; *S. aureus* and coagulase-negative staphylococci also are common. Gram-negative bacilli and *Candida* spp. are seen less frequently in late PVE than in early PVE. The abnormal hemodynamic environment and the foreign material of a prosthetic valve make it susceptible to a large variety of organisms that rarely infect a native valve.

Endocarditis associated with intravenous drug use has a distinct clinical picture. Most notably in this population, the right side of the heart is often infected because of repeated damage to this site from contaminants injected with the drug. Contaminants such as talc, quinine, or cotton fibers damage the endothelial surface, particularly on the tricuspid valve. These damaged areas are more susceptible to infection by transient bacteremia.[49] Heavy colonization of the skin and frequent skin infections caused by numerous injections with poor sterile technique are sources for transient bacteremias in drug users. Studies suggest that the injected drug is rarely contaminated. The skin of drug users is often colonized with *S. aureus,* which causes most cases of right-sided endocarditis in this group.[50] Methicillin-resistant *S. aureus*, which is usually a cause of nosocomial infection, may present as a community-acquired infection in intravenous drug users.[51] Other skin organisms such as *Bacillus* spp. and *Candida parapsilosis* are also common causes of endocarditis in this population.[52–54] Although it is less common than right-sided endocarditis, left-sided endocarditis may be seen. It may be caused by *S. aureus* or, more commonly, by gram-negative bacilli. *P. aeruginosa* is also a frequent cause of endocarditis in these patients.[55]

Pathologic Changes

The classic vegetation of infective endocarditis consists of fibrin, platelet aggregates, and bacteria. Red blood cells and white blood cells are not common.[56–58] Single or multiple vegetations may be present and may range in size from a few millimeters to several centimeters. These vegetations, which are often friable, may embolize at any time with potentially devastating effects. In addition, vegetations may be large enough to cause valvular stenosis. The underlying valve is often destroyed, especially by virulent organisms such as *S. aureus*. Furthermore, the infection may cause perforation of the valve leaflet or rupture of the chordae tendineae, interventricular septum, or papillary muscle. These complications often lead to acute congestive heart failure. Other complications include abscess of the valve ring with the formation of a fistula that extends into the myocardium or pericardium and results in myocarditis or pericarditis, respectively. Aneurysms of the valve leaflets or the sinus of Valsalva are also common. The vegetations are usually located along the line of closure of the valve leaflet on the atrial surface of the mitral or tricuspid valve or on the ventricular surface of the aortic or pulmonic valve. With treatment, healing occurs by fibrosis and occasional calcification. The healing process may leave a residual valvular stenosis and may increase the risk of subsequent episodes of endocarditis.

Involvement of the peripheral vascular system is common in patients with endocarditis. Mycotic aneurysms usually develop during active endocarditis but may also develop months later. Mechanisms postulated for the development of mycotic aneurysms are (1) direct bacterial invasion of the arterial wall with abscess formation, (2) septic or bland emboli to the vaso vasorum, or (3) the deposition of immune complexes in the arterial wall, with resultant injury. These aneurysms, usually seen at bifurcation points, are often found in the cerebral vessels, especially at the peripheral branches of the middle cerebral artery. Other common locations are the vaso vasorum of the aorta, the splenic arteries, the mesenteric arteries, the pulmonary arteries, and occasionally, the coronary arteries.[59]

The kidney, with its high blood flow, is often affected in patients with endocarditis. The common pathologic processes seen in the kidney include infarction, abscess formation, or glomerulonephritis. Renal infarction, present in 56% of untreated cases, is the most common kidney lesion seen in patients with infective endocarditis.[1] Usually, small multiple infarctions are found at autopsy. However, these lesions are uncommon in patients with right-sided endocarditis. Glomerulonephritis, the second most common lesion, may occur as focal or diffuse disease.[60, 61] Focal glomerulonephritis is found in 50% of cases of infective endocarditis and is more common in subacute disease than in acute endocarditis. Diffuse glomerulonephritis, seen in 30% to 60% of cases, is found more frequently in subacute endocarditis.[62] Abscesses, the least frequently occurring renal complication, are usually associated with suppurative infections such as *S. aureus*.

The central nervous system is another common site for complications of infective endocarditis. Lesions such as cerebral emboli, cerebral infarction, arteritis, abscesses, mycotic aneurysm, intracerebral or subarachnoid hemorrhage, encephalomalacia, cerebritis, and meningitis have been reported.[63, 64] Cerebral emboli, occurring in up to 30% of all cases of infective endocarditis, usually involve the middle cerebral artery or its branches. Hemorrhage into an ischemic infarction from septic emboli is common in endocarditis; therefore, anticoagulants must be used with caution.

The lungs are rarely affected except in patients with right-sided endocarditis, where emboli (bland or septic) may present as infarctions, acute pneumonia, pleural effusions, or empyema.[65] *S. aureus* is an unusual cause of community-acquired pneumonia; if the organism is seen in an otherwise healthy individual, right-sided endocarditis should be considered.

Cutaneous manifestations of infective endocarditis are common and result from bacterial invasion of the skin, from septic or bland emboli, or from immune complex disease. In the preantibiotic era, the classic peripheral lesion associated with endocarditis was present in about 85% of patients; now these lesions are found in only 18% to 50% of patients.[66, 67] Petechiae, seen in 20% to 40% of cases, are usually found in the conjunctiva of the eyelids, the dorsum of the hands and feet, the anterior chest wall, the abdominal wall, and the soft palate or pharyngeal mucosa. Subungual hemorrhages or splinter hemorrhages, often seen in trauma patients, are less common in patients with endocarditis. Osler's nodes are small, raised, tender nodules that occur in the pulp spaces of the terminal phalanges of fingers, backs of toes, soles of feet, and the thenar or hypothenar eminences of the hand. Before the introduction of antibiotics, Osler's nodes were present in 70% of patients with infective endocarditis but are now found in only 10% to 23% of cases. These nodes are believed to be a localized vasculitis resulting from the deposition of immune complexes rather than from direct bacterial invasion. Janeway lesions, flat, painless lesions ranging from 1 to 4 mm in diameter, are usually present on the thenar and hypothenar eminences of the hands and the soles of the feet. Rarely, these lesions may present as diffuse, macular lesions over the trunk. Unlike Osler's nodes, Janeway lesions are microabscesses that form secondary to septic emboli, and the bacteria can be seen on histologic examination.

The Roth spot, another classic lesion associated with endocarditis, is also occurring less frequently. Seen in 2% to 10% of patients with endocarditis, the Roth spot is a cotton wool–like exudate in the retina composed of a perivascular collection of lymphocytes in the nerve layer. Edema or hemorrhage also may be present. Other eye lesions seen with infective endocarditis include so-called white spots and optic neuritis.

CLINICAL MANIFESTATIONS

Infective endocarditis is a systemic disease with protean clinical signs and symptoms. Four basic processes contribute to the clinical presentation: (1) the infectious process on the valve, (2) bland or septic embolization, (3) continuous bacteremia, and (4) circulating immune complexes. Because of these multiple simultaneous processes, the clinical presentation of infective endocarditis is highly variable, and the differential diagnosis is often broad.

Patients usually present with nonspecific signs and symptoms, such as low-grade fever, chills, malaise, anorexia, myalgias, night sweats, or a flulike illness, characteristic of a subacute case. Presentation of acute endocarditis is more fulminant, with high fevers, severe prostration, or septic shock.

Heart murmurs are present in more than 85% of cases; however, the classic changing murmur or new murmur of infective endocarditis occurs in less than 16% of cases.[68, 69] Heart murmurs may be absent in right-sided or mural infection. Frequently, regurgitant murmurs may signify a perforated valve or a ruptured chordae tendineae. Of those patients who develop a new regurgitant murmur, more than 90% will develop congestive heart failure (CHF). The incidence of CHF associated with endocarditis appears to be increasing; CHF is now the leading cause of death in patients with infective endocarditis.[70] Although a regurgitant murmur has the greatest hemodynamic significance in patients with endocarditis, a murmur of valvular stenosis may signify a valve obstruction by a vegetation. This situation requires emergent surgery. Perivalvular or myocardial abscesses are often difficult to detect clinically, even with echocardiography. Often, the only sign is a conduction defect found on electrocardiography.

Major emboli can involve any organ system and are second only to CHF as a significant complication of infective endocarditis. The clinical presentation depends on the organ involved. Emboli are usually characterized by the sudden onset of pain. If in the left upper quadrant of the abdomen, the pain may suggest an embolus to the splenic artery with a splenic infarction. A sudden loss of vision in one eye may suggest an embolism of the retinal artery. Chest pain may suggest an embolus to a coronary artery in a patient with left-sided infective endocarditis or a pulmonary infarction in a patient with right-sided endocarditis. Gross hematuria suggests an embolus to the kidney. Patients who have fungal endocarditis, which is characterized by large, bulky vegetations, are more likely to have emboli in major vessels.

Neurologic manifestations of infective endocarditis develop in 20% to 40% of cases.[62, 63] Cerebral emboli, occurring in 10% to 30% of patients, usually present as hemiplegia, sensory loss, ataxia, aphasia, or a change in mental status. Less common features include seizures, severe headache, visual changes, and cranial nerve palsies. Toxic encephalopathy, which is particularly common in the elderly, ranges in presentation from mild confusion to psychosis. Often, neurologic complications may be the first manifestation of infective endocarditis and should be considered in young patients with sudden neurologic complications.

Febrile illnesses requiring hospitalization often develop in intravenous drug users. Endocarditis is responsible for 5% to 8% of these hospital admissions.[49] Diagnosis may be difficult in these patients; only 35% have heart murmurs because the right side of the heart is often involved. In patients who have endocarditis associated with drug use, the tricuspid valve is infected alone or in combination in 52.2%; the aortic valve in 18.5%; the mitral valve in 10.8%; and both the aortic and mitral valves in 12.5%.[71] Pulmonary symptoms predominate in patients with right-sided infection. Abnormalities on chest radiographs are found in 75% to 85% of patients and include pneumonia, septic emboli, effusions, and empyema. Cough, productive sputum, hemoptysis, and pleuritic chest pain are frequent pulmonary symptoms in patients with right-sided endocarditis. Only one third of patients have any signs of tricuspid insufficiency (e.g., a systolic regurgitant murmur that is louder with inspiration, large V waves, or a pulsatile liver).[64] The age and gender of these patients is helpful in making a diagnosis: Most patients are men (4 to 6:1) between the ages of 20 and 40 years.

DIAGNOSIS

The hallmark of the diagnosis of infective endocarditis is persistent bacteremia in the appropriate clinical setting. The bacteremia is usually continuous and yields a low colony count (<100 colony-forming units [CFU]/ml blood).[72] In patients who have not been treated with antibiotics, the first two sets of blood cultures yield the pathogen in more than 90% of cases.[73] The most common cause of culture-negative endocarditis is prior antibiotic therapy. The rate of positive blood cultures is 36% less in patients pretreated with antibiotics than in patients who have not received antibiotics.[41] Three sets of blood cultures (aerobic and anaerobic) should be drawn from different sites over a 24-hour period. The diagnostic success may be improved if 10 ml of blood is obtained. Most pathogens grow within 1 week. If cultures are negative at 1 week and endocarditis is still suspected, the cultures should be held for 3 weeks to detect fastidious or slow-growing organisms. Techniques that have been developed to increase the yield of blood cultures include adding antibiotic-binding resins to the culture medium or the lysis-centrifugation technique to detect intracellular organisms.[74, 75]

Routine laboratory studies, such as a complete blood cell count or urinalysis, are not usually helpful in diagnosing infective endocarditis.[67] Most patients (70% to 90%) have a normochromic, normocytic anemia, and thrombocytopenia is unusual. Leukocytosis with a left shift, which is seen in only 20% to 30% of the cases, is most common in acute endocarditis. The white cell and differential counts are normal in patients with subacute endocarditis. The erythrocyte sedimentation rate is elevated in 90% to 100% of patients.[70] Hypergammaglobulinemia, hypocomplementemia, and a positive rheumatoid factor are seen only when the illness lasts longer than 6 weeks. In most cases, proteinuria and microscopic hematuria are seen on urinalysis.

Several indirect diagnostic tests have been developed for the diagnosis of infective endocarditis. Echocardiography, the most useful of those tests, was first employed to diagnose endocarditis in 1973.[76] Initially, M-mode echocardiography gave a unidimensional "ice pick" view of the heart. Several years later, two-dimensional echocardiography was shown to be better than the M-mode technique at defining spatial relationships and configuration of cardiac structures.[77] Several studies have shown that the two-dimensional technique, with sensitivity ranging from 45% to 88%, is more useful than the M-mode technique in visualizing valvular vegetations.[78–80] Nevertheless, some technical problems were associated with the traditional two-dimensional echocardiogram, which was performed transthoracically. Acoustical interference from the chest wall and lungs often reduced the quality of the results, and visualizing the right side of the heart was difficult. Moreover, vegetations on prosthetic valves were not easily detected with the two-dimensional technique because the prosthesis disrupted the transducer's beam. However, the introduction of transesophageal echocardiography (TEE) resolved many of those technical difficulties.[81, 82] Placing the transducer in the esophagus eliminates the need to find a window for adequate visualization and improves resolution and detail. Both the posterior aspect and the right side of the heart are more easily visualized, and TEE's sensitivity ranges from 83% to 100%. TEE also improves the visualization of vegetations on prosthetic valves. In fact, TEE can identify 75% of the vegetations on a prosthetic valve compared with 35% identified by transthoracic echocardiography.[82] Furthermore, TEE is more useful in identifying myocardial and perivalvular abscesses. Daniel and coworkers[83] reported that the sensitivity and specificity of TEE in detecting abscesses ranges from 87% to 95%.

Universally accepted diagnostic criteria have been difficult to develop because of the protean manifestations of infective endocarditis. The most widely accepted diagnostic criteria, developed by von Reyn and colleagues,[84] categorize the diagnosis of infective endocarditis as definite, probable, possible, or rejected. Under these guidelines, a definite case of infective endocarditis requires positive blood cultures, histologic evidence of infection in the valve, or a major embolus. When these criteria were applied, most cases of endocarditis were defined as probable because most patients with endocarditis do not undergo surgery. Moreover, von Reyn's criteria did not make allowances for other diagnostic techniques such as echocardiography commonly used in the clinical diagnosis of infective endocarditis. Given these limitations, von Reyn's criteria were rarely used clinically. Recently, the Duke Endocarditis Service has developed new criteria for the diagnosis of infective endocarditis.[85] Like von Reyn's criteria, a diagnosis is categorized as definite, probable, possible, or rejected. Unlike the von Reyn criteria, however, clinical criteria (major and minor) are used in addition to the histologic and culture criteria. Further, Duke's criteria include the use of echocardiographic findings as well as microbiologic data. In a comparative study of the two criteria, the diagnostic sensitivity of the Duke criteria was 82% and that of von Reyn's criteria was 44%.[86]

MEDICAL MANAGEMENT

Before the development of antibiotics, infective endocarditis was a fatal disease; even with modern antibiotic therapy, it is difficult to cure and requires weeks of therapy. Moreover, relapses are common. Because the infection is located in a tight fibrin meshwork, the bacteria are protected from attack by phagocytic cells. Often, the bacterial counts in vegetations are high (10^9 to 10^{10} CFU/g).[87] Because these organisms may be in a state of reduced metabolic activity and cell division, they may be less susceptible to agents such as the beta-lactam antibiotics that affect cell wall synthesis. Antimicrobial penetration into the vegetation and its effect on therapy is an unresolved issue. Although studies have shown a great variability in antibiotic penetration into a vegetation, three basic patterns have emerged. In the first pattern, the antibiotic (teicoplanin) is only detected at the periphery and does not penetrate to the core. In the second pattern, the antibiotic (ceftriaxone) penetrates slowly to the core of the vegetation with a large gradient from the periphery to the center. Finally, certain fluoroquinolones diffuse evenly throughout the vegetation.[88] The predictive value of these findings in determining therapeutic efficacy is unknown.

Certain principles have evolved for the antibiotic treatment of infective endocarditis. Parenteral antibiotics are recommended because sustained antibacterial activity is important. The potential for erratic absorption and patient noncompliance has made oral medications less desirable. Bacteriostatic agents do not easily control the initial infection and are generally not recommended because of frequent relapses. Prolonged antibiotic therapy in a hospital setting has traditionally been recommended.

Although these recommendations have been used for more than 50 years, modern medical techniques and medical economics have brought some of them into question. The two areas of greatest study in the management of endocarditis are the use of short-term therapy and the use of outpatient treatment.

Geraci and Martin[89] first reported on the use of short-course therapy for uncomplicated penicillin-sensitive streptococcal endocarditis in 1953. Further studies by Geraci[90] and Wilson and associates[91] have supported the use of 2 weeks of combination therapy with a penicillin and an aminoglycoside. In these studies, 98% to 99% of patients who had uncomplicated endocarditis with penicillin-sensitive (<0.2 μg/ml) viridans streptococci or *S. bovis* were cured.[90, 91] These findings were comparable to those seen in patients who had been treated with 4 weeks of penicillin. Penicillin alone for 2 weeks had an unacceptably high relapse rate of up to 50%.[92, 93] Other antibiotic combinations have also been evaluated. Francioli and associates[94] cured 42 of 48 patients who had streptococcal endocarditis with a 2-week course of ceftriaxone and netilmicin, with only one relapse. New guidelines developed by the American Heart Association (AHA) now include short-course therapy for native valve endocarditis caused by penicillin-susceptible viridans streptococci and *S. bovis*.[95]

Short-course therapy may also be effective in uncomplicated right-sided endocarditis caused by *S. aureus*. In initial studies, a combination of nafcillin and tobramycin was used in a hospital setting for 2 weeks.[96] The overall success rate was 94% with three relapses. These patients had no evidence of renal failure, extrapulmonary infection, aortic or mitral valve involvement, meningitis, or infection with methicillin-resistant *S. aureus*. Similar results with an acceptably low rate of relapse were reported in subsequent studies.[97, 98] These patients should be treated in a hospital setting to monitor for complications. Vancomycin is not recommended for short-course therapy for right-sided endocarditis because of an unacceptably high relapse rate attributed to a less rapid bactericidal effect than beta-lactam antibiotics in vitro, especially in the high numbers of bacteria seen in a vegetation.[99, 100]

The second area of investigation involves the use of outpatient therapy. Traditionally, patients who have endocarditis have been admitted to the hospital or the intensive care unit for close monitoring. However, patients in stable condition may be candidates for outpatient therapy. Parenteral agents with long half-lives and new portable infusion devices make it practical to administer antibiotics in an outpatient setting. Stamboulian and associates[101] treated 30 stable patients with uncomplicated streptococcal endocarditis with single daily injections of ceftriaxone for 4 weeks. This regimen allowed patients to be discharged early from the hospital for treatment on an outpatient basis. The results were comparable to those obtained with traditional penicillin therapy; no relapses or complications were attributed to outpatient therapy. Stamboulian and colleagues estimated that 380 hospital days were saved because of outpatient therapy. Francioli and coworkers[102] presented similar data on 59 patients treated with a 4-week course of daily ceftriaxone injections for uncomplicated streptococcal endocarditis. Again, no complications were attributed to outpatient management. In a study of right-sided endocarditis caused by *S. aureus* in intravenous drug users, Heldman and associates[103] reported that a 4-week course of oral ciprofloxacin and rifampin was as effective as 4 weeks of parenteral therapy. Outpatient treatment of this population is difficult; however, these patients may be treated outside of the hospital in a supervised environment such as a drug-treatment facility. It must be emphasized that only certain patients are candidates for short-course therapy or outpatient management of endocarditis.

Transient bacteremia is a known risk factor for infection of a previously damaged valve. Physicians often prescribe antibiotics to prevent the development of endocarditis in patients who are to undergo a procedure that may cause bacteremia; however, only 4% to 19% of cases of endocarditis are associated with these high-risk procedures.[104, 105] Thus, only an estimated 6% of cases can be prevented by antibiotic prophylaxis.[104, 105]

No case-controlled study has proved that antibiotic prophylaxis prevents infective endocarditis. However, most authorities agree that prophylaxis should be offered to high-risk patients during procedures known to be associated with bacteremia. To determine which patients should receive antibiotic prophylaxis, two factors should be known: the procedure's risk of causing bacteremia and the susceptibility of the cardiac lesion to developing endocarditis. There are extensive data on the frequency of bacteremia after various procedures.[106] Generally, dental procedures such as tooth extraction or periodontal surgery carry the greatest risk of bacteremia. The risk of developing endocarditis after a genitourinary procedure is greatest when an active infection is present. The risk of bacteremia and subsequent endocarditis during normal vaginal delivery is low,[106] and the AHA guidelines do not recommend routine antibiotic prophylaxis during uncomplicated deliveries including cesarean delivery.[107] Antibiotic prophylaxis is recommended during an obstetric or gynecologic procedure only when an active infection is present.

The relative risk of a patient's underlying heart condition leading to endocarditis is based on the frequency with which that lesion is found in patients with endocarditis. MVP is estimated to be the underlying cardiac lesion in 15% to 25% of cases of infective endocarditis.[108] MVP increases the risk for endocarditis by five to eight times, and it is found in 3% to 4% of the general population and in 6% to 10% of women.[18, 109] However, recommending prophylaxis for endocarditis in patients with MVP is difficult because of its frequency in the population and because patients have a variable susceptibility to infection. The greatest risk of infection is in patients with a systolic murmur and in those who have thickening and redundancy of the mitral valve leaflets seen on echocardiography. The AHA guidelines recommend prophylaxis for patients who have MVP and a systolic murmur or redundant leaflets on echocardiography. However, these recommendations have been criticized because the systolic murmur of MVP may be present intermittently, and the absence of a murmur does not exclude redundancy of the mitral valve.[110] Based on findings from a cost-benefit analysis, Clemens and Ransohoff[111] have argued that antibiotic prophylaxis for MVP is not cost effective. They suggest that the relative risk of infective endocarditis after a dental procedure is so low that the years of life lost because of endocarditis may be exceeded by the years of life lost because of anaphylaxis related to penicillin, which is used for prophylaxis.

References

1. Lerner PI, Weinstein L: Infective endocarditis in the antibiotic era. N Engl J Med 274:199, 1966.
2. Seaworth BJ, Durack MB: Infective endocarditis in obstetric and gynecologic practice. Am J Obstet Gynecol 154:180, 1986.
3. Newsom SW: The treatment of endocarditis by vancomycin. J Antimicrob Chemother 14(Suppl):D79, 1984.
4. Griffin M, Wilson W, Edwards W, et al: Infective endocarditis. Olmstead County, Minnesota, 1950 through 1981. JAMA 254:1199, 1985.
5. Thayer WS: Studies on bacterial (infective) endocarditis. Johns Hopkins Hosp Rep 22:1, 1926.
6. Durack DT, Petersdorf RG: Changes in the epidemiology of endocarditis. In Kaplan EL, Taranta AV (eds): Infective Endocarditis. An American Heart Association Symposium. American Heart Association, Dallas, 1977, p 3.
7. Morgan WL, Bland EF: Bacterial endocarditis in antibiotic era. Circulation 19:753, 1959.
8. Durack DT, Petersdorf RG: Changes in epidemiology of endocarditis. Infective endocarditis. Am Heart Assoc Monogr 52:3, 1977.
9. Stimmel B, Donoso E, Dack S: Comparison of infective endocarditis in drug addicts and nondrug users. Am J Cardiol 32:924, 1973.
10. Pastorek JG 2nd, Plauche WC, Faro S: Acute bacterial endocarditis in pregnancy. A report of three cases. J Reprod Med 28:611, 1983.
11. MacDonald RA, Robbins SL: The significance of nonbacterial thrombotic endocarditis: An autopsy and clinical study of 78 cases. Ann Intern Med 46:255, 1957.
12. Weinstein L, Brusch JL: Epidemiology. In Weinstein L, Brusch JL (eds): Infective Endocarditis. Oxford University Press, New York, 1996, p 23.
13. McKinsey DS, Ratts TE, Bisno AL: Underlying cardiac lesions in adults with infective endocarditis. The changing spectrum. Am J Med 82:681, 1987.
14. Szekely P, Turner R, Snaith L: Pregnancy and the changing pattern of rheumatic heart disease. Br Heart J 35:1293, 1973.
15. Barlow JB, Pocock WA, Marchand P, Denny M: The significance of late systolic murmurs. Am Heart J 66:443, 1963.
16. Savage DD, Garrison RJ, Devereux RB, et al: Mitral valve prolapse in the general population. 1. Epidemiologic features: The Framingham Study. Am Heart J 106:571, 1983.
17. Levy D, Savage D: Prevalence and clinical features of mitral valve prolapse. Am Heart J 113:1281, 1987.
18. Procacci PM, Savran SV, Schreiter SL, Bryson AL: Prevalence of clinical mitral-valve prolapse in 1169 young women. N Engl J Med 294:1086, 1976.
19. Devereux RB, Hawkins I, Kramer-Fox R, et al: Complications of mitral valve prolapse. Disproportionate occurrence in men and older patients. Am J Med 81:751, 1986.

20. Zuppiroli A, Rinaldi M, Kramer-Fox R, et al: Natural history of mitral valve prolapse. Am J Cardiol 75:1028, 1995.
21. Everett ED, Hirschmann JV: Transient bacteremia and endocarditis prophylaxis. A review. Medicine 56:61, 1977.
22. Roudaut R, Lartigue MC, Texier-Maugein J, Dallocchio M: Incidence of bacteraemia or fever during transoesophageal echocardiography: A prospective study of 82 patients. Eur Heart J 14:936, 1993.
23. Shyu KG, Hwang JJ, Lin SC, et al: Prospective study of blood culture during transesophageal echocardiography. Am Heart J 124:1541, 1992.
24. Nikutta P, Mantey-Stiers F, Becht I: Risk of bacteremia induced by transesophageal echocardiography: Analysis of 100 consecutive procedures. J Am Soc Echocardiogr 5:168, 1992.
25. Livengood CH 3rd, Land MR, Addison WA: Endometrial biopsy, bacteremia, and endocarditis risk. Obstet Gynecol 65:678, 1985.
26. Cox SM, Leveno KJ: Pregnancy complicated by bacterial endocarditis. Clin Obstet Gynecol 32:48, 1989.
27. Felice PV, Salom IL, Levine R: Bivalvular endocarditis complicating pregnancy. A case report and literature review. Angiology 46:441, 1995.
28. Hughes LO, McFadyen IR, Raftery EB: Acute bacterial endocarditis on a normal aortic valve following vaginal delivery. Int J Cardiol 18: 261, 1988.
29. Blanco JD, Gibbs RS, Castaneda YS: Bacteremia in obstetrics: Clinical course. Obstet Gynecol 58:621, 1981.
30. Smith RH, Radford DJ, Clark RA, Julian DG: Infective endocarditis: A survey of cases in the South-East region of Scotland 1969–72. Thorax 31:373, 1976.
31. Boggess KA, Watts DH, Hillier SL, et al: Bacteremia shortly after placental separation during cesarean delivery. Obstet Gynecol 87: 779, 1996.
32. Summary of the workshop on perinatal infections due to group B streptococcus. J Infect Dis 136:137, 1977.
33. Schwartz B, Schuchat A, Oxtoby MJ, et al: Invasive group B streptococcal disease in adults. A population-based study in metropolitan Atlanta. JAMA 266:1112, 1991.
34. Sexton DJ, Rockson SG, Hempling RE, Cathey CW: Pregnancy-associated group B streptococcal endocarditis: A report of two fatal cases. Obstet Gynecol 66(Suppl):S44, 1985.
35. Scully BE, Spriggs D, Neu HC: *Streptococcus agalactiae* (group B) endocarditis—a description of twelve cases and review of the literature. Infection 15:169, 1987.
36. Cherubin CE, Neu HC: Infective endocarditis at the Presbyterian Hospital in New York City from 1938–1967. Am J Med 51:83, 1971.
37. Tuazon CU, Perez A, Kishaba T, Sheagren JN: *Staphylococcus aureus* among insulin-injecting diabetic patients. An increased carrier rate. JAMA 231:1272, 1975.
38. Kirmani N, Tuazon CU, Murray HW, et al: *Staphylococcus aureus* carriage rate of patients receiving long-term hemodialysis. Arch Intern Med 138:1657, 1978.
39. Tuazon CU, Sheagren JN: Increased rate of carriage of *Staphylococcus aureus* among narcotic addicts. J Infect Dis 129:725, 1974.
40. Tuazon CU, Sheagren JN: Teichoic acid antibodies in the diagnosis of serious infections with *Staphylococcus aureus*. Ann Intern Med 84: 543, 1976.
41. Gallagher PG, Watanakunakorn C: *Listeria monocytogenes* endocarditis: A review of the literature 1950–1986. Scand J Infect Dis 20: 359, 1988.
42. Pazin GJ, Saul S, Thompson ME: Blood culture positivity: Suppression by outpatient antibiotic therapy in patients with bacterial endocarditis. Arch Intern Med 142:263, 1982.
43. Karchmer AW, Archer GL, Dismukes WE: *Staphylococcus epidermidis* causing prosthetic valve endocarditis: Microbiologic and clinical observations as guides to therapy. Ann Intern Med 98:447, 1983.
44. Calderwood SB, Swinski LA, Waternaux CM, et al: Risk factors for the development of prosthetic valve endocarditis. Circulation 72:31, 1985.
45. Kluge RM, Calia FM, McLaughlin JS, Hornick RB: Sources of contamination in open heart surgery. JAMA 230:1415, 1974.
46. Fang G, Keys TF, Gentry LO, et al: Prosthetic valve endocarditis resulting from nosocomial bacteremia. A prospective, multicenter study. Ann Intern Med 119:560, 1993.
47. Grignon A, Spencer H, Robson HG, et al: Prosthetic valve infections. Can J Surg 24:615, 1981.
48. Masur H, Johnson WD Jr: Prosthetic valve endocarditis. J Thorac Cardiovasc Surg 80:31,1980.
49. Cannon NJ, Cobbs NG: Infective endocarditis in drug addicts. In Kaye D (ed): Infective Endocarditis. University Park Press, Baltimore, 1976, p 11.
50. Levine DP, Crane LR, Zervos MJ: Bacteremia in narcotic addicts at the Detroit Medical Center. II. Infectious endocarditis: A prospective comparative study. Rev Infect Dis 8:374, 1986.
51. Crane LR, Levine DP, Zervos MJ, Cummings G: Bacteremia in narcotic addicts at the Detroit Medical Center. I. Microbiology, epidemiology, risk factors, and empiric therapy. Rev Infect Dis 8:364, 1986.
52. Banks T, Fletcher R, Ali N: Infective endocarditis in heroin addicts. Am J Med 55:444, 1973.
53. Cherubin CE, Baden M, Kavaler F: Infective endocarditis in narcotic addicts. Ann Intern Med 69:1091, 1968.
54. Weems JJ Jr: *Candida parapsilosis:* Pathogenicity, clinical manifestations, and antimicrobial susceptibility. Clin Infect Dis 14:756, 1992.
55. Shekar R, Rice TW, Zierdt CH, Kallick CA: Outbreak of endocarditis caused by *Pseudomonas aeruginosa* serotype 011 among pentazocine and tripelennamine abusers in Chicago. J Infect Dis 151:203, 1985.
56. Weinstein L, Schlesinger JJ: Pathoanatomic, pathophysiologic and clinical correlations in endocarditis. N Engl J Med 291:832, 1974.
57. Arnett EN, Roberts WC: Active infective endocarditis: A clinicopathologic analysis of 137 necropsy cases. Curr Probl Cardiol 1:2, 1976.
58. Roberts WC, Buchbinder NA: Healed left-sided infective endocarditis: A clinicopathological study of 59 patients. Am J Cardiol 40:876, 1977.
59. Anderson CB, Butcher HR Jr, Ballinger WF: Mycotic aneurysms. Arch Surg 109:712, 1974.
60. Villareal H, Somoloff J: The occurrence of renal insufficiency in subacute bacterial endocarditis. Ann Intern Med 87:754, 1977.
61. Eknoyan G, Lister BJ, Kim HS, Greenberg SD: Renal complications of bacterial endocarditis. Am J Nephrol 5:457, 1985.
62. Weinstein L: Infective endocarditis. In Braunwald E (ed): Heart Disease: A Textbook of Cardiovascular Medicine, 3rd Ed. Saunders, Philadelphia, 1988, p 1108.
63. Pruitt AA, Rubin RH, Karchmer AW, Duncan GW: Neurologic complications of bacterial endocarditis. Medicine (Baltimore) 57:329, 1978.
64. Greenlee JE, Mandell GL: Neurological manifestations of infective endocarditis: A review. Stroke 4:958, 1973.
65. Chambers HF, Korzeniowski OM, Sande MA: *Staphylococcus aureus* endocarditis: Clinical manifestations in addicts and nonaddicts. Medicine (Baltimore) 62:170, 1983.
66. Libman E, Freidberg CK: Subacute Bacterial Endocarditis. Oxford University Press, Oxford, 1948.
67. Scheld WM, Sande MA: Endocarditis and intravascular infections. In Mandell GL, Douglas RG Jr, Bennett JE (eds): Principles and Practice of Infectious Diseases, 4th ed. Churchill Livingstone, New York, 1995, p 740.
68. Pankey GA: Subacute bacterial endocarditis at University of Minnesota Hospitals, 1939–1959. Ann Intern Med 55:550, 1961.
69. Pankey GA: Acute bacterial endocarditis at University of Minnesota Hospitals, 1939–1959. Am Heart J 64:583, 1962.
70. Pelletier LL Jr, Petersdorf RG: Infective endocarditis: A review of 125 cases from the University of Washington Hospitals, 1963–1972. Medicine (Baltimore) 56:287, 1977.
71. Watanakunakorn C: Changing epidemiology and newer aspects of infective endocarditis. Adv Intern Med 22:21, 1977.
72. Beeson PB, Bannon ES, Warren JV: Observations on the sites of removal of bacteria from the blood of patients with bacterial endocarditis. J Exp Med 81:9, 1945.
73. Werner AS, Cobbs CG, Kaye D, Hook EN: Studies on the bacteremia of bacterial endocarditis. JAMA 202:199, 1967.
74. Lichtlen P: General principles of conservative treatment of infective endocarditis. In Horstkotte D, Bodnar E (eds): Infective Endocarditis. ICR Publishers, London, 1991, p 85.
75. Washington JA: The microbiological diagnosis of infective endocarditis. J Antimicrob Chemother 20(Suppl):A29, 1987.
76. Dillon JC, Feigenbaum H, Konecke LL, et al: Echocardiographic manifestations of valvular vegetations. Am Heart J 86:698, 1973.
77. Gilbert BW, Haney RS, Crawford F, et al: Two-dimensional echocardiographic assessment of vegetative endocarditis. Circulation 55:346, 1977.
78. Martin RP, Meltzer RS, Chia BL, et al: Clinical utility of two dimensional echocardiography in infective endocarditis. Am J Cardiol 46: 379, 1980.
79. Melvin ET, Berger M, Lutzker LG, et al: Noninvasive methods for detection of valve vegetations in infective endocarditis. Am J Cardiol 47:271, 1981.

80. Mintz GS, Kotler MN: Clinical value and limitations of echocardiography. Its use in the study of patients with infectious endocarditis. Arch Intern Med 140:1022, 1980.
81. Daniel WG, Schroeder E, Mugge A, et al: Transesophageal echocardiography in infective endocarditis. Am J Card Imaging 2:78, 1988.
82. Daniel WG, Mugge A: Transesophageal echocardiography. N Engl J Med 332:1268, 1995.
83. Daniel WG, Mugge A, Martin RP, et al: Improvement in the diagnosis of abscesses associated with endocarditis by transesophageal echocardiography. N Engl J Med 324:795, 1991.
84. von Reyn CF, Levy BS, Arbeit RD, et al: Infective endocarditis: An analysis based on strict case definitions. Ann Intern Med 94:505, 1981.
85. Durack DT, Lukes AS, Bright DK: New criteria for diagnosis of infective endocarditis: Utilization of specific echocardiographic findings. Duke Endocarditis Service. Am J Med 96:200, 1994.
86. Hoen B, Selton-Suty C, Danchin N, et al: Evaluation of the Duke criteria versus the Beth Israel criteria for the diagnosis of infective endocarditis. Clin Infect Dis 21:905, 1995.
87. Durack DT, Beeson PB: Experimental bacterial endocarditis. II. Survival of a bacteria in endocardial vegetations. Br J Exp Pathol 53: 50, 1972.
88. Cremieux AC, Carbon C: Pharmacokinetic and pharmacodynamic requirements for antibiotic therapy of experimental endocarditis. Antimicrob Agents Chemother 36:2069, 1992.
89. Geraci JE, Martin WJ: Antibiotic therapy of bacterial endocarditis. IV. Successful short-term (two weeks) combined penicillin-dihydrostreptomycin therapy in subacute bacterial endocarditis caused by penicillin-sensitive streptococci. Circulation 8:494, 1953.
90. Geraci JE: The antibiotic therapy of bacterial endocarditis. Therapeutic data on 172 patients seen from 1951 through 1957; additional observations on short-term therapy (two weeks) for penicillin-sensitive streptococcal endocarditis. Med Clin North Am 42:1101, 1958.
91. Wilson WR, Thompson RL, Wilkowske CJ, et al: Short-term therapy for streptococcal infective endocarditis. Combined intramuscular administration of penicillin and streptomycin. JAMA 245:360, 1981.
92. Karchmer AW, Moellering RC Jr, Maki DG, Swartz MN: Single-antibiotic therapy for streptococcal endocarditis. JAMA 241:1801, 1979.
93. Malacoff RF, Frank E, Andriole VT: Streptococcal endocarditis (non-enterococcal, non-group A): Single vs combination therapy. JAMA 241:1807, 1979.
94. Francioli P, Ruch W, Stamboulian D: Treatment of streptococcal endocarditis with a single daily dose of ceftriaxone and netilmicin for 14 days: A prospective multicenter study. Clin Infect Dis 21: 1406, 1995.
95. Wilson WR, Karchmer AW, Dajani AS, et al: Antibiotic treatment of adults with infective endocarditis due to streptococci, enterococci, staphylococci, and HACEK microorganisms. American Heart Association. JAMA 274:1706, 1995.
96. Chambers HF, Miller RT, Newman MD: Right-sided *Staphylococcus aureus* endocarditis in intravenous drug abusers: Two-week combination therapy. Ann Intern Med 109:619, 1988.
97. Torres-Tortosa M, deCueto M, Vergara A, et al: Indications and therapeutic results of an antibiotic regimen lasting two weeks in intravenous drug users with right-sided *S. aureus* infective endocarditis: A multicentre study of 139 consecutive cases. Eur J Clin Microbiol Infect Dis 13:533, 1994.
98. Espinosa FJ, Valdes M, Martin-Luego F, et al: [Right endocarditis caused by *Staphylococcus aureus* in parenteral drug addicts: Evaluation of a combined therapeutic scheme for 2 weeks versus conventional treatment.] Enferm Infecc Microbiol Clin 11:235, 1993.
99. Levine DP, Fromm BS, Reddy BR: Slow response to vancomycin or vancomycin plus rifampin in methicillin-resistant *Staphylococcus aureus* endocarditis. Ann Intern Med 115:674, 1991.
100. Small PM, Chambers HF: Vancomycin for *Staphylococcus aureus* endocarditis in intravenous drug users. Antimicrob Agents Chemother 34:1227, 1990.
101. Stamboulian D, Bonvehi P, Arevalo C, et al: Antibiotic management of outpatients with endocarditis due to penicillin-susceptible streptococci. Rev Infect Dis 13(Suppl):S160, 1991.
102. Francioli P, Etienne J, Hoigne R, et al: Treatment of streptococcal endocarditis with a single daily dose of ceftriaxone sodium for 4 weeks. Efficacy and outpatient treatment feasibility. JAMA 267:264, 1992.
103. Heldman AW, Hartert TV, Ray SC, et al: Oral antibiotic treatment of right-sided staphylococcal endocarditis in injection drug users: Prospective randomized comparison with parenteral therapy. Am J Med 101:68, 1996.
104. Van der Meer JT, Van Wijk W, Thompson J, et al: Efficacy of antibiotic prophylaxis for the prevention of native-valve endocarditis. Lancet 339:135, 1992.
105. Van der Meer JT, Thompson J, Valkenburg HA, et al: Epidemiology of bacterial endocarditis in the Netherlands. II. Antecedent procedures and use of prophylaxis. Arch Intern Med 152:1869, 1992.
106. Durack DT: Prevention of infective endocarditis. N Engl J Med 332: 38, 1995.
107. Dajani AS, Bisno AL, Chung KJ, et al: Prevention of bacterial endocarditis. Recommendations by the American Heart Association. JAMA 264:2919, 1990.
108. Nolan CM, Kane JJ, Grunow WA: Infective endocarditis and mitral prolapse: A comparison with other types of endocarditis. Arch Intern Med 141:447, 1981.
109. Devereux RB, Kramer-Fox R, Kligfield P: Mitral valve prolapse: Causes, clinical manifestations, and management. Ann Intern Med 111:305, 1989.
110. Marks AR, Choong CY, Sanfilippo AJ, et al: Identification of high-risk and low-risk subgroups of patients with mitral-valve prolapse. N Engl J Med 320:1031, 1989.
111. Clemens JD, Ransohoff DF: A quantitative assessment of pre-dental antibiotic prophylaxis for patients with mitral-valve prolapse. J Chronic Dis 37:531, 1984.

SECTION V

CARDIOMYOPATHY

CHAPTER 16

Dilated Cardiomyopathy

16.1 Pathophysiology, Clinical Recognition, and Medical Therapy

Edward K. Massin

Dilated cardiomyopathy is a clinicopathologic disease process typically characterized by dilation of the cardiac chambers, with secondary dilation of the annuli of the atrioventricular valves. Thrombi may be present in both the atria and in the ventricles. The clinical presentation is most often congestive heart failure.[1, 2] Cardiac arrhythmias, systemic and pulmonary emboli, and sudden or premature death are characteristic of the process. Major features seen on histologic examination include hypertrophy and degeneration of myocytes and interstitial fibrosis.

ETIOLOGY

Whereas the etiology of dilated cardiomyopathy is often obscure, specific causative factors can sometimes be identified. Data from the Framingham studies suggest that hypertension and coronary artery disease are the most common processes leading to the clinical picture of congestive heart failure.[3, 4] A large percentage of dilated cardiomyopathy cases are diagnosed as idiopathic and are frequently presumed to be viral in origin. The presence of enteroviral and adenoviral genomes has been described in the myocardium of adult patients with dilated cardiomyopathy.[5] Viral infection may result in an autoimmune process leading to myocardial damage. Detection of high titers of antibody to Coxsackie B virus in patients with idiopathic dilated cardiomyopathy and with myocarditis implicates Coxsackie B virus as a causative agent in some cases.[6, 7] Genetic defects (e.g., mutations in genes encoding cardiac cytoskeletal proteins and sarcomere proteins) account for an estimated 25% to 35% of idiopathic dilated cardiomyopathy cases.[8–10]

Depending on the factors responsible for dilated cardiomyopathy, the condition may sometimes be reversed. For example, dilated cardiomyopathy caused by alcohol abuse can sometimes be reversed by abstention.[11, 12] Dilated cardiomyopathy caused by renal failure is sometimes reversible by renal transplantation.

In cancer patients, a toxic dilated cardiomyopathy may sometimes result from the use of the chemotherapeutic agent doxorubicin hydrochloride (Adriamycin).[13, 14] A small percentage of pregnancies are complicated by a peripartum dilated cardiomyopathy.[15, 16] Cardiomyopathy in such cases may improve or return to normal with standard therapy for heart failure (diuretics, vasodilators, and digoxin as needed), though hospitalization and more aggressive support may sometimes be needed.[17] Angiotensin-converting enzyme (ACE) inhibitors should be avoided prenatally. Left ventricular dysfunction may recur during a subsequent pregnancy in women with a history of peripartum cardiomyopathy even though normal or near normal function was restored after the initial episode.[18] Whereas, in biopsy specimens, the transition from myocarditis to dilated cardiomyopathy is poorly documented, patients with myocarditis may present with a clinical picture of dilated cardiomyopathy.[19, 20] Neuromuscular and familial diseases account for a small portion of patients presenting with dilated cardiomyopathy, and in these situations, the cardiac process may not be the principal concern.[21]

Gender differences both in the etiology and in the clinical course of various forms of dilated cardiomyopathy are recognized (see Chapter 17). Although dilated cardiomyopathy generally has been addressed as a single process, etiology and gender have prognostic implications and may be bases for selection of specific treatment modalities.[22, 23]

CLINICAL CHARACTERISTICS

Presenting symptoms of dilated cardiomyopathy result from low cardiac output (e.g., fatigue and weakness) or pulmonary and visceral congestion (e.g., dyspnea, cough, abdominal distention, and edema). Initially, about 86% of patients present with exertional dyspnea; 30% present with palpitations, and 29% with edema.[24] Anginal chest pain is a presenting symptom in 8% to 20% of patients, and it will ultimately affect more than one third of patients with dilated cardiomyopathy.[1] By the time of diagnosis, advanced heart failure will have developed in most patients. Presenting symptoms may be similar to those of pneumonia, gastrointestinal disease, or myocardial infarction.

Although the onset of symptoms may be gradual—over weeks to months—patients may seek medical care only after an acute exacerbation. Cardiac arrhythmias, either atrial or ventricular, may precipitate acute decompensation of congestive heart failure and may, rarely, cause dizziness, syncope, or sudden death as presenting manifestations.[1, 2] Fewer than 5% of patients present with an embolic event.[1, 12] Thrombus formation in the left atrium or left ventricle may embolize systemically; venous thrombus may embolize to the lungs or, paradoxically, through a patent foramen ovale to the systemic circulation.

Upon physical examination, the severity of left ventricular dysfunction will be confirmed by findings of hypotension, low pulse pressure, and pulsus alternans. Other signs of dilated cardiomyopathy include elevated jugular venous pressure, rales, and leftward displacement of the cardiac apex with a broad apical thrust and a ventricular gallop.

There may be audible systolic murmurs of atrioventricular valve regurgitation. Hepatomegaly, ascites, and peripheral edema reflect increasingly severe right-sided heart failure. Cachexia may be apparent in end-stage patients with poor caloric intake and increased metabolic demands.

DIAGNOSTIC STUDIES

Laboratory studies in the course of dilated cardiomyopathy are important for establishing the correct diagnosis, disclosing possible etiologies and aggravating factors, determining disease severity and prognosis, and following the disease process and response to treatment. Assays of endogenous brain natriuretic peptide (BNP), which is synthesized in the cardiac ventricles, may confirm the presence of congestive heart failure in patients who present with dyspnea and may provide a measure of the severity of heart failure.[25, 26]

Pulmonary evaluation (i.e., chest x-ray, CT scan) can rule out adult respiratory distress syndrome, pneumonia, asthma, and infiltrative malignancy from the differential diagnosis. Renal function parameters (e.g., blood urea nitrogen, serum creatinine, and creatinine clearance) can identify renal failure as a cause of dilated cardiomyopathy or as a factor aggravating congestive heart failure. Blood counts will assess the role of anemia as a causative or aggravating factor in congestive heart failure. Hypocalcemia and hypophosphatemia are causes of congestive heart failure that can be successfully treated.

Clues to the etiology of congestive heart failure can also be found in the chest x-ray when it reveals pericardial or valvular calcification. Recognition of cardiomegaly and specific chamber enlargement, as well as prominence of pulmonary vascular markings, are basic data used in establishing the diagnosis, estimating severity, explaining symptoms, and following the response to treatment and progression of disease.

In cases of dilated cardiomyopathy, the electrocardiogram often shows sinus tachycardia. Left bundle branch block and left anterior hemiblock patterns are common, especially in later stages of the disease.[27–30] Bradycardia may be a sign of chronotropic incompetence and may prevent an appropriate response to a need for increased cardiac output. Persistent tachyarrhythmias, e.g., atrial fibrillation or flutter, supraventricular tachycardia, or ventricular tachycardia, can be causes of congestive heart failure reversible by restoring normal rhythm or by controlling ventricular rate. Atrioventricular dissociation with slow ventricular response limits cardiac output and can cause syncope.

Although Q waves on the electrocardiogram may reflect myocardial infarction and ischemic heart disease as a cause of dilated cardiomyopathy, Q waves are also seen in cases of idiopathic dilated cardiomyopathy in the absence of coronary disease. Arrhythmias and abnormal QRS patterns may be associated with cardiomyopathies of muscular dystrophies and storage diseases.[31]

Doppler echocardiography provides useful data such as chamber sizes, left ventricular ejection fraction and wall motion abnormalities, right-sided heart function, and estimation of pulmonary pressures.[32] Congenital heart lesions, such as atrial septal defect, or valvular lesions may be apparent by echocardiographic examination though obscure on physical examination. In patients with severely depressed left ventricular function, a murmur of aortic stenosis may be unimpressive, and low flow across a stenotic mitral valve may be inaudible; however, Doppler echocardiographic studies should be diagnostic. Diastolic ventricular function can often be assessed by echocardiography.

Radionuclide ventriculography is useful in evaluating ventricular function, especially when a good-quality echocardiogram cannot be obtained: ventricular volume and ejection fraction have prognostic significance. Perfusion imaging provides data regarding myocardial viability and the potential benefit of revascularization procedures when coronary artery disease is present and ischemia is suspected as the cause of dilated cardiomyopathy. The usefulness of such data may be enhanced by a variety of special techniques. Reinjection of isotope with repeat scanning at a later time may uncover viable tissue. Exercise stress testing and, if that is not advisable, dobutamine infusion or administration of dipyridamole may assist in distinguishing viable tissue suitable for revascularization. One caveat, however, is that idiopathic dilated cardiomyopathy can be associated with perfusion defects.[33]

Cardiac magnetic resonance imaging is useful in assessing myocardial viability and ventricular function in patients with cardiomyopathies.[34] The role of positron emission tomography (PET) in determining tissue viability remains unclear. PET is not routinely used because of its limited availability and high cost (compared with nuclear imaging).

Cardiac catheterization and angiography are valuable in the evaluation of dilated cardiomyopathy. In addition to confirming the status of the coronary arteries, knowledge of right heart pressures and pulmonary vascular resistance is necessary to evaluate the potential for use of mechanical support devices and the possibility of heart transplantation. Because little evidence exists for effective treatment of myocarditis (though immunoadsorption shows promise in this regard[35, 36]), the value of myocardial biopsy is limited.[37]

Gender-specific data related to normal cardiac function are sparse. Echocardiographic data have generally demonstrated a smaller left ventricular chamber size and left ventricular mass in women than in men. Framingham data suggest that left ventricular mass declines as men age; however, it increases slightly as women age.[38, 39] Animal studies indicate that hormonal influences account for the gender differences in cardiac function; it is not clear whether this occurs by altering blood pressure or intravascular volume.[40] Women are reported to have higher heart rates than men, both at rest and during exercise, as well as a lower MVO_2 even when adjusted for age and lean body mass.[41–43] While not specifically addressing dilated cardiomyopathy, Framingham data regarding congestive heart failure indicate only a slight predominance in men, although coronary artery disease was much more frequent in men.[44] Systolic hypertension was the strongest predictor of congestive heart failure in women. Framingham data[3, 4] and data from the Coronary Artery Surgery Study (CASS)[45] suggest a high incidence of left ventricular systolic dysfunction in both men and women with congestive heart failure, but a higher incidence of diastolic left ventricular dysfunction in women than in men with the disease.

Framingham data continue to report significantly improved survival after onset of congestive heart failure for women compared with men. Median survival time after onset of congestive heart failure was 1.7 years for men and 3.2 years for women. One- and 5-year survival rates for men were 57% and 25%, compared with 64% and 38% for women.[44] Population-based data from the Scottish National Health Service indicate that, over a 10-year period, the median survival time after a first hospitalization for heart failure increased from 1.23 to 1.64 years.[22] Thirty-day case fatality rates fell by 26% in men and 17% in women; longer term rates fell by 18% in men and 15% in women. The median survival time was 1.47 years in men and 1.39 years in women. In contrast, a population-based study of data from the Rochester Epidemiology Project revealed that survival rates of patients presenting with new-onset congestive heart failure remained poor and did not significantly improve between 1981 and 1991 (72% and 77% at 1 year and 34% and 33% at 5 years).[46] The Rochester study found no sex difference in long-term survival.

RISK FACTORS

Risk factors for dilated cardiomyopathy in women were examined by the Washington, DC, Dilated Cardiomyopathy Study.[47] There were positive correlations with asthma, diabetes mellitus, hypertension, and black race. The influence of hypertension was especially strong among women under 50 years of age. There was a negative correlation with use of oral contraceptives. The Italian Multicenter Cardiomyopathy Study Group examined clinical, laboratory, and prognostic differences in men and women with idiopathic dilated cardiomyopathy. A number of variables were significantly different between men and women (Table 16–1).[48] Women presented at a more advanced stage of disease, and their prognosis was no different from that of men.[48] Women had more severe symptoms (above NYHA class III in 48% of women versus 39% of men), presented more frequently with heart failure signs (63% versus 41%), and had a higher cardiothoracic ratio and a higher frequency of left bundle branch block. By Cox multivariate analysis, left ventricular ejection fraction was a significant independent predictor of cardiac death or heart transplantation in both sexes ($p < .05$ in men; $p < .005$ in women). Andersson and Waagstein reported that among their hospitalized study group, women presented more frequently than did men for dilated cardiomyopathy associated with systemic disease, valvular heart disease, or diabetes mellitus.[49]

Table 16–1. LABORATORY FINDINGS ACCORDING TO SEX*

	WOMEN (*n* = 65)	MEN (*n* = 238)	*p* Value
Electrocardiogram			
Left bundle branch block	27 (41%)	68 (29%)	<0.05
Left anterior hemiblock	3 (4%)	45 (19%)	<0.05
Cardiothoracic ratio	0.56 ± 0.06	0.53 ± 0.06	<0.05
Exercise stress test (*n* = 251)			
Duration of exercise (min)	7 ± 3	10 ± 4	< 0.001
Echocardiography			
LV end-diastolic diameter index (mm/m²)	42 ± 7	39 ± 6	<0.01
LV end-systolic diameter index (mm/m²)	36 ± 7	33 ± 6	<0.05
Mean myocardial thickness index (mm/m²)	11 ± 2	10 ± 2	<0.05
LV mass index (g/m²)	196 ± 120	152 ± 73	0.001
Catheterization			
Mean right atrial pressure (mm Hg)	4 ± 3	5 ± 4	<0.05

*All findings listed in this table represent statistically significant differences between men and women in the study.

Abbreviations: LV, left ventricular.

Source: Adapted from De Maria R, Gavazzi A, Recalcati F, et al on behalf of The Italian Multicenter Cardiomyopathy Study Group (SPIC): Comparison of clinical findings in idiopathic dilated cardiomyopathy in women versus men. Am J Cardiol 72: 580, 1993.

Prognosis of a specific patient with dilated cardiomyopathy is difficult to determine. It is clearly impossible to ascertain how many patients may have undetected, asymptomatic cardiomegaly or the duration of such status prior to presentation. Survival with treated dilated cardiomyopathy has improved in recent years with the use of newer agents for management of congestive heart failure and cardiac arrhythmias and with the availability of mechanical support devices and improvements in the management of heart transplant recipients; yet the prognosis remains poor.[50–52] Data published in 1994 from the Heart Muscle Study Group in Italy[50] suggest that during 15 years of data acquisition, the 1-year survival rate increased from 73.8% to 90.3%, and the 4-year survival rate increased from 53.8% to 82.9%. Improved survival may be based on earlier disease detection, better treatment, or studies based on populations at risk rather those referred to major medical centers. Some patients may experience long periods of clinical stability; even spontaneous clinical improvement and increase of ejection fraction may occur. Choices of therapy should address quality-of-life issues as well as survival.

A variety of clinical features have been used to stratify risk among patients with dilated cardiomyopathy. Young age and female sex seem to predict a better prognosis.[44] Functional class IV,[29] syncope,[1] persistent ventricular gallop, and right-sided heart failure[53] are predictive of poor outcome. Evidence of atrioventricular conduction block[54] or left bundle branch block also suggest poor prognosis.[30] The Veterans Administration Vasodilator Heart Failure Trials (VHeFT-I[55] and VHeFT-II[56]) concluded that prognosis was influenced by left ventricular ejection fraction, maximal oxygen consumption, cardiothoracic ratio, ventricular arrhythmias, and history of antiarrhythmic drug use. The later trial also reported that an accelerated heart rate and low systolic and diastolic blood pressures were predictive of high mortality rate.

In the VHeFT-I study, the mortality rate was 19.5% for patients in the control group (functional classes II and III),[55] whereas in the Cooperative North Scandinavian Enalapril Survival Study (CONSENSUS-1), the mortality rate was 52% for patients in the control group (functional class IV).[57]

Although left ventricular ejection fraction is a good general predictor of mortality rate, it is not sufficiently specific to guide therapy for an individual patient.[58] Right ventricular ejection may be an independent prognostic indicator.[53]

Measurement of serum levels of several vasoactive substances has proved predictive of survival in patients with chronic heart failure. Cohn and associates in 1984 reported that levels of plasma norepinephrine were predictive of subsequent risk of death[59]; levels were found to be higher in patients who died of progressive heart failure than in those who died suddenly. Since then, studies have suggested that serum sodium levels may provide a simply obtained surrogate for plasma norepinephrine level.[60]

Since Cohn's description of the value of plasma norepinephrine as a prognostic indicator, other vasoactive hormones have been found to be effective indices of prognosis (e.g., levels of plasma atrial natriuretic factor).[58] Changes in BNP levels during treatment are strong predictors of mortality in patients with congestive heart failure.[61]

Measurements of functional capacity are probably the best prognostic indices for a specific patient. Maximal oxygen consumption appears to be predictive of 1-year survival in individual patients.[62] MVO_2 of less than 10 ml/kg body weight per minute suggests a 1-year mortality rate of over 50% and should prompt consideration of heart transplantation.[63] Peak exercise systolic blood pressure and percent predicted peak exercise VO_2 may be used to prognostically stratify patients with congestive heart failure.[64] A 6-minute walk test can be standardized to provide similar useful prognostic data.[65] Whereas hemodynamic data are almost always assessed in the evaluation of dilated cardiomyopathy patients, the relation to long-term outlook remains unclear. Elevated right-sided heart pressures, low cardiac output, high pulmonary vascular resistance, and high transpulmonary gradient have been cited as predictive of poor long-term outlook.[12] Loss of cardiac myofilaments on endomyocardial biopsy specimens is predictive of a poor prognosis.[66] The timing of prognostic indices remains in question: should testing be done early after diagnosis or following achievement of maximal clinical response to treatment?

TREATMENT

The management of dilated cardiomyopathy is multifaceted. First, congestive heart failure must be treated. Anticoagulation and the use of antiarrhythmic agents should be considered. Patient education regarding the nature of the disease, including its symptoms and its prognosis, is important. Patients should receive careful instructions about their medications and the possible side effects of each, as well as information regarding proper nutrition, particularly the need for sodium and fluid restrictions. Patients should be instructed about sodium content of prepared foods, fast foods, and canned foods. They should be encouraged to weigh regularly and to report weight changes outside fixed parameters, and they should learn to measure liquid intake. Some patients should be advised regarding caloric restrictions, whereas others may require nutritional supplements. In general, patients with dilated cardiomyopathy, especially those with severe heart failure, should receive prophylaxis against influenza and pneumonia.

Congestive heart failure is associated with changes in the peripheral circulation and skeletal muscle.[67] Vasodilator capacity is reduced. Force of sustained muscle contractility and decreased endurance with repetitive contractions are characteristic. Muscle fiber changes occur, and there are alterations of mitochondria within the skeletal muscle cells. Exercise training, even at low levels, can contribute to reversal of these problems.[68, 69]

Drug Therapy for Congestive Heart Failure

The most common presentation of dilated cardiomyopathy is congestive heart failure.[24] Diuretics, ACE inhibitors, beta blockers, and digoxin all have an acknowledged role to play in the management of congestive heart failure. Several other classes of drugs (i.e., calcium-channel agonists, inotropic agents, angiotensin receptor blockers, endothelin receptor antagonists, BNP, and tumor necrosis factor-α competitors) have also been used as therapy, though their benefit to patients is still being studied.[70] Intravenous immunoglobulin (IVIG) has been used as therapy, but with conflicting results. In a placebo-controlled study in patients with recent-onset idiopathic dilated cardiomyopathy, IVIG did not improve cardiac function.[71] Conversely, in a placebo-controlled study in patients with congestive heart failure, it induced a significant 26% to 31% increase in cardiac function.[72] (For more discussion of drug therapies for congestive heart failure, see Chapter 17.)

Cardiac Arrhythmias

The management of cardiac arrhythmias in dilated cardiomyopathy patients remains the subject of investigation. Thirty percent of patients presenting with dilated cardiomyopathy have palpitations.[19] Both atrial and ventricular arrhythmias can be documented in dilated cardiomyopathy patients; bradyarrhythmias and tachycardias occur; atrioventricular block is indicative of poor prognosis.[2] About 12% of patients with dilated cardiomyopathy die suddenly, and about 28% of all deaths are sudden.[73] A large percentage of dilated cardiomyopathy patients have premature ventricular beats and nonsustained ventricular tachycardia. The presence of ventricular ectopy tends to correlate with poor ventricular function, but the value of treating the abnormal rhythm is yet to be defined.[74] Use of many antiarrhythmic agents is associated with pro-arrhythmias and with negative inotropic effects. Electrophysiologic studies have some prognostic value in patients with ischemic cardiomyopathy; inability to induce ventricular tachycardia is predictive of low risk of arrhythmic death.[75] Electrophysiologic studies are not predictive when applied to heart failure patients with nonsustained ventricular tachycardia. The predictive value of signal-averaged ECG is higher in postinfarction patients than in dilated cardiomyopathy.

Since the CAST[76] studies of antiarrhythmic drug usage post-infarction, there has been reluctance to prescribe drugs for asymptomatic arrhythmias. Use of class I agents has been felt to be associated with increased risk. Amiodarone, an agent with multiple activities, has been tested in two large trials for benefit in management of dilated cardiomyopathy patients. The GESICA trial was an Argentine study of over 500 patients, in which about half received 300 mg amiodarone daily and the other half received placebo.[77] Treated patients had decreased risk of sudden death, fewer hospitalizations, and less progression of congestive heart failure. Subsequently, the Congestive Heart Failure–Survival Trial of Antiarrhythmic Therapy (CHF-STAT) in the United States reported no change of total mortality rate or of sudden death, although there was a trend toward decreased mortality rate among patients with nonischemic dilated cardiomyopathy.[78] Ventricular arrhythmias were suppressed and left ventricular ejection fraction was increased in treated patients. The role of amiodarone is yet to be defined. However, more recent data from the CHF-STAT database demonstrate that amiodarone can convert atrial fibrillation to sinus rhythm and control ventricular response, suggesting that it may lower mortality in patients converted to sinus rhythm.[79]

Another approach to the management of life-threatening ventricular arrhythmia is implantation of a cardioverter/defibrillator with pacing capability. These devices can be implanted transvenously without thoracotomy at relatively low risk. If high-degree heart block is documented, a pacemaker can be implanted with the same criteria for installation as would apply in other clinical situations. Several clinical studies—e.g., the Sudden Cardiac Death Heart Failure Trial (SCD-HeFT), the Multicenter Automatic Defibrillator Implantation Trial II (MADIT II), and a substudy of the Coronary Artery Bypass Graft (CABG)-Patch—are investigating the role of implantable defibrillator therapy in patients with heart failure.[80] The Marburg Cardiomyopathy Study (MACAS), a prospective 5-year study, is assessing the value of several noninvasive arrhythmia risk predictors in predicting sudden cardiac death in over 200 patients with idiopathic dilated cardiomyopathy.[81] Its results should have important implications for the design of future studies of prophylactic defibrillator therapy in idiopathic dilated cardiomyopathy. Biventricular pacing is an emerging therapy for congestive heart failure that, according to data from the Ventak CHF trial, may lessen the need for therapy with an implantable cardioverter/defibrillator.[82, 83]

Embolic Complications

The increased frequency of embolic complications in dilated cardiomyopathy has led to the recommendation for anticoagulation. There are no published prospective trials of anticoagulation in this setting. Retrospective analysis of data gathered in the VHeFT-I and -II trials suggests that anticoagulation may not be beneficial for patients with NYHA class II or III heart failure: treatment with warfarin did not reduce the incidence of thromboembolism. The authors concluded that the incidence of major bleeding in other trials approached the risk of thromboembolism in patients with class II or III congestive heart failure. Initial data from Studies of Left Ventricular Dysfunction (SOLVD) similarly indicated no benefit for patients receiving warfarin.[84, 85] However, a retrospective study indicated that in patients with moderate to severe left ventricular dysfunction resulting from coronary artery disease, antiplatelet and anticoagulant therapy are each associated with a reduction in the risk of sudden cardiac death.[86] Nevertheless, when anticoagulation therapy is used, there is always the danger of harmful drug interactions. The efficacy of warfarin, clopidogrel, and aspirin is being compared prospectively in the Warfarin and Antiplatelet Therapy in Chronic Heart Failure (WATCH) trial now underway.[87]

CONCLUSIONS

Questions remain regarding optimal treatment of arrhythmias and optimal use of anticoagulation in dilated cardiomyopathy patients. Long-term prospective studies involving large patient populations will be necessary to resolve the issues. Meanwhile, investigations proceed in search of new approaches for successful management of congestive heart failure. Will angiotensin II receptor blockade add to the benefits of ACE inhibitors? The Evaluation of Losartan in the Elderly (ELITE) study and its ELITE II offshoot showed that the angiotensin receptor blocker losartan was better tolerated than the ACE inhibitor captopril but that it did not significantly improve outcome.[88, 89] A large randomized multicenter trial called Candesartan in Heart Failure—Assessment of Reduction in Mortality and Morbidity (CHARM) is currently investigating the clinical usefulness of a long-acting angiotensin II type 1 receptor blocker, candesartan cilexetil, in patients with symptomatic heart failure.[90] The Valsartan Heart Failure Trial (Val-HeFT) has shown valsartan to be clinically efficacious in patients receiving standard therapy for heart failure.[91] Will blockade of endothelin-1 activity be useful in management of patients with congestive heart failure? Several large clinical studies of endothelin receptor antagonists have been undertaken in this regard.[70] Will inhibition of central nervous system sympathetic activity by agents such as clonidine confirm recent studies indicating benefits in treatment of congestive heart failure? Can inhibition of atrial natriuretic factor degradation result in improved hemodynamics in congestive heart failure patients?

Historically, we have addressed heart failure management by trying to enhance the performance of remaining viable myocytes, by optimizing load on the heart (reducing preload and afterload), by salvaging jeopardized myocardium (e.g., revascularization procedures for ischemic disease), and by modulation of growth (an effect of ACE inhibitors and aldosterone). New research is being focused on different and more imaginative approaches to the problem.[92] Attempts are being made to implant fetal myocytes into failing hearts. Genetic manipulations may be able to alter differentiation of cells within the heart, e.g., causing fibroblasts to develop into myocardial cells. Genetic alterations may also be able to prevent the suppression of mitosis of adult myocytes to allow the heart to replace damaged contractile cells. Conversely, prevention or inhibition of programmed cell death, apoptosis, might prolong the availability of viable and contractile myocytes. Stem cell research may lead to new therapies for failing hearts.

Pending improved medication for management of end-stage dilated cardiomyopathy, patients whose disease is refractory to therapy should be considered for circulatory support devices or for heart transplantation.

References

1. Komajda M, Jais JP, Reeves F, et al: Factors predicting mortality in idiopathic dilated cardiomyopathy. Eur Heart J 11:824, 1990.
2. Sugrie DD, Rodeheffer RJ, Codd MB, et al: The clinical course of idiopathic dilated cardiomyopathy: A population based study. Ann Intern Med 117:117, 1992.
3. McKee PA, Castelli WP, McNamara PM, Kannel WB: The natural history of congestive heart failure: The Framingham Study. N Engl J Med 285:1441, 1971.
4. Kannel WB: Vital epidemiologic clues in heart failure. J Clin Epidemiol 53:229, 2000.
5. Pauschinger M, Bowles NE, Fuentes-Garcia FJ, et al: Detection of adenoviral genome in the myocardium of adult patients with idiopathic left ventricular dysfunction. Circulation 99:1348, 1999.

6. Orchard LC, Bowles NE, Olsen EGJ, Richardson PJ: Detection of persistent Coxsackie B virus RNA in dilated cardiomyopathy and myocarditis. Eur Heart J 8 (Suppl J):437, 1987.
7. Muir P, Nicholson F, Tilzey AJ, et al: Chronic relapsing pericarditis of dilated cardiomyopathy: serological evidence of persistent enterovirus infection. Lancet 1:804, 1989.
8. Michels VV, Moll PP, Miller FA, et al: The frequency of familial dilated cardiomyopathy in a series of patients with idiopathic dilated cardiomyopathy. N Engl J Med 326:77, 1992.
9. Grunig E, Tasman JA, Kucherer H, et al: Frequency and phenotypes of familial dilated cardiomyopathy. J Am Coll Cardiol 32:1136, 1998.
10. Kamisago M, Sharma SD, DePalma SR, et al: Mutations in sarcomere protein genes as a cause of dilated cardiomyopathy. N Engl J Med 343: 1688, 2000.
11. Regan JT: Alcoholic cardiomyopathy. Prog Cardiovasc Dis 28:141, 1984.
12. Fuster V, Gersh BJ, Giulianni ER, et al: The natural history of idiopathic dilated cardiomyopathy. Am J Cardiol 47:525, 1981.
13. Haq MM, Legha SS, Cholesi J, et al: Doxorubicin-induced congestive heart failure in adults. Cancer 56:1361, 1985.
14. Kapoor AS: Doxorubicin toxicity. In Kapoor AS (ed): Cancer and the Heart. Springer-Verlag, New York, 1986, p 228.
15. Veille JC: Peripartum cardiomyopathy: A review. Am J Obstet Gynecol 148:805, 1984.
16. O'Connell JB, Costanzo-Nordin MR: Peripartum cardiomyopathy: Clinical, hemodynamic, histologic, and prognostic characteristics. J Am Coll Cardiol 8:52, 1986.
17. Pearson GD, Veille JC, Rahimtoola S, et al: Peripartum cardiomyopathy: National Heart, Lung, and Blood Institute and Office of Rare Diseases (National Institutes of Health) workshop recommendations and review. JAMA 283:1183, 2000.
18. Elkayam U, Tummala PP, Rao K, et al: Maternal and fetal outcomes of subsequent pregnancies in women with peripartum cardiomyopathy. N Engl J Med 344:1567, 2001.
19. Dec GW Jr, Palacios JF, Fallon JT, et al: Active myocarditis in the spectrum of acute dilated cardiomyopathies, clinical features, histologic correlates, and clinical outcome. N Engl J Med 312:885, 1985.
20. MacArthur CG, Tarin D, Goodwin JF, Hallidie-Smith KA: The relationship of myocarditis to dilated cardiomyopathy. Eur Heart J 5:1023, 1984.
21. Michels VV, Moll PP, Miller FA, et al: The frequency of familial dilated cardiomyopathy in a series of patients with idiopathic cardiomyopathy. N Engl J Med 326:77, 1992.
22. MacIntyre K, Capewell S, Stewart S, et al: Evidence of improving prognosis in heart failure: Trends in case fatality in 66,547 patients hospitalized between 1986 and 1995. Circulation 102:1126, 2000.
23. Felker GM, Thompson RE, Hare JM, et al: Underlying causes and long-term survival in patients with initially unexplained cardiomyopathy. N Engl J Med 342:1077, 2000.
24. Diaz RA, Obasohan A, Oakley CM: Prediction of outcome in dilated cardiomyopathy. Br Heart J 58:393, 1987.
25. Maisel A: B-type natriuretic peptide levels: A potential novel "white count" for congestive heart failure. J Card Fail 7:183, 2001.
26. Maisel A, Koon J, Krishnaswamy P, et al: Utility of B-natriuretic peptide as a rapid, point-of-care test for screening patients undergoing echocardiography to determine left ventricular dysfunction. Am Heart J 141: 367, 2001.
27. Roberts WC, Siegel RJ, McManus BM, et al: Idiopathic dilated cardiomyopathy: Analysis of 152 necropsy patients. Am J Cardiol 60:1540, 1987.
28. Wilensky RL, Yudelman P, Cohen AL, et al: Serial electrocardiographic changes in dilated cardiomyopathy confirmed at autopsy. Am J Cardiol 62:276, 1988.
29. Kelly TL, Cremo R, Nielsen C, Shabetai R: Prediction of outcome in late-stage cardiomyopathy. Am Heart J 119:1111, 1990.
30. Huang X, Shen W, Gong L: Clinical significance of complete left bundle branch block in dilated cardiomyopathy. Chinese Med Sci J 10: 158, 1995.
31. Cannes RO III, Cummins RE, Parrillo JE, et al: Dynamic limitation of coronary vasodilator reserve in patients with dilated cardiomyopathy and chest pain. J Am Coll Cardiol 10:1190, 1987.
32. Shah PM: Echocardiography in congestive or dilated cardiomyopathy. J Am Soc Echocardiogr 1:20, 1988.
33. Dilsizian V, Bonow RO: Current diagnostic techniques of assessing myocardial viability in patients with hibernating and stunned myocardium. Circulation 87:1, 1993.
34. Schulz-Menger J, Friedrich MG: Magnetic resonance imaging in patients with cardiomyopathies: When and why. Herz 25:384, 2000.
35. Müller J, Wallukat G, Dandel M, et al: Immunoglobulin adsorption in patients with idiopathic dilated cardiomyopathy. Circulation 101: 385, 2000.
36. Staudt A, Schäper F, Stangl V, et al: Immunohistological changes in dilated cardiomyopathy induced by immunoadsorption therapy and subsequent immunoglobulin substitution. Circulation 103:2681, 2001.
37. Mason JW, O'Connell JB: Clinical merit of endomyocardial biopsy. Circulation 79:971, 1989.
38. Levy D, Savage DD, Garrison RJ, et al: Echocardiographic criteria for left ventricular hypertrophy: The Framingham Heart Study. Am J Cardiol 59:956, 1987.
39. Dannenberg AL, Levy D, Garrison CJ: Impact of age on echocardiographic left ventricular mass in a healthy population (The Framingham Study). Am J Cardiol 64:1066, 1989.
40. Schaible TF, Malhotra A, Ciambrone G, Scheurer J: The effect of gonadectomy on left ventricular function and cardiac contractile proteins in male and female rats. Circ Res 54:38, 1984.
41. Becklake MR, Frank H, Dagenais GR, et al: Influence of age and sex on exercise cardiac output. J Appl Physiol 20:938, 1965.
42. Hossack KF, Bruce RA: Maximal cardiac function in normal sedentary men and women: Comparison of age-related changes. J Appl Physiol 53:799, 1982.
43. Drinkwater BL: Women and exercise: Physiological aspects. Exer Sport Sci Rev 12:21, 1984.
44. Ho KK, Anderson KM, Kannel WB, et al: Survival after the onset of congestive heart failure in Framingham Heart Study subjects. Circulation 88:107, 1993.
45. Davis KB, Chaitman B, Ryan T, et al: Comparison of 15-year survival for men and women after initial medical or surgical treatment for coronary artery disease: A CASS Registry study. J Am Coll Cardiol 25: 1000, 1995.
46. Senni M, Tribouilloy CM, Rodeheffer RJ, et al: Congestive heart failure in the community: trends in incidence and survival in a 10-year period. Arch Intern Med 159:29, 1999.
47. Coughlin SS, Tefft MC: The epidemiology of dilated cardiomyopathy in women: The Washington DC Dilated Cardiomyopathy Study. Epidemiology 5:449, 1994.
48. De Maria R, Gavazzi A, Recalcati F, et al on behalf of The Italian Multicenter Cardiomyopathy Study Group (SPIC): Comparison of clinical findings in idiopathic dilated cardiomyopathy in women versus men. Am J Cardiol 72:580, 1993.
49. Andersson B, Waagstein F: Spectrum and outcome of congestive heart failure in a hospitalized population. Am Heart J 126:632, 1993.
50. DiLenarda A, Secoli G, Perkan A, et al: Changing mortality in dilated cardiomyopathy. The Heart Muscle Disease Study Group. Br Heart J 72(6 Suppl)S46, 1994.
51. Stevenson WG, Stevenson LW, Middlekauff HR, et al: Improving survival for patients with advanced heart failure: A study of 757 consecutive patients. J Am Coll Cardiol 26:1417, 1995.
52. Konstam MA: Progress in heart failure management? Lessons from the real world [editorial]. Circulation 102:1076, 2000.
53. Likoff MJ, Chandler SL, Kay HR: Clinical determinants of mortality in chronic congestive heart failure secondary to idiopathic dilated or ischemic cardiomyopathy. Am J Cardiol 59:634, 1987.
54. Unverferth DV, Magorien RD, Moeschberger ML, et al: Factors influencing the one-year mortality of dilated cardiomyopathy. Am J Cardiol 54:147, 1984.
55. Cohn JN, Archibald DG, Ziesche S, et al: Effect of vasodilator therapy on mortality in chronic congestive heart failure: Results of a Veterans Administration Cooperative Study. N Engl J Med 314:1547, 1986.
56. Cohn JN, Johnson G, Ziesche S, et al: A comparison of enalapril with hydralazine-isosorbide dinitrate in the treatment of chronic congestive heart failure. N Engl J Med 325:303, 1991.
57. The CONSENSUS Trial Study Group: Effects of enalapril on mortality in severe congestive heart failure: Results of The Cooperative North Scandinavian Enalapril Survival Study (CONSENSUS). N Engl J Med 316:1429, 1987.
58. Keogh AM, Baron DW, Hickie JB: Prognostic guides in patients with idiopathic or ischemic dilated cardiomyopathy assessed for cardiac transplantation. Am J Cardiol 65:903, 1990.
59. Cohn JN, Levine TB, Olivari MT, et al: Plasma norepinephrine as a guide to prognosis in patients with chronic congestive heart failure. N Engl J Med 311:819, 1984.

60. Lee WH, Pacher M: Prognostic importance of serum sodium concentration and its modification by converting enzyme inhibition in patients with severe chronic heart failure. Circulation 75:257, 1986.
61. Cheng V, Kazanagra R, Garcia A, et al: A rapid bedside test for B-type peptide predicts treatment outcomes in patients admitted for decompensated heart failure: A pilot study. J Am Coll Cardiol 37: 386, 2001.
62. Stelken AM, Younis LT, Jennison SH, et al: Prognostic value of cardiopulmonary exercise testing using percent achieved of predicted peak oxygen uptake for patients with ischemic and dilated cardiomyopathy. J Am Coll Cardiol 27:345, 1996.
63. Mancini DM, Eisen H, Kussmaul W, et al: Value of peak exercise oxygen consumption for optimal timing of cardiac transplantation in ambulatory patients with heart failure. Circulation 83:778, 1991.
64. Osada N, Chaitman BR, Miller LW, et al: Cardiopulmonary exercise testing identifies low risk patients with heart failure and severely impaired exercise capacity considered for heart transplantation. J Am Coll Cardiol 33:577, 1998.
65. Guyatt GH, Sullivan MJ, Fellen EL, et al: The six minute walk: A new measure of exercise capacity in patients with chronic heart failure. Can Med Assoc J 132:919, 1985.
66. Figulla HR, Rahlf G, Nieger M, et al: Spontaneous hemodynamic improvement of stabilization and associated biopsy findings in patients with congestive cardiomyopathy. Circulation 71:1095, 1985.
67. Drexler H: Changes in the peripheral circulation in heart failure. Curr Opin Cardiol 10:268, 1995.
68. Belardinelli R, Georgiou D, Cianci G, et al: Exercise training improves left ventricular diastolic filling in patients with dilated cardiomyopathy: Clinical and prognostic implications. Circulation 91:2775, 1995.
69. Minotti JR, Massie BM: Exercise training in heart failure patients: Does reversing the peripheral abnormalities protect the heart? [editorial]. Circulation 85:2323, 1992.
70. Krum H: New and emerging pharmacologic strategies in the management of chronic heart failure [review]. Clin Cardiol 23:724, 2000.
71. McNamara DM, Holubkov R, Starling RC, et al: Controlled trial of intravenous immune globulin in recent-onset dilated cardiomyopathy. Circulation 103:2254, 2001.
72. Gullestad L, Aass H, Fjeld JG, et al: Immunomodulating therapy with intravenous immunoglobulin in patients with chronic heart failure. Circulation 103:220, 2001.
73. Dec GW, Fuster V: Idiopathic dilated cardiomyopathy. N Engl J Med 331:1564, 1994.
74. Meinertz T, Hofmann T, Kagre W, et al: Significance of ventricular arrhythmias in idiopathic dilated cardiomyopathy. Am J Cardiol 53: 902, 1984.
75. Das SK, Morady F, DiCarlo L Jr, et al: Prognostic usefulness of programmed ventricular stimulation in idiopathic dilated cardiomyopathy without symptomatic ventricular arrhythmias. Am J Cardiol 58: 998, 1986.
76. Wyse DG, Morganroth J, Hallstrom A for the CAST Investigators: Analysis of early ventricular proarrhythmias in CAST [abstract]. J Am Coll Cardiol 19:77A, 1992.
77. Doval HC, Nul DR, Grancelli HO, et al, and The GESICA Investigators: Randomized trial of low-dose amiodarone in severe congestive heart failure. Grupo de Estudio de la Sobrevida en la Insuficiencia Cardiaca. Lancet 344:493, 1994.
78. Singh SN, Fletcher RD, et al for The Survival Trial of Antiarrhythmic Therapy for Congestive Heart Failure: Amiodarone in patients with congestive heart failure and asymptomatic ventricular arrhythmia. N Engl J Med 333:77, 1995.
79. Deedwania PC, Singh BN, Ellenbogen K, et al for the Department of Veterans Affairs CHF-STAT Investigators: Spontaneous conversion and maintenance of sinus rhythm by amiodarone in patients with heart failure and atrial fibrillation: Observations for the Veterans Affairs Congestive Heart Failure Survival Trial of Antiarrhythmic Therapy (CHF-STAT). Circulation 98:2574, 1998.
80. Cannom DS: Other primary prevention trials—what is clinically and economically necessary? [review]. J Interv Card Electrophysiol 4(Suppl 1):109, 2000.
81. Grimm W, Hoffmann J, Menz V, Muller HH, Maisch B: Prediction of major arrhythmic events and sudden cardiac death in dilated cardiomyopathy: The Marburg Cardiomyopathy Study design and description of baseline clinical characteristics. Herz 25:189, 2000.
82. Saxon LA, Boehmer JP, Hummel J, et al: Biventricular pacing in patients with congestive heart failure: Two prospective randomized trials. The VIGOR CHF and VENTAK CHF Investigators. Am J Cardiol 83(5B):120D, 1999.
83. Higgins SL, Yong P, Sheck D, et al: Biventricular pacing diminishes the need for implantable cardioverter defibrillator therapy. Ventak CHF Investigators. J Am Coll Cardiol 36:824, 2000.
84. The SOLVD Investigators: Effect of enalapril on survival in patients with reduced left ventricular ejection fractions and congestive heart failure. N Engl J Med 325:293, 1991.
85. The SOLVD Investigators: Effect of enalapril on mortality and the development of heart failure in asymptomatic patients with reduced left ventricular ejection fractions [published erratum appears in N Engl J Med 327:1768, 1992]. N Engl J Med 327:685, 1992.
86. Dries DL, Domanski MJ, Waclawiw MA, Gersh BJ: Effect of antithrombotic therapy on risk of sudden coronary death in patients with congestive heart failure. Am J Cardiol 79:909, 1997.
87. Cleland JG, Alamgir F, Nikitin NP, Clark AL, Norell M: What is the optimal medical management of ischemic heart failure? Prog Cardiovasc Dis 43:433, 2001.
88. Pitt B, Segal R, Martinez FA, et al: Randomised trial of losartan versus captopril in patients over 65 with heart failure (Evaluation of Losartan in the Elderly Study, ELITE). Lancet 349(9054):747, 1997.
89. Pitt B, Poole-Wilson PA, Segal R, et al: Effect of losartan compared with captopril on mortality in patients with symptomatic heart failure: randomised trial—the Losartan Heart Failure Survival Study ELITE II. Lancet 355(9215):1582, 2000.
90. Swedberg K, Pfeffer M, Granger C, et al: Candesartan in Heart Failure—Assessment of Reduction in Mortality and morbidity (CHARM): Rationale and design. CHARM-Programme Investigators. J Card Fail 5:276, 1999.
91. Cohn JN, Tognoni G for the Val-HeFT Investigators. Effect of the angiotensin receptor blocker valsartan on morbidity and mortality in heart failure: the Valsartan Heart Failure Trial (Val-HeFT) [abstract]. Circulation 102(21):2672-b, 2000.
92. Schneider MD: Myocardial infarction as a problem of growth control: Cell cycle therapy for cardiac myocytes? In Therapies for heart failure: A glimpse into the future. Discovery International Symposium, Otsuka America Pharmaceutical, Inc. Orlando, FL, March 23, 1996.

16.2 Mechanical Circulatory Assistance

Timothy J. Myers and O. H. Frazier

The prevalence of congestive heart failure (CHF) in the United States has been estimated to exceed 4 million people.[1] As our population ages, the number of CHF cases is continuing to rise, with 400,000 new cases reported annually. CHF remains a major health concern in the United States and other industrialized nations. As with other forms of heart disease, the incidence of and mortality rate for CHF are considerably greater in men than in women.[2] The median survival time from diagnosis of class IV stage disease is 1.7 years in men and 3.2 years for women.[3] New medical and surgical therapies are continually being developed to reduce the morbidity and mortality rates associated with this disease. Medical therapy, heart transplantation, and mechanical circulatory support (MCS) all play important roles in treating CHF, yet the effectiveness of each is limited.

Medical therapy is largely supportive, in that it aims to reduce the workload of the heart but does not address the underlying pathology and malfunction. Because CHF is a progressive disease, dilated cardiomyopathy is progressive, and there is a point at which medical therapy fails to sustain adequate cardiac function. The use of heart transplantation is very limited not only because of the imbalance between the number of transplant candidates and available donor hearts, but also because of the limited life-span of the transplantable heart owing to graft, atherosclerosis, and the acute and chronic mortality rate for transplantation and immunosuppression. Moreover, it does not appear that the number of heart transplant donors will increase substantially in the future.

MCS encompasses a variety of devices that are either connected to the heart or placed within the heart to assume some degree of cardiac function. These devices range from a total artificial heart that completely replaces the natural heart with a mechanical pump to small catheter-mounted pumps that minimally augment cardiac function. The MCS systems that are used clinically or are under development have the common goals of assisting circulation to prolong the patient's life with an acceptable quality and at a cost that will be acceptable to society. It has been estimated that each year somewhere between 35,000 and 70,000 Americans benefit from some form of MCS therapy.[4]

The use of MCS systems to support CHF patients continues to gain greater acceptance. However, refinement in MCS system designs, improved patient selection criteria, and optimized supportive medical care are necessary before the use of MCS will significantly affect CHF morbidity and mortality rates. The efficacy of MCS as a bridge to heart transplantation has been well demonstrated,[5–7] and studies to evaluate the long-term use of MCS are under way.[8] As more experience is gained, the appropriate use of MCS in CHF patients continues to evolve in certain settings (e.g., in idiopathic dilated cardiomyopathy and its variant, peripartum cardiomyopathy).

Idiopathic dilated cardiomyopathy (IDC), a form of CHF, is a disease of the myocardium that is mainly characterized by left ventricular dilation with poor systolic function. Poor myocardial contractility leads to a decreased left ventricular ejection fraction and to increased left ventricular end-diastolic volume. IDC occurs in 3 to 10 persons per 100,000 population, with 20,000 new cases reported annually.[9] The mortality rate for patients with class IV disease is approximately 25% at 1 year, 40% at 2 years, and 80% at 5 years. IDC may occur at any age but is most prevalent in midlife. The etiology of IDC has not been specifically identified, but evidence suggests that genetic alteration of the immune system or viral infections may be responsible. Factors often associated with a diagnosis of IDC are alcoholism, pregnancy, and a family history of IDC. Symptoms of IDC may be very subtle, developing slowly over months to years, but some patients may experience acute symptoms. As the symptoms progress to pulmonary, systemic, and hepatic congestion, IDC patients often require intensive care with maximal medical therapy and intra-aortic balloon pump support. Spontaneous improvement in heart failure symptoms has been observed, but complete resolution of IDC is rare. Patients whose IDC is refractory to conventional medical therapy often die, but some may be fortunate enough to receive a heart transplant or MCS. MCS may function as a temporary measure before heart transplantation, or in some cases, sufficient reversal of heart failure may occur, allowing removal of the MCS device.

Peripartum cardiomyopathy is a variation of IDC that afflicts only parturient women. The pathologic features of peripartum cardiomyopathy are very similar to those of general IDC; however, the clinical course of the former may result in a worse outcome.[10] Although rare, peripartum cardiomyopathy is devastating because it has a high mortality rate and afflicts young mothers at an age when they are needed most by their families. Its incidence appears to be somewhat dependent on geographic region and is somewhere between 1:3,000 and 1:15,000 births.[11] In the United States, the peak incidence is reported to be 1:4000 births.[12] The etiology of peripartum cardiomyopathy is unknown; however, the mother's advanced age, multiparity, birthing of twins, and African descent are all risk factors. The mortality rate for peripartum cardiomyopathy can be as high as 50%, but nearly 50% of patients who have it demonstrate a significant improvement in cardiac function and have a good long-term prognosis.[13] When medical therapy fails to reverse the disease process, heart transplantation can be a viable option. However, owing to the shortage of donor hearts and the acute nature of peripartum cardiomyopathy, MCS is necessitated in some patients with this disease.

MCS use in women is reported to occur in only 16% of all patients requiring this therapy.[14] Specific studies of MCS in women are nonexistent, with the exception of anecdotal reports on the use of MCS in young women with peripartum cardiomyopathy. This chapter will describe some of the MCS systems used to support patients with IDC and, where applicable, will present specific information on the use of MCS in women.

MECHANICAL CIRCULATORY SUPPORT SYSTEMS

Over the past three decades, MCS systems have undergone extensive research and development. Like many other technologies, new MCS technology is developing rapidly in an attempt to meet an enormous demand. The ideal MCS system would be small, portable, reliable, and minimally invasive and could be used in all heart failure populations. Because this ideal system does not exist, there are a variety of MCS system designs. Currently available MCS systems are relatively large and most often are not used in children and small adults. Some MCS systems have been designed to be portable, but others remain very cumbersome. In vitro and in vivo studies have demonstrated good reliability for short-term MCS use; however, the long-term reliability over periods of years has not been tested. Some MCS systems require cardiac surgery with cardiopulmonary bypass, whereas small catheter pumps, such as the intra-aortic balloon pump (IABP), can be inserted percutaneously.

Since the total artificial heart was first used as a bridge to heart transplantation in 1969,[15] numerous MCS systems have evolved.[16] Collectively, the currently available MCS systems can be used to treat the vast majority of patients with heart failure. However, as a result of regulatory and financial barriers, the use of MCS is limited to major cardiovascular institutions, and most users do not have all types of MCS devices available. By 1999 there were four commercially available bridge-to-transplant MCS systems, and one more system is being tested under a U.S. Food and Drug Administration (FDA) Investigational Device Exemption (IDE). MCS system designs vary widely, depending on the intended clinical application. There are three MCS systems commercially available for short-term circulatory support in patients with acute heart failure. These systems are generally designed either for short-term or for long-term use. Table 16–2 summarizes the basic designs and intended uses of currently available MCS systems. The short-term MCS systems can be either implantable or extracorporeal and are most commonly used in acute heart failure. The short-term systems also tend to be smaller or are configured for use in relatively small patients. Long-term MCS systems, typically used for chronic heart failure patients, are designed to be implantable for support periods ranging from months to years. Implantable MCS devices allow for mobility and reduce the likelihood of infection that is often associated with devices incorporating percutaneous components.

Cardiomyopathy patients may develop acute decompensation, which requires prompt intervention with MCS. Others may suffer from slow progressive heart failure and may undergo MCS implantation electively prior to developing severe multisystem dysfunction. The two primary goals of MCS therapy in cardiomyopathy patients are to support circulation until sufficient cardiac recovery occurs and, in those who do not recover, to serve as a bridge to heart transplantation. Patients supported by short-term MCS systems after cardiac surgery or other acute heart failure episodes may become suitable candidates for a heart transplant during support. Short-term MCS systems are not usually the device of choice for bridge-to-heart transplant use, but numerous patients have undergone heart transplantation after being supported by these devices. In this chapter the short-term MCS systems are briefly described, followed by a more detailed description of the long-term MCS systems designed to support cardiomyopathy patients.

SHORT-TERM MECHANICAL CIRCULATORY SUPPORT SYSTEMS

Intra-aortic Balloon Pump

The intra-aortic balloon pump (IABP) was developed in the early 1960s and was first introduced clinically in 1967[17] (Fig. 16–1). The IABP continues to be the most widely used MCS system because of its relative ease of use and its longstanding acceptance. The IABP is normally easy to insert, and many medical professionals are trained to apply this device. Thus, it can be used in many hospital settings, such as the cardiac catheterization laboratory, the intensive care unit, and the operating room. In the treatment of many forms of heart failure, the IABP is usually the first MCS system applied. The IABP is most frequently used in acute heart failure situations, such as acute myocardial infarction and failure to wean from cardiopulmonary bypass. Patients who are dependent on IABP support but are otherwise in good condition may undergo heart transplantation or implantation of a long-term MCS device.

The IABP balloon catheter is normally inserted percutaneously via the femoral artery or through a sternotomy incision and is then positioned within the descending thoracic aorta. The major advantages of the IABP are that it can be inserted rapidly and that operation of the control system is relatively easy. A good-quality ECG signal is necessary for proper operation of the IABP system. The IABP provides counterpulsation support by inflating during diastole and deflating at the start of systole. Inflation of the balloon during diastole increases the coronary perfusion pressure by increasing the diastolic aortic pressure. As systole begins, the balloon deflates, lowering the resistance to left ventricular ejection. The effect of increasing coronary perfusion pressure and decreasing the left ventricular afterload improves the balance between myocardial oxygen delivery and myocardial oxygen consumption.[18] The IABP has several limitations: (1) the maximum amount of cardiac output support under optimal conditions is approximately 1.5 L/min, (2) cardiac output and rhythm must be stable, and (3) since patients are not ambulatory, the duration of IABP use must be relatively short. Despite these limitations, there are numerous heart failure patients whose status can be improved with IABP support. The IABP will continue to be in common use in the future and likely will not be replaced by newer MCS systems.

The IABP is often used to support cardiomyopathy patients during periods of acute decompensation. Maximal medical therapy plus IABP support is useful not only to sustain patients but also to optimize a patient's condition prior to MCS insertion or heart transplantation. The post–heart transplantation survival of patients supported by a pretransplant IABP is comparable to survival of patients treated medically or those supported with an MCS system.[19]

Table 16–2. MECHANICAL CIRCULATORY SUPPORT SYSTEMS

	PLACEMENT	FLOW TYPE	APPLICATION
Short-term MCS			
IABP	Intra-aortic	Pulsatile	Bridge to TX/postcardiotomy/AMI
ABIOMED BVS 5000	Extracorporeal	Pulsatile	Postcardiotomy/AMI
Centrifugal pumps	Extracorporeal	Nonpulsatile	CPB/postcardiotomy
Long-term MCS			
HeartMate IP and VE LVAS	Intra-abdominal/preperitoneal	Pulsatile	Bridge to TX/alternative to TX
Thoratec VAD	Paracorporeal	Pulsatile	Bridge to TX/postcardiotomy
Novacor VAS	Preperitoneal	Pulsatile	Bridge to TX
CardioWest TAH	Intrathoracic	Pulsatile	Bridge to TX

Abbreviations: AMI, acute myocardial infarction; CPB, cardiopulmonary bypass; IABP, intra-aortic balloon pump; IP, implanted pneumatic; LVAS, left ventricular assist system; MCS, mechanical circulatory support; TX, transplantation; VAD, ventricular assist device; VAS, ventricular assist system; VE, vented electric; TAH, total artificial heart.

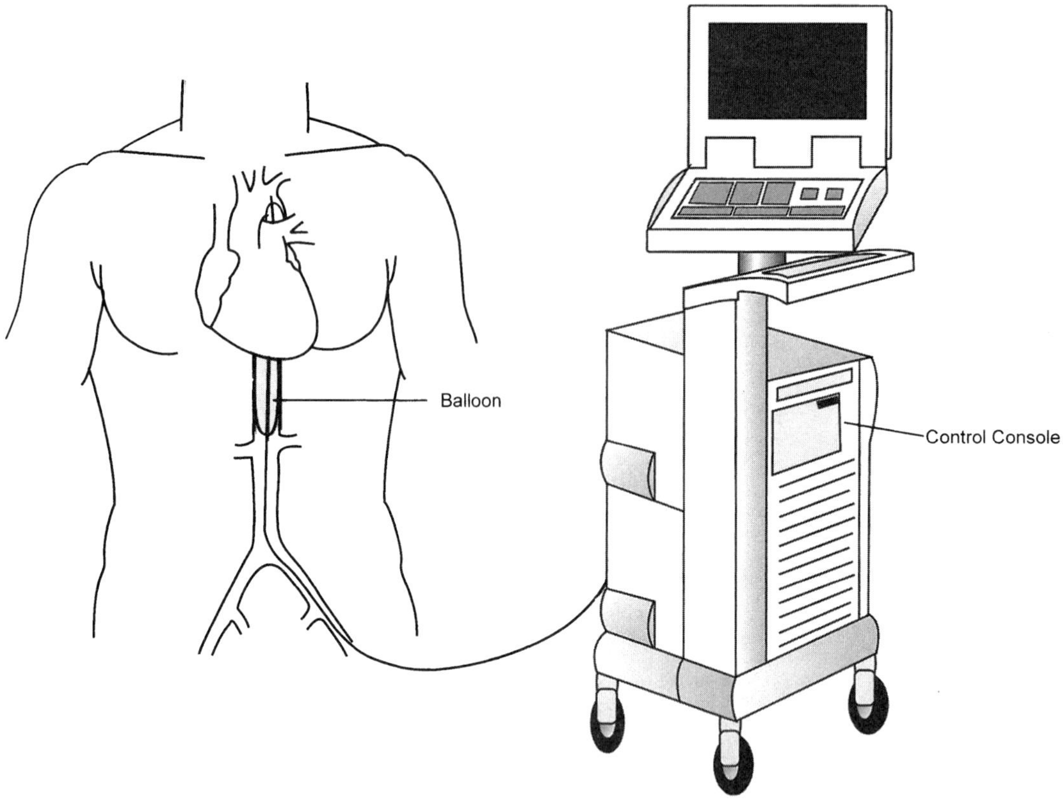

FIGURE 16–1. The intra-aortic balloon pump (IABP) external console causes inflation and deflation of the intra-aortic balloon by shuttling helium between the balloon and the console. A microprocessor within the console uses the patient's electrocardiogram to time inflation and deflation of the balloon properly. The IABP system requires a continuous source of electrical power and helium gas. (Courtesy of the Texas Heart Institute, Houston.)

Although the IABP is a useful adjunct for the treatment of heart failure, the mortality rate for IABP-supported patients is reportedly as high as 86%.[20] The IABP can support patients adequately to survive acute heart episodes; however, many patients remain in a state of severe failure and succumb to multisystem failure. In one reported case,[21] a 43-year-old women with peripartum cardiomyopathy received IABP support for 7 weeks and then was weaned from the device. Her heart failure did not resolve, and she died 3 weeks after IABP removal. In this case, because there was not complete reversal of the heart failure, heart transplantation or an MCS device providing a higher level of support might have resulted in a better outcome. Patients with marginal heart function after 1 to 2 weeks of IABP support should be considered for implantation of a long-term MCS system.

ABIOMED BVS 5000

The BVS 5000 (ABIOMED Inc., Danvers, MA) is an extracorporeal pulsatile ventricular assist system that may be used for univentricular or biventricular support (Fig. 16–2).[22] This system was designed to support patients with postcardiotomy heart failure until their native heart function recovers sufficiently to allow removal of the device. The blood pumps normally are placed at the bedside and are mounted on an intravenous pole. The gravity-filled blood pumps are kept at a constant level below the patient's chest to ensure adequate filling of the atrial chamber of the pump. The pump inflow cannulas are placed in the right or left atrium or in both if biventricular support is required. The outflow cannulas have a 14-mm Dacron graft at one end for anastomosis to the ascending aorta or the pulmonary artery. The Dacron-covered cannulas are externalized through the chest wall and connected to the blood pump tubing. A pneumatic dual-drive console provides power and control for one or two blood pumps. The BVS 5000 can provide up to 5 L/min of cardiac output support. A microprocessor within the drive console monitors the filling status of the blood pump and automatically adjusts the pumping rate to maximize cardiac output. This automated system does not require constant attention by specially trained medical personnel. The user may manually adjust the pump rate to decrease pump flows for weaning purposes.

In 1992, the BVS 5000 received commercial approval from the FDA for use as a postcardiotomy circulatory assist device. In 1996 over 500 patients supported by the BVS had been reported to a voluntary registry.[23] The majority of these patients (53%) received this support in response to postcardiotomy heart failure. Extensive experience has also been gained in Europe using the BVS to support patients as a bridge to heart transplantation. Patients who are supported by the BVS 5000 for postcardiotomy heart failure and fail to be weaned from the device may become heart transplant candidates. Patients who were bridged to heart transplant had a 40% hospital discharge rate.[23] Biventricular support was used in the majority of the cardiomyopathy cases. The major complication experienced in these patients was excessive bleeding, which is a result of the required anticoagula-

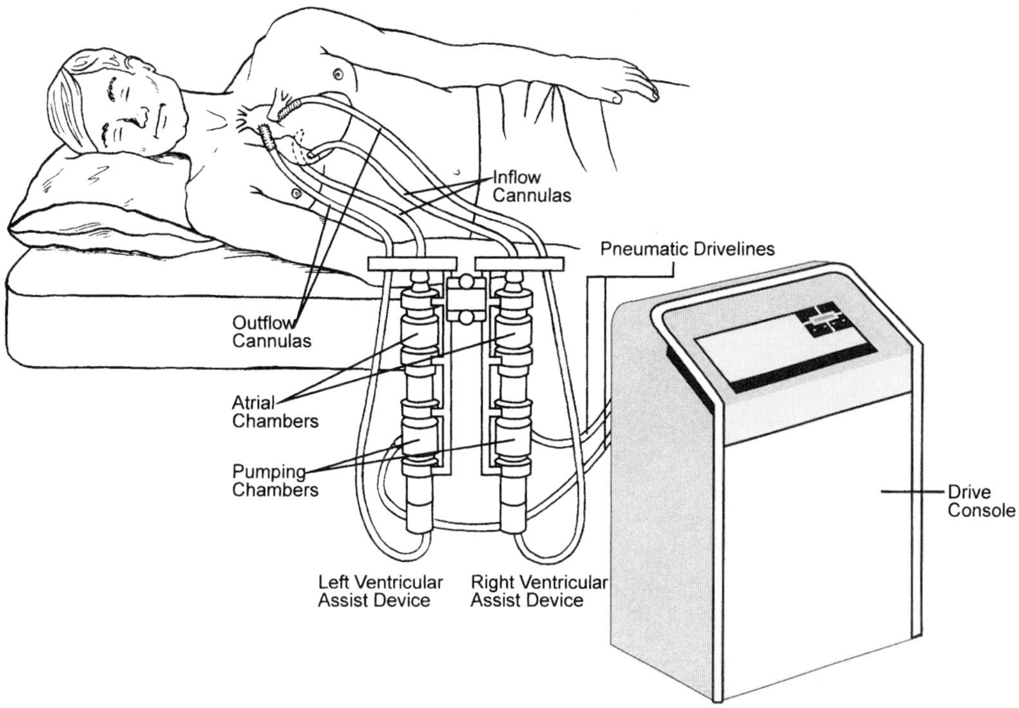

FIGURE 16–2. ABIOMED BVS 5000 blood pump(s) and console normally reside at the patient's bedside. A pneumatic driveline connects the console and blood pump or pumps. An atrial chamber in the upper portion of the blood pump serves as a reservoir for the lower ventricular chamber. Air from the console compresses the ventricular bladder, which causes ejection of blood from the pump. Two trileaflet polyurethane valves ensure unidirectional blood flow through the pump. (Courtesy of the Texas Heart Institute, Houston.)

tion therapy. An evolving use of the BVS 5000 is for right ventricular support in patients with right ventricular failure following implantation of a left ventricular assist device (LVAD).[21] Some potential advantages of the BVS 5000 over the more commonly used centrifugal pumps for right ventricular support are improved cannulation techniques and a reduced cost due to the system's ease of operation.[22] Because the blood pumps are not implantable, another potential advantage is this system's ability to be used in patients of various sizes. This system can be used to support some children and small adults. A disadvantage of the BVS 5000 is that patients must remain in bed during support, which disallows ambulation and physical rehabilitation.

The BVS 5000 requires anticoagulation therapy to prevent device-related thromboembolism. In patients with abnormal clotting, maintaining the proper balance between the control of bleeding and anticoagulation can be extremely difficult. One such case[25] was reported in a 32-year-old woman with peripartum cardiomyopathy who required BVS 5000 support. She was treated for disseminated intravascular coagulation and then received continuous heparin. She underwent heart transplantation but prior to removal of the BVS 5000 experienced systemic and cerebral embolization, which led to brain death. Careful monitoring of the patient's coagulation status and transfusion of blood products is essential for successful support. Meticulous attention to control of surgical bleeding is also critical. The external blood pumps and tubing have a fairly large surface area, which can result in excessive heat loss. The external tubing should be covered by an insulating material to help maintain body temperature.

Centrifugal Pumps

There are three types of centrifugal continuous-flow pumps that are routinely used for cardiopulmonary bypass that may be used for temporary circulatory support (Fig. 16–3) (Biomedicus, Eden Praire MN; 3M Sarns, Minneapolis, MN; and St Jude Medical, St Paul, MN). These pumps are widely available in many institutions in which cardiovascular surgery is performed, where they are often used for postcardiotomy support. These systems have been applied as a short-term bridge to heart transplantation and for right ventricular support following the implantation of an LVAD.[16, 26] Pediatric and adult-sized pumps are available, and the systems can provide up to 10 L/min of cardiac output support. Advantages of centrifugal pumps are availability, versatility with regard to use in patients of different physical sizes, ability to provide biventricular or univentricular circulatory support, and maximum flow rates of greater than 10 L/min. Proper operation of the pump requires nearly constant monitoring by trained personnel. The pump motor speed must be manually adjusted as a patient's intravascular volume changes. Cannulas are placed in either atria, in the aorta, or in the pulmonary artery. Control of surgical bleeding and appropriate blood component replacement are always necessary to avoid life-threatening blood loss. Heparin infusion is often used after the bleeding rate has slowed and weaning from the pump is attempted. Because of the likelihood of infection from the externalized cannulas, the centrifugal pumps should only be used for short-term support. Because of the externalized cannula and the cumbersome console, patients are unable to walk during support with this pump.

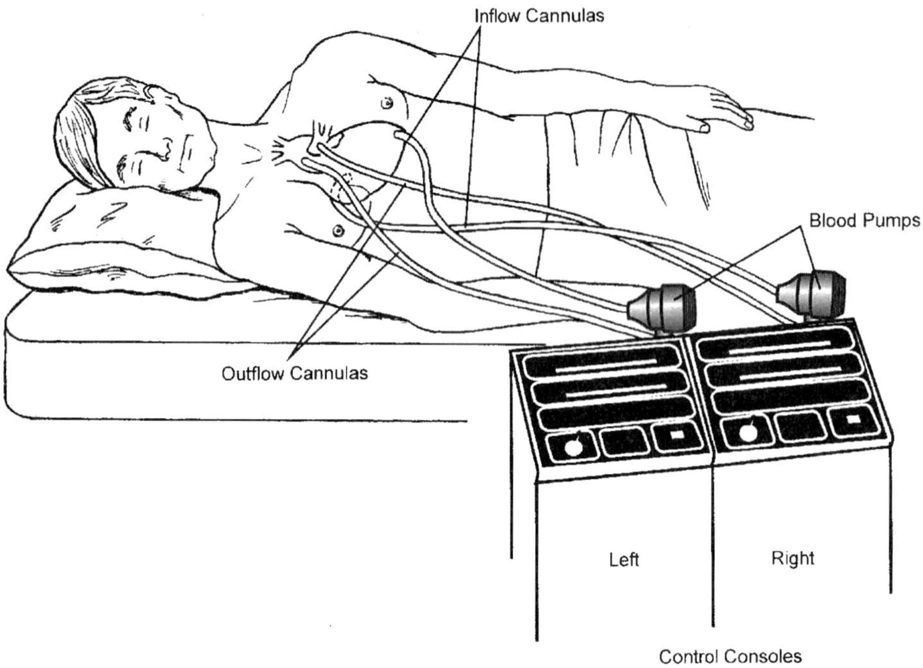

FIGURE 16–3. The centrifugal blood pump is controlled by an external drive console and is powered by a rotating magnetic motor. Externalized cannulas are connected to the pump tubing from the bedside pump or pumps. Blood is drawn into the center portion of the cone-shaped blood pump and exits the outlet on the side of the pump. (Courtesy of the Texas Heart Institute, Houston.)

Centrifugal blood pumps are incorporated into extracorporeal membrane oxygenation (ECMO)[27] or cardiopulmonary support (CPS)[28] systems. Extended cardiopulmonary support with ECMO or CPS can be complicated by excessive bleeding and thrombus formation within the pump. The centrifugal pumps are somewhat nonthrombogenic, and hemolysis is less than with conventional roller pumps. Centrifugal pump systems are compact enough to allow transport of patients within and between hospitals. The CPS system resides on a portable cart to allow implementation in various areas of the hospital.

Recent regulatory approvals of pulsatile ventricular assist device systems are making these devices more available, which is decreasing the frequency of use of centrifugal pumps. Use of centrifugal pumps for cardiopulmonary bypass, ECMO, and CPS is now standard, but their use for extended cardiac support is declining. Centrifugal pumps have not undergone controlled clinical trials to evaluate their safety and efficacy for postcardiotomy or other acute heart failure applications.

LONG-TERM MECHANICAL CIRCULATORY SUPPORT SYSTEMS

HeartMate Left Ventricular Assist Systems

The HeartMate left ventricular assist systems (LVAS) (Thermo Cardiosystems Inc., Woburn, MA) are powered either pneumatically or electrically. The Implantable Pneumatic LVAS (IP LVAS) and the Vented Electric LVAS (VE LVAS) both use an identical blood pump, but each has very different external hardware requirements. The HeartMate blood pump housing is constructed from a titanium alloy. Within this housing, a flexible polyurethane diaphragm separates the blood chamber from either an air chamber, as in the IP LVAS, or a motor chamber, as in the VE LVAS. During pump ejection, the diaphragm moves upward, causing pressurization of the blood chamber. The inflow and outflow conduits each contain 25-mm porcine xenograft valves that are sewn within a woven Dacron graft and contained in a titanium cage. The valves ensure unidirectional blood flow through the pump. With the exception of the valves, all blood-contacting surfaces in the HeartMate blood pumps are textured to allow adherence of circulating cells. Platelets, macrophages, smooth muscle cells, and endothelial cells make up a continuous tissue lining that runs throughout the pump[29, 30] and aids in preventing infection and thrombus formation within the blood pump.[31, 32]

The HeartMate blood pump is surgically placed in the upper left quadrant of the abdomen and connected to the left ventricle and aorta. The pump inflow cannula is placed in the left ventricle through a Silastic sewing ring. The outflow graft is anastomosed to the ascending aorta. The Dacron-covered driveline is externalized through the abdominal wall. The maximum stroke volume of the HeartMate blood pump is 83 ml. The IP LVAS can pump at rates up to 140 strokes per minute, which allows for a maximum flow rate of 11.6 L/min. The VE LVAS has a maximum pump rate of 120 strokes per minute and a maximum flow rate of 10 L/min. Both HeartMate systems can be operated in either an automatic mode or a fixed-rate mode. The automatic mode will continuously maximize pump output by adjusting the pump rate with variations in pump filling, which is primarily dependent on left ventricular volume. The automatic mode is typically used for the majority of the support time. In the fixed-rate mode, the operator sets a rate that remains constant regardless of pump filling. The fixed-rate mode is used whenever it is desirable to limit pump output, such as during weaning from the pump or at startup of the system.

The IP LVAS (Fig. 16–4) uses an external drive console that sends programmed pulses of air to the implanted blood pump. An interconnect cable provides the pneumatic and

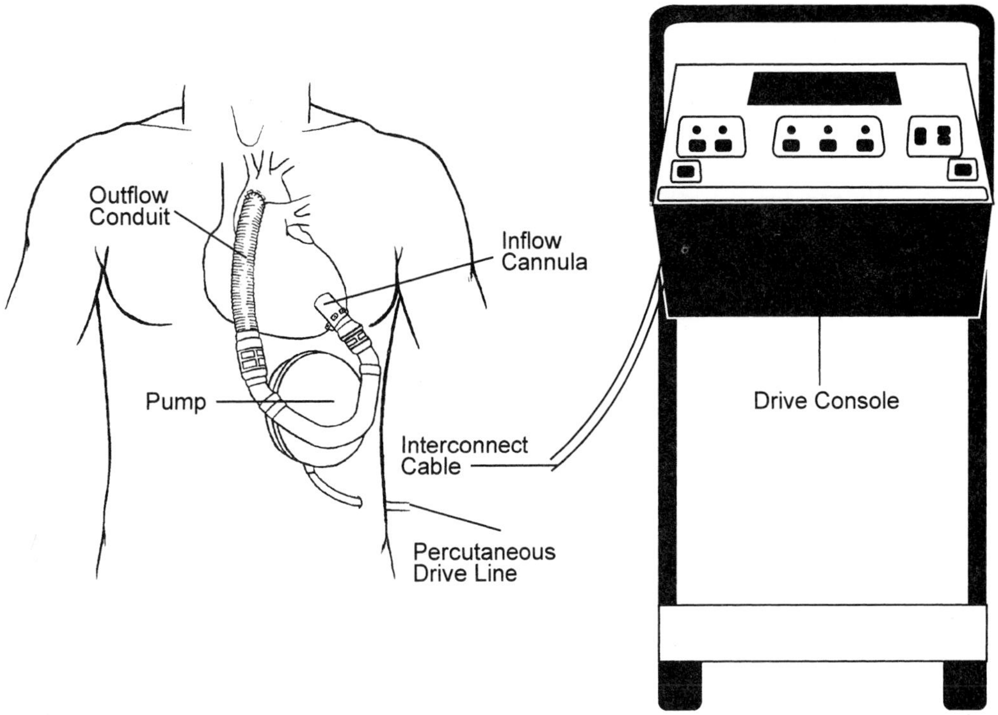

FIGURE 16–4. The HeartMate implantable pneumatic (IP) left ventricular assist system consists of the implanted blood pump, an interconnect cable, and a console. This portable system is designed for ease of use and is normally operated by ambulating patients. Use of room air and battery power allows for full mobility. (Courtesy of the Texas Heart Institute, Houston.)

electrical connection between the implanted blood pump and the drive console. A microprocessor within the drive console continuously monitors the filling status of the pump and then adjusts the pump rate accordingly. Displays on the front panel of the console give continuous readouts of the stroke volume, pump rate, and total flow. The console resides on a wheeled cart that allows for fairly easy mobility. The size and weight of the console limits patient activity; however, a small, lightweight portable drive console is undergoing clinical testing.[33]

The VE LVAS (Fig. 16–5) is actuated by an electric motor contained within the housing of the implanted blood pump. The VE LVAS is very portable because of its small external components. A microprocessor-based system controller provides continuous control and monitoring of the implanted electric motor. Visual and audible signals from the system controller alert the operator to abnormal conditions in the motor. A mode switch on the system controller allows the operator to toggle between the fixed-rate and automatic modes. A dual 12-volt DC power supply connected to the system controller provides the energy necessary to move the diaphragm and cause pump ejection. A vent is necessary to allow for proper diaphragm movement and provides a means of backup pneumatic power. In case of motor failure, the operator attaches a hand pump to manually move the diaphragm and eject blood from the pump. For ambulatory operation, a pair of conventional lead acid gel cell batteries are connected to the system controller, which is then conveniently placed in a shoulder holster or waist pouch. During periods of rest, the power supply is switched to a 20-foot cable attached to a bedside power base unit. This unit converts 120-volt AC power to 12-volt DC power, which allows for continuous operation using a wall power source. The power base unit also tests and recharges up to six batteries at a time. A small display module can be attached to the power base unit to display stroke volume, pump rate, total pump flow, and any alert messages.

From the beginning of the clinical trials in January 1996 through January 1998, nearly 1100 IP LVAS were implanted. Clinical trials to test the safety and efficacy of the IP LVAS as a bridge to heart transplantation were concluded in October 1994.[5] At the conclusion of the trials, the IP LVAS received

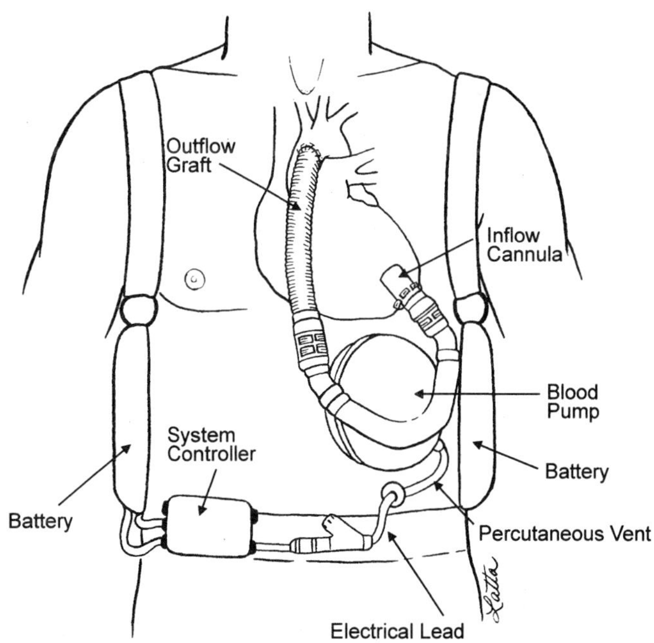

FIGURE 16–5. The HeartMate vented electric (VE) left ventricular assist system uses a system controller that is connected to either a pair of batteries or a 20-foot power cable. A table-top power base unit charges the batteries and provides an interface for pump performance monitoring. (Courtesy of the Texas Heart Institute, Houston.)

commercial approval from the FDA. One hundred eight heart transplant candidates meeting the study criteria (90 men [83.3%] and 18 women [16.7%]) were enrolled in the trials: 75 patients (64 men [85%] and 11 women [15%]) received the IP LVAS, and 33 patients were retrospective control subjects. In the total IP LVAS experience (1100 patients), 15% of the patients were women. This gender difference is somewhat inconsistent with the one seen in patients on the United Network for Organ Sharing (UNOS) transplant waiting list (Fig. 16–6) but is consistent with the one seen in a larger population of patients receiving various types of MCS.[14] A factor that may limit use of the HeartMate in women is the size of the implanted blood pump and the requirement that the patient's body surface area (BSA) be greater than 1.5 m^2.

Compared with nontreated control subjects, the IP LVAS group had better rates of survival to transplant (71% versus 36%) and post-transplant survival at 1 year (91% versus 67%). Complications observed in the IP LVAS group included bleeding, infection, renal dysfunction, and right ventricular failure. Less frequent complications were embolic events and hemolysis. One of the most important results of this study was the degree of rehabilitation noted in patients implanted with this device. Patients with end-organ dysfunction at the time of the IP LVAS implant surgery generally demonstrated subsequent significant improvement in renal, hepatic, and pulmonary function.[34] This improvement in end-organ function resulted from improved hemodynamics. The average pump flow was 42% greater than the preimplant cardiac output. Many patients supported by the IP LVAS for periods exceeding 30 days achieved a class I New York Heart Association classification by the time of heart transplantation and had a survival rate of 100% at 1 and 2 years.[35]

Clinical trials for bridge-to-transplant use of the VE LVAS were initiated in 1991[36] and were concluded in September 1998 with FDA commercial approval. There were nearly 500 implants of the VE LVAS during this period. The results of the VE LVAS clinical trials are similar to results of the IP LVAS trials except that VE LVAS implant patients were discharged to go home while they waited for a suitable heart donor. Improved hemodynamic function resulted in normalization of the patient's physical status prior to heart transplantation in nearly 70% of cases. Once patients recovered from the VE LVAS implant surgery and attained a class I NYHA classification, they were allowed to leave the hospital.[37] While away from the hospital, VE LVAS patients are expected to follow a protocol designed to monitor safety. Medical personnel are not required to continuously attend the patients but are "on call" for any emergencies. These patients have resumed a fairly normal lifestyle, which includes returning to work, traveling, and performing their usual daily activities.[38] Allowing these patients to leave the hospital while awaiting heart transplantation has a potential for tremendous cost savings.[39] These results have led investigators to evaluate the feasibility of using long-term VE LVAS support for patients who have end-stage heart failure and are not heart transplant candidates.[8] An ongoing FDA-approved study, which is partially funded by the National Institutes of Health, is a multicenter trial intended to compare 2-year mortality rates of patients treated medically with rates of patients supported by the VE LVAS.

Thoratec Ventricular Assist Device

The Thoratec ventricular assist device (VAD) system (Thoratec Laboratories Corp., Berkeley, CA) is a paracorporeal, pneumatically powered system that can provide univentricular or biventricular circulatory support (Fig. 16–7).[40] The blood pump sac and cannulas are fabricated from a polyurethane elastomer that is designed to be durable and thromboresistant.[41] The pump sac is contained within a transparent polycarbonate housing. The stroke volume is 65 ml, and the maximum pump output is 7.0 L/min. For left ventricular support, an inflow cannula is placed either into the left ventricle or the left atrium, and the outflow cannula is anastomosed to the ascending aorta. For right ventricular support, the inflow cannula is placed in the right atrium and the outflow cannula is anastomosed to the main pulmonary artery. The cannulas are externalized through the anterior chest wall and connected to the pump, which resides on the abdomen. The external drive console can power one or two pumps, depending on the need for univentricular or biventricular support. During pump ejection, the drive console sends pressurized air to the pump, causing the sac to compress the blood. During the filling phase, the console

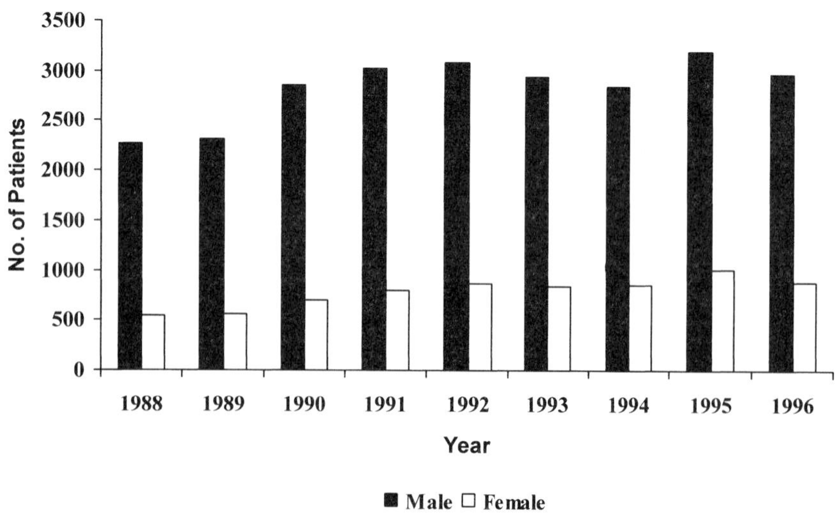

FIGURE 16–6. Number of patients, by gender and year, added to the United Network for Organ Sharing (UNOS) heart transplant waiting list.

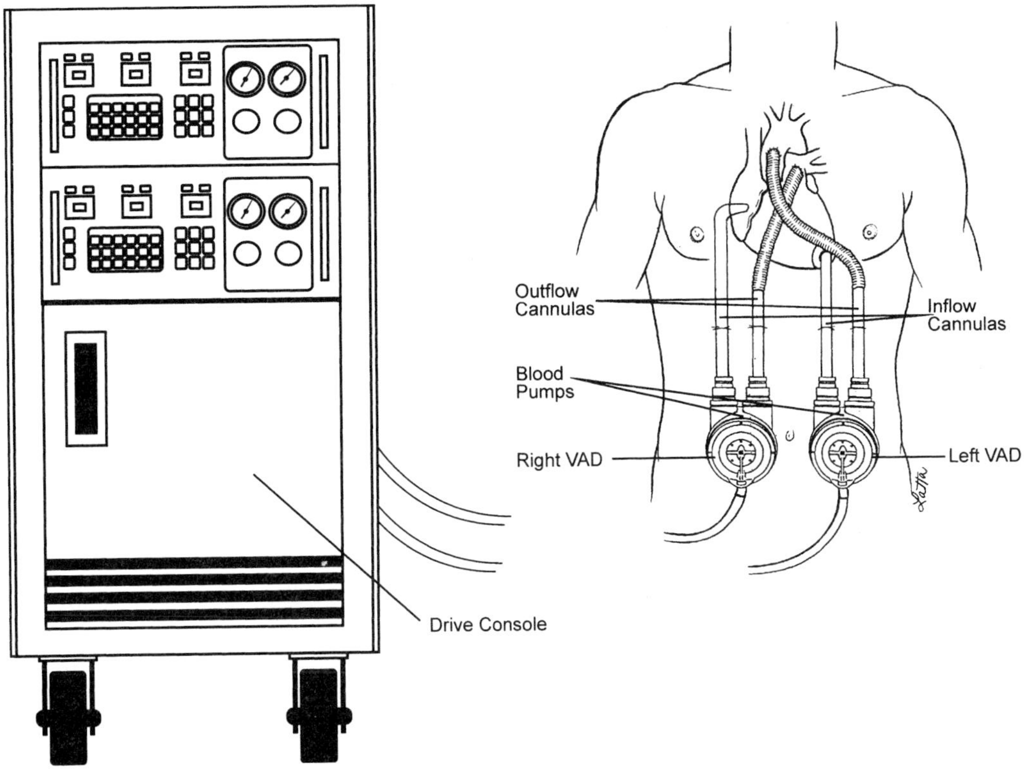

FIGURE 16–7. The Thoratec ventricular assist device (VAD) uses one or two paracorporeal blood pumps that are powered pneumatically by an external drive console. (Courtesy of the Texas Heart Institute, Houston.)

draws a vacuum around the pump sac, which aids in filling the pump with blood. Although patients can be ambulatory during support, mobility is limited by the large size of the console.

The Thoratec VAD system can be operated in one of three different modes.[42] The first is the asynchronous mode, which pumps at a rate set by the operator and is not synchronized with the patient's heart rhythm. Total pump flow in the asynchronous mode will vary, depending on the stroke volume or pump preload from the left ventricle. The second mode of operation is the volume mode, which operates on the fill-to-empty principle and results in varying pump rates depending on the filling status. More rapid filling results in a higher pump rate and maximization of the total pump flow. Finally, the synchronous mode operates based on the patient's ECG signal, which is sent to the console from the patient's bedside monitor. The synchronous mode can be used to maximize unloading of the ventricle and possibly to reduce the workload of the heart. The synchronous mode can also be used for weaning from VAD support.

Clinical trials with the Thoratec VAD began in 1976. Initially, the Thoratec VAD was used to support patients with cardiogenic shock[43]; however, its primary use has evolved as a bridge to heart transplant,[40] and it is used less often for postcardiotomy support. The FDA granted marketing approval for use of the Thoratec VAD system as a bridge to heart transplantation in 1995 and for postcardiotomy heart failure in 1997. As of June 1998, the Thoratec VAD registry reported that this system had supported 906 patients (77% men and 23% women).[44] The majority of the cases (536; 59%) involved bridge-to-heart transplantation with a 61% transplant rate and 87% post-transplant survival rate. IDC was the most common diagnosis (43%) in the patients bridged to heart transplantation. There were 151 patients (17%) supported for failure to wean from cardiopulmonary bypass; 24 (16%) of them underwent heart transplantation and 18 of those 24 (75%) survived. Of the 127 postcardiotomy failure patients, only 33 (26%) were weaned from the VAD and discharged from the hospital. The remaining 219 patients received univentricular Thoratec VAD support along with LVAD support with another type of VAD system.

The major advantage of the Thoratec VAD system is the ability to support a variety of patient sizes. The smallest patient supported by a Thoratec VAD weighed 17 kg and had a BSA of 0.73 m^2.[45] Forty-seven patients with a BSA less than 1.5 m^2 have been supported by the Thoratec VAD. The majority of these small patients were women, and the ages ranged from 7 to 73 years. This system has been used on a number of occasions to support young women with peripartum cardiomyopathy.[45, 46] The outcomes for this group of small patients is similar to those of the general MCS population.

The Thoratec VAD system is continuing to undergo refinements to expand its clinical uses. Modifications will be made to the pump housing, which will allow for implantation into preperitoneal or peritoneal spaces. The implantation of this device should optimize conditions for its longer-term use. The average length of support in the Thoratec VAD bridge-to-transplant patient group was 32 days, and the longest was over 350 days. The duration of VAD use may lengthen for Thoratec VAD patients as more evidence accumulates in support of its use for longer periods to allow improvement in end-organ function.[5, 35, 47, 48] Another related system in development is the TLC-II portable pneumatic drive unit. The TLC-II is small and lightweight and uses rechargeable batteries for extended battery operation. The TLC-II should eventually allow Thoratec VAD–supported patients to live outside the hospital while they await heart transplantation. Clinical trials to evaluate the TLC-II are ongoing in Europe and the United States. Ambulatory and out-of-hospital use of VAD systems in the transplant population is necessary to meet the financial constraints in health care and to improve the quality of life for heart failure patients.

Novacor Left Ventricular Assist System

The Novacor N100 LVAS is an electrically actuated, portable system intended for bridge-to-transplant use (Fig. 16–8).[6] Clinical trials with this system have been ongoing since 1984. The blood pump consists of a seamless polyurethane sac that is adhered to two opposing pusher-plates. Ejection of blood from the pump is achieved by electromagnetically compressing the two pusher-plates, which results in pressurization of the blood. The inflow and outflow connections are made of a Dacron graft that contains bovine pericardial valves. The blood pump is surgically placed in a preperitoneal pocket in the left upper quadrant of the abdomen. A median sternotomy and cardiopulmonary bypass are required for implantation of this LVAS. The inflow conduit is placed within the left ventricle, and the outflow is anastomosed to the ascending aorta. The externalized driveline allows for venting and provides the electrical connection to the control console. The maximum stroke volume is 70 ml, and the system can provide up to 10 L/min of cardiac output. Pumping parameters and the patient's ECG signal and blood pressure are displayed on the front panel of the drive console.

The Novacor LVAS has three modes of operation. The synchronized mode uses the patient's ECG signal to fill the pump during cardiac systole. This maximizes ventricular unloading by allowing the heart to fill the pump with minimal effort. The fill-to-empty or automatic mode functions asynchronously with the heart and maximizes output by adjusting the pump rate depending on the filling of the pump. The last mode is the fixed-rate mode, in which the operator sets a constant pumping rate that is independent of filling.

The Novacor LVAS was originally intended for short-term use; therefore, the drive console was configured for in-hospital use and weighs 150 kg. The original drive console also required frequent monitoring by medical or engineering personnel. As transplant candidates became ambulatory during LVAS support and as transplant waiting times lengthened, the Novacor LVAS was redesigned to be more portable.[49] The controller and external batteries weigh approximately 3 pounds and can be worn on a belt or contained in a shoulder bag. The batteries will allow up to 6 hours of continuous untethered operation.

Clinical trials for bridge-to-transplant application with the new wearable system began in 1993. Patients have been rehabilitated following surgery and eventually discharged from the hospital. Patients who recover from the implant surgery often recover from end-organ dysfunction. Patients leaving the hospital follow a strict protocol to monitor safety.[50] One patient who received Novacor LVAS support for 220 days spent 147 days out of the hospital without experiencing malfunction of the LVAS system components.[51] Novacor LVAS patients discharged from the hospital have demonstrated improvement in their quality of life at less cost.[52] Clinical trial results of the console and wearable versions have been very similar. Through 1994, a total of 221 patients have been supported by both LVAS versions.[49] The average duration of support was 44 days, with a maximum duration of 370 days. Sixty-one percent of supported patients have subsequently received a heart transplant and had a 92% post-transplant survival rate. Reported complications with the Novacor LVAS include bleeding, infection, and thromboembolism.[6, 53] Because the Novacor LVAS is an implantable system, fitting the device in small-statured patients may become a problem. In one case report, a small woman with peripartum cardiomyopathy was successfully supported by the Novacor LVAS despite a significant size mismatch between the pump and the patient.[54] The implantation was done even though the size problem was known preoperatively. The duration of support was relatively short in this patient, but a long duration of support may have been very difficult because of the size mismatch.

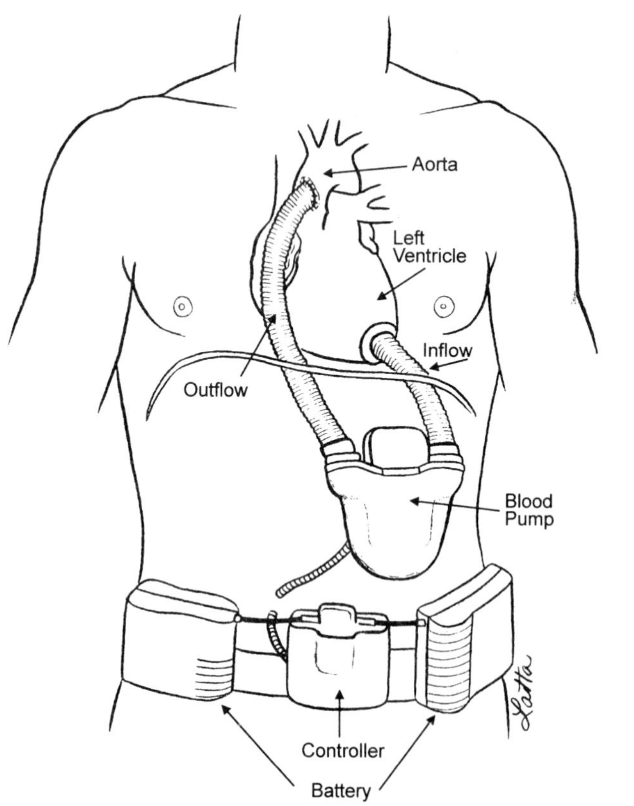

FIGURE 16–8. The Novacor N100 left ventricular assist system uses an external control unit and power supply. The small external components allow for easy mobility. (Courtesy of the Texas Heart Institute, Houston.)

CardioWest Total Artificial Heart

The CardioWest total artificial heart (TAH) is a cardiac replacement system that uses two blood pumps in place of the natural ventricles (Fig. 16–9).[55] The TAH is intended to

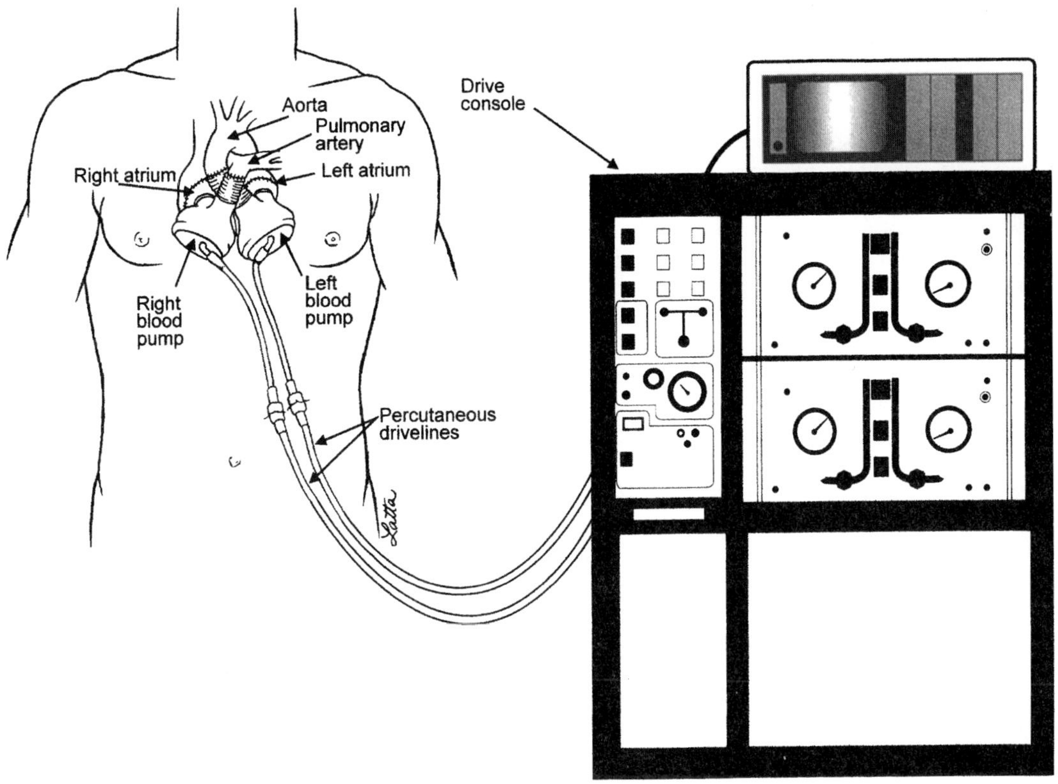

FIGURE 16–9. The CardioWest total artificial heart completely replaces both ventricles with two air-driven blood pumps. The large bedside drive console controls and monitors pump function and pneumatically powers the blood pumps. (Courtesy of the Texas Heart Institute, Houston.)

be used in patients who have biventricular heart failure and have an elevated pulmonary vascular resistance. Patients with profound right ventricular failure and a high pulmonary vascular resistance often cannot be supported by an LVAD alone. In the 1980s, the CardioWest TAH was known as the Jarvik 7 or Symbion TAH. The original clinical trials involved both bridge-to-heart transplant and permanent implantation. The clinical trials sponsored by Symbion ended in 1991 without FDA approval. The FDA suspended the clinical trials for reasons of regulatory issues. CardioWest then resumed the clinical trials in 1993 to study safety and efficacy in patients waiting for heart transplantation.

The TAH blood pumps are constructed of a rigid polyurethane housing that contains a segmented flexible polyurethane diaphragm. The diaphragm separates the blood and air chambers within the pump. During pump systole, compressed air from the drive console pressurizes the air chamber, causing the diaphragm to move upward and eject blood from the blood chamber. There are two mechanical valves within each blood pump that provide unidirectional blood flow. The maximum stroke volume of the blood pump is 70 ml and the maximum flow rate is 15 L/min. Adjusting the percentage of systole, pump rate, and driving pressure optimizes the TAH cardiac output.

The TAH is surgically placed in the mediastinal space following excision of the ventricles. Cuffs that are sewn to the right and left atria provide the blood pump inflow connections, and outflow grafts are anastamosed to the aorta and pulmonary artery. Two pneumatic drivelines are externalized through the lower anterior chest wall and are then connected to cables from the drive console. The large and cumbersome drive console limits patient activity; however, patients may be ambulatory during support. The smooth surfaces of the blood pump and the junctions with the atrial cuffs make this pump susceptible to thrombus formation. Throughout the duration of TAH support, patients receive anticoagulation therapy with a combination of heparin, warfarin, aspirin, and dipyridamole.

In the initial clinical trials, which took place from 1982 to 1991, 176 patients with end-stage heart failure were supported by this TAH.[56] Five of the 176 patients received the TAH as a permanent implant, with the longest period of support being 603 days. The successful bridge-to-transplant rate was 66%. The most significant causes of death were sepsis and multiple organ failure. This early experience demonstrated that the TAH could adequately support patients for extended periods of time. In the more recent clinical experience,[55] the successful heart transplant rate is 70%, with a hospital discharge rate of 65%. The most common complications associated with the TAH are bleeding, infection, renal failure, and thromboembolism. The overall results with the TAH have been comparable to those achieved with various VAD systems in the total MCS population.[57]

SELECTION OF MECHANICAL CIRCULATORY SUPPORT DEVICES

With regards to MCS in women, patient size is a major consideration when selecting the appropriate device to implant. The Novacor and HeartMate LVASs are implanted within the abdominal cavity or a preperitoneal pocket and are usually too large for people with a BSA of less than 1.5 m^2. The CardioWest TAH also can only be used in adults that are of average or large size, but proper fitting is limited in small patients. These three implantable MCS systems are most often used as a bridge to heart transplantation in large adult males. The Thoratec VAD is more suitable for smaller adults and large children who require extended MCS. The Thoratec VAD is a paracorporeal device that resides on the exterior anterior abdominal surface, rather than within a body cavity. The only size limitation is that due to the diameter of the required cannulas. Of all the available implantable MCS systems, the Thoratec VAD has the highest percentage of use in women and children because it is more accommodating to small patients.

The duration of MCS application is an important factor in MCS device selection. Patients who are likely to need extended MCS support are those who need extensive physical rehabilitation and those who are not likely to be matched with an appropriate heart donor. Fully implantable systems such as the HeartMate and Novacor devices are most suitable for long-term use. These two systems use fully implantable blood pumps with actuators and have one percutaneous driveline. This configuration allows for easy mobility and should minimize the risk of infection. Patients supported by the HeartMate VE LVAS and the Novacor LVAS have been supported for extended periods of time as outpatients. Patients with very long expected transplant waiting times should be supported by a HeartMate or Novacor system to allow them to wait at home. The Thoratec VAD and the CardioWest TAH have been used for long-term support while allowing patients to be fully ambulatory; however, the large drive console for these systems limits mobility. The CardioWest TAH and the HeartMate and Novacor LVASs have all been used in a small number of patients as permanent MCS support.

The ABIOMED BVS 5000 and the IABP and centrifugal systems are generally used only for short-term application because of the very limited mobility patients are allowed. In most cases, patients supported by these short-term systems must remain immobile and in bed. These short-term devices should be used in patients that are expected to experience recovery of native cardiac function within days. Although these devices have been used for many weeks, use for less than 1 week is more common.

Patients with significant right ventricular failure and who have an elevated pulmonary vascular resistance may require circulatory support with a TAH or a biventricular Thoratec VAD. Preimplant assessment of pulmonary hypertension reversal with prostaglandin E_1 or nitric oxide inhalation may be useful in assessing the need for biventricular support. Hybrid VAD systems, such as a HeartMate or Novacor for left ventricular assistance and an ABIOMED BVS or a centrifugal VAD for right ventricular assistance, are used occasionally for prolonged biventricular support. In some cases, the right ventricular assist device may be used only temporarily and left ventricular support is extended.

THE FUTURE OF MECHANICAL CIRCULATORY SUPPORT SYSTEMS

MCS systems for future clinical use are now under development in many laboratories. The newer designs are smaller and fully implantable. The smaller devices will allow their use in a wider range of patient sizes. Because of their size, the MCS systems in clinical use in the 1990s are somewhat sex- and age-biased in their designs. The MCS systems described above were all developed to primarily treat adult men, the largest population of patients with heart failure. In 1997, there were no readily available MCS systems for long-term use in pediatric or small adult patients. This bias is partly due to the marketing influence on medical product development. The market for any manufacturer developing an MCS system for small people is very limited; therefore, the return on the manufacturer's investment will likely be low or none. Future MCS systems are being designed to be anatomically suitable for many patient sizes and to have a wide range of pump-flow capabilities. Downsizing of the current MCS technology will be very difficult to accomplish. New systems will have very different mechanisms of pumping.

The next generation of blood pumps to be clinically applied is likely to be axial flow pumps. Axial flow pumps have a number of advantages over existing systems. These pumps are typically the size of a conventional D cell battery and can be placed in smaller hearts. The blood flow is continuous, which eliminates the need for valves and significantly reduces the complexity and costs. Because there is no pumping sac or diaphragm within the axial flow pumps, a compliance chamber is not required, and thus, these systems are more suitable for total implantation. Because totally implanted systems do not require percutaneous tubes, the problem of driveline infection will be eliminated. These pumps are easily implanted; the blood pump is placed into the left ventricle, and the outflow conduit is anastomosed to the aorta. The simplicity of the axial flow pump design will allow for easy operation.[58] The axial flow pumps should be durable because of the few movable parts within the blood pump; however, the longevity of bearings remains questionable. The effects of blood on the bearings in axial flow pumps is an important engineering problem that will need to be overcome before long-term applications are attempted. Early in vivo studies have demonstrated good reliability of axial flow pumps for many months.[59, 60] The future applications of axial flow pumps will be broad and will include both short- and long-term support in children and small adults.

An evolving use of MCS for the treatment of cardiomyopathy is as a bridge to recovery.[61] Prior to the modern age of heart transplantation and MCS, a treatment used for heart failure was bed rest.[62] Bed rest decreases blood pressure, heart rate, cardiac output, and cardiac size, all of which result in less work by the heart. Less work by the cardiomyopathic heart results in ventricular remodeling. MCS can achieve these same goals more efficiently and in an acceptable manner. Ventricular assist devices can unload the left ventricle to a larger degree than bed rest can, and patients can resume a normal, active lifestyle. The second patient to be supported by a HeartMate VE LVAS in 1992 demonstrated this concept.[36] The patient was a 32-year-old man who had been supported by the VE LVAS for 503 days when he suffered a stroke and eventual brain death. When the VE LVAS was turned off, his blood pressure and cardiac output remained normal until he became a liver and kidney donor 16 hours later. In the authors' recent experience, there have been three young patients with IDC who were supported by the LVAS for prolonged periods and who demonstrated a significant degree of improvement in native cardiac function. They have had the LVAS removed and continue to do well 32, 29, and 11 months later. All three patients are NYHA class I and have returned to active lifestyles without undergoing heart transplantation. It appears that patients with IDC will have at least as much improvement in native cardiac function as will those patients with ischemic disease. Identifying patients who are suitable to undergo MCS removal following myocardial recovery is a difficult challenge. Continued research is important to define patient populations, to establish methods for monitoring cardiac recovery, and to determine the most appropriate type of ventricular support.

There are a number of reasons that bridge to recovery is important for patients with IDC. Heart transplantation is an option for only a small number of candidates, and survival rates are poor for long-term allograft patients. In 1995, nearly 500 patients died while on the active heart transplant waiting list.[63] The post–heart transplant survival rate at 11 years is 36.9% in the United States and 37.1% outside this country.[64] With a less than 50% chance of survival beyond one decade, young patients with IDC may not have a good long-term outlook with transplantation. Instead, the best option for some young IDC patients may be to support them with an MCS system until heart function recovers and then to remove the MCS device, thus avoiding heart transplantation. Avoiding heart transplantation would also significantly reduce financial costs for some individual patients. Costs of the heart transplant procedure and post-transplant care can be substantial in many patients.

Cost containment in health care may be limiting the expanded use of MCS systems. As managed care contains health costs further, the need for inexpensive cardiovascular devices becomes more significant. It is difficult for manufacturers to develop inexpensive MCS systems because of the extensive research and development costs and the regulatory constraints in the manufacturing of medical devices. The next generation of MCS systems theoretically can be manufactured at a lower cost, but if research and development costs are high and managed care reduces the potential marketplace, there will be little incentive for manufacturers to market these systems. One existing MCS system has been removed from clinical trials because the manufacturer determined that the cost of manufacturing it would be greater than the potential market returns. Shorter research and development time and a more efficient regulatory process, along with less expensive system designs, will enable some MCS devices to meet the future needs. Used properly, MCS systems can help reduce the overall cost of care for some heart failure patients.

The experience gained in recent years using MCS systems for the treatment of CHF is leading to a new generation of devices that hold great promise. A single device that is durable and can be used for long and short durations in patients of various physical sizes will offer hope to many critically ill patients. A very important recent advancement is the ability of patients to live outside the hospital while being supported by MCS systems. Future patients may electively receive a device implant, return to their usual routine, and then electively remove the device. In some cases, a device may be placed during an acute episode of heart failure, and even without a return of native cardiac function, the MCS system may sustain the patient for many years with a reasonable quality of life. Acceptance of MCS systems by the general population and the medical community will depend on achieving a proper balance between survival, quality of life, and cost. With funding and expanded research and development efforts, the new MCS systems have the potential to positively affect the morbidity and mortality rates associated with heart failure.

References

1. Funk M: Epidemiology of end-stage heart disease. In Hogness JR, Van Antwerp M (eds): The Artificial Heart: Prototypes, Policies, and Patients. Appendix D. Institute of Medicine. National Academy Press, Washington, DC, 1991, pp 251–261.
2. Schocken DD, Arrieta MI, Leaverton PE, Ross EA: Prevalence and mortality rate of congestive heart failure in the United States. J Am Coll Cardiol 20:301, 1992.
3. Ho KK, Pinsky JL, Kannel WB, Levy D: The epidemiology of heart failure: The Framingham study. J Am Coll Cardiol 22(4 Suppl A): 6A, 1993.
4. Hogness JR, Van Antwerp M (eds): The Artificial Heart: Prototypes, Policies and Patients. Institute of Medicine. National Academy Press, Washington, DC, 1991, p 4.
5. Frazier OH, Rose EA, McCarthy P, et al: Improved mortality and rehabilitation of transplant candidates treated with a long-term implantable left ventricular assist system. Ann Surg 222(3):327, 1995.
6. Vetter HO, Kaulbach HG, Schmitz C, et al: Experience with the Novacor left ventricular assist system as a bridge to cardiac transplantation, including the new wearable system. J Thorac Cardiovasc Surg 109: 74, 1995.
7. Dew MA, Kormos RL, Roth LH, et al: Life quality in the era of bridging to cardiac transplantation. Bridge patients in an outpatient setting. ASAIO J 39(2):145, 1993.
8. Rose EA, Goldstein DJ: Wearable long-term mechanical support for patients with end-stage heart disease: A tenable goal. Ann Thorac Surg 61(1):399, 1996.
9. Gilbert EM, Bristow MR: Idiopathic dilated cardiomyopathy. In Schlant RC, Alexander RW (eds): The Heart, 8th ed. McGraw-Hill, New York, 1995, Chap 17, pp 191–201.
10. van Hoeven KH, Kitsis RN, Katz SD, Factor SM: Peripartum versus idiopathic dilated cardiomyopathy in young women—comparison of clinical, pathologic and prognostic features. Int J Cardiol 40(1):57, 1993.
11. Lampert MB, Lang RM: Peripartum cardiomyopathy. Am Heart J 130(4):860, 1995.
12. Ventura HO: Peripartum cardiomyopathy: Clinical and therapeutic characteristics. J La State Med Soc 143(5):45, 1991.
13. O'Connell JB, Costanzo-Nordin MR, Subramanian R, et al: Peripartum cardiomyopathy: Clinical, hemodynamic, histologic and prognostic characteristics. J Am Coll Cardiol 8(1):52, 1986.
14. Mehta SM, Aufiero TX, Pae WE, et al: Combined registry for the clinical use of mechanical ventricular assist pumps and the total artificial heart in conjunction with heart transplantation: Sixth official report. J Heart Lung Transplant 14:585, 1995.
15. Cooley DA, Liotta D, Hallman GL, et al: Orthotopic cardiac prothesis for two-staged cardiac replacement. Am J Cardiol 24:723, 1969.
16. Frazier OH, Short HD, Wampler RK, et al: Mechanical circulatory support in the transplant population. In Frazier OH (ed): Support and Replacement of the Failing Heart. Lippincott-Raven, Philadelphia, 1996, Chap 11.
17. Kantrowitz A, Tjonneland S, Freed PS, et al: Initial clinical experience with intraaortic balloon pumping in cardiogenic shock. JAMA 203(2): 113, 1968.
18. Igo SR, Hibbs CW, Trono R, et al: Intra-aortic balloon pumping: Theory and practice. Artif Organs 2:249, 1978.
19. Birovljev S, Radovancevic B, Burnett CM, et al: Heart transplantation after mechanical circulatory support: Four years' experience. J Heart Lung Transplant 11:240, 1992.
20. Creswell LL, Rosenbloom M, Cox JL, et al: Intraaortic balloon counterpulsation: Patterns of usage and outcome in cardiac surgery patients. Ann Thorac Surg 54:11, 1992.

21. Brantigan CO, Grow JB, Schoonmaker FW: Extended use of intra-aortic balloon pumping in peripartum cardiomyopathy. Ann Surg 183: 1, 1976.
22. Shook BJ: The Abiomed BVS 5000 biventricular support system; system description and clinical summary. Cardiac Surgery: State of the Art Reviews. Vol. 7, No. 2. Hanley and Belfus, Philadelphia, 1993.
23. Jett GK: ABIOMED BVS 5000: Experience and potential advantages. Ann Thorac Surg 61:301, 1996.
24. Chen JM, Levin HR, Rose EA, et al: Experience with right ventricular assist devices for perioperative right-sided circulatory failure. Ann Thorac Surg 61:305, 1996.
25. Resano FG, Goldstain SA, Boyce SW: Thromboembolic complications in a peripartum cardiomyopathy patient supported with the Abiomed BVS 5000 ventricular assist device. ASAIO J 42:240, 1996.
26. Noon GP, Ball JW, Papaconstantinou MS: Clinical experience with Biomedicus centrifugal ventricular support in 172 patients. Artif Organs 19(7):756, 1995.
27. Pesenti A, Gattinoni L, Kolobow T, Damia G: Extracorporeal circulation in adult respiratory failure. ASAIO Trans 34:43, 1988.
28. Bavin TK, Cohen SE: Bard cardiopulmonary support system. In Quaal SJ (ed): Cardiac Mechanical Assistance beyond Balloon Pumping. Mosby, St Louis, 1993, pp 144–156.
29. Dasse KA, Chapman SD, Sherman CW, et al: Clinical experience with textured blood-contacting surfaces in ventricular assist devices. ASAIO Trans 33:418, 1987.
30. Frazier OH, Baldwin RT, Eskin SG, Duncan JM: Immunochemical identification of human endothelial cells on the lining of a ventricular assist device. Tex Heart Inst J 20:78, 1993.
31. Myers TJ, McGee MG, Zeluff BJ, et al: Frequency and significance of infections in patients receiving prolonged LVAD support. ASAIO Trans 37:M283, 1991.
32. Slater JP, Rose EA, Levin HR, et al: Low thromboembolic risk without anticoagulation using advanced-design left ventricular assist devices. Ann Thorac Surg 62:1321, 1996.
33. Tamez D, Myers TJ, Inman RW, et al: Clinical evaluation of the HeartPak: A new pneumatic portable driver for use with the HeartMate implantable pneumatic left ventricular assist system. ASAIO J 43: M797, 1997.
34. Dasse KA, Frazier OH, Lesniak JM, et al: Clinical responses to ventricular assistance versus transplantation in a series of bridge to transplant patients. ASAIO J 38:M622, 1992.
35. Frazier OH, Macris MP, Myers TJ, et al: Improved survival after extended bridge to cardiac transplantation. Ann Thorac Surg 57:1416, 1994.
36. Frazier OH: First use of an untethered, vented electric left ventricular assist device for long-term support. Circulation 89:2908, 1994.
37. Myers TJ, Dasse KA, Macris MP, et al: Use of a left ventricular assist device in an outpatient setting. ASAIO J 40:M471, 1994.
38. Myers TJ, Cantanese KA, Vargo RL, Dressler DK: Extended cardiac support with a portable left ventricular assist device in the home. ASAIO J 42:M576, 1996.
39. Cloy MJ, Myers TJ, Stutts LA, et al: Hospital charges for conventional therapy versus left ventricular assist system therapy in heart transplant patients. ASAIO J 41:M535, 1995.
40. Farrar DJ, Hill D: Univentricular and biventricular Thoratec VAD support as a bridge to transplantation. Ann Thorac Surg 55:276, 1993.
41. Farrar DJ, Lawson JH, Lawson JH, et al: In vivo evaluations of a new thromboresistant polyurethane for artificial heart blood pumps. J Thorac Cardiovasc Surg 95:191, 1988.
42. Farrar DJ, Litwak P, Lawson JH, et al: Control modes of a clinical ventricular assist device. Institute of Electrical and Electronics Engineers Eng Med Biol 5:19, 1986.
43. Pae WE, Rosenberg G, Donachy JH, et al: Mechanical circulatory assistance for postoperative cardiogenic shock: A three year experience. Trans Am Soc Artif Intern Organs J 26:256, 1980.
44. Thoratec's Heartbeat Newsletter 12(2):1, June 1998.
45. Thoratec's Heartbeat Newsletter 12(3):1, September 1998.
46. Hovsepian PG, Ganzel B, Sohi GS, et al: Peripartum cardiomyopathy treated with a left ventricular assist device as a bridge to cardiac transplantation. South Med J 82(4):527, 1989.
47. Kormos RL, Murali S, Dew MA, et al: Chronic mechanical circulatory support: Rehabilitation, low morbidity, and superior survival. Ann Thorac Surg 57:51, 1994.
48. Ashton RC, Goldstein DJ, Rose EA, et al: Duration of left ventricular assist device support affects transplant survival. J Heart Lung Transplant 15:1151, 1996.
49. Miller PJ, Billich TJ, LaForger DH, et al: Initial clinical experience with a wearable controller for the Novacor left ventricular assist system. ASAIO J 40:M465, 1994.
50. Pristas JM, Winowich S, Nastala CJ, et al: Protocol for releasing Novacor left ventricular assist system patients out-of-hospital. ASAIO J 41: M539, 1995.
51. Winowich S, Nastala CJ, Pristas JM, et al: Discharging patients who are undergoing mechanical circulatory support. Ann Thorac Surg 61: 478, 1996.
52. Arabia FA, Smith RG, Jaffe C, et al: Cost analysis of the Novacor left ventricular assist system as an outpatient bridge to heart transplantation. ASAIO J 42:M546, 1996.
53. McCarthy PM, Portner PM, Tobler HG, et al: Clinical experience with the Novacor ventricular assist system. Bridge to transplantation and the transition to permanent application. J Thorac Cardiovasc Surg 102: 578, 1991.
54. Tandler R, Schmid C, Weyand M, Scheld HH: Novacor LVAD bridge to transplantation in peripartum cardiomyopathy. Eur J Cardiothorac Surg 11(2):394, 1997.
55. Copeland JG, Pavie A, Duveau D, et al: Bridge to transplantation with the CardioWest total artificial heart: The international experience 1993 to 1995. J Heart Lung Transplant 15(pt 1):94, 1996.
56. Johnson KE, Prieto M, Joyce LD, et al: Summary of the clinical use of the Symbion Total Artificial Heart: A registry report. J Heart Lung Transplant 11:103, 1992.
57. Arabia FA, Smith RG, Rose DS, et al: Success rates of long-term circulatory assist devices used currently for bridge to heart transplantation. ASAIO J 42:M542, 1996.
58. Macris MP, Myers TJ, Jarvik R, et al: In vivo evaluation of an intraventricular electric axial flow pump assist device. ASAIO J 40:M719, 1994.
59. Macris MP, Jarvik R, Parnis SM, et al: Five-month survival in a calf supported with an intraventricular axial flow pump. ASAIO J 41(1): 42, 1995.
60. Macha M, Litwak P, Yamazaki K, et al: Survival for up to six months in calves supported with an implantable axial flow ventricular assist device. Am Soc Artif Internal Organs J 43(4):311, 1997.
61. Frazier OH, Benedict CR, Radovancevic B, et al: Improved left ventricular function after chronic left ventricular unloading. Ann Thorac Surg 62:675, 1996.
62. Burch GE, DePasquale NP: On resting the human heart. Am Heart J 71:422, 1966.
63. United Network for Organ Sharing, on-line address: http//www.unos.org/frame-default.asp
64. Keck BM, Bennett LE, Fiol BS, et al: Worldwide thoracic organ transplantation: A report from the UNOS/ISHLT International Registry for Thoracic Organ Transplantation. Clin Transplant 35, 1995.

CHAPTER 17

Congestive Heart Failure

Beverly H. Lorell and Lynne W. Stevenson

WOMEN AND HEART FAILURE

Congestive heart failure continues to be a major public health challenge in the United States. National health statistics indicate that there is an annual incidence of about 400,000 new cases of heart failure per year, with a prevalence of nearly 5 million persons in the United States, of whom over half are 65 years of age or older.[1–3] The number of hospitalizations for heart failure is rising, accounting for 787,000 hospital discharges in 1991 and an estimated 1 million in 2001, more than six times the number in 1970. The increasing prevalence of heart failure and hospitalizations for heart failure may be related to both the increasing age of the population, better salvage of patients with acute myocardial infarction, and the longer survival of patients with chronic heart disease.[4] Recent epidemiologic and observational studies suggest that there are possible differences in the etiology and outcome of heart failure in women compared with men. In addition, observations based on patients participating in clinical trials as well as cardiac transplant programs raise the possibility that there may be gender-related differences in outcome in response to current therapies for heart failure. In this chapter we review current data that address these controversial issues.

EPIDEMIOLOGY OF HEART FAILURE IN WOMEN

Much of our understanding of the natural history of heart failure in the United States is derived from the initial Framingham Heart Study, which began enrollment in 1949, and the follow-up of the 5209 index subjects and their 5135 offspring.[5, 6] In this database, a diagnosis of heart failure was established by presence of two major clinical criteria (paroxysmal nocturnal dyspnea, neck vein distension, rales, radiologic cardiomegaly, acute pulmonary edema, S3 gallop, prolonged circulation time, hepatojugular reflux, pulmonary or visceral congestion, or cardiomegaly at autopsy) or one major and two minor criteria (ankle edema, nocturnal cough, exertional dyspnea, hepatomegaly, pleural effusion, reduction in vital capacity, or tachycardia). Quantitation of left ventricular ejection fraction was not performed in this database such that cases of heart failure may include patients with predominant left ventricular systolic dysfunction as well as diastolic dysfunction with preserved left ventricular ejection fraction. During the 1980s, the overall annual incidence of heart failure was 4.7/1000 women and 2.3/1000 men, whereas among people aged 45 years or older, the age-adjusted annual incidence was 4.7/1000 women and 7.2/1000 men. Among people aged 45 years or older, the prevalence of heart failure was the same in women and men: 2.5% and 2.4%, respectively.

ETIOLOGIES OF HEART FAILURE

The etiologies of heart failure in men and women enrolled in the Framingham Heart Study are somewhat different. Although hypertension and coronary artery disease were the most common causes, coronary artery disease was less common in women than in men with heart failure (48% versus 59%, respectively) and known prior infarction was less common in women with coronary artery disease than in men (57% versus 80%, respectively). Data over the past 40 years suggests that although the incidence of coronary artery disease is declining in the general population of women and men, the prevalence of coronary artery disease in subjects with heart failure is increasing in both genders. This suggests a rise in coronary heart disease as the cause of heart failure in the United States and a declining contribution of hypertension, valvular heart disease, alcoholism, and idiopathic cardiomyopathy. Valvular heart disease, with or without hypertension, accounts for 20% of heart failure cases in women and 12% in men, whereas hypertension without coronary or valvular heart disease was the attributable cause in 26% of women and 21% of men.

In the Framingham Heart Study, heart failure of unknown etiology (including idiopathic dilated cardiomyopathy) is very rare and equally common in men and women with heart failure (7%). However, in other U.S. and European databases idiopathic dilated cardiomyopathy appears to be more common in men than in women, with a prevalence of male gender of about 80%.[7–9] The explanation for the apparent lower prevalence of women in registry studies of idiopathic dilated cardiomyopathy is unknown and is not readily explained by the current paucity of information regarding autoimmune mechanisms or subtle patterns of familial inheritance. Interestingly, the Washington DC Dilated Cardiomyopathy Study,[10] which examined risk factors for development of cardiomyopathy using a neighborhood case-control method, found that idiopathic dilated cardiomyopathy was strongly associated with history of asthma, diabetes, black race, and hypertension, particularly among women younger than 50 years of age. An unexpected finding was a strong inverse association with oral contraceptive use independent of pregnancy history; the possible protective effect from oral contraceptive use (and female reproductive hormones) on the risk of developing dilated cardiomyopathy is provocative but not yet confirmed. (See Chapter 16 for more discussion of dilated cardiomyopathy.)

Diabetes independently increases the risk of heart failure in both men and women; however, the prevalence of diabetes is twofold higher in women with heart failure than in men (26% versus 14%, respectively). The excess risk of developing heart failure in diabetics appears to be present in insulin-requiring diabetics and is independent of hypertension, age, and lipid status.[11] Some studies suggest that there is an excess age-independent risk of developing heart failure in obese female diabetics, especially in the postinfarction setting.[12]

ALCOHOL AND HEART FAILURE IN WOMEN

Alcohol use and its contribution to heart failure may also differ in men and women. The Framingham Heart Study database does not directly examine alcohol as a direct etiologic or confounding variable. However, recent observations among male and female alcoholics employing quantitative measurements of muscle strength, left ventricular function, and muscle biopsies suggest that there is a greater risk of developing cardiomyopathy and skeletal myopathy among women than among men.[13] Furthermore, the threshold cumulative alcohol dose for the development of cardiomyopathy was significantly lower in women and the decline in left ventricular ejection fraction with increasing alcohol dose was significantly steeper. These findings suggest that women may be more sensitive than men to toxic effects of alcohol on the heart; in this regard, studies are needed to examine potential gender-related effects of alcohol on ventricular function as well as survival in patients with heart failure due to the more common primary causes of coronary artery disease and hypertension.

CLINICAL PRESENTATION OF HEART FAILURE

There are apparent differences in the clinical presentation of heart failure in women and men. The Framingham Heart Study database demonstrates that women are older at the time of diagnosis than men (71.9 versus 68.1 years) and that the trend over the past four decades is for both women and men to be older at the time of diagnosis of heart failure (mean age at diagnosis, 57.3 years in the 1950s and 76.4 years in the 1980s). Among patients with idiopathic dilated cardiomyopathy enrolled in a European multicenter registry, the mean age at presentation was younger than in the Framingham Heart Study database and similar in women and men (45 versus 42 years).[9] In this data set, women tended to present with more severe symptoms of heart failure, more severe left ventricular dilatation measured by echocardiography, and shorter exercise time. It is not yet clear if these differences are related to social or cultural differences in access to or seeking of medical care such that women seek attention at a later stage of the disease, or to biologic gender-related differences in the relationship between exercise hemodynamics and ventricular remodeling.

GENDER DIFFERENCES IN HYPERTROPHY AND HEART FAILURE

There are also differences in the clinical presentation and outcomes of women and men with congestive failure due to pressure overload from valvular heart disease. Among elderly patients with valvular aortic stenosis and a similar degree of outflow obstruction, women have a greater preservation of fractional shortening (ejection fraction) and generate significantly higher left ventricular pressure and cardiac index than men and are much less likely to have depressed ejection performance (18% of women versus 64% of men).[14] Although the absolute magnitude of left ventricular hypertrophy was greater in men than in women, women tended to develop a pattern of hypertrophy with concentric wall thickening with a small left ventricular cavity (low radius/wall thickness ratio) such that end-systolic wall stress was lower with better preservation of systolic shortening. Interestingly, men and women were equally symptomatic with regard to complaints of dyspnea, presyncope, and angina. These data raise the possibility that diastolic dysfunction, related to impaired filling of a small stiff left ventricular cavity, may contribute to symptoms of heart failure in women in the absence of overt depression of left ventricular systolic function. Because most patients were treated with valve replacement, this study did not address the favorable or adverse effects of this female pattern of hypertrophic remodeling on long-term morbidity and survival. However, these observations support the hypothesis that women may develop a more favorable geometric pattern of left ventricular remodeling, leading to a lower systolic wall stress and better preservation of systolic ventricular performance.[15] Observations by Aurigemma and associates in patients with pressure overload hypertrophy also support the hypothesis of gender-related differences in hypertrophic remodeling.[16] In the Treatment of Mild Hypertension Study (TOMHS), which examined echocardiographic correlates of left ventricular structure in minimally hypertensive men and women, the frequency of echocardiographically determined hypertrophy indexed by body surface area or height was significantly higher in women than in men, independent of other variables.[17]

Because the prevalence of heart failure increases during aging, a potential biologic mechanism that could contribute to differences in cardiac remodeling is gender-related differences in preservation of myocytes relative to apoptotic loss during aging itself. A morphometric study of myocytes obtained from male and female human hearts raised the hypothesis that aging in female hearts is associated with better preservation of myocyte number and structure than is seen in aging male hearts, which are characterized by greater loss of myocytes (implicitly via apoptosis) with reactive changes in volume in remaining myocytes.[18] If this hypothesis is correct, gender-related differences in preservation of myocardial cell number and structure would set the stage during the insult of chronic pressure overload for more pronounced chamber dilatation without the favorable pattern of concentric hypertrophic remodeling in men compared with women. Gender-related differences in cell loss by apoptosis during normal aging, and during pathologic heart failure, merit further study in both humans and experimental models of heart failure.

In addition, basic science studies strongly suggest that female and male animals exhibit differences in the left ventricular response to pressure overload and the transition to overt heart failure. Pfeffer and colleagues[19] reported that spontaneously hypertensive male rats developed cardiac failure evident as a decrease in left ventricular developed pressure, stroke volume, and ejection fraction earlier than age-matched female rats. More recently, our team has examined potential gender-related differences in the response to severe pressure overload from ascending aortic banding in rats. Preliminary data suggest that female banded animals exhibit more favorable hypertrophic remodeling (lower radius/wall thickness ratio)[20] in association with gender-related differences in the expression of left ventricular genes that regulate contractility and calcium homeostasis.[21] Taken together, these observations support the notion that there are gender-related differences in hypertrophic remodeling and gene expression in response to pressure overload that contribute to the development of heart failure. Because these differences in hypertrophic remodeling are observed in postmenopausal women as well as young experimental animals, it is likely that the underlying cellular mechanism is not solely related to differing trophic effects of female versus male reproductive hormones on cardiac growth.

The presentation of women and men for surgery for aortic regurgitation, a problem of predominant volume overload, also appears to differ in women and men. Klodas and coworkers[22] observed that women are twice as likely to have severe heart failure symptoms (class II to IV) preoperatively as men despite comparable depression of ejection fractions, increase in left ventricular wall stress, and increase in ventricular dimensions, normalized for body surface area. Age-adjusted late mortality was also worse in women. Thus, these data raise the possibility that the favorable "female" pattern of hypertrophic remodeling that helps to preserve ventricular ejection indices in response to *pressure* overload does not occur in response to valvular lesions causing chronic *volume* overload. No data are yet available regarding potential gender differences in ventricular remodeling and clinical manifestations of heart failure in the volume overload due to mitral regurgitation.

SURVIVAL IN WOMEN WITH HEART FAILURE

Epidemiologic Studies

The population-based Framingham Heart Study results, which are based on clinical criteria for the diagnosis of heart failure, suggest that survival is better in women than in men.[6, 23] In the Framingham Heart Study, 652 participants developed heart failure between 1948 and 1988. In the later decades of the study, subjects were older at the time of initial diagnosis of heart failure (57 years in the 1950s, 65.9 years in the 1960s, 71.6 years in the 1970s, and 76.4 years in the 1980s). The median survival after the onset of clinical heart failure was 1.7 years in men and 3.2 years in women. The overall 1-year and 5-year survival rates were 57% and 25% in men and 64% and 38% in women. As expected, mortality increased with age for both sexes; however, age-adjusted survival was better in women than in men. There was a significant gender difference in the frequency of attributable causes. Coronary heart disease was less common in women with heart failure than in men, and valvular heart disease was more frequent in women, whereas hypertension was equally common as the attributable cause of heart failure. Although heart failure attributable to unknown cause (idiopathic cardiomyopathy) or valvular disease carried a worse prognosis than heart failure due to coronary disease in men, survival in women was not distinctly affected by any of the attributable causes. Curiously, the prognosis of heart failure did not change appreciably between 1948 and 1988, although it should be noted that this time interval may not yet register the full impact of the use of angiotensin-converting enzyme (ACE) inhibitors. Within the Framingham Heart Study cohort, heart failure carries a poorer prognosis than many cancers, including breast cancer. The epidemiology of congestive heart failure was also studied by Gillum,[24] who examined data from the National Center for Health Statistics to determine the number of deaths between 1970 and 1985 whose underlying cause was coded as congestive heart failure, left ventricular failure, or heart failure. He reported that for each decade of age between ages 35 to older than 75 years, men had higher mortality rates than women.

A limitation of the Framingham Heart Study and data from the National Center for Health Statistics is that heart failure was defined by clinical symptoms and signs and left ventricular systolic function parameters (ejection fraction) were not characterized. Thus, this study cohort is likely to include patients with predominant left ventricular systolic dysfunction from ischemic and nonischemic dilated cardiomyopathies, as well as patients with preserved ejection fraction and predominant diastolic dysfunction due to hypertensive heart disease, coronary artery disease without prior infarction, or diabetic heart disease. In this regard, in a small echocardiographic study of 50 patients with clinical symptoms of heart failure, Echeverria and associates[25] identified depressed systolic performance in 72% of the men and only 40% of the women, implicating abnormalities of left ventricular diastolic relaxation and distensibility as factors underlying the clinical syndrome of heart failure in the majority of the women.

Heart Failure Registries and Clinical Trials

The conclusion that women with heart failure have a better survival than men contrasts with several earlier, and smaller, series of patients referred to heart failure units at academic centers. In contrast to the Framingham Heart Study, in which the heart failure cohort was 51% male, each of these small series was skewed toward a preponderance (70 to 75%) of male subjects. Unverferth and colleagues[26] determined prognostic indicators in 69 patients with nonischemic dilated cardiomyopathy. Although univariate analysis suggested that left ventricular ejection fraction, conduction delay, mean right atrial pressure, and ventricular arrhythmias were predictive of mortality, gender was not a prognostic risk factor. Likoff and coworkers[27] prospectively followed 201 patients with ischemic or idiopathic cardiomyopathy. A proportional hazards model identified an ischemic etiology of heart failure, left ventricular ejection fraction, and maximal oxygen uptake during exercise as independent variables that predicted mortality, but not gender. Although women may be more likely than men to develop heart failure after myocardial infarction, they do appear to have similar survival after the diagnosis of heart failure. The Worcester Heart Attack Study of 4100 patients after myocardial infarction or cardiac arrest showed equivalent long-term survival for men and women among the subgroup of patients who developed heart failure.[28] Matoba and colleagues[29] studied the prognosis of Japanese patients with new-onset heart failure and also found no difference in 1-year, 5-year, or 10-year survival between men and women.

In contrast, the Study of Left Ventricular Dysfunction (SOLVD) Registry database reported a *worse* 1-year outcome in women.[30] This registry enrolled 6273 consecutive patients over a period of 14 months who were characterized by a left ventricular ejection fraction less than 45% (79% of the subjects) or a hospital discharge diagnosis of congestive heart failure confirmed by chest roentgenographic evidence of pulmonary venous congestion (14%) or both (7%). Heart failure was mild (class I or II) in 80% of patients. This registry was also skewed toward males, who comprised 74% of the study cohort. Ischemic cardiomyopathy was the underlying cause in approximately 70% of the subjects. Consistent with other series, women were older than men (66 versus 61 years). Women had significantly higher rates of all adverse endpoints at 1 year compared with men: 22% versus 17% all-cause mortality, 12% versus 9% congestive heart failure–related death, and 22% versus 17% hospital admissions for heart failure. The apparent advantage of male gender on mortality (relative risk 0.7) may result largely from the older age of the women (67 years versus 62 years). In fact, the relative risk of mortality for patients older than 65 years was 1.48. Notably, these gender-related differences were found in white patients only; in contrast, the incidence of all-cause death or hospitalization was similar in black males and females. In the multivariate analysis, age, ejection fraction, female gender, diabetes, and atrial fibrillation (but not black versus white race) were independent predictors of mortality.

To examine the prognostic impact of gender and etiology of heart failure, Adams and associates[31] examined the short-term outcome in 380 men and 177 women with symptomatic heart failure enrolled in the University of North Carolina heart failure database. Patients were followed for an average of 2.4 years. The ejection fraction was slightly higher in women (29 ± 1%) than in men (24 ± 0.6%). In comparison with the Framingham Heart Study database, the mean age of the patients at the onset of heart failure was younger in both men and women (age 52 and 59 years, respectively). By life-table analysis, survival of women was significantly better than that of men with regard to both all-cause mortality and cardiovascular mortality. Women were also less likely to undergo urgent cardiac transplantation. Mortality was still lower in women after adjusting for baseline differences in left ventricular function. However, multivariate proportional hazards analysis suggested that the favorable association between all-cause mortality and female gender was dependent on the attributable etiology of heart failure. In men and women with coronary heart disease, the risk of death was similar. In contrast, among patients with nonischemic causes of heart failure, men had a significantly greater risk of death compared with women. In the nonischemic group, women had a significantly higher left ventricular ejection fraction, which was over 40% in some patients. The apparently better survival in these relatively young women without coronary artery disease may have reflected the inclusion of some patients with predominant diastolic dysfunction.

The most recent analysis of gender and survival was done in the Cardiac Insufficiency Bisoprolol Study (CIBIS) II trial in patients with predominantly class III heart failure (an average LVEF of 27% and average systolic blood pressure of 130 mm Hg).[32] The average age of enrolled patients was 65 years for women (n = 515) compared with 60 years for men (n = 2132). The women were found less likely to have documented ischemia and more likely to have hypertension. When adjusted for known predictors (relative risks of 0.64 for all cardiovascular deaths, 0.11 for noncardiovascular deaths, and 0.30 for pump failure), overall survival was significantly higher for women than men. This better survival for women was statistically significant for heart failure attributed to coronary artery disease, but not for patients with nonischemic heart failure. Although survival remained greater for women than for men when they were grouped by different multiple predictors of mortality, no significant interaction was found between gender and any of these predictors.

It is of interest to examine separately the outcome in patients with very advanced heart failure due to left ventricular systolic dysfunction referred for evaluation for cardiac transplantation. We analyzed the outcome of 698 patients with advanced heart failure referred for consideration of cardiac transplantation, all with an ejection fraction less than 35% (mean 20%).[33] Only 34 of the 138 women had coronary artery disease, with severity of illness and 2-year survival (considering urgent transplantation as an endpoint) of 52% equivalent to that for men with ischemic cardiomyopathy. For the 278 men and 104 women with nonischemic cardiomyopathy, mean New York Heart Association class was greater than III in both groups, and the left ventricular ejection fraction, hemodynamic parameters, magnitude of valvular regurgitation, and serum sodium level indicated equivalent severity of illness. The 2-year survival (including urgent transplantation as an endpoint) was 60% for women and 57% for men (Fig. 17–1).

Thus, review of current information regarding survival of women with heart failure shows discrepant results, some of which may be explained by differences in the populations studied. Women tend to develop heart failure at older ages but are less likely than men to have coronary artery disease and more likely to have left ventricular hypertrophy and relative preservation of left ventricular ejection fraction. The Framingham Heart Study database and the National Center for Health Statistics database, which both suggest a better survival in women, identify patients with heart failure by clinical criteria that cannot distinguish between systolic and diastolic heart failure. Age, coronary artery disease, systolic left ventricular dysfunction, and clinical severity of disease are all clear predictors of worse outcome. To assess the impact of gender on survival, each of these variables must be closely matched between cohorts of men and women with heart failure.

GENDER-RELATED DIFFERENCES IN TREATMENT OF HEART FAILURE

Angiotensin-Converting Enzyme Inhibitors

The outcome of major trials suggesting benefit of therapies for men with heart failure and the potential impact for

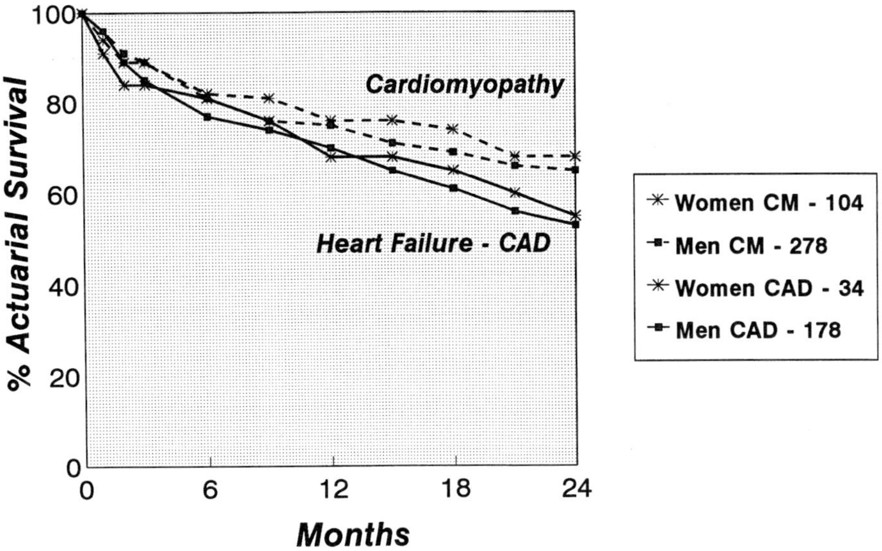

FIGURE 17–1. Actuarial survival determined for 698 patients after referral for evaluation at a cardiac transplant center.[33] All patients had a left ventricular ejection fraction ≤30% (19 ± 5%). Patient characteristics are similar between men and women, as shown in Table 17–2. Survival for women and men is equivalent when considered in terms of the presence or absence of coronary artery disease, which is a more common cause of heart failure in men. CM, cardiomyopathy; CAD, coronary artery disease.

women is summarized in Table 17–1. Further study is needed to determine if the apparent lack of benefit of some therapies reflects inadequate sample size of women, different dosing requirements, or fundamental difference in response to therapy. Determination of the contribution of gender will require control for other related variables such as age, etiology, and left ventricular function.

The major advance of the past decade in the treatment of heart failure is the use of ACE inhibitors. ACE inhibitors have been shown to improve survival in patients with left ventricular systolic dysfunction and advanced symptoms of heart failure and in patients with left ventricular systolic dysfunction and acute myocardial infarction. ACE inhibitors have also been shown to favorably modify the progression to symptomatic heart failure in asymptomatic patients with left ventricular systolic dysfunction (SOLVD). In all of these placebo-controlled randomized trials, women have comprised a minority (< 30%) of the study population. At present, the available data from these clinical trials support the use of ACE inhibitor therapy in both men and women with left ventricular systolic dysfunction who are symptomatic or asymptomatic. However, the benefits of ACE inhibitor treatment of heart failure have been less well demonstrated in women than in men. In one review, which examined the role of gender in clinical trials of ACE inhibition in heart failure, Kimmelstiel and Konstam[34] cautioned, "Some data suggest the possibility that angiotensin-converting enzyme inhibition may be less beneficial in women as compared with men. However, the small number of women and lack of direct comparison with men in these studies prevent firm interpretation of the observed data and highlights the need for greater recruitment of women into clinical heart failure trials."

In the SOLVD prevention trial, which examined the effects of enalapril on the development of heart failure in asymptomatic patients with reduced left ventricular ejection fraction, only 11% of the study patients were women, and in both the SOLVD prevention and treatment trials no data were presented regarding outcome for each gender.[35,36] Distinct from major study endpoints of mortality, the frequency of possible drug-related side effects has been reported for men and women enrolled in the SOLVD prevention and treatment trials.[37] Therapy with the ACE inhibitor enalapril causes a higher rate of side effects in women than in men, owing largely to the difference in incidence of cough, which occurred in 10% of women and 4.2% of men

Table 17–1. MAJOR TRIALS SHOWING BENEFIT OF THERAPIES FOR MEN WITH HEART FAILURE: IMPACT FOR WOMEN

	TOTAL NO.	PROPORTION OF WOMEN	NO. WOMEN	TREND IN WOMEN	IMPACT FOR WOMEN
V-HeFT I and II	642 + 804	0	0		
CONSENSUS I	253	30%	76	Less benefit	NS*
SAVE (Captopril)	2231	18%	402	Less benefit	NS*
TRACE (Trandolapril)	2606	29%	501	Less benefit	NS*
SOLVD (Enalapril)	2569	20%	514	Less benefit	NS*
DIG trial	7788	25%	1947	No benefit	Absence of benefit†
GESICA	516	20%	101	Benefit	(0.076)
Carvedilol	1094	23%	256	Benefit	Benefit
CIBIS II (Bisoprolol)	2827	18%	515	Benefit	Benefit
RALES (Spironolactone)	1663	27%	446	Benefit	Benefit

*Further study will be needed to determine if the apparent lack of benefit reflects inadequate sample size of women, different dosing requirements, or fundamental difference in response to therapy. Determination of the contribution of gender will require control for other related variables such as age, etiology, and left ventricular function.

†With the large sample sizes in the DIG trial, it can be demonstrated that the benefit of digoxin to decrease hospitalization in men was not present in women who received digitalis in this protocol.

treated with the ACE inhibitor compared with 3% of women and 1.8% of men treated with placebo. This difference in side effects may have been related to the older age of the women in the SOLVD trial data set. Patients older than age 65 years showed a 33% rate of side effects on enalapril compared with 23% for patients younger than age 56 years, with higher incidence of hypotension, cough, azotemia, and hyperkalemia.

The Cooperative North Scandinavian Enalapril Survival (CONSENSUS) trial demonstrated a significant benefit of enalapril versus placebo on survival in patients with advanced congestive heart failure.[38] Kimmelstiel and Goldberg subsequently reported outcomes in the subgroups of men and women.[39] In this trial, only 30% were women; and because of the small number of women entered into the trial, a statistically significant benefit of enalapril treatment was *not* shown in women. Men randomized to therapy with enalapril showed a 51% reduction in 6-month mortality compared with controls, whereas enalapril-treated women experienced only a 6% reduction in mortality. No data are available distinguishing the outcome of men versus women in the other long-term randomized clinical trials of ACE inhibition in symptomatic patients with advanced heart failure.

The Survival and Ventricular Enlargement (SAVE) trial studied the effect of captopril therapy on survival and morbidity in patients with left ventricular systolic dysfunction after myocardial infarction.[40] In this landmark study, only 17% of the subjects were women. Among the placebo-treated patients, the frequency of the two major endpoints was similar in males and females with regard to death from all causes (25.7% versus 20.1%, respectively) and cardiovascular death and morbidity (40.2% versus 39.7%, respectively), which suggests that men and women were at comparable risk for serious long-term adverse events, including death. Among men, death from all causes occurred in 25.7% of the placebo group and 20.6% of the captopril group, a 22% risk reduction (confidence limits 6 to 36). In contrast, among women, death from all causes occurred in 20.1% of the placebo group and 19.9% of the captopril group, a 2% risk reduction (confidence limits −53 to 37). Similarly, captopril-treated men experienced a 28% risk reduction (confidence limits 16 to 38) in the endpoint of cardiovascular death and morbidity, whereas the risk reduction was only 4% (confidence limits −32 to 30) in captopril-treated women. The study of the ACE inhibitor trandolapril in 2606 patients with left ventricular ejection fractions less than or equal to 35% after myocardial infarction (Trandolapril Cardiac Evaluation [TRACE]) showed very similar results.[41] Mortality was 26% lower in men but only 10% lower in women, a reduction that was not significant, although the group of 501 women had a placebo mortality that was slightly higher than that for men.

On the other hand, available data raise the speculation that ACE inhibition may be of comparable or greater benefit in preventing late ischemic events in female patients with low ejection fractions. A retrospective analysis of patients who were randomized to enalapril or placebo in the SOLVD treatment and prevention trials was performed to study the effects of enalapril on the development of myocardial infarction and hospitalization for unstable angina.[42] Overall, this analysis showed that enalapril treatment significantly reduced the risk of myocardial infarction, unstable angina, and cardiac mortality. Subgroup analysis of men and women enrolled in the placebo group suggested a similar frequency of myocardial infarction or hospitalization for unstable angina (28.8% versus 24.6%, respectively), whereas the reduction in risk in men and women treated with enalapril raised the possibility of comparable or greater benefit in women (risk reduction [95% confidence limits], 19% [10 to 27] versus 35% [16 to 49], respectively). A more recent trial studied the effect of the ACE inhibitor ramipril to prevent myocardial infarction, stroke, and cardiovascular death in patients without heart failure or low ejection fraction at enrollment.[43] The frequency of this endpoint was reduced from 17.8% to 14% over a 5-year period. Of the 9297 patients enrolled, women comprised 27% and demonstrated a risk reduction equivalent to that of the men.

It is unclear whether these possible gender-related differences are related solely to the small number of women patients analyzed in these trials or to possible biologic gender-related differences in the role of ACE and angiotensin in the progression of heart failure and development of late ischemic events. The lower degree of confidence regarding efficacy of ACE inhibition in women with heart failure and left ventricular systolic dysfunction underscores the need to recruit substantive numbers of women into future clinical trials to permit a direct analysis of efficacy of the intervention in women.

Newer trials addressing inhibition of the renin-angiotensin system in heart failure have included the same proportions of women but more patients overall, providing more information regarding the impact of these interventions in women. The Assessment of Treatment with Lisinopril and Survival (ATLAS) trial compared low and high doses of the ACE inhibitor lisinopril.[44] Over approximately 4 years, mortality was 44.9% in the low-dose arm and 42.5% in the high-dose arm, representing a nonsignificant 8% reduction in relative risk. The rate of death or hospitalization was reduced from 83.8% to 79.7%. The confidence interval of hazard for death in women included 1.0, while the intervals around the hazard for death or rehospitalization were less than 1, indicating similar relative benefits for men and women. The ELITE II Study (Losartan Heart Failure Survival Study) compared the ACE inhibitor captopril and the angiotensin II receptor blocker losartan.[45] Of the 3152 patients enrolled, 30% (966) were women. Captopril was found to be equivalent to or better than losartan for both men and women. In the Randomized Aldactone Evaluation Study (RALES), the aldosterone inhibitor spironolactone was added to other standard therapies, including ACE inhibitors, in 1663 patients with class IIIB or IV heart failure.[46] Women (n = 446) made up 27% of the study population, and the relative risk for death on the spironolactone regimen was approximately 0.70 for both men and women.

Beta-Adrenergic Blocking Agents

The benefit of beta-adrenergic blocking agents for patients with heart failure has been demonstrated in numerous studies.[47–49] A consistent reduction of 25% to 35% in mortality for class II–III patients has been noted, a benefit all the more remarkable for being evident over a background of

ACE inhibitor therapy. In the four trials constituting the United States carvedilol experience, women (n = 256) represented 23% of enrolled patients. In this short experience, only 14 adverse cardiac events occurred in women, but there was no evidence of any difference in benefit for men versus women.[47] The Cardiac Insufficiency Bisoprolol Study (CIBIS) trial enrolled 515 women, who demonstrated significant survival benefit from bisoprolol (Table 17–1).[32] Although multivariate analysis revealed no significant interaction between gender and treatment effect in this study, there was a trend for even greater benefit in women for most causes of death.

Inotropic Agents for Heart Failure

Inotropic agents for heart failure have generally increased mortality. The phosphodiesterase inhibitor milrinone was associated with increased risk in men and women (relative risk 1.33).[50] The positive inotropic drug vesnarinone is thought to act through multiple mechanisms including ion-channel effects as well as phosphodiesterase inhibition. Although an earlier small trial suggested a survival benefit from a moderate dose of vesnarinone, a larger trial demonstrated an increase in mortality from 18.9% to 22.9% in patients with class III or IV heart failure followed for an average of 9 months.[51] This increase in mortality was seen in both men and women.

While traditionally considered an inotropic agent, digoxin may have effects on central autonomic function that contribute to its clinical effects. In the Digitalis Investigation Group (DIG) trial, which enrolled 7788 patients (22% women),[52] digoxin had no net impact on mortality but did reduce the rate of overall hospitalization and hospitalization for worsening heart failure. Yet, despite the relatively large number of women enrolled in the study, this benefit did not extend to them.

Cardiac Transplantation in Women

Heart transplantation has been performed in over 35,000 patients, approximately 20% of whom are women.[53] This is comparable to the proportion of women of appropriate age and left ventricular systolic dysfunction who are evaluated for transplantation.[33, 54] The differences between this proportion of women and the larger proportion of women in broader heart failure populations results from the relatively older age of women at the onset of heart failure, the frequent association of heart failure in women with severe diabetes that may contraindicate transplantation, and the higher frequency of hypertrophic hypertensive diastolic dysfunction in women.

The observed proportion of women referred to transplantation does not appear to reflect a pattern of referral later in the course of disease, because the severity of clinical and hemodynamic decompensation is similar to that of men undergoing evaluation (Table 17–2). Although absolute values of peak oxygen consumption predict survival in advanced heart failure and tend to be lower in women candidates, such assessment is less useful for comparison of women to men, owing to gender-related differences in normal exercise capacity. Adjustment of measurements to "% predicted maximal values" may improve these comparisons but suffers from limited databases characterizing normal and mildly impaired exercise in women. Although overall numbers suggest equally timely referral of women and men for transplantation, there may be smaller regions where there is gender bias regarding assessment of symptoms and disease severity.

Once referred, women are as likely as men to be found acceptable for transplantation.[33, 54] When analyzing other experiences, it remains necessary to consider etiology of heart failure. The Los Angeles experience[33] demonstrated a trend to higher acceptance of patients with heart failure due to coronary artery disease regardless of gender. The likelihood of acceptance of patients with nonischemic cardiomy-

Table 17–2. GENDER, ETIOLOGY, AND COMPENSATION IN 698 PATIENTS REFERRED FOR TRANSPLANTATION

	MALE CM	FEMALE CM	MALE CAD	FEMALE CAD
No. Patients	278	104	282	34
Age	48 ± 13	44 ± 15	56 ± 9	52 ± 19
NYHA	3.4 ± 0.6	3.6 ± 0.6	3.4 ± 0.6	3.5 ± 0.7
LVEF	19 ± 5	19 ± 6	20 ± 6	20 ± 5
LVDD	76 ± 10*	72 ± 9*	75 ± 9†	70 ± 8†
LVDI	40 ± 6*	43 ± 7*	39 ± 6†	42 ± 6†
MR (0–3)	1.9 ± 0.9	2.0 ± 0.9	1.9 ± 0.8	1.8 ± 0.8
CI_i	2.1 ± 0.7	2.1 ± 0.8	2.1 ± 0.6	2.1 ± 0.5
CI_{Rx}	2.6 ± 0.6	2.7 ± 0.7	2.5 ± 0.5	2.6 ± 0.5
PCW_i	26 ± 10*	22 ± 10*	25 ± 9	23 ± 9
PCW_{Rx}	16 ± 6*	14 ± 6*	16 ± 6	15 ± 5
RAP_i	13 ± 7*	11 ± 7*	11 ± 6	11 ± 7
RAP_{Rx}	7 ± 4	7 ± 4	7 ± 4	6 ± 3
PAP_i	52 ± 15*	44 ± 16	53 ± 17*	50 ± 16
PAP_{Rx}	41 ± 12*	36 ± 12	41 ± 12*	40 ± 15
HR	94 ± 19	96 ± 19	87 ± 16	90 ± 13
Na	135 ± 5	135 ± 5	135 ± 5	136 ± 5
Vo_2 (n = 300)	14 ± 5	12 ± 3	12 ± 4	12 ± 4

*Differences ($p < .05$) between men and women with nonischemic cardiomyopathy after revision of therapy during initial evaluation.

†Differences ($p < .05$) between men and women with heart failure due to coronary artery disease.

CM, nonischemic cardiomyopathy; CAD, coronary artery disease; NYHA, New York Heart Association; LVEF, left ventricular ejection fraction; LVDD, left ventricular diastolic dimension; LVDI, left ventricular diastolic index; MR, mitral regurgitation; CI, cardiac index; i, initial reading; R_X, after therapy; PCW, pulmonary capillary wedge pressure; RAP, right atrial pressure; PAP, pulmonary artery pressure; HR, heart rate; Na, sodium; Vo_2, oxygen consumption.

opathy was the same in both groups. Once accepted, there was a trend for women with coronary artery disease to require urgent transplantation more often than men. The rate of urgent transplantation was lower, approximately 15%, for both women and men with nonischemic cardiomyopathy.

In examining trends in transplant evaluation, the distinction between "acceptable" and "accepted" becomes increasingly important, as physicians and/or patients may elect to defer transplantation until greater urgency develops. The University of Pennsylvania demonstrated that women candidates at home were more likely than men at home to decline transplantation but were slightly less likely to be considered "too well."[51]

The decision to accept transplantation involves weighing of multiple risks, both in terms of immediate versus delayed risk of death and the anticipated improvement in activity level versus immunosuppression side effects and biopsy requirements that accompany transplantation. There may be a tendency for younger women with small children to shun the up-front risk of transplantation and the logistic difficulties of child care during hospitalization and frequent clinic visits. Older women may be more likely to prefer a restricted activity level to the anticipated side effects of immunosuppression. Current information does not allow evaluation of potential differences in the way that options are presented to patients.

Survival after transplantation is comparable for men and women—approximately 85% at 1 year and 60% at 6 years.[55–57] Early information from the international database suggested lower survival for women, but more recent data indicate no difference. Women do have a shorter time to first rejection and a higher rejection rate than men. This appears to occur largely in women who have a history of previous pregnancies, which sensitize them to HLA antigens. This sensitization is often not detectable on the routine antibody screenings done before listing for transplantation. Although most programs have had experience with a multiparous patient suffering early fatal rejection unpredicted by the usual prospective donor-recipient crossmatches, these cases are rare.

Men and women enjoy comparable improvement in functional status after transplantation. The side effects of immunosuppression cause more concern in women. The facies and centripetal weight gain due to use of corticosteroids are often more intense for women early after transplantation, owing to the greater need for augmentation of dosing to prevent rejection. Many women need to use depilatories for the excess facial and body hair arising from cyclosporine use. The most debilitating side effect is osteoporosis, which is more common in postmenopausal women but can occur in any transplant recipient. Although aggressive prophylactic therapy may decrease the incidence, vertebral fracture can lead to a wheelchair-bound existence, which is more restricting than heart failure.

CONCLUSION

Multiple factors may contribute to differences between overall survival and efficacy of therapeutic interventions in men and women with heart failure. It is clear from the confusion already generated, however, that such future analyses should control for age, coronary artery disease, magnitude of left ventricular systolic dysfunction, and clinical severity of disease. As the population ages, promoting a focus on the enlarging group of heart failure patients over the age of 65 years, additional factors such as diabetes, other comorbidities, and living status (alone or with spouse partner) may need to be analyzed before concluding that there are specific differences in the biology and outcome of heart failure in women.

References

1. Garg R, Packer M, Pitt B, Yusuf S: Heart failure in the 1990s: Evolution of a major public health problem in cardiovascular medicine. J Am Coll Cardiol 22:3–5A, 1993.
2. National Heart, Lung, and Blood Institute: Report of the Task Force on Research in Heart Failure. U.S. Department of Health and Human Services, National Institutes of Health, Bethesda, MD, May 1994.
3. Shocken DD, Arrieta MI, Leaverton PE, Ross EA: Prevalence and mortality rate of congestive heart failure in the United States. J Am Coll Cardiol 20:301–306, 1992.
4. Ghali JK, Cooper R, Ford E: Trends in hospitalization rates for heart failure in the United States, 1973–1986. Arch Intern Med 150:769–773, 1990.
5. Ho KKL, Pinsky JL, Kannel WB, Levy D: Epidemiology of heart failure: The Framingham Study. J Am Coll Cardiol 22:6A–13A, 1993.
6. Ho KKL, Anderson KM, Kannel WB, et al: Survival after the onset of congestive heart failure in Framingham Heart Study subjects. Circulation 88:107–115, 1993.
7. Codd MB, Sugrue DD, Gersh BJ, Melton J: Epidemiology of idiopathic dilated and hypertrophic cardiomyopathy. Circulation 80:564–572, 1989.
8. Bagger JP, Bandruup U, Rasmussen K: Cardiomyopathy in western Denmark. Br Heart J 52:327–331, 1984.
9. DeMaria R, Gavassi A, Recalcati F, et al, on behalf of the Italian Multicenter Cardiomyopathy Study Group: Comparison of clinical findings in idiopathic dilated cardiomyopathy in women versus men. Am J Cardiol 72:580–585, 1993.
10. Coughlin SS, Teffft MC: The epidemiology of idiopathic dilated cardiomyopathy in women: The Washington DC Dilated Cardiomyopathy Study. Epidemiology 5:449–455, 1994.
11. Kannell WB, Hjortland M, Castelli WP: Role of diabetes in congestive heart failure: The Framingham Study. Am J Cardiol 68:85–89, 1991.
12. Tansey MJB, Opie LJ, Kennelly BM: High mortality in obese women diabetics with acute myocardial infarction. BMJ i:1624–1626, 1977.
13. Urbano-Marquez A, Estruch R, Fernandez-Sola J, et al: The greater risk of alcoholic cardiomyopathy and myopathy in women compared with men. JAMA 274:149–154, 1995.
14. Carroll JD, Carroll EP, Feldman T, et al: Sex-associated differences in left ventricular function in aortic stenosis of the elderly. Circulation 86: 1099–1107, 1992.
15. Buttrick P, Scheuer J: Sex-associated differences in left ventricular function in aortic stenosis of the elderly. Circulation 86:1336–1338, 1992.
16. Aurigemma GP, Silver KH, McLaughlin M, et al: Impact of chamber geometry and gender on left ventricular systolic function in patients > 60 years of age with aortic stenosis. Am J Cardiol 74:794–798, 1994.
17. Liebson PR, Grandits G, Prineas R, et al: Echocardiographic correlates of left ventricular structure among 844 mildly hypertensive men and women in the Treatment of Mild Hypertension Study. Circulation 87: 476–486, 1993.
18. Olivetti G, Giordano G, Corradi D, et al: Gender differences and aging: Effects on the human heart. J Am Coll Cardiol 26:1068–1079, 1995.
19. Pfeffer JM, Pfeffer MA, Fletcher P, et al: Favorable effects of therapy on cardiac performance in spontaneously hypertensive rats. Am J Physiol 242 (Heart Circ Physiol 11):H776–H784, 1982.
20. Katz SE, Chen MH, Weinberg EO, et al: Hypertrophic remodeling: Gender differences in response to pressure overload. (Abstract). Circulation 94:I-547, 1996.
21. Weinberg EO, Thienelt CD, Katz SE, et al: Gender differences in left ventricular gene expression in pressure overload hypertrophy. (Abstract). Circulation 94:I-187, 1996.

22. Klodas E, Enriquez-Sarano M, Tajik AJ, et al: Surgery for aortic regurgitation in women: Contrasting indications and outcomes compared with men. Circulation 94:2472–2478, 1996.
23. McKee PA, Castelli WP, McNamara PM, Kannel WB: Natural history of congestive heart failure: The Framingham Study. N Engl J Med 285:1441–1446, 1971.
24. Gillum RF: Heart failure in the United States 1970–1985. Am Heart J 113:1043–1045. 1987.
25. Echeverria HH, Bilsker MS, Myerburg RJ, Kessler KM: Congestive heart failure: Echocardiographic insights. Am J Med 75:750–755, 1983.
26. Unverferth DV, Magorien RD, Moeschberger M, et al: Factors influencing the one-year mortality of dilated cardiomyopathy. Am J Cardiol 54:147–152, 1984.
27. Likoff MJ, Chandler SL, Kay HR: Clinical determinants of mortality in chronic congestive heart failure secondary to idiopathic dilated or to ischemic cardiomyopathy. Am J Cardiol 59:634–638, 1987.
28. Goldberg RJ, Gore JM, Alpert JS, Dalen JE: Incidence and case fatality rates of acute myocardial infarction (1975–1984): The Worcester Heart Attack Study. Am Heart J 115:761–767, 1988.
29. Matoba MM, Matsui S, Hirakawa T, et al: Long-term prognosis of patients with congestive heart failure. Jpn Circ J 54:57–61, 1990.
30. Bourassa MG, Gurne O, Bangdiwala SI, for the Studies of Left Ventricular Dysfunction (SOLVD) Investigators: Natural history and patterns of current practice in heart failure. J Am Coll Cardiol 22(Suppl A):14A–19A, 1993.
31. Adams KF, Dunlap SH, Sueta CA, et al: Relation between gender, etiology and survival in patients with symptomatic heart failure. J Am Coll Cardiol 28:1781–1788, 1996.
32. Simon T, Mary-Krause M, Funck-Brentano C, Jaillon P: Sex differences in the prognosis of congestive heart failure. Circulation 103:375–380, 2001.
33. Stevenson WG, Stevenson LW, Middlekauff HR, et al: Improving survival for patients with advanced heart failure: A study of 737 consecutive patients. J Am Coll Cardiol 26:1417–1423, 1995; Stevenson LW: Personal communication, 1997.
34. Kimmelstiel CD, Konstam MA: Heart failure in women. Cardiology 86:304–309, 1995.
35. The SOLVD Investigators: Effect of enalapril on mortality and the development of heart failure in asymptomatic patients with reduced left ventricular ejection fractions. N Engl J Med 327:685–691, 1992.
36. The SOLVD Investigators: Effect of enalapril on survival in patients with reduced left ventricular ejection fractions and congestive heart failure. N Engl J Med 325:293–302, 1991.
37. Kostis JB, Shelton B, Gosselin G, et al, for the SOLVD Investigators: Adverse effects of enalapril in the Studies of Left Ventricular Dysfunction (SOLVD). Am Heart J 131:350–355, 1996.
38. Consensus Trial Study Group. Effects of enalapril on mortality in severe congestive heart failure: Results of the Cooperative North Scandinavian Survival Study. N Engl J Med 316:1429–1435, 1987.
39. Kimmelstiel C, Goldberg RJ: Congestive heart failure in women: Focus on heart failure due to coronary artery disease in diabetes. Cardiology 77(Suppl 2):71–79, 1990.
40. Pfeffer MA, Braunwald E, Moye LA, et al, on behalf of the SAVE Investigators: Effect of captopril on mortality and morbidity in patients with left ventricular dysfunction after myocardial infarction. N Engl J Med 327:669–677, 1992.
41. Kober L, Trop-Pedersen C, Carlsen JE, et al, for the Trandolapril Cardiac Evaluation (TRACE) Study Group: A clinical trial of the angiotensin-converting enzyme inhibitor trandolapril in patients with left ventricular dysfunction after myocardial infarction. N Engl J Med 333:1670–1676, 1995.
42. Yusef S, Pepine CJ, Garces C, et al: Effect of enalapril on myocardial infarction and unstable angina in patients with low ejection fractions. Lancet 340:1173–1178, 1992.
43. The Heart Outcomes Prevention Evaluation Study Investigators: Effects of an angiotensin-converting-enzyme inhibitor, ramipril, on cardiovascular events in high-risk patients. N Engl J Med 342:145–153, 2000.
44. Packer M, Poole-Wilson PA, Armstrong PW, et al: Comparative effects of low and high doses of the angiotensin converting enzyme inhibitor, lisinopril, or morbidity and mortality in chronic heart failure. Circulation 100:2312–2318, 1999.
45. Pitt B, Poole-Wilson PA, Segal R, et al: Effect of losartan compared with captopril on mortality in patients with symptomatic heart failure: Randomized trial—the Losartan Heart Failure Survival Study ELITE II. Lancet 355:1582–1587, 2000.
46. Pitt B, Zannad F, Remme WJ, et al: The effect of spironolactone on morbidity and mortality in patients with severe heart failure. N Engl J Med 341:709–717, 1999.
47. Packer M, Bristow MR, Cohn JN, et al: The effect of carvedilol on morbidity and mortality in patients with chronic heart failure. U.S. Carvedilol Heart Failure Study Group. N Engl J Med 334:1349–1355, 1996.
48. The Cardiac Insufficiency Bisoprolol Study II (CIBIS-II): A randomized trial; CIBIS investigators. Lancet 353:9–13, 1999.
49. Effect of metoprolol CR/XL in chronic heart failure: Metoprolol CR/XL Randomised Intervention Trial in Congestive Heart Failure (MERIT-HF). Lancet 353:2001–2007, 1999.
50. Packer M, Carver JR, Rodeheffer RJ, et al: Effect of oral milrinone on mortality in severe chronic heart failure. The PROMISE Study Research Group. N Engl J Med 325:1468–1475, 1991.
51. Cohn JN, Goldstein SO, Greenberg BH, et al: A dose-dependent increase in mortality with vesnarinone among patients with severe heart failure. N Engl J Med 339:1810–1816, 1998.
52. Digitalis Investigation Group: The effect of digoxin on mortality and morbidity in patients with heart failure. N Engl J Med 336:525–533, 1997.
53. Hosenpud JD, Novick RJ, Bennett LE, et al: The Registry of the International Society for Heart and Lung Transplantation: Thirteenth official report 1996. J Heart Lung Transplant 15:655–674, 1996.
54. Aaronson KD, Schwartz JS, Goin JE, Mancini DM: Sex differences in patient acceptance of cardiac transplant candidacy. Circulation 91:2752–2761, 1995.
55. Bourge RC, Naftel DC, Constanzo-Nordin MR, et al: Pretransplantation risk factors for death after heart transplantation: A multi-institutional study. J Heart Lung Transplant 12:549–562, 1993.
56. Kobashigawa JA, Kirklin JK, Naftel DC, et al: Pretransplantation risk factors for acute rejection after heart transplantation: A multi-institutional study. J Heart Lung Transplant 12:355–366, 1993.
57. Johnson MR, Naftel DC, Hobbs RE, et al, and the Cardiac Transplant Research Database Group: The incremental risk of female gender in cardiac transplantation: A multi-institutional study of peripartum cardiomyopathy and pregnancy. J Heart Lung Transplant 16:801–812, 1997.

CHAPTER
18
Hypertrophic Cardiomyopathy

Anna Woo, Grace L. Chua, E. Douglas Wigle, and Harry Rakowski

INTRODUCTION AND EPIDEMIOLOGY

Hypertrophic cardiomyopathy (HCM) is a primary cardiac disorder characterized by distinct genetic abnormalities, unique morphologic features, and a diverse clinical profile. HCM may be defined as the presence of unexplained ventricular hypertrophy, which is usually asymmetric and predominantly involves the interventricular septum.[1] The histopathologic hallmark of HCM is the finding of myocyte hypertrophy and myocyte disarray.[2–4] HCM can be associated with arrhythmias and premature death.

The early studies that described the clinical course of HCM were largely derived from data obtained at tertiary referral centers investigating highly selected patients. These studies suggested a male predominance in this disorder (Table 18–1).[3, 5–7] More recent reports also demonstrate a preponderance of male subjects in studies of HCM. A review of 78 studies published in the mid 1980s determined that 62% of the patients included in studies of HCM were male and 38% were female.[8] Studies derived from unselected outpatient populations of HCM indicate a similar male-to-female ratio, with males constituting 68% and females constituting 32% of the study cohorts.[8, 9]

Prevalence of Hypertrophic Cardiomyopathy

Studies of the epidemiology of HCM in the general population are suggestive of a lower prevalence and incidence in women. Data from a retrospective study of known cases of HCM in the general population of Olmsted County, Minnesota, showed a sex- and age-adjusted prevalence of 19.7/100,000. The age-adjusted prevalence of HCM in males was nearly twice as high as the prevalence in females (25.8/100,000 vs. 13.0/100,000, respectively).[10] Data from the Coronary Artery Risk Development in Adults (CARDIA) study, a prospective study of 4111 apparently healthy adults aged younger than 40 years from a community-based general population, provide a reasonable estimate of the frequency of HCM in a population of young adults.[11] The prevalence of HCM detected by echocardiographic examination was 0.17%. HCM was more common in men compared with women (0.26% vs. 0.09%). A recent study of 33,735 young athletes (85% male, 15% female) who underwent preparticipation medical screening in Italy detected 22 cases of HCM (0.07%). The frequency of HCM was higher in males (20/28,539, or 0.07%) than in females (2/5196, or 0.04%).[12]

In contrast, prospective studies of more selected subjects, who were identified by electrocardiographic screening or who were referred for echocardiography, have yielded different results. A study of 12,841 Japanese workers reported a prevalence of 0.17% for HCM. The prevalence of this disorder was similar in men and women. However, this study cohort consisted of an overwhelming proportion of male subjects (84%).[13] An Icelandic study reported a prevalence of 1.1% for HCM, which was identified after electrocardiographic screening or at autopsy. This study examined the prevalence of HCM only in men.[14] The prevalence of HCM in 714 consecutive patients referred for echocardiography was reported as 0.5%. There was no significant difference in the frequency of HCM between men and women.[15]

Incidence

Data from the general population in Olmsted County, Minnesota, between the years 1975 and 1984 showed a sex- and age-adjusted incidence rate of 2.5/100,000 person-years for HCM. The male age-adjusted incidence rate was 3.1/100,000 person-years, and the female age-adjusted incidence rate was 1.8/100,000 person-years.[10] The incidence rates were greater for men than for women in all age groups until age 75. In contrast, the crude annual incidence of HCM in Western Denmark from 1980 to 1981 was only 0.4/100,000 person-years. There was no significant difference in the incidence of HCM between males and females.[16]

PATHOPHYSIOLOGY

Genetics

Molecular genetic studies have permitted the identification of various molecular defects responsible for HCM, which has increased our understanding of the clinical heterogeneity of this condition. HCM can be caused by a mutation in one of the genes encoding proteins of the myofibrillar apparatus (Table 18–2).[17–21]

More than 100 individual disease-causing mutations in these genes have been identified. The majority of these genetic defects are missense mutations. HCM is transmitted

Table 18–1. MALE VERSUS FEMALE PREDOMINANCE OF HYPERTROPHIC CARDIOMYOPATHY

STUDY	NO. PATIENTS	MALES (%)	FEMALES (%)
Braunwald et al.[3]	64	43 (67)	21 (33)
Frank and Braunwald[5]	126	84 (67)	42 (33)
Adelman et al.[6]	60	38 (63)	22 (37)
Shah et al.[7]	190	114 (60)	76 (40)

Table 18–2. GENETIC CAUSES OF HYPERTROPHIC CARDIOMYOPATHY

PROTEIN	CHROMOSOMAL LOCUS
Myofilament Proteins	
β-Myosin heavy chain (β-MHC)[18, 19]	14q11.2-q12
Ventricular myosin essential light chain 1	3p21.2-p21.3
Ventricular myosin regulatory light chain 2	12q23-q24.3
Thin-Filament Proteins	
Cardiac troponin T[20]	1q3
Cardiac troponin I	19p13.2-q13.2
α-Tropomyosin	15q22
α-Cardiac actin	15q14
Myosin-Binding Protein	
Myosin-binding protein C[21]	11p11.2

as an autosomal dominant trait. The approximate incidence of mutations in these genes is represented in Figure 18–1.[22] The hypertrophy in HCM is believed to be compensatory in response to the abnormalities induced by these mutations.[17]

Molecular genetic techniques have led to the identification of patients with a delayed penetrance of HCM and patients with phenotypically silent HCM. These findings have provided insight to previous conflicting reports of differences in the gender distribution of known cases of familial HCM. Braunwald's two classic series describing the clinical course of HCM highlighted statistically significant differences in the gender of patients with the familial versus the nonfamilial forms of HCM.[3, 5] There was a higher proportion of female patients with familial HCM (52% in the first series and 45% in the second series) than with nonfamilial HCM (22% in the first series and 28% in the second series). In contrast, an M-mode and echocardiographic study of first-degree relatives from 70 families with HCM suggested that genetic transmission was more likely in males. This study identified significantly more cases of HCM in male relatives than in female relatives (26% vs. 17%).[23] These findings likely reflect the limitations of the methods of diagnosis and recognition of HCM in these studies.

Penetrance of Hypertrophic Cardiomyopathy

Genetic studies suggest that there are gender differences in the penetrance of mutations causing HCM. The HCM phenotype was detected in 62 of 90 individuals with known HCM mutations. The overall penetrance of HCM was 69%. However, the penetrance of HCM was greater in male than in female subjects (77.5% vs. 58.5%, respectively). The male-to-female odds ratio for age-adjusted penetrance was 3.98.[24]

Genetic Abnormalities and Stratification of Risk

There is increasing evidence that the overall long-term outcome of patients with HCM is related to the underlying genotype. The β-myosin heavy chain (β-MHC) mutations Arg403Gln, Arg453Cys, and Arg719Cys are associated with a high penetrance, a high incidence of sudden death, and a poor prognosis. In contrast, the β-MHC mutations Val606Met and Leu908Val are associated with a low penetrance, a low incidence of sudden death, and a more benign course.[25–27] It is surmised that mutations that involve a change in the charge of the amino acid residue, which likely cause associated conformational structural changes and functional abnormalities of the sarcomeric protein, are associated with a worsened prognosis.[28, 29] A study of individuals with six types of β-MHC mutations did not demonstrate a relationship between the underlying β-MHC missense mutation and a specific degree or pattern of hypertrophy.[30]

The manifestations of patients with cardiac troponin T mutations differ from those with β-MHC mutations. Patients

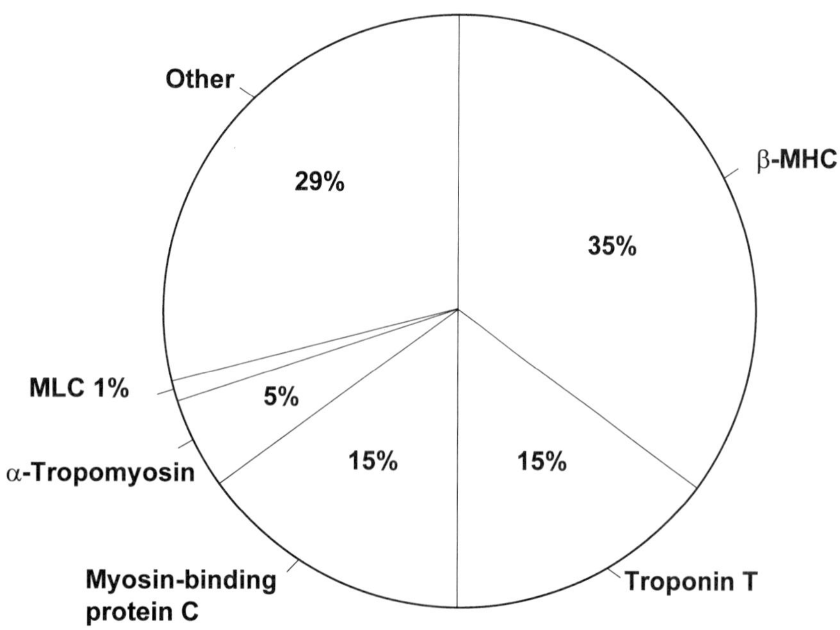

FIGURE 18–1. Estimated frequencies of mutations responsible for HCM. (MHC, myosin heavy chain; MLC, myosin light chain.)

with cardiac troponin T mutations had a lower disease penetrance, a milder degree of left ventricular (LV) hypertrophy, and a significantly higher risk of sudden death compared with patients with β-MHC missense mutations that were considered benign and not associated with an amino acid charge change.[31] In contrast, near-normal life expectancy was found in patients with the α-tropomyosin mutation Asp175Asn. Long-term survival was comparable to that of patients with the benign β-MHC mutation Val606Met.[32] Patients with mutations in the cardiac myosin-binding protein C often have delayed phenotypic expression until middle or old age. The majority of cardiac deaths in affected patients occurred suddenly. However, survival is significantly better than that observed among patients with HCM caused by other mutations in the genes for cardiac sarcomeric proteins.[33]

The angiotensin I–converting enzyme (ACE) insertion/deletion polymorphism has been shown to modify the phenotypic expression of HCM. The ACE genotype DD has been associated with a higher LV mass index, more extensive hypertrophy, and a higher rate of sudden death.[34, 35] Other modifier genes such as the endothelin-1 gene may have a significant influence on the expression of LV hypertrophy in HCM.[36]

Importantly, the associations between an unfavorable prognosis and specific genotypes are based on findings obtained from a limited number of patients, and key exceptions to the above findings have been reported.[37] This highlights the need for larger studies and the need for further identification of genetic markers for premature and sudden death. It is foreseen that the application of molecular genetic tools will enhance the ability of investigators and clinicians to optimize the diagnosis and risk stratification of patients, provide informative genetic counseling, and develop more definitive therapy.

Left Ventricular Hypertrophy

Asymmetric septal hypertrophy is the gross anatomic marker and one of the principal determinants of the manifestations of HCM (Fig. 18–2). There is considerable variation in the degree, distribution, and pattern of LV hypertrophy.[38] The factors that influence the phenotypic expression of HCM are incompletely understood but include gender, modifier genes, environmental differences, blood pressure, and acquired traits (e.g., exercise, differences in lifestyle).

Gender differences in the phenotypic expression of LV hypertrophy have been demonstrated in patients with HCM.[36] In this study, male patients had a significantly greater LV mass index and extent of hypertrophy compared with female patients. Another study that examined a unique subset of 34 patients with extreme increases in LV wall thickness, defined as a maximal thickness of at least 35 mm, showed that the majority of affected patients were male (71%).[39] These findings are contrary to the findings of a

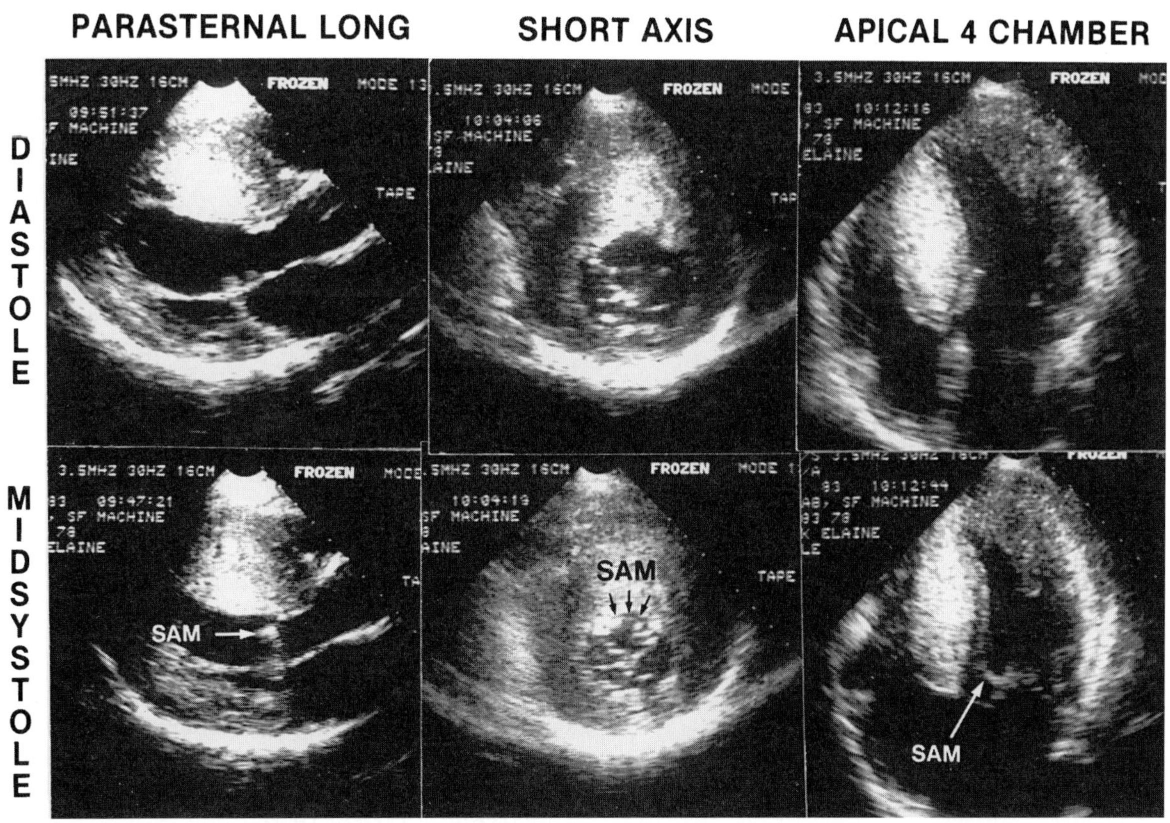

FIGURE 18–2. Diastolic and midsystolic parasternal and apical four-chamber frames from a young woman with HCM, severe asymmetric hypertrophy, and obstruction at rest. SAM of mitral apparatus involves the chordae and anterior leaflet, severely narrowing the LV outflow tract. SAM septal contact is extensive, involving much of the circumference *(short axis arrows)* of LV outflow tract. (From Rakowski H, Fulop J, Wigle ED: The role of echocardiography in the assessment of hypertrophic cardiomyopathy. Postgrad Med J 62:557–561, 1986.)

large echocardiographic study of 600 patients, which did not demonstrate differences between men and women in the maximal wall thickness, in extent of LV hypertrophy, or in the number of involved hypertrophied segments.[40]

Experimental models have provided additional insight into the nature of the gender differences in the phenotypic expression of HCM. A transgenic model of α-MHC[403/+] mice showed a milder phenotype in female compared with male mice, with less pronounced histologic and morphologic findings and a later age at onset of these abnormalities.[41] Another transgenic mice model of HCM demonstrated preservation of LV hypertrophy and systolic function in female mice, whereas there was progressive LV wall thinning, LV cavity dilatation, and reduced LV systolic function in the male mice.[42]

Studies have demonstrated that gender may modulate the development of other forms of pathologic LV hypertrophy. In a rat model of pressure overload created by banding of the ascending aorta, male but not female rats showed an early transition to heart failure, with cavity dilatation, loss of concentric remodeling, elevated wall stress, higher LV systolic pressures, and abnormal diastolic filling.[43] These gender differences have been corroborated by studies in humans, which have shown that women with aortic stenosis have a greater degree of LV hypertrophy, more concentric remodeling, and better LV function than men.[44–46]

There are multiple possible mechanisms for the influence of gender on the process of hypertrophic remodeling. Estrogen and androgen receptors have been demonstrated in the myocardium.[47, 48] Sex hormones modulate myocardial mass, myocardial function, and myosin isoenzyme and adenosine triphosphatase patterns.[49] There are gender-related differences in gene expression in the sarcomeric and structural proteins of the myocardium. Estrogen may act as a transcriptional regulator of genes implicated in LV hypertrophy, including myosin heavy-chain isoforms and extracellular matrix proteins.[50] Preliminary data suggest that there are gender differences in the upregulation of β-MHC messenger RNA levels in a rat model of pressure overload.[51] In addition, estrogen may induce changes in hypertrophic remodeling via its effects on the renin-angiotensin system.[52, 53]

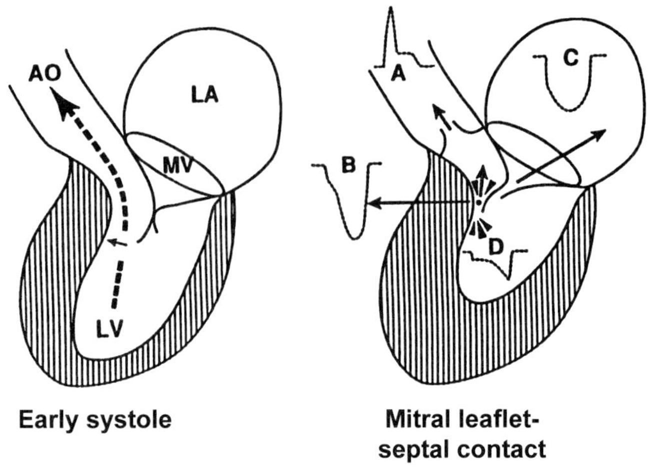

FIGURE 18–3. Diagram of pathophysiology of the obstruction to outflow and mitral regurgitation in subaortic obstructive HCM. Early systole *(left)*: The left ventricular outflow tract is narrowed by septal hypertrophy, anterior displacement of the papillary muscles, and the mitral leaflets. The point of coaptation of the elongated mitral leaflets occurs in the body of the leaflets. The portion of the anterior leaflet beyond the coaptation point is carried anteriorly and superiorly (SAM) by Venturi and/or drag forces and results in mitral leaflet–septal contact, causing the subaortic obstruction (indicated by converging and diverging lines, right). Mitral leaflet–septal contact *(right)*: The SAM of the anterior leaflet results in malcoaptation of the mitral leaflets and the onset of mitral regurgitation, which is directed posteriorly into the left atrium, through the inter-leaflet gap. A, B, C, and D indicate Doppler velocity recordings throughout systole in the ascending aorta (A), at the level of mitral leaflet-septal contact (B), in the left atrium (C), and near the LV apex (D). (From Wigle ED, Rakowski H, Kimball BP, Williams WG: Hypertrophic cardiomyopathy: Clinical spectrum and treatment. Circulation 92:1680–1692, 1995.)

Left Ventricular Outflow Tract Obstruction

HCM may be classified according to its hemodynamic features (Table 18–3).[54]

Subaortic (or LV outflow tract) obstruction is far more common than midventricular or right ventricular outflow tract obstruction. The morphologic factors that contribute to the development of subaortic obstruction include narrowing of the LV outflow tract, caused by ventricular septal hypertrophy, anterior displacement of the papillary muscles, and the anterior position of the elongated mitral leaflets, which coapt abnormally in the body of the leaflets.[55, 56] Therefore, the anterior mitral leaflet distal to the coaptation point is subjected to Venturi and/or drag forces,[57] resulting in systolic anterior motion (SAM) with subsequent mitral leaflet-septal contact and the production of subaortic obstruction. The concomitant mitral regurgitation seems to be related both to the degree of SAM of the anterior leaflet and to the length and mobility of the posterior leaflet,[58] which determine the size of the interleaflet gap and the degree of midsystolic malcoaptation of the mitral leaflets (Fig. 18–3).

One study showed that there was no difference in the distribution of gender in HCM patients with and without SAM.[57] This finding was supported by a study of 149 consecutive HCM patients, consisting of 84 men and 65 women, referred for cardiac catheterization.[59] This study showed no gender differences either in the prevalence of LV obstruction or in left- and right-sided intracavitary pressures.

Table 18–3. HEMODYNAMIC CLASSIFICATION OF HYPERTROPHIC CARDIOMYOPATHY

I. Obstructive HCM
  A. Subaortic obstruction
    1. Resting obstruction
    2. Latent obstruction
  B. Midventricular obstruction
  C. Right ventricular outflow tract obstruction
II. Nonobstructive HCM
  A. Normal systolic function
  B. Impaired systolic function (end-stage HCM)

Diastolic Dysfunction

Studies of LV diastolic function have identified abnormalities in relaxation, compliance, and filling in the majority of pa-

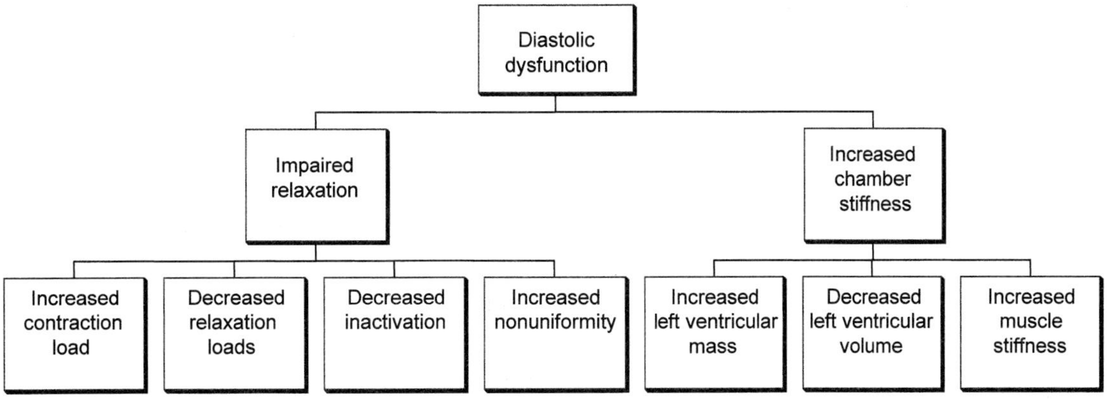

FIGURE 18–4. The factors that contribute to diastolic dysfunction in HCM.

tients with the nonobstructive and the obstructive forms of HCM. Abnormal relaxation, manifested by a prolonged isovolumic relaxation period and a reduced rate of decline in LV pressure, is evident in most patients.[60, 61] Mechanisms influencing relaxation include the inactivation process, several load-dependent processes (including LV end-systolic pressure and volume), afterload, wall stress, coronary blood flow, and regional asynchrony.[62] The factors that contribute to diastolic dysfunction in HCM are outlined in Figure 18–4.

There may be gender differences in LV diastolic function. Sex hormones likely influence LV filling because gonadectomy in rats results in abnormal diastolic filling.[63] Differences between normal male and female subjects have been demonstrated in Doppler-derived pulmonary venous flow patterns and LV inflow velocities.[64, 65] Multiple studies have examined the abnormal diastolic patterns seen in HCM. A study of 149 HCM patients (84 men and 65 women) showed a significant difference in the transmitral E/A ratio (early diastolic/atrial contraction velocity) between the men (1.2 ± 0.4) and the women (0.8 ± 0.3), suggestive of abnormal diastolic filling and impaired ventricular relaxation.[59] These findings were associated with significantly greater symptoms and a worsened functional status in women.

Myocardial Ischemia

The potential mechanisms that may contribute to myocardial ischemia in HCM are outlined in Table 18–4.

Patients with HCM may have abnormal intramural coronary arterioles,[66] with thickened walls, increased amounts of intimal and medial collagen, and a narrowed lumen. Septal perforator artery compression[67] and myocardial bridging have been associated with myocardial ischemia and sudden death.[68] In addition, impairment in LV relaxation may itself result in ischemia.[69]

Table 18–4. POTENTIAL MECHANISMS OF MYOCARDIAL ISCHEMIA IN HYPERTROPHIC CARDIOMYOPATHY

• Small vessel disease with decreased vasodilator capacity
• Septal perforator artery compression
• Myocardial bridging
• Decreased coronary artery perfusion pressure
• Left ventricular outflow tract obstruction
• Decreased capillary myocardial fiber ratio

CLINICAL RECOGNITION

Symptoms

The pathophysiologic components that contribute to symptom production in HCM include LV hypertrophy, diastolic dysfunction, myocardial ischemia, and outflow tract obstruction. The symptoms in any given patient reflect the complex interactions among these factors. Patients with HCM may complain of dyspnea, angina, and presyncope or syncope on exertion. The chest pain experienced by patients with HCM often has atypical features for myocardial ischemia, because it can be nonexertional, prolonged, and not relieved with nitrates.[70] Therefore, the diagnosis of HCM may be particularly difficult in women in whom the evaluation of chest pain is generally more controversial.[71]

There are gender differences both in the age at onset of symptoms and in the age at presentation of HCM. A study of 94 patients (55 men and 39 women) divided the age at onset of symptoms in patients with HCM into four groups: (1) younger than 15 years (and premenarche), (2) 15 to 29 years, (3) 30 to 39 years, and (4) older than 40 years.[72] Female patients with HCM developed symptoms later than males (31.3 years vs. 26.7 years). There was no significant difference between the genders in the youngest age group. There was a predominance of male patients in the 15- to 29-year and the 30- to 39-year age groups, whereas there was a significant predominance of female patients with symptom onset after the age of 40 years.

In addition, there appears to be a gender gap in the timing of presentation and in the referral of patients with HCM. Teare's original case series of 8 patients included six males and two females.[2] The two females in his series had the longest duration of symptoms, whereas the males predominantly presented with sudden death or died shortly after symptom onset. Braunwald's series of 64 patients reported a significant gender difference in the age of patients at the time of their initial referral, with a mean age of 22.8 years in males and 31.7 years in females.[3] An Italian study of 84 men and 65 women addressed gender differences in the manifestations of HCM. This study reported that women were significantly older (44 vs. 35 years) and had a longer duration of symptoms (23 vs. 11 months) than their male counterparts at the time of referral for hemodynamic evaluation.[59]

There may be gender differences in the degree of symptoms experienced by patients with HCM. One early study reported a significant gender difference in the proportion of severely symptomatic patients, with 41% of female patients versus 13% of male patients reporting class III or IV symptoms.[5] A more recent study showed that women had a statistically significant higher frequency of dyspnea (58% vs. 30%), chest pain (46% vs. 23%), and presyncope or syncope (42% vs. 21%) compared with men.[59] In addition, women had reduced exercise capacity on stress testing, with an exercise time of 4.5 minutes versus 7.4 minutes in men. These clinical manifestations were not associated with differences between the genders in LV mass, prevalence of subaortic obstruction, ejection fraction, or cardiac index. As previously mentioned, there was a significant difference in measured diastolic filling parameters in this study cohort.

Physical Examination

Patients with HCM and LV outflow tract obstruction can be distinguished from those with nonobstructive HCM by a number of distinctive physical findings (Table 18–5).[54]

The presence of right ventricular outflow tract obstruction may be identified by a prominent A wave in the jugular venous waveform, a right-sided gallop, and a systolic ejection murmur along the left sternal border. Patients with obstruction at the midventricular level have a distinguishing long apical diastolic rumble, which reflects the midventricular narrowing and asynchronous relaxation in diastole.[73]

Diagnosis

HCM was first well characterized through hemodynamic studies and angiography.[74, 75] In the past three decades such imaging modalities as echo-Doppler,[76–78] nuclear imaging,[79, 80] magnetic resonance imaging,[81] and positron emission tomography[82] have emerged and have contributed to the understanding, detection, management, and follow-up of this condition. The diagnosis of HCM may be complicated because some individuals with HCM may have delayed phenotypic expression of the disorder.

Table 18–5. DISTINGUISHING SIGNS IN HYPERTROPHIC CARDIOMYOPATHY WITH OUTFLOW TRACT OBSTRUCTION

- Bifid carotid pulse
- Double systolic to triple apex beat
- Reversed splitting of the second heart sound
- Systolic murmur at the left sternal border
- Systolic murmur radiating to the axilla
- Mitral diastolic inflow rumble
- Mitral leaflet–septal contact sound

Echo-Doppler is an invaluable tool in the management of patients with HCM, because it can determine the location and extent of hypertrophy; the level and severity of obstruction; the direction, timing, and degree of mitral regurgitation; the presence of diastolic filling abnormalities; and the presence of additional valvular lesions.[76, 78] Echo-Doppler allows for the serial noninvasive assessment of HCM in response to physiologic and pharmacologic maneuvers (supine and upright exercise, dobutamine infusion, amyl nitrite inhalation) and in response to therapeutic interventions. Transesophageal echocardiography can be used intraoperatively in planning the surgical procedure(s), in characterizing the degree and level(s) of obstruction, and in assessing the degree of obstruction, SAM, and mitral regurgitation after surgical myectomy.[56, 83] A recent indication for echocardiography has been the use of contrast echocardiography to guide ethanol septal reduction.[84]

There are no data to suggest that there are gender differences in the echocardiographic evaluation of HCM. The echocardiographic finding of a septal/posterior wall thickness ratio of greater than 1.3 is strongly associated with HCM.[76] One study has demonstrated that there are gender- and age-related differences in septal wall thickness between normal male and female subjects. Septal thickness in female subjects was least in the third to fifth decades of life and greatest in those in the eighth decade and older. There were no appreciable changes in septal thickness in normal male subjects from the third to the eighth decades of life. Left ventricular posterior wall thickness in both males and females was least in the third decade of life and greatest in the eighth decade and older.[65] However, there was no difference in the mean ratios of septal/posterior wall thickness ratio between males and females in early M-mode studies of HCM.[85]

Nuclear angiography has been useful in the assessment of diastolic filling in patients with HCM. Myocardial perfusion scintigraphy and positron emission tomography allow for the evaluation of myocardial ischemia. Magnetic resonance imaging is helpful in characterizing the site and extent of hypertrophy when echocardiographic studies are suboptimal, especially in apical HCM.[86]

HCM and Reproductive Issues

Pre-pregnancy Counseling

Patients with HCM should have counseling regarding the inheritance of HCM, the maternal and fetal risks of pregnancy, and the overall implications of a diagnosis of HCM. Female patients of childbearing age can then make an informed decision about proceeding with pregnancy. Patients with obstructive HCM should ideally be managed in a tertiary center staffed by obstetricians, cardiologists, neonatologists, and anesthesiologists experienced in the management of pregnant patients with cardiac disorders.

Hemodynamic Considerations During Pregnancy in HCM

The physiologic changes that occur in pregnancy may have an important impact on patients with HCM. This is a particular concern in case of dynamic outflow tract obstruction, in which the severity of the gradient is significantly affected by alterations in preload, afterload, and contractility. Pregnancy is a hyperdynamic circulatory state with multiple accompanying changes in the maternal cardiovascular system. An increase in cardiac output and stroke volume (secondary to increases in plasma volume and red blood cell mass), beginning at the sixth week of gestation and plateauing in the third trimester, generally decreases the severity of the outflow tract obstruction. An incremental increase in the heart rate in the last 20 weeks of pregnancy contributes to the increased cardiac output. The outflow tract obstruction of HCM may be worsened by a decrease in the systemic vascular resistance during pregnancy, which has been attributed to circulating estrogen and progesterone levels, heat production by the fetus, and low-resistance arteriovenous shunting in the placenta. In the third trimester the outflow tract obstruction may be further aggravated by decreased venous return secondary to uterine compression and displacement of the inferior vena cava.[87]

Active labor is associated with increases in heart rate, maternal systolic blood pressure, and cardiac output. Patients may experience large fluctuations in preload. There is an autotransfusion of blood with uterine contractions. However, the performance of the Valsalva maneuver during labor increases LV outflow obstruction by decreasing venous return and LV volume. In addition, there may be significant bleeding associated with the delivery—an average blood loss of 300 to 500 ml during a vaginal delivery and 1000 ml during a cesarean section. In the immediate postpartum period there is a further increase in blood volume as a result of autotransfusion from the empty uterus and the relief of vena caval compression.

Maternal and Fetal Risks of Pregnancy

Several case reports and case series have demonstrated that pregnancy can be safely completed by patients with HCM.[88–91] Reviews of the literature[92, 93] have described the outcomes of 109 pregnancies in 52 patients since 1967. Many patients experienced the onset or the worsening of symptoms such as palpitations, dizziness, syncope, chest pain, and congestive heart failure. There have been two reported cases of maternal death and one case of a patient who survived cardiac arrest.[94, 95] Additional significant complications have included two cases of pulmonary edema in the peripartum period in women who ultimately had successful deliveries.[96]

Reviews of the fetal outcomes of pregnant patients with HCM suggest a 17% rate of midtrimester spontaneous abortion. Premature delivery was reported in 7% of pregnancies. Neonatal complications occurred in 13 of 89 pregnancies (15%), including fetal bradycardia, fetal distress, hypoglycemia, or small weight for gestational age.[93]

Risk Assessment in Pregnant Patients with Hypertrophic Cardiomyopathy

The development of cardiovascular complications in pregnant patients with HCM has not been attributed to a specific risk factor. A recent study examining the outcomes of pregnancy in 221 patients with various cardiac lesions included 7 patients with HCM.[97] Poor maternal functional class or cyanosis was predictive of neonatal events. The risk factors predictive of maternal cardiac complications (defined as new-onset heart failure, symptomatic arrhythmias, cerebrovascular events, or cardiac death) in the study cohort are outlined in Table 18–6.

Table 18–6. RISK FACTORS FOR MATERNAL CARDIAC COMPLICATIONS

- Poor maternal functional class or cyanosis
- Myocardial dysfunction (HCM or restrictive cardiomyopathy or systolic dysfunction)
- Left-sided heart obstruction (defined as an outflow tract gradient of >30 mm Hg in HCM)
- Prior arrhythmias
- Prior cardiac events

Antepartum Drug Therapy

The asymptomatic patient with mild disease does not usually require any specific treatment. Advice should be given to avoid situations that adversely increase the LV outflow tract gradient in patients with the obstructive form of HCM. Symptomatic patients may be considered for drug therapy. The use of β-adrenergic blockers such as propranolol in pregnant patients with increasing symptoms has been reported anecdotally by many authors.[98] The fetal risks of β-adrenergic blocker therapy are controversial. The reported fetal effects include an increased incidence of intrauterine growth retardation, bradycardia, hypoglycemia, hypoxemia, and depressed respirations.[99] However, a placebo-controlled study of the use of atenolol in the treatment of pregnancy-associated hypertension showed that neonatal bradycardia was the only significant side effect in the fetus.[100]

β-Adrenergic blockers are the drugs of choice in pregnant patients with HCM and intolerable symptoms. There is no evidence that the routine use of β-adrenergic blockers in asymptomatic patients will increase maternal or fetal complications. There is little experience with the use of calcium channel blocking agents in pregnant patients with HCM. One sudden death has been reported in a pregnant HCM patient who was taking verapamil.[95]

There has been much less experience with the use of disopyramide during pregnancy. No fetal anomalies have been attributed to disopyramide in teratology studies performed in rats and rabbits. Disopyramide has been reported to stimulate uterine contractions in women.[101, 102] It is unknown whether the use of disopyramide during labor or delivery increases maternal or fetal complications. Studies in rats and humans indicate that disopyramide can cross the placenta[103, 104] and is excreted in breast milk.[105]

Many animal and human studies have examined the maternal and fetal effects of amiodarone use during pregnancy.[106] A study in pregnant rats demonstrated placental transfer of amiodarone and its principal metabolite, desethylamiodarone, to the newborn. Levels of amiodarone and desethylamiodarone were detected in the newborn liver and lung, but there were no gross developmental defects.[107] Gestational exposure to amiodarone has been reported to cause fetal bradycardia, fetal thyroid dysfunction, intrauterine growth retardation, and neurologic abnormalities.[108] However, the use of amiodarone is not absolutely contraindicated in pregnancy. It should be reserved for the management of life-threatening ventricular arrhythmias or for significant supraventricular arrhythmias that are not adequately controlled by other agents. No adverse effects have been reported with amiodarone in breast-fed infants.[109]

Management During Labor and Delivery

A left lateral decubitus position is favored in obstructive HCM to limit vena caval compression and to increase venous return to the heart. Antibiotics should be administered to prevent infective endocarditis. Prostaglandins have vasodilatory properties and should be used with caution. The slow infusion of oxytocin, which can also cause vasodilatation, has been well tolerated in previous reports.[90, 110] The use of intravenous β-adrenergic blockers at the time of delivery has been described.[111] The short-term use of beta blockers has also been associated with transient fetal hypoglycemia, hypotension, hypotonia, and bradycardia.

Adequate pain relief and anesthesia is required to decrease circulating catecholamine levels, which can potentially worsen the outflow tract gradient in patients with obstructive HCM. Epidural and spinal anesthesia with sympathetic blockade should be avoided in patients with obstructive HCM, because it may significantly decrease afterload.[112] However, analgesia through the epidural or spinal routes can be achieved with minimal sympathetic blockade using such narcotic agents as fentanyl. In addition, patients with HCM can receive intravenous analgesics (e.g., meperidine [Demerol], fentanyl).

Most pregnant patients with obstructive HCM are able to tolerate a vaginal delivery well. Some authors recommend the use of forceps to shorten the second stage of labor.[90, 94] There is no demonstrated benefit with delivery by means of cesarean section in patients with obstructive HCM. Invasive hemodynamic monitoring with a Swan-Ganz catheter is rarely indicated and should be reserved for patients with significant symptoms, hemodynamic impairment, and a high resting outflow tract gradient.[96] One recent report has described the use of echo-Doppler during labor and delivery in a 35-year-old woman with resting outflow tract obstruction. Echo-Doppler allowed for the serial real-time evaluation of the patient's outflow tract gradient in response to the administration of fluids, oxytocin, and propranolol.[113]

In general, volume loss during and after delivery should be corrected with intravenous fluids. Crossmatched blood should be readily available. Vasopressors without significant inotropic effects (e.g., phenylephrine) are favored for the management of significant hypotension. The use of β-sympathomimetic agents for tocolysis is not recommended.

Hypertrophic Cardiomyopathy in the Elderly Patient

Hypertrophic cardiomyopathy in the elderly patient (HCME) forms a unique subset of this condition and has multiple distinguishing clinical and morphologic features. The majority of patients with HCME are women, with female subjects forming 51% to 75% of study cohorts of HCME.[114–117] Systemic hypertension is more common in elderly patients, and it may be difficult to distinguish elderly patients with hypertensive heart disease[118] from those with HCM. Elderly patients with HCM are more likely to have concentric hypertrophy and a milder degree of hypertrophy. The pattern of hypertrophy tends to be focal and localized to the anterior or posterior portion of the septum.[116, 119] A study of normal male and female subjects has shown that women had increases in their mean septal wall thickness from 8.6 to 10.2 mm between the third and the eighth decades of life. The corresponding septal to posterior wall ratios in these normal subjects increased from 1.0 to 1.13; these changes were not identified in men.[65] The presence of a sigmoid-shaped septum is an age-related phenomenon and may be seen in many patients with HCME. Its presence may facilitate the development of outflow tract obstruction.[120]

Mitral annular calcification (MAC) in association with HCM was detected in 30% of patients older than 40 years in an autopsy series.[121] In this study, 70% of the patients with MAC were women. Patients with MAC were more likely to develop calcific deposits in the epicardial coronary arteries and on aortic valve cusps. The annular calcium distorts the mitral apparatus, and significant MAC is usually accompanied by an independent jet of mitral regurgitation, which is often centrally directed and distinct from the posteriorly directed jet of mitral regurgitation caused by SAM.

The mechanisms of outflow tract obstruction in HCME are different from those seen in younger patients. Patients with HCME typically have a relatively small heart, distorted LV outflow tract geometry, and a higher prevalence of MAC. The presence of MAC displaces the mitral apparatus more anteriorly, resulting in narrowing of the outflow tract and less angulation of the mitral leaflets. In addition, there is restricted SAM of the anterior leaflet, with mitral leaflet/septal contact occurring in the body of the leaflet rather than at the tip as in younger patients. Outflow tract obstruction, either at rest or with provocation, is seen in the majority of patients with HCME.[116]

The treatment of HCME is similar to that in younger patients (see later). Treatment is targeted to the cause of the patient's symptoms and may include antianginal agents, antiarrhythmic agents, or drugs that improve diastolic filling. However, calcium channel blockers are generally not favored in HCME, because elderly patients may have compromised atrioventricular node function and significant outflow tract obstruction. Dual-chamber pacing may have an important role in the management of patients with HCME, because elderly patients tend to have longer PR intervals, making complete ventricular capture more easily achieved, and because many elderly patients are not good candidates for surgical myectomy.

The long-term prognosis of HCME is generally favorable. One study of 95 patients with HCM diagnosed after the age of 65 showed 1- and 5-year survival rates of 95% and 76%, respectively. Gender was not associated with a difference in survival on univariate analysis. Significant risk factors associated with a worsened prognosis were advanced (class III) dyspnea and left atrial size.[122]

Table 18–7. REPORTED BENEFITS OF DUAL-CHAMBER PACING IN HYPERTROPHIC CARDIOMYOPATHY

- Reduction in LV outflow tract obstruction
- Reduction in mitral regurgitation
- Reduction in LV filling pressures
- Reduction in drug-refractory symptoms
- Improvement in exercise tolerance

time.[54] The most common adverse side effects of disopyramide are related to its anticholinergic properties and are dose dependent. The most common reactions were a dry mouth (32%), urinary hesitancy (16%), blurred vision (3% to 9%), gastrointestinal symptoms (3% to 9%), and urinary retention (2%). Urinary retention is reported to occur less commonly in women than in men. One case series of nine patients with disopyramide-induced urinary retention included seven men and two women.[150]

Dual-Chamber Pacing

The previously reported benefits of dual-chamber pacing are outlined in Table 18–7.[140]

Dual-chamber pacing reduces LV outflow tract obstruction by inducing both acute and chronic changes.[151–153] In the acute phase, RV apical pacing causes (1) paradoxic or diminished inward movement of the ventricular septum, which increases LV outflow tract dimensions; (2) asynchronous and late activation at the base of the septum, which may contribute to opening the LV outflow tract during systole; and (3) decreased myocardial contractility. The atrioventricular delay must be optimized to achieve complete ventricular capture. Radiofrequency ablation of the atrioventricular node may be required to improve ventricular preexcitation. Acute studies have revealed impairment of both systolic and diastolic function, possibly related to asynchronous contraction and relaxation.[154]

Initial reports suggested that dual-chamber pacing could result in an improvement in symptoms and in favorable LV remodeling and LV mass regression.[155] This mode of therapy was believed to be a particularly important option for women, who are generally older than men with HCM and who may not be good candidates for surgery. Recent studies of the benefits of pacing have been less encouraging. A double-blind crossover trial involving 19 patients (10 men, 9 women) randomized subjects to DDD followed by AAI pacing or AAI followed by DDD pacing. DDD pacing resulted in a significant reduction in the severity of the LV outflow tract gradient. However, this hemodynamic benefit was not accompanied by an objective improvement in exercise capacity. In addition, although DDD pacing resulted in fewer symptoms in 63%, subjective improvement was also experienced in 42% of patients with AAI programming. The results of this study suggest that the perceived reduction in symptoms may largely be due to a placebo effect. An analysis of variables predictive of subjective improvement during DDD pacing showed no significant association with gender. Younger age was associated with a perceived higher functional capacity during DDD pacing.[156]

Alcohol Septal Ablation

A more recently described nonsurgical intervention is chemical septal ablation. This procedure involves the infusion of ethanol through a catheter into one or more septal perforator branches of the left anterior descending artery. This results in the infarction and thinning of a portion of the proximal interventricular septum.[157] Possible benefits include a reduction in LV pressure gradients, reduced symptoms, and improved exercise tolerance. However, potential early complications include conduction abnormalities and heart block, ventricular arrhythmias, and death. Potential late complications include an increased incidence of arrhythmias.

Chemical septal ablation may become a particularly important option for women with HCM, because they are more likely to be older and less ideal candidates for surgery. One study of 18 patients, which had an equal number of male and female subjects, included eight women with class III symptoms and less symptomatic men, with six men reporting class II symptoms and three men reporting class III symptoms.[157] Alcohol septal ablation resulted in a significant reduction in the mean outflow tract gradient from 67 to 25 mm Hg. The majority of women, 8 of 9 patients, experienced an improvement in functional capacity from class III to class I or II. The majority of male patients also experienced an improvement in functional class. The only patient who had no symptomatic benefit at 3 months of follow-up was a 41-year-old woman. Another study of alcohol septal ablation involved 25 patients, including 13 women and 12 men with a mean age of 55 years. This study showed a significant reduction in the LV outflow tract gradient and clinical improvement in 88% of patients. No gender differences were reported. The only death in this series occurred in an 86-year-old woman.[158]

Surgery

Surgery for HCM was first performed in 1958.[159] Ventricular septal myectomy consists of the resection of a portion of the basal septum (2 to 5 g). This results in enlargement of the LV outflow tract, a decrease in SAM, and its associated mitral regurgitation. Surgery abolishes or significantly reduces the resting outflow tract gradient in more than 90% of patients.[160–162] Data involving more than 1500 patients show substantial and persistent symptomatic improvement in approximately 70 percent of patients 5 or more years after operation. The operative mortality of this procedure has progressively decreased. However, there is a 1% to 2% cumulative annual mortality. Other potential complications include a 5% risk of heart block requiring permanent pacing, ventricular septal defect, mild aortic regurgitation, arrhythmias, and progressive LV dysfunction. Surgical mortality appears to be higher among elderly patients and those undergoing both myectomy and coronary artery bypass grafting.[163–165]

A review of the patients who underwent myectomy in highly specialized referral centers shows that the majority of surgical series have included a substantial number of female patients. The proportion of female patients in key studies ranges from 34% to 49%.[160–162] No significant gender differences have been reported for perioperative complications or for long-term outcome.

CONCLUSION

Hypertrophic cardiomyopathy is a genetic disorder that demonstrates many gender-related differences. Studies suggest that there is a male predilection for the penetrance of genetic defects and that there is a higher frequency of HCM in males. Experimental and clinical studies have demonstrated that the phenotypic expression of hypertrophy is modulated by gender-related differences. There are clinically relevant gender differences in the age and symptomatic status of patients with HCM. Special considerations are required in the management of the pregnant patient with HCM, especially in cases of LV outflow tract obstruction. Therapeutic options in symptomatic patients with HCM include pharmacotherapy, dual-chamber pacing, alcohol septal ablation, or surgical myectomy. Long-term management strategies in patients with HCM may differ between men and women, who may be less suitable candidates for surgery.

References

1. Richardson P, McKenna W, Bristow M, et al: Report of the 1995 World Health Organization/International Society and Federation of Cardiology Task Force on the Definition and Classification of Cardiomyopathies. Circulation 93:841–842, 1996.
2. Teare RD: Asymmetrical hypertrophy of the heart in young adults. Br Heart J 20:1–8, 1958.
3. Braunwald E, Lambrew C, Rockoff SD, et al: Idiopathic hypertrophic subaortic stenosis: I. Description of the disease based upon an analysis of 64 patients. Circulation 29(Suppl IV):IV-3–IV-119, 1964.
4. Maron BJ: Hypertrophic cardiomyopathy. Lancet 350:127–133, 1997.
5. Frank S, Braunwald E: Idiopathic hypertrophic subaortic stenosis: Clinical analysis of 126 patients with emphasis on the natural history. Circulation 37:759–788, 1968.
6. Adelman AG, Wigle ED, Ranganathan N, et al: The clinical course in muscular subaortic stenosis: A retrospective and prospective study of 60 hemodynamically proved cases. Ann Intern Med 77:515–525, 1972.
7. Shah PM, Adelman AG, Wigle ED, et al: The natural (and unnatural) history of hypertrophic obstructive cardiomyopathy. Circ Res 34(Suppl II):II-179–195, 1974.
8. Spirito P, Chiarella F, Carratino L, et al: Clinical course and prognosis of hypertrophic cardiomyopathy in an outpatient population. N Engl J Med 320:749–755, 1989.
9. Cecchi F, Olivotto I, Montereggi A, et al: Hypertrophic cardiomyopathy in Tuscany: Clinical course and outcome in an unselected regional population. J Am Coll Cardiol 26:1529–1536, 1995.
10. Codd MB, Sugure DD, Gersh BJ, Melton LJ III: Epidemiology of idiopathic dilated and hypertrophic cardiomyopathy: A population-based study in Olmsted County, Minnesota, 1975–1984. Circulation 80:564–572, 1989.
11. Maron BJ, Gardin JM, Flack JM, et al: Prevalence of hypertrophic cardiomyopathy in a general population of young adults: Echocardiographic analysis of 4111 subjects in the CARDIA study. Circulation 92:785–789, 1995.
12. Corrado D, Basso C, Schiavon M, Thiene G: Screening for hypertrophic cardiomyopathy in young athletes. N Engl J Med 339:364–369, 1998.
13. Hada Y, Sakamoato T, Amano K, et al: Prevalence of hypertrophic cardiomyopathy in a population of adult Japanese workers as detected by echocardiographic screening. Am J Cardiol 59:183–184, 1987.
14. Agnarsson UT, Hardarson T, Hallgrimsson J, Sigfusson N: The prevalence of hypertrophic cardiomyopathy in men: An echocardiographic population screening study with a review of death records. J Intern Med 232:499–506, 1992.
15. Maron BJ, Peterson EE, Maron MS, et al: Prevalence of hypertrophic cardiomyopathy in an outpatient population referred for echocardiographic study. Am J Cardiol 73:577–580, 1994.
16. Bagger JP, Baandrup U, Rasmussen K, et al: Cardiomyopathy in Western Denmark. Br Heart J 52:327–331, 1984.
17. Seidman C. Hypertrophic cardiomyopathy. From man to mouse. J Clin Invest 106:509–513, 2000.
18. Jarcho JA, McKenna W, Pare JAP, et al: Mapping a gene for familial hypertrophic cardiomyopathy to chromosome 14q1. N Engl J Med 321:1372–1378, 1989.
19. Geisterfer-Lowrance AAT, Kass S, Tanigawa G, et al: A molecular basis for familial hypertrophic cardiomyopathy: A β-myosin heavy chain gene missense mutation. Cell 62:999–1006, 1990.
20. Thierfelder L, Watkins H, MacRae C, et al: α-Tropomyosin and cardiac troponin T mutations cause familial hypertrophic cardiomyopathy: A disease of the sarcomere. Cell 77:701–712, 1994.
21. Watkins H, Conner D, Thierfelder L, et al: Mutations in the cardiac myosin binding protein-C gene on chromosome 11 cause familial hypertrophic cardiomyopathy. Nat Genet 11:434–437, 1995.
22. Spirito P, Seidman CE, McKenna WJ, Maron BJ: The management of hypertrophic cardiomyopathy. N Engl J Med 336:775–785, 1997.
23. Maron BJ, Nichols PF III, Pickle LW, et al: Patterns of inheritance in hypertrophic cardiomyopathy: Assessment by M-mode and two-dimensional echocardiography. Am J Cardiol 53:1087–1094, 1984.
24. Charron P, Carrier L, Dubourg O, et al: Penetrance of familial hypertrophic cardiomyopathy. Genet Couns 8:107–114, 1997.
25. Watkins H, Rosenzweig A, Hwang D-S, et al: Characteristics and prognostic implications of myosin missense mutations in familial hypertrophic cardiomyopathy. N Engl J Med 326:1108–1114, 1992.
26. Epstein ND, Cohn GM, Cyran F, Fananapazir L: Differences in clinical expression of hypertrophic cardiomyopathy associated with two distinct mutations in the β-myosin heavy chain gene: A $908^{Leu \rightarrow Val}$ mutation and a $403^{Arg \rightarrow Gln}$ mutation. Circulation 86:345–352, 1992.
27. Marian AJ, Roberts R: Recent advances in the molecular genetics of hypertrophic cardiomyopathy. Circulation 92:1336–1347, 1995.
28. Anan R, Greve G, Thierfelder L, et al: Prognostic implications of novel beta cardiac myosin heavy chain gene mutations that cause familial hypertrophic cardiomyopathy. J Clin Invest 93:280–285, 1994.
29. Marian AJ, Mares A Jr, Kelly DP, et al: Sudden cardiac death in hypertrophic cardiomyopathy: Variability in phenotypic expression of β-myosin heavy chain mutations. Eur Heart J 16:368–376, 1995.
30. Solomon SD, Wolff S, Watkins H, et al: Left ventricular hypertrophy and morphology in familial hypertrophic cardiomyopathy associated with mutations of the beta-myosin heavy chain gene. J Am Coll Cardiol 22:498–505, 1993.
31. Watkins H, McKenna WJ, Thierfelder L, et al: Mutations in the genes for cardiac troponin T and α-tropomyosin in hypertrophic cardiomyopathy. N Engl J Med 332:1058–1064, 1995.
32. Coviello DA, Maron BJ, Spirito P, et al: Clinical features of hypertrophic cardiomyopathy caused by mutation of a "hot spot" in the alpha-tropomyosin gene. J Am Coll Cardiol 29:635–640, 1997.
33. Niimura H, Bachinski LL, Sangwatanaroj S, et al: Mutations in the gene for cardiac myosin-binding protein C and late-onset familial hypertrophic cardiomyopathy. N Engl J Med 338:1248–1257, 1998.
34. Marian AJ, Yu QT, Workman R, et al: Angiotensin-converting enzyme polymorphism in hypertrophic cardiomyopathy and sudden cardiac death. Lancet 342:1085–1086, 1993.
35. Lechin M, Quinones MA, Omran A, et al: Angiotensin-I converting enzyme genotypes and left ventricular hypertrophy in patients with hypertrophic cardiomyopathy. Circulation 92:1808–1812, 1995.
36. Brugada R, Kelsey W, Lechin M, et al: Role of candidate modifier genes on the phenotypic expression of hypertrophy in patients with hypertrophic cardiomyopathy. J Invest Med 45:542–551, 1997.
37. Fananapazir L, Epstein ND: Genotype-phenotype correlations in hypertrophic cardiomyopathy: Insights provided by comparisons of kindreds with distinct and identical β-myosin heavy chain gene mutations. Circulation 89:22–32, 1994.
38. Maron BJ, Gottdiener JS, Epstein SE: Patterns and significance of distribution of left ventricular hypertrophy in hypertrophic cardiomyopathy: A wide-angle, two-dimensional echocardiographic study of 125 patients. Am J Cardiol 48:418–428, 1981.
39. Louie EK, Maron BJ: Hypertrophic cardiomyopathy with extreme increase in left ventricular wall thickness: Functional and morphologic features and clinical significance. J Am Coll Cardiol 8:57–65, 1986.
40. Klues HG, Schiffers A, Maron BJ: Phenotypic spectrum and patterns of left ventricular hypertrophy in hypertrophic cardiomyopathy: Morphologic observations and significance as assessed by two-dimensional echocardiography in 600 patients. J Am Coll Cardiol 26:1699–1708, 1995.
41. Geisterfer-Lowrance AAT, Christe M, Conner DA, et al: A mouse

model of familial hypertrophic cardiomyopathy. Science 272:731–734, 1996.
42. Weinberger HD, Vikstrom KL, Knudson OA, et al: Gender specific dilation in transgenic mice with hypertrophic cardiomyopathy: An echocardiographic study. (Abstract). J Am Soc Echocardiogr 10:427, 1997.
43. Douglas PS, Katz SE, Weinberg EO, et al: Hypertrophic remodeling: Gender differences in the early response to left ventricular pressure overload. J Am Coll Cardiol 32:1118–1125, 1998.
44. Carroll JD, Carroll EP, Feldman T, et al: Sex-associated differences in left ventricular function in aortic stenosis of the elderly. Circulation 86:1099–1107, 1992.
45. Douglas PS, Otto CM, Mickel MC, et al: Gender differences in left ventricle geometry and function in patients undergoing valvuloplasty for isolated aortic stenosis. Br Heart J 73:548–554, 1995.
46. Aurigemma GP, Gaasch WH: Gender differences in older patients with pressure-overload hypertrophy of the left ventricle. Cardiology 86:310–317, 1995.
47. Stumpf WE, Sar M, Aumuller G: The heart: A target organ for estradiol. Science 196:319–321, 1977.
48. McGill HC Jr, Anselmo VC, Buchanan JM, Sheridan PJ: The heart is a target organ for androgen. Science 207:775–777, 1980.
49. Scheuer J, Malhotra A, Shaible TF, Capasso J: Effects of gonadectomy and hormonal replacement on rat hearts. Circ Res 61:12–19, 1987.
50. Rosenkranz-Weiss P, Tomek RJ, Mathew J, Eghbali M: Gender-specific differences in expression of mRNAs for functional and structural proteins in rat ventricular myocardium. J Mol Cell Cardiol 26:261–271, 1994.
51. Weinberg EO, Thienelt CD, Katz SE, et al: Gender differences in left ventricular gene expression in pressure overload hypertrophy. (Abstract). Circulation 94:I-187, 1996.
52. Proudler AJ, Ahmed AH, Crook D, et al: Hormone replacement therapy and serum angiotensin-converting enzyme activity in postmenopausal women. Lancet 346:89–90, 1995.
53. Schundert H, Danser AH, Hense H-W, et al: Effects of estrogen replacement therapy on the renin-angiotensin system in postmenopausal women. Circulation 95:39–45, 1997.
54. Wigle ED, Rakowski H, Kimball BP, Williams WG: Hypertrophic cardiomyopathy: Clinical spectrum and treatment. Circulation 92: 1680–1692, 1995.
55. Henry WL, Clark CE, Griffith JM, Epstein SE: Mechanism of left ventricular outflow obstruction in patients with obstructive asymmetric septal hypertrophy (idiopathic hypertrophic subaortic stenosis). Am J Cardiol 35:337–345, 1975.
56. Grigg LE, Wigle ED, Williams WG, et al: Transesophageal Doppler echocardiography in obstructive hypertrophic cardiomyopathy: Clarification of pathophysiology and importance in intraoperative decision making. J Am Coll Cardiol 20:42–52, 1992.
57. Jiang L, Levine RA, King ME, Weyman AE: An integrated mechanism for systolic anterior motion of the mitral valve in hypertrophic cardiomyopathy based on echocardiographic observations. Am Heart J 113: 633–644, 1987.
58. Schwammenthal E, Nakatani S, He S, et al: Mechanism of mitral regurgitation in hypertrophic cardiomyopathy: Mismatch of posterior to anterior leaflet length and mobility. Circulation 98:856–865, 1998.
59. Pelliccia F, Cianfrocca C, De Castro S, Critelli G: Is there a gender gap in clinical presentation and outcome of hypertrophic cardiomyopathy? J Am Coll Cardiol 25:107A, 1995.
60. Takenaka K, Dabestani A, Gardin JM, et al: Left ventricular filling in hypertrophic cardiomyopathy: A pulsed Doppler echocardiographic study. J Am Coll Cardiol 7:1263–1271, 1986.
61. Spirito P, Maron BJ: Relation between extent of left ventricular hypertrophy and diastolic filling abnormalities in hypertrophic cardiomyopathy. J Am Coll Cardiol 15:808–813, 1990.
62. Brutsaert DL, Rademakers FE, Sys SU: Triple control of relaxation: Implications in cardiac disease. Circulation 69:190–196, 1984.
63. Schaible TF, Malhotra A, Ciambrone G, Scheuer J: The effects of gonadectomy on left ventricular function and cardiac contractile proteins in male and female rats. Circ Res 54:38–49, 1984.
64. Voutilainen S, Kupari M, Hippeläinen M, et al: Factors influencing Doppler indexes of left ventricular filling in healthy persons. Am J Cardiol 68:653–659, 1991.
65. Klein AL, Burstow DJ, Tajik AJ, et al: Effects of age on left ventricular dimensions and filling dynamics in 117 normal persons. Mayo Clin Proc 69:212–224, 1994.
66. Maron BJ, Wolfson JK, Epstein SE, Roberts WC: Intramural ("small vessel") coronary artery disease in hypertrophic cardiomyopathy. J Am Coll Cardiol 8:545–557, 1986.
67. Pichard AD, Meller J, Teichholz LE, et al: Septal perforator compression (narrowing) in idiopathic hypertrophic subaortic stenosis. Am J Cardiol 40:310–314, 1977.
68. Yetman AT, McCrindle BW, MacDonald C, et al: Myocardial bridging in children with hypertrophic cardiomyopathy—a risk factor for sudden death. N Engl J Med 339:1201–1209, 1998.
69. Cannon RO, Rosing DR, Maron BJ, et al: Myocardial ischemia in patients with hypertrophic cardiomyopathy: Contribution of inadequate vasodilator reserve and elevated left ventricular filling pressures. Circulation 71:234–243, 1985.
70. Maron BJ, Bonow RO, Cannon RO, et al: Hypertrophic cardiomyopathy: Interrelations of clinical manifestations, pathophysiology, and therapy. N Engl J Med 316:780–789; 844–852, 1987.
71. Wenger NK, Speroff L, Packard B: Cardiovascular health and disease in women. N Engl J Med 329:247–256, 1993.
72. Dimitrow PP, Czarnecka D, Jaszcz KK, Dubiel JS: Sex differences in age at onset of symptoms in patients with hypertrophic cardiomyopathy. J Cardiovasc Risk 4:33–35, 1997.
73. Woo A, Wigle ED, Rakowski RC, et al: Long-term outcome of hypertrophic cardiomyopathy with mid-ventricular obstruction. J Am Coll Cardiol 31:182A, 1998.
74. Ross J Jr, Braunwald E, Gault JH, et al: The mechanism of the intraventricular pressure gradient in idiopathic hypertrophic subaortic stenosis. Circulation 34:558–578, 1966.
75. Simon A, Ross J Jr, Gault JH: Angiographic anatomy of the left ventricle and mitral valve in idiopathic hypertrophic subaortic stenosis. Circulation 36:852–867, 1967.
76. Henry WL, Clark CE, Epstein SE: Asymmetric septal hypertrophy: Echocardiographic identification of the pathognomonic anatomic abnormality of IHSS. Circulation 47:225–233, 1973.
77. Pollick C, Rakowski H, Wigle ED: Muscular subaortic stenosis: The quantitative relationship between systolic anterior motion and the pressure gradient. Circulation 69:43–49, 1984.
78. Rakowski H, Sasson Z, Wigle ED: Echocardiographic and Doppler assessment of hypertrophic cardiomyopathy. J Am Soc Echocardiogr 1:31–47, 1988.
79. Bonow RO, Frederick RM, Bacharach SL, et al: Atrial systole and left ventricular filling in hypertrophic cardiomyopathy: Effect of verapamil. Am J Cardiol 51:1386–1391, 1983.
80. Cannon RO, Dilsizian V, O'Gara PT, et al: Impact of surgical relief of outflow obstruction on thallium perfusion abnormalities in hypertrophic cardiomyopathy. Circulation 85:1039–1045, 1992.
81. Higgins CB, Byrd BF, Stark D, et al: Magnetic resonance imaging in hypertrophic cardiomyopathy. Am J Cardiol 55:1121–1126, 1985.
82. Nienaber CA, Gambhir SS, Mody FV, et al: Regional myocardial blood flow and glucose utilization in symptomatic patients with hypertrophic cardiomyopathy. Circulation 87:1580–1590, 1993.
83. Marwick TH, Stewart WJ, Lever HM, et al: Benefits of intraoperative echocardiography in the surgical management of hypertrophic cardiomyopathy. J Am Coll Cardiol 20:1066–1072, 1992.
84. Lakkis NM, Nagueh SF, Kleiman NS, et al: Echocardiography-guided ethanol septal reduction for hypertrophic obstructive cardiomyopathy. Circulation 98:1750–1755, 1998.
85. Clark CE, Henry WL, Epstein SE: Familial prevalence and genetic transmission of idiopathic hypertrophic subaortic stenosis. N Engl J Med 289:709–714, 1973.
86. Suzuki J, Watanabe F, Takenaka K, et al: New subtype of apical hypertrophic cardiomyopathy identified with nuclear magnetic resonance imaging as an underlying cause of markedly inverted T-waves. J Am Coll Cardiol 22:1175–1181, 1993.
87. Pritchard JA: Changes in the blood volume during pregnancy and delivery. Anesthesiology 26:393–399, 1965.
88. Turner GM, Oakley CM, Dixon HG: Management of pregnancy complicated by hypertrophic obstructive cardiomyopathy. BMJ 4:281–284, 1968.
89. Oakley GDG, McGarry K, Limb DG, Oakley CM: Management of pregnancy in patients with hypertrophic cardiomyopathy. BMJ 1:1749–1750, 1979.
90. Kolibash AJ, Ruiz DE, Lewis RP: Idiopathic hypertrophic subaortic stenosis in pregnancy. Ann Intern Med 82:791–794, 1975.
91. Van Kasteren YM, Kleinhout J, Smit MA, et al: Hypertrophic cardiomyopathy and pregnancy: A report of three cases. Eur J Obstet Gynecol Reprod Biol 38:63–67, 1990.

92. Kumar A, Elkayam U: Hypertrophic cardiomyopathy in pregnancy. In Elkayam U, Gleicher N (eds): Cardiac Problems in Pregnancy, Diagnosis and Management of Maternal and Fetal disease, 2nd ed. Alan R. Liss, New York, 1990, p 129.
93. Benitez RM: Hypertrophic cardiomyopathy and pregnancy: Maternal and fetal outcomes. J Matern Fetal Invest 6:51–55, 1996.
94. Shah DM, Sunderji GS: Hypertrophic cardiomyopathy and pregnancy: Report of a maternal mortality and review of the literature. Obstet Gynecol Surv 40:444–448, 1985.
95. Pelliccia F, Cianfrocca C, Gaudio C, Reale A: Sudden death during pregnancy in hypertrophic cardiomyopathy. Eur Heart J 13:421–423, 1992.
96. Tessler MJ, Hudson R, Naugler-Colville M, Biehl DR: Pulmonary oedema in two parturients with hypertrophic obstructive cardiomyopathy (HOCM). Can J Anaesth 37:469–473, 1990.
97. Siu SC, Sermer M, Harrison DA, et al: Risk and predictors for pregnancy-related complications in women with heart disease. Circulation 96:2789–2794, 1997.
98. Sabom MB, Curry RC, Wise DE: Propranolol therapy during pregnancy in a patient with idiopathic hypertrophic subaortic stenosis: Is it safe? South Med J 71:328–329, 1978.
99. Rubin PC: Beta blockers in pregnancy. N Engl J Med 305:1323–1326, 1981.
100. Rubin PC, Clark DM, Sumner EJ, et al: Placebo-controlled trial of atenolol in treatment of pregnancy-associated hypertension. Lancet 1: 431–434, 1983.
101. Leonard RF, Braun TE, Levy AM: Initiation of uterine contractions by disopyramide during pregnancy. N Engl J Med 299:84–85, 1978.
102. Tadmor OP, Keren A, Rosenak D, et al: The effect of disopyramide on uterine contractions during pregnancy. Am J Obstet Gynecol 162: 482–486, 1990.
103. Karim A, Cook C, Campion J: Placental and milk transfer of disopyramide and its metabolites in rats. Drug Metab Dispos 6:346–348, 1978.
104. Echizen H, Nakura M, Saotome T, et al: Plasma protein binding of disopyramide in pregnant and postpartum women, and in neonates and their mothers. Br J Clin Pharmacol 29:423–430, 1990.
105. Barnett DB, Hudson SA, McBurney A: Disopyramide and its N-monodesalkyl metabolite in breast milk. Br J Clin Pharmacol 14: 310–312, 1982.
106. Widerhorn J, Bhandari AK, Bughi S, et al: Fetal and neonatal adverse effects profile of amiodarone treatment during pregnancy. Am Heart J 122:1162–1166, 1991.
107. Hill DA, Reasor MJ: Effects of amiodarone administration during pregnancy in Fischer 344 rats. Toxicology 65:259–269, 1991.
108. Magee LA, Downar E, Sermer M, et al: Pregnancy outcome after gestational exposure to amiodarone in Canada. Am J Obstet Gynecol 172:1307–1311, 1995.
109. Strunge P, Frandsen J, Andreasen F: Amiodarone during pregnancy. Eur Heart J 9:106–109, 1988.
110. Boccio RV, Chung JH, Harrison DM: Anesthetic management of cesarean section in a patient with idiopathic hypertrophic subaortic stenosis. Anesthesiology 65:663–665, 1986.
111. Fairley CJ, Clarke JT: Use of esmolol in a parturient with hypertrophic obstructive cardiomyopathy. Br J Anaesth 75:801–804, 1995.
112. Minnich ME, Quirk JG, Clark RB: Epidural anaesthesia for vaginal delivery in a patient with idiopathic hypertrophic subaortic stenosis. Anesthesiology 67:590–592, 1987.
113. Wilansky S, Belcik T, Osborn R, Carpenter R: Hypertrophic cardiomyopathy in pregnancy: The use of two-dimensional and Doppler echocardiography during labor and delivery. A case report. J Heart Valve Dis 7:355–357, 1998.
114. Whiting RB, Powell JW, Dinsmore RE, Sanders C: Idiopathic hypertrophic subaortic stenosis in the elderly. N Engl J Med 285:196–200, 1971.
115. Krasnow N, Stein RA: Hypertrophic cardiomyopathy in the aged. Am Heart J 96:326–336, 1978.
116. Lewis JF, Maron BJ: Clinical and morphologic expression of hypertrophic cardiomyopathy in patients ≥ 65 years of age. Am J Cardiol 73: 1105–1111, 1994.
117. Rakowski H, Freedman D, Wigle ED: Echocardiographic evaluation of hypertrophic cardiomyopathy in the elderly. Cardiol Elderly 3: 415–422, 1995.
118. Topol EJ, Traill TA, Fortuin NJ: Hypertensive hypertrophic cardiomyopathy of the elderly. N Engl J Med 312:277–283, 1985.
119. Chikamori T, Doi Y, Yonazawa Y, et al: Comparison of clinical features of patients > 60 years of age to those < 40 years of age with hypertrophic cardiomyopathy. Am J Cardiol 66:875–877, 1990.
120. Lever HM, Karam RF, Currie PJ, Healy BP: Hypertrophic cardiomyopathy in the elderly. Circulation 79:580–589, 1989.
121. Motamed HE, Roberts WC: Frequency and significance of mitral annular calcium in hypertrophic cardiomyopathy: Analysis of 200 necropsy patients. Am J Cardiol 60:877–884, 1987.
122. Fay WP, Taliercio C, Histrup DM, et al: Natural history of hypertrophic cardiomyopathy in the elderly. J Am Coll Cardiol 18:821–826, 1990.
123. Robinson K, Frenneaux MP, Stockins B, et al: Atrial fibrillation in hypertrophic cardiomyopathy: A longitudinal study. J Am Coll Cardiol 15:1279–1285, 1990.
124. Furlan AJ, Craciun AR, Raju NR, Hart N: Cerebrovascular complications associated with idiopathic hypertrophic subaortic stenosis. Stroke 15:282–284, 1984.
125. Russell JW, Biller J, Hajduczok ZD, et al: Ischemic cerebrovascular complications and risk factors in idiopathic hypertrophic subaortic stenosis. Stroke 22:1143–1147, 1991.
126. McKenna WJ, Harris L, Rowland E, et al: Amiodarone for long-term management of patients with hypertrophic cardiomyopathy. Am J Cardiol 54:802–810, 1984.
127. Watson DC, Henry WL, Epstein SE, Morrow AG: Effects of operation on left atrial size and the occurrence of atrial fibrillation in patients with hypertrophic subaortic stenosis. Circulation 55:178–181, 1977.
128. Kofflard MJ, Waldstein DJ, Vos J, ten Cate FJ: Prognosis in hypertrophic cardiomyopathy: A retrospective study. Am J Cardiol 72:939–943, 1993.
129. McKenna W, Deanfield J, Faruqui A, et al: Prognosis in hypertrophic cardiomyopathy: Role of age and clinical, electrocardiographic and hemodynamic features. Am J Cardiol 47:534–538, 1981.
130. McKenna WJ, Franklin RC, Nihoyanopoulos P, et al: Arrhythmia and prognosis in infants, children and adolescents with hypertrophic cardiomyopathy. J Am Coll Cardiol 11:147–153, 1988.
131. Fananapazir L, McAreavey D: Hypertrophic cardiomyopathy: Evaluation and treatment of patients at high risk for sudden death. PACE 20[pt II]:478–501, 1997.
132. Fananapazir L, Chang AC, Epstein SE, McAreavey D: Prognostic determinants in hypertrophic cardiomyopathy: Prospective evaluation of a therapeutic strategy based on clinical, Holter, hemodynamic, and electrophysiological findings. Circulation 86:730–740, 1992.
133. McKenna WJ, Oakley CM, Krikler DM, Goodwin JF: Improved survival with amiodarone in patients with hypertrophic cardiomyopathy and ventricular tachycardia. Br Heart J 53:412–416, 1985.
134. Spirito P, Maron BJ, Bonow RO, Epstein SE: Occurrence and significance of progressive left ventricular wall thinning and relative cavity dilatation in patients with hypertrophic cardiomyopathy. Am J Cardiol 59:123–129, 1987.
135. Maron BJ, Isner JM, McKenna WJ: Hypertrophic cardiomyopathy, myocarditis and other myopericardial disease, and mitral valve prolapse: Task Force 3. In Maron BJ, Mitchell JH (eds): 26th Bethesda Conference: Recommendations for Determining Eligibility for Competition in Athletes with Cardiovascular Abnormalities. J Am Coll Cardiol 24:880–885, 1994.
136. Maron BJ, Thompson PD, Puffer JC, et al: Cardiovascular preparticipation screening of competitive athletes: A statement for health professionals from the Sudden Death Committee (Clinical Cardiology) and Congenital Cardiac Defects Committee (Cardiovascular Disease in the Young), American Heart Association. Circulation 94:850–856, 1996.
137. Maron BJ, Roberts WC, Epstein SE: Sudden death in hypertrophic cardiomyopathy: A profile of 78 patients. Circulation 65:1388–1394, 1982.
138. Pelliccia A, Maron BJ, Culasso F, et al: Athlete's heart in women: Echocardiographic characterization of highly trained elite female athletes. JAMA 276:211–215, 1996.
139. Maron BJ: Heart disease and other causes of sudden death in young athletes. Curr Probl Cardiol 23:482–529, 1998.
140. Fananapazir L, McAreavey D: Therapeutic options in patients with obstructive hypertrophic cardiomyopathy and severe drug-refractory symptoms (editorial comment). J Am Coll Cardiol 31:259–264, 1998.
141. Thompson DS, Naqvi N, Juul SM, et al: Effects of propranolol on myocardial oxygen consumption, substrate extraction, and haemodynamics in hypertrophic obstructive cardiomyopathy. Br Heart J 44: 488–498, 1980.

142. Rosing DR, Kent KM, Maron BJ, Epstein SE: Verapamil therapy: A new approach to the pharmacologic treatment of hypertrophic cardiomyopathy: II. Effects on exercise capacity and symptomatic status. Circulation 60:1208–1213, 1979.
143. Bonow RO, Rosing DR, Bacharach SL, et al: Effects of verapamil on left ventricular systolic function and diastolic filling in patients with hypertrophic cardiomyopathy. Circulation 64:787–796, 1981.
144. Lorell BH, Paulus WJ, Grossman W, et al: Modification of abnormal left ventricular diastolic properties by nifedipine in patients with hypertrophic cardiomyopathy. Circulation 64:499–507, 1982.
145. Iwase M, Sotobata I, Takagi S, et al: Effects of diltiazem on left ventricular diastolic behavior in patients with hypertrophic cardiomyopathy: Evaluation with exercise pulsed Doppler echocardiography. J Am Coll Cardiol 9:1099–1105, 1987.
146. Epstein SE, Rosing DR: Verapamil: Its potential for causing serious complications in patients with hypertrophic cardiomyopathy. Circulation 64:437–441, 1981.
147. Rosing DR, Idänpään-Heikkilä U, Maron BJ, et al: Use of calcium-channel blocking drugs in hypertrophic cardiomyoapthy. Am J Cardiol 55(Suppl):185B–195B, 1985.
148. Pollick C: Muscular subaortic stenosis: Hemodynamic and clinical improvement after disopyramide. N Engl J Med 307:997–999, 1982.
149. Sherrid M, Delia E, Dwyer E: Oral disopyramide therapy for obstructive hypertrophic cardiomyopathy. Am J Cardiol 62:1085–1088, 1988.
150. Danziger LH, Horn JR: Disopyramide-induced urinary retention: Report of nine cases and review of the literature. Arch Intern Med 143: 1683–1686, 1983.
151. Fananapazir L, Cannon RO, Tripodi D, Panza JA: Impact of dual-chamber permanent pacing in patients with obstructive hypertrophic cardiomyopathy with symptoms refractory to verapamil and β-adrenergic blocker therapy. Circulation 85:2149–2161, 1992.
152. Jeanrenaud X, Goy JJ, Kappenberger L: Effects of dual-chamber pacing in hypertrophic obstructive cardiomyopathy. Lancet 339:1318–1323, 1992.
153. Slade AKB, Sadoul N, Shapiro L, et al: DDD Pacing in hypertrophic cardiomyopathy: A multicentre clinical experience. Heart 75:44–49, 1996.
154. Nishimura RA, Hayes DL, Ilstrup DM, et al: Effect of dual-chamber pacing on systolic and diastolic function in patients with hypertrophic cardiomyopathy. J Am Coll Cardiol 27:421–430, 1996.
155. Fananapazir L, Epstein ND, Curiel RV, et al: Long-term results of dual-chamber (DDD) pacing in obstructive hypertrophic cardiomyopathy: Evidence for progressive symptomatic and hemodynamic improvement and reduction of left ventricular hypertrophy. Circulation 90:2731–2742, 1994.
156. Nishimura RA, Trusty JM, Hayes DL, et al: Dual-chamber pacing for patients with hypertrophic obstructive cardiomyopathy: A prospective randomized, double-blind cross-over study. J Am Coll Cardiol 29: 435–441, 1997.
157. Knight C, Kurbaan AS, Seggewiss H, et al: Nonsurgical septal reduction for hypertrophic obstructive cardiomyopathy: Outcome in the first series of patients. Circulation 95:2075–2081, 1997.
158. Seggewiss H, Gleichmann U, Faber L, et al: Percutaneous transluminal myocardial ablation (PTSMA) in hypertrophic obstructive cardiomyopathy: Acute results and 3-month follow-up in 25 patients. J Am Coll Cardiol 31:252–258, 1998.
159. Cleland WP: The surgical management of obstructive cardiomyopathy. J Cardiovasc Surg 4:489–491, 1963.
160. Maron BJ, Merrill WH, Freier PA, et al: Long-term clinical course and symptomatic status of patients after operation for hypertrophic subaortic stenosis. Circulation 57:1205–1213, 1978.
161. Williams WG, Wigle ED, Rakowski H, et al: Results of surgery for hypertrophic obstructive cardiomyopathy. Circulation 76(Suppl V): V-104–V-108, 1987.
162. Robbins RC, Stinson EB: Long-term results of left ventricular myotomy and myectomy for obstructive hypertrophic cardiomyopathy. J Thorac Cardiovasc Surg 11:586–594, 1996.
163. McCully RB, Nishimura RA, Tajik AJ, et al: Extent of clinical improvement after surgical treatment of hypertrophic cardiomyopathy. Circulation 94:467–471, 1996.
164. Cooper MM, McIntosh CL, Tucker E, Clark RE: Operation for hypertrophic subaortic stenosis in the aged. Ann Thorac Surg 44: 370–378, 1987.
165. Siegman IL, Maron BJ, Permut LC, et al: Results of operation for coexistent obstructive hypertrophic cardiomyopathy and coronary artery disease. J Am Coll Cardiol 13:1527–1533, 1989.

SECTION

VI

HYPERTENSION

CHAPTER 19

Pathophysiology, Clinical Recognition, Therapy, and Prevention of Hypertension

Susan Wilansky

Hypertension is considered a significant public health issue, largely owing to its prevalence and associated complications. In the United States alone, this condition affects approximately 50 million people and constitutes a major risk factor for the development of cardiovascular, renal, and cerebrovascular disease in industrialized countries worldwide.[1, 2] By definition, hypertension is systolic blood pressure greater than 140 mm Hg and/or diastolic blood pressure greater than 90 mm Hg.

EPIDEMIOLOGY

Of the general population with hypertension, nearly 60% are women.[1] Furthermore, the prevalence of hypertension in women increases significantly after menopause.[3, 4] Staessen and colleagues reported a fourfold increase in the prevalence of hypertension in postmenopausal women compared with that in premenopausal women.[5] Even after adjusting the data for body mass index and age, postmenopausal women were still more than twice as likely to have hypertension as premenopausal women were.[5] Hypertension prevalence among elderly women approaches 75%, according to the Third National Health and Nutrition Examination Survey (NHANES III).[6]

In general, blood pressure tends to increase throughout adult life in both sexes; however, the *patterns* of increase differ between the sexes.[1] Systolic blood pressure rises with age in both men and women,[7] but the absolute increase in women over age 60 is as great as or greater than that in men.[1] Diastolic blood pressure also increases with age but is lower in women than in men at all ages.[1, 2]

PATHOPHYSIOLOGY

Hypertension is classified into two basic types: essential and secondary. Essential hypertension, that is, hypertension having no known etiology, accounts for over 90% of all cases in the United States. Secondary hypertension, or hypertension having a well-defined etiology, comprises the remaining 5 to 10% of cases.[3]

Among the etiologic factors associated with secondary hypertension (Table 19–1), several are more gender-specific. For example, renal artery stenosis due to fibromuscular dysplasia is predominantly a condition of young women.[1–3] It should therefore be considered a possible cause of hypertension in young women (under 40 years of age) who have hypertension or in women whose blood pressure is difficult to control.[1]

Oral contraceptives also can cause hypertension. It appears that the degree of increase in blood pressure is directly related to the dose of estrogen and progestin in the birth control pills.[1–3] The older preparations were associated with a 5% incidence of pill-induced hypertension.[1] The newer, lower-dose pills still confer some increase in risk, but the relative risk (RR) is reportedly lower (RR = 1.8).[1] Overall, the risk of hypertension in women using oral contraceptives increases with prolonged pill use, older user age, and high body mass.[4]

It has recently been demonstrated that hormone replacement therapy (estrogen and/or progesterone) does not cause a significant increase in blood pressure.[8] Essential hypertension is dependent upon a complex interplay of the endocrine system and hemodynamic characteristics. One such characteristic, plasma renin activity, is reportedly lower in hypertensive women than in hypertensive men.[3] Investigators who recently examined this issue in women receiving estrogen replacement therapy concluded that this therapy may modulate plasma renin activity.[9]

Several gender-specific differences in hemodynamic properties also have been described. Premenopausal women tend to have higher heart rates, cardiac indexes, and left ventricular ejection times than men do.[1, 10] Furthermore, women experience a greater rise in blood pressure in response to isometric exercise[8, 10]; this phenomenon is even more pronounced after menopause. Several studies have suggested that hormone replacement therapy may improve vascular function, at least acutely.[1, 11–14] More long-term studies are needed to assess the duration of this effect.

HYPERTENSION AS A CARDIOVASCULAR RISK FACTOR

There are significant gender differences in the risk for all cardiovascular complications of hypertension. The Chicago

Table 19–1. ETIOLOGIC FACTORS ASSOCIATED WITH SECONDARY HYPERTENSION IN WOMEN

Vascular	Endocrine
Renal artery stenosis	Pheochromocytoma
Coarctation of aorta	Cushing's disease
Renal	Thyroid
Polycystic kidney disease	Hyperaldosteronism
Glomerulonephritis	Connective tissue disease
	Lupus

Heart Association Project in Industry[15] demonstrated that at all levels of blood pressure greater than 120/80 mm Hg, the relative risk of death from coronary artery disease was significantly (twofold) higher in white women than in white men, regardless of the extent of blood pressure elevation.

Left ventricular mass is consistently greater in men than in women, even with adjustments for an individual's height, weight, and body mass index.[1, 16–19] Weight is an important factor in the development of left ventricular hypertrophy (LVH) in women,[20] and this effect is magnified in obese women with hypertension. The incidence of LVH in obese women is 58% compared with 29% in the nonobese.[1, 21] LVH in women portends a much greater risk than does LVH in men. The incidence of stroke also is higher in hypertensive women than in hypertensive men (59% versus 39%), as is the incidence of congestive heart failure.[1, 22]

DIAGNOSIS

Table 19–2 outlines appropriate laboratory and other tests to evaluate hypertension in women.

TREATMENT

Lifestyle Changes

Lifestyle modifications have been advocated as the first-line therapeutic approach in women who have mild hypertension. These modifications include weight loss, sodium restriction in salt-sensitive women (those with low plasma-renin activity, the elderly, and black women),[4] and reduction of alcohol intake. Unfortunately, women do not lose weight as effectively as men do.

No gender-specific prospective trials of treatment of hypertension have yet been published. Thus, what currently exists are post hoc analyses of major hypertension trials that have included significant numbers of women.[20, 23] Women have been substantially represented in two such large trials. The Hypertension Detection and Follow-up Program (HDFP)[20] compared the effects of "stepped care" (predetermined protocol treatment to reach the target blood pressure) with those of "usual care" (determined by the primary care physician). In doing so, this trial amassed comprehensive data on the effects of gender and race on hypertension.[2] A major reduction in all-cause mortality rate was reported for black men and women and for white men randomized to receive "stepped care." There was, however, a 2.5% *increase* in the 5-year mortality rate among white women receiving the "stepped-care" protocol.[1, 23] Criticisms of this study maintained that the white women represented a low-risk group that had blood pressures almost comparable with those of the control group.[1] Nevertheless, the Australian Therapeutic Trial, which randomized patients to receive placebo or stepped care, did find a 36% reduction in cardiovascular endpoints.[23] There was a 26% reduction in all endpoints among treated men, whereas women sustained no treatment benefit after control for other cardiac risk factors. Subsequent smaller trials have demonstrated varying reductions of risk for cardiovascular and cerebrovascular events in both men and women.[10]

Table 19–2. LABORATORY TESTS TO EVALUATE HYPERTENSION IN WOMEN

General screening
Blood—electrolytes, BUN, creatinine, lipids, fasting blood sugar levels
Urine—urinalysis
ECG
Screening for secondary causes
Pheochromocytoma—24-hr urinalysis for vanillymandelic acid, catecholamines, and metanephrines
Cushing's disease—AM and PM cortisol; if elevated, dexamethasone suppression test
Thyroid—thyroid panel
Hyperaldosteronism—serum aldosterone, magnetic resonance imaging
Renal artery stenosis—renal angiography, magnetic resonance angiography
Connective tissue disease—antinuclear antibody

Medical Therapy

No large-scale trials have yet been conducted that specifically address drug therapy for hypertension in women. Women and older individuals tend to have lower plasma-renin activity, and theoretically, beta-blockers and angiotensin-converting enzyme (ACE) inhibitors may be less effective in those groups. The Amlodipine Cardiovascular Community Trial (ACCT) Study Group reported better blood pressure control in women than in men.[24] Thiazide diuretics exert a favorable effect on bone mineral density,[1] and their use has been associated with a decrease in the risk of hip fracture.[3] Use of these diuretics may, however, be less appropriate in the elderly, who have lower plasma volumes.[3]

Finally, the side effects of antihypertensive drugs differ between the genders. Among patients receiving thiazides, hyponatremia and hypokalemia are more commonly seen side effects in women,[1, 3] whereas the incidence of gout as a side effect is higher in men. Cough induced by ACE inhibitors is reported to be two to three times more common among women than men.[1, 3, 25] In most cases, however, this did not result in cessation of therapy.[3]

CONCLUSION

In summary, there are significant gender-specific differences in the epidemiology, pathophysiology, and treatment of hypertension. The result of the Women's Health Initiative Study is awaited with great anticipation.

References

1. Hayes SN, Taler SJ: Hypertension in women: Current understanding of gender differences. Mayo Clin Proc 73:157–165, 1998.
2. Reynolds E, Baron RB: Hypertension in women and the elderly: Some puzzling and some unexpected findings of treatment studies. Women and the Elderly 100(4):58–70, 1996.
3. Lewis CE: Characteristics and treatment of hypertension in women: A review of the literature. Am J Med Sci 311(4):193–199, 1996.
4. August P, Oparil S: Hypertension in women. J Clin Endocrinol Metab 84(6):1862–1866, 1999.

5. Staessen J, Bulpitt CJ, Fagard R, et al: The influence of menopause on blood pressure. J Hum Hypertens 3:427–433, 1989.
6. Burt VL, Whelton P, Roccella EJ, et al: Prevalence of hypertension in the US adult population: Results of the Third National Health and Nutrition Examination Survey, 1988–1991. Hypertension 25:305–313, 1995.
7. Messerli FH: Hypertension in special populations. Med Clin North Am 81(6):1335–1345, 1997.
8. Writing Group for the PEPI Trial: Effects of estrogen or estrogen/progestin regimens on heart disease risk factors in postmenopausal women. The Postmenopausal Estrogen/Progestin Interventions (PEPI) Trial. JAMA 273(3):199–208, 1995.
9. Schunkert H, Danser AH, Hense HW, et al: Effects of estrogen replacement therapy on the renin-angiotensin system in postmenopausal women. Circulation 95:39–45, 1997.
10. Hanes DS, Weir MR, Sowers JR: Gender considerations in hypertension pathophysiology and treatment. Am J Med 101(suppl 3A):10S–21S, 1996.
11. Gangar KF, Vyas S, Whitehead M, et al: Pulsatility index in the internal carotid artery in relation to transdermal oestradiol and time since menopause. Lancet 338:839–842, 1991.
12. Mercuro G, Zoncu S, Pilia I, et al: Effects of acute administration of transdermal estrogen on postmenopausal women with systemic hypertension. Am J Cardiol 80:652–655, 1997.
13. Gilligan DM, Badar DM, Panza JA, et al: Effects of estrogen replacement therapy on peripheral vasomotor function in postmenopausal women. Am J Cardiol 75:264–268, 1995.
14. Rajkumar C, Kingwell BA, Cameron JD, et al: Hormonal therapy increases arterial compliance in postmenopausal women. J Am Coll Cardiol 30:350–356, 1997.
15. Stamler J, Stamler R, Neaton JD: Blood pressure, systolic and diastolic, and cardiovascular risks. US population data. Arch Intern Med 153(5):598–615, 1993.
16. Levy D, Garrison RJ, Savage DD, et al: Prognostic implications of echocardiographically determined left ventricular mass in the Framingham Heart Study. N Engl J Med 322:1561–1566, 1990.
17. Hinderliter AL, Light KC, Willis PW IV: Gender differences in left ventricular structure and function in young adults with normal or marginally elevated blood pressure. Am J Hypertens 5:32–36, 1992.
18. Marcus R, Krause L, Weder AB, et al: Sex-specific determinants of increased left ventricular mass in the Tecumseh Blood Pressure Study. Circulation 90:928–936, 1994.
19. Gardin JM, Wagenknecht LE, Anton-Culver H, et al: Relationship of cardiovascular risk factors to echocardiographic left ventricular mass in healthy young black and white adult men and women: The CARDIA study. Circulation 92:380–387, 1995.
20. Hypertension Detection and Follow-up Program Cooperative Group: Five-year finding of the hypertension detection and follow-up program. II. Mortality by race-sex and age. JAMA 242(23):2572–2577, 1979.
21. de Simone G, Devereux RB, Roman MJ, et al: Relation of obesity and gender to left ventricular hypertrophy in normotensive and hypertensive adults. Hypertension 23:600–606, 1994.
22. Levy D, Larson MG, Vasan RS, et al: The progression from hypertension to congestive heart failure. JAMA 275:1557–1562, 1996.
23. Australian National Blood Pressure Management Committee: The Australian therapeutic trial in mild hypertension. Lancet 1(8181):1261–1267, 1980.
24. Kloner RA, Sowers JR, DiBona GF, et al: Sex- and age-related antihypertensive effects of amlodipine. The Amlodipine Cardiovascular Community Trial Study Group. Am J Cardiol 77(9):713–722, 1996.
25. Os I, Bratland B, Dahlof B, et al: Female sex as an important determinant of lisinopril-induced cough. Lancet 339:372, 1992.

SECTION

VII

ARTERIAL DISEASE

CHAPTER 20

Aortic Diseases and Aortic Dissection

20.1 Pathophysiology, Diagnosis, and Medical Treatment

Dianna M. Milewicz and James T. Willerson

ANATOMY

The aorta arises from the heart at the base of the left ventricle, providing the body with oxygenated blood. Anatomically, the aorta may be divided into the following sections: aortic root, ascending aorta, arch, and descending and abdominal aorta. The three sinuses of Valsalva and the aortic valve form the aortic root, which is slightly dilated compared with the ascending aorta. The ascending aorta is a continuation of the root and has a lumen of constant caliber. The tubular structure of the ascending aorta extends 5 to 6 cm from the root to the level of the innominate artery, where it becomes the aortic arch (Fig. 20–1). Three large arterial branches—innominate, left common carotid, and left subclavian—emerge from the aortic arch as it curves to the subclavian artery to become the descending aorta. The diameter of the aortic arch becomes smaller after the origin of the innominate artery. The descending aorta continues from the aortic arch to the diaphragm at the level of intercostal space T12. During its descending course, the thoracic aorta provides blood to multiple small branches and intercostal branches. As it passes through the diaphragm, the aorta becomes the abdominal aorta, which descends through the abdominal cavity, ending at the bifurcation of the iliac arteries. As it descends, the abdominal aorta progressively decreases in size, owing to the number of large branches. At the level of the diaphragm, the aorta is typically 25 mm in diameter; at the iliac bifurcation, the aorta is approximately 15 mm in diameter.

HISTOLOGY

The elastic properties of the aorta are conferred by the structure of the aortic wall, which consists of three layers: the inner layer (the intima), the middle layer (the media), and the outer layer (the adventitia) (Fig. 20–2). The strength of the aorta lies in the media, which is composed of elastic fibers, smooth muscle cells, and collagen. The elastic fibers are organized in concentric plates called lamellae, which are connected by finer elastic fibers (elastin). Collagen and smooth muscle cells are interspersed circumferentially between the elastic lamellae. In the thoracic aorta, the elastin content is greater than the collagen content; in the abdominal aorta, however, the collagen content is greater than the elastin content.[1] The structural properties of elastin and collagen are complementary. Elastin acts as the main load-bearing component and provides elastic recoil; collagen gives powerful but inextensible strength at high loads.

IMAGING OF THE AORTA

Chest radiography provides limited assessment of the thoracic aorta but may be used to detect secondary signs of aortic disease. Chest radiography may show mediastinal widening related to a thoracic aortic aneurysm. Hemothorax, apical pleural capping, and rib fractures may be seen in association with aortic trauma. Abdominal radiography occasionally shows the densely calcified wall of an abdominal aortic aneurysm, leading to the correct diagnosis. Accurate diagnosis of aortic disease typically requires additional imaging by means of angiography, computed tomographic (CT) scanning, magnetic resonance imaging (MRI), or ultrasonography (Fig. 20–3).

Echocardiography and ultrasonography are noninvasive techniques that accurately assess the size and structure of the aorta. Transthoracic echocardiography allows visualization of the aortic root and the ascending aorta. Transesophageal echocardiography provides more details of these structures and of the descending aorta, allowing for assessment of the size and structure of the aorta in the thoracic cavity.

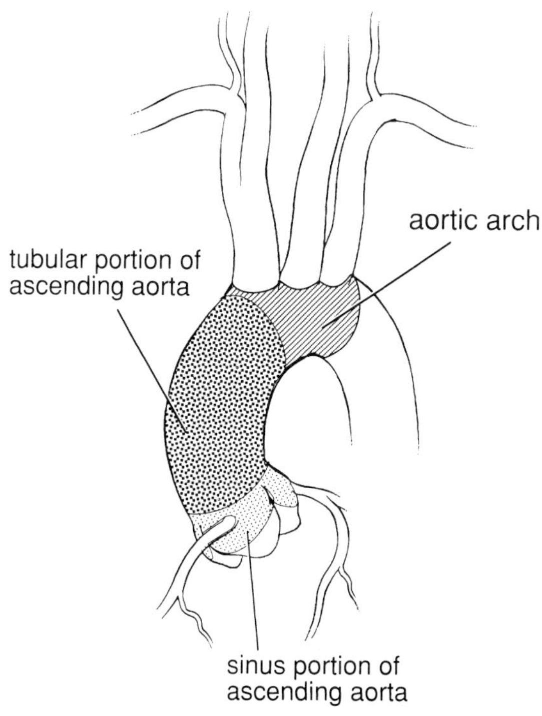

FIGURE 20–1. Anatomy of the aortic root, ascending aorta, and aortic arch.

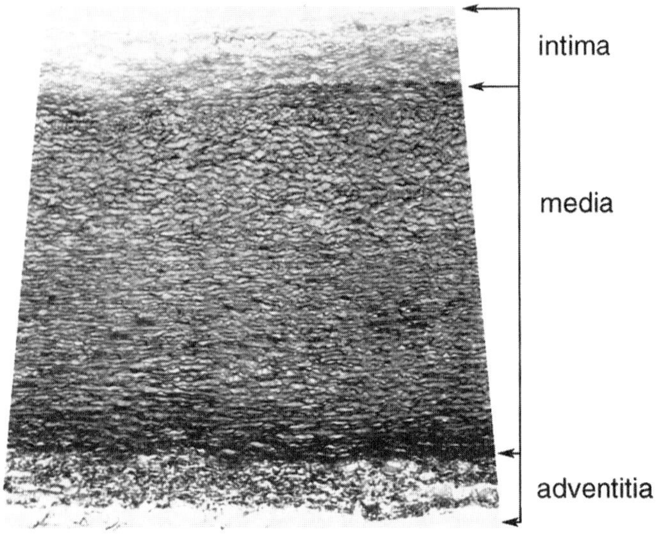

FIGURE 20–2. Histology of the normal aorta.

Studies have shown that transesophageal echocardiography may also efficiently diagnose aortic dissection.[2] Abdominal ultrasonography allows assessment of the abdominal aorta.

MRI and CT scanning are also useful for diagnostic imaging of the aorta. Angiography is the traditional invasive method used for evaluating the aorta, particularly when surgical intervention is anticipated.

DISEASES OF THE AORTA

On the basis of etiology, diseases of the aorta can be categorized into acquired, congenital, and genetic conditions (Table 20–1). Some of the diseases that are categorized as acquired have been shown to involve both genetic and environmental predisposing factors. This discussion focuses on acquired and genetic disorders of the aorta, with particular emphasis on the pathogenesis and progression of these disorders in women.

Acquired Diseases of the Aorta

Aortic Aneurysms

An aortic aneurysm is a pathologic enlargement of the aorta, loosely defined as a 50% increase in the normal aortic diameter. Normal variation in the size of the aorta is based on the patient's body surface area, age, and sex.[3] Variations in the size of the aortic root and ascending aorta, based on body surface area and age, are well established.[4] Nomograms for the infrarenal abdominal aorta, acquired from ultrasono-

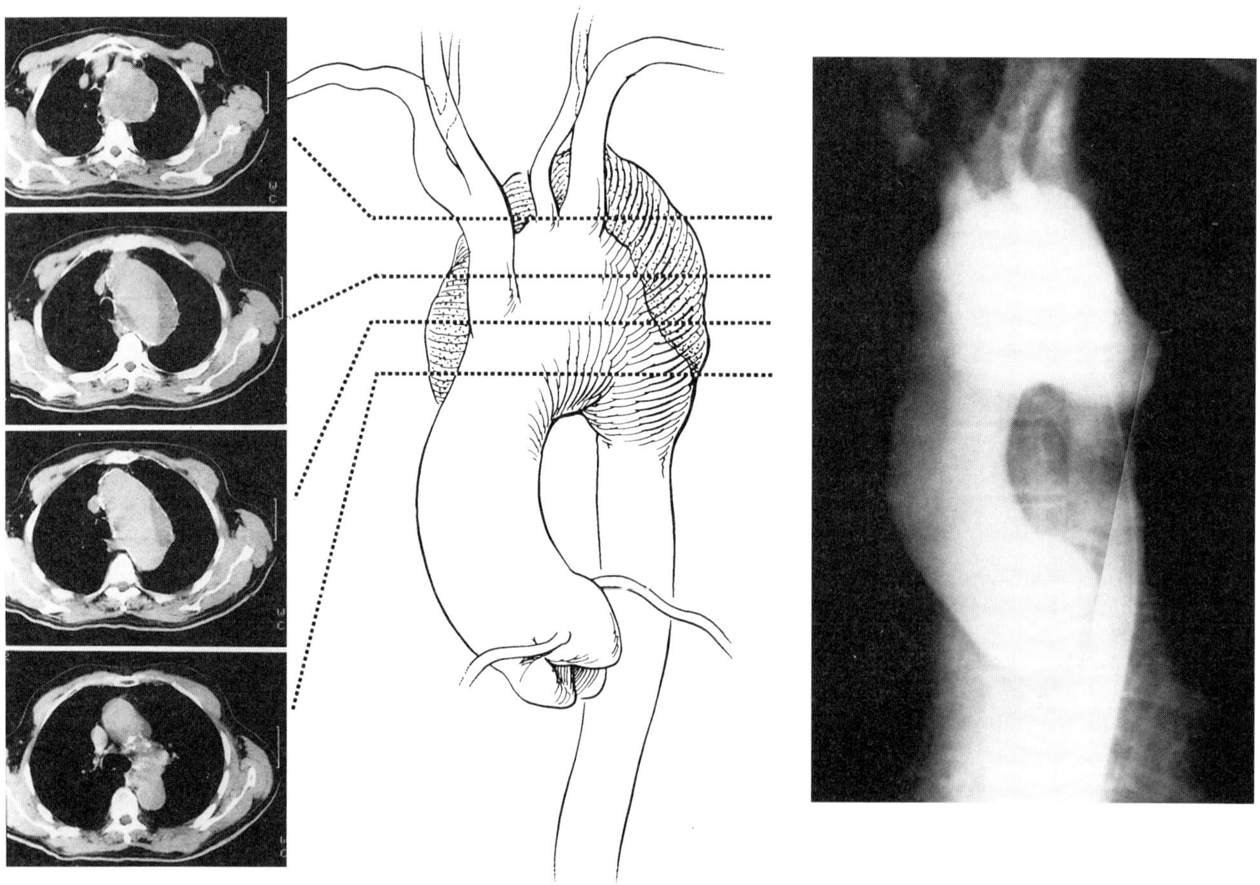

FIGURE 20–3. Computed tomograph (*left*), artist's rendition (*middle*), and aortogram (*right*) of an aneurysm of the ascending aorta, transverse aortic arch, and descending thoracic aorta.

Table 20–1. DISEASES OF THE AORTA

- Acquired
  - Aortic aneurysms
    - Abdominal aortic aneurysms
    - Thoracic aortic aneurysms
  - Aortic dissections
  - Aortitis
    - Takayasu's arteritis
    - Giant cell arteritis
  - Syphilitic aortitis
  - Aortic embolism
  - Aortic bacterial infections
  - Aortic tumors
- Congenital
  - Right-sided aortic arch
  - Anomalous arterial branches
  - Double aortic arches
  - Coarctation
  - Pseudocoarctation
  - Congenital aneurysms
- Genetic
  - Marfan's syndrome
  - Supravalvular aortic stenosis
  - Turner's syndrome

graphic analysis, have been determined from body surface area and sex.[3, 5] Data regarding variations in the size of the descending aorta are sparse.[3]

Classification of aneurysms relies on site, origin, histologic features, and clinical manifestations.[3] Aortic aneurysms are typically classified according to their anatomic location, that is, the ascending thoracic aorta, aortic arch, descending thoracic aorta, thoracoabdominal aorta (involving the descending thoracic aorta as it enters the abdominal cavity), and abdominal or infrarenal aorta. This division is based on the different operative approaches and operative risks associated with aneurysms in these locations.

Aneurysms within the thoracoabdominal aorta are labeled as types I through V (Fig. 20–4). Type II (from the left subclavian artery to below the left renal artery) is the most extensive thoracoabdominal aortic aneurysm and one of the greatest risk factors for the development of neurologic deficit.[6] Previously, type I (from distal to the left subclavian artery to above the renal arteries) was also considered a statistically significant risk factor for a neurologic deficit. However, the operative adjuncts of cerebrospinal fluid drainage and distal aortic perfusion have reduced the risk of a neurologic deficit from 15% to less than 1% for type I thoracoabdominal aortic aneurysms. The less extensive types of aneurysms (III, IV, and V) are considered to involve a relatively low risk. Type III descends from the sixth intercostal space to below the left renal artery; type IV (total abdominal aortic aneurysm), from the 12th intercostal space to the iliac bifurcation; and type V, from the sixth intercostal space to just above the renal arteries.

The pathogenesis of aneurysms varies with the anatomic location. The terms fusiform and saccular describe the configuration of aneurysms. *Fusiform* aneurysms have a stellate shape, gradually changing in size. *Saccular* aneurysms are balloon-shaped and are typically mycotic or syphilitic. *True* aneurysms are dilatations of the entire vessel wall. A *false* aneurysm is created when a full-thickness defect in the aortic wall allows blood to circulate out of the confines of the artery. This circulating blood is contained only by the soft tissues that surround the vessel. *Arteriomegaly* is a diffuse enlargement involving several arterial segments. *Mega-aorta* denotes an aneurysmal formation involving most or all of the aorta. *Ectasia* is characterized by a dilatation that does not exceed 50% of the normal diameter.[7–9]

Abdominal Aortic Aneurysms

Abdominal aortic aneurysms (AAAs) involve the abdominal aorta below the renal arteries. Well-established associated

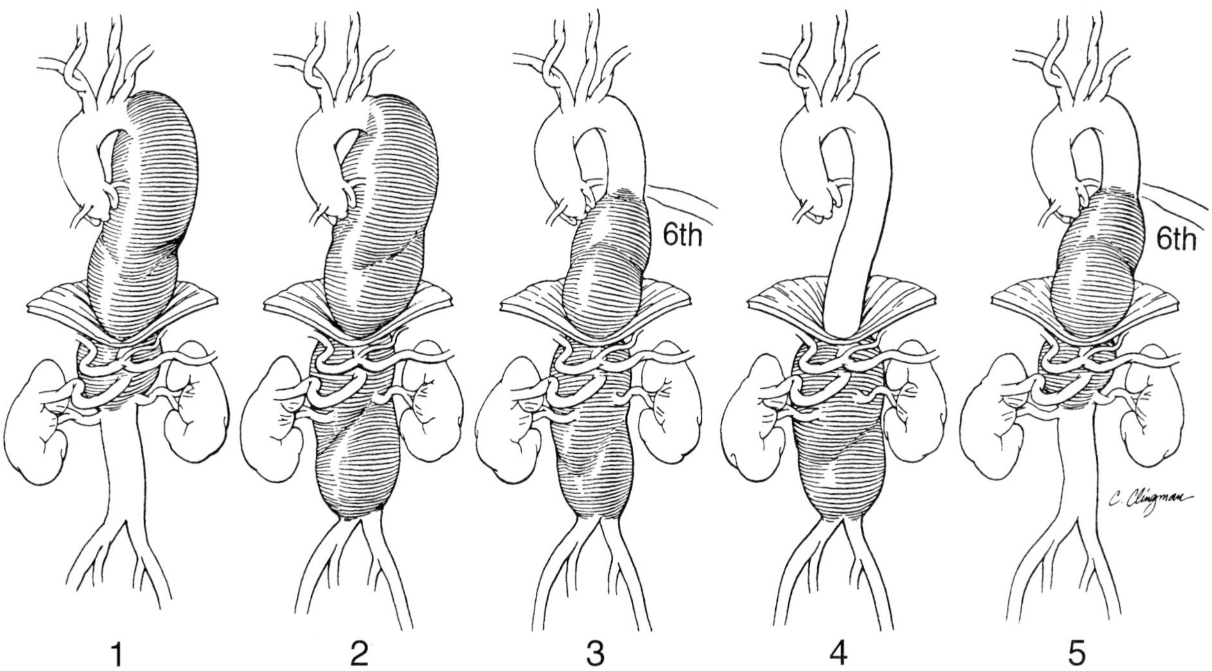

FIGURE 20–4. Thoracoabdominal aortic aneurysm classification, types I through V.

risk factors are male sex, smoking, hypertension, and advanced age. Studies indicate that white men are at highest risk for development of AAAs. The prevalence of these aneurysms depends on the definition of an aneurysm, but most studies define an AAA as an enlargement of the infrarenal aorta to a diameter of greater than 40 mm. Abdominal aortic aneurysms are very unusual in men younger than 55 years. In women, such aneurysms occur 10 to 15 years later than in men.[5, 10–12] In men, the prevalence increases at 55 years and reaches a peak (greater than 10%) after age 80 (when an aneurysm is defined as 30 mm or larger in diameter); in women, the highest prevalence (5%) is in those 85 years and older. Rupture of an AAA is rare in either sex before age 65 years, the median age being 75 years in men and 76 years in women. In women younger than 80 years, the risk of death from rupture of an AAA is one fifth that in men. This fact has led to the recommendation that women younger than 80 years should not be routinely screened for such aneurysms. However, epidemiologic studies show a possible trend toward an increase in the age-standardized incidence of AAAs.[13, 14] Whether this trend reflects a true modification in the incidence or better awareness and diagnosis because of improved imaging techniques is not certain.

The structure of the aortic wall depends primarily on the connective tissue components, mainly elastic fibers and collagen.[1] Abdominal aortic aneurysms are associated with (1) intimal atherosclerosis and medial destruction of the elastic lamellae, (2) medial neovascularization, (3) a decrease in vascular smooth muscle cells, and (4) a chronic immune or inflammatory response. The chronic atherosclerotic process erodes the aortic wall, leading to the formation of a fusiform aneurysm. Most AAAs originate below the renal arteries and extend to involve the aortic bifurcation.

Studies have shown familial aggregation of AAAs and a higher frequency of such lesions in identical twins, indicating that genetic influences play a role.[15–19] Whereas earlier studies showed that familial AAAs tended to affect women,[17, 20] later studies demonstrated higher incidence in men.[19, 21] A genetic etiology is clearly established, but neither the genes that are responsible nor their modes of inheritance have been identified.[11, 19]

Symptoms

The majority of AAAs are asymptomatic and are incidentally detected during imaging studies. Aneurysmal symptoms are usually the result of expansion or rupture. Expansion can result in back, abdominal, or flank pain, including a sense of fullness in the epigastric region. Rupture causes severe pain and rapid circulatory collapse.

Examination

The retroperitoneal location of the aorta can make examination difficult, particularly in obese patients. With the patient supine, the knees flexed, and the abdominal musculature relaxed, the abdominal aorta should be palpable. The transverse diameter can be estimated by straddling the aorta with both hands, but this maneuver should be performed with extreme caution. Occasionally, a bruit is heard over the aneurysm. The peripheral pulses also should be palpated, because many patients with AAAs have peripheral occlusive disease. Ultrasonography of the abdomen is a sensitive test for confirming the presence of an abdominal aneurysm.

Treatment

The natural history of an AAA involves expansion and rupture, which are the basis for surgical treatment. Control of hypertension may be valuable in retarding the progression of aneurysmal dilatation. Aneurysms measuring more than 5 cm must be surgically repaired. Otherwise, the 5-year risk of rupture is 25%.[22] Rupture typically occurs into the retroperitoneal space, although some aneurysms rupture into the peritoneal cavity.

Controversy exists regarding the treatment of asymptomatic aneurysms that are 4 to 5 cm in diameter. If repair of such an aneurysm is postponed, a surveillance program should be undertaken, with follow-up ultrasonography every 6 months. Symptomatic or rapidly expanding AAAs should be surgically repaired, as should those that present with complications (distal embolism, thrombosis, fistulization, or distal ischemia secondary to associated occlusive disease).

Thoracic Aortic Aneurysms

At the turn of the century, syphilitic aortitis, with subsequent aneurysm formation involving the thoracic aorta, caused thoracic aortic aneurysms (TAAs) to be more common. However, with the later advent of an effective treatment for syphilis, along with improved control of hypertension, the incidence of TAAs decreased, so that it is currently estimated to be one third that of AAAs. In 1982, Bickerstaff and colleagues[23] reported that the prevalence of TAAs in Rochester, Minnesota, was 5.9/100,000 person-years. Those aneurysms involved the ascending aorta in 52% of cases, the descending thoracic aorta in 37%, and the aortic arch in 11%. In contrast to AAAs, TAAs affect women almost as commonly as men. Studies have shown a male-female ratio of between 1:1 and 2:1. The average age of patients with TAAs tends to be younger than that of patients with AAAs, being 64 years for men and 67 years for women.[24]

With TAAs, the histopathology is more diverse than with AAAs. Atherosclerosis is the cause of many descending TAAs and some ascending aortic aneurysms; the pathogenesis and risk factors are similar to those for AAAs. Many TAAs that involve the ascending aorta involve a pathologic lesion termed *idiopathic cystic medial necrosis*.[23] This lesion is characterized by degeneration of the aortic media with deterioration of the elastic tissue. The loss of elastic fibers is associated with higher quantities of basophilic ground substances that on microscopic examination appear to be cyst-like structures. These pathologic changes in the aortic media can be observed in nonaneurysmal elderly individuals or those with long-standing hypertension but are more severe and more extensive in individuals with aortic aneurysms or dissections.[25]

Cystic medial necrosis is the pathologic lesion observed in patients with Marfan's syndrome, which raises the risk of aneurysms or dissections involving the ascending aorta.

Interestingly, certain congenital abnormalities are associated with cystic medial necrosis of the ascending aorta, including bicuspid aortic valve and coarctation of the aorta. Therefore, these lesions may represent related developmental defects involving the cardiovascular system. Aortitis or syphilis is found in a minority of cases.

Clinical Manifestation

Like AAAs, many TAAs are asymptomatic and are identified only during routine imaging (Fig. 20–5). The clinical features of these aneurysms are due to compression, distortion, erosion of surrounding structures, dissection, or rupture. The presenting symptoms are diffuse and include wheezing, hemoptysis, dyspnea, dysphagia, hoarseness, and segmental pneumonitis. Pain is rarely associated with TAAs; when it occurs, it often heralds rupture or dissection of the aneurysm. Aortic valve insufficiency can occur if the aneurysm distorts the aortic annulus.

Higher rates of aneurysmal expansion are seen either in patients with larger aortic diameters (greater than 5 cm) or in those who smoke.[26] Rupture of an aneurysm causes a severe, substernal, knifelike pain that radiates to the back. Rupture also leads to rapid circulatory collapse. The mortality and morbidity associated with rupture of a TAA are high.[27, 28]

Diagnosis

On chest radiographs, a TAA is often evident as a widening of the mediastinum. More accurate means of imaging the aorta are usually needed to assess the size and extent of the aneurysm. Transthoracic echocardiography can be used to assess the ascending thoracic aorta. Transesophageal echocardiography can give better images of the descending thoracic aorta. Both CT scanning and MRI are adequate for assessing the entire thoracic aorta. Before surgical repair of a TAA, angiography is usually necessary to determine the size and extent of the aneurysm.

Treatment

Surgical repair is usually necessary for patients with TAAs (see Chapters 27.2 and 27.3).

Aortic Dissection

Aortic dissection is caused by a sudden tear in the aortic intima, which diverts the blood stream into the aortic media. Blood flows through the media, along the aortic wall, in a course parallel to that of normal blood flow, causing the inner and outer layers of the vessel to separate. Dissection can lead to weakening of the outer wall, which can result in

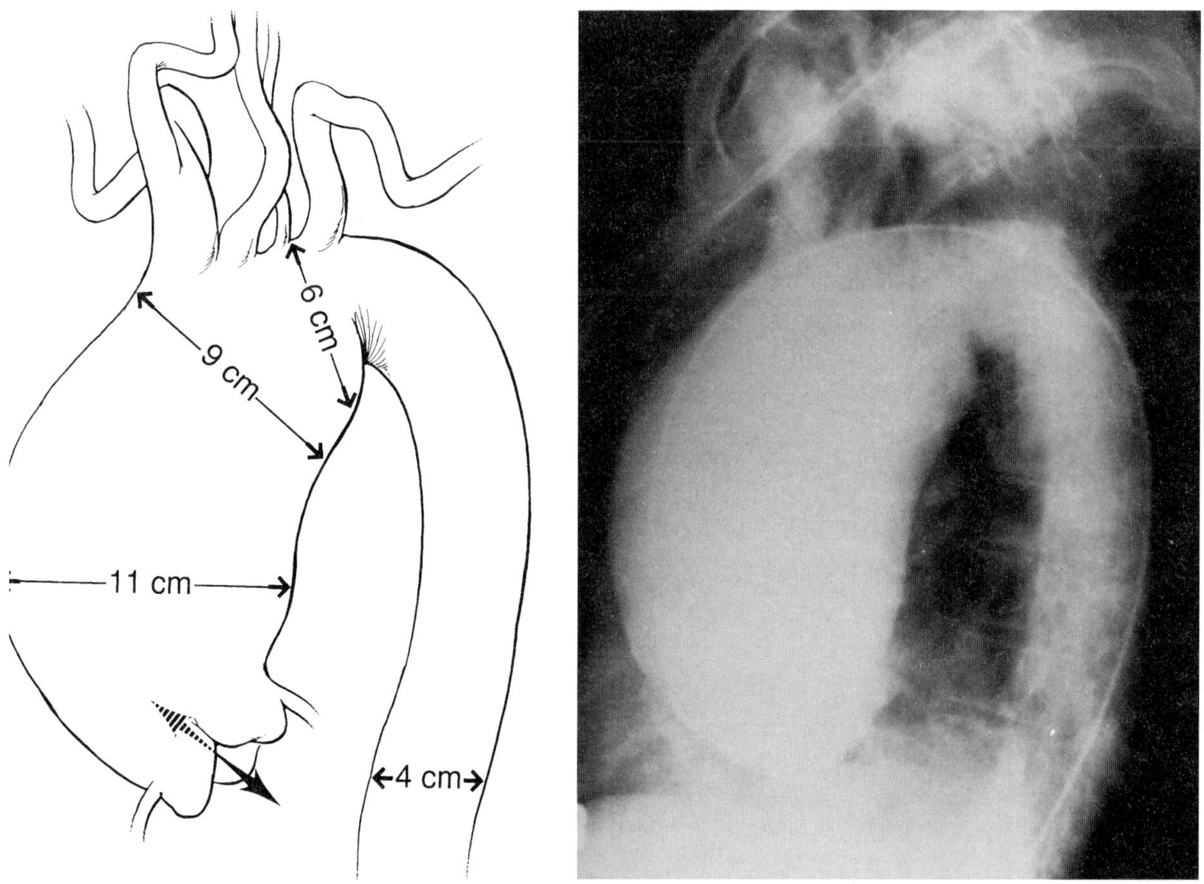

FIGURE 20–5. Drawing and aortogram of an aneurysm of the ascending aorta and aortic arch. The descending thoracic aorta has a normal diameter.

rupture, aneurysm formation, and occlusion of vessels that branch from the aorta (causing a variety of symptoms); alternatively, dissection can lead to disruption of the aortic valve, which results in aortic regurgitation. Most aortic dissections originate in one of two locations (Fig. 20–6).[29]

According to a classification system originally proposed by DeBakey and colleagues,[30] aortic dissections are designated types I through III, depending on the site of the intimal tear and the extent of the dissection.[30] In types I and II, the intimal tear involves the ascending aorta, usually immediately above the aortic valve. The dissection extends distal to the ascending portion in a type I dissection but is limited to the ascending aorta in a type II dissection. In type III dissections, the intimal tear involves the descending thoracic aorta and usually occurs immediately after the origin of the left subclavian artery. The dissection extends retrograde into the ascending aorta in type IIIa and antegrade in type IIIb. In contrast to the entry tear, a reentry tear is identified far less frequently. In half of cases, reentry occurs in the aorta, and in the other half, in a peripheral artery. In the Stanford classification system, DeBakey type I and type II dissections are grouped together because they both involve the ascending aorta; proximal (type A) dissections involve the ascending aorta and distal (type B) dissections involve the descending aorta (corresponding to DeBakey type III).[31]

The most common type of dissection is DeBakey type I, which occurs in more than half of cases. The remaining dissections are equally divided between types II and III. Systemic hypertension is present in approximately half of patients with dissecting aneurysms; most patients with type III dissections have systemic hypertension.[32] Eighty percent of patients with aortic dissections are hypertensive. Furthermore, the incidence of cystic medial necrosis is higher in hypertensive than in nonhypertensive people.[29] Men are more commonly affected than women, in an approximately 2:1 ratio. Dissection typically occurs in persons in their early 60s, although it can occur in young adults and teenagers. Because aortic dissection often results in sudden death, its true prevalence is difficult to determine. If an autopsy is not performed, many deaths caused by aortic dissection are attributed to heart attack or arrhythmia.

Etiology

In dissection, histopathology of the aorta shows medial degeneration (cystic medial necrosis) and, in many cases, loss

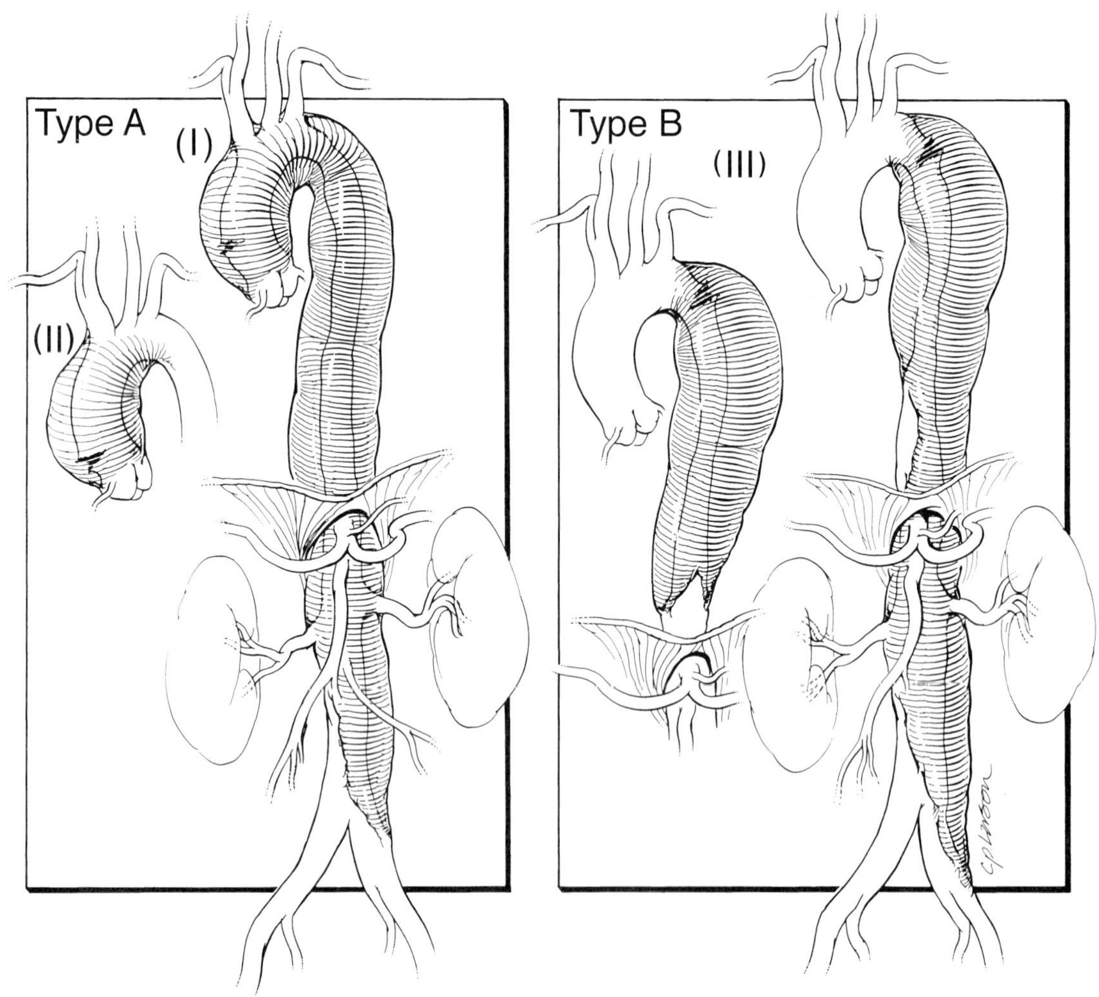

FIGURE 20–6. Classification of aortic dissections. Type A (types I and II) originates in the ascending aorta; type B (type III) arises in the descending aorta.

of elastic fibers and smooth muscle cells, particularly in the ascending aorta. Although these changes could also be seen in the nonaneurysmal aging aorta and in individuals with longstanding hypertension, medial degeneration is often more extensive and severe in persons with aortic dissection. Medial degeneration is observed in ascending aortic dissection but rarely in type III dissection. By contrast, extensive aortic atherosclerosis is seen in most type III dissections but less commonly in types I and II.

Congenital bicuspid aortic valve is also associated with a higher risk of aortic dissection.[32] In addition, dissection tends to occur at a younger age in people with bicuspid aortic valves than in those with tricuspid aortic valves. The disorder associated with bicuspid aortic valve is medial degeneration, leading some researchers to suggest that bicuspid aortic valve and medial degeneration represent a common developmental defect of the cardiovascular system. People with a bicuspid aortic valve have a ninefold greater risk of aortic dissection than those with a tricuspid aortic valve.

Individuals with either Marfan's or Turner's syndrome are at increased risk of aortic dissection, as described later. Additionally, individuals with a family history of aortic dissection are themselves at higher risk of dissection.

Clinical Findings

Acute type I or II (type A) aortic dissections of the proximal aorta should be treated as surgical emergencies to avoid rupture into the pericardium and subsequent cardiac tamponade. Before surgical treatment is initiated, acute type III (type B) dissections can be treated medically, the objective being to correct hypertension and stabilize the patient's condition.[33] Of note, whereas acute type I or II dissections may rupture in a matter of hours, type III dissections essentially follow the pattern of nondissecting aneurysms, having a median period of 1 to 3 years.[34] Antihypertensive treatment, however, does not obviate the need for close monitoring of affected patients. The hospital mortality associated with primary medical treatment remains relatively high, and a substantial percentage of patients require surgery during the initial hospitalization. The main causes of death in both medical and surgical groups are rupture and abdominal malperfusion.

Symptoms

In the vast majority of patients with an acute aortic dissection, the presenting symptom is severe pain with an acute onset.[35, 36] With dissection of the ascending aorta, the pain is typically in the anterior chest and penetrates from front to back (in the midscapular region). Conversely, the posterior portion of the chest, usually the interscapular area, is the major site of pain with type III dissections. The pain can be migratory, corresponding to the path of the dissection. Other, less common symptoms are syncope, stroke, and congestive heart failure with or without associated chest pain. A very small percentage of patients (less than 5%) present with painless dissection. At presentation, other rare findings are hemoptysis, oliguria, Horner's syndrome, stroke, bowel ischemia, paraplegia, limb ischemia, and acute myocardial infarction (MI).

Physical Findings

Patients with distal dissections are likely to be hypertensive at presentation. Conversely, patients with proximal dissections are more likely to be initially hypotensive, perhaps because of cardiac tamponade or interpleural or intraperitoneal rupture. Approximately half of patients with proximal dissection have pulse deficits involving the brachiocephalic vessels, most commonly the right carotid or subclavian arteries. With proximal dissections, a murmur indicating aortic regurgitation can be heard if the dissection distorts the aortic valve. Neurologic deficits can occur, including cerebrovascular accidents, ischemic peripheral neuropathy, and disturbances of consciousness.

Diagnosis

Imaging of the aorta is needed when a dissection is suspected. Standard transthoracic echocardiography may be useful for excluding a proximal dissection of the aorta. Other imaging techniques, such as transesophageal echocardiography, CT scanning (with contrast injection), MRI, and angiography, are more powerful diagnostic tools that are needed to identify a type III dissection or to determine the extent of a proximal dissection.[2]

Treatment

In patients with an acute dissection, blood pressure needs to be lowered immediately.[37] Oxygen and intravenous fluid should be given, and an arterial line should be started. The patient should be monitored continuously in an intensive care setting. Medical therapy is directed at decreasing the force and velocity of myocardial contractility. The blood pressure should be lowered to 100 mm Hg (systolic) with intravenous nitroprusside, beta blockers, or a combined alpha-beta–adrenergic blocker. When no contraindication exists, beta blockers should be given to decrease the heart rate and the velocity of the pulse increase in the arteries.

Chronic dissection is believed to be the stabilized consequence of an acute dissection. Although chronic dissection is not as urgent as the acute form, complications such as aneurysm formation and rupture remain serious possibilities. The 30-day surgical mortality for this type of aortic dissection is 5% to 10%, and the stroke rate for chronic type I or II dissection is 4%.

Operations for acute type III dissection are performed selectively and only if complications arise. Indications for surgery are persistent pain, aneurysmal dilatation (5 cm or greater), end organ (kidney, bowel) or limb ischemia, bleeding from the aneurysm, and evidence of retrograde dissection to the ascending aorta. Cases that do not meet these criteria are treated with aggressive medical therapy aimed at achieving the lowest systolic blood pressure that can be tolerated. Chest radiographs are obtained daily and CT scans weekly during hospitalization. Patients in stable condition are discharged after 10 to 14 days. At the follow-up visit, patients are urged to undergo quarterly CT scans for the first year, semiannual CT scans for the next 2 years, and annual CT scans thereafter. Any changes in symptoms or aortic diameter are considered indications for surgical reevaluation.

PREGNANCY

Pregnancy is associated with an increased risk of aortic dissection, although this complication rarely occurs. Early studies indicated that approximately half of the aneurysms in women of childbearing age occurred during pregnancy. More recent studies, however, suggest that the causal relationship between pregnancy and acute aortic dissection has been markedly overestimated and that most women younger than 40 years are not pregnant at the time of acute aortic dissection.[38] Pregnancy-related acute dissection occurs most commonly during the third trimester, although there are reports of dissections occurring during delivery or postpartum.

Medical treatment of aortic dissection in pregnancy is the same as for any other form of acute dissection.[38] The pain should be relieved with narcotics, and the blood pressure and pulse pressure should be controlled with intravenous hydralazine and a beta-adrenergic blocking agent. Hydralazine should be used instead of sodium nitroprusside because of possible adverse fetal effects related to the cyanide and thiocyanate toxicity of nitroprusside. Nitroprusside itself should be used only in refractory cases. If the fetus can survive, immediate delivery by means of cesarean section with the aid of epidural anesthesia is generally indicated. If the fetus is too premature for delivery, surgical repair can be attempted; in general, however, fetuses tolerate cardiopulmonary bypass poorly, even with short bypass times and high flow rates.[39]

Aortitis

Takayasu's Arteritis

Takayasu's arteritis (pulseless disease) is a chronic inflammatory arteritis of unknown etiology that primarily affects young women and results in stenosis and aneurysm formation in the aorta and its major branches. Takayasu's arteritis was first described in Japanese women and is more prevalent in Asia than in Western countries.[40] The estimated prevalence in the United States is 2.6 cases per 1 million person-years, and more than 90% of the affected individuals are women. The median age at onset is 25 years.[41, 42]

ETIOLOGY

Although the specific etiology of Takayasu's arteritis is unknown, the bulk of evidence favors an autoimmune etiology. Early in the disease, histopathologic examination of the aorta and arteries shows granulomatous panarteritis and transmural inflammation. The cellular infiltrate, seen primarily in the media, consists of lymphocytes and plasma cells. The late stage of the disease is characterized by progressive intimal and adventitial fibrosis and extensive medial scarring, which produces stenosis of the affected vessel. A link between Takayasu's arteritis and HLA antigens, specifically HLA-B52 and HLA-B39, has been reported.[43] Later studies have determined that anti–endothelial cell antibodies are frequently present in patients with Takayasu's arteritis, perhaps playing a role in the pathogenesis of the disease.[44]

CLINICAL MANIFESTATIONS

The symptoms of Takayasu's arteritis reflect both the arteritis and the systemic inflammatory state. Patients often experience weight loss, headache, fatigue, arthralgia, myalgia, and fever. The arteritis can lead to vascular insufficiency or localized tenderness over the affected vessels, especially the carotid arteries. Systemic hypertension often occurs because of renal artery stenosis. Takayasu's arteritis is primarily characterized by progressive stenosis, but fusiform or saccular arterial aneurysms can occur.

The disease can also involve the parenchyma of various organs.[45] Specific glomerular lesions include mesangial proliferative, membranoproliferative, crescentic glomerulonephritis, and amyloidosis. Dermatologic manifestations include erythema nodosum, a facial lupus rash, and erythema induratum. Rarely, interstitial lung disease, idiopathic ulcerative colitis, rheumatoid arthritis, and polymyositis are associated with Takayasu's arteritis.

DIAGNOSIS

The American College of Rheumatology has identified six major criteria for the diagnosis of Takayasu's arteritis.[46] Arteriography is necessary to confirm the diagnosis and to define the disease's extent. Classification of the disease is based on the extent of angiographic involvement.[47, 48] In type I, only the aortic arch and its branches are involved. In type II, the disease involves both the descending aorta and the abdominal segments. Type III combines the first two types. In type IV, there is pulmonary artery involvement.

TREATMENT

Most patients with Takayasu's arteritis require medical therapy, but a minority have a monophasic, self-limiting disease. Immunosuppressive treatment with glucocorticoids, alone or in combination with a cytotoxic agent, usually induces remission.[49] Approximately half of patients in whom remission is achieved have a relapse. The mortality is low, but the morbidity is substantial.

Giant Cell Arteritis

Giant cell arteritis, or temporal arteritis, is a systemic disease that occurs predominantly in elderly women, is more common in white women than African American women, and is rare in Hispanic women.[50] The average age at diagnosis is 69 years, and approximately twice as many women as men are affected.[51] The main manifestation of the disorder is granulomatous arteritis involving the temporal vessels. The typical triad of presenting symptoms comprises temporal headache, malaise, and fever. The superficial temporal arteries can be so inflamed and swollen that affected individuals cannot wear a hat or comb the hair. Claudication of the jaw is also common and suggests the diagnosis. Amaurosis is the most frequent ischemic complication and the main cause of permanent disability.[52] Premonitory symptoms include amaurosis fugax, diplopia, partial field defects, and blurry vision, which, if left untreated, can lead to permanent visual defects in a substantial number of patients. Up to 15% of patients with giant cell arteritis experience visual impairment. Other constitutional symptoms are night sweats, malaise, anorexia, weight loss, and myalgia. Several studies have shown that the survival rate is not lower in patients with giant cell arteritis than in the age-matched general population.

Extracranial vessel involvement typically affects medium-sized arteries but can also affect the aorta.[51,53] Aortic complications include aneurysm and dissection. A review of 72 cases of aortic involvement in patients with temporal arteritis indicated that the ascending aorta and aortic arch were more frequently involved than the abdominal aorta.[51] It is difficult to determine the true incidence of aortic involvement, because arteriosclerotic cardiovascular complications also occur in elderly people without giant cell arteritis; however, the incidence of aortic involvement is estimated to range from 3% to 15%. Some patients with giant cell arteritis also experience limb girdle pain and stiffness characteristic of polymyalgia rheumatica.

Etiology

The etiology of giant cell arteritis is poorly understood. The underlying pathologic alteration is granulomatous inflammation of the media. An inflammatory infiltrate that includes eosinophils, plasma cells, and other mononuclear cells is present.[54] The inflammatory nature of the arterial lesions strongly implicates the arterial wall as the site of a local cell-mediated immune response. Familial aggregation and racial differences in disease incidence suggest that a predisposition for giant cell arteritis is genetically determined. This condition has not been consistently linked with any class I HLA antigen but is clearly associated with HLA-DR4, the frequency of which is increased twofold in patients with giant cell arteritis.

Diagnosis

A markedly elevated sedimentation rate (usually 50 mm/h or higher) reflects the active inflammatory process in affected individuals. A normochromic, normocytic anemia is often present. The diagnosis of giant cell arteritis is confirmed by biopsy of the temporal artery or another involved artery.

Treatment

Treatment of giant cell arteritis involves administration of high-dose steroids. Reductions in symptoms and the sedimentation rate are useful indicators that the disease has decreased in activity. The steroid dosage can be tapered off when the active inflammatory process begins to wane.

Cardiovascular Syphilis

In the past, syphilitic aortitis was a major cause of cardiovascular death. However, with the advent of an effective treatment, syphilitic aortitis is now rarely observed. Syphilis is a systemic disease caused by *Treponema pallidum.* Patients may present with symptomatic primary, secondary, or tertiary manifestations, or an asymptomatic infection may be detected by means of serologic testing during the latent stage.[55–57] Cardiovascular complications occur in approximately 10% of patients with untreated syphilis and appear long after the initial infection, usually at the end of a 10- to 25-year latent period. Syphilitic aortitis results from direct infection of the aortic media by *T. pallidum.* In "uncomplicated" cases, there are no complicating syphilitic lesions, that is, aneurysm, insufficiency, and ostial stenosis.[58] Subsequent inflammation leads to scarring and destruction of the musculoelastic medial tissue. These changes are found in the ascending aorta and extend distally for varying distances. At autopsy, the intimal surface of the ascending thoracic aorta demonstrates wrinkles, ridges, and pearly plaques characteristic of syphilitic aortitis. This weakening leads to the formation of aortic aneurysms, which usually involve the ascending aorta and are saccular. The aortic valve can be infected by *T. pallidum,* leading to aortic insufficiency. Syphilitic aortitis can also lead to coronary ostial stenosis. Serologic test results are negative in 15% to 30% of patients with syphilitic aortitis, making diagnosis difficult.[59] Individuals who die of cardiovascular syphilis most often succumb to rupture of an ascending TAA.

Genetic Diseases of the Aorta

A limited number of single-gene disorders affect the aorta. Because these syndromes are inherited in an autosomal dominant manner, men and women usually are affected equally. Turner's syndrome, however, is a chromosome aneuploidy that occurs only in women and specifically affects the aorta.

Marfan's Syndrome

Marfan's syndrome is an autosomal dominant disorder that has pleiotropic manifestations involving the skeletal, ocular, and cardiovascular systems. The skeletal manifestations are outwardly apparent in people with Marfan's syndrome. Such manifestations include arachnodactyly (spider-like fingers), dolichostenomelia (long, thin extremities), scoliosis, pectus deformities (pectus excavatum and pectus carinatum), pes planus, and a highly arched palate. Ocular manifestations include lens dislocation, myopia, and, rarely, retinal detachment. Cardiovascular complications are life-threatening and manifest primarily as ascending TAAs or dissections. If left untreated, the aortic complications will shorten the patient's life expectancy. Marfan's syndrome occurs in approximately

1 in 10,000 persons, affecting men and women equally, in all ethnic groups. The condition results from mutations in the fibrillin-1 gene (*FBN1*), which encodes a component of the elastic fiber system in the extracellular matrix.

The major cardiovascular complications associated with Marfan's syndrome are ascending aortic aneurysms and dissections. Aortic involvement is characterized by progressive enlargement of the ascending aorta.[60, 61] This enlargement typically begins with dilatation of the aorta at the sinus of Valsalva, which is often enlarged in children with Marfan's syndrome.[62] The rate of progression of aortic dilatation varies among affected individuals; therefore, careful monitoring of the aortic root with transthoracic echocardiography is recommended. Because nomograms are available for the aortic root diameter (based on age and body surface area), determining whether an individual has a dilated aortic root can be easily done.[4] Transesophageal echocardiography, CT scanning, and MRI can also be used to monitor the size of the proximal aorta.[63, 64] Patients with Marfan's syndrome rarely present with involvement of the descending thoracic aorta. Initially, monitoring can be done annually, but as the aorta enlarges, the frequency of monitoring should be increased.

Aortic regurgitation that occurs because of the distortion of the aortic annulus resulting from dilatation of the root is usually not a major complication until the aortic root is larger than 60 mm. The risk of dissection rises as the aorta progressively dilates but is low until the aortic root reaches 50 to 55 mm in diameter. For this reason, surgical repair of the ascending aorta is recommended when the aorta reaches 55 mm. Type I dissections (DeBakey classification) are the most common, originating in the ascending aorta and extending to involve the descending aorta. Fewer than 10% of patients with Marfan's syndrome present with type III dissections that originate distal to the left subclavian artery and involve the descending aorta (sparing the ascending aorta).

To decrease the stress on the proximal aorta, it is recommended that individuals with Marfan's syndrome avoid contact sports and isometric exercises. Use of beta-adrenergic blocking agents has been proposed because their negative chronotropic and inotropic actions slow the progressive enlargement of the aortic root. A randomized trial examining the prophylactic use of beta-adrenergic blocking agents in adolescents and adults with classic Marfan's syndrome and mild to moderate dilatation of the aorta showed that these agents slow the rate of aortic dilatation and reduce the development of aortic complications in some patients.[65] A retrospective study also found a reduced rate of aortic root dilatation among children and adolescents.[66] Therefore, medical treatment with beta-adrenergic blocking agents appears to slow the rate of aortic dilatation.

Medical and surgical therapy for aortic complication has had a significant impact on the survival of patients with Marfan's syndrome. A life expectancy study published in 1972, before medical treatment and composite graft repair became widespread, indicated that the average age at death for patients with this disorder was 32 years.[67] Later studies have shown that the life expectancy has improved and is consistent with the greater survival of this population. Patients with Marfan's syndrome are now living 9 to 14 years longer than similar patients did 30 years ago, and there is no significant difference between the survival rates of men and women.[68, 69]

Pregnancy and Marfan's Syndrome

Pregnancy in patients with Marfan's syndrome increases the risk of cardiovascular complications. Pregnancy is known to impose substantial cardiovascular stress and to raise the risk of dissection. Although the literature contains a number of case reports of cardiovascular complications in women with Marfan's syndrome during pregnancy, a prospective study of pregnancy outcomes indicates that women with aortic root diameters less than 40 mm have favorable maternal and fetal outcomes.[70] The current recommendation is that a woman with Marfan's syndrome consider having children before the aortic root diameter exceeds 40 mm. In addition, transthoracic echocardiography should be performed every 6 to 10 weeks during pregnancy and immediately postpartum. Delivery should be achieved by means of the least hemodynamically stressful method. The higher risk of dissection persists for 8 weeks after delivery, until the circulatory changes associated with pregnancy resolve. The use of beta-adrenergic blocking agents during pregnancy has been recommended, but the teratogenic risk of these agents has not been established.

Supravalvular Aortic Stenosis

Supravalvular aortic stenosis is an autosomal dominant vascular disorder in which congenital narrowing of the ascending aorta occurs at the sinotubular ridge. Males and females are equally affected, and the incidence of the disorder is estimated to be 1 in 25,000 live births. Although most patients are asymptomatic, the lesion is usually progressive. In addition, other arteries, including the pulmonary artery, are often affected.[71] The disorder usually occurs as a discrete hourglass deformity but also may consist of diffuse hypoplasia of the entire ascending aorta. Occasional complications include bacterial endocarditis, aortic aneurysm, MI, and sudden death. A genetic defect that contributes to supravalvular aortic stenosis is a mutation in the gene encoding elastin on the long arm of chromosome 7.

Familial Thoracic Aortic Aneurysms and Dissections (Erdheim's Cystic Medial Necrosis)

The literature contains reports of families that have multiple members with thoracic aortic aneurysms, dissection, or both in the absence of manifestations of a genetic syndrome (such as Marfan's syndrome). Later reports contain more thorough clinical information and delineate a condition involving familial thoracic aortic aneurysms and dissection. In 1967, Hanley and Jones[72] described dissecting aortic aneurysms in two sisters and the son of one of the sisters. None of the affected individuals had any stigmata of Marfan's syndrome. Subsequently, a number of similar cases have been reported.[73–76] The features of this condition include dominant inheritance, some families showing male-to-male inheritance indicative of an autosomal gene defect.

This familial condition can present as asymptomatic enlargement of the aortic root or as acute dissection. In some cases, the dissection occurs without evidence of aortic root dilatation. Other systems do not appear to be affected by this condition; specifically, there is no evidence of a generalized connective tissue abnormality as is observed in Marfan's syndrome and Ehlers-Danlos syndrome type IV. Systemic hypertension may be present in affected people in some families but is notably absent in others.[73, 75] In these families, the aortic disease associated with the disorder is similar to the aortic disease found in Marfan's syndrome or the aged aorta. Histologic examination of the aorta typically shows disruption of elastic fibers and medial necrosis, with increased mucopolysaccharide deposition. The genetic defect responsible for familial thoracic aortic aneurysms and dissection is not known.

Turner's Syndrome

Turner's syndrome is a chromosomal syndrome in which one of the two X chromosomes is missing, and the karyotype is 45,X. Individuals with Turner's syndrome are girls who have a proportionately short stature, sexual infantilism with ovarian dysgenesis, webbing of the neck, a broad and shieldlike chest, and cubitus valgus. Cardiovascular anomalies occur in 20% to 44% of affected patients, the most common abnormalities being coarctation of the aorta and bicuspid aortic valve.[58, 77] Additionally, numerous case reports in the literature describe women with Turner's syndrome who have dilated or dissecting aneurysms involving the ascending thoracic aorta.[78–80] In some of these cases, there is associated hypertension. Cystic medial necrosis is typically found on histopathologic examination of the aorta. Aortic dissection can occur in these patients in the absence of either coarctation of the aorta or a bicuspid aortic valve. A high rate of unrecognized aortic root dilatation has been observed in patients with Turner's syndrome (8.8%).[79, 81] Therefore, patients with the disorder should be alerted to their higher risk of aortic dissection and should be made aware of the symptoms.

References

1. Fine LG: Abdominal aortic aneurysm. Lancet 341:215, 1993.
2. Erbel R, Engberding R, Daniel W, et al: Echocardiography in diagnosis of aortic dissection. Lancet 1(8636):457, 1989.
3. Johnston KW, Rutherford RB, Tilson MD, et al: Suggested standards for reporting on arterial aneurysms. Subcommittee on Reporting Standards for Arterial Aneurysms, Ad Hoc Committe on Reporting Standards, Society for Vascular Surgery and North American Chapter, International Society for Cardiovascular Surgery. J Vasc Surg 13:452, 1991.
4. Roman MJ, Devereux RB, Kramer-Fox R, et al: Two-dimensional echocardiographic aortic root dimensions in normal children and adults. Am J Cardiol 64:507, 1989.
5. Bengtsson H, Sonesson B, Bergqvist D: Incidence and prevalence of abdominal aortic aneurysms, estimated by necropsy studies and population screening by ultrasound. Ann N Y Acad Sci 800:1, 1996.
6. Safi HJ, Miller CC 3rd, Reardon MJ, et al: Operation for acute and chronic aortic dissection: Recent outcome with regard to neurologic deficit and early death. Ann Thorac Surg 66:402, 1998.
7. Gore I, Hirst AE, Jr. Arteriosclerotic aneurysms of the abdominal aorta: A review. Prog Cardiovasc Dis 16:113, 1973.
8. The Abdominal Aorta Aneurysm: Genetics, Pathophysiology, and Molecular Biology. Proceedings of a Conference, New York City, March 79, 1996. Ann N Y Acad Sci 800:1, 1996.
9. Belkin M, Donaldson MC, Whittemore AD: Abdominal aortic aneurysms. Curr Opin Cardiol 9:581, 1994.
10. Bickerstaff LK, Hollier LH, Van Peenen HJ, et al: Abdominal aortic aneurysms: The changing natural history. J Vasc Surg 1:6, 1984.
11. Collin J: The Oxford Screening Program for aortic aneurysm and screening first-order male siblings of probands with abdominal aortic aneurysm. Ann N Y Acad Sci 800:36, 1996.
12. Reilly JM, Tilson MD: Incidence and etiology of abdominal aortic aneurysms. Surg Clin North Am 69:705, 1989.
13. Lilienfeld DE, Gunderson PD, Sprafka JM, et al: Epidemiology of aortic aneurysms. I: Mortality trends in the United States, 1951 to 1981. Arteriosclerosis 7:637, 1987.
14. Lilienfeld DE, Baxter J, Sprafka JM: Prevalence of aortic aneurysms in the Twin Cities metropolitan area, 1979–84. Public Health Rep 108: 506, 1993.
15. Tilson MD, Seashore MR: Fifty families with abdominal aortic aneurysms in two or more first-order relatives. Am J Surg 147:551, 1984.
16. Cole CW, Barber GG, Bouchard AG, et al: Abdominal aortic aneurysm: Consequences of a positive family history. Can J Surg 32:117, 1989.
17. Darling RCD, Brewster DC, Darling RC, et al: Are familial abdominal aortic aneurysms different? J Vasc Surg 10:39, 1989.
18. Tilson MD, Seashore MR: Human genetics of the abdominal aortic aneurysm. Surg Gynecol Obstet 158:129, 1984.
19. Verloes A, Sakalihasan N, Limet R, Koulischer L: Genetic aspects of abdominal aortic aneurysm. Ann N Y Acad Sci 800:44, 1996.
20. Johnston KW, Scobie TK: Multicenter prospective study of nonruptured abdominal aortic aneurysms. I: Population and operative management. J Vasc Surg 7:69, 1988.
21. Salo JA, Soisalon-Soininen S, Bondestam S, et al: Familial occurrence of abdominal aortic aneurysm. Ann Intern Med 130:637, 1999.
22. Darling RC, Messina CR, Brewster DC, et al: Autopsy study of unoperated abdominal aortic aneurysms: The case for early resection. Circulation 56:II161, 1977.
23. Bickerstaff LK, Pairolero PC, Hollier LH, et al: Thoracic aortic aneurysms: A population-based study. Surgery 92:1103, 1982.
24. Biddinger A, Rocklin M, Coselli J, et al: Familial thoracic aortic dilatations and dissections: A case control study. J Vasc Surg 25:506, 1997.
25. Carlson RG, Lillehei CW, Edwards JE: Cystic medial necrosis of the ascending aorta in relation to age and hypertension. Am J Cardiol 25: 411, 1970.
26. Dapunt OE, Galla JD, Sadeghi AM, et al: The natural history of thoracic aortic aneurysms. J Thorac Cardiovasc Surg 107:1323, 1994.
27. Johansson G, Markstrom U, Swedenborg J: Ruptured thoracic aortic aneurysms: A study of incidence and mortality rates. J Vasc Surg 21: 985, 1995.
28. McNamara JJ, Pressler VM: Natural history of arteriosclerotic thoracic aortic aneurysms. Ann Thorac Surg 26:468, 1978.
29. Roberts WC: Aortic dissection: Anatomy, consequences, and causes. Am Heart J 101:195, 1981.
30. DeBakey ME, McCollum CH, Crawford ES, et al: Dissection and dissecting aneurysms of the aorta: Twenty-year follow-up of five hundred twenty-seven patients treated surgically. Surgery 92:1118, 1982.
31. Daily PO, Trueblood HW, Stinson EB, et al: Management of acute aortic dissections. Ann Thorac Surg 10:237, 1970.
32. Larson EW, Edwards WD: Risk factors for aortic dissection: A necropsy study of 161 cases. Am J Cardiol 53:849, 1984.
33. Wheat MW Jr: Current status of medical therapy of acute dissecting aneurysms of the aorta. World J Surg 4:563, 1980.
34. Perko MJ, Norgaard M, Herzog TM, et al: Unoperated aortic aneurysm: A survey of 170 patients. Ann Thorac Surg 59:1204, 1995.
35. Slater EE, DeSanctis RW: The clinical recognition of dissecting aortic aneurysm. Am J Med 60:625, 1976.
36. Wheat MW Jr: Acute dissecting aneurysms of the aorta: Diagnosis and treatment—1979. Am Heart J 99:373, 1980.
37. Fuster V, Ip JH: Medical aspects of acute aortic dissection. Semin Thorac Cardiovasc Surg 3:219, 1991.
38. Oskoui R, Lindsay J Jr: Aortic dissection in women < 40 years of age and the unimportance of pregnancy. Am J Cardiol 73:821, 1994.
39. Mabie WC, Freire CM: Sudden chest pain and cardiac emergencies in the obstetric patient. Obstet Gynecol Clin North Am 22:19, 1995.

40. Kerr G: Takayasu's arteritis. Curr Opin Rheumatol 6:32, 1994.
41. Takayasu Arteritis II. Proceedings of an international conference. Singapore, 12–13 October 1995. Int J Cardiol 54(Suppl):S1, 1996.
42. Hoffman GS: Takayasu arteritis: Lessons from the American National Institutes of Health experience. Int J Cardiol 54(Suppl):S99, 1996.
43. Kimura A, Kitamura H, Date Y, et al: Comprehensive analysis of HLA genes in Takayasu arteritis in Japan. Int J Cardiol 54(Suppl):S61, 1996.
44. Eichhorn J, Sima D, Thiele B, et al: Anti–endothelial cell antibodies in Takayasu arteritis. Circulation 94:2396, 1996.
45. Sharma BK, Jain S, Sagar S: Systemic manifestations of Takayasu arteritis: The expanding spectrum. Int J Cardiol 54(Suppl):S149, 1996.
46. Lightfoot RW Jr, Michel BA, Bloch DA, et al: The American College of Rheumatology 1990 criteria for the classification of polyarteritis nodosa. Arthritis Rheum 33:1088, 1990.
47. Sharma BK, Jain S, Suri S, et al: Diagnostic criteria for Takayasu arteritis. Int J Cardiol 54(Suppl):S141, 1996.
48. Moriwaki R, Noda M, Yajima M, et al: Clinical manifestations of Takayasu arteritis in India and Japan—new classification of angiographic findings. Angiology 48:369, 1997.
49. Hoffman GS, Leavitt RY, Kerr GS, et al: Treatment of glucocorticoid-resistant or relapsing Takayasu arteritis with methotrexate. Arthritis Rheum 37:578, 1994.
50. Gonzalez EB, Varner WT, Lisse JR, et al: Giant-cell arteritis in the southern United States: An 11-year retrospective study from the Texas Gulf Coast. Arch Intern Med 149:1561, 1989.
51. Lie JT: Aortic and extracranial large vessel giant cell arteritis: A review of 72 cases with histopathologic documentation. Semin Arthritis Rheum 24:422, 1995.
52. Font C, Cid MC, Coll-Vinent B, et al: Clinical features in patients with permanent visual loss due to biopsy-proven giant cell arteritis. Br J Rheumatol 36:251, 1997.
53. Klein RG, Hunder GG, Stanson AW, et al: Large artery involvement in giant cell (temporal) arteritis. Ann Intern Med 83:806, 1975.
54. Stevens RJ, Hughes RA: The aetiopathogenesis of giant cell arteritis. Br J Rheumatol 34:960, 1995.
55. Nandwani R: Modern diagnosis and management of acquired syphilis [see comments]. Br J Hosp Med 55:399, 1996.
56. Sanchez MR: Infectious syphilis. Semin Dermatol 13:234, 1994.
57. Rolfs RT: Treatment of syphilis, 1993. Clin Infect Dis 20(Suppl 1): S23, 1995.
58. Van der Hauwaert LG, Fryns JP, Dumoulin M, et al: Cardiovascular malformations in Turner's and Noonan's syndrome. Br Heart J 40: 500, 1978.
59. Gormsen H: Postmortem diagnosis of syphilitic aortitis, including serological verification on postmortem blood. Forensic Sci Int 24:51, 1984.
60. McKusick VA: The cardiovascular aspects of Marfan's syndrome: A heritable disorder of connective tissue. Circulation 11:321, 1955.
61. Roberts WC, Honig HS: The spectrum of cardiovascular disease in the Marfan syndrome: A clinico-morphologic study of 18 necropsy patients and comparison to 151 previously reported necropsy patients. Am Heart J 104:115, 1982.
62. Sisk HE, Zahka KG, Pyeritz RE: The Marfan syndrome in early childhood: Analysis of 15 patients diagnosed at less than 4 years of age. Am J Cardiol 52:353, 1983.
63. Simpson IA, de Belder MA, Treasure T, et al: Cardiovascular manifestations of Marfan's syndrome: Improved evaluation by transoesophageal echocardiography. Br Heart J 69:104, 1993.
64. Schaefer S, Peshock RM, Malloy CR, et al: Nuclear magnetic resonance imaging in Marfan's syndrome. J Am Coll Cardiol 9:70, 1987.
65. Shores J, Berger KR, Murphy EA, et al: Progression of aortic dilatation and the benefit of long-term beta-adrenergic blockade in Marfan's syndrome [see comments]. N Engl J Med 330:1335, 1994.
66. Salim MA, Alpert BS, Ward JC, et al: Effect of beta-adrenergic blockade on aortic root rate of dilation in the Marfan syndrome. Am J Cardiol 74:629, 1994.
67. Murdoch JL, Walker BA, Halpern BL, et al: Life expectancy and causes of death in the Marfan syndrome. N Engl J Med 286:804, 1972.
68. Finkbohner R, Johnston D, Crawford ES, et al: Marfan syndrome: Long-term survival and complications after aortic aneurysm repair. Circulation 91:728, 1995.
69. Silverman DI, Burton KJ, Gray J, et al: Life expectancy in the Marfan syndrome. Am J Cardiol 75:157, 1995.
70. Rossiter JP, Repke JT, Morales AJ, et al: A prospective longitudinal evaluation of pregnancy in the Marfan syndrome. Am J Obstet Gynecol 173:1599, 1995.
71. Kumar A, Stalker HJ, Williams CA: Concurrence of supravalvular aortic stenosis and peripheral pulmonary stenosis in three generations of a family: A form of arterial dysplasia [see comments]. Am J Med Genet 45:739, 1993.
72. Hanley WB, Jones NB: Familial dissecting aortic aneurysm: A report of three cases within two generations. Br Heart J 29:852, 1967.
73. Nicod P, Bloor C, Godfrey M, et al: Familial aortic dissecting aneurysm. J Am Coll Cardiol 13:811, 1989.
74. Toyama M, Amano A, Kameda T: Familial aortic dissection: A report of rare family cluster. Br Heart J 61:204, 1989.
75. McManus BM, Cassling RS, Soundy TJ, et al: Familial aortic dissection in absence of ascending aortic aneurysms: A lethal syndrome associated with precocious systemic hypertension. Am J Cardiovasc Pathol 1: 55, 1987.
76. Conte MR, Restagno G, Mangiardi L, et al: [Another case of dissecting aortic aneurysm with familial incidence]. Cardiologia 37:513, 1992.
77. Miller MJ, Geffner ME, Lippe BM, et al: Echocardiography reveals a high incidence of bicuspid aortic valve in Turner syndrome. J Pediatr 102:47, 1983.
78. Lie JT: Aortic dissection in Turner's syndrome. Am Heart J 103:1077, 1982.
79. Lin AE, Lippe BM, Geffner ME, et al: Aortic dilation, dissection, and rupture in patients with Turner syndrome. J Pediatr 109:820, 1986.
80. Rubin K: Aortic dissection and rupture in Turner syndrome [letter]. J Pediatr 122:670, 1993.
81. Subramaniam PN: Turner's syndrome and cardiovascular anomalies: A case report and review of the literature. Am J Med Sci 297:260, 1989.

20.2 Surgical Treatment of Aortic Disease and Aortic Dissection

Denton A. Cooley

During the last century, the surgical treatment of aortic aneurysms and dissections evolved to such an extent that these lesions can now be successfully repaired in most cases. An important factor in the current success of aortic repair was the introduction of synthetic vascular grafts in the late 1950s. Previously, the surgical treatment of aortic aneurysms had depended on obliteration or excision of the diseased segment. The latter approach often caused hemorrhagic complications and trauma to nearby mediastinal structures. Now that sturdy, low-porosity synthetic grafts are available, the main goals of repair are to prevent rupture and restore unobstructed pulsatile flow through the aorta. The operation can be accomplished with minimal loss of blood and minimal risk of ischemic or neurologic complications. The operative method of choice and the results of the procedure depend on (1) the portion of the aorta in which the lesion is located,

(2) the type of aneurysm involved (saccular versus fusiform), and (3) the presence or absence of dissection.

Operative methods used to repair aneurysms in the various anatomic locations in the aorta are the same for women and men, although the propensity of aortic aneurysms to affect the different anatomic locations does vary somewhat with gender. This discussion describes the surgical technique my colleagues and I at the Texas Heart Institute use to repair aortic aneurysms. When pertinent, issues specific to women will be described.

ANATOMIC LOCATION

At the Texas Heart Institute, nondissecting aneurysms are classified into the following four categories:

- Type A aneurysms affect mainly the ascending aorta and the proximal transverse arch.
- Type B aneurysms are localized, sacciform lesions that affect the transverse arch alone.
- Type C lesions are transverse arch aneurysms that may have spread to the proximal descending aorta.
- Type D aneurysms involve mainly the descending thoracic aorta, including the thoracoabdominal segment.

Of course, an aneurysm may affect more than one anatomic site. For convenience, however, these four sites are described separately in the discussion of treatment.

SACCULAR VERSUS FUSIFORM ANEURYSMS

Saccular aneurysms involve a localized outpouching of the aorta and are generally closed with a fabric patch. This approach leaves the walls of the lesion intact and eliminates the need for excision. In contrast, fusiform aneurysms involve the entire aortic circumference and may be quite extensive. Repair of fusiform aneurysms, for which we use the technique of endoaneurysmorrhaphy, is described here.

DISSECTING ANEURYSMS

Dissecting aneurysms result when a layer of the aortic wall (most often the medial layer) becomes detached from the rest of the aorta. They are especially common in patients with Erdheim's cystic medial necrosis. The initial lesion may involve either a tear in the intima or an intramural hemorrhage that perforates into the aortic lumen. The most common sites of dissection are the ascending aorta and the proximal descending aorta, at the so-called isthmus; at our institution, dissecting aneurysms in these two locations are classified as types A and B, respectively. Because of their propensity to result in tamponade and death from intrapericardial rupture, type A lesions necessitate emergency surgery.

Although aortic dissections more often affect men (4:1 in our series), the chance of dissection increases with age in women, most likely as a result of the higher incidence of hypertension in women older than 50 years. In women younger than 40 years, dissection primarily affects patients with Marfan's syndrome, especially if they are pregnant. Approximately one half of women affected by dissection before age 40 are pregnant; most are in their last trimester.[1] In pregnant women, dissection most likely results from the hypercirculatory state, hypertension, connective tissue changes induced by the hormonal changes of pregnancy, or a combination of these factors.

SYNTHETIC GRAFTS

Today the synthetic grafts used in repair of aortic aneurysms are safer and more effective than ever before. Their low porosity minimizes operative bleeding, promotes healing, and resists infection. Because these grafts are also quite durable, the incidence of pseudoaneurysm formation has decreased. Finally, the newer grafts are easier to handle, facilitating the technical portion of the procedure. One such improved conduit is the Hemashield Microvel double-velour vascular graft (Meadox Medicals, Inc., Oakland, NJ), which is made of woven or knitted polyester fibers impregnated with collagen.

CARDIOPULMONARY BYPASS

Cardiopulmonary bypass is routinely used in the repair of aneurysms in the ascending aorta and proximal arch. Lesions that involve only the distal arch may be repaired with or without cardiopulmonary bypass. In preparation for cardiopulmonary bypass, the arterial cannula is placed in the ascending aorta, transverse arch, or femoral artery, depending on the extent of the aneurysm and the presence or absence of dissection. The right atrium or venae are also cannulated. For return of oxygenated blood, I prefer to cannulate the femoral artery, because this arrangement allows full access to the ascending aorta, transverse arch, and brachiocephalic vessels. Of course, cannulation of the femoral artery is mandatory for aortic dissections and transverse arch aneurysms. In these cases, cannulation of the arch might cause atherosclerotic particles or other debris to embolize to the brain; likewise, in acute cases, the ascending aorta should not be cross-clamped because of the friability of tissue. An "open" anastomosis with the aorta dissected is preferred during hypothermic circulatory arrest.

In most cases, cardiopulmonary bypass is instituted with moderate systemic hypothermia (28 to 30°C). For cerebral protection during repair of a type A dissection or a transverse arch aneurysm, however, I recommend more profound hypothermia (20 to 22°C) and total circulatory arrest.[2]

During aortic repair, excessively high or low pressures proximal to the aortic clamp must be avoided. If the proximal pressure does become elevated (greater than 150 mm Hg), hypotensive drugs such as nitroprusside and trimethaphan camsylate (Arfonad) may be administered. These drugs should be given with caution, however, because they may hinder the resumption of normal pressure upon release of the proximal aortic clamp. As the clamp is released, the surgeon should carefully observe the effect on the proximal aortic pressure. I recommend the use of a properly occluding clamp with a long ratchet, which permits the clamp to be released gradually.

SPINAL CORD PROTECTION

I use an "open" technique for the distal anastomosis during repair of descending thoracic lesions. A single cross-clamp is placed proximal to the aneurysm to exsanguinate the lower body.[3–6] This partial exsanguination (1) adequately controls proximal hypertension by reducing nitrate vasodilator requirements, (2) helps protect the spinal cord by maintaining the autoregulatory mechanisms of spinal blood flow and by preventing spinal cord edema, and (3) decreases the central venous and cerebrospinal fluid (CSF) pressures, thereby improving spinal cord perfusion despite critically low abdominal aortic pressure. Details of this method are discussed later.

BLOOD LOSS

During aortic resection, shed blood is replaced through use of a cell saver. To control bleeding, protamine sulfate is given as the proximal aortic clamp is released.

TREATMENT OF NONDISSECTING ANEURYSMS

Nondissecting aneurysms are repaired by means of the following methods, which are described according to anatomic site.

Aneurysms of the Ascending Aorta and the Proximal Transverse Arch (Type A)

The ascending aorta is the most vulnerable portion of the entire vascular system. Nevertheless, repair of an ascending aortic aneurysm can restore a patient with this condition to a relatively normal life. The preferred treatment varies, depending on whether the lesion involves the aortic root, the transverse arch, or both. In many cases, ascending aortic aneurysms are of the diffuse fusiform type, and surgical repair entails relining the aneurysmal cavity with a fabric graft. The aorta is approached through a median sternotomy incision.

In repairing aneurysms of the proximal ascending aorta and transverse arch, we have tried various methods for preventing cerebral ischemia during aortic circulatory arrest. We found that deep hypothermic arrest (12 to 14°C) sometimes caused bleeding and cerebral injury. Therefore, we now prefer a compromise technique that involves hypothermic arrest with partial exsanguination (Fig. 20–7).[1, 2] Once cardiopulmonary bypass has been instituted in a routine manner, a heat exchanger in the circuit is used to lower the patient's temperature to 20 to 22°C. The aneurysm (Fig. 20–7*A*), is incised and only enough blood is aspirated to allow the distal extent of the aneurysm to be visualized (Fig. 20–7*B*). The distal anastomosis between the graft and the aorta rarely takes more than 20 to 30 minutes to create (Fig. 20–7*C*).

Upon completion of the anastomosis, arterial perfusion in the femoral cannula is begun. The patient may be placed in the head-down position during the period of reperfusion. Perfusion of the aorta and the proximal portion of the graft causes air to be removed from the arch. The graft is then clamped (Fig. 20–7*D*), and if the arch vessels have been occluded, the occluding clamp is released. As perfusion continues, the patient is rewarmed to 36°C, after which cardiopulmonary bypass is no longer necessary. The rewarming phase may take 30 minutes to an hour to complete.

Meanwhile, the proximal anastomosis is created. To create the distal and proximal anastomoses, I use polypropylene or braided polyester sutures in a continuous technique. Valvular or coronary procedures are performed next, if necessary (Fig. 20–7*E*). Although women's coronary vessels are smaller than men's, coronary bypass concomitant with repair of an aortic aneurysm can be accomplished successfully in women.

Aneurysms Involving the Aortic Root and Valve

In patients with annuloaortic ectasia and aortic valve regurgitation, I prefer to insert a valved conduit according to a modified Bentall technique, which simplifies graft implantation. In the original Bentall technique, the native aortic valve is excised, and the valved conduit is attached to the aortic annulus with a continuous 2-0 polypropylene suture (Fig. 20–8*A* and *B*).[7] A disposable cautery is then used to excise two "buttons" from the conduit (Fig. 20–8*C*). These openings are connected to the left and right coronary ostia (Fig. 20–8*D*), respectively, with a continuous 4-0 polypropylene suture. It is most important that the stitches be placed in the aorta, not in the coronary ostia themselves. If no dissection is present and the rest of the aorta is healthy, the distal anastomosis is created according to the inclusion technique,[8] with the aortic cross-clamp in place.

Because the Bentall technique can result in postoperative bleeding, I often use the following modification: To control postoperative bleeding, a fistula is created between the enclosed perigraft space and the right atrium, as described by Cabrol and colleagues[9] (Fig. 20–9). The retained aortic wall is then wrapped securely around the conduit. This technique offers an extremely physiologic type of autotransfusion, because any blood shed from the mediastinum is returned to the right atrium. It is especially appropriate for use in Jehovah's Witnesses. Unlike Bentall's original technique, this modified approach causes no postoperative bleeding or false aneurysm formation.

Ascending Aortic Aneurysms Involving the Proximal Transverse Arch

For aneurysmal disease that extends to the base of the innominate artery or to the proximal transverse arch, we recommend a "hemiarch" repair,[3] in which a beveled graft is sutured to the aorta and around the origin of the innominate artery. While the proximal anastomosis is being created

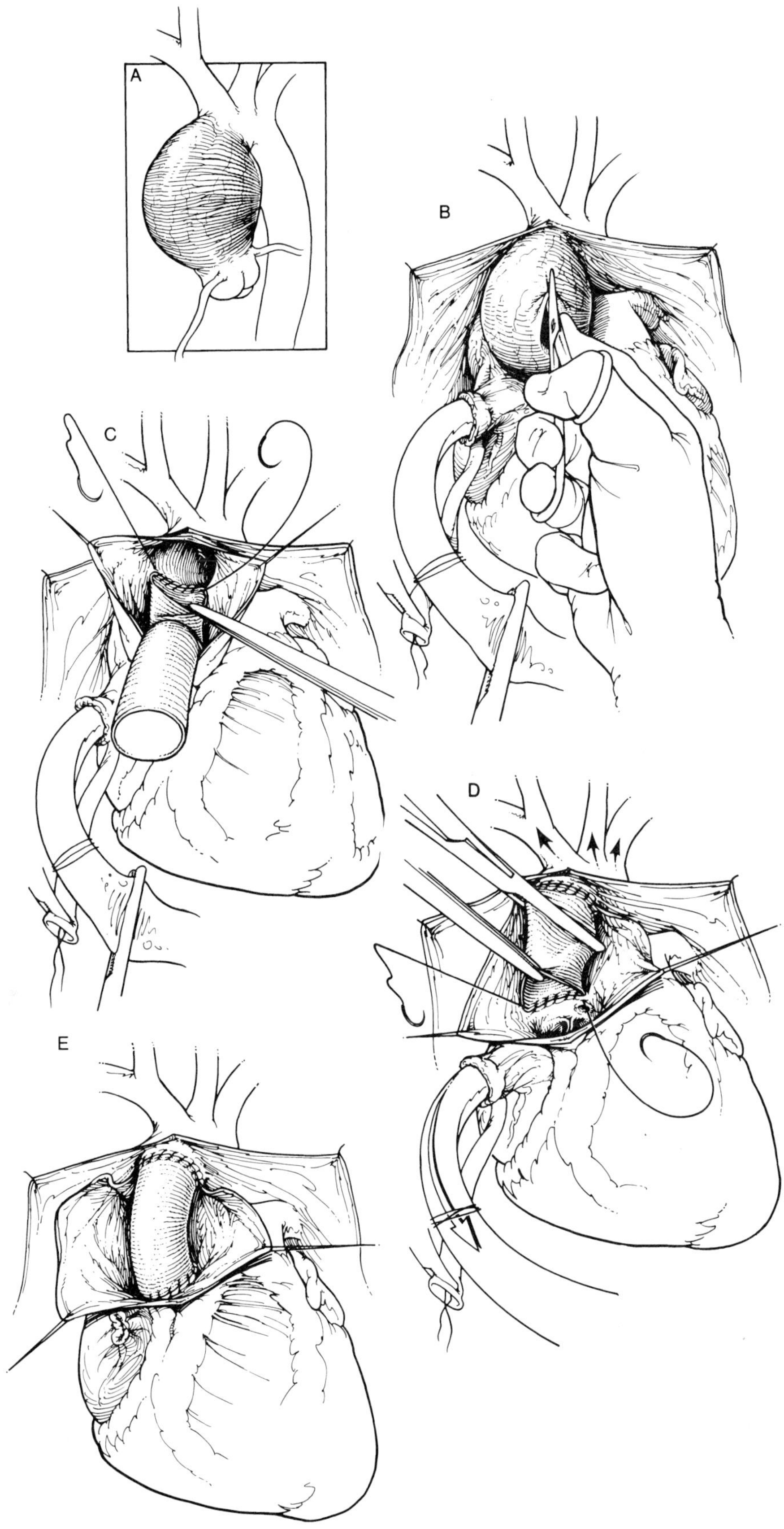

FIGURE 20–7. Open distal anastomosis for repair of aneurysms of the ascending aorta and transverse arch. *A* and *B*, After the aneurysm is exposed, it is opened widely to expose the transverse arch. *C*, The open distal anastomosis is performed first with a continuous polypropylene suture. *D*, Entrapped air is eliminated as blood gradually fills the aorta and the proximal segment of the graft as the proximal anastomosis is completed. *E*, Completed repair. (From Cooley DA: Surgical Treatment of Aortic Aneurysms, W.B. Saunders, Philadelphia, 1986.)

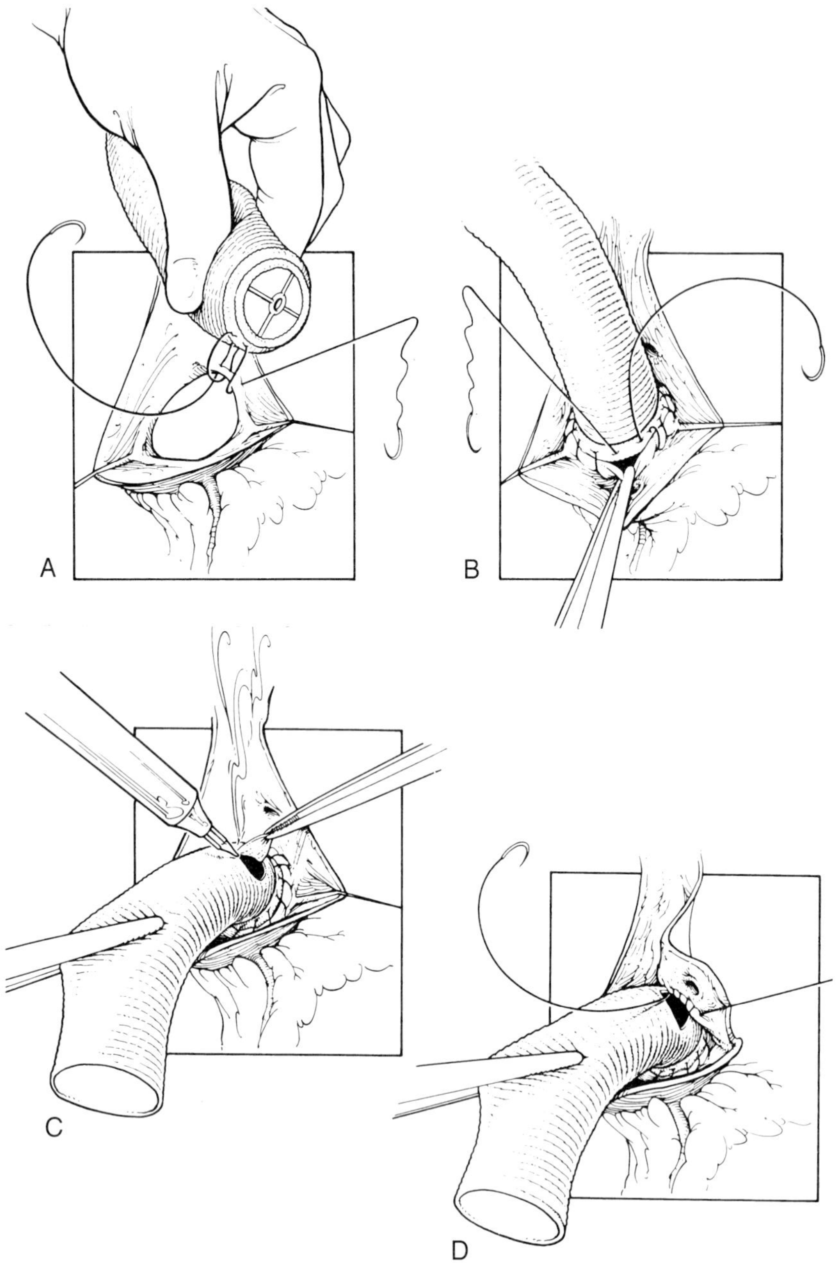

FIGURE 20–8. Insertion of a valved conduit by using a modified Bentall technique. *A* and *B*, After the native aortic valve is excised, the valved conduit is attached to the aortic annulus with a continuous 2-0 polypropylene suture. *C*, Openings in the graft are made by disposable hot cautery adjacent to the left coronary ostium. *D*, The graft is then anastomosed to the coronary orifices. (From Cooley DA, Surgical Treatment of Aortic Aneurysms, W.B. Saunders, Philadelphia, 1986.)

and the left coronary ostium reimplanted, hypothermia (20 to 22°C) is induced. Circulatory arrest is then begun, and the patient is placed in a steep Trendelenburg position. The aorta is unclamped, and the distal anastomosis is created. The aortic arch is replaced tangentially along its lesser curvature. To achieve this goal, the surgeon must tailor a long "tongue" of graft to fit the aorta (Fig. 20–10). After rewarming of the patient has been initiated and the right coronary artery has been reimplanted, the procedure is concluded as in the modified Bentall operation.

Aneurysms of the Transverse Arch (Types B and C)

During repair of the transverse arch, the surgeon must use some means of protecting the brain from ischemia while the circulation is interrupted. We have found hypothermic circulatory arrest to be invaluable for this purpose.[10] Once cardiopulmonary bypass with profound hypothermia has been instituted, the ascending aorta is cross-clamped, and the heart is stopped. Cold cardioplegic solution is injected into the ascending aorta, and cold saline solution is applied topically. A sump is inserted into the right superior pulmonary vein. If the distal extent of the aneurysm is proximal to the level of the ligamentum arteriosum, a median sternotomy is performed. If the aneurysm spreads beyond the ligamentum arteriosum, however, a transverse incision may be necessary.

In most cases, the orifices of the great vessels are free of disease, and the aortic wall alone is affected. Therefore, repair involves implanting the major arch vessels into the graft as a unit (Fig. 20–11). Usually, the graft anastomoses can be created without a need for individual graft connection. This technique is relatively simple, and the risk of postoperative bleeding or thrombosis is minimal, so occlusion of the cerebral arteries is not necessary during circulatory arrest. Moreover, air embolism is not a threat in these vessels.

Aneurysms of the Descending Thoracic Aorta (Type D)

Aneurysms of the descending thoracic aorta account for about half of all thoracic aneurysms.[11] These lesions are usually of the fusiform type and involve much of the circumference of the aorta. Occasionally, the entire descending thoracic aorta, including the thoracoabdominal region, is affected.

Prevention of Spinal Cord Ischemia

Repair of the descending aorta is fraught with difficulty because of the need for aortic cross-clamping, which interrupts blood flow through the aneurysm. If the cross-clamp period is excessively prolonged, spinal cord ischemia may result, leading to postoperative paraplegia or renal failure (incidence, 40% or less).[12, 13] Although hypothermia offers some protection for the brain and spinal cord,[14] it can also cause its own complications,[15] especially when the hypothermia is profound. As an alternative, some surgeons have provided adjunctive intraoperative perfusion with temporary arterial shunts[16] and partial extracorporeal bypass[17–19] or retrograde cerebral perfusion during hypothermic circulatory arrest.[20, 21] Other techniques that have been tried include preoperative radiographic assessment of critical intercostal arteries,[22] intraoperative monitoring of somatosensory and motor evoked potentials,[23, 24] use of oxygen free radical scavengers to prevent reperfusion injury,[25] administration of intrathecal agents to improve collateral flow to the spinal cord,[26–29] and use of neuroplegic solutions such as calcium channel blockers.[29]

Having tried many adjunctive techniques, including some of those just listed, I have decided that the best approach is simple aortic cross-clamping without distal support. Our results have shown that prolonged aortic cross-clamping (longer than 30 minutes) is the most important cause of spinal cord injury.[30] Therefore, to expedite repair, we have simplified the surgical approach to descending aortic resection. We use an operative strategy that we discovered somewhat by accident in 1989,[5] when we treated a difficult descending thoracic aneurysm. In that case, we were unable to apply a distal clamp below the aneurysm. Therefore, to create the distal anastomosis to the supraceliac artery, we used only a proximal aortic clamp (see next section for details).[4–6] This technique would have been impossible without continuous autotransfusion, which permitted back-bleeding through the open distal aorta and segmental spinal arteries, thereby decompressing the distal aorta. The open technique yielded such satisfactory neurologic results that we began to use it in other cases. By combining moderate hypothermia with the open technique when necessary, the period of spinal cord ischemia can be lengthened, which may further protect against postoperative complications.

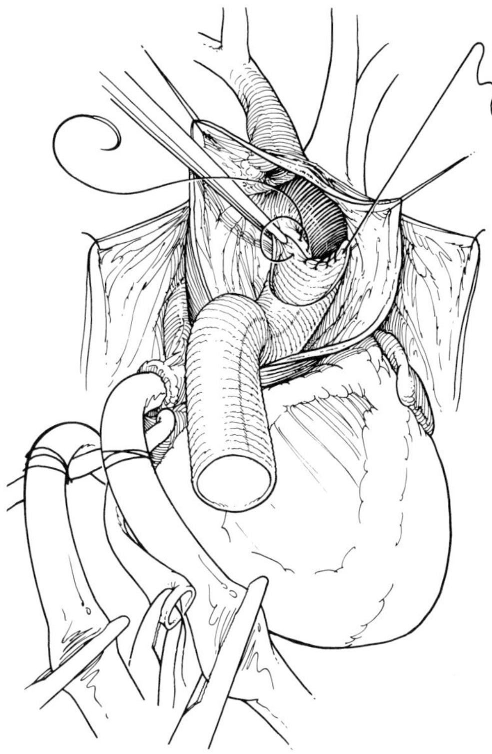

FIGURE 20–10. Open anastomosis performed to the transverse arch during hypothermic circulatory arrest. (From Lewis CTP, Cooley DA, Murphy MC, et al: Surgical repair of aortic root aneurysms in 280 patients. Ann Thorac Surg 53:38, 1992.)

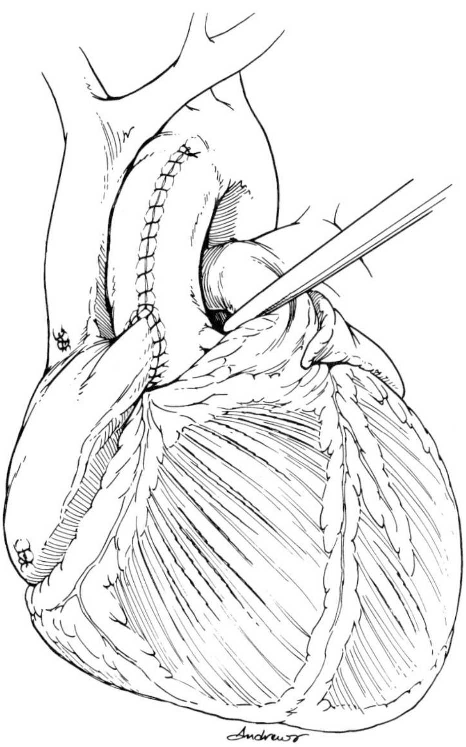

FIGURE 20–9. Fistula created between the perigraft space and right atrium. (From Lewis CTP, Cooley DA, Murphy MC, et al: Surgical repair of aortic root aneurysms in 280 patients. Ann Thorac Surg 53:38, 1992.)

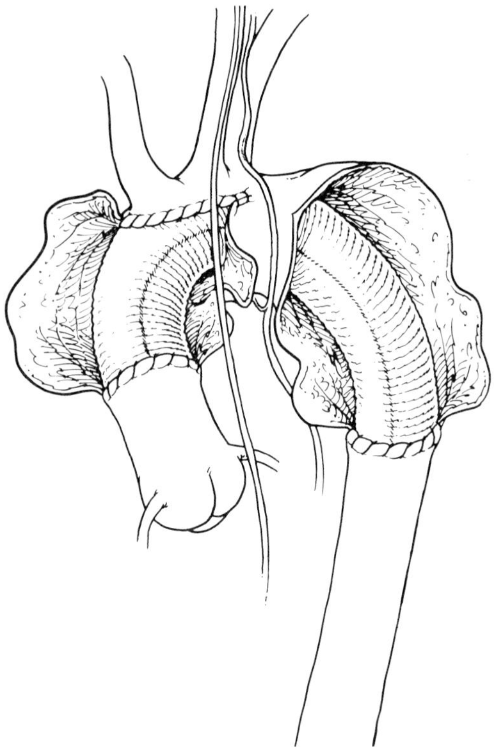

FIGURE 20–11. Implantation of the arch vessels as a unit into the side of the graft in the transverse aorta. (From Cooley DA: Surgical Treatment of Aortic Aneurysms. W.B. Saunders, Philadelphia, 1986.)

Repair Techniques

The open method of resection and graft replacement is appropriate for aneurysms of the descending thoracic and thoracoabdominal sections of the aorta. To approach the proximal segment of the descending aorta, I make a routine left posterolateral incision in the fourth intercostal space. In cases that involve an extensive aneurysm, the distal portion can be accessed through a second incision in the seventh intercostal space.

Dissection is carried out at the proposed site of proximal aortic cross-clamping. The patient is then given systemic heparin (1 mg/kg body weight). The clamp is applied, and a longitudinal incision is made in the aneurysm (Fig. 20–12*A*). Once intraluminal thrombus has been removed, the proposed anastomotic sites are cleared of atheromatous debris. Throughout the cross-clamping period, blood is continuously drawn into the autotransfusion device. Back-bleeding from the distal aorta and from exposed segmental vessels within the aneurysmal lumen is allowed to occur freely. Because the blood is processed and returned to the patient as necessary, the ascending aortic pressure remains near normal.

A woven Dacron tube graft of appropriate size is sewn to the distal aorta with 2-0 polypropylene sutures (Fig. 20–12*B*). For this step, I prefer a large MH double-armed needle (No. 8853H; Ethicon, Somerville, NJ). Whenever possible, I also create an oblique suture line. This approach allows me to incorporate back-bleeding segmental vessels into the new lumen, thereby maintaining intercostal flow and avoiding reattachment of individual vessels.

After the distal anastomosis is completed, the graft is anastomosed to the proximal aorta with 2-0 or 3-0 polypropylene sutures (Fig. 20–12*C*). During aortic cross-clamping, sodium nitroprusside may be given as necessary to regulate the blood pressure. At the end of the cross-clamping period, the sodium nitroprusside infusion is tapered off, and the proximal clamp is slowly loosened. Circulatory stability is restored with appropriate drugs, and the segmental vessels are oversewn. The leftover aneurysmal wall is then tailored and sewn over the Dacron graft (Fig. 20–12*D*). Once the procedure is finished, all remaining aspirated blood is processed and autotransfused.

Thoracoabdominal or suprarenal aneurysms are ap-

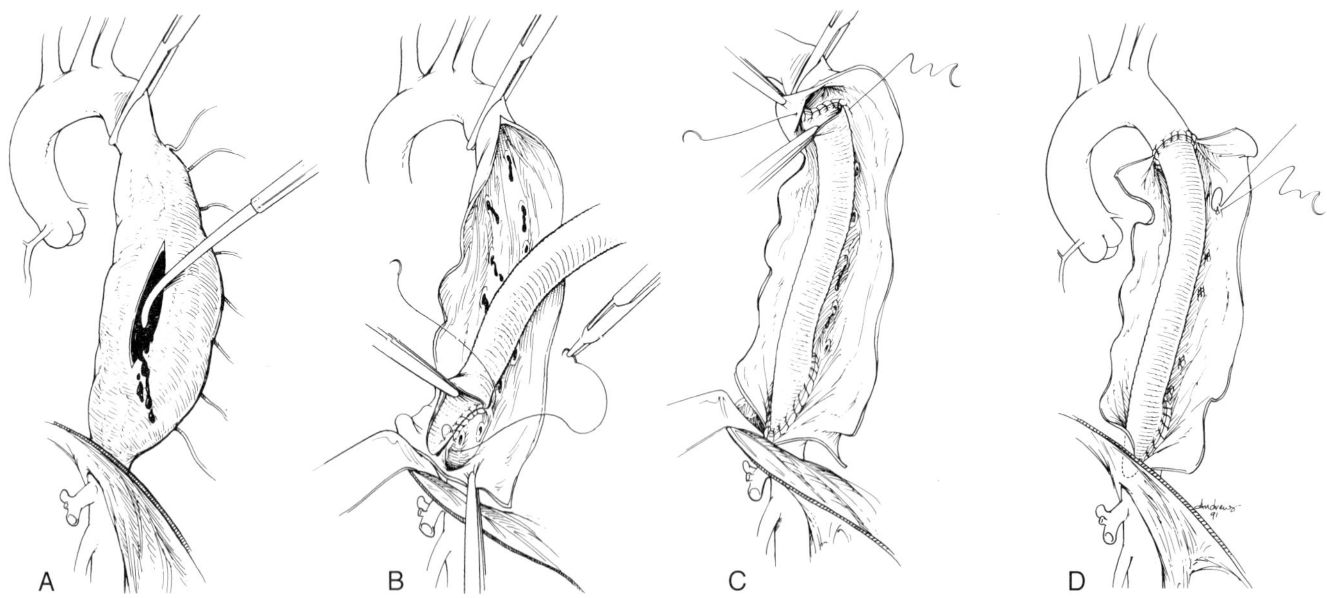

FIGURE 20–12. Technique for repair of aneurysms of the descending thoracic aorta. *A,* Longitudinal incision is made after the proximal clamp is applied. *B,* The distal anastomosis is completed without an aortic clamp in the open fashion. *C,* The proximal anastomosis is then completed. *D,* Finally, the aneurysmal wall is sutured over the graft. (From Cooley DA, Baldwin RT: Technique of open distal anastomosis for repair of descending thoracic aortic aneurysms. Ann Thorac Surg 54:932, 1992.)

proached through a thoracoabdominal incision. The distal anastomosis is created first. Then, a single Carrel patch, containing the superior mesenteric, celiac, and both renal arteries, is reattached to the aorta. Once the proximal anastomosis has been finished, distal flow is resumed.

Other Options

In selected cases involving small, multiple, or moderately sized fusiform aneurysms, the lesion may be wrapped with a double velour fabric to prevent expansion and rupture. This approach is recommended mainly for elderly or severely debilitated patients who would be poor candidates for a more definitive surgical procedure. For patients in whom surgery cannot be tolerated at all, percutaneous insertion of an intravascular stent or graft may be a lifesaving alternative.[31–33]

TREATMENT OF DISSECTING ANEURYSMS

Because dissections of the ascending aorta are separate clinical entities from those of the descending aorta, the two types require different operative approaches. If the disease involves more than one portion of the aorta, surgical priority should be given to whichever areas pose the greatest risk. In rare cases, the entire aorta may have to be replaced (see later).

In cases of acute dissection, the involved tissues are friable and delicate. Therefore, creating secure anastomoses can be technically challenging. To seal the dissected aortic layers, some surgeons resort to polytetrafluoroethylene felt reinforcement, intraluminal sutureless prostheses,[34, 35] or biologic gelatin-resorcinol glue, which has not been approved yet for use in the United States.[36, 37] Chronic dissections do not pose as much of a problem because the tissues are better able to hold sutures.

Dissections of the Ascending Aorta (Type A)

Both acute and chronic ascending aortic dissections are repaired in the same manner. Because acute dissections can rapidly cause severe complications or even death, they are viewed as surgical emergencies. Women who experience acute dissections or rupture often have Ehlers-Danlos syndrome or Marfan's syndrome or are pregnant. Pregnant women with these syndromes are particularly prone to dissection or rupture during their last trimester or during labor and delivery, especially when their aortic root exceeds 40 mm in diameter,[38] although dissection may also occur in the absence of dilatation. In most cases, the dissection occurs proximally and must be managed aggressively. A cesarean section should be performed, followed immediately by aortic repair. If the dissection occurs during the first two trimesters of pregnancy, repair will probably need to be undertaken but may be delayed if the mother's condition is stable. Cardiopulmonary bypass may induce placental dysfunction and, thus, increase the chance for spontaneous abortion.

For acute dissecting aneurysms in the ascending aorta, we repair the distal section of the aneurysm by the open technique (as previously described). The aorta should be completely transected distally, however, to ensure that both layers of the aortic wall involved in the dissection are included in the suture line. Repair of the dissection at the aortic arch level usually involves no more than 20 minutes of circulatory arrest.

When the proximal portion of the dissection involves the aortic valve, we try to repair the valve first, especially if it is only modestly insufficient. In the patient with severe aortic regurgitation, we replace the valve or perform a modified Bentall procedure with hemiarch repair. The repair is performed as described previously, except for the following differences: The aorta is completely transected distal to the intimal tear.[39] To eradicate the false lumen, the surgeon creates an end-to-end distal anastomosis. A nerve hook may be used to enhance hemostasis at the anastomotic site. The right coronary artery is reimplanted during rewarming of the patient. In this type of repair, use of the inclusion technique or Cabrol fistula is precluded. Therefore, the retained aortic wall is placed loosely over the repair, and the distal anastomosis is covered with a 12-mm Dacron tube graft.

Dissections of the Descending Aorta (Type B)

Most patients with descending aortic dissections (type B), including women, are treated medically until symptoms or complications supervene. Unfortunately, however, the presence of complications is associated with an extremely high operative mortality. Both chronic and acute dissections are treated in the same manner, although we believe that most acute lesions should be operated on during the original period of hospitalization. In pregnant women, conservative treatment is continued as long as possible. However, the patient should undergo cesarean delivery followed by aortic repair if life-threatening complications or the potential for such complications exists. It is important to normalize blood pressure in pregnant women, especially during delivery, to avoid the increased risk of dissection and rupture. When surgery is indicated, the procedure of choice is excision of the diseased segment and replacement with a synthetic graft. Some experts believe that early surgical replacement of the proximal descending aorta may reduce the likelihood of false aneurysm formation in other portions of the aorta or of late ischemic complications.[32, 38, 40]

Many patients with acute type B dissections are elderly, seriously ill, or otherwise unsuitable candidates for standard operative intervention. In these cases, when dissection results in limb or organ ischemia, direct surgical fenestration of the false aneurysm's flap may be performed through a retroperitoneal approach.[41] This procedure results in little blood loss and minimal compromise of the patient's overall condition. Alternatively, fenestration may be performed with a balloon catheter[32, 42]; the device may be used either to enlarge a previously existing opening in the aneurysmal flap or to create such an opening. Experience with balloon fenestration remains limited, however, and long-term results are not yet available. Another catheter technique that may relieve ischemic complications associated with acute type B

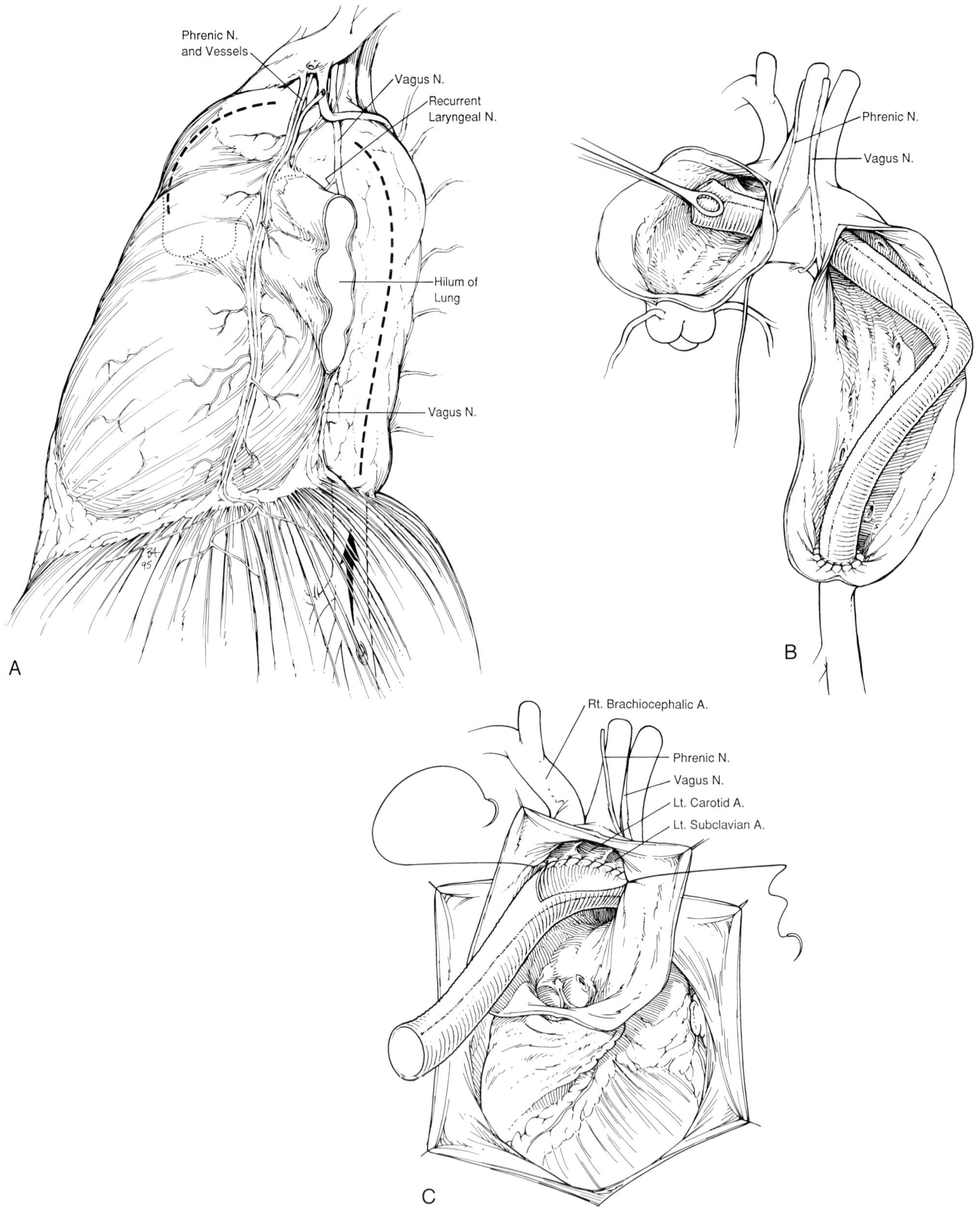

FIGURE 20–13. Retrograde replacement of the thoracic aorta. *A,* Aneurysm is incised upward, to the level of the transverse arch. *B,* Graft is passed through the pedicle containing the vagus and phrenic nerves. *C,* Elliptical portion of the graft is excised for anastomosis to the brachiocephalic arteries.

dissections is insertion of a balloon-expandable intravascular stent[32] or graft.[33]

For expansion or impending rupture of the dissected aorta, some experts recommend a thromboexclusion technique,[41] in which the thoracic aorta is bypassed with a large-caliber Dacron graft. The descending aorta is then permanently occluded with a surgical stapler just beyond the left subclavian artery. This procedure was first described by Carpentier and associates[43] in 1981. Once the diseased segment has been excluded, it undergoes gradual thrombosis, which prevents rupture or extension of the dissection. Moreover, blood flow to the spine is augmented by the formation of collateral arteries.

TREATMENT OF ANEURYSMS INVOLVING MOST OF THE AORTA

For aneurysms that extend from the ascending aorta or transverse arch well into the descending aorta, one may replace the aorta by means of a two-staged "elephant-trunk" operation.[44] During the first stage of the procedure, the descending aorta is replaced. The distal anastomosis is created in end-to-end fashion, just beyond the left subclavian artery. The graft is then telescoped and drawn into the descending thoracic aorta. Repair of the ascending and transverse sections is then completed. The second stage of the repair is performed several weeks later through a posterolateral incision.

In contrast, I prefer a one-stage retrograde "pull-through" procedure that, in my opinion, is simpler and more effective.[45] For this operation, the patient is positioned at a 45-degree angle. The aneurysm is accessed through an anterolateral incision in the fourth, fifth, or sixth intercostal space, and the ascending aorta is accessed via a median sternotomy. Cardiopulmonary bypass is then begun routinely, and hypothermia (18 to 20°C) is induced, usually transfemorally. Once the ascending aorta has been cross-clamped, cold crystalloid cardioplegic solution is administered. Cardiopulmonary bypass is interrupted, and a clamp is placed on the venous line. The distal aneurysm is incised upward through the intercostal incision (Fig. 20–13*A*), and blood within the lesion is aspirated. Care should be taken to avoid transecting the vagus and phrenic nerves. The distal anastomosis is created with a continuous 2-0 or 3-0 monofilament polypropylene suture. Next, the ascending aorta is incised through the sternotomy as far as the middle segment of the transverse arch. The surgeon then brings the graft through the pedicle that contains the vagus and phrenic nerves (Fig. 20–13*B*). An elliptical opening is made in the graft for anastomosis of the brachiocephalic vessels (Fig. 20–13*C*).

Once this step is completed, cardiopulmonary bypass is slowly resumed, and the patient is repositioned with his or her head down. Upon application of the proximal clamp, the graft is de-aired (Fig. 20–13*D*). The proximal anastomosis is performed during the rewarming period. When all the repairs have been completed, hemostasis is obtained by oversewing of the segmental vessels in the descending aorta (Fig. 20–13*E*). These vessels may or may not be reimplanted. When the abdominal or thoracoabdominal segments of the aorta are involved, they may be repaired through an expansion of the lateral thoracotomy. In the presence of hypothermia, this expeditious retrograde approach reduces the threat

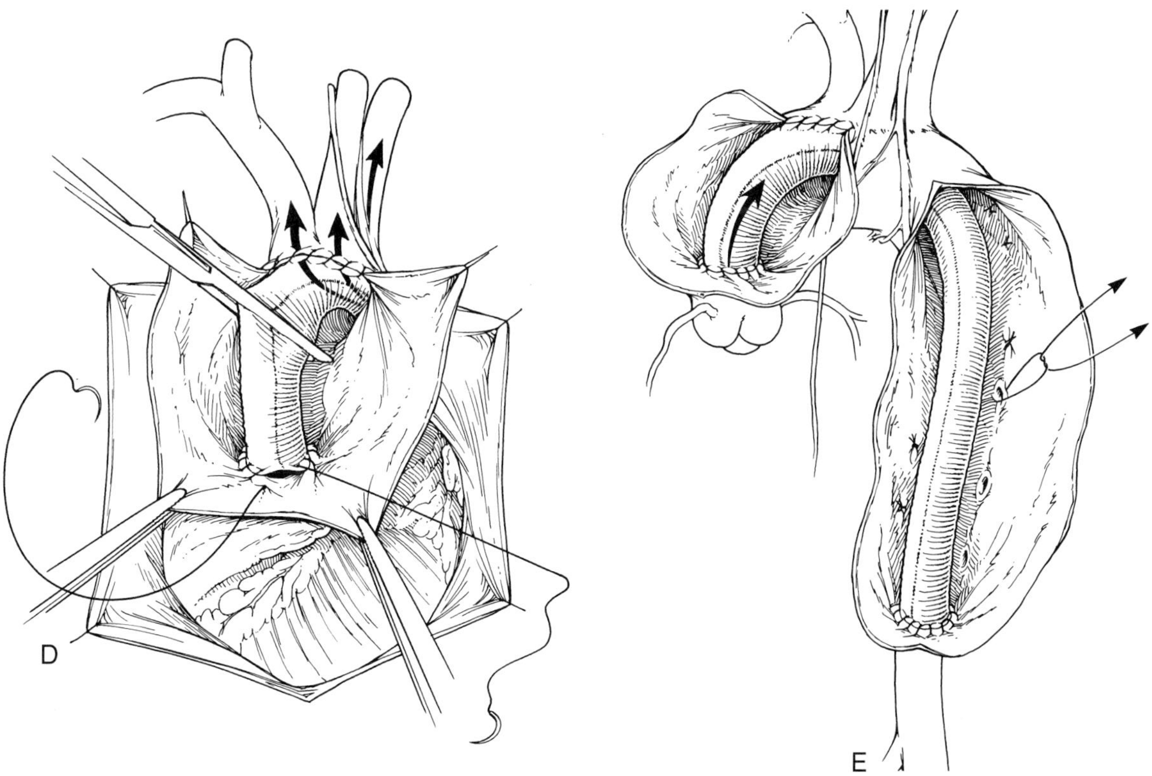

FIGURE 20–13 *Continued. D,* With the patient in the head-down position, the graft is clamped proximally to eliminate air. *E,* Segmental vessels in the descending aorta are oversewn to achieve hemostasis. (From Cooley DA: Retrograde replacement of the thoracic aorta. Tex Heart Inst J 22:162, 1992.)

of ischemia and necrosis of the spinal cord and brain, allowing safe replacement of the entire thoracic aorta.

CONCLUSION

During the last century, much progress was made in treating aortic disease and dissection. Nevertheless, further advances are needed in several areas, particularly in protecting the central nervous system during aortic repair. In the future, even better methods will become available for diagnosing aneurysms noninvasively. Treatment will also become less invasive as surgeons gain experience with stented grafts and other intraluminal devices for aortic repair. Meanwhile, the methods described in this chapter will continue to offer the most definitive repair possible while subjecting the patient to the least degree of risk.

Although there have been reports that women have been treated less often for abdominal aneurysms and with poorer results,[46] the percentage of women in our entire series of aortic aneurysms has remained stable—21% of approximately 7000 cases, which includes abdominal aneurysms. When risk factors are accounted for, the percentage of early deaths in women has also remained similar.

References

1. Borst HG, Heinemann MK, Stone CD (eds): Surgical Treatment of Aortic Dissection. Churchill Livingstone, New York, 1996, p 15.
2. Ott DA, Frazier OH, Cooley DA: Resection of the aortic arch using deep hypothermia and temporary circulatory arrest. Circulation 58(Suppl 1):227, 1978.
3. Livesay JJ, Cooley DA, Duncan JM, et al: Open aortic anastomosis: Improved results in the treatment of aneurysms of the aortic arch. Circulation 66(Suppl 1):1, 1982.
4. Scheinin SA, Cooley DA: Graft replacement of the descending thoracic aorta: Results of "open" distal anastomosis. Ann Thorac Surg 58:19, 1994.
5. Cooley DA, Baldwin RT: Technique of open distal anastomosis for repair of descending thoracic aortic aneurysms. Ann Thorac Surg 54: 932, 1992.
6. Cooley DA: Distal exsanguination in aortic aneurysm surgery. Eur J Cardiothorac Surg 6:459, 1992.
7. Bentall H, De Bono A: A technique for complete replacement of the ascending aorta. Thorax 23:338, 1968.
8. Creech O Jr: Endoaneurysmorrhaphy and treatment of aortic aneurysms. Ann Surg 164:935, 1966.
9. Cabrol C, Pavie A, Mesnildrey P: Long-term results with total replacement of the ascending aorta and reimplantation of the coronary arteries. J Thorac Cardiovasc Surg 91:17, 1986.
10. Cooley DA, Ott DA, Frazier OH, Walker WE: Surgical treatment of aneurysms of the transverse aortic arch: Experience with 25 patients using hypothermic techniques. Ann Thorac Surg 32:260, 1981.
11. Bojar RM: Thoracic aneurysms. In Bojar RM (ed): Adult Cardiac Surgery. Blackwell Scientific, Boston, 1992, p 274.
12. Crawford ES, Crawford JL, Safi HJ, et al: Thoracoabdominal aortic aneurysms: Preoperative and intraoperative factors determining immediate and long-term results of operations in 605 patients. J Vasc Surg 3:389, 1986.
13. Schepens MAAM, Defauw JJAM, Hamerlijnck RPHM, et al: Surgical treatment of thoracoabdominal aortic aneurysms by simple crossclamping. Risk factors and late results. J Thorac Cardiovasc Surg 107:134, 1994.
14. Colon R, Frazier OH, Cooley DA, McAllister HA: Hypothermic regional perfusion for protection of the spinal cord during periods of ischemia. Ann Thorac Surg 43:639, 1987.
15. Svensson LG, Crawford ES, Hess KR, et al: Deep hypothermia with circulatory arrest. Determinants of stroke and early mortality in 656 patients. J Thorac Cardiovasc Surg 106:19, 1993.
16. Gott VL: Heparinized shunts for thoracic vascular operations [editorial]. Ann Thorac Surg 14:219, 1972.
17. Bloodwell RD, Hallman GL, Cooley DA: Partial cardiopulmonary bypass for pericardiectomy and resection of descending thoracic aortic aneurysms. Ann Thorac Surg 6:46, 1968.
18. Connolly JE, Wakabayashi A, German JC, et al: Clinical experience with pulsatile left heart bypass without anticoagulation for thoracic aneurysms. J Thorac Cardiovasc Surg 62:568, 1971.
19. Yasuura K, Okamoto H, Ogawa Y, et al: Resection of aortic aneurysms without aortic clamp technique with the aid of hypothermic total body retrograde perfusion. J Thorac Cardiovasc Surg 107:1237, 1994.
20. Frist WH, Baldwin JC, Starnes VA, et al: A reconsideration of cerebral perfusion in aortic arch replacement. Ann Thorac Surg 42:273, 1986.
21. Ueda Y, Miki S, Kusuhara K, et al: Surgical treatment of aneurysm or dissection involving the ascending aorta and aortic arch, utilizing circulatory arrest and retrograde cerebral perfusion. J Cardiovasc Surg 31:553, 1990.
22. Kieffer E, Thierry R, Chiras J, et al: Preoperative spinal cord arteriography in aneurysmal disease of the descending thoracic and thoracoabdominal aorta: Preliminary results in 45 patients. Ann Vasc Surg 3: 34, 1989.
23. Laschinger JC, Cunningham JN, Cooper MM, et al: Monitoring of somatosensory evoked potentials during surgical procedures on the thoracoabdominal aorta. I: Relationship of aortic cross-clamping duration, SEPs, and incidence of neurologic dysfunction. J Thorac Cardiovasc Surg 94:260, 1987.
24. Laschinger JC, Cunningham JN, Baumann FG, et al: Monitoring of somatosensory evoked potentials during surgical procedures on the thoracoabdominal aorta. III: Intraoperative identification of vessels critical to spinal cord blood supply. J Thorac Cardiovasc Surg 94:271, 1987.
25. Gerhardt EB, Stewart JR, Morrison JG, et al: Spinal cord protection during ischemia: Comparison of mannitol, thiopental, and free-radical scavengers. Surg Forum 4:197, 1987.
26. Breckwoldt WL, Genco CM, Connolly RJ, et al: Spinal cord protection during aortic occlusion: Efficacy of intrathecal tetracaine. Ann Thorac Surg 51:959, 1991.
27. Del Rossi AJ, Cernaianu AC, Cilley KH, et al: Preventive effect of Fluosol-DA for paraplegia encountered after surgical treatment of the thoracic aorta: Preliminary results in a dog model. J Thorac Cardiovasc Surg 99:665, 1990.
28. Svensson LG, Grum DF, Bednarski M: Appraisal of cerebrospinal fluid alterations during aortic surgery with intrathecal papaverine administration and cerebrospinal fluid drainage. J Vasc Surg 11:423, 1990.
29. Svensson LG, von Ritter CM, Groeneveld HT, et al: Cross-clamping of the thoracic aorta: Influence of aortic shunts, laminectomy, papaverine, calcium channel blockers, allopurinol, and superoxide dismutase on spinal cord blood flow and paraplegia in baboons. Ann Surg 204: 38, 1986.
30. Livesay JJ, Cooley DA, Ventemiglia RA, et al: Surgical experience in descending thoracic aneurysmectomy with and without adjuncts to avoid ischemia. Ann Thorac Surg 39:37, 1985.
31. Ruiz CE, Zhang HP, Douglas JT, et al: A novel method for treatment of abdominal aortic aneurysms using percutaneous implantation of a newly designed endovascular device. Circulation 91:2470, 1995.
32. Miller DC: The continuing dilemma concerning medical versus surgical management of patients with acute type B dissections. Semin Thorac Cardiovasc Surg 5:33, 1993.
33. Inoue K, Iwase T, Sato M, et al: Clinical application of transluminal endovascular graft placement for aortic aneurysms. Ann Thorac Surg 63:522, 1997.
34. Lemole GM, Strong MD, Spagna PM, Karmilowicz NP: Improved results for dissecting aneurysms: Intraluminal sutureless prosthesis. J Thorac Cardiovasc Surg 83:249, 1982.
35. Barner HB, Willman VL: Intraluminal graft for acute dissection of the ascending aorta. Ann Thorac Surg 17:58, 1974.
36. Carrel T, Maurer M, Tkebuchava T, et al: Embolization of biologic glue during repair of aortic dissection. Ann Thorac Surg 60:1118, 1995.
37. Bachet J, Goudot B, Teodori G: Surgery of type A acute aortic dissection with gelatin-formol biological glue: A twelve year experience. J Thorac Cardiovasc Surg 31:263, 1990.
38. Lindsay J Jr: In Diseases of the Aorta. Lea & Febiger, Philadelphia, 1994, p 65.
39. Lewis CTP, Cooley DA, Murphy MC, et al: Surgical repair of aortic root aneurysms in 280 patients. Ann Thorac Surg 53:38, 1992.

40. Roberts CS, Roberts WC: Aortic dissection with entrance tear in the descending thoracic aorta: Analysis of 40 necropsy patients. Ann Surg 231:356, 1991.
41. Elefteriades JA, Hartleroad J, Gusberg RJ, et al: Long-term experience with descending aortic dissection: The complication-specific approach. Ann Thorac Surg 53:11, 1992.
42. Williams DM, Brothers TE, Messina LM: Relief of mesenteric ischemia in type III aortic dissection with percutaneous fenestration of the aortic septum. Radiology 174:450, 1990.
43. Carpentier AF, Deloche A, Fabiani JN, et al: New surgical approach to aortic dissection: Flow reversal and thromboexclusion. J Thorac Cardiovasc Surg 81:659, 1981.
44. Borst HG, Frank G, Schaps D: Treatment of extensive aortic aneurysm by a new multiple stage approach. J Thorac Cardiovasc Surg 95:11, 1988.
45. Cooley DA: Retrograde replacement of the thoracic aorta. Tex Heart Inst J 22:162, 1992.
46. Katz DJ, Stanley JC, Zelenock GB: Gender differences in abdominal aortic aneurysm prevalence, treatment, and outcome. J Vasc Surg 25: 561, 1997.

20.3 Treatment of Aortic Disease and Aortic Dissection: Other Surgical Approaches and Endovascular Interventions

Hazim J. Safi

During the previous half century, growing experience with aortic aneurysm has led to the standardization of preoperative assessment, operative procedures, and graft materials. Today, it is possible to treat nearly all aneurysms, including leaking or ruptured lesions that require emergency repair. Outcomes can be fairly well predicted, and complications can often be anticipated and prevented. Although surgical repair is still the mainstay of treatment, the advent of endovascular repair has expanded the therapeutic options, especially for high-risk patients who would otherwise be poor surgical candidates.

The previous subchapter presented Dr. Denton Cooley's open techniques for the repair of ascending and descending aortic aneurysms and for one-stage repair of the entire diseased aorta. This section describes other approaches that may be used to repair aortic aneurysms in both women and men. For diagrams of the various types of aortic aneurysms (Crawford types I through V, DeBakey types I through III, and Stanford types A and B), see Chapter 20.1, Figures 20–4 and 20–6.

SURGICAL REPAIR

Nondissecting Aneurysms

The preferred surgical technique differs greatly, depending on whether the aneurysm is located in (1) the ascending aorta, aortic arch, or both or (2) the descending thoracic or thoracoabdominal aorta. The patient's sex does not affect the surgical technique. Whichever technique is used, protection of the brain (during ascending aortic and arch procedures) and of the spinal cord (during descending thoracic and thoracoabdominal aortic operations) is imperative to prevent neurologic deficits. For this purpose, surgeons use various adjunctive methods (see later), which may differ from one institution to another.

Ascending Aorta

For aneurysms of the ascending aorta, aortic arch, or both, the chest is entered through a median sternotomy incision. If aneurysmal disease is limited to the tubular portion of the ascending aorta, it is possible to clamp the aorta, resect the diseased portion, and insert a synthetic graft without using profound hypothermia. For aneurysms that extend from the ascending aorta into the arch, see later discussion.

In patients with Marfan's syndrome, the indications for repair of the ascending aorta are an aortic root diameter of 55 mm or more or proximal aortic dissection (type I or II). For ascending aortic aneurysms, the method of choice is a composite graft repair. Many reports have delineated the success of aortic repair in patients with Marfan's syndrome. Major centers have reported not only a low perioperative mortality with elective repair of the ascending aorta but also a low mortality with emergency replacement of the ascending aorta for either ruptured or dissecting aneurysms.[1–4] These centers have also documented a 5-year survival rate of 93% and a 10-year survival rate of 76%.[1] Cardiovascular complications continue to be the most common causes of death in patients with Marfan's syndrome who have undergone aortic graft repair. Death may be related to endocarditis, rupture or dissection of the aorta, congestive heart failure, stroke, or arrhythmia, or it may occur perioperatively during subsequent aortic repair.[1, 5]

Aortic Arch

If the aneurysm extends from the ascending aorta into the arch, the patient must undergo deep hypothermia, cardiopulmonary bypass, and circulatory arrest. I use adjunctive retrograde cerebral perfusion (RCP) to protect the brain. In this method, oxygenated blood is perfused in a retrograde direction through the superior vena cava and the internal jugular veins. The ascending aorta and the transverse arch are excised, with preservation of an island that comprises

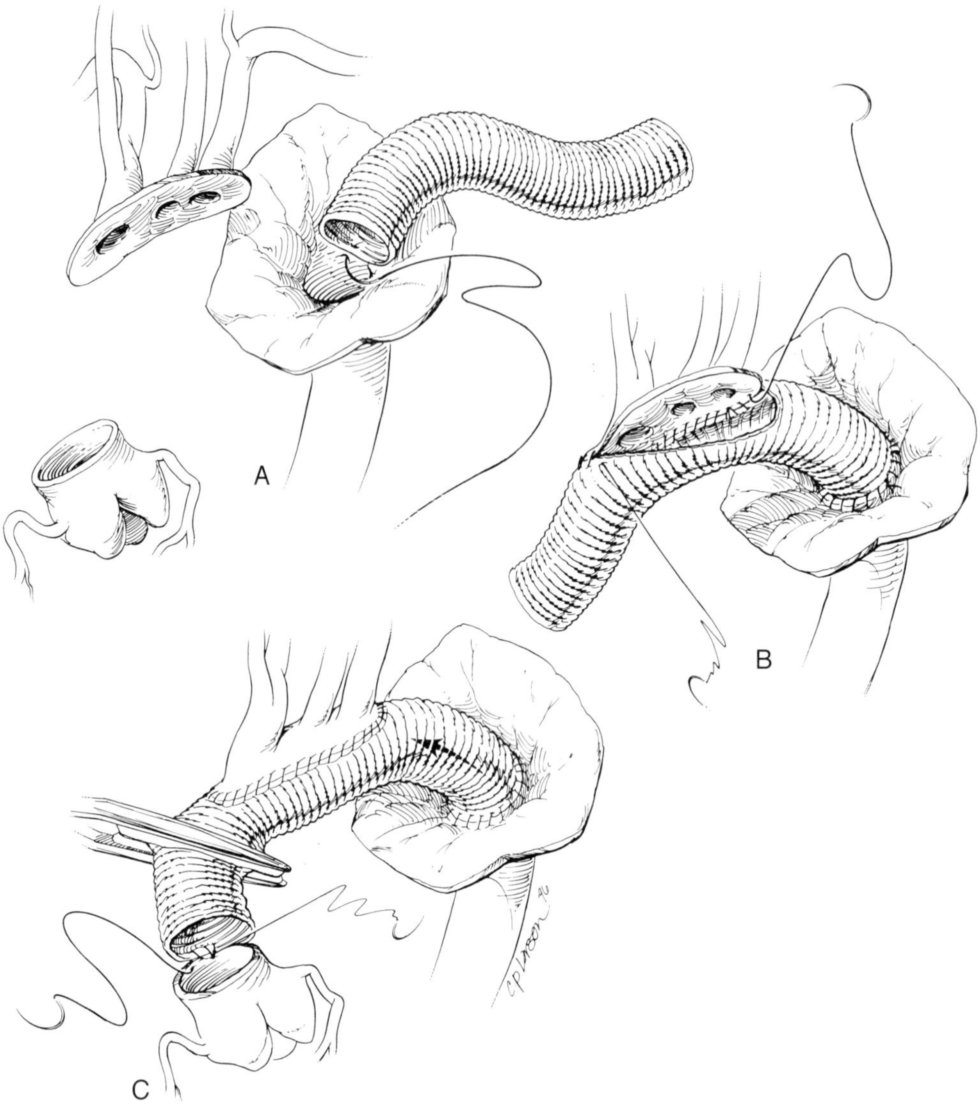

FIGURE 20–14. *A*, Distal anastomosis after excision of the ascending aorta and arch; *B*, anastomosis of the preserved island, comprising the brachiocephalic arteries, to the graft; *C*, the proximal anastomosis.

the brachiocephalic arteries (Fig. 20–14*A*). After the graft is sutured to the descending thoracic aorta just distal to the left subclavian artery, the island is anastomosed to a sidehole cut in the superior arch portion of the graft (Fig. 20–14*B*). The aortic valve and aortic sinuses are inspected and repaired if necessary. The graft is then sutured to the supracoronary ascending aorta (Fig. 20–14*C*).

The major potential complications of ascending aortic and arch repair are stroke and encephalopathy. The rate of stroke is approximately 9% without RCP but only 3% with RCP (Table 20–2).[6]

Descending Thoracic and Thoracoabdominal Aorta

For aneurysms of the descending and thoracoabdominal aorta, the incision begins on the patient's left side, between the shoulder blades, then curves around the chest and proceeds downward toward the umbilicus. The site of termination of the incision depends on the extent of the aneurysm. Of course, the aorta must be clamped long enough to allow graft placement. Cessation of the blood flow increases the risk of neurologic dysfunction. Aortic pressure distal to the upper clamp decreases greatly, leading to reduced spinal

Table 20–2. ASCENDING AORTIC AND AORTIC ARCH ANEURYSMS: RATES OF POSTOPERATIVE STROKE AND EARLY MORTALITY ASSOCIATED WITH SURGICAL TECHNIQUE

TECHNIQUE*	RATE OF POSTOPERATIVE STROKE (%)	30-DAY MORTALITY (%)
Normothermia[6]	Not reported	25–75
Circulatory arrest and profound hypothermia[6]	2–10	5–10
Antegrade cerebral perfusion[6]	5–6	0–20
Retrograde cerebral perfusion[6]	3	5

*Superscript numbers indicate references.

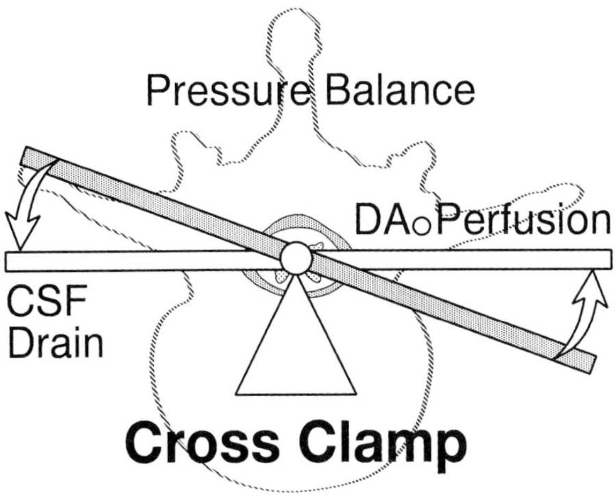

FIGURE 20–15. Distal aortic (DA) perfusion and cerebrospinal fluid (CSF) drainage protect the spinal cord by balancing the spinal-cord pressure during aortic crossclamping.

artery perfusion pressure and increased cerebrospinal fluid (CSF) pressure. Adjunctive left atrial–to–left femoral bypass (distal aortic perfusion) and CSF drainage work together to counteract this imbalance (Fig. 20–15).

During the last 10 to 15 years, these adjuncts have made a notable difference in the operative outcome. The rate of paraplegia and paraparesis for the most extensive and troublesome thoracoabdominal aortic aneurysms (Crawford type II) has decreased from 30%-40% to 10%-12% (Table 20–3).[7] Currently, these operations entail a short-term mortality rate of 5% to 10%, as opposed to the 20% to 25% observed 10 years ago. Reimplantation of intercostal arteries, which became practical with the introduction of perfusion adjuncts, has also dramatically improved the results of these operations.[8] In the repair of type II aneurysms, visceral perfusion protects the kidneys and negates a postoperative increase in liver function values. In this technique, the left kidney is cooled by perfusion via a catheter passed through an ice bath. The left renal artery temperature is kept below 15°C. Warming of the lower circulation keeps the body temperature at 32 to 33°C.

Table 20–3. THORACOABDOMINAL AORTIC ANEURYSMS: RATES OF MAJOR COMPLICATIONS AND MORTALITY ASSOCIATED WITH SURGICAL TECHNIQUE

TYPE OF ANEURYSM*	MAJOR COMPLICATIONS (%)	30-DAY MORTALITY (%)	5-YEAR MORTALITY (%)
Thoracoabdominal, types I–IV[7, 9–12]	Neurologic deficit (0–15) Renal failure (5–25)	5–10	25–40
Thoracoabdominal, type II, without adjuncts†[7, 10–13]	Neurologic deficit (30–40) Renal failure (17)	22	65
Thoracoabdominal, type II, with adjuncts†[7, 10, 11, 13]	Neurologic deficit (10–12) Renal failure (7)	10	30–40

*Crawford classification. Superscript numbers indicate references.
†Distal aortic perfusion and CSF drainage.

In thoracoabdominal aortic aneurysm repair, the main risk factors for a poor outcome are an extensive aneurysm (particularly type II), poor preoperative renal function, and a prolonged aortic cross-clamping time. Paraplegia, paraparesis, and renal failure are relatively uncommon complications but nonetheless remain a threat. Other important issues related to the repair of thoracoabdominal aneurysms are described elsewhere.[9–14]

Abdominal Aorta

Surgical repair of abdominal aortic aneurysms has been practiced for nearly half a century, and many reports describe follow-up periods of at least 10 years. In large, single-center reports, the mortality rates for the repair of unruptured abdominal aortic aneurysms range from 0% to 4%, with a mean of 2%.[15] Multicenter reports generally cite slightly higher mortality rates (3% to 5%; mean, 4%), and population-based reports cite a rate of 7%.[15] These advances in survival have occurred despite the fact that a growing number of surgical patients are older and have severe comorbid conditions. Preoperative detection and treatment of significant cardiac disease have been important factors in improving the outcome. In contrast, the operative results for patients with ruptured abdominal aortic aneurysms are not nearly as favorable, and almost half of such patients die postoperatively.

Mega Aorta

The most far-reaching aneurysm is the so-called mega aorta, which involves the ascending aorta, transverse aortic arch, and thoracoabdominal aorta (Figs. 20–16 and 20–17). In the widely used "elephant-trunk" procedure, surgical repair is performed in two separate stages (see Fig. 20–17).[16] The replacement graft is partially inverted onto itself and is inserted 7 to 10 cm downward into the descending aorta. The inverted edge of the graft is sutured to the descending thoracic aorta just distal to the left subclavian artery. When this distal anastomosis is completed, the inner portion of the tube graft is retrieved, and the outer portion (elephant trunk) is left in the descending aorta. The island formed by the left common carotid, subclavian, and innominate arteries is then anastomosed to a sidehole cut in the superior arch portion of the graft. After a 6- to 8-week recovery period, the second-stage repair is performed on the descending thoracic or thoracoabdominal aorta. A second graft is sewn to the dangling original graft and then to the distal portion of the aorta. Table 20–4 compares the one- and two-staged approaches with respect to major complications and early mortality.[17–19]

Dissecting Aneurysms

Acute Dissection

Type I or II

In DeBakey type I or II aortic dissection, which corresponds to Stanford type A, patients who present in a moribund state

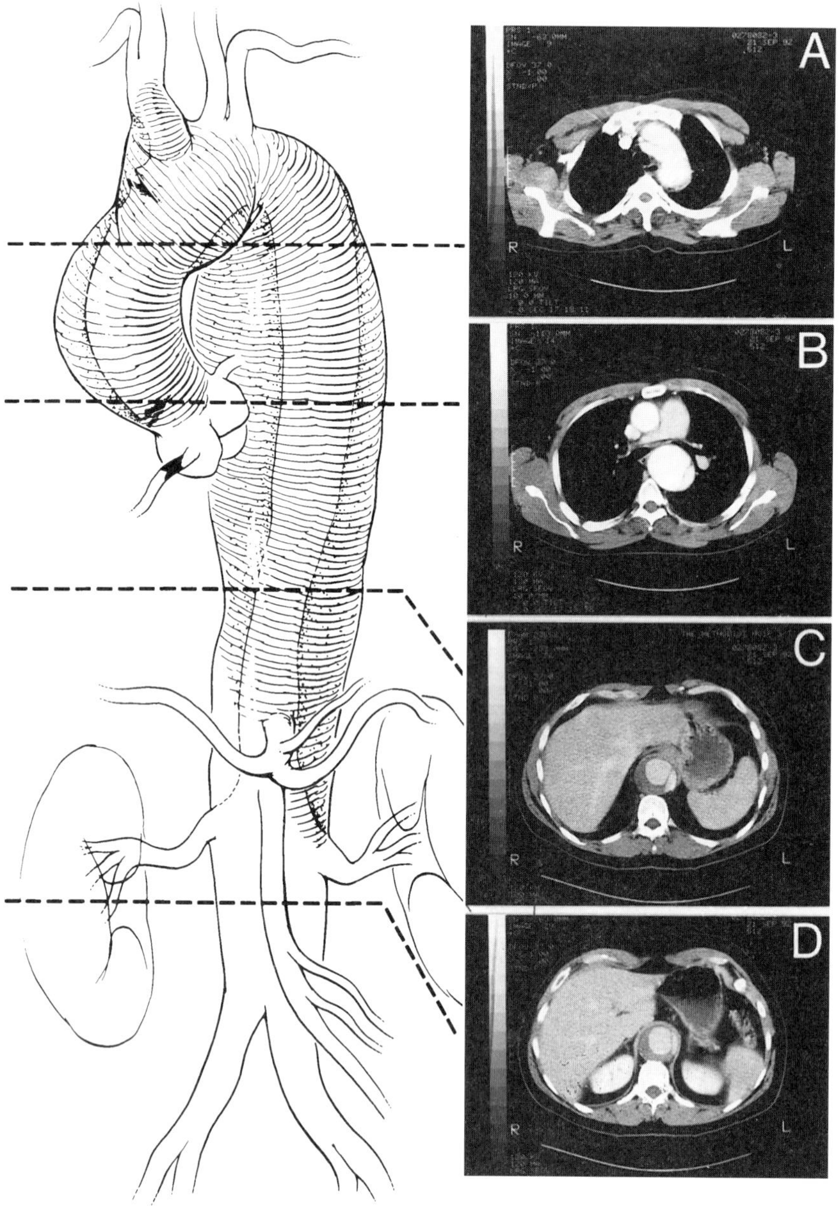

FIGURE 20–16. Drawing and corresponding computed tomogram of a mega-aorta.

Table 20–4. EXTENSIVE OR TOTAL AORTIC ANEURYSMS: RATES OF MAJOR COMPLICATIONS AND EARLY MORTALITY ASSOCIATED WITH SURGICAL TECHNIQUE

TECHNIQUE*	MAJOR COMPLICATIONS (%)	30-DAY MORTALITY (%)
Single-stage repair†[16]	Pulmonary (67) Stroke (13) Neurologic deficit (13)	30
Two-stage repair‡[14, 16]	Stroke (0) Neurologic deficit (0)	3–6

*Superscript numbers indicate references.

†Single-stage repair: The entire extensive aortic aneurysm is repaired during one surgical session, through a left thoracotomy incision.

‡Two-stage repair: The extensive aortic aneurysm is repaired in two separate operations. In stage 1, the ascending aorta and arch are repaired with the aid of profound hypothermia. In stage 2, the descending thoracic and/or thoracoabdominal aorta is repaired with the aid of moderate hypothermia, distal aortic perfusion, and CSF drainage.

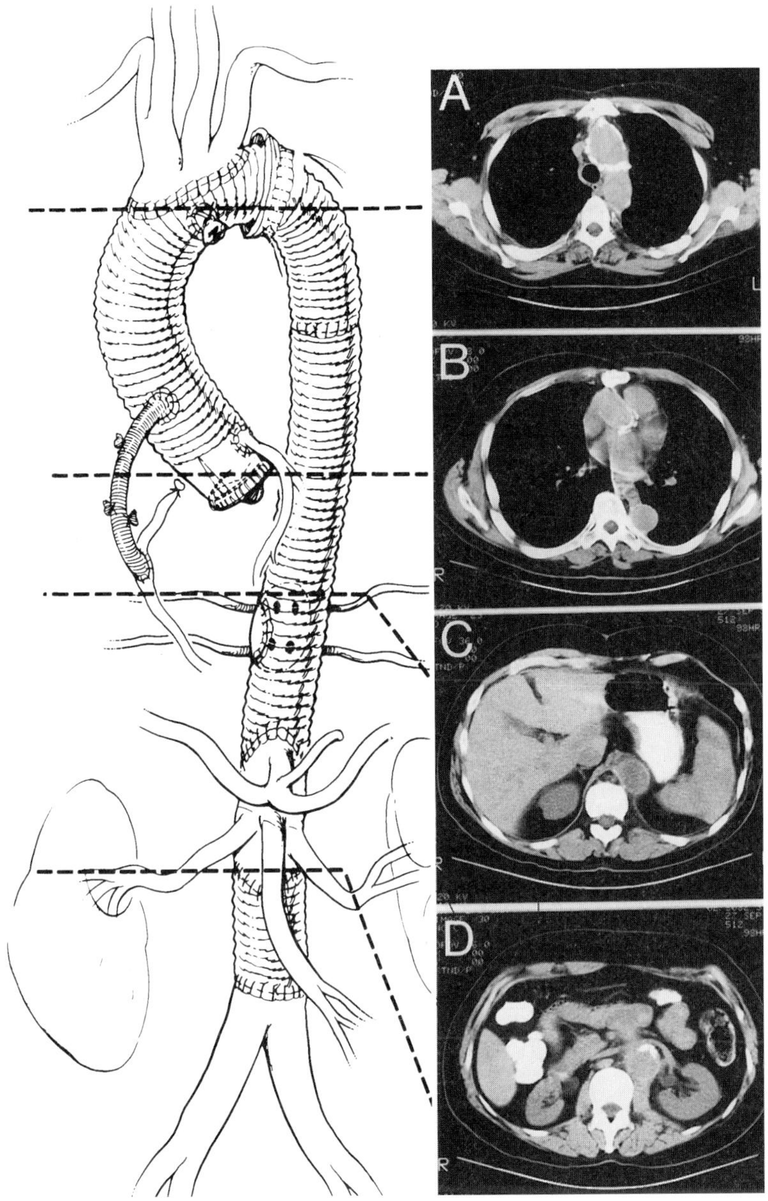

FIGURE 20–17. Drawing and corresponding computed tomogram of an elephant trunk repair.

are sent directly to the emergency department or to the operating room for anesthesia induction and transesophageal echocardiography to identify the site and extent of the intimal disruption. Non-moribund patients with acute symptoms are admitted to the surgical intensive care unit, where they are evaluated with transesophageal echocardiography and are prepared for operation as soon as possible.

The surgical procedure is the same as that previously described for aneurysms of the ascending aorta or arch (Fig. 20–18). After a median sternotomy has been performed, cardiopulmonary bypass is initiated, and profound hypothermia is induced. Cannulation is done via the femorofemoral approach for cardiopulmonary bypass and via the superior vena cava for retrograde cerebral perfusion. Throughout the procedure, myocardial protection is provided by cardioplegic solution, which is perfused via the coronary sinus to keep the myocardial temperature below 15°C. Venting through the left superior pulmonary vein or artery prevents ventricular distention and allows optimal decompression of the left ventricle. Once the intima and adventitia have been sutured together, the surgeon attaches a graft that is reinforced both inside and outside with pledgeted sutures (Fig. 20–18*D*). The aortic valve may be resuspended (Fig. 20–18*F*) or replaced.

For untreated, acute type I or II aortic dissection, the mortality rate exceeds 48% within 48 hours of presentation and is approximately 75% within 2 weeks.[17] In the 1960s, when the first successful operations were performed, the 30-day surgical mortality was 40%. By the late 1980s, the rate had fallen to less than 20%, and it currently hovers in the range of 20% to 30%, depending on risk factors (Table 20–5).[17, 18] Today, mortality is unlikely to be due to technical limitations but, instead, results from underlying end organ ischemic injury related to the dissection itself. The most prevalent major complication is stroke, which occurs in approximately 9% of patients.[12] Major risk factors for postoper-

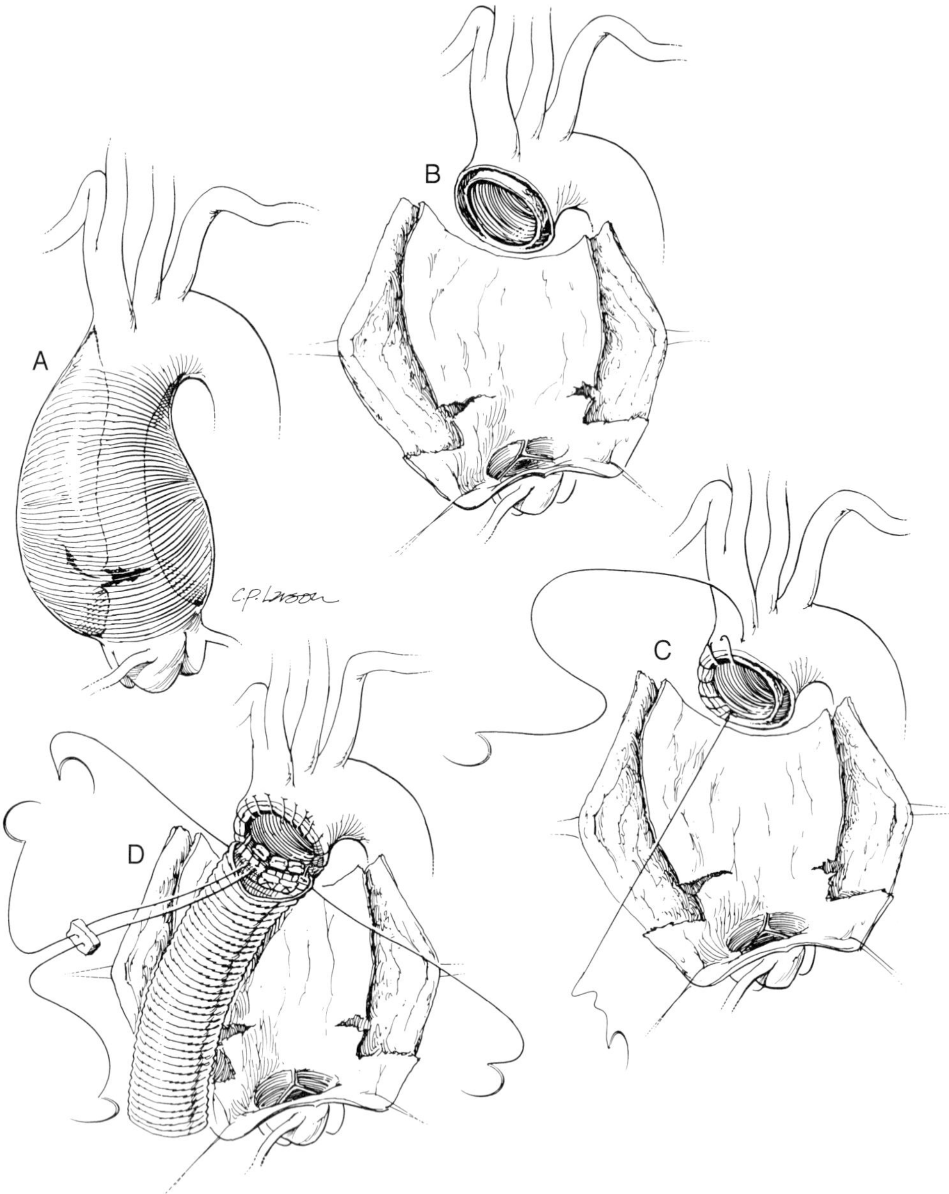

FIGURE 20–18. *A*, Dissection and aneurysm of the ascending aorta (DeBakey type I-II, Stanford type A); *B*, excision of the aneurysm; *C*, suturing of the aortic walls; *D*, graft placement with the aid of pledgeted sutures; *E*, distal anastomosis, including reinforcement with pledgeted sutures; *F*, resuspension of the aortic valve; *G*, proximal anastomosis with the aid of pledgeted sutures.

ative stroke are a prolonged pump time and the presence of severe hypotension (such as occurs with rupture).[18]

Type III

The operative technique for acute DeBakey type III (Stanford type B) aortic dissection is the same as that previously described for descending thoracic or thoracoabdominal aneurysms. When the descending thoracic graft is sutured to the reinforced distal aorta, blood is rechanneled into the true aortic lumen. At my institution, adjunctive CSF drainage and distal aortic perfusion are used in all cases. The visceral vessels and renal arteries are attached to the graft either directly or with the aid of a woven Dacron graft. In acute dissections, all the intercostal and lumbar arteries are ligated, because friable tissue is likely to lead to a fatal hemorrhage. In patients with a chronic dissection, intercostal arteries T9 through T12 are reimplanted into either a sidearm graft or a graft with a sidehole to which the arteries are reattached directly.

The optimal treatment is more debatable for an acute DeBakey type III (Stanford type B) dissection than for an acute type I or II dissection. With proficient intensive care and aggressive blood pressure control, the results are equal to, or probably better than, the results of immediate operation.[18, 20–22] The 30-day postoperative mortality is 25% to 50% (see Table 20–5), compared with 7% to 32% after initial medical treatment.[12, 18] The comparability of the various series is difficult to judge, but the literature contains many published results, and the trends appear to be reproducible. The major potential complication is ischemic spinal cord injury. If the dissection is as extensive as a type II thoracoabdominal aneurysm, the incidence of neurologic deficits is as high as 32%.[18] As with acute type I or II dissection, the high morbidity and mortality are due mainly to ischemic sequelae related to the underlying disease.

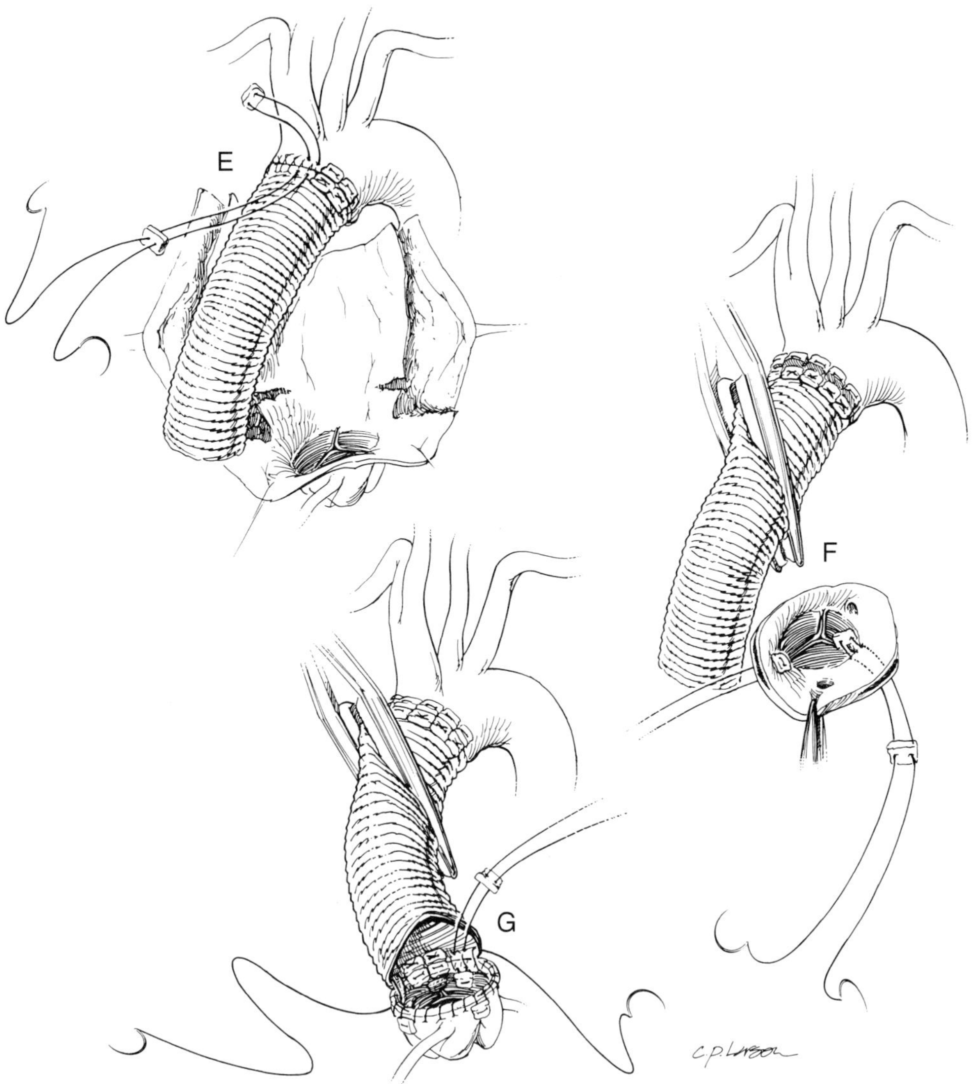

FIGURE 20–18 *Continued*

Chronic Dissection

A chronic dissection is the stabilized result of a previous acute event. Surgical repair of chronic dissection yields results similar to those associated with the repair of aneurysms of the descending thoracic and thoracoabdominal aorta; the best outcome is obtained when the aneurysm involves the upper one half to one third of the aorta. The 30-day mortality ranges from 10% to 25% (see Table 20–5), and a neurologic deficit occurs in approximately 9% of cases.[12, 18]

Table 20–5. AORTIC DISSECTION: RATES OF MAJOR COMPLICATIONS AND EARLY MORTALITY ASSOCIATED WITH SURGICAL TECHNIQUE

TYPE OF ANEURYSM*	MAJOR COMPLICATIONS (%)	30-DAY MORTALITY (%)
Type I or II:		
Acute dissection[17, 18]	Stroke (9)	20–30
Chronic dissection[12]	Stroke (4)	4
Type III:		
Acute dissection[12, 18]	Neurologic deficit (30) Renal failure (30)	25–50
Chronic dissection[12, 18]	Neurologic deficit (9) Renal failure (14)	10–25†

*DeBakey classification: types I and II correspond to Stanford type A; type III corresponds to Stanford type B. Superscript numbers indicate references.

†The 5-year mortality is 44%.

ENDOVASCULAR REPAIR

Because of the risks associated with the surgical repair of aortic aneurysms, particularly in older, sicker patients, an interventional approach using endoluminal stent-grafts is growing in favor. Endovascular repair may be used for aneurysms of the descending thoracic or thoracoabdominal aorta.

All endovascular procedures involve femoral artery exposure for the insertion of a guidewire and subsequent introduction of a stent-graft into the aortic lumen to exclude the aneurysmal sac. Intraoperative imaging by means of fluoroscopy, angiography, or intravascular ultrasonography is essential.

A prospective, nonrandomized, multicenter trial comparing endoluminal and surgical aneurysm repair has revealed no significant differences in operative mortality.[1] Endovascular treatment is also associated with a significantly shorter hospital stay. This approach entails the best outlook for high-risk patients, particularly the very elderly, who may have an unreconstructible aorta, poor left ventricular function with congestive heart failure, or severe obstructive disease.

In a small percentage of cases, an attempted endovascular repair is unsuccessful and must be converted to an open operation. In such cases, the morbidity and mortality are greater than those associated with elective surgical repair. Fortunately, the risk of conversion is decreasing because of growing interventional experience, better selection of candidates, and the advent of improved endovascular devices.

Once a stent-graft has been successfully deployed, the most common potential problem is "endoleakage," in which an incomplete seal around the edges of the graft allows blood flow to continue to pressurize the aneurysm. This continued flow raises the risk of late graft thrombosis, migration, dysfunction, or even rupture.

Descending Thoracic Aorta

Endovascular repair of the thoracic aorta is controversial. A problem with the use of stent-grafts in the thoracic aorta is the exclusion of intercostal arteries, which increases the spinal cord's vulnerability to ischemic injury. In a 1998 series, the early mortality after thoracic endovascular stent-grafting was 9%.[23] Major complications were stroke (7%) and paraplegia (3%). Twenty-four percent of the grafts developed an early endoleak, for which 18% required additional intervention. Approximately 5% of the grafts had to be removed or otherwise excluded.

The lack of long-term data should rule out the use of endovascular grafts in patients who are younger or are expected to survive for more than 5 years. Also, if a patient is too ill to undergo surgical graft replacement and has a short life expectancy, the merit of endovascular repair must be carefully evaluated.

Abdominal Aorta

Endovascular repair of the abdominal aorta is much less controversial than that of the descending thoracic aorta. The first definitive abdominal aortic aneurysm repair involving the transfemoral insertion of a prosthetic graft was reported in 1991.[24] Since then, a number of improved devices and strategies have been developed and evaluated. Although clinical experience with endovascular abdominal aortic aneurysm repair is growing rapidly, the precise risk, particularly the long-term risk, of such repair is unknown. Published clinical series vary widely with respect to mortality, graft failure rate, and other measures of outcome. The rate of successful aneurysm exclusion approaches 90%,[25–27] but a number of problems are possible, including vessel perforation, inability to advance the device through the iliac artery, inability to seal the aneurysm, and need to convert the procedure to an open surgical repair.

Not all patients with infrarenal aortic aneurysms are candidates for an endovascular procedure. Morphologic features that may contraindicate endovascular graft repair include severe vessel tortuosity, accessory renal arteries, iliac aneurysms and occlusions, and associated branch vessel stenoses.

Before endovascular abdominal aortic aneurysm repair can be widely applied, follow-up results from ongoing trials will have to be analyzed.

References

1. Gott VL, Pyeritz RE, Cameron DE: Composite graft repair of Marfan aneurysm of the ascending aorta: Results in 100 patients. Ann Thorac Surg 52:38, 1991.
2. Kouchoukos NT, Wareing TH, Murphy SF, et al: Sixteen-year experience with aortic root replacement: Results of 172 operations. Ann Surg 214:308, 1991.
3. Murdoch JL, Walker BA, Halpern BL, et al: Life expectancy and causes of death in the Marfan syndrome. N Engl J Med 286:804, 1972.
4. Coselli JS, LeMaire SA, Buket S: Marfan syndrome: The variability and outcome of operative management. J Vasc Surg 21:432, 1995.
5. Finkbohner R, Johnston D, Crawford ES, et al: Marfan syndrome: Long-term survival and complications after aortic aneurysm repair. Circulation 91:728, 1995.
6. Safi HJ, Letsou GV, Iliopoulos DC, et al: Impact of retrograde cerebral perfusion on ascending aortic and arch aneurysm repair. Ann Thorac Surg 63:1601, 1997.
7. Safi HJ, Campbell MP, Miller CC 3rd, et al: Cerebral spinal fluid drainage and distal aortic perfusion decrease the incidence of neurological deficit: The results of 343 descending and thoracoabdominal aortic aneurysm repairs. Eur J Vasc Endovasc Surg 14:118, 1997.
8. Safi HJ, Miller CC 3rd, Carr C, et al: Importance of intercostal artery reattachment during thoracoabdominal aortic aneurysm repair. J Vasc Surg 27:58, 1998.
9. Galloway AC, Miller JS, Spencer FC, et al: Thoracic aneurysms and aortic dissection. In Schwartz SI (ed): Principles of Surgery, 7th ed. McGraw-Hill, New York, 1999, p 909.
10. Safi HJ, Miller CC 3rd, Iliopoulos D, et al: Long-term results following thoracoabdominal aortic aneurysm repair. In Branchereau A, Jacobs M (eds): Long-term Results of Arterial Interventions. Futura, Armonk, NY, 1997, p 181.
11. Safi HJ, Harlin SA, Miller CC, et al: Predictive factors for acute renal failure in thoracic and thoracoabdominal aortic aneurysm surgery [published erratum appears in J Vasc Surg 25:93, 1997]. J Vasc Surg 24:338, 1996.
12. Svensson LG, Crawford ES, Hess KR, et al: Experience with 1509 patients undergoing thoracoabdominal aortic operations. J Vasc Surg 17:357, 1993.
13. Safi HJ, Miller CC 3rd, Yawn DH, et al: Impact of distal aortic and visceral perfusion on liver function during thoracoabdominal and descending thoracic aortic repair. J Vasc Surg 27:145, 1998.
14. Borst HG, Frank G, Schaps D: Treatment of extensive aortic aneurysms by a new multiple-stage approach. J Thorac Cardiovasc Surg 95:11, 1988.
15. Zarins CK, White RA, Schwarten D, et al: AneuRx stent graft versus open surgical repair of abdominal aortic aneurysms: Multicenter prospective clinical trial. J Vasc Surg 29:292, 1999.
16. Safi HJ, Miller CC 3rd, Iliopoulos DC, et al: Staged repair of extensive aortic aneurysm: Improved neurologic outcome. Ann Surg 226.599, 1997.
17. Borst HG, Heinemann MK, Stone CD: Surgical Treatment of Aortic Dissection. Churchill Livingstone, New York, 1996, p 103.
18. Safi HJ, Miller CC 3rd, Reardon MJ, et al: Operation for acute and chronic aortic dissection: Recent outcome with regard to neurologic deficit and early death. Ann Thorac Surg 66:402, 1998.
19. Perko MJ, Norgaard M, Herzog TM, et al: Unoperated aortic aneurysm: A survey of 170 patients. Ann Thorac Surg 59:1204, 1995.
20. Masuda Y, Yamada Z, Morooka N, et al: Prognosis of patients with medically treated aortic dissections. Circulation 84:III7, 1991.
21. Crawford ES, Svensson LG, Coselli JS, et al: Aortic dissection and dissecting aortic aneurysms. Ann Surg 208:254, 1988.
22. Glower DD, Fann JI, Speier RH, et al: Comparison of medical and surgical therapy for uncomplicated descending aortic dissection. Circulation 82:IV39, 1990.

23. Dake MD, Miller DC, Mitchell RS, et al: The "first generation" of endovascular stent-grafts for patients with aneurysms of the descending thoracic aorta. J Thorac Cardiovasc Surg 116:689, 1998.
24. Parodi JC, Palmaz JC, Barone HD: Transfemoral intraluminal graft implantation for abdominal aortic aneurysms. Ann Vasc Surg 5:491, 1991.
25. Blum U, Voshage G, Lammer J, et al: Endoluminal stent-grafts for infrarenal abdominal aortic aneurysms. N Engl J Med 336:13, 1997.
26. May J, White GH, Waugh R, et al: Life-table analysis of primary and assisted success following endoluminal repair of abdominal aortic aneurysms: The role of supplementary endovascular intervention in improving outcome. Eur J Vasc Endovasc Surg 19:648, 2000.
27. Howell MH, Zaqqa M, Villareal RP, et al: Endovascular exclusion of abdominal aortic aneurysms: Initial experience with stent-grafts in cardiology practice. Tex Heart Inst J 27:136, 2000.

CHAPTER 21

Peripheral Vascular Disease

21.1 Overview

Zvonimir Krajcer and Kathryn Dougherty

EPIDEMIOLOGY OF PERIPHERAL ARTERIAL DISEASE

Few trials have specifically addressed the issue of gender and how it affects the outcome of peripheral arterial disease (PAD). The prevalence of vascular disease in women is greater than previously reported. PAD, however, is a cause of considerable morbidity especially in older women. Current estimates in the United States indicate that at least 20% to 25% of elderly women in the United States are affected by PAD and that as many as 90% of these women remain untreated.[1] Often, older women believe leg pain is a normal part of aging and so do not report cramping ischemic pain to their physician. Therefore, PAD commonly is unrecognized and remains untreated.[2]

The prevalence of PAD, as determined through the use of noninvasive objective measures such as ankle-brachial index (ABI), is several-fold higher than previously reported and increases sharply after age 60 years.[3] In the Edinburgh Artery Study, prevalence of claudication increased with age, and by age 65 to 69 years, men and women were affected equally.[4] In another study using ABI in 275 women, PAD was present in 3% of those younger than 60 years and in 20% of those older than 75 years.[5] In the Cardiovascular Health study, ABI was measured in more than 5000 people older than 65 years; men and women were affected equally, and there was a strong association of PAD with increased age.[6]

RISK FACTORS FOR DEVELOPMENT OF PERIPHERAL ARTERIAL DISEASE

Hyperlipidemia

Most of the modifiable risk factors for development of PAD are similar for men and women. Elevated plasma low-density lipoprotein (LDL) levels, decreased high-density lipoprotein (HDL) levels, and raised blood pressure are associated with development and progression of atherosclerosis.[7]

Nicotine Effects

Cigarette smoking is firmly established as the most avoidable cause of morbidity and mortality for both genders.[8, 9] Cigarette smoking is associated with an increased risk and progression of advanced atherosclerotic disease in the peripheral as well as the coronary arteries. The likelihood of claudication, amputation, stroke, abdominal aortic aneurysm (AAA), and failure of vascular reconstruction is higher in smokers than nonsmokers.[10] Several studies have revealed that at least 90% of patients with symptomatic PAD have a history of cigarette smoking.[8, 9, 11] Furthermore, a diagnosis of PAD is commonly established a decade earlier in smokers than in nonsmokers. Smoking increases the risk of development of claudication significantly more frequently in women than in men.[12] In a report from the Mayo Clinic, all women older than 46 years who were examined prior to a peripheral artery revascularization procedure were smokers.[13]

Smoking induces a wide variety of physiologic responses, some of which appear likely to be involved in accelerating atherogenesis or increasing the probability of thrombosis. Fortunately, a rapid amelioration of the physiologic changes and a dramatic reduction in the risk of atherosclerotic progression occur after cessation of smoking, suggesting that these processes are readily reversible. In addition, these benefits accrue regardless of age at the time of cessation.[8, 9]

Despite the publicized health risks of smoking, the number of female smokers continues to increase while the number of male smokers is rapidly decreasing.[14, 15] Recent reports indicate that smoking is more common among women than men, particularly among teenagers and people in their early 20s.[16, 17] This trend will contribute substantially to the future of cardiovascular disease, PAD, and other smoking-related illnesses among U.S. women.[17, 18]

Arterial Hypertension

Hypertension also raises the risk of PAD. The Framingham Study provides the most convincing epidemiologic evidence linking hypertension and PAD. Elevated systolic blood pressure was an independent predictor of claudication, with women experiencing a relative risk ratio twice as high as that in men.[17] After menopause, the incidence of arterial hypertension progressively rises in women compared with men.[17, 19] Hypertensive women are four times more likely than age-matched normotensive men to develop cardiovascular diseases.[20]

The benefits of pharmacologic treatment of hypertension are also very clear.[18–20] In the past, however, the benefits of treatment to lower mild elevations in blood pressure had been less certain. In a meta-analysis of several pharmacologic treatment trials, an average decrease of 6 mm Hg in diastolic blood pressure reduced the risk of stroke for 42% of subjects, myocardial infarction for 14%, and vascular death for 21%.[19]

Menopause and Hormone Replacement Therapy

The incidence of cardiovascular disease is lower in women before menopause than in men but rises dramatically after menopause.[21] This risk is further increased by both premature menopause and oophorectomy.[22–24] In a review of operative records for nondiabetic women undergoing lower extremity revascularization over a period of 24 years, aortoiliac occlusion occurred twice as frequently among those in whom the onset of menopause came before age 43.[25] Premenopausal women, compared with men and postmenopausal women, have higher HDL cholesterol (HDL-C) levels, lower LDL cholesterol (LDL-C) levels, and higher estrogen levels. These differences are likely to contribute to their protection from atherosclerosis.[26] On the other hand, postmenopausal estrogen deficiency induces metabolic and hemodynamic changes that can accelerate atherosclerosis, hypertension, and peripheral vasomotor instability.

Estrogen replacement therapy, initially administered to prevent osteoporosis and attenuate fastidious symptoms of menopause, is proposed to be a beneficial cardioprotective agent. There is a wealth of epidemiologic evidence indicating that postmenopausal estrogen therapy can significantly reduce cardiovascular risks. Several observational studies support the concept that estrogens play a protective role by increasing endothelial regrowth after vascular injury,[27, 28] thus delaying the onset of cardiovascular symptoms. In addition, estrogen replacement raises HDL-C, lowers LDL-C and total cholesterol,[29] and decreases levels of both lipoprotein (a)[30] and homocysteine.[31] Elevations in fibrinogen and factor VII have been associated with cardiovascular disease. In the Atherosclerosis Risk in Communities Study, women who were taking estrogen or estrogen and progestin had lower levels of fibrinogen than those who were not.[26]

Progestins are also thought to have several effects on the cardiovascular system, mainly related to their androgenic activity, and are capable of antagonizing the favorable impact of estrogens. Estrogen replacement therapy is also associated with a reduction in plasminogen activator inhibitor-1 (PAI-1) levels, which is consistent with enhanced fibrinolysis.[32] In a double-blind, placebo-controlled crossover trial, improved arterial dilatation with reactive hyperemia was seen in postmenopausal women taking estrogen with or without progestin.[33] This observed improvement in endothelium-dependent vasodilatation suggests that estrogen may also improve the bioavailability of nitric oxide, a potent antiatherogenic molecule.

Although the potential effects of estrogen therapy on the peripheral vascular system are unknown, the data thus far suggest that they would be beneficial and that such therapy is the one obvious unique gender difference in the reduction of cardiovascular risk factors.

Diabetes Mellitus

Numerous studies have demonstrated an association between diabetes mellitus and the development of PAD.[34, 35] The role of intensive blood glucose control in the prevention of microcirculatory complications has been well established. Diabetes, however, is an even greater risk factor in women than in men, as revealed in the Framingham Study. Women with an impaired glucose tolerance had a fourfold increase in risk for symptomatic PAD, compared with a 2.4-fold increase in men, and glycosuria raised the risk even further in women, by eightfold.[35, 36] Furthermore, people with diabetes have a sevenfold higher rate of lower extremity amputation than people without the disease.[36] Despite the prominence of PAD in diabetic women, far fewer women than men complain of or receive hospital treatment for their disease.[35, 36]

Hypothyroidism

Hypothyroidism is common among elderly women and has been observed in almost one fourth of women with symptomatic claudication.[36] Patients with hypothyroidism have a lower metabolic rate, which contributes to reduced activity and increased lipid levels. This condition in combination with smoking can accelerate the development of PAD.

Obesity

Obesity is also known to be a strong predictor of atherosclerosis-related events in both men and women. Several other risk factors, including hypertension, diabetes, and hypercholesterolemia, are worsened in the presence of obesity. Data from the Third National Health and Nutrition Examination Survey (NHANES III) indicate that marked increases in the prevalence of obesity have occurred among the U.S. population.[37] An estimated 35% of all women in the United States (32 million) are overweight, marking a dramatic increase from the rates recorded in previous national surveys.

In the Nurses' Health Study, women in the highest category of overweight experience a more than threefold greater risk of cardiovascular disease.[38] However, there are not enough data available to support the hypothesis that weight loss can cause significant reduction in the risk for cardiovascular events.

INFLAMMATORY AND AUTOIMMUNE CAUSES OF PERIPHERAL ARTERIAL DISEASE

Takayasu's Arteritis

Takayasu's arteritis is a chronic inflammatory arteritis affecting large vessels, primarily the aorta and its main branches. Marked intimal proliferation and fibrosis with elastic degeneration of the media can lead to stenosis, occlusion, aneurysmal dilation of the affected vessels, or a combination of these conditions.[39–41] Takayasu's arteritis occurs predominantly in Asian women, with onset usually between 10 and 40 years of age.[42] The pathogenesis and cause of the disease are not known, although autoimmunity appears to play an important role. Many patients are asymptomatic, and the diagnosis is first suspected during an evaluation of an abnormal physical finding (e.g., unequal arm blood pressures, absent pulses, or a bruit). Inflammation initially leads to patchy thickening of the affected arterial walls, causing direct injury and leading over time to fibrosis.

Treatment of Takayasu's Arteritis

Corticosteroids are considered first-line therapy for the treatment of active Takayasu's arteritis. However, revasculari-

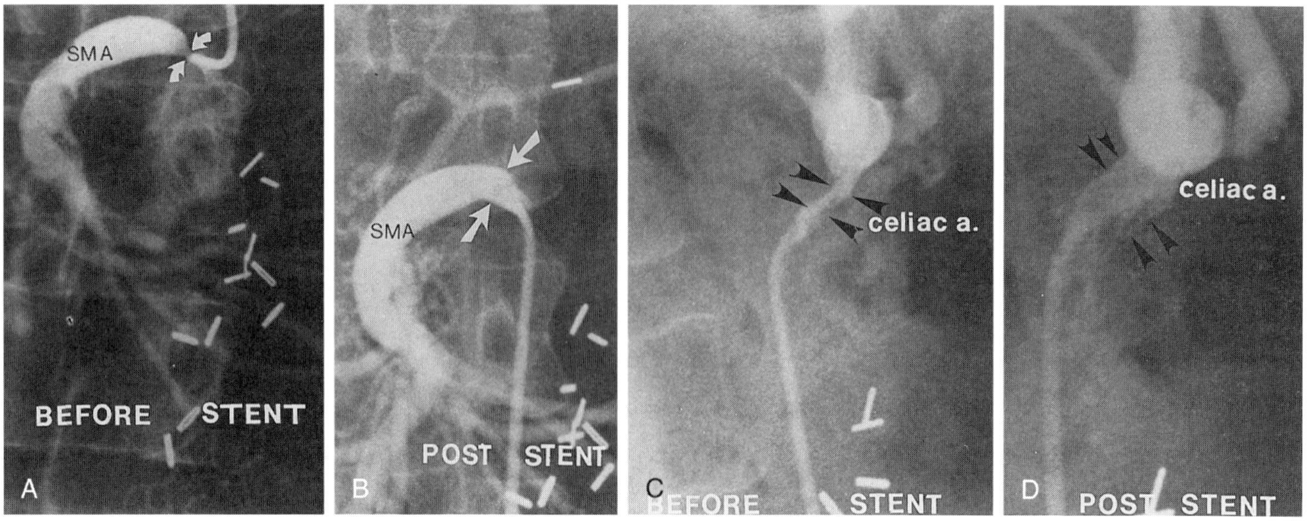

FIGURE 21–1. *A,* Selective superior mesenteric artery angiography in a 42-year-old women with Takayasu's arteritis showing at least 80% stenosis of the ostium. *B,* After stent implantation. *C,* Celiac angiography in the same patient showing a long ostial stenosis. *D,* Follow-up angiography after stent placement.

zation procedures are frequently required during the chronic occlusive phase of the disease. Multivessel involvement, graft occlusion, and high mortality rates have complicated surgical revascularization. Several small series have reported success of and low associated morbidity for the use of balloon angioplasty to treat stenotic lesions of Takayasu's arteritis.[43–45] Stent-supported angioplasty of the mesenteric and celiac arteries has also resulted in significant symptomatic relief (Fig. 21–1).[46]

Giant Cell Arteritis

Giant cell arteritis is another poorly understood chronic inflammatory vascular disease. It involves medium to large arteries, especially the thoracic aorta, large cervical arteries, and branches of the external carotid artery. As in Takayasu's arteritis, autoimmunity appears to play a role in the cause and pathogenesis of the disease. Giant cell arteritis occurs almost exclusively in white women older than 50 years, with a geographic predilection for individuals from the northern United States and Scandinavian countries.[47–49]

The mainstay of treatment for the disease is corticosteroid therapy, which should be administered immediately once the diagnosis is suspected and maintained for up to 2 years.[50] A temporal artery biopsy remains the standard for diagnosis. Histologic examination reveals granulomatous inflammatory lesions with necrosis of the internal elastic lamina, often with multinucleated giant cells.[51]

Fibromuscular Dysplasia

Fibromuscular dysplasia is a noninflammatory, nonatherosclerotic vascular disease affecting small to medium-sized vessels. It is most commonly found in the renal arteries (60% to 75%), although it has been described in many other vascular beds.[49] Fibromuscular disease is classified according to primary sites of involvement in the arterial wall, and histologic findings are correlated with angiographic appearances. Lesions are categorized according to the layer of arterial wall involved.[52] The classifications are intimal fibroplasias, medial fibroplasias, fibromuscular hyperplasia, and subadventitial fibroplasias.

Fibromuscular disease is most commonly seen in women between the ages of 25 and 50 years and accounts for approximately 40% of all renovascular disorders. The lesions are considered congenital dysplasias with maldevelopment of the fibrous, muscular, and elastic tissues of the renal artery. Medial fibroplasia is the most common of the fibrous lesions and generally occurs in both renal arteries but may appear in other vessels, such as the carotid, mesenteric, or iliac arteries.

Angiographically, medial fibroplasias demonstrate a typical "string of beads" appearance involving the distal two thirds of the main renal artery and branches. The degree of stenosis is sometimes difficult to assess, because saccular aneurysms are larger than the normal vessel and areas of stenosis are overshadowed by contrast medium.

Perimedial fibroplasias occur predominantly in women between 15 and 30 years of age. These lesions make up 10% to 15% of all fibrous lesions and are characterized by collagen deposits in the outer border of the media. The angiographic appearance is that of arterial beading, but the beading does not exceed the caliber of the normal vessel. Perimedial fibroplasias produce severe stenosis with progressive obstruction and require intervention before ischemic renal atrophy occurs.

Fibromuscular dysplasia is not as common as perimedial and medial fibroplasias, constituting only 1% to 2% of fibrous lesions. Fibromuscular dysplasia is most commonly seen in children and young adults. It involves concentric smooth muscle cell proliferation and fibrous tissue in variable quantities. Progressive obstruction develops, appearing angiographically as a smooth stenosis that may be indistinguishable from intimal fibroplasias.

Treatment of Fibromuscular Dysplasia

Surgical revascularization for the lesions of fibromuscular dysplasia has declined significantly, a reflection of the fact

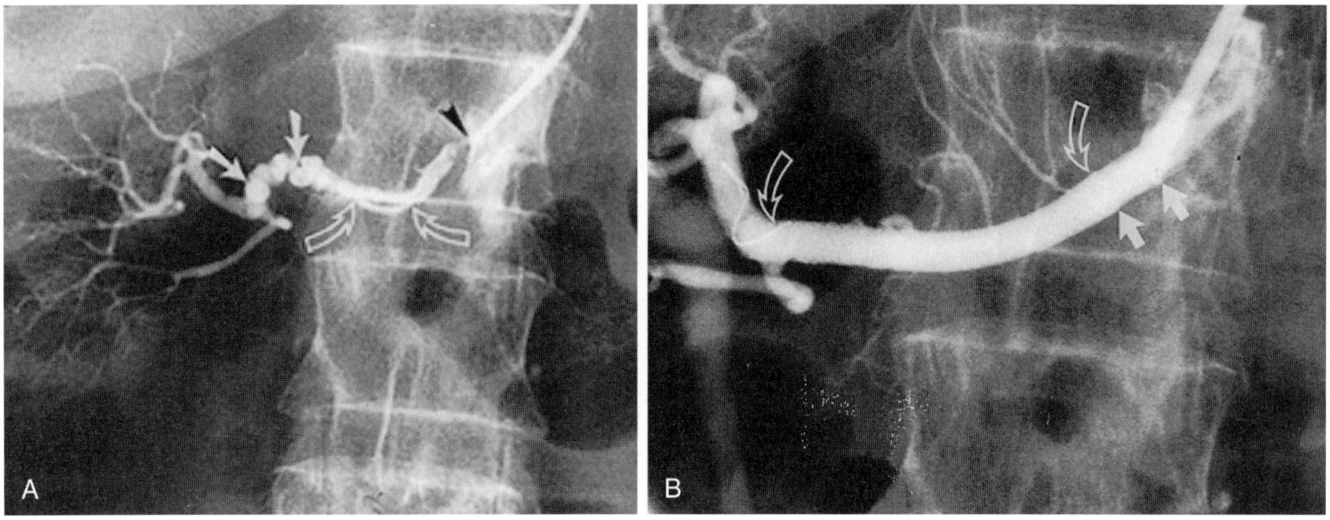

FIGURE 21–2. *A,* Before stent implantation in the right renal artery in a patient with fibromuscular disease. *B,* After stent implantation in the same patient.

that they can be treated quite effectively with percutaneous intervention (Fig. 21–2). The rate of initial technical success exceeds 90%, and up to 87% of patients experience elimination or a significant reduction of hypertension at 6 months.[53–55] Klinge and coworkers[53] reported an initial clinical success rate (success defined as cure or significant improvement of hypertension) of 87%. During 5 years of follow-up, only 6% of patients experienced recurrences.[53]

Medial fibroplasia responds most favorably to percutaneous transluminal renal angioplasty (PTRA).[54] Low inflation pressures usually result in a normal appearance on follow-up angiography. Intimal fibroplasia, medial hyperplasia, and adventitial fibroplasia cause eccentric stenosis, require higher inflation pressures, and less commonly permit complete dilatation.[55]

ANATOMIC FACTORS ASSOCIATED WITH DEVELOPMENT OF PERIPHERAL ARTERIAL DISEASE

Previous studies have revealed that 96% of patients with PAD also have arteriographic evidence of coronary artery disease (CAD).[11] Patients with PAD have widespread arterial disease and a significantly higher risk of stroke, myocardial infarction, and cardiovascular death. At least 10% of patients with PAD have cerebral vascular disease.[2] Patients with PAD should be viewed as having potentially diffuse arterial disease and at higher risk of cardiovascular death.

Cerebrovascular Disease

Epidemiology

The number of women affected by cerebrovascular disease is unknown because women have rarely been included in previous studies of the disorder. A 10-year population study showed, however, that the incidences of stroke and transient ischemic attacks were equal in men and women.[56] Diabetes mellitus was an independent risk factor for large vessel infarction in both genders, and obesity in women was associated with a higher incidence of basilar infarction.[57] The influence of gender on the distribution of cerebrovascular disease was also evaluated in a longitudinal study of patients admitted to a community hospital: Men were found to be more likely than women to have intracranial arterial disease.[58]

Surgical Treatment of Carotid Atherosclerosis

Of all the studies published on carotid endarterectomy during the 1980s, none emphasized the impact of female gender on the operative results. However, far fewer carotid endarterectomies were performed on women despite the fact that their mean age was nearly identical to that of men.[59] A multiple regression analysis by the European Carotid Surgery Trial (ECST) collaborators found an association between female gender and operative risk.[60] Others have reported that rates of perioperative neurologic events were higher in women.[58, 59, 61]

Endoluminal Treatment of Extracranial Carotid Artery Disease

Stent-supported carotid angioplasty continues to evolve as an endovascular alternative to carotid endarterectomy and is currently being investigated in multicenter clinical trials.[62] Carotid endarterectomy has many limitations, especially in high-risk patients with multiple comorbid conditions such as advanced age, diabetes, and recurrent carotid stenosis. Female gender has been implicated as a predisposing factor in the development of recurrent stenosis after carotid endarterectomy. This might be related to the smaller arteries more often encountered in women.[60, 61] The complications after "redo" carotid surgery are significantly higher than after the first operation. Stent-supported carotid angioplasty for treatment of restenosis after carotid endarterectomy has

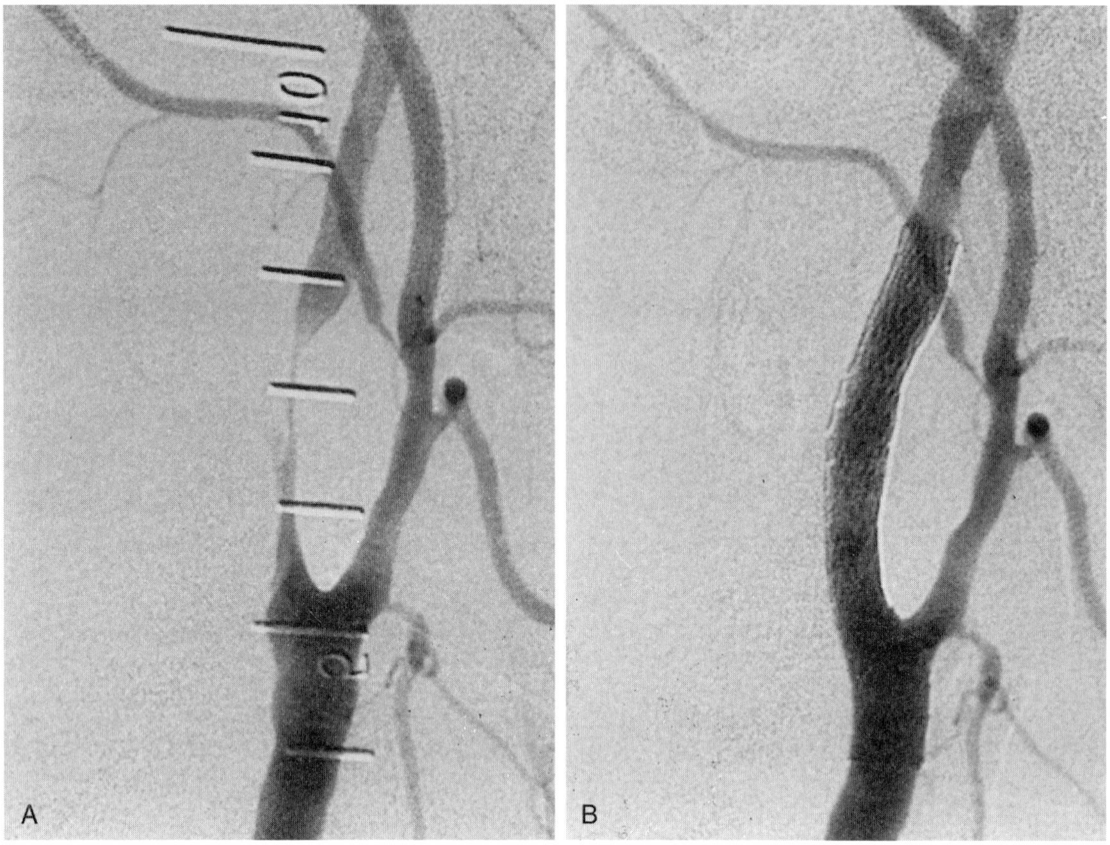

FIGURE 21–3. *A*, Before angioplasty and stent implantation in a 57-year-old woman who had radical neck surgery and radiation-induced stenosis of the right internal carotid artery. *B*, After stent implantation in the same patient.

become very popular.[63, 64] It has also shown very encouraging preliminary results (Fig. 21–3).

ATHEROSCLEROTIC RENOVASCULAR DISEASE

Prevalence and Natural History of Renovascular Disease

Renovascular hypertension is usually caused by partial or complete occlusion of one or both renal arteries. The overall incidence of hypertension due to renal artery stenosis (RAS) is less than 5%.[65] It is estimated, however, that 2 to 4 million people in the United States have renovascular disease.

Atherosclerosis accounts for two thirds of all cases of RAS.[66] Atherosclerotic renovascular disease typically manifests in patients older than 40 years and most commonly affects the renal ostium, proximal third of the renal artery, or both. The disease appears to affect men twice as often as women.[66–68] The incidence of end-stage renal disease due to hypertension has risen sharply in the United States over the last two decades, especially in elderly white patients undergoing dialysis.[69]

Indications for Revascularization

The presence of RAS is not always associated with hypertension. Many patients with RAS have normal or mildly elevated blood pressure. The following clinical features are commonly present in patients with renovascular hypertension:

- Onset of diastolic hypertension after age 55 years
- Refractory hypertension
- Development of uncontrolled hypertension
- Malignant hypertension
- Rapid deterioration of renal function
- Recurrent "flash" pulmonary edema with no readily explainable cause

Revascularization for Atherosclerotic Renal Artery Stenosis

Renal revascularization is indicated only in cases of inadequate control of arterial hypertension with optimal medical therapy.[70] Although revascularization in atherosclerotic RAS is rarely curative, considerable improvement in blood pressure control is expected in most patients. Clinical predictors of cure by revascularization include a duration of hypertension of less than 5 years, significant elevation of preprocedural diastolic blood pressure, and a significant difference between renal vein renins.[71]

There is abundant evidence that revascularization by surgery or angioplasty can result in the improvement or stabilization of arterial hypertension and renal function. In a study by Hansen and coworkers,[71] 90% of 152 patients with atherosclerotic renovascular hypertension demonstrated improvement in blood pressure control after surgical renal artery revascularization.

The surgical mortality rates in reported studies range from 3% to 17%, with an average mortality of 6%.[71–74] Novick and associates,[73] however, have shown that surgical revascularization in patients with diffuse aortic atheromatosis can significantly worsen the outcome of the procedure. In their series of 241 patients, after a mean follow-up period of 39 months, thrombosis or restenosis had occurred in 4.3% of operated arteries and mortality was 11.2%.[73]

The average improvement in renal function occurred in 41% to 43% of patients.[73, 74] The longevity of surgical repair procedures in the form of endarterectomy or bypass varies significantly among the published reports. Several studies have revealed that patients in whom end-stage renal disease has recently developed may also benefit from revascularization.[72–74]

On the basis of the existing evidence in published studies, patients who experience a progressive decline in renal function, accelerated hypertension, hypertension that is difficult to control, congestive heart failure, or a combination of these conditions are likely to benefit from renal revascularization.

Percutaneous Transluminal Angioplasty or Stenting for Treatment of Atherosclerotic Renal Artery Stenosis

Since Gruntzig's original description in 1978 of successful renal PTRA, there has been an ongoing controversy regarding the relative benefits of PTRA and surgical revascularization procedures.[75] Unfortunately, only one prospective randomized trial has compared the results of these two revascularization alternatives.[76] Weibull and colleagues[76] reported that in their randomized trial, there was no statistically significant difference in acute outcomes between PTRA and surgical revascularization procedures.[76] After 24 months of follow-up, the primary patency rates in the surgical and PTRA groups were 97% and 62%, respectively. The secondary patency rate in the PTRA group was 90% after repeat PTRA or surgery. Weibull and colleagues[76] also reported similar results in the two groups regarding the cure of or improvement in hypertension and complications. Their analysis revealed that with the use of PTRA, 60% of patients would require additional treatment in the form of repeat PTRA or surgery.

Several predictors of initial failure or restenosis following PTRA have been identified.[77–79] The most important predictor of restenosis after PTRA is lesion location.[77–79] PTRA of ostial stenosis, particularly when calcified, has had disappointing results. The initial success rates range from 24% to 35%, and the restenosis rates range from 15% to 42%.[77–79]

To overcome the problem of elastic recoil after angioplasty, several investigators have recommended the use of intravascular stents for treatment of ostial renal artery stenosis.[77–80] These investigators have also demonstrated greater augmentation in luminal diameter and reduction of the trans-stenotic pressure gradient after stent implantation than after PTRA alone. Several types of stents have been successfully used for renal artery revascularization.[77–80] Damaraju and Krajcer[80] have shown a benefit from using the combination of a self-expandable stent and a balloon-expandable stent for treatment of an iatrogenic renal artery dissection in a patient with atherosclerotic and fibromuscular disease (Fig. 21–4).

In a prospective study of 68 patients in whom PTRA for ostial renal artery stenosis failed, Blum and associates[81] reported a 100% initial technical success rate for Palmaz stent deployment. The restenosis rate in this study after 24 months of follow-up was 11%. A second intervention resulted in a secondary patency rate of 92%. Renal function remained stable, even in patients with abnormal baseline renal functional parameters. Arterial hypertension improved in 62% of patients. Dorros and associates[82] reported encouraging results of renal artery stenting in patients with normal baseline renal function. Their results, however, revealed high mortality in patients with bilateral renal artery disease and baseline serum creatinine levels of 2.0 mg/dl or higher. These researchers proposed that early diagnosis and revascularization before the onset of renal dysfunction could beneficially affect hypertension control, preserve or prevent deterioration of renal function, and improve patient survival.

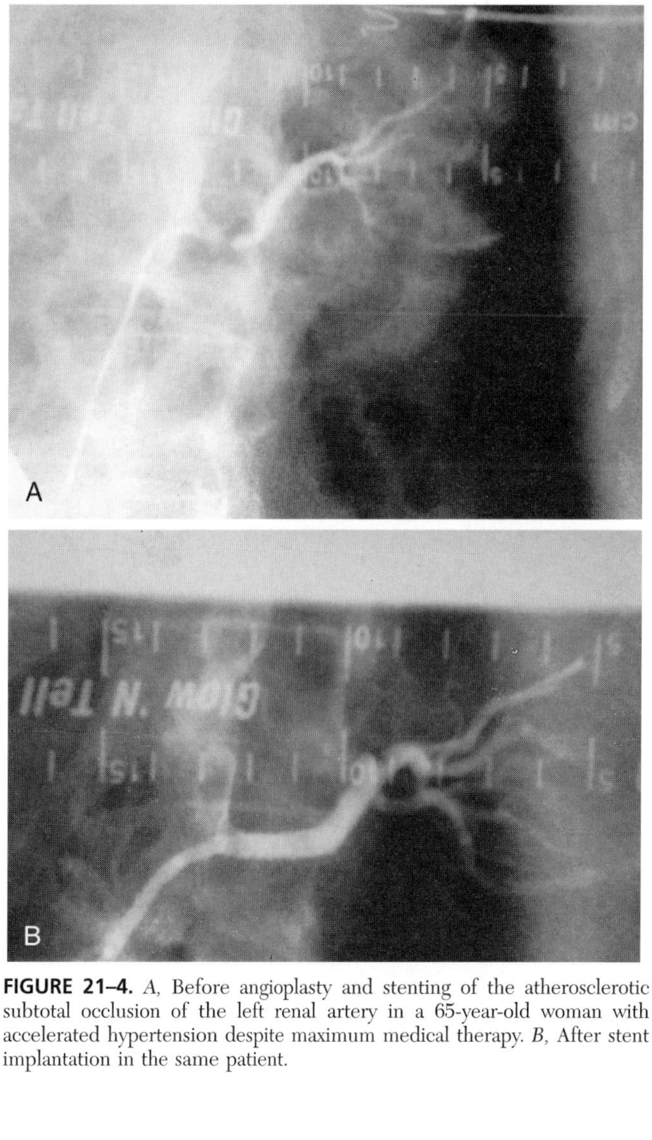

FIGURE 21–4. *A*, Before angioplasty and stenting of the atherosclerotic subtotal occlusion of the left renal artery in a 65-year-old woman with accelerated hypertension despite maximum medical therapy. *B*, After stent implantation in the same patient.

AORTOILIAC DISEASE

Almost one half of the patients who present with localized aortoiliac disease are women.[83] They commonly present with a characteristic clinical picture termed "hypoplastic aortoiliac syndrome."[84] This syndrome is observed exclusively in women, usually hypercholesterolemic heavy smokers between the ages of 40 and 55 years.[84] Hypoplastic aortic syndrome may be a variation on the pattern of peripheral occlusive disease seen in most female smokers, for which the average age at onset of claudication is 42 years. Atherosclerotic lesions are primarily located in the aortoiliac segment, with narrowing from the infrarenal aorta to less than 14 mm and the iliac and common femoral arteries to less than 7 mm. Affected women are generally small in stature and present with intermittent claudication. There is also a high incidence of single bifurcating lumbar arteries at the fourth and fifth lumbar vertebrae, suggesting that aortic hypoplasia results from embryonic overfusion of the dorsal aortas.

Surgical and Endovascular Revascularization of Aortoiliac Disease

Previously, bypass grafting has been the standard method of aortoiliac repair.[85] Morbidity associated with aortoiliac disease is significant. In a small series of 19 patients, 75% of patients with disabling claudication required aortobifemoral bypass, and 20% of those required reoperation.[84] Results of balloon angioplasty and stenting of aortoiliac stenosis are comparable to those of surgical reconstruction,[86] but unlike surgery, balloon angioplasty with stenting avoids major late complications (Fig. 21–5).[85] Covered endoprosthetic grafts have also been used to improve the restenosis rate after stenting by preventing fibrointimal hyperplasia and tissue growth within the stent.[87]

ABDOMINAL AORTIC ANEURYSM

As the population ages, the overall incidence of AAA increases; however, women remain in the minority for development of aneurysmal disease. In a large screening study of hypertensive patents, AAA was detected in 4% of men and only 0.9% of women.[88, 89] Consequently, routine screening is not recommended in hypertensive women, even though (1) female aortas are three times more likely to rupture[89] and (2) less than 10% of women will survive emergency surgery after rupture.[90] Adverse outcome is thought to be due, in part, to the smaller arteries seen in women. It is also due to recommendations for repair that are based on studies involving mostly men. In the United Kingdom Small Aneurysm Trial, for instance, the average size of the female aorta at the time of rupture was a full centimeter less than that of the male aorta (5 cm versus 6 cm).[90]

Endovascular Treatment of Abdominal Aortic Aneurysms

Endovascular stent grafts are a promising alternative to surgical repair of AAA. Stent grafts are a less invasive alternative to surgical AAA repair.[91–93] The first-generation endovascular endoluminal grafts were large-bore, rigid tubular grafts (Color Plate 21–1). Later aortomonoiliac, bifurcated one-piece and modular grafts were developed (Color Plate 21–2). Stent grafts have undergone a variety of modifications and improvements so that they are now more flexible and available in smaller diameters to accommodate smaller female arteries.[94–97] The prosthetic wall of such a graft is made of a polyethylene terephthalate textile in woven or knitted form, or of an expanded polytetrafluoroethylene material. The stent grafts are either self-expandable or balloon-expandable. Fixation of the stent graft is achieved through the radial force of the stent or by a specific attachment system including barbs (see Fig. 21–7). Unfortunately, given the small

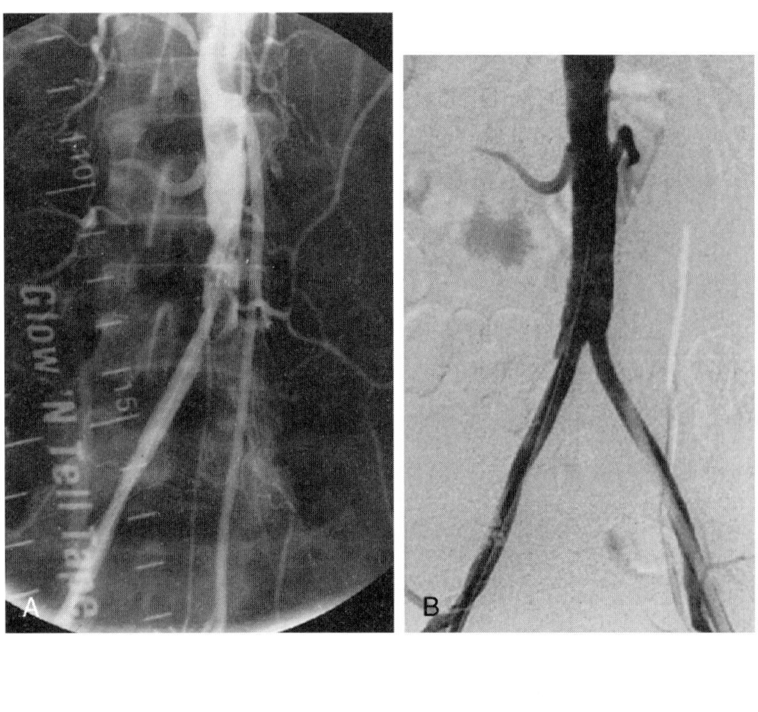

FIGURE 21–5. *A*, Before angioplasty and stent implantation in a 46-year-old woman with hypoplastic aorta syndrome who had a totally occluded left iliac and multiple filling defects in the abdominal aorta and right iliac. *B*, After stent implantation in the same patient.

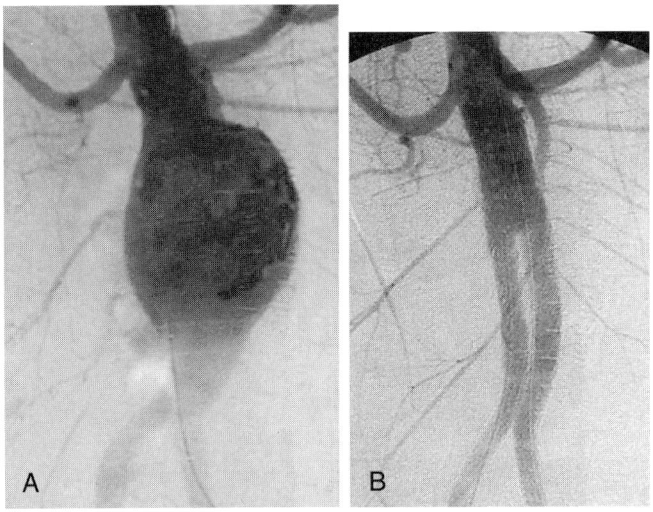

FIGURE 21–6. *A*, Abdominal aortic aneurysm measuring 5.2 cm in a 67-year-old woman. *B*, After endoluminal exclusion with a modular stent graft system.

number of women who experience AAA, it may be quite some time before it is known whether endoluminal stent grafts perform well in the smaller female anatomy (Fig. 21–6).

MEDICAL MANAGEMENT AND PHARMACOLOGIC THERAPY OF PERIPHERAL ARTERIAL DISEASE

Standard medical management of patients with PAD includes risk factor reduction by smoking cessation, lipid-lowering therapy, estrogen replacement therapy, hypertension control, antiplatelet therapy, and a walking exercise program. Few studies have evaluated the impact of lipid-lowering therapy, antiplatelet therapy, and estrogen therapy on claudication or reduction of the risk of PAD. Several studies, however, clearly show the impact of these therapies on reducing overall cardiovascular risks.

Walking distance can be increased as much as 40% in women with claudication who stop smoking.[98] In addition, antiplatelet therapy and cilostazol therapy are beneficial for treating PAD. Therapy with cilostazol, a phosphodiesterase inhibitor, significantly improved walking distances in patients with intermittent claudication and also improved ABI.[98]

LOWER EXTREMITY REVASCULARIZATION

Approximately one third of all distal revascularization procedures and amputations are performed on women. In all of the literature published on the outcome of lower extremity revascularization and graft failure, few reports have clearly addressed the issue of gender. Two studies of graft patency have identified female gender as an independent predictor of graft failure.[99, 100] Arterial size appears to have a significant effect on the success of the reconstruction. In a randomized, multicenter controlled trial comparing prosthetic above-knee femoropopliteal bypass grafts, the use of a smaller graft was associated with a decrease in 5-year patency from 69.1% to 37.9%.[101]

Balloon angioplasty has been effective in treating lower limb ischemia. Acceptable 5-year patency rates have been achieved following angioplasty of iliac artery occlusions (Fig. 21–7).[102] Angioplasty of tibial-peroneal disease offers the highest technical success rate and long-term patency rates

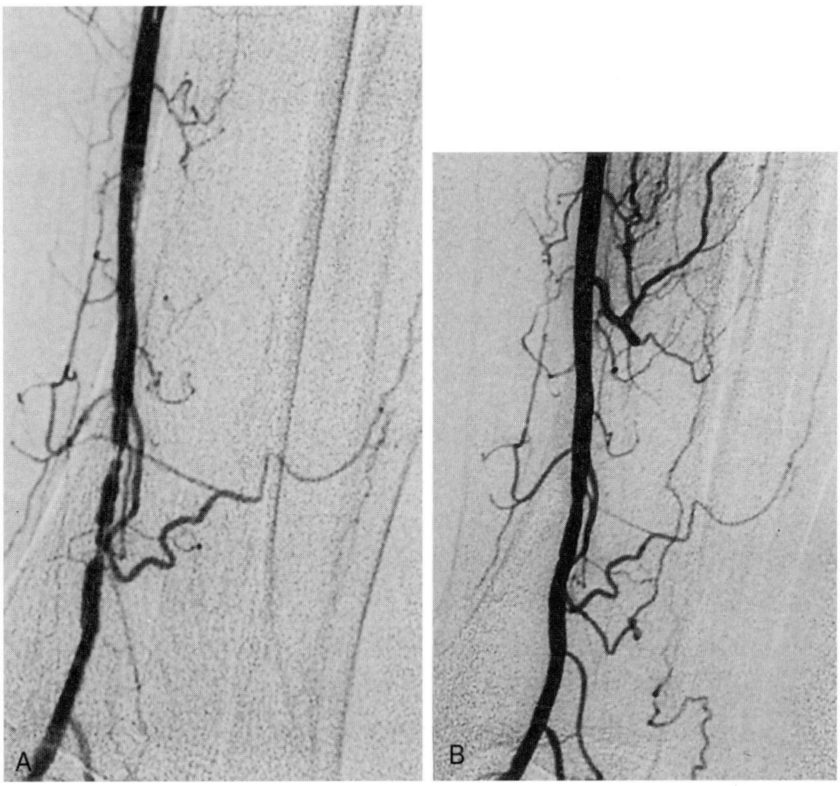

FIGURE 21–7. *A*, Femoral angiogram showing tandem lesions in the posterior tibial artery after thrombolysis and rheolytic therapy in a 58-year-old woman with severe right leg claudication. *B*, Follow-up angiogram after balloon angioplasty showing minimal residual stenosis.

for treatment of short, focal, and concentric atherosclerotic lesions.[103–107] Using life-table analysis, Horvath and coworkers[105] reported cumulative patency rates after balloon tibial-peroneal angioplasty of 79.8% at 1 year and 75.3% at 3 years of follow-up. In a later study, Bull and coworkers reported a cumulative 3-year clinical success rate of 83% for angioplasty when it was performed for single stenosis and 76% when it was performed for multilevel lesions.[106]

THROMBOLYTIC THERAPY FOR ACUTE LOWER EXTREMITY ISCHEMIA

A principal goal of treatment for acute limb ischemia is rapid restoration of blood flow to the ischemic region before irreversible changes occur. Surgical treatment of acute limb ischemia plus comorbid conditions carries a 30-day mortality of 15% to 25%.[108]

Intravenous infusion of exogenous plasminogen activators, specifically streptokinase, was attempted about three decades ago for the treatment of peripheral arterial occlusion.[109] Several studies have shown that thrombolysis can be effective initial treatment for many patients with acute arterial occlusions.[109–112] One of the advantages of thrombolysis over surgical intervention is that after thrombolysis, angiographic evaluation can uncover any underlying cause that played a role in thrombus formation.[109–112] Any underlying lesions thus identified can be treated either by balloon angioplasty or by elective surgical revascularization.

Thrombolytic agents that have been used are streptokinase, urokinase, recombinant tissue plasminogen activator (r-tPA), anisoylated plasminogen-streptokinase complex (APSAC), and pro-urokinase (pro-UK) (Fig. 21–8). All these agents induce a systemic fibrinolytic state. In comparative studies on the treatment of arterial thrombosis, streptokinase, urokinase, r-tPA, and pro-UK have been shown to be more effective than heparin alone in lysing the thrombus.[109–112] A retrospective study from the Cleveland Clinic revealed clinical success rates of 60% for streptokinase, 95% for urokinase, and 91% for r-tPA.[112] Urokinase is no longer available.[109–112]

SUMMARY

The incidence of PAD is rising as the population ages, and the total prevalences are similar in women and men. Insufficient emphasis has been placed on evaluating the complex mechanisms and causes of PAD in women. The treatment strategies currently being used to treat men with PAD have not been adequately tested in women. Greater efforts and additional studies are necessary to test current and future modalities of treatment for this condition in women.

Women with CAD very frequently have comorbid illnesses that significantly increase the risk of general anesthesia and surgery. It has also been established that disease in one region commonly influences other regions.

The endovascular treatment of peripheral vascular disease has undergone a dramatic expansion in the last few decades. Peripheral vascular interventions have been developed with the intention of avoiding the risk of general or regional anesthesia, reducing the risk of surgery, decreasing patient discomfort, and shortening recovery time. The enthusiasm for these therapies has been growing rapidly among specialists in cardiology, interventional radiology, and vascular surgery.

The introduction of balloon angioplasty, stents, stent

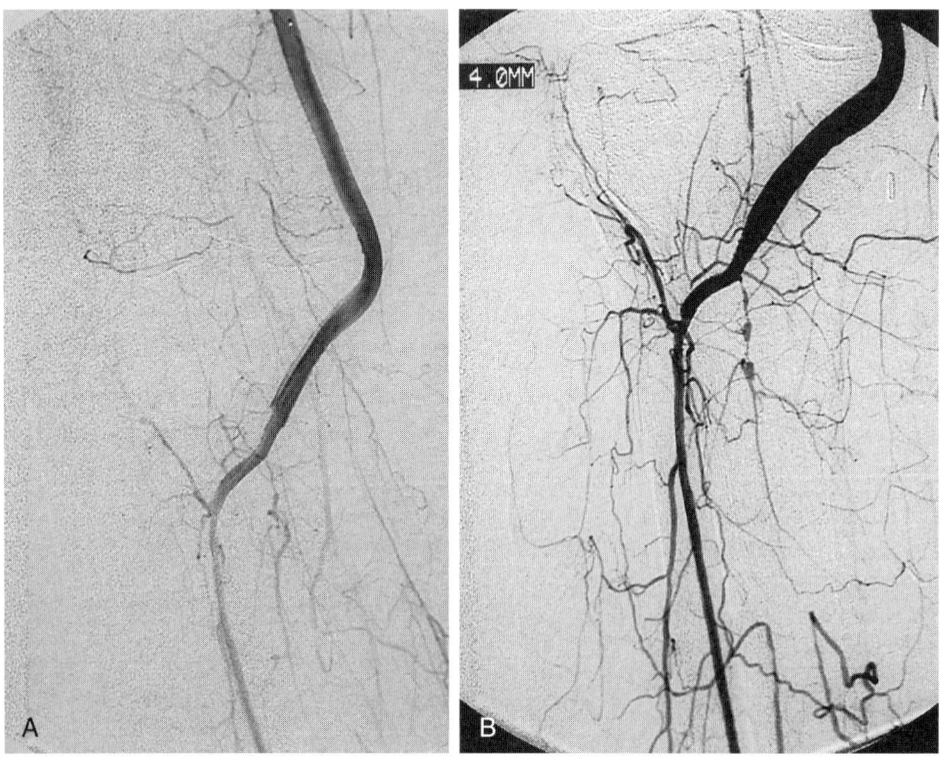

FIGURE 21–8. *A,* Run-off angiogram in a 63-year-old woman with rest pain showing a large filling defect at the distal anastomosis of the popliteal-tibial bypass. *B,* After intra-arterial urokinase (250,000 U) therapy and balloon angioplasty.

grafts, atherectomy devices, and intra-arterial thrombolysis for treatment of CAD has offered physicians the opportunity to apply these techniques as treatments in patients with PAD. Because the results of vascular surgery are less optimal in women than in men, it is essential to evaluate whether endovascular treatment of PAD in women might produce better results.

References

1. McDermott MM, Fried L, Simonsick E, et al: Asymptomatic peripheral arterial disease is independently associated with impaired lower extremity functioning: The Women's Health and Aging Study. Circulation 101:1007, 2000.
2. Morbidity Statistics from General Practice 1991–1992 (OPCS Series MB5 No 3). HMSO, London, 2000.
3. Vogt MT, Wolfson SK, Kuller LH: Lower extremity arterial disease and the aging process: A review. J Clin Epidemiol 45:529, 1992.
4. Fowkes FGR: Epidemiology of atherosclerotic arterial disease in the lower limbs. Eur J Vasc Surg 2:283, 1988.
5. Criqui MH, Fronek A, Barrett-Connor E, et al: The prevalence of peripheral arterial disease in a defined population. Circulation 71: 510, 1985.
6. Newman AB, Siscovick DS, Manolio TA, et al, for the Cardiovascular Health Study Collaborative Research Group: Ankle-arm index as a marker of atherosclerosis in the Cardiovascular Health Study. Circulation 88:837, 1993.
7. Greenhalgh RM, Lewis B, Rosengarten DS, et al: Serum lipids and lipoproteins in peripheral vascular disease. Lancet 2(7731):947, 1971.
8. Willett WC, Manson JE, Stampfer MJ, et al: Relative and absolute excess risks of coronary heart disease among women who smoke cigarettes. N Engl J Med 317:1303, 1987.
9. LaCroix AZ, Lang J, Scherr P, et al: Smoking and mortality among older men and women in three communities. N Engl J Med 324: 1619, 1991.
10. Hughson WG, Mann JI, Woods HF, Walton I: Intermittent claudication: Factors influencing outcome. Br Med J 1(6124):1377, 1978.
11. American Heart Association: 2000 Heart and Stroke Statistical Update. American Heart Association, Dallas, 1999.
12. Kannel WB, Shurtleff D: Framingham Study: Cigarettes and the development of intermittent claudication. Geriatrics 28:61, 1973.
13. Holmes DR, Burbank MK, Fulton RE, Bernatz PE: Arteriosclerosis obliterans in young women. Am J Med 66:997, 1979.
14. Mellstrom D, Svanborg A: Tobacco smoking—a major cause of sex differences in health. Compr Gerontol 1:34, 1987.
15. Powell JT, Edwards RJ, Worrell PC, et al: Important risk factors for the development of peripheral arterial disease in smokers. Br J Surg 81:607, 1994.
16. Peto R, Lopez AD, Broeham J, et al: Mortality from tobacco in developed countries: Indirect estimates from national vital statistics. Lancet 339:1268, 1992.
17. Collins R, Peto R, MacMahon S, et al: Blood pressure, stroke and coronary heart disease. Part 2: Short-term reductions in blood pressure: Overview of randomized drug trials in their epidemiologic context. Lancet 335:827, 1990.
18. U.S. Department of Health and Human Services: Health United States, 1991. National Center for Health Statistics, Hyattsville, MD, 1992.
19. Bradshaw K: Hormone replacement therapy in hypertensive postmenopausal women: Role of the gynecologist. In Safar M, Stimpel M, Zanchetti A (eds): Hypertension in Post-menopausal Women. Springer-Verlag, Berlin, 1994, p 45.
20. Kitler ME: Difference in men and women in coronary artery disease, systemic hypertension and their treatment. Am J Cardiol 70:1077, 1992.
21. Colditz GA, Willett WC, Stampfer MJ, et al: Menopause and the risk of coronary heart disease in women. N Engl J Med 340:1801, 1999.
22. Stampfer MJ, Colditz GA, Willett WC, et al: Postmenopausal estrogen therapy and cardiovascular disease: Ten-year follow-up from the Nurses' Health Study. N Engl J Med 325:756, 1991.
23. Barrett-Connor E, Bush T: Estrogen and coronary heart disease in women. J Am Med Assoc 265:1861, 1991.
24. Parris HM, Carr LA, Hall DG: Time interval from castration in premenopausal women to development of excessive coronary atherosclerosis. Am J Obstet Gynecol 99:155, 1967.
25. Weiss NS: Premature menopause and aortoiliac occlusive disease. J Chronic Dis 25:133, 1972.
26. Cronenwett JL, Davis JT Jr, Gooch JB, Garrett ME: Aortoiliac occlusive disease in women. Surgery 88:775, 1980.
27. Mendelsohn ME, Karas RH: The protective effect of estrogen on the cardiovascular system. N Engl J Med 340:1801, 1999.
28. Krasinski K, Spyridopoulos I, Asahara T, et al: Estradiol accelerates functional endothelial recovery after arterial injury. Circulation 95: 1768, 1997.
29. Walsh BW, Schiff I, Rosner R, et al: Effects of post-menopausal estrogen replacement on concentrations and metabolism of plasma proteins. N Engl J Med 325:1196, 1991.
30. Moliterno DJ, Jokinen EV, Miserez AR, et al: No association between plasma lipoprotein(a) concentration and the presence or absence of coronary atherosclerosis in African-Americans. Arterioscler Thromb Vasc Biol 15:850, 1995.
31. van der Mooren MJ, Wouters MG, Blom HJ, et al: Hormone replacement therapy may reduce high serum homocysteine in post-menopausal women. Eur J Clin Invest 25:333, 1994.
32. Koh KK, Mincemoyer R, Bui MN, et al: Effects of hormone-replacement therapy on fibrinolysis in postmenopausal women. N Engl J Med 336:683, 1997.
33. Gerhard MD, Walsh BW, Tawakol A, et al: Estradiol therapy combined with progesterone and endothelium-dependent vasodilatation in postmenopausal women. Circulation 98:1158, 1998.
34. Caes F, Cham B, Van den Brande P, Welch W: Small artery syndrome in women. Surg Gynecol Obstet 161:165, 1985.
35. McConathy WJ, Greenhalgh RM, Alauporic P, et al: Plasma lipid and apolipoprotein profiles of women with two types of peripheral arterial disease. Atherosclerosis 50:295, 1984.
36. Orchard TJ, Dorman JS, Maser RE, et al: Prevalence of complications in IDDM by sex and duration. Pittsburgh Epidemiology of Diabetes Complications Study II. Diabetes 39:1116, 1990.
37. Kuczmarski RJ, Flegel KM, Campbell SM, et al: Increasing prevalence of overweight among U.S. adults: The National Health and Nutrition Examination Surveys, 1960–1991. JAMA 272:205, 1994.
38. Mason JE, Golditz GA, Stamfler MJ, et al: A prospective study of obesity and coronary heart disease in women. N Engl J Med 322: 882, 1990.
39. Lupi-Herrera E, Sanchez-Torres G, Marcushamer J, et al: Takayasu's arteritis: Clinical study of 107 cases. Am Heart J 93:94, 1977.
40. Ishikawa K: Natural history and classification of occlusive thromboaortopathy (Takayasu's disease). Circulation 57:27, 1978.
41. Kerr G, Hallahan C, Giordano J, et al: Takayasu arteritis. Ann Intern Med 120:919, 1994.
42. Arend WP, Michel BA, Bloch DA, et al: The American College of Rheumatology 1990 criteria for classification of Takayasu arteritis. Arthritis Rheum 33:1129, 1990.
43. Sharma S, Rajani M, Kaul U, et al: Initial experience with percutaneous angioplasty in the management of Takayasu's arteritis. Br J Radiol 63:517, 1990.
44. Tyagi S, Kaul U, Nair M, et al: Balloon angioplasty of the aorta in Takayasu's arteritis: Initial and long-term results. Am Heart J 124: 876, 1992.
45. Kumar S, Mandalam R, Rao V, et al: Percutaneous transluminal angioplasty in non-specific aortoarteritis (Takayasu's disease): Experience of 16 cases. Cardiovasc Intervent Radiol 12:321, 1990.
46. Ozdil E, Parikh DK, Krajcer Z: Stent placement in a patient with Takayasu's arteritis. Cathet Cardiovasc Diagn 38:373, 1996.
47. Hunder GG, Bloch DA, Michel BA, et al: The American College of Rheumatology 1990 criteria for the classification of giant cell arteritis. Arthritis Rheum 33:1122, 1990.
48. Machado EBV, Michet CJ, Ballard DJ, et al: Trends in the incidence and clinical presentation of temporal arteritis in Olmsted County, Minnesota, 1950–1985. Arthritis Rheum 31:745, 1988.
49. Gray BH, Young JR, Olin JW: Miscellaneous arterial diseases. In Young JR, Olin JW, Bartholomew JR (eds): Peripheral Vascular Diseases, 2nd edition, Mosby-Year Book, St. Louis, 1996, p 425.
50. Hunder GG: Giant cell arteritis and polymyalgia rheumatica. In Kelly WN, Ruddy S, Harris ED Jr, et al (eds): Textbook of Rheumatology, 5th edition, vol 2. WB Saunders, Philadelphia, 1997, p 1123.
51. Begelman SM, Olin JW: Nonatherosclerotic arterial disease of the extracranial cerebrovasculature. Semin Vasc Surg 13:153, 2000.

52. Zierler RE, Bergelin RO, Isaacson JA, Strandness DE Jr: Natural history of atherosclerotic renal artery stenosis: A prospective study with duplex ultrasonography. J Vasc Surg 19:250, 1994.
53. Klinge J, Mali WP, Puijlaert CB, et al: Percutaneous transluminal renal angioplasty: Initial and long-term results. Radiology 171:501, 1989.
54. Sos TA, Pickering TG, Phil D: Percutaneous transluminal renal angioplasty in renovascular hypertension due to atheroma or fibromuscular dysplasia. N Engl J Med 309:274, 1983.
55. Tegmeyer CJ, Dyer R, Teates CD, et al: Percutaneous transluminal dilatation of the renal arteries. Radiology 135:589, 1980.
56. Vogt MT, Wolfson SK, Kuller LH: Lower extremity arterial disease and the aging process: A review. J Clin Epidemiol 45:529, 1992.
57. Lemesle M, Milan C, Faivre J, et al: Incidence of trends of ischemic stroke and transient ischemic attacks in a well-defined French population from 1985 through 1994. Stroke 30:371, 1999.
58. Kim JS, Choi-Kwon S: Risk factors for stroke in different levels of cerebral arterial disease. Eur Neurol 42:150, 1999.
59. Wityk RJ, Lehman D, Klag M, et al: Race and sex differences in the distribution of cerebral atherosclerosis. Stroke 27:1974, 1996.
60. Schneider J, Droste J, Golan J: Carotid endarterectomy in women versus men: Patient characteristics and outcomes. J Vasc Surg 25: 890, 1997.
61. Rothwell P, Slattery J, Warlow C: Clinical and angiographic predictors of stroke and death from carotid endarterectomy: A systematic review. Br Med J 315:1571, 1997.
62. Hobson RW: CREST (Carotid Revascularization Endarterectomy versus Stent Trial): Background, design, and current status. Semin Vasc Surg 13:139, 2000.
63. Yadav JS, Roubin GS, King P, et al: Angioplasty and stenting for restenosis after carotid endarterectomy: Initial experience. Stroke 27: 2075, 1996.
64. Lanzino G, Mericle RA, Loes DK, et al: Percutaneous transluminal angioplasty and stent placement for recurrent carotid artery stenosis. J Neurosurg 90:688, 1999.
65. Kaplan NM: Hypertension. In Willerson JT, Cohn JN (eds): Cardiovascular Medicine, 3rd ed. Churchill Livingstone, New York, 2000, p 2234.
66. Harding MB, Smith LR, Himmelstein SI, et al: Renal artery stenosis: Prevalence and associated risk factors in patients undergoing routine cardiac catheterization. J Am Soc Nephrol 2:1608, 1992.
67. Ploth DW: Renovascular hypertension. In Jacobson HR, Striker GE, Klahr S (eds): The Principles and Practice of Nephrology, 2nd ed. Mosby, St. Louis, 1995, p 379.
68. Tollefson DF, Ernst CB: Natural history of atherosclerotic renal artery stenosis associated with aortic disease. J Vasc Surg 14:327, 1991.
69. Barri YM, Davidson RA, Senler S, et al: Prediction of cure of hypertension in atherosclerotic RAS. South Med J 89:679, 1996.
70. Novick AC, Ziegelboum M, Vidt DG, et al: Trends in surgical revascularization for renal artery disease: Ten years' experience. JAMA 257: 498, 1987.
71. Hansen KJ, Starr SM, Sands RE, et al: Contemporary surgical management of renovascular disease. J Vasc Surg 16:319, 1992.
72. Jamieson GG, Clarkson AR, Woodroffe AJ, Faris I: Reconstructive renal vascular surgery for chronic renal failure. Br J Surg 71:338, 1984.
73. Novick AC, Textor SC, Bodie B, Khauli RB: Revascularization to preserve renal function in patients with atherosclerotic renovascular disease. Urol Clin North Am 11:477, 1984.
74. Libertino JA, Bosco PJ, Ying CY, et al: Renal revascularization to preserve and restore renal function. J Urol 147:1485, 1992.
75. Gruntzig A, Kuhlmann U, Lutolf U, et al: Treatment of renovascular hypertension with percutaneous transluminal dilatation of a renal-artery stenosis. Lancet 1(8068):801, 1978.
76. Weibull H, Berquist D, Bergantz SE, et al: Percutaneous transluminal renal angioplasty versus surgical reconstruction of atherosclerotic renal artery stenosis: A prospective randomized study. J Vasc Surg 18: 841, 1993.
77. Martin LG, Cork RD, Kaufman SL. Long-term results of angioplasty in 110 patients with renal artery stenosis. J Vasc Interv Radiol 3: 619, 1992.
78. Rees CR, Palmaz JC, Becker GJ, et al: Palmaz stent in atherosclerotic stenoses involving the ostia of the renal arteries: Preliminary report of a multicenter study. Radiology 181:507, 1991.
79. Eldrup-Jorgensen J, Harvey HR, Sampson LN, et al: Should transluminal renal angioplasty be applied to ostial artery atherosclerosis? J Vasc Surg 21:909, 1995.
80. Damaraju S, Krajcer Z: Successful Wallstent implantation for extensive iatrogenic renal artery dissection in a patient with fibromuscular dysplasia. J Endovasc Surg 6:297, 1999.
81. Blum U, Krumme B, Flügel P, et al: Treatment of ostial renal-artery stenosis with vascular endoprosthesis after unsuccessful balloon angioplasty. N Engl J Med 336:459, 1997.
82. Dorros G, Jaff M, Mathiak L, et al: Four-year follow-up of Palmaz-Schatz revascularization as treatment for atherosclerotic renal artery stenosis. Circulation 98:642, 1998.
83. Caes F, Cham B, Van den Brande P, Welch W: Small artery syndrome in women. Surg Gynecol Obstet 161:165, 1985.
84. Jernigan WR, Fallat ME, Hatfield DR: Hypoplastic aortoiliac syndrome: An entity peculiar to women. Surgery 94:752, 1983.
85. Brewster DC: Clinical and anatomical considerations for surgery in aortoiliac disease and results of surgical treatment. Circulation 83: I42, 1991.
86. Palmaz JC, Laborde JC, Rivera FJ, et al: Stenting of the iliac arteries with the Palmaz stent: Experience from a multicenter trial. Cardiovasc Intervent Radiol 15:291, 1992.
87. Krajcer Z, Sioco G, Reynolds T: Comparison of Wallgraft and Wallstent for treatment of complex iliac artery stenosis and occlusion: Preliminary results of a prospective randomized study. Tex Heart Inst J 24:193, 1997.
88. Williams IM, Hughes OD, Townsend E, et al: Prevalence of abdominal aortic aneurysm in a hypertensive population. Ann R Coll Surg Engl 78:501, 1996.
89. Brown L, Powell J: Risk factors for aneurysm rupture in patients kept under ultrasound surveillance. United Kingdom Small Aneurysm Trial Participants. Ann Surg 230:289, 1999.
90. Semmens J, Norman P, Lawrence-Brown M, Holman C: The influence of gender on the outcome of ruptured abdominal aortic aneurysm. Br J Surg 87:191, 2000.
91. Parodi JC, Palmaz JC, Barone HD: Transfemoral intraluminal graft implantation for abdominal aortic aneurysms. Ann Vasc Surg 5:491, 1991.
92. Zarins CK, Haris EJ: Operative repair for aortic aneurysms: The gold standard. J Endovasc Surg 4:232, 1997.
93. Beebe HG: Imaging modalities for aortic endografting. J Endovasc Surg 4:111, 1997.
94. Fogarty TJ: The Medtronic-AneuRx Modular Bifurcated Graft. Presented at Techniques in Vascular and Endovascular Surgery, December 11, 1997, Chicago.
95. Taheri SA, Leonhardt HJ, Greenan T: The TALENT™ endoluminal graft placement system. In Yao JST, Pearce WH (eds): Techniques in Vascular Surgery. Appelton and Lange, Stamford, CT, 1998, p 433.
96. Beebe HG: The Meadox Vanguard Endovascular Graft. Presented at Techniques in Vascular and Endovascular Surgery, December 11, 1997, Chicago.
97. Rhee RY, Eskandari MK, Zaihko AB, Makaroun MS: Long-term fate of the aneurysmal sac after endoluminal exclusion of abdominal aortic aneurysms. J Vasc Surg 32:689, 2000.
98. Dawson DL, Cutler BS, Hiatt WR, et al: A comparison of cilostazol and pentoxifylline for treating intermittent claudication. Am J Med 109:523, 2000.
99. Enzler M, Ruoss M, Seifert B, Berger M: The influence of gender on the outcome of arterial procedures in the lower extremity. Eur J Vasc Endovasc Surg 11:446, 1996.
100. Magnant J, Cronenwett J, Walsh D, et al: The surgical treatment of infrainguinal arterial occlusive disease in women. J Vasc Surg 17: 67, 1993.
101. Green RM, Abbott WM, Matsumoto T, et al: Prosthetic above-knee femoropopliteal bypass grafting: Five year results of a randomized trial. J Vasc Surg 31:417, 2000.
102. Tegmeyer CJ, Hartwell GD, Selby JB, et al: Results and complications of angioplasty in aortoiliac disease. Circulation 83:I53, 1991.
103. Rutherford RB, Becker GJ: Standards for evaluating and reporting the results of surgical and percutaneous therapy for peripheral arterial disease. J Vasc Interv Radiol 2:169, 1991.
104. Gruntzig A: Die perkutane rekanalisation chronischer arterialler verschlusse (Dotter-Prinzip) mit einem neuem dopplelumigen dilatationkatheter. Rofo Fortsch Geb Rontgenstr Nuklearmed 124:80, 1976.
105. Horvath W, Oertl M, Haidinger D: Percutaneous transluminal angioplasty of crural arteries. Radiology 177:565, 1990.
106. Bull PG, Mendel H, Hold M, et al: Distal popliteal and tibioperoneal

transluminal angioplasty: Long-term follow-up. J Vasc Interv Radiol 3: 522, 1992.
107. Brown RT, Moore ED, Getrajdman GI, Sadekni S: Infrapopliteal angioplasty: Long term follow-up. J Vasc Interv Radiol 4:139, 1993.
108. Yeager RA, Moneta GL, Taylor LM, et al: Surgical management of severely acute lower extremity ischemia. J Vasc Surg 15:358, 1992.
109. Ouriel K, Veith FJ, Sasahara AA: A comparison of recombinant urokinase with vascular surgery as initial treatment for acute arterial occlusion of the legs. N Engl J Med 338:1105, 1998.
110. McNicol GB, Reid W, Bain WH, Douglas AS: Treatment of peripheral arterial occlusions by streptokinase perfusion. Br Med J 1:1508, 1963.
111. Goldhaber SZ, Kessler CM, Heit JA, et al: Recombinant tissue-type plasminogen activator versus a novel dosing regimen of urokinase in acute pulmonary embolism: A randomized controlled multicenter trial. J Am Coll Cardiol 20:24, 1992.
112. Groar RA, Olin J, Bartholomew JR, et al: Efficacy and safety of intraarterial local infusion of streptokinase, urokinase, or tissue plasminogen activator for peripheral arterial occlusion: A retrospective review. J Vasc Med Biol 2:310, 1990.

|21.2| Clinical Recognition

Maria C. Henderson-Everhardus and J. Hajo van Bockel

Peripheral vascular arterial disease is defined as obstructive arteriosclerotic disease of the aorta or its branches. Most commonly, PAD comprises occlusive disease of the infrarenal abdominal aorta and renal arteries as well as the iliac, femoral, tibial, and peroneal arteries. Occlusive lesions of the carotid arteries also are classified as PAD. In this discussion, we concentrate on PAD below the inguinal ligament.

Most of the epidemiologic information on PAD and its complications has been obtained from studies in predominantly white men. However, this information is not necessarily accurate for women. More focus has now been placed on evaluating studies of cardiac disease conducted in women. These clinical and epidemiologic studies have determined that there are clinical differences between the genders with regard to cardiac disease. This review concentrates on PAD in women.

It is generally believed that women have the same manifestations of PAD as men. However, studies have shown that PAD occurs 10 years later in life in women. Most manifestations of lower extremity arteriosclerosis in women typically occur after menopause. The prevalence of lower extremity atherosclerotic disease, as diagnosed by noninvasive assessment methods (including an ABI less than 0.80 [normal = 1.00, or 100%]), was found to be 3% in women younger than 60 years and more than 20% in women 75 years and older.[1] An overview by Gerhard and associates[2] of the epidemiology of PAD in women describes the risk factors.

The clinical recognition of PAD in women is not essentially different from that in men. PAD is a marker of CAD, cerebrovascular disease, and AAA. Among individuals with severe, asymptomatic large-vessel PAD, there is an increase in mortality due to cardiovascular disease and coronary heart disease.[3, 4] PAD can be very incapacitating, especially when limb loss is imminent. The ABI, a universally accepted method for evaluating blood flow in the legs, is an independent predictor of mortality in women (relative risk, 1 in 9).[5] Early identification of risk factors for PAD, as well as early diagnosis and treatment, may help reduce morbidity and mortality in selected patients. Therefore, the focus should be on prevention of cardiovascular events through reduction of the risk in patients with claudication. Once the disease has developed, recognizing it is the starting point for therapy, which should be primarily conservative.[6]

CLINICAL PRESENTATION

It has been stated that "There are few areas in medicine in which the conditions encountered lend themselves so readily to diagnosis solely on the basis of thoughtful history and careful physical examination as does vascular disease."[7] In other words, PAD is usually identified from classic manifestations elicited through the search for specific signs and symptoms.

A comprehensive patient history includes information about the patient and family. The family history should provide information about heart and vascular disease. If any significant risk factors for PAD are present, the patient should be evaluated for nicotine use, high blood pressure, hypercholesteremia, obesity, physical activity, and diabetes. A significant risk marker for women is postmenopausal status.

Certain physical differences between women and men should also be noted. Women generally weigh less, have less body surface area, and have smaller blood vessels than men. The diameter of the aorta has been directly related to body surface area[8] and may have an effect on both obstructive disease and vessel patency after arterial reconstruction.[9] Although blood velocities within the aorta are not significantly less in women than in men,[10] premenopausal women have significantly lower brachial and ankle systolic pressures and lower ankle-arm pressure index than age-matched men.[11]

Differentiating PAD from other diseases is usually not difficult. However, on occasion, several problems (such as arthrosis, venous disease, and neurologic disorders) may occur simultaneously in a patient. The signs and symptoms of PAD vary with the location and severity of the disease (Table 21–1). It is imperative that PAD be differentiated from venous disease. The signs and symptoms of PAD result from arterial obstruction in the arteries as well as in the microcirculation, whereas peripheral venous disease occurs with venous obstruction or chronic venous insufficiency.

Signs and Symptoms of Mild Peripheral Arterial Disease

The main symptom typically described by patients with claudication is pain in the thighs, hips, or calves when they walk

Table 21–1. SIGNS AND SYMPTOMS OF PERIPHERAL ARTERIAL DISEASE

Mild to Moderate Peripheral Arterial Disease
Muscular pain in legs, directly related to exercise and relieved with a short period of rest
Diminution or absence of peripheral pulses
Normal temperature of extremities and an immediate capillary refill time
Severe Peripheral Arterial Disease
Persistent throbbing pain in feet, relieved with dangling of the feet
Inability to walk short distances owing to severe leg pain and cramping
Absence of peripheral pulses at knee and ankle level
Color changes: pale leg, dependent rubor, cyanosis or gangrene
Temperature changes: cool leg and foot
Ulcerative lesion on toes, feet, and/or heels
Tissue Loss or Threatened Limb Loss
Excruciating pain in leg, foot, and toes
Color changes: pale and mottled extremity
Temperature changes: cool leg and foot
Tissue necrosis and gangrene of toes
Loss of nerve sensation (predominantly sensory loss)

a specific distance. The leg pain is relieved when at rest and recurs when exercise is resumed. Intermittent claudication occurs when the demand for blood in the limb increases with exercise and a lack of sufficient blood volume causes oxygen deprivation in skeletal muscle. Secondary symptoms associated with claudication include cramping within a specific area of the leg or a generalized tiredness, tightness, or aching in the legs.

Physical examination may reveal the peripheral pulses to be diminished or absent, but the extremities to be warm and capillary refill time immediate. Mild arterial obstruction is present, with ABIs of 0.80 to 0.90.

Signs and Symptoms of Moderate to Severe Peripheral Arterial Disease

When obstructive PAD has advanced, leg pain is more persistent. During this phase, the obstruction usually has occluded one or more vessels, resulting in a greater than 50% reduction in lumen diameter. In long-standing occlusive disease, collateral flow may develop. Patients complain of a distinct pain or tiredness in the leg. When one or more major vessels are obstructed, blood flow and oxygen delivery to the lower extremities decrease significantly, resulting in continuous pain. This pain, characterized by a throbbing or burning sensation, is referred to as *rest pain*. Rest pain may be relieved by placing the limb in a dependent position, such as hanging the affected leg over the side of the bed. In rest pain, arterial obstruction involves the leg, the foot, and the toes.

Other secondary symptoms associated with rest pain are dependent rubor, hair loss, skin color changes such as cyanosis, tissue necrosis or gangrene, and temperature changes (Color Plates 21–3 through 21–5). Ulcerative lesions on the toes, feet, or heels may occur with long-standing disease. If the arterial obstruction has progressed to a moderate level, the ABI falls into the 0.80 to 0.60 range; severe arterial obstruction is compatible with an ABI of 0.40 to 0.60 or lower. Another physical finding observed in PAD is distal embolization of arterial debris following AAA reconstruction (Color Plate 21–6).

By contrast, acute or chronic venous disease presents with pain, swelling, redness, and tenderness of the affected extremity. In people who have chronic venous insufficiency, venous ulcerations appear, located on the medial aspect of the ankle (Color Plate 21–7). Venous gangrene manifests as a swollen leg with bluish discoloration, shiny skin, and, often, multiple blisters (Color Plate 21–8). People with long-standing diabetes also present with ulceration and neurotrophic skin changes. These skin changes are a result of small vessel obstruction affecting the larger arteries and the vessels of the nerves and skin.

Signs and Symptoms of Tissue Loss and Threatened Limb Loss

In advanced PAD, a major artery or, more often, several vessels are obstructed, and blood supply to the limb is minimal. The foot and especially the toes become cyanotic; in progressive, long-standing disease, they become necrotic. The patient experiences excruciating pain with no relief from a change of position. The severity of PAD with threatened limb loss is evident once systolic blood pressure drops below 40 mm Hg. Yao[12] reported an average ABI of 0.26 in patients who had rest pain. Other investigators have shown that the natural history of a patient with claudication who has an ABI less than or equal to 0.35 is poor.[13]

Palpation of the pulse at the distal arteries is a routine procedure to detect any abnormality in blood flow. The description of peripheral pulses can be characterized by the following five-category scales:

- 0 = absent
- 1 = markedly impaired
- 2 = moderately impaired
- 3 = slightly impaired or almost normal
- 4 = normal

Upon auscultation, a bruit can be detected, indicating turbulent flow. Palpation can be performed at the common femoral, popliteal, dorsalis pedis, and posterior tibial arteries.[14] However, it should be noted that the accuracy of pulse palpation varies among physicians.[15]

CLASSIFICATION OF PERIPHERAL ARTERIAL DISEASE

Classification of lower extremity arteriosclerosis is clinically important because it leads to therapy and provides information on the specific (with regard to the limb involved) and general (with regard to overall morbidity and mortality) prognosis. Various methods are used to classify the severity of lower extremity arterial disease.

The simplest method is the Fontaine classification, which is based exclusively on history and physical examination and is used by many clinicians, mainly in Europe.[16, 17] Briefly, disease is categorized into four stages. In stage I, the patient is asymptomatic with no clinical symptoms of arterial occlusive disease. In stage II, the patient experiences symptoms of intermittent claudication. In stage III, there is PAD leading to pain at rest. In stage IV, there is arterial disease associated with ulceration, gangrene, or both caused by arterial disease. Because of the variation in the interpretation of stage III disease, or "critical limb ischemia," many attempts have been made to propose a more precise definition.[18] Currently, most clinicians prefer the classification proposed by the Ad Hoc Committee on Reporting Standards of the Society for Vascular Surgery and the North American Chapter of the International Society for Cardiovascular Surgery.[19] However, this classification method requires additional noninvasive testing and is particularly suitable for reports dealing with lower extremity ischemia.

Measurement of the ABI also provides important information about the patient's general prognosis. The risk of mortality is inversely proportional to the ABI[20]; the lower the ABI, the greater the risk for cardiovascular disease. Even patients with a modestly reduced ABI (0.8 to 0.97) appear to be at risk for cardiovascular complications.[21]

DIAGNOSTIC TESTS

Ankle-Brachial Index

A simple way to evaluate the limb for arterial obstruction is to measure ankle pressure and calculate the ABI. Ankle pressure is a reliable indicator of the severity of disease.[12] Doppler ankle pressure measurements rely on signals from the posterior tibial and the dorsalis pedis arteries (Color Plate 21–9). The ABI is a simple test to perform. First, inflating pressure cuffs are placed around the ankles to determine blood flow in the arteries. Then a continuous-wave Doppler velocity detector is used as a "stethoscope" to measure the ankle blood pressure and to quantify a decrease in blood pressure in the ankle. In addition, analysis of Doppler signal blood flow characteristics to determine triphasic, biphasic, or monophasic flow provides information on distal circulation. Subsequently, the ankle pressure value is divided into the highest arm pressure value to determine the ABI.

An ABI of less than 0.90 is considered positive for PAD. Limb viability is threatened if the ABI is less than 0.40 or if arterial pressure is less than 50 mm Hg in a patient who does not have diabetes. In the comparative correlation study conducted by Ouriel and colleagues,[22] the ABI was normally greater than 0.97. This value proved accurate for discriminating between the presence and absence of occlusive disease. Other investigators have demonstrated that inherent variabilities in techniques may produce a normal variation in ABI of 0.12 in either direction.[23, 24]

Certain criteria are utilized to interpret the ABI. An ABI of 1.00 to 0.90 is associated with normal flow and no evidence of disease. Minimal or mild arterial disease is evident with an ABI of 0.89 to 0.80. Moderate disease is present with an ABI of 0.79 to 0.60. Once the obstruction becomes severe, the ABI has decreased to the range 0.59 to 0.45. The final category, tissue ischemia and limb loss, is compatible with an ABI less than 0.40. An ABI greater than 1.10 is characteristic of calcified vessels that cannot be compressed during cuff inflation.

Segmental Leg Pressure Measurements

Arterial pressure of segments in the leg may be measured when an extensive examination is indicated and if arterial disease is detected from an ABI less than 0.90. To obtain these measurements, cuffs are applied over segments of the arteries (high thigh, thigh, calf, ankle) in the legs. With use of continuous-wave Doppler velocity, the ABIs between the highest arm pressure and arterial pressure in each leg segment are determined. No evidence of significant arterial obstruction is considered present if the pressure in each leg segment equals that of the highest arm pressure. A gradient of 30 mm Hg between cuffs on the same leg indicates significant arterial obstruction. A significant decrease in the high thigh pressure indicates arterial obstruction in the aorta and aortoiliac arteries; however, this indication is not reliable for evaluating the significance of the obstruction. Multisegment disease is often apparent when arterial pressures are decreased significantly at all segmental regions.[25, 26]

Segmental pressure measurements can be used to detect PAD; however, it should be noted that these measurements are commonly unreliable in the presence of calcified, incompressible arterial walls, which are often found in patients with diabetes. Currently, segmental pressure measurements are used less frequently because of the aforementioned disadvantages. Although intended to localize the level of occlusive disease, these tests have been replaced by duplex ultrasonography, which invariably has higher precision, sensitivity, and specificity.

Toe Pressure Measurements

Toe pressure measurement is used to evaluate arterial flow in the toes and thereby quantify the overall extent of occlusive disease in the lower limb. Arterial pressures in the toe are obtained by placing photoplethysmographic sensors on the toes and measuring loss of the arterial signal when a toe occlusion cuff is inflated (Color Plate 21–10).

Toe pressures are of special value in assessing the extent and severity of disease (even if ankle pressure is normal). In normal subjects, toe pressures are always lower than ankle pressures and are usually lower than brachial systolic pressures. In the study by Carter and Lezack,[27] the lower limit of normal for toe pressure was 50 mm Hg and 64% of the brachial systolic pressure. For the ankle-toe gradient, the upper limit of normal was 70 mm Hg. Correlation of toe pressure measurements with angiographic findings from 102 extremities showed abnormal pressures in 97% of limbs having arterial occlusion and in 74% of extremities having stenotic lesions, indicating that these pressure values represent a valid index of the occlusive process.

Toe pressure measurements are a very beneficial method of evaluating the extent of arterial disease in diabetic patients. Toe pressure of no less than 55 mm Hg and greater than 70% of the arm pressure indicates normal arterial flow. Once toe pressure falls below 70% (range, 64% to 70%) of the arm pressure, the flow is noted to be marginal or borderline for arterial obstruction. Abnormal flow is signified by a toe pressure less than 60% of the arm pressure.[28]

Exercise Stress Testing

Segmental pressure gradients may indicate the level of disease, but they may overestimate or underestimate the extent of obstruction or functional impairment. The treadmill stress test is reliable for assessing functional impairment because it demonstrates the location, severity, and time of onset of the pain. Treadmill stress testing adds little to the sensitivity or specificity of detecting disease[29, 30] but can help differentiate between vascular and neuromuscular abnormalities. Treadmill stress testing can also be useful in patients with a normal or borderline (higher than 0.80) resting ABI and symptoms of occlusive disease.

Treadmill stress testing should be performed carefully while the patient is monitored for cardiac or pulmonary complications. If the patient experiences leg pain within 5 minutes of standardized exercise and shows a decrease in ankle pressures, a conclusive diagnosis of arterial obstruction can be made. Along with symptoms of claudication, treadmill stress testing is a reliable indicator of a causal relationship between the vascular disease and the symptoms. Decreases in both ankle pressure and recovery time constitute a reliable indicator of not only the extent of functional impairment but also the presence of multisegmental disease.[31]

Interpretation of the exercise stress test is as follows. The two characteristics observed are (1) the magnitude of the immediate drop in ankle pressure and (2) the time it takes for the ankle pressure to recover to resting ankle pressure levels. Single-segmental occlusive disease is indicated when ankle pressures fall to a low or unrecordable level immediately after exercise and return to resting pressure state between 2 and 6 minutes later. Multisegmental disease is associated with ankle pressures that remain low or unrecordable for up to 12 minutes. Severe ischemia is associated with ankle pressures that rarely recover to resting state after 15 minutes (Fig. 21–9).[32]

Color-Flow Duplex Ultrasonography

Duplex ultrasonography is superior to segmental pressure measurements for detecting hemodynamically significant stenosis because of its ability to directly evaluate the vessel as well as the flow within the vessel.[33] Duplex scanning can differentiate severe stenosis from occlusion and can distinguish multiple lesions from single, focal lesions; it is useful in providing information specific to the selection of appropriate interventional therapy (Color Plate 21–11).

Evaluation of the femoropopliteal arteries with duplex ultrasonography is less demanding than that of the aortoiliac arteries because of the superficial location of the former arteries. Color-flow duplex ultrasonography facilitates the identification of lesions, bruits, and collateral vessels.[34, 35] Diagnostic criteria developed and prospectively tested by the University of Washington Vascular Laboratory indicate that this method has a sensitivity of 82% and a specificity of 92%.[36] Some studies of femoropopliteal disease also suggest that valid clinical decisions can be made on the basis of duplex scans and that these decisions are similar to those based on arteriography.[37] Other studies indicate that duplex scanning has the potential to replace arteriography for evaluating femoropopliteal lesions.[38]

Kohler[39] evaluated normal subjects to determine normal arterial flow and vessel diameter for each segment of the arterial circulation in the leg. Jager and associates[40] also studied normal values in both men and women and found that the peak aortic velocity diminishes with increasing age. Arteries in women are smaller than those in men; however, the flow velocities do not differ with gender.

Normal flow is characterized by a triphasic waveform with no noted spectral broadening. A 1% to 19% reduction of lumen diameter is characterized by a normal waveform with slight spectral broadening and an increase in peak velocity of less than 30% over that in the proximal segment. A 20% to 40% reduction in diameter is characterized by enhanced spectral broadening and a peak velocity that is less than 100% greater than in the proximal segment. A 50% to 90% reduction of lumen diameter is characterized by an increase in peak systolic velocity that is more than 100% of that in the proximal segment as well as by monophasic or reduced post-stenosis flow. An occlusion is characterized by absence of flow within the artery or by a monophasic preocclusive "thump" heard proximal to the occlusion. The velocities are markedly diminished beyond the stenosis.[41]

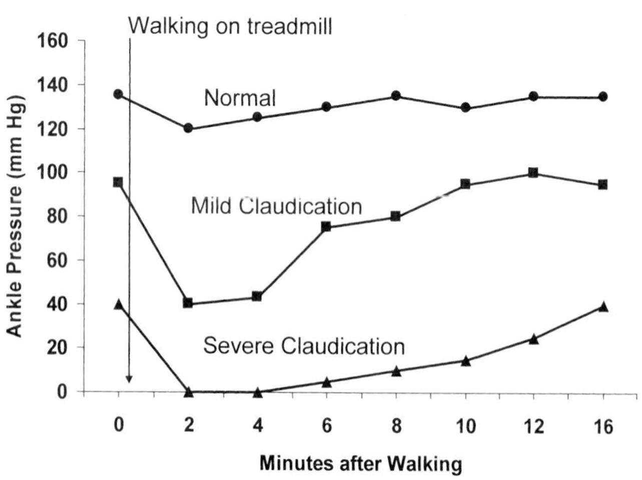

FIGURE 21–9. Exercise stress testing. The effect of severity of occlusive disease on recovery of ankle pressures.

Invasive Diagnostic Methods

Arteriography provides an anatomic road map, defining the vessel size, the length of the stenosis, and the presence of any vessel's collateral circulation. A complete complement of noninvasive and invasive tests can determine the arterial inflow and outflow circulation and can aid the choice of appropriate interventional therapy. Arteriography also clearly demonstrates arterial wall calcification, a condition manifested in people with diabetes.

ALGORITHM FOR DIAGNOSIS AND THERAPEUTIC IMPLICATIONS

The stage of PAD can be classified on the basis of the patient's history, physical examination, Doppler-derived ABIs, and duplex ultrasonography. This information allows one to formulate an idea of the severity of disease and the prognosis for the limb and the patient's life. For people who have ischemic pain at rest and in whom gangrene is present, the indication for surgical intervention is clear, but for those people who have intermittent claudication, conservative treatment is usually the first step. Intervention may be performed at a later stage, depending on the effect of the disease on the person's lifestyle or work.

Arterial disease of the femoropopliteal artery has a benign course as far as the limb is concerned. In one report, the risk for intervention for an isolated femoral artery lesion appeared to be 11% at 5 years and 14% at 10 years.[42] In patients who mainly have intermittent claudication, a conservative walking exercise program for 3 to 6 months is started. Usually, the pain-free walking distance can be more than doubled if the patient is on a walking program.[43] In addition, anticoagulation therapy is beneficial to prevent progression of arterial disease.[44] If the symptoms are still incapacitating after an exercise program, progressive intervention is indicated.[45] Factors reported to predict a worse outcome in patients with intermittent claudication are a low initial ABI, a reduced ABI at a subsequent visit, and continued smoking by the patient.[46, 47]

If intervention is indicated, the standard is still the femoropopliteal bypass operation using an autologous vein.[48, 49] Other options are endarterectomy and percutaneous interventional procedures. Duplex ultrasonographic examination can help determine whether a less invasive intervention with angioplasty is possible. Noninvasive diagnostic assessment using both ABI and duplex ultrasonography are routinely utilized in evaluating all interventions, including percutaneous transluminal angioplasty (PTA), placement of peripheral

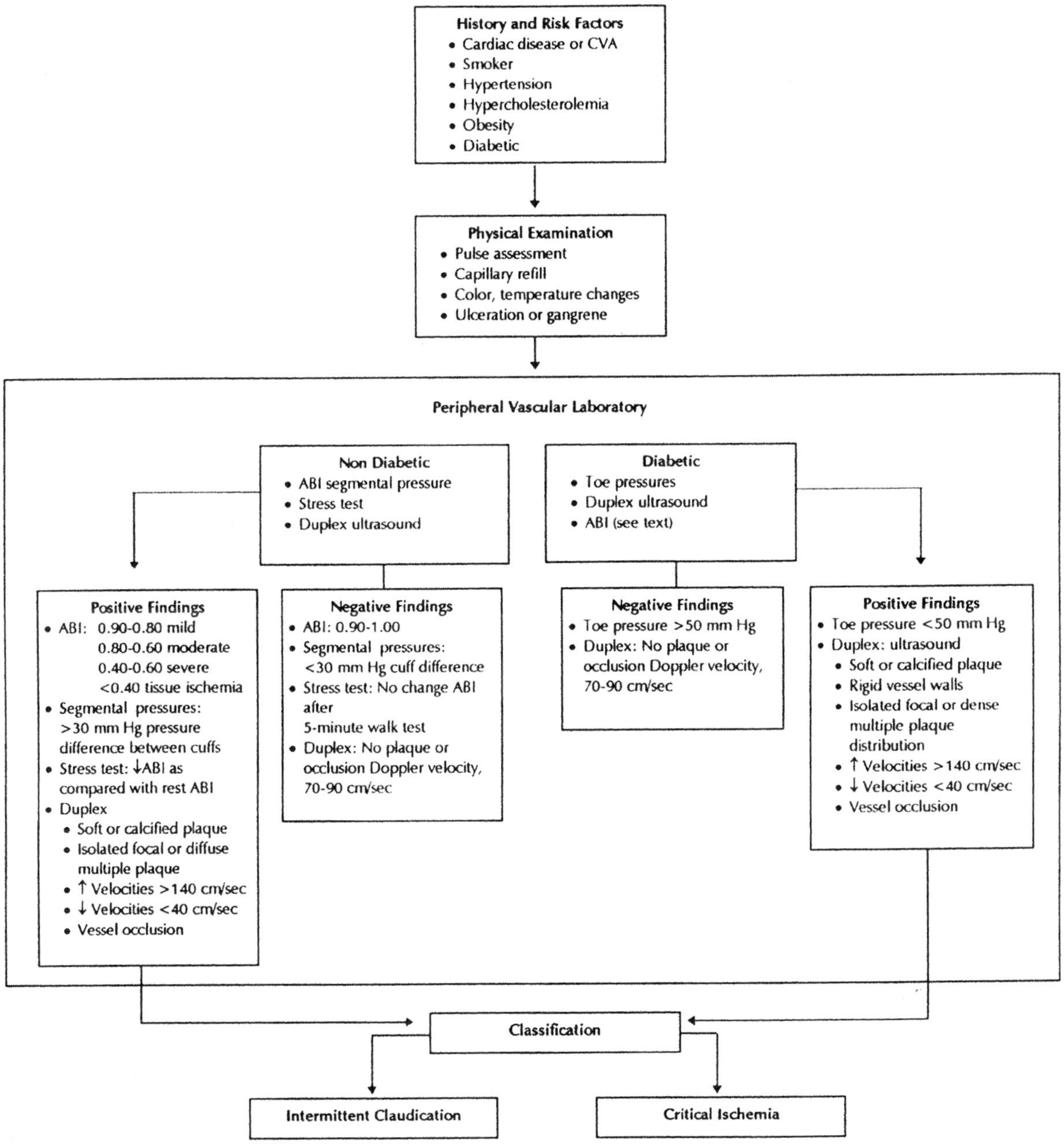

FIGURE 21–10. Peripheral vascular assessment and classification.

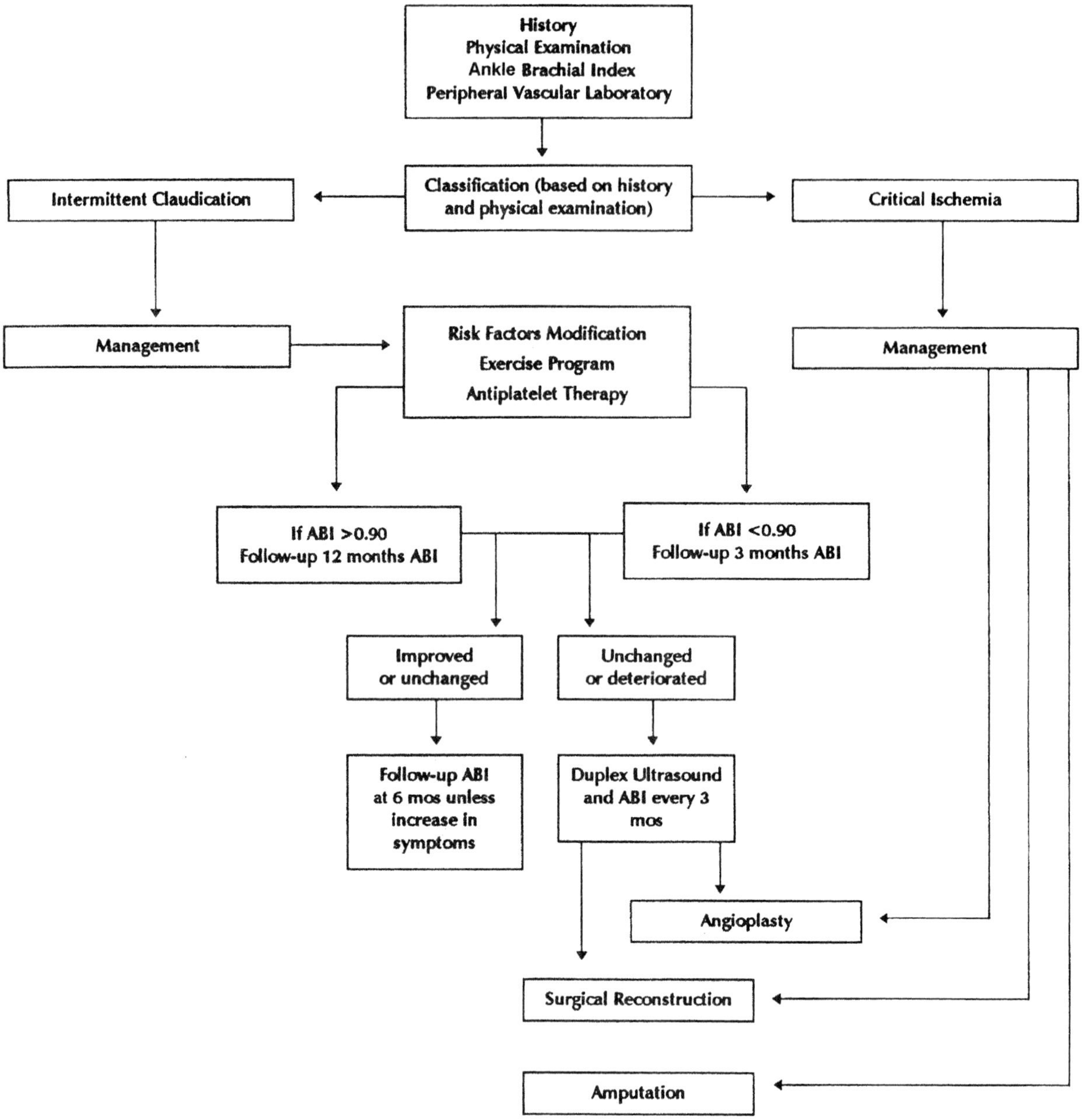

FIGURE 21–11. Management of peripheral vascular disease.

stents, and bypass graft surgery. Routine surveillance at frequent intervals is recommended to ensure patency of the arteries as well as to detect any disease progression or restenosis.

There is still much debate about PTA for femoropopliteal disease, especially of infrapopliteal vessels.[50, 51] Although PTA is clearly less invasive than surgical reconstruction, the results with PTA are inferior to those obtained with surgery.[52, 53] Moreover, some investigators have indicated that PTA is not clearly superior to an exercise program.[54]

A decision analysis may help to define the optimal treatment strategy for intermittent claudication.[55] An algorithm for the assessment of, and suggested therapy for, femoropopliteal occlusive disease based on findings from the patient's history, physical examination, and noninvasive tests is provided in Figures 21–10 and 21–11.

References

1. Criqui MH, Fronek A, Barrett-Connor E, et al: The prevalence of peripheral arterial disease in a defined population. Circulation 71: 510, 1985.
2. Gerhard M, Baum P, Raby KE: Peripheral arterial-vascular disease in women: Prevalence, prognosis, and treatment. Cardiology 86:349, 1995.
3. Criqui MH, Langer RD, Fronek A, et al: Mortality over a period of 10 years in patients with peripheral arterial disease. N Engl J Med 326: 381, 1992.
4. Smith GD, Shipley MJ, Rose G: Intermittent claudication, heart disease risk factors, and mortality. The Whitehall Study. Circulation 82:1925, 1990.
5. Vogt MT, McKenna M, Wolfson SK, Kuller LH: The relationship between ankle brachial index, other atherosclerotic disease, diabetes, smoking and mortality in older men and women. Atherosclerosis 101: 191, 1993.
6. Coffman JD: Intermittent claudication—be conservative. N Engl J Med 325:577, 1991.

3|

Medical/Interventional Therapy

Neil E. Strickman and James M. Wilson

of peripheral vascular disease appear when an owing reduces the capacity for maximal blood h that it is insufficient to meet the demands of scle. If the lumen size is further reduced, maxi- acity may fall below the needs of resting tissue, mptoms even in the absence of stress and, in enario, tissue death. The presence of atheroscle- eripheral vasculature signifies advanced disease, doubtedly present in the coronary and carotid . Therefore, the goals of therapy for peripheral ase are (1) to impede the progression of athero- (2) to improve blood flow to the affected limb

t of peripheral vascular disease extends beyond ut claudication and limb loss. Affected women ost fourfold increase in mortality during a 10- [2] Most of the deaths are the result of cardiovas- [2, 3] Of women with peripheral vascular disease, die of complications from coronary heart dis- impact of coronary disease is most prominent men with claudication, 50% of whom will die f myocardial ischemia, compared with 5% of age-matched controls.[8] A further 7% to 17% of deaths are the result of cerebrovascular disease.[3] Therefore, any intervention that would affect the natural history of atherosclerosis, in any distribution, would be beneficial in terms of mortality and disability (Table 21–3).

OALS OF THERAPY IN PERIPHERAL ASCULAR DISEASE

RECOGNITION OF COMORBIDITY

- Carotid stenosis
- Coronary stenosis
- Renal artery stenosis
- Aortic aneurysm

ALTERATION OF NATURAL HISTORY

- Risk factor identification/reduction:
  - Smoking
  - Menopause
  - Diabetes
  - Hypertension
  - Hyperhomocysteinemia
- Medical therapy:
  - Antiplatelet therapy (aspirin)
  - Hormone replacement
  - Glucose control
  - Blood pressure control
  - Vitamin E
  - Vitamin C
  - Folate/pyridoxine
  - Ticlopidine

YMPTOM REDUCTION

- Exercise
- Pentoxifylline
- Revascularization:
  - Angioplasty/stent
  - Surgical bypass/endarterectomy

MB SALVAGE

- Thrombolysis
- Angioplasty/stent
- Surgical bypass/endarterectomy

In the patient with coronary or carotid vascular disease, anatomic investigation is often performed at the first appearance of symptoms to detect and correct abnormalities associated with high risk of death or severe disability. In contrast, acute, life-threatening events in the peripheral vascular beds are rare.

Preemptive revascularization therapy is not superior to conservative measures in the unthreatened limb, and symptomatic relief is achievable by use of conservative measures. Physiologic testing, in addition to clinical factors, may confirm a diagnosis of peripheral vascular disease and guide the judicious use of angiography (Table 21–4). Patients with resting ischemic pain, ulceration, and gangrene are at a substantial risk for limb loss, mandating angiography and some form of intervention. Current options for revascularization include lysis of embolus or clot, angioplasty, stent implantation, and surgical bypass or endarterectomy. Additionally, in patients with disabling symptoms of claudication but not at immediate risk for limb loss, the physician can substantially improve the quality of life with revascularization by making diagnostic angiography an early step in the overall evaluation (see Table 21–4).

RISK FACTORS

A review of medical therapy should include a discussion of risk and prevention that cannot be properly emphasized by a contrast angiogram and an aesthetically pleasing arterial lumen. Whereas the immediate gratification of successful angioplasty reinforces its popularity, it is perhaps more important to apply therapies on the basis of systemic value and long-term goals (see Table 21–4). Most women with peripheral vascular disease have one or several risk factors for atherosclerosis that should be addressed to decrease the likelihood of disease progression.

Smoking

Long-term smoking affects both the risk of development of symptomatic atherosclerosis and the distribution of harmful lesions. For example, a rather distinct form of peripheral vascular disease can be seen in the distal aorta in women as young as 40 to 50 years who are heavy smokers. These women are also frequently hyperlipidemic and have experienced surgical menopause. Severe narrowing or obstruction occurs at the aortic bifurcation, which is unusually high and accompanied by small iliac and femoral vessels (Fig. 21–12). This grouping has been named the "hypoplastic aorto-iliac

7. Rutherford RB, Johnson G Jr, Moore WS, et al (eds): Vascular Surgery, 3rd ed. WB Saunders, Philadelphia, 1989.
8. Pearce WH, Slaughter MS, Le Maire S, et al: Aortic diameter as a function of age, gender, and body surface area. Surgery 114:691, 1993.
9. Valentine RJ, Hansen ME, Myers SI, et al: The influence of sex and aortic size on late patency after aortofemoral revascularization in young adults. J Vasc Surg 21:296, 1995.
10. Gardin JM, Davidson DM, Rohan MK, et al: Relationship between age, body size, gender, and blood pressure and Doppler flow measurements in the aorta and pulmonary artery. Am Heart J 113:101, 1987.
11. London GM, Guerin AP, Pannier B, et al: Influence of sex on arterial hemodynamics and blood pressure: Role of body height. Hypertension 26:514, 1995.
12. Yao JST: Haemodynamic studies in peripheral arterial disease. Br J Surg 57:761, 1970.
13. Fowl RJ, Gewirtz RJ, Love MC, Kempczinski RF: Natural history of claudicants with critical hemodynamic indices. Ann Vasc Surg 6: 31, 1992.
14. Gerlock AJ, Giyanani VL, Krebs C: Noninvasive vascular examinations of the lower extremity arteries. In: Applications of Noninvasive Vascular Techniques. WB Saunders, Philadelphia, 1988, p 299.
15. Brearley S, Shearman CP, Simms MH: Peripheral pulse palpation: An unreliable physical sign. Ann R Coll Surg Engl 74:169, 1992.
16. Fontaine R, Buck P, Riveaux R, et al: Sur le traitement des oblitérations artérielles: De la valuer respective des thrombectomies et thromendartériectomies, des shunts arterio-veneux et des greffes vasculaires (autogreffes veineuses fra3/4ches). Lyon Chir 46:73, 1951.
17. Second European Consensus Document on Chronic Critical Leg Ischaemia. Eur J Vasc Surg 6(Suppl A):1, 1992.
18. Jamieson C: The definition of critical ischaemia of a limb [editorial]. Br J Surg 69(Suppl):S2, 1982.
19. Rutherford RB, Flanigan DP, Gupta SK, et al: Suggested standards for reports dealing with lower extremity ischemia. Prepared by the Ad Hoc Committee on Reporting Standards, Society for Vascular Surgery/North American Chapter, International Society for Cardiovascular Surgery. J Vasc Surg 4:80, 1986.
20. Vogt MT, McKenna M, Anderson SJ, et al: The relationship between ankle-arm index and mortality in older men and women. J Am Geriatr Soc 41:523, 1993.
21. Newman AB, Siscovick DS, Manolio TA, et al: Ankle-arm index as a marker of atherosclerosis in the Cardiovascular Health Study. Cardiovascular Heart Study (CHS) Collaborative Research Group. Circulation 88:837, 1993.
22. Ouriel K, Zarins CK: Doppler ankle pressure: An evaluation of three methods of expression. Arch Surg 117:1297, 1982.
23. Baker JD, Dix DE: Variability of Doppler ankle pressures with arterial occlusive disease: An evaluation of ankle index and brachial-ankle pressure gradient. Surgery 89:134, 1981.
24. Johnston KW, Hosang MY, Anders DF: Reproducibility of noninvasive vascular laboratory measurements of the peripheral circulation. J Vasc Surg 6:147, 1987.
25. Carter SA: Clinical measurement of systolic pressures in limbs with arterial occlusive disease. JAMA 207:1869, 1969.
26. Rutherford RB, Lowenstein DH, Klein MF: Combining segmental systolic pressures and plethysmography to diagnose arterial occlusive disease of the legs. Am J Surg 138:211, 1979.
27. Carter SA, Lezack JD: Digital systolic pressures in the lower limb in arterial disease. Circulation 43:905, 1971.
28. Gerlock AJ, Giyanani VL, Krebs C: Toe pressures and digital photoplethysmography. In: Applications of Noninvasive Vascular Techniques. WB Saunders, Philadelphia, 1988, p 413.
29. Clyne CAC, Tripolitis A, Jamieson CW, et al: The reproducibility of the treadmill walking test for claudication. Surg Gynecol Obstet 149: 727, 1979.
30. Ouriel K, McDonnell AE, Metz CE, Zarins CK: A critical evaluation of stress testing in the diagnosis of peripheral vascular disease. Surgery 91:686, 1982.
31. Sumner DS, Strandness DE Jr: The relationship between calf blood flow and ankle blood pressure
Surgery 65:763, 1969.
32. Strandness DE, Zierler RE: I
arterial disease. In Bernstein
Mosby-Year Book, St. Louis,
33. Moneta GL, Yeager RA, Lee
of arterial occlusive disease:
sures and arterial duplex map
34. Stedge KG, Hannan LJ, Ka
mode ultrasound to study art
ities. Bruit 9:71, 1985.
35. Salles-Cunha SX, Andros C
infrainguinal revascularizatio
36. Kohler TR, Nance DR, Cran
sis of aortoiliac and femorop
lation 76:1074, 1987.
37. Kohler TR, Andros G, Port
arteriography for lower ext
280, 1990.
38. Legemate DA, Teeuwen C,
scanning to replace aorto-il
Vasc Surg 3:49, 1989.
39. Kohler T: Duplex scannin
disease. In Bernstein EF (
Book, St. Louis, 1993, p 5
40. Jager KA, Ricketts HJ, S
evaluation of lower limb a
vasive Diagnostic Techniq
Louis, 1985, p 619.
41. Kohler TR: Duplex scann
disease. In Bernstein EF
Louis, 1993.
42. Cox GS, Hertzer NR, Y
superficial femoral artery
172, 1993.
43. Gardner AW, Poehlman
treatment of claudication
44. Goldhaber SZ, Manson J
subsequent peripheral ar
Lancet 340(8812):143, 1
45. Lundgren F, Dahllof
claudication—surgical re
tive randomized trial of
46. Rosenbloom MS, Flanig
the natural history of i
1988.
47. McDaniel MD, Cronen
of intermittent claudicat
48. Taylor LM Jr, Edwards
bypass grafting: Five-ye
193, 1990.
49. Dalman RL, Taylor LM
larization procedures.
50. Fraser SCA, Al-Kutoul
angioplasty of the infra
33, 1996.
51. Bakal CW, Cynamon J,
luminal angioplasty: W
52. Johnston KW: Femora
balloon angioplasty. R
53. Wilson SE, Sheppard
plasty for peripheral
1990.
54. Creasy TS, McMillan
nal angioplasty better
from a prospective ra
55. Troeng T, Bergqvist I
treatment of intermit
J Vasc Surg 7:438, 19

21.

Symptoms
arterial na
flow so mu
working m
mal flow c
producing
the worst s
rosis in the
which is u
beds as we
vascular dis
sclerosis an
(Table 21–2
The imp
concerns ab
have an alı
year period.
cular diseas
35% to 57%
ease.[4–7] The
in elderly w
as a result

Table 21–2.

Table 21–3. MEDICAL THERAPY FOR PERIPHERAL VASCULAR DISEASE

AGENT	ACTION	BENEFIT	COMMENTS
Aspirin	Platelet inhibition	Reduced likelihood of amputation	GI ulceration
Ticlopidine (Ticlid)	Platelet inhibition	Less need for revascularization, symptom reduction	Neutropenia, GI intolerance, rash
Pentoxifylline (Trental)	Improved RBC deformability	Symptom reduction	Minor benefit
Statins	Cholesterol lowering	Decreased probability of AMI	GI intolerance, myositis, hepatitis
Fibrates	Cholesterol, triglyceride lowering	Decreased probability of AMI	Gallstones, myositis
Resins	Cholesterol lowering	Decreased probability of AMI	GI intolerance
Niacin	Cholesterol lowering, HDL increase	Decreased probability of AMI	Gout, flushing, hyperglycemia, peptic ulcer
Estrogens	Hormone replacement	Decreased probability of AMI	Increase in breast/uterine cancer?
Vitamin E	Antioxidant	Decreased probability of AMI	Benefit unproven
Vitamin C	Antioxidant	Slowing of disease progression	Diminished LDL oxidation in smokers, benefit unproven
Folate/pyridoxine	Cofactor for cystathionine beta-synthase activity	Decreased plasma homocysteine concentrations	Presumptive benefit

AMI, acute myocardial infarction; GI, gastrointestinal; LDL, low-density lipoprotein; RBC, red blood cell.

syndrome."[9, 10] Unfortunately for women with this condition, risk reduction through smoking cessation does not improve symptoms; thus, some form of mechanical revascularization is required. However, for the remaining majority of patients with symptomatic disease, or for patients who are at risk for development of peripheral vascular disease, smoking cessation has important benefits.

Smoking is the most important risk factor for accelerated progression of atherosclerosis, and it is associated with a higher risk of death, amputation, and the need for limb salvage therapy.[9, 11–16] Nine of 10 women with claudication who continue to smoke eventually require some form of revascularization.[9]

Positive effects of smoking cessation include a reduction of plasma fibrinogen concentration, oxidation of LDL cholesterol, and enhanced vasomotor tone. These effects translate into clinical benefits as a reduced rate of progression to critical limb ischemia and a substantial improvement of symptoms.[11, 13, 17–19] Most patients who stop smoking enjoy a twofold to threefold increase in symptom-free walking time.

Hyperlipidemia

Various forms of hyperlipidemia are strongly associated with the development and progression of atherosclerosis.[1, 3] The few studies that have addressed lipid-lowering therapy for peripheral atherosclerosis have shown beneficial results.[20, 21]

Table 21–4. PERIPHERAL VASCULAR DISEASE: PHYSIOLOGIC STATUS AND INDICATED THERAPY

SYMPTOMS	FONTAINE CLASS	ANKLE-BRACHIAL INDEX	THERAPY
None	I	>0.95	Conservative
Pain upon walking:			
At >200 meters	IIa	_0.9	Conservative/consider revascularization
At <200 meters	IIb	_0.7	Revascularization
Rest/nocturnal pain	III	_0.5	Urgent revascularization
Necrosis/gangrene	IV	<0.3	Revascularization/ amputation

The effect of cholesterol lowering upon coronary events, and perhaps stroke, is extensive and compelling in both men and women.[22–25] The association of peripheral vascular disease with advanced coronary atherosclerosis strongly suggests that affected women realize substantial benefit from lipid-lowering therapy. Drug choice and dosing must be individualized according to the specific lipid abnormality. Correction of coexistent maladies that influence lipid abnormalities, such as hypothyroidism, obesity, and diabetes mellitus, may also be of value.

Hormonal Status

Women usually manifest symptoms of peripheral vascular disease at a later age than men.[1, 3] In younger age groups, there is a marked discrepancy in the prevalence of disease, with women beginning to close the gap at about age 65 years. The most probable source of this delay is the protective effect of female reproductive hormones, which are lost in most women by their mid-50s. A large body of epidemiologic evidence supports the hypothesis that early estrogen deprivation accelerates the progression of atherosclerosis, leading to the suggestion that hormone replacement after menopause may be protective.[26] In one of the largest studies to date, the Nurses' Health Study, women treated with hormone replacement therapy, including progestins, had a relative risk of coronary events of 0.39.[27] However, no effect on the incidence of stroke was detected, and no effect related to claudication was reported. There are no data to support the idea that women affected by peripheral vascular disease benefit from hormone replacement therapy. Nonetheless, the implied benefits to women with peripheral atherosclerosis are substantial; hormone replacement therapy should be *strongly* considered in such patients.

Other Risk Factors

Whereas the exact interaction between hypertension and atherosclerosis is unknown, the adverse effect of hypertension is unquestionable. Unlike the natural history of coronary

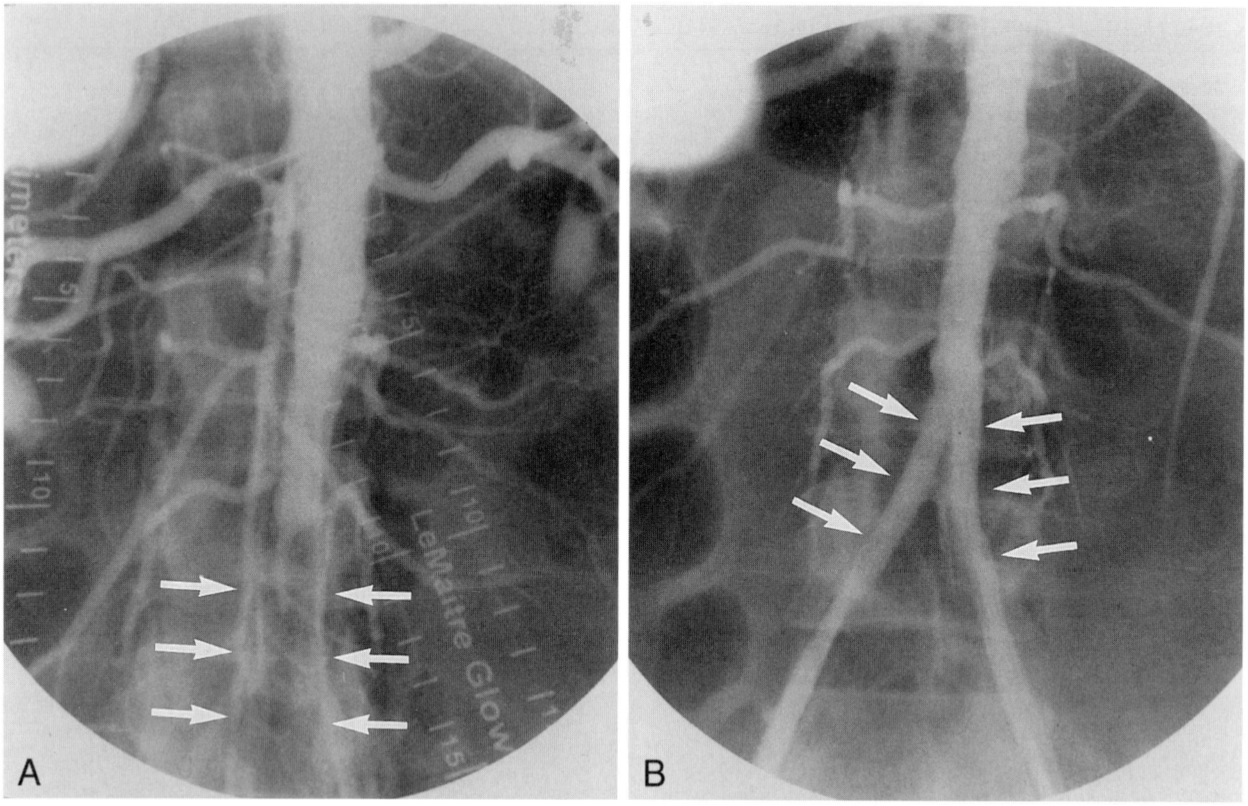

FIGURE 21–12. A 45-year-old woman with a history of heavy smoking was diagnosed with bilateral hip claudication, which occurred after she walked approximately 50 feet. Diagnostic angiography revealed occlusion of the aorta just above the bifurcation (*A*). Angiographic and clinical results were excellent after angioplasty and stenting of both common iliac arteries (*B*).

and carotid disease, that of peripheral vascular disease is not known to be affected by antihypertensive therapy. Antihypertensive therapy has not been shown to greatly influence symptoms of claudication. Vasodilators, such as calcium channel blockers and nitrates, have no proven beneficial effect.[28] Meanwhile, concerns about the detrimental effect of beta blockade have not been confirmed in controlled trials.[29]

Diabetes strongly influences the probability of development and the distribution of atherosclerosis.[1, 3, 12, 30] Vascular disease in diabetic patients is usually more distal, diffuse, and calcified, making treatment of any sort somewhat problematic. Patients with diabetes are almost 20 times more likely to need revascularization and five times more likely to undergo amputation.[31] The effects of coexistent microvascular disease may lower the threshold for revascularization by detrimentally affecting wound healing and infection. Intense glycemic control will prevent or delay the onset of microvascular complications and may improve coexistent hyperlipidemia. Currently, however, its effect on the progression of atherosclerosis is presumptive.

Another risk factor for which recognition is slowly growing is hyperhomocysteinemia. Inheritance of a defective gene coding for the enzyme cystathionine beta-synthase results in an accumulation of homocysteine. Homocysteine is a reactive molecule that may injure endothelial cells. The homozygous condition is marked by ocular, skeletal, and neurologic complications, the development of premature atherosclerosis, and a prothrombotic state. Women with a single abnormal gene for cystathionine beta-synthase have a higher prevalence of elevated homocysteine concentrations than do heterozygous men. This appears to be an independent risk factor for the development of peripheral vascular disease.[32, 33] For many of these patients, the response to high doses of pyridoxine and folate is a reduction in homocysteine concentration.

THERAPY OPTIONS

Antithrombotic Therapy

Clinically apparent atherosclerosis consists mostly of complex lesions that have reached the stage of rapid progression, meaning that plaque fracture or ulceration is not uncommon and that thrombosis has become the most important and dramatic event in plaque evolution. Inhibition of thrombosis should therefore slow the progression of disease and prevent clinical events such as the development of critical limb ischemia.

Under arterial flow conditions, the primary effector of thrombosis is the blood platelet, whose inhibition has become an important target for therapy. Aspirin irreversibly inhibits platelet cyclooxygenase, impairing production of thromboxane A_2 and, thereby, the processes of activation and aggregation. Its effect on the progression of peripheral vascular disease in women has not been established. However, the administration of aspirin effectively lowers the incidence of complications of coronary and carotid atherosclerosis and, in treated men, reduces the need for lower extremity revascularization.[34]

Like aspirin, ticlopidine impairs platelet activation pathways, reducing the likelihood of thrombotic complications. Unlike treatment with aspirin, however, treatment with ticlopidine may actually lengthen the duration of symptom-free exercise.[35] Unfortunately, the use of this agent is associated with the development of reversible neutropenia in about 1% to 5% of treated patients. The risk-benefit ratio for the long-term use of ticlopidine in patients with peripheral vascular disease has not been established, relegating it to second-line therapy for patients with aspirin intolerance or short-term therapy for those undergoing revascularization procedures. Triflusal is an experimental antiplatelet drug that is similar to ticlopidine in its effect on the duration of symptom-free exercise, suggesting that this may be a class effect of potent platelet antagonists.[36]

Clopidogrel, an oral platelet aggregation inhibitor similar to ticlopidine, appears to be more effective than aspirin in preventing the thrombotic complications of atherosclerosis. In one study, patients with symptomatic peripheral atherosclerosis who were treated with clopidogrel experienced a 24% reduction of risk for stroke, myocardial infarction, or vascular death compared with patients who received aspirin. Neutropenia was not a significant side effect of the drug, and gastrointestinal bleeding was actually less common in clopidogrel-treated patients than in aspirin-treated patients.[37]

Lastly, the glycoprotein IIb/IIIa antagonists are theoretically promising and are undergoing trials at present for the treatment of peripheral atherosclerosis.

Rheologic Therapy

According to Poiseuille's law, the flow capacity of a vessel is proportional to the fourth power of the vessel radius and inversely proportional to lesion length and blood viscosity. The most effective method to increase flow capacity is therefore to enlarge the vessel lumen. Fixed lesions cannot be dilated medically. Vasodilator therapy has been disappointing when used in attempts to reduce claudication, leaving mechanical revascularization as the only effective method of enlarging the vessel lumen.

Although complex, the viscous resistance of whole blood can be thought of in terms of the amount and properties of (1) the cellular element, erythrocytes, and (2) the fluid element, the major contributor of which is fibrinogen. Pentoxifylline is a methylxanthine derivative that improves erythrocyte deformability and may reduce fibrinogen concentrations. Its administration has been shown to prolong treadmill walking times. Unfortunately, only a small proportion of treated patients realize any symptomatic benefit, and long-term administration may be necessary to achieve these benefits.[38, 39]

Exercise

A woman with mild to moderate claudication may experience a remarkable improvement in symptoms with medical therapy and a consistent exercise routine.[40–48] In fact, exercise and balloon angioplasty have similar rates of long-term effectiveness for reducing symptoms in patients with mild claudication.[48]

In addition to an improved sense of well-being, regular exercise has an interesting effect on the genesis of claudication. During exercise, mean arterial pressure rises slightly, and rhythmic muscle activity assists limb venous outflow, raising the pressure gradient for limb blood flow. Arteriolar dilatation produced by accumulation of muscle metabolites reduces resistance, further augmenting blood flow. In a patient with peripheral vascular disease, the diseased conductance vessel becomes the site of maximal resistance, usurping the regulatory role of precapillary arterioles. During exercise, muscular arterioles behave normally. However, the lesion in the conductance vessel becomes the site of maximal resistance. As a result, muscles fed by vessel branches arising proximal to the lesion site provide the path of least resistance and are fed preferentially. Aerobic conditioning of these muscle beds delays the onset of arteriolar dilatation and the "steal" phenomenon that produces claudication.[49, 50]

A reasonable exercise prescription is flat-surface or treadmill walking for at least 30 minutes five times per week. Walking speed should be brisk, about 3 to 5 miles per hour. Severe claudication may be relieved by periods of rest, but the occurrence of mild claudication should not interrupt exercise.

PERCUTANEOUS REVASCULARIZATION

Percutaneous balloon angioplasty has been used to improve blood flow to ischemic limbs since Gruentzig introduced it in 1974.[51] It is a remarkably successful method of revascularization, with benefits including short hospital stays and low complication rates. Because of the ease and relative safety of angioplasty, the benefit of revascularization has been extended to patients with mild symptoms who might not otherwise have been treated. There are few contraindications to angioplasty, and the list is getting shorter. They include uncontrolled coagulopathy,[9] absence of reliable vascular access, and renal insufficiency. The risk of permanent renal damage may be greater when the serum creatinine level is higher than 1.8 mg/dL. Angioplasty is most effective for short, discrete lesions in larger vessels such as the common iliac artery.[52]

Several technologic advances have produced methods to assist in the mechanical enlargement of diseased vessels (Table 21–5). Although many of these technologies have found a niche, only the endovascular stent has truly improved upon the balloon procedure, allowing attempts at percutaneous therapy for long, chronically occluded lesions and as a "bailout" procedure for circumstances that previously would have required surgical bypass (Fig. 21–13).[53–59] Percutaneous methods are now the treatment of choice when possible. With the help of stenting, the success rate is excellent and the risks are low. In the case of more difficult lesions, and when interventional treatment fails, surgical bypass may be preformed with a minor increase in morbidity.

The indications for revascularization therapy are symptoms that impair lifestyle, rest discomfort, poor wound healing in the presence of moderate to severe ischemia, and gangrene (see Table 21–4).[52] This philosophy, which arose from experiences with surgical bypass and endarterectomy, is firmly grounded in risk-benefit analysis. However, the

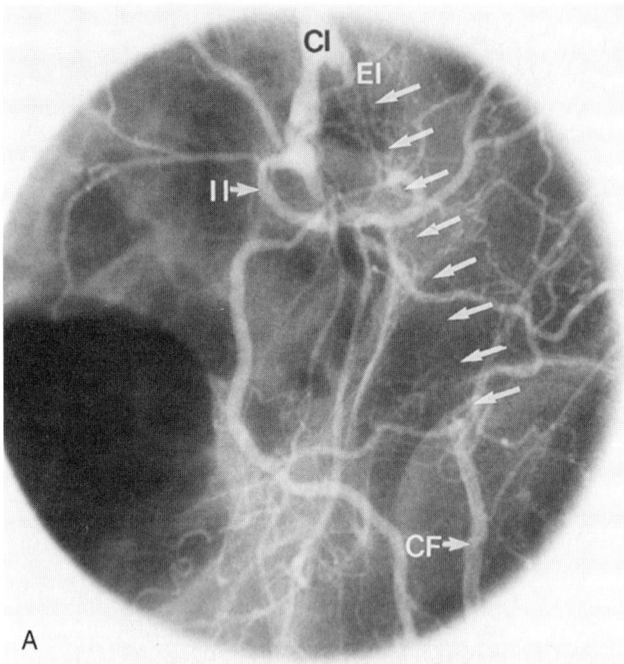

FIGURE 21–13. Complaints of rest discomfort prompted angioplasty in this 80-year-old woman. The external iliac artery is completely occluded over an 8-cm span (*A*). Although wire passage was accomplished without difficulty, angioplasty results were suboptimal (*B*). The implantation of a Wallstent (Boston Scientific Corporation) produced excellent results obviating the need for surgical bypass (*C*). CI, common iliac artery; EI, external iliac artery; II, internal iliac artery; CF, common femoral artery.

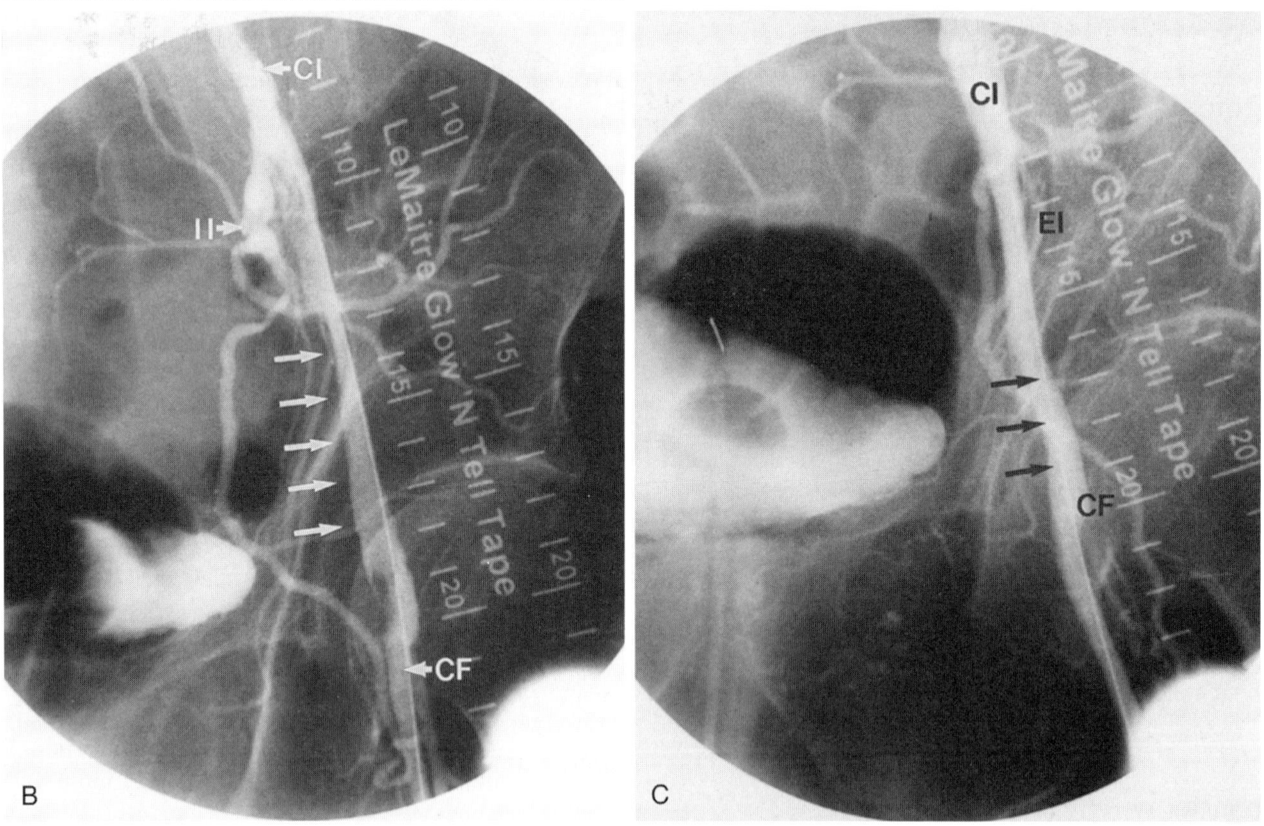

Table 21–5. PERCUTANEOUS REVASCULARIZATION DEVICES FOR PERIPHERAL VASCULAR DISEASE

DEVICE	USE	COMMENTS
Balloon	Most lesions	Remains the standard
Stent	Long lesions Calcified lesions Total occlusions After inadequate balloon result	Best results in aorta and iliac arteries
Rotablation device	Debulking of hard, calcified lesions	Limited use, expensive
Transluminal extraction catheter	Severely diseased segments of graft	Rarely used, perforation risk
Directional atherectomy device	Debulking of eccentric lesions	Rarely used, embolization risk
Rheolytic thrombectomy device	Extraction of acute thrombus	Helpful if clot burden is small and < 2 wk old
Excimer laser	Debulking; total occlusions	Perforation risk

prescription for therapy must be individualized. The goal is to avoid attempts at intervention in patients with marginal indications in whom the risk of complication is high. For example, the sedentary, elderly diabetic with renal insufficiency and moderate to severe claudication would meet strict indications for revascularization but would be best served by conservative care unless ischemia endangers her limb. On the other hand, the young or middle-aged woman whose lifestyle is inhibited by claudication should be offered the chance for percutaneous revascularization.

Mechanism

Balloon angioplasty fractures the diseased arterial intima and stretches the surrounding media. Newly exposed surfaces provide purchase for platelets and initiate the thrombotic process. Large-volume accumulation of thrombus may be prevented by the administration of aspirin and heparin at the time of the procedure and by the improvements in blood flow resulting from the procedure. With time, the treated site heals and develops a new endothelial lining. In some proportion of treated lesions an overexuberant healing process or contracture of surrounding tissues produces lesion recurrence.[60] Fortunately, restenosis lesions may be treated with second angioplasty procedures, offering a reasonable chance of long-term success (Fig. 21–14).

Results

The results of angioplasty in women are equivalent to those in men.[61] Angioplasty is most effective for discrete lesions in larger vessels. It is less successful in long, heavily calcified lesions, in chronic total occlusions, and in severe diffuse disease with poor runoff, as is frequently seen when limb

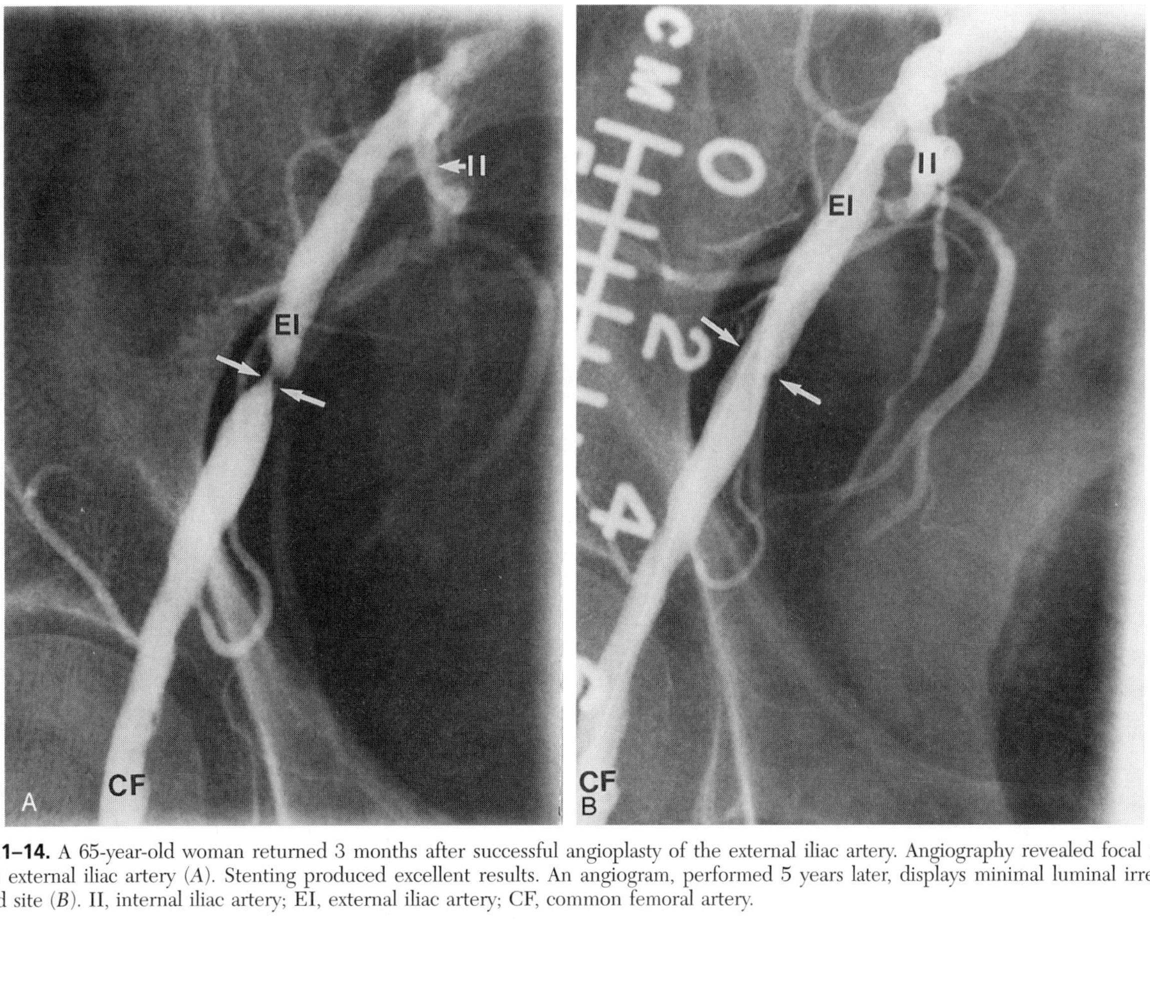

FIGURE 21–14. A 65-year-old woman returned 3 months after successful angioplasty of the external iliac artery. Angiography revealed focal recurrence within the external iliac artery (*A*). Stenting produced excellent results. An angiogram, performed 5 years later, displays minimal luminal irregularity at the treated site (*B*). II, internal iliac artery; EI, external iliac artery; CF, common femoral artery.

Table 21–6. RESULTS OF ANGIOPLASTY FOR PERIPHERAL VASCULAR DISEASE

SEGMENT	ACUTE (% SUCCESS)	LONG-TERM PATENCY (% SUCCESS)	COMMENTS
Aortoiliac	92–100	75–85	Improved by stenting
Femoropopliteal	85–90	40–65	Increased risk of stent thrombosis
Tibioperoneal	86	25–40*	Limb salvage

*Limb salvage and clinical success rather than true angiographic patency.

salvage is attempted.[52] Patients with severe distal disease and those who are diabetic are less likely to have successful procedures. The greatest hindrance of angioplasty procedures has historically been intima-media dissection and vessel recoil, both of which can result in immediate recurrence of stenosis and vessel closure. A significant step forward was made with the introduction and refinement of the endovascular stent. The application of an expandable metal buttress prevents recoil and prolapse of dissected tissue into the vessel lumen. As a result, both immediate and long-term results are substantially improved.

Balloon angioplasty is quite successful in both short-term and long-term follow-up for the treatment of aortoiliac stenosis. Quoted patency rates range from slightly more than 50% in patients with diffuse distal atherosclerosis to more than 90% in patients with focal disease (Table 21–6).[62–68] Primary or "bailout" implantation of stents increases initial success rates to almost 100% and provides excellent long-term patency with less than 10% recurrence of stenosis at the treated site.[53–55, 69–77] Although stents are a remarkable advance in percutaneous therapy, their long-term performance is not as good in women as in men[62]; the reason for this discrepancy is unknown.

Femoral and popliteal segments also respond well to angioplasty, although long-term results are not as good as those seen in aortoiliac stenosis (see Table 21–6).[55, 63–65, 78, 79] This difference is in part due to the character of disease affecting those vessels. The adductor canal, also known as Hunter's canal, is a long segment of the superficial femoral artery traversing the midthigh above the popliteal artery, which has a predilection for development of atherosclerosis (Fig. 21–15).[30, 63–65, 78, 79] This segment usually has regions of diffuse disease that tend to be totally occluded, raising the risk of late progression of disease and failure of angioplasty. Unfortunately, stents have not performed as well in these segments and are best reserved for treatment of a suboptimal angioplasty result.[56, 71, 77, 80–82]

Technologic advances have improved the outcome of infrapopliteal angioplasty, expanding its scope. In the past, because of complication rates and poor results in these vessels, angioplasty was relegated to use only in attempts at limb salvage. Whereas a patient with diffuse disease should still be treated only for limb salvage, therapy for more focal disease with good runoff is acceptable (Fig. 21–16) and may be increasingly used to help patients with disabling claudication (see Table 21–6).[63, 81, 83–89]

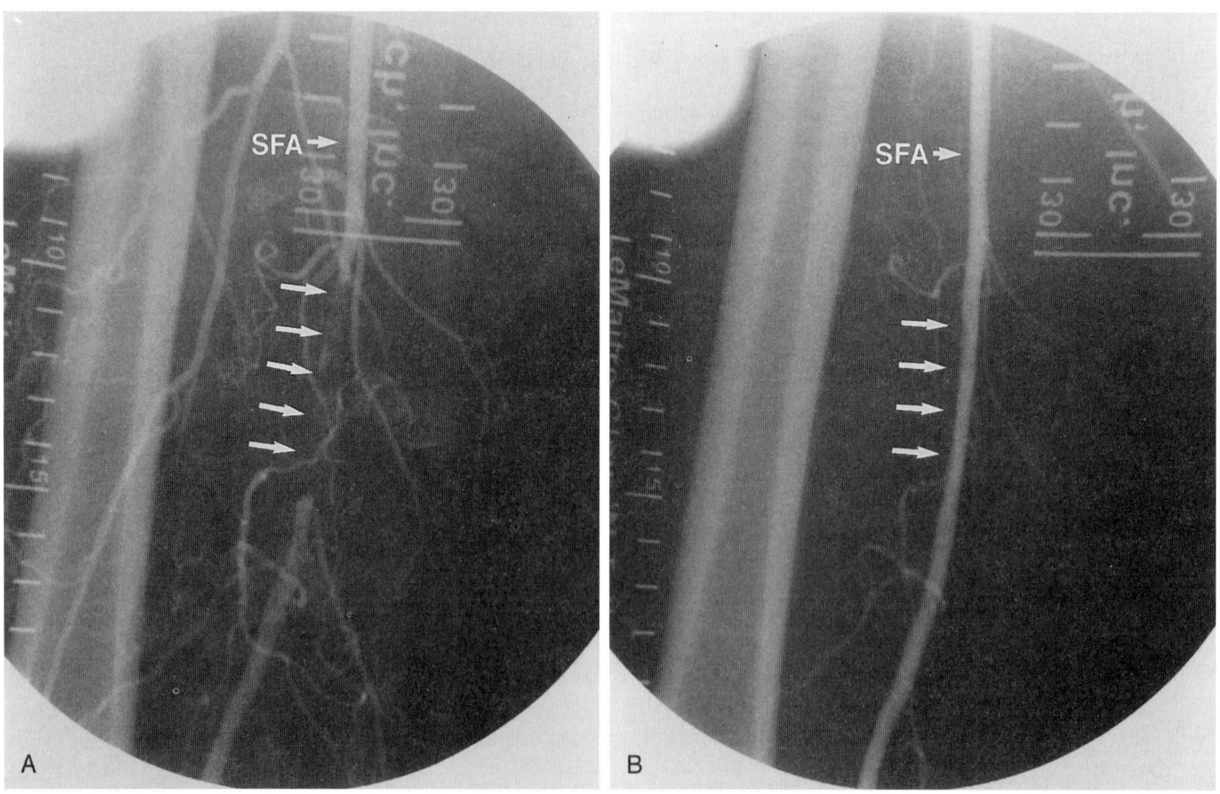

FIGURE 21–15. The adductor canal is frequently the site of disease affecting the superficial femoral artery. The value of antithrombotic therapy is emphasized in this lesion, which has an undulated surface and sharply demarcated distal border, suggesting a recent thrombotic complication (*A*). After intraarterial urokinase, balloon angioplasty produced excellent results with minimal residual narrowing (*B*). SFA, superficial femoral artery.

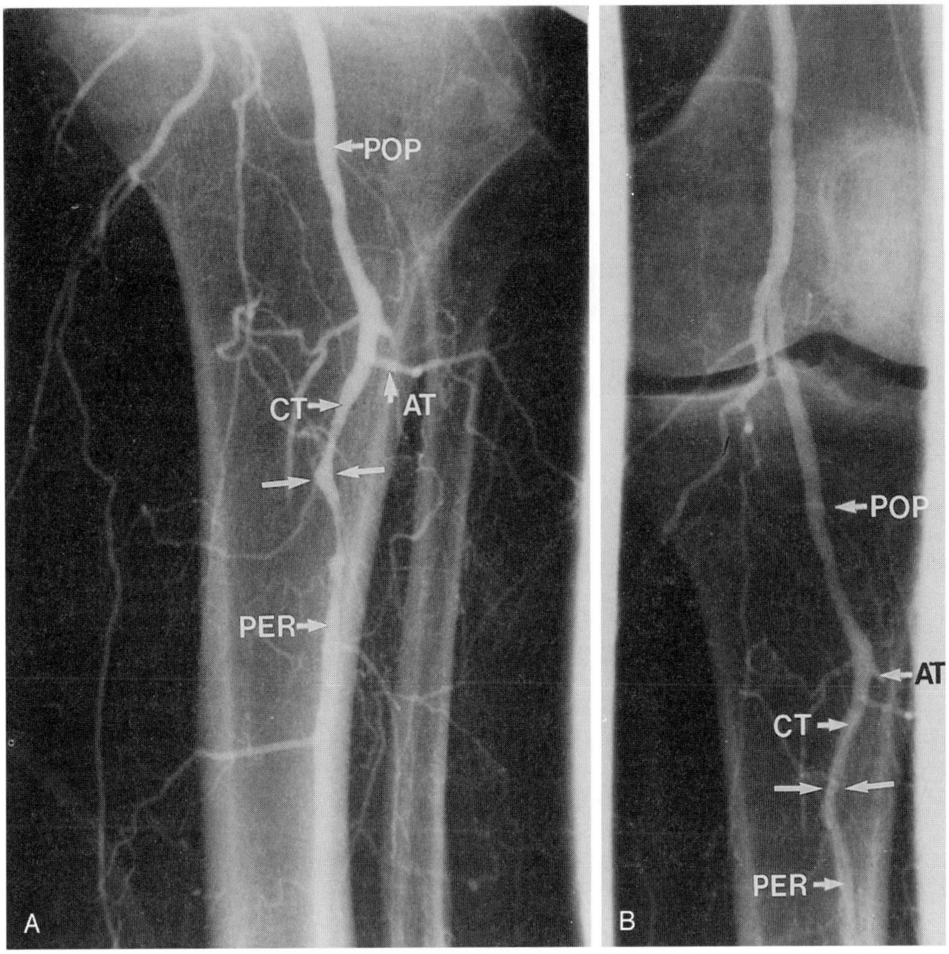

FIGURE 21–16. Historically, percutaneous revascularization below the knee has met with discouraging short- and long-term results. Most clinicians avoid revascularization attempts unless the limb is in jeopardy. However, technologic advances have improved the acute results of angioplasty and may expand the scope of percutaneous procedures in this distribution. The diagnostic angiogram in this 75-year-old diabetic woman displays complete occlusion of all but the peroneal artery (*A*). An extensive collateral network can be seen originating above a 90% diameter stenosis of the single remaining vessel supplying the foot. Angioplasty results were excellent (*B*). POP, popliteal artery; CT, tibioperoneal trunk; AT, anterior tibial artery; PER, peroneal artery.

Complications

Severe complications of percutaneous angioplasty include vessel rupture or perforation, abrupt closure, and acute renal failure. They are fortunately rare and in many cases can be avoided with meticulous attention to detail. Minor complications include hematoma and pseudoaneurysm at the site of vessel entry. Pseudoaneurysm, the more serious of the two, occurs in less than 1% of percutaneous procedures and often resolves with ultrasound-guided external compression. It appears to occur with greater frequency in patients who are receiving excessive anticoagulant therapy. Other complications are bleeding, arteriovenous fistula, thrombosis, intimal dissection, distal embolization, myocardial infarction, and cerebrovascular accident.

THROMBOLYSIS

Thrombolytic therapy provides a third option for revascularization, working best in cases of acute occlusion of bypass grafts or thromboemboli. It is also useful in selected occlusions of longer duration and in native vessel atherosclerosis complicated by large-volume thrombosis. A variety of agents are available for use. Technical success rates vary from 65% to 97%, often requiring prolonged infusions (longer than 24 hours).[90–102] Newer infusion protocols have been developed that may prove faster and require lower drug doses. The time required to achieve lysis limits the usefulness of thrombolytic agents in cases in which urgent revascularization is required. The frequency (10% to 20%) of hemorrhagic complications further limits the use of this modality. There is no evidence to suggest the different efficacy of these agents in women versus men.

THE FUTURE

The short- and long-term outcomes of percutaneous angioplasty will undoubtedly improve with the development of better stent technology, including covered stents, which may also be of value for aneurysmal disease (Fig. 21–17). Great strides have been made in understanding the mechanism of restenosis, which is the last major limitation of balloon procedures.

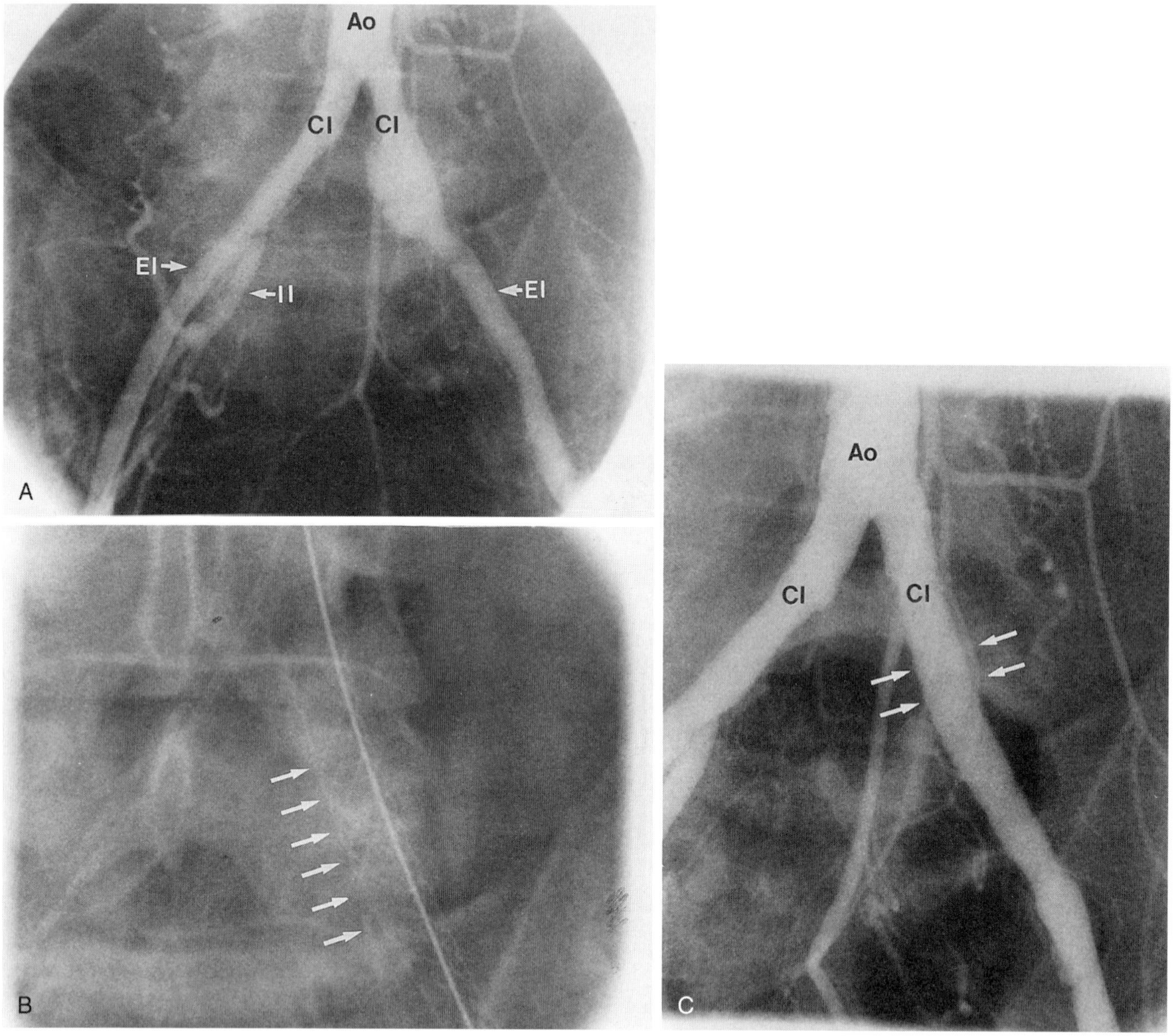

FIGURE 21–17. Whereas aneurysms of the common iliac artery may rupture, the more common clinical presentation is that of peripheral embolization. Similar events prompted the need for intervention in this vessel (*A*). A wish to avoid major abdominal surgery prompted the placement of 2 graft-covered Palmaz iliac stents completely excluding the aneurysmal segment of the vessel (*B* and *C*). CI, common iliac artery; EI, external iliac artery; II, internal iliac artery.

Several new medical therapies are currently being tested (Table 21–7). Goals include improving muscular energy efficiency, thrombosis, and blood rheology. The latest and most exciting development has been in the field of molecular biology. Vascular endothelial growth factor (VEGF) is a protein that promotes the growth of new blood vessels. The gene for VEGF has been successfully delivered to and expressed in a patient with critical limb ischemia for whom no revascularization procedure was available. Delivered by a hydrogel-coated balloon catheter, VEGF appeared to promote the development of new collateral vessels.[103]

SUMMARY

Peripheral vascular disease occurs in older women, mostly those more than 65 years old. It is strongly associated with the presence of risk factors for atherosclerosis, namely smoking, hyperlipidemia, and premature menopause. The greatest concern in these women is the association of death and disability due to coronary and cerebrovascular disease in

Table 21–7. NEW DRUGS WITH POTENTIAL BENEFIT FOR PERIPHERAL VASCULAR DISEASE

DRUG	EFFECT
Fibans*	Inhibits platelets
Naftidrofuryl	Improves muscle metabolic efficiency
Carnitine	Improves muscle metabolic efficiency
Vascular endothelial growth factor	Develops collateral channels

*A family of platelet glycoprotein IIb/IIIa inhibitors, including tirofiban, orbofiban, and xemlofiban.

those afflicted with peripheral vascular disease. Therefore, the goals of therapy include altering the progression of atherosclerosis in addition to relieving symptoms of limb ischemia.

Most patients show good response to medical therapy with aspirin, hormone replacement, smoking cessation, lipid lowering, and a consistent exercise regimen. In patients with limb ischemia that impairs lifestyle, occurs at rest, or endangers limb viability, percutaneous angioplasty is the first approach to revascularization. With the assistance of stenting, even the most complex lesions may be treated with success.

References

1. Kannel WB, McGee DL: Update on some epidemiologic features of intermittent claudication: The Framingham study. J Am Geriatric Soc 33:13, 1985.
2. Criqui MH, Langer RD, Fronek A, et al: Mortality over a period of ten years in patients with peripheral arterial disease. N Engl J Med 326:381, 1992.
3. Vogt MT, Wolfson SK, Kuller LH: Lower extremity arterial disease and the aging process: A review. J Clin Epidemiol 45:529, 1992.
4. Kallero KS: Mortality and morbidity in patients with intermittent claudication as defined by venous occlusion plethysmography: A ten year follow-up study. J Chron Dis 34:455, 1981.
5. Criqui MH, Coughlin SS, Fronek A: Non-invasively diagnosed peripheral arterial disease as a predictor of mortality: Results from a prospective study. Circulation 72:768, 1985.
6. Jelnes R, Gaardsring O, Hougard-Jensen K, et al: Fate in intermittent claudication: Outcome and risk factors. Br Med J 293:1137, 1986.
7. McKenna M, Wolfson S, Kuller L: The ratio of ankle and arm pressure as an independent predictor of mortality. Atherosclerosis 87:119, 1991.
8. Agner E: Natural history of angina pectoris, possible previous myocardial infarction and intermittent claudication during the eighth decade. Acta Med Scand 210:271, 1981.
9. Cronenwett JL, Davis JT, Gooch JB, Garrett HE: Aorto-iliac occlusive disease in young women. Surgery 88:775, 1980.
10. Brewster DC: Aorto-iliac, aortofemoral, and iliofemoral arteriosclerotic occlusive diseases. In Haimovici H (ed): Haimovici's Vascular Surgery. Blackwell Science, Cambridge, 1996, p 582.
11. Cronenwett JL, Warner KG, Zelenock GB, et al: Intermittent claudication: Current results of nonoperative management. Arch Surg 119: 430, 1984.
12. Hughson WG, Mann JL, Tibbs DJ, et al: Intermittent claudication: Factors determining outcome. Br Med J 1:1379, 1978.
13. Jonason T, Bergstrom R: Cessation of smoking in patients with intermittent claudication: Effects on the risk of peripheral vascular complications, myocardial infarction and mortality. Acta Med Scand 221: 253, 1987.
14. Fowkes FG, Housley E, Cawood EHH, et al: Edinburgh Artery Study: Prevalence of asymptomatic and symptomatic peripheral arterial disease in the general population. Int J Epidemiol 20:384, 1991.
15. Holmes DR, Burbank MK, Fulton RE, Bernatz PT: Arteriosclerosis obliterans in young women. Am J Med 66:997, 1979.
16. Vogt MT, Cauley JA, Kuller LH, Halley SB: Prevalence and correlates of lower extremity arterial disease in elderly women. Am J Epidemiol 137:559, 1993.
17. Krupski WC, Rapp JH: Smoking and atherosclerosis. Perspect Vasc Surg 1:103, 1989.
18. Couch NP: On the arterial consequences of smoking. J Vasc Surg 3: 807, 1986.
19. Quick CR, Catton LT: The measured effect of stopping smoking on intermittent claudication. Br J Surg 69(Suppl):524, 1982.
20. Blankenhorn DH, Hodis HN: George Lyman Duff Memorial Lecture: Arterial imaging and arteriosclerosis reversal. Arterioscler Thromb 14: 177, 1994.
21. Cooke JP, Ma AD: Medical management of peripheral arterial occlusive disease. In Ouriel K (ed): Lower Extremity Vascular Disease. WB Saunders, Philadelphia, 1995, p 37.
22. Scandinavian Simvistatin Survival Study Group: Randomized trial of cholesterol lowering in 4444 patients with coronary heart disease: the Scandinavian Simvistatin Survival Study (4S). Lancet 344:1383, 1994.
23. Shepherd J, Cobbe SM, Ford I, et al: Prevention of coronary heart disease with pravastatin in men with hypercholesterolemia. N Engl Med 333:1301, 1995.
24. National Cholesterol Education Program: Second report of the expert panel on detection, evaluation and treatment of high blood cholesterol in adults. Circulation 89:1333, 1994.
25. Sacks FM, Pfeffer MA, Moye LA, et al, for the Cholesterol and Recurrent Events Trial Investigators: The effect of pravastatin on coronary events after myocardial infarction in patients with average cholesterol levels. N Engl J Med 335:1001, 1996.
26. Grodstein F, Stampfer MJ: The epidemiology of coronary heart disease and estrogen replacement in postmenopausal women. Prog Cardiovasc Dis 38:199, 1995.
27. Grodstein F, Stampfer MJ, Manson JE, et al: Postmenopausal estrogen and progestin use and the risk of cardiovascular disease. N Engl J Med 335:453, 1996.
28. Duprey D, Clement DL: Medical treatment of peripheral vascular disease: Good or bad. Eur Heart J 13:149, 1992.
29. Solomon SA, Ramsay LE, Yeo WW, et al: Beta blockade and intermittent claudication: Placebo controlled trial of atenolol and nifedipine and their combination. BMJ 303:1100, 1991.
30. Haimovici H: Arteriographic patterns of atherosclerotic occlusive disease of the lower extremity. In Haimovici H (ed): Haimovici's Vascular Surgery. Blackwell Science, Cambridge, 1996, p 531.
31. The Diabetes Control and Complications Trial Research Group: The effect of intensive treatment of diabetes on the development and progression of long-term complications in insulin-dependent diabetes mellitus. N Engl J Med 329:977, 1993.
32. Clarke R, Daly L, Robinson K, et al: Hyperhomocystinemia: An independent risk factor for vascular disease. N Engl J Med 324: 1149, 1991.
33. Malinow MR, Kang SS, Taylor LM, et al: Prevalence of hyperhomocystinemia in patients with peripheral arterial occlusive disease. Circulation 79:1180, 1989.
34. Goldhaker S, Manson J, Henekens C, et al: Low dose aspirin and subsequent peripheral arterial surgery in the Physicians' Health Study. Lancet 340:143, 1992.
35. Janson L, Bergvist D, Bokerg D, et al: Prevention of myocardial infarction and stroke in patients with intermittent claudication: Effects of ticlopidine. Results from STIMS, the Swedish Ticlopidine Multicentre Study. J Intern Med 227:301, 1990.
36. Auteri A, Angaroni A, Borgatti E, et al: Triflusal in the treatment of patients with chronic peripheral arteriopathy: Multicenter double-blind clinical study vs placebo. Int J Clin Pharmacol Res 15:57, 1995.
37. Gent M, Beaumont D, Blanchard J, et al: A randomized, blinded, trial of Clopidogrel versus Aspirin in Patients at Risk of Ischemic Event (CAPRIE). Lancet 348:1329, 1996.
38. Porter JM, Cutler BS, Lee By, et al: Pentoxifylline efficacy in the treatment of intermittent claudication: Multicenter controlled double-blind trial with objective assessment of chronic occlusive arterial disease patients. Am Heart J 104:66, 1982.
39. Accetto B: Beneficial hemorheologic therapy of chronic peripheral arterial disorders with pentoxifylline: Results of a double-blind study versus vasodilator-nylidrin. Am Heart J 103:864, 1982.
40. Hiatt WR, Regensteiner JG, Hargarten ME, et al: Benefit of exercise conditioning for patients with peripheral arterial disease. Circulation 81:602, 1990.
41. Lundgren F, Dahlof G, Lundholm K, et al: Intermittent claudication in surgical reconstruction or physical training. A prospective randomized trial of treatment efficiency. Ann Surg 209:346, 1989.
42. Carter SA, Hamel ER, Patersen JM, et al: Walking ability and ankle systolic pressures: Observations in patients with intermittent claudication in a short-term walking exercise program. J Vasc Surg 10:642, 1989.
43. Larsen OA, Lassen NA: Effect of daily muscular exercise in patients with intermittent claudication. Lancet 2:1093, 1966.
44. Ericsson B, Haeger K, Lindell SE: Effect of physical training on intermittent claudication. Angiology 21:188, 1970.
45. Dahllof AG, Bjointorp P, Holm J, et al: Metabolic activity of skeletal muscles in patients with peripheral arterial insufficiency. Eur J Clin Invest 4:9, 1974.
46. Ernst EE, Matrai A: Intermittent claudication, exercise and blood rheology. Circulation 76:1110, 1987.
47. Mannarino E, Pasqualini L, Menna M, et al: Effects of physical training on peripheral vascular disease: A controlled study. Angiology 40:5, 1989.

48. Creasy TS, McMillan PJ, Fletcher EWL, et al: Is percutaneous transluminal angioplasty better than exercise for claudication? Preliminary results from a prospective randomized trial. Eur J Vasc Surg 4:135, 1990.
49. Ernst E, Fialka V: A review of the clinical effectiveness of exercise therapy for intermittent claudication. Arch Intern Med 153:2357, 1993.
50. Shepherd JT: Historical aspects. In Clement DL, Shepherd JT (eds): Vascular Diseases in the Limbs: Mechanism and Principles of Treatment. Mosby-Year Book, St. Louis, 1993, p 1.
51. Grüntzig A, Hopff H: Perkkutane rekanalisation chronischer arterieller verschluesse mit cinem neven dilationskatheter. Dtsch Med Wochenschr 99:2502, 1974.
52. Pentecost MJ, Criqui MH, Dorros G, et al: Guidelines for peripheral percutaneous transluminal angioplasty of the abdominal aorta and lower extremity vessels. Circulation 89:511, 1994.
53. Henry M, Amar M, Ethevenot G, et al: Palmaz stent placement in iliac and femoropopliteal arteries: Primary and secondary patency in 310 patients with two to four years follow-up. Radiology 197:167, 1995.
54. Rosenblum JD, Leef JA, Kostelic JK, Boyle CM: Angioplasty and intravascular stents in peripheral vascular disease. Surg Clinic North Am 75:621, 1995.
55. Murray JG, Apthorp LA, Wilkins RA: Long-segment (> or = 10 cm) femoropopliteal angioplasty: Improved technical success and long-term patency. Radiology 195:158, 1995.
56. Gunther RW, Vorwer KD, Bohndorf K, et al: Iliac and femoral artery stenosis and occlusions: Treatment with intravascular stents. Radiology 172:725, 1989.
57. Becker GJ, Palmaz JC, Rees CR, et al: Angioplasty-induced dissections in human iliac arteries: Management with Palmaz balloon-expandable intraluminal stents. Radiology 176:31, 1990.
58. Gunther RW, Vorwerk D, Antonucci F, et al: Iliac artery stenosis or obstruction after unsuccessful balloon angioplasty: Treatment with a self-expandable stent. AJR Am J Roentgenol 156:389, 1991.
59. Rees CR, Palmaz JC, Garcia O, et al: Angioplasty and stenting of completely occluded iliac arteries. Radiology 172:953, 1989.
60. Becker GJ, Waller BF: Mechanisms of balloon angioplasty and restenosis. In Baum S, Pentecost MJ (eds): Abrams' Angiography: Interventional Radiology. Little, Brown, Boston, 1996, p 3.
61. Gerhard M, Baum P, Raby KE: Peripheral arterial vascular disease in women: Prevalence, prognosis and treatment. Cardiology 86:349, 1995.
62. Laborde JC, Palmaz JC, Rivera FJ, et al: Influence of anatomic distribution of atherosclerosis on the outcome of revascularization with iliac stent placement. J Vasc Int Radiol 6:513, 1995.
63. Johnston KW, Rae M, Hogg-Johnston SA, et al: Five-year results of a prospective study of percutaneous transluminal angioplasty. Ann Surg 206:403, 1987.
64. Gallino A, Mahler F, Probst P, Nachbur B: Percutaneous transluminal angioplasty of the arteries of the lower limbs: A five year followup. Circulation 70:619, 1984.
65. Spence RK, Freiman DB, Gatenby R, et al: Long-term results of transluminal angioplasty of the iliac and femoral arteries. Arch Surg 116:1377, 1981.
66. Kadir S, White RI Jr, Kaufman SL, et al: Long-term effects of aorto-iliac angioplasty. Surgery 94:10, 1983.
67. Rooke TW, Stanson AW, Johnson CM, et al: Percutaneous transluminal angioplasty in the lower extremities: A five-year experience. Mayo Clin Proc 62:85, 1987.
68. Cambria RP, Faust G, Gusberg R, et al: Percutaneous angioplasty for peripheral arterial occlusive disease: Correlates of clinical success. Arch Surg 122:283, 1987.
69. Palmaz JC, Laborde JC, Rivera FJ, et al: Stenting of the iliac arteries with the Palmaz stent: Experience from a multicenter trial. Cardiovasc Intervent Radiol 15:291, 1992.
70. Vorwerk D, Gunther RW: Stent placement in iliac arterial lesions: Three years of clinical experience with the Wallstent. Cardiovasc Intervent Radiol 15:28, 1992.
71. Zollikofer CL, Antonucci F, Pfyffer M, et al: Arterial stent placement with use of the Wallstent: Midterm results of clinical experience. Radiology 179:449, 1991.
72. Raillat C, Rousseau H, Joffre F, Roux D: Treatment of iliac artery stenoses with the Wallstent endoprosthesis. AJR Am J Roentgenol 154:613, 1990.
73. Palmaz JC, Garcia OJ, Schatz RA, et al: Placement of balloon-expandable intraluminal stents in iliac arteries: First 171 procedures. Radiology 174:969, 1990.
74. Cikrit DF, Becker GJ, Dalsing MC, et al: Early experience with the Palmaz expandable intra-luminal stent in iliac artery stenosis. Ann Vasc Surg 5:150, 1991.
75. Long AL, Gaux JC, Raynaud AC, et al: Infrarenal aortic stents: Initial clinical experience and angiographic followup. Cardiovasc Intervent Radiol 16:203, 1993.
76. Dyet JF, Shaw JW, Cook AM, Nicholson AA: The use of the Wallstent in aorto-iliac vascular disease. Clin Radiol 48:227, 1993.
77. Martin EC, Katzen BT, Deithrich EB, et al: A multicenter trial of the Wallstent in the iliac and femoral arteries. J Vasc Intervent Radiol 6: 843, 1995.
78. Hewes RC, White RI Jr, Murray RR, et al: Long-term results of superficial femoral artery angioplasty. AJR Am J Roentgenol 146: 1025, 1986.
79. Krepel VM, van Andel GJ, van Erp WF, Breslau RJ: Percutaneous transluminal angioplasty of the femoropopliteal artery: Initial and long-term results. Radiology 156:325, 1985.
80. Saproval MR, Long AL, Raynaud RC, et al: Femoropopliteal stent placement: Long-term results. Radiology 184:833, 1992.
81. Rousseau HP, Raillat CR, Joffre FG, et al: Treatment of femoropopliteal stenoses by means of self-expandable endoprostheses: Mid-term results. Radiology 172:961, 1989.
82. Do-dai-Do, Triller J, Walpoth BH, et al: A comparison study of self-expandable stents vs balloon angioplasty alone in femoropopliteal artery occlusions. Cardiovasc Intervent Radiol 15:306, 1992.
83. Bull PG, Mendel H, Hold M, et al: Distal popliteal and tibioperoneal transluminal angioplasty: Long-term followup. J Vasc Interv Radiol 3: 45, 1992.
84. Capek P, McLean G, Berkowitz H: Femoropopliteal angioplasty: Factors influencing long-term success. Circulation 83(2 Suppl):170, 1991.
85. Schwarten DE: Clinical and anatomical considerations for nonoperative therapy in tibial disease and the results of angioplasty. Circulation 83(2 Suppl):86, 1991.
86. Schwarten DE, Cutliff WB: Arterial occlusive disease below the knee: Treatment with percutaneous transluminal angioplasty performed with low profile catheters and steerable guidewires. Radiology 169:71, 1988.
87. Bakal CW, Sprayregan S, Scheinbaum K, et al: Percutaneous transluminal angioplasty of the infrapopliteal arteries: Results in 53 patients. AJR Am J Roentgenol 154:171, 1990.
88. Brown KT, Moore ED, Gefiajdman GI, Saddekni S: Infrapopliteal angioplasty: Long-term follow-up. J Vasc Interv Radiol 4:139, 1993.
89. Saeb MH, Smith DC, Aka PK, et al: Percutaneous transluminal angioplasty of tibial arteries for limb salvage. Cardiovasc Intervent Radiol 15:211, 1992.
90. McNamara TO, Fischer JR: Thrombolysis of peripheral arteries and bypass grafts: Improved results using high dose urokinase. AJR Am J Roentgenol 144:769, 1985.
91. Koltun WA, Gardiner GA, Harrington DP, et al: Thrombolysis in the treatment of peripheral arterial vascular occlusions. Arch Surg 122: 901, 1987.
92. Cragg AH, Smith TD, Carson JD, et al: Two urokinase dose regimens in native arterial and graft occlusions: Initial results of a prospective, randomized clinical trial. Radiology 178:681, 1991.
93. Pernes JM, de Almeida Augusto M, Vitoux JF, et al: Local thrombolysis in peripheral arteries and bypass grafts. J Vasc Surg 6:372, 1987.
94. Motarjeme A: Thrombolytic therapy in arterial occlusion and graft thrombosis. Semin Vasc Surg 2:155, 1989.
95. Eisenbud DE, Brener BJ, Shoenfeld R, et al: Treatment of acute vascular occlusions with intra-arterial urokinase. Am J Surg 160:160, 1990.
96. Brookstein JJ, Volji K: Pulse spray pharmacomechanical thrombolysis: Updated clinical and laboratory observations. Semin Intervent Radiol 9:174, 1992.
97. LeBlang SD, Becker GJ, Benenati JF, et al: Low-dose urokinase regimen for the treatment of lower extremity arterial and graft occlusions: Experience in 132 cases. J Vasc Interv Radiol 3:475, 1992.
98. Ouriel K, Veith FJ, Saashara AA: Thrombolysis or peripheral arterial surgery: Phase I results. Thrombolysis or Peripheral Arterial Surgery (TOPAS) Investigators. J Vasc Surg 23:64, 1996.
99. Meyerovatz MF, Didier D, Vogel JJ, et al: Thrombolytic therapy compared with mechanical recanalization in nonacute peripheral arterial occlusions: A randomized trial. J Vasc Interv Radiol 6:775, 1995.

100. Bero CJ, Carsella JF, Reddy K, et al: Recombinant tissue plasminogen activator for the treatment of lower extremity peripheral vascular occlusive disease. J Vasc Interv Radiol 6:571, 1995.
101. Huehl EA, Soulen MC: Thrombolysis of lower extremity embolic occlusions: A study of the results of the STAR registry. Radiology 197: 141, 1995.
102. Vanderschueren S, Stockx L, Wilms G, et al: Thrombolytic therapy of peripheral arterial occlusion with recombinant staphylokinase. Circulation 92:2050, 1995.
103. Isner JM, Peiczek A, Schainfeld R, et al: Clinical evidence of angiogenesis after arterial gene transfer of ph $VEGF_{165}$ in patient with ischaemic limb. Lancet 348:370, 1996.

21.4 Surgical Therapy

Thomas J. Takach and George J. Reul, Jr

In the United States, 10% of all people older than 70 years and 2% of all those aged 37 to 69 years have symptoms of claudication secondary to atherosclerotic occlusive disease of the aorta and lower extremity vessels.[1] This disease has resulted in compromised lifestyle and has been associated with an increased risk of amputation as well as shortened life expectancy.[2–8] Each year, approximately 100,000 operations are performed as treatment for the sequelae of atherosclerotic compromise of the lower extremities.[9] As the population of the United States ages, a growing number of people will be affected. Hence, the prevention, detection, and treatment of peripheral vascular occlusive disease (PVOD) constitute an issue of increasing importance in both men and women.

The early literature regarding PVOD was biased toward men; however, during the past two decades, the literature has been more focused on gender-based differences in the epidemiology and natural history of the disease, a change that has had a profound effect on the approach to treatment in women.

EPIDEMIOLOGY

In early studies reviewing the natural history and incidence of atherosclerosis of the aorta and lower extremities, 10% to 15% of all people undergoing treatment for aortoiliac and infrainguinal occlusive disease were women.[10, 11] Although European studies continue to report a significant male predominance among patients undergoing operative intervention,[12–14] American investigators have documented that females constitute 40% of their patients who undergo procedures for aortoiliac occlusive disease (AIOD) and infrainguinal occlusive disease (IIOD).[15–17] The basis for this greater prevalence of PVOD in women in the American studies is multifactorial and has been identified as (1) a higher incidence of tobacco use by women,[18–20] (2) the greater survival rate of older women,[21] (3) improved recognition and treatment of vascular disease in women,[17, 22] and (4) changes in the referral patterns of primary care physicians.[23]

The growing incidence of PVOD in women, as noted by multiple reports, parallels the increased incidence of lung cancer and other tobacco-related diseases occurring in women.[18, 19] The negative influence of tobacco use has been reported to be additive with other risk factors prevalent in women, including diabetes and small-diameter vessels.[24, 25]

Cronenwett and colleagues[17, 26] have reported that aortoiliac hypoplasia is more commonly documented in women (9% to 38%) than in men (1% to 4%) after development of lower extremity claudication or ischemia. Using angiographic data, these investigators have defined aortoiliac hypoplasia as aortic measurements less than 19 mm above and less than 13 mm below the renal arteries and less than a 10-mm diameter at the aortic bifurcation (Fig. 21–18).[26–29] It is believed that aortoiliac hypoplasia represents one end of the developmental spectrum of vessel diameter rather than a specific disease entity. It may be secondary to excessive fusing of the two dorsal aortae during intrauterine development.[30] The smaller-diameter vessels are susceptible to an earlier and more severe progression of a given amount of atherosclerotic plaque on an already smaller lumen.[31] Therefore, this predominantly female group of patients is at increased risk for development of the negative sequelae associated with progression of atherosclerosis. Furthermore, the presence of aortoiliac hypoplasia and other risk factors, such as cigarette smoking, appear to be additive as risk factors for development of symptomatic PVOD.[31, 32]

Women who have AIOD without hypoplasia tend to have localized areas of atherosclerotic involvement with fewer superficial femoral artery occlusions, less iliac artery involvement, and lower angiographic outflow scores.[17, 33] In contrast, the type of AIOD seen in men and in women *with* hypoplasia consists of diffuse atherosclerotic involvement of the aorta and outflow vessels. This finding influences potential operative interventions, because diffuse disease is less likely to be amenable to treatment by endarterectomy and patch angioplasty.[34]

Some reports have suggested that women receive different treatment for both CAD[35–37] and PVOD.[23] Specifically, it appears that women are less likely to be referred by primary caregivers for invasive treatment. For women with PVOD, this bias occurs for non–limb-threatening indications but not for limb-threatening indications.[23] On the basis of outcomes data (which are reviewed later in this discussion) as well as analysis of severity of ischemia in men and women and procedures undertaken, it does not appear that this bias from referring physicians is justified.

Mild to moderate claudication in women tends to remain stable or improve over time. Approximately 75% of affected patients have stable or decreased symptoms 5 years after diagnosis.[6, 7] However, in the remainder of the group, increasingly severe symptoms develop, and 5% to 7% ulti-

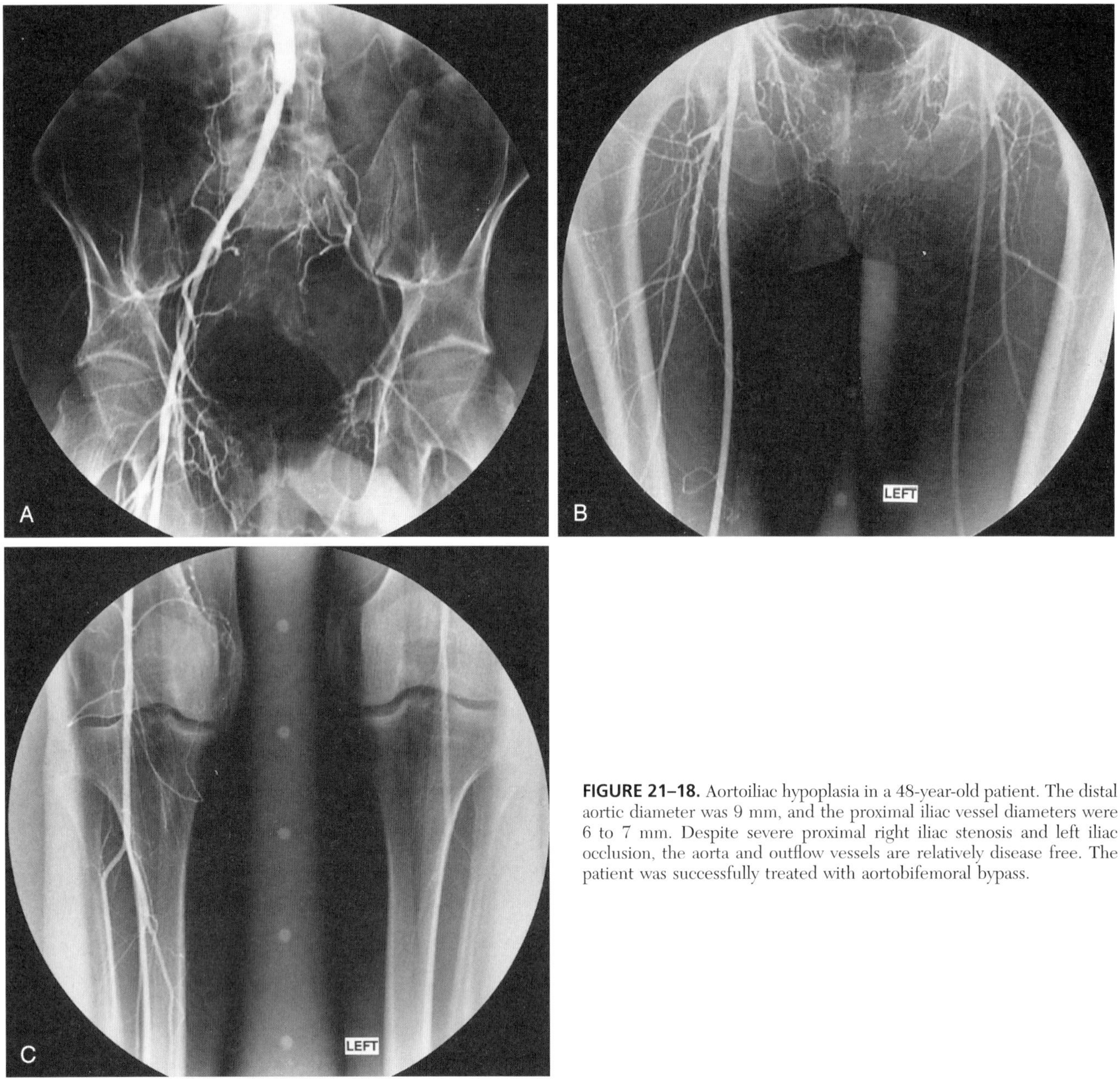

FIGURE 21–18. Aortoiliac hypoplasia in a 48-year-old patient. The distal aortic diameter was 9 mm, and the proximal iliac vessel diameters were 6 to 7 mm. Despite severe proximal right iliac stenosis and left iliac occlusion, the aorta and outflow vessels are relatively disease free. The patient was successfully treated with aortobifemoral bypass.

mately require limb amputation.[6, 7] The consequences of the atherosclerosis, in general, have a greater impact on life expectancy than on long-term limb viability. Primarily because of the effects of generalized atherosclerosis, men and women with claudication have been noted to have 5- and 10-year survival rates of 72% and 50%, respectively.[8] The 5-year survival rate for age-matched control subjects is 90%.

Women with concomitant cerebrovascular disease and those with CAD and claudication have 5-year survival rates of 61% and 59%, respectively. Most deaths (75%) in these patients are a direct consequence of CAD.[38, 39] CAD occurs concomitantly with PVOD in 40% to 50% of patients requiring revascularization. Of these patients, 10% to 20% may be asymptomatic, primarily because of an inability to exercise.[40]

RISK MANAGEMENT AND NONOPERATIVE THERAPY

Although approximately 100,000 operative interventions are performed annually for PVOD in the United States, most patients are managed nonoperatively. The effective management of risk factors can successfully influence the course of the disease and halt its progression. Thus, amputation, surgery, and a decreased life expectancy are not inevitable consequences once the diagnosis of PVOD has been made.

Most risk factors for CAD are independent predictors for claudication.[21] However, diabetes mellitus is a more powerful predictor for development of claudication and PVOD in women than in men.[21] Population-based studies have shown that a growing incidence of PVOD in females is more closely associated with an increasing use of tobacco than with any other single factor.[20, 41]

Higher survival rates in women are also an independent risk factor for lower extremity atherosclerosis. Postmenopausal women have been noted to be at greater risk for progressive development of CAD that parallels changes in serum lipids and that can be modified by replacement estrogen therapy.[42] Findings are less clear for PVOD. Gender has not been demonstrated to be predictive of disease progression in people with claudication. However, compared with women of the same age, men are twice as likely to die after diagnosis of PVOD.[43]

Risk factors are generally additive. In a study of 520 patients with PVOD, Juergens and associates[8] demonstrated that patients with claudication who smoke have an 11.4% risk of eventual amputation, compared with a 0% risk in patients with claudication who abstain from smoking. Silbert and Zazeela[25] reported that in patients with claudication, 34% of those who had diabetes but only 8% of those who did not have diabetes underwent amputation. Because these risk factors are additive, the prognosis is worse in diabetic patients who continue to smoke. Continued tobacco use, diabetes, and the presence of symptomatic coronary or cerebrovascular disease are independent risk factors predicting a higher mortality in patients with claudication.[2, 40, 44, 45]

Smokers are nine times more likely than nonsmokers to experience claudication and represent 98% of all patients who actually have claudication that leads to amputation.[46–48] Cessation of tobacco use is an essential step in the nonoperative treatment of chronic lower extremity ischemia. Patients with claudication who quit smoking demonstrate better ankle pressures, treadmill walking distance, and severity of claudication than smokers.[49] In several studies, greater long-term patency of aortoiliac and femoropopliteal grafts was shown in patients who quit smoking than in those who continued to smoke.[50–52] Of major importance, a lower incidence of limb loss was also shown in patients who quit smoking than in those who continued to smoke.[53]

Important factors in risk management, in addition to elimination of tobacco use and control of diabetes, are lipid normalization, blood pressure control, weight control, and exercise. Modification of risk factors continues to be an important facet of management of PVOD and is especially effective if combined with a program of regular exercise to tolerance. Multiple studies using exercise programs consisting of walking report improvement in walking distances of 80% to 234%.[54, 55] These studies have effectively established exercise as a foundation for nonoperative management of PVOD. A study by Creasy and associates[56] randomly assigned patients to either walking therapy or percutaneous balloon dilatation of atherosclerotic lesions. They found that at the end of 1 year, the noninvasive therapy group had better exercise tolerance, decreased ankle-pressure indices, and diminished severity of claudication. These results underscore the effectiveness of exercise in an integrated nonoperative program for the treatment of PVOD.

Exercise and modification of risk factors must be combined with foot care, especially in diabetic patients. Pharmacologic therapy, including rheologic agents, calcium channel blockers, and prostaglandins, have demonstrated only modest efficacy in multiple studies.[57–60]

AORTOILIAC OCCLUSIVE DISEASE

The successful outcomes following aortoiliac and aortofemoral bypass surgery for the treatment of AIOD have made bypass the most common mode of operative therapy and the standard by which other modes of therapy must be judged. Indications for operative intervention are similar for men and women; they include critical limb ischemia threatening limb viability, claudication compromising lifestyle, and distal emboli originating from proximal atherosclerotic lesions.

In specific situations, axillofemoral bypass, femorofemoral bypass, or endarterectomy with patch angioplasty may be considered as an alternative mode of therapy. However, as noted in a previous section, aortoiliac hypoplasia, which tends to occur more often in women, is usually characterized by a diffuse distribution of atherosclerosis. There is therefore a higher incidence of postoperative restenosis in patients in whom endarterectomy with patch angioplasty is performed.[34]

Aortoiliac hypoplasia is characterized by the presence of a small aorta. End-to-end anastomoses with a Dacron or polytetrafluoroethylene graft below the renal arteries is the usual mode of reconstruction.[34] For the patient with an aorta of 10 mm, a 10-mm graft would be an appropriate fit and would avoid problems associated with size mismatch. However, the limbs of a 10-mm graft are small (5 mm) and may predispose to postoperative restenosis secondary to myointimal hyperplasia. Therefore, some investigators suggest modifying a 12-mm graft to fit end-to-end to a 10-mm aorta by beveling both the graft and vessel. Others suggest proceeding with an end-to-side anastomosis with a 12-mm graft.[34] A definitive advantage has not been established for either technique.

As opposed to different infrainguinal bypass results in men and women, long-term patency and survival rates appear to be equal.[13, 61, 62] Primary and secondary patency rates in the Dartmouth experience at 3 years were 84% and 96%, respectively, for women and 86% and 92%, respectively, for men. Limb salvage rates at 3 years were 89% for women and 93% for men. Survival rates were also comparable, at 88% for women and 86% for men.[61]

Results of percutaneous balloon angioplasty of iliac lesions have been similar for the two genders.[63, 64] For treatment of PVOD, angioplasty of isolated, short iliac lesions is the only technique for which results approximate those achieved by surgical bypass.[63, 64] Both angioplasty and surgery result in greater than 80% primary patency rates at 3 years.

INFRAINGUINAL OCCLUSIVE DISEASE

In contrast to similar survival and patency rates in men and women following revascularization for AIOD, gender has been found to have an important influence on the outcome of infrainguinal bypass surgery. In data from three large surgical groups, women undergoing infrainguinal bypass procedures had shorter survival and lower patency rates than men receiving the same interventions.[65–68] However, limb salvage rates for the two genders were similar. These findings have important implications for the management of PVOD in women.

Both operative and late mortality rates are higher in females. In a study of more than 7000 patients at the Cleve-

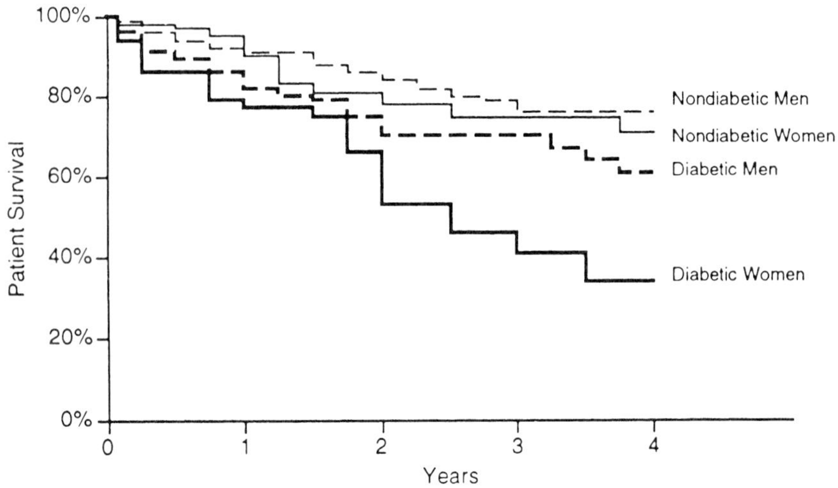

FIGURE 21–19. Life-table analysis of survival after infrainguinal bypass in women and men stratified by diabetic status. Survival in women with diabetes was significantly reduced compared with that in women without diabetes ($p < .01$). Although there was a trend toward worse survival in men with diabetes, this was not statistically significant. (From Magnant JG, Cronenwett JL, Walsh DB, et al: Surgical treatment of infrainguinal arterial occlusive disease in women. J Vasc Surg 17:67, 1993.)

land Clinic, the operative mortality was 3.9% in women and 2.5% in men.[69] These findings were confirmed by Cronenwett and colleagues,[65, 66] who reported an operative mortality rate of 3.8% in women and 2.0% in men. Although the reasons for these findings are speculative, it is believed that concomitant CAD plays a major role.[70, 71]

Late survival at 4 years is also markedly reduced in women compared with age-matched male controls (54% versus 72%). In a study from Dartmouth-Hitchcock Medical Center, diabetes appeared to completely explain the lower survival observed in women (Fig. 21–19).[65, 72] Diabetes was an independent predictor of late mortality whether a multivariate or univariate analysis was used.

All three of the large studies of infrainguinal bypass in women reported a lower graft patency rate in women (Fig. 21–20).[65–68] This figure included primary patency, assisted primary patency, and secondary patency. Women appear to be at increased risk for vein graft failure, especially when infrapopliteal bypasses are performed for limb salvage.

Studies by Cronenwett and colleagues[65, 66] have shown that after 3 years, rates for primary patency (54% versus 70%), assisted primary patency (59% versus 77%), and secondary patency (69% versus 86%) are lower in women than in men treated with similar infrainguinal bypass procedures. Evaluation of all patients showed that independent predictors of graft failure were female gender and small vein graft diameter. When graft diameter was assessed by duplex ultrasonography, a 1.2-fold increase in failure rate occurred for every millimeter decrease in diameter of the saphenous vein graft. The failure rate of grafts within the first postoperative year was also found to be higher in women than men. This higher failure rate was independent of graft diameter and was believed to be secondary to decreased arterial outflow due to smaller distal arterial diameters. The investigators ultimately concluded that a combination of more diffuse distal arterial disease in diabetic women and smaller arterial diameters was primarily responsible for the diminished graft patency.[65] Despite the lower graft patency rates for women in the three studies noted earlier, the rate of limb salvage at 3 years after surgery was similar for men and women (82% versus 89%).

The clinical implications of the preceding findings are important. Reduced graft patency rate in the first preoperative year and in late follow-up following infrainguinal bypass in females suggests the need for frequent, noninvasive postoperative surveillance. Potential graft defects that are detected by noninvasive surveillance can be further evaluated with arteriography and aggressively corrected with surgical

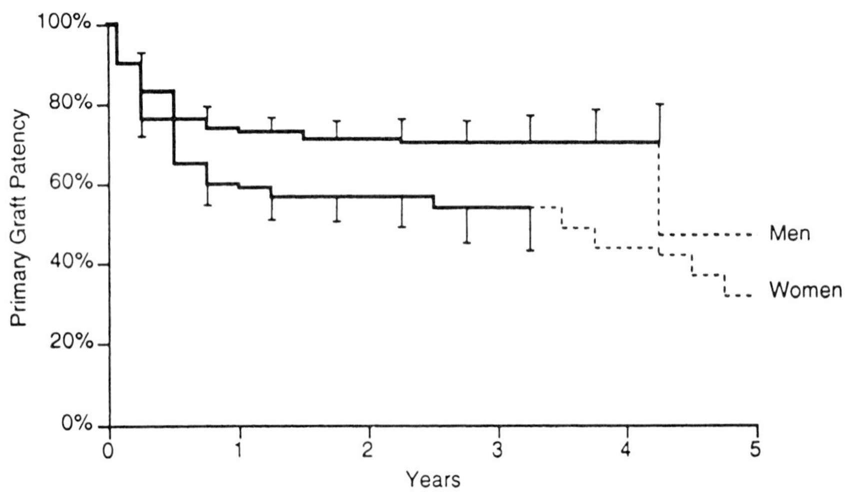

FIGURE 21–20. Primary graft patency after infrainguinal bypass was significantly lower in women compared with that in men ($p < .005$). (From Magnant JG, Cronenwett JL, Walsh DB, et al: Surgical treatment of infrainguinal arterial occlusive disease in women. J Vasc Surg 17:67, 1993.)

intervention. The profound impact of diabetes on late survival reinforces the importance of careful medical management for diabetic control. Although late survival is influenced by the presence of diabetes in women, the high limb salvage rates demonstrated by the preceding studies justify aggressive intervention in all women.

SUMMARY

Regardless of gender, PVOD is a challenging problem that will increase in importance as the population of the United States continues to age. During the past two decades, the incidence of PVOD in females has risen dramatically. Despite multifactorial causes, the increase in tobacco smoking among women has been identified as the most important factor contributing to that rise.

Smaller diameter of the aorta, runoff vessels, and potential vein grafts in women profoundly influence both the occurrence and treatment of PVOD. Aortoiliac hypoplasia occurs primarily in females and may predispose to development of AIOD. Smaller arterial and vein graft diameters profoundly influence both immediate and late patency rates after infrainguinal bypass in women. Diabetes is associated with a lower late survival rate following bypass for treatment of IIOD in women.

The gender-based differences demonstrated by an evolving body of literature emphasize the importance of a continued analysis of the effect of gender on the prevention, detection, and treatment of PVOD. Furthermore, these same findings have several important clinical implications. The initiation of smoking cessation programs for women can potentially decrease the incidence of PVOD in women and result in better outcomes of treatment for PVOD. The lower patency rate of grafts in women treated with infrainguinal bypass strongly suggests the need for aggressive noninvasive, postoperative surveillance. This approach may, in turn, improve secondary and assisted primary patency rates. Diabetes has a great influence on survival following treatment of PVOD in women, and an aggressive program for optimal medical management of this disease is essential. Finally, the outcomes for treatment of limb salvage justify aggressive treatment for this indication in all women.

References

1. Spencer G: Projections of the Population of the United States, by Age, Sex, and Race: 1983–2080. Current Population Reports Series P-25. Population Estimates and Projections, No. 952. US Dept of Commerce, Bureau of the Census, Washington, DC, 1984.
2. Malone JM, Moore WS, Goldstone J: Life expectancy following aortofemoral arterial grafting. Surgery 81:551, 1977.
3. Reunanen A, Takkunen H, Aromaa A: Prevalence of intermittent claudication and its effect on mortality. Acta Med Scand 211:249, 1982.
4. Veith FJ, Gupta SK, Samson RH, et al: Progress in limb salvage by reconstructive arterial surgery combined with new or improved adjunctive procedures. Ann Surg 194:386, 1981.
5. Edwards JE, Taylor LM Jr, Porter JM: Treatment of failed lower extremity bypass grafts with new autogenous vein bypass. J Vasc Surg 11:136, 1990.
6. Boyd AM: Natural course of arteriosclerosis of lower extremities. Proc R Soc Med 53:591, 1962.
7. Imparato AM, Kim GE, Davidson T, Crowley JG: Intermittent claudication: Its natural course. Surgery 78:795, 1975.
8. Juergens JC, Barker NW, Hines EA: Arteriosclerosis obliterans: Review of 520 cases with special reference to pathogenic and prognostic factors. Circulation 21:188, 1960.
9. Rutkow IM, Ernst CB: An analysis of vascular surgical manpower requirements and vascular surgical rates in the United States. J Vasc Surg 3:74, 1986.
10. Boyd AM: The natural course of arteriosclerosis of the lower extremities. Angiology 11:10, 1960.
11. Alinaji, Barker CF, Berkowitz HD, et al: Femoropopliteal vein grafts for claudication: Analysis of 100 consecutive cases. Ann Surg 188: 79, 1978.
12. van den Akker PJ, van Schilfgaarde R, Brand R, et al: Aortoiliac and aortofemoral reconstruction of obstructive disease. Am J Surg 167: 379, 1994.
13. Polterauer P, Prager M, Holzenbein T, et al: Dacron versus polytetrafluoroethylene for Y-aortic bifurcation grafts: A six-year prospective, randomized trial. Surgery 111:626, 1992.
14. Nevelsteen A, Wouters L, Suy R: Aortofemoral Dacron reconstruction for aorto-iliac occlusive disease: A 25-year survey. Eur J Vasc Surg 5: 179, 1991.
15. Schneider JR, McDaniel MD, Walsh DB, et al: Axillofemoral bypass: Outcome and hemodynamic results in high-risk patients. J Vasc Surg 15:952, 1992.
16. Schneider JR, Zwolak RM, Walsh DB, et al: Lack of diameter effect on short-term patency of size-matched Dacron aortobifemoral grafts. J Vasc Surg 13:785, 1991.
17. Cronenwett JL, Davis JT Jr, Gooch JB, Garrett HE: Aortoiliac occlusive disease in women. Surgery 88:775, 1980.
18. Pollin W: The role of the addictive process as a key step in causation of all tobacco related diseases. JAMA 252:2874, 1984.
19. Sherman CB: Health effects of cigarette smoking. Clin Chest Med 12: 643, 1991.
20. Berman BA, Gritz ER: Women and smoking: Current trends and issues for the 1990s. J Subst Abuse 3:221, 1991.
21. Kannel WB, McGee DL: Update on some epidemiologic features of intermittent claudication: The Framingham Study. J Am Geriatr Soc 33:13, 1985.
22. Schneider JR, Besso SR, Walsh DB, et al: Femorofemoral versus aortobifemoral bypass: Outcome and hemodynamic results. J Vasc Surg 19:43, 1994.
23. Feinglass J, McDermott MM, Foroohar M, Pearce WH: Gender differences in interventional management of peripheral vascular disease: Evidence from a blood flow laboratory population. Ann Vasc Surg 8: 343, 1994.
24. Vlietstra RE, Kronmal RA, Oberman A, et al: Effect of cigarette smoking on survival of patients with angiographically documented coronary artery disease: Report from the CASS registry. JAMA 255:1023, 1986.
25. Silbert S, Zazeela H: Prognosis in arteriosclerotic peripheral vascular disease. JAMA 166:1816, 1958.
26. Cronenwett JL, Garrett HE: Arteriographic measurement of the abdominal aorta, iliac, and femoral arteries in women with atherosclerotic occlusive disease. Radiology 148:389, 1983.
27. Burke PM Jr, Herrmann JB, Cutler BS: Optimal grafting methods for the small abdominal aorta. J Cardiovasc Surg (Torino) 28:420, 1987.
28. DeLaurentis DA, Freidman SP, Wolferth CC Jr, et al: Atherosclerosis and the hypoplastic aortoiliac system. Surgery 83:27, 1978.
29. Jernigan WR, Fallat ME, Hatfield DR: Hypoplastic aortoiliac syndrome: An entity peculiar to women. Surgery 94:752, 1983.
30. Arnot RS, Louw JH: The anatomy of the posterior wall of the abdominal aorta: Its significance with regard to hypoplasia of the distal aorta. S Afr Med J 2:899, 1973.
31. Hoogendam IJ, Van Rinsum AC, Olyslager J: The diameter of the distal abdominal aorta and the aetiology of local atheroma. J Cardiovasc Surg (Torino) 25:408, 1984.
32. Lallemand RC, Brown KG, Boulter PS: Vessel dimensions in premature atheromatous disease of aortic bifurcation. Br Med J 2:255, 1972.
33. Rutherford RB, Flanigan DP, Gupta SK, et al: Suggested standards for reports dealing with lower extremity ischemia. J Vasc Surg 20:195, 1994.
34. Schneider JR, Cronenwett JL: Aortoiliac hypoplasia. In Ernst CB, Stanley JC (eds): Current Therapy in Vascular Surgery, 2nd ed. BC Decker, Philadelphia, 1991, p 394.
35. Khan SS, Nessim S, Gray R, et al: Increased mortality of women in coronary artery bypass surgery: Evidence for referral bias. Ann Intern Med 112:561, 1990.

36. Loop FD, Golding LR, MacMillan JP, et al: Coronary artery surgery in women compared with men: Analyses of risks and long-term results. J Am Coll Cardiol 1:383, 1983.
37. Tobin JN, Wasserteil-Smoller S, Wexler JP, et al: Sex bias in considering coronary artery bypass surgery. Ann Intern Med 107:19, 1987.
38. Brewster DC, Edwards JP: Cardiopulmonary complications related to vascular surgery. In Bernhard VM, Towne JB (eds): Complications in Vascular Surgery. Quality Medical Publishing, St. Louis, 1991, p 23.
39. Yeager RA, Moneta FL: Assessing cardiac risk in vascular surgical patients: Current status. Perspect Vasc Surg 2:18, 1990.
40. Hertzer NR, Beven EG, Young JR, et al: Coronary artery disease in peripheral vascular patients: A classification of 1000 coronary angiograms and results of surgical management. Ann Surg 199:223, 1984.
41. Witteman JC, Grobbee DE, Valkenburg HA, et al: Cigarette smoking and the development and progression of aortic atherosclerosis: A 9-year population-based follow-up study in women. Circulation 88:2156, 1993.
42. Eaker ED, Chesebro JH, Sacks FM, et al: Cardiovascular disease in women. Circulation 88:1999, 1993.
43. Jelnes R, Gaardsting O, Hougaard Jensen K, et al: Fate in intermittent claudication: Outcome and risk factors. Br Med J (Clin Res Ed) 293: 1137, 1986.
44. Szilagyi DE, Elliott JP Jr, Smith RF, et al: A thirty-year survey of the reconstructive surgical treatment of aortoiliac occlusive disease. J Vasc Surg 3:421, 1986.
45. Crawford ES, Bomberger RA, Glaeser DH, et al: Aortoiliac occlusive disease: Factors influencing survival and function following reconstructive operation over a twenty-five-year period. Surgery 90:1055, 1981.
46. Hughson WG, Mann JI, Garrod A: Intermittent claudication: Prevalence and risk factors. Br Med J 1(6124):1379, 1978.
47. Eastcott HHG: Arterial Surgery, 2nd ed. Pitman Medical Publishers, London, 1973.
48. Lithell H, Hedstrand H, Karlsson R: The smoking habits of men with intermittent claudication. Acta Med Scand 197:473, 1975.
49. Quick CR, Cotton LT: The measured effect of stopping smoking on intermittent claudication. Br J Surg 69(Suppl):S24, 1982.
50. Robicsek F, Daugherty HK, Mullen DC, et al: The effect of continued cigarette smoking on the patency of synthetic vascular grafts in Leriche syndrome. J Thorac Cardiovasc Surg 70:107, 1975.
51. Greenhalgh RM, Laing SP, Colap V, et al: Progressing atherosclerosis following revascularization. In Bernhard VM, Towne JB (eds): Complications in Vascular Surgery. Grune & Stratton, New York, 1980, p 39.
52. Provan JL, Sojka SG, Murnaghan JJ, Jaunkalns R: The effect of cigarette smoking on the long term success rates of aortofemoral and femoropopliteal reconstructions. Surg Gynecol Obstet 165:49, 1987.
53. Jurgens IL, Barker NW, Hines EA: Arteriosclerosis obliterans: A review of 520 cases with special reference to pathogenic and prognostic factors. Circulation 21:188, 1960.
54. Ekroth R, Dahllof AG, Gundevall B, et al: Physical training of patients with intermittent claudication: Indications, methods and results. Surgery 84:640, 1978.
55. Clifford PC, Davies PW, Hayne JA, Baird RN: Intermittent claudication: Is a supervised exercise class worthwhile? Br Med J 280:1503, 1980.
56. Creasy TS, McMillan PJ, Fletcher EW, et al: Is percutaneous transluminal angioplasty better than exercise for claudication? Preliminary results from a prospective randomized trial. Eur J Vasc Surg 4:135, 1990.
57. Bollinger A, Frel C: Double-blind study of pentoxifylline against placebo in patients with intermittent claudication. Pharmatherapeutica 1: 557, 1977.
58. Nizankowski R, Krolikowski W, Bielatowicz J, Szczeklik A: Prostacyclin for ischemic ulcers in peripheral arterial disease: A random-assignment, placebo-controlled study. Thromb Res 37:21, 1985.
59. Porter JM, Cutler BS, Lee BY, et al: Pentoxifylline efficacy in the treatment of intermittent claudication: Multicenter controlled double-blind trial with objective assessment of chronic occlusive arterial disease patients. Am Heart J 104:66, 1982.
60. Snyder SH, Reynolds IJ: Calcium-antagonist drugs: Receptor interactions that clarify therapeutic effects. N Engl J Med 313:995, 1985.
61. Schneider JR: Aortoiliac occlusive disease. Semin Vasc Surg 8:277, 1995.
62. Valentine RJ, Hansen ME, Myers SI, et al: The influence of sex and aortic size on late patency after aortofemoral revascularization in young adults. J Vasc Surg 21:296, 1995.
63. Tunis SR, Bass EB, Steinberg EP: The use of angioplasty, bypass surgery, and amputation in the management of peripheral vascular diseases. N Engl J Med 325:556, 1991.
64. Johnston KW, Rae M, Hogg-Johnston SA, et al: 5-year results of a prospective study of percutaneous transluminal angioplasty. Ann Surg 206:403, 1987.
65. Cronenwett JL: Infrainguinal occlusive disease. Semin Vasc Surg 8: 284, 1995.
66. Magnant JG, Cronenwett JL, Walsh DB, et al: Surgical treatment of infrainguinal arterial occlusive disease in women. J Vasc Surg 17: 67, 1993.
67. Clark LT, Veith FJ, Sanchez LA, et al: Impact of gender, race, and diabetes on graft patency, limb salvage and survival following infrainguinal arterial reconstruction. Presented at the Peripheral Vascular Surgery Society meeting in Seattle, WA, June 5, 1994.
68. Belkin M, Conte MS, Donaldson MC, et al: The impact of gender on the results of arterial bypass with in situ greater saphenous vein. Am J Surg 170:97, 1995.
69. Harris EJ Jr, Taylor LM Jr, Moneta GL, Perter JM: Outcome of infrainguinal arterial reconstruction in women. J Vasc Surg 18:627, 1993; see N Hertzer's remarks in discussion, 634–636.
70. Killen DA, Reed WA, Arnold M, et al: Coronary bypass in women: Long-term survival. Ann Thorac Surg 34:559, 1982.
71. Eysmann SB, Douglas PS: Reperfusion and revascularization strategies for coronary artery disease in women. JAMA 268:1903, 1992.
72. Kannel WB, McGee DL: Diabetes and cardiovascular disease: The Framingham study. JAMA 241:2035, 1979

CHAPTER 22

Cerebrovascular Disease

22.1 Pathophysiology, Clinical Recognition, and Medical Therapy

Carlos Villar-Cordova, Reeta Achari, and Frank M. Yatsu

Cardiovascular diseases are a major cause of death in women, despite misconceptions to the contrary.[1, 2] Nearly a half-million women die each year in the United States of cardiovascular diseases, primarily from myocardial infarction and stroke. Although the onset of cardiovascular disease occurs at a later age in women than in men, the problem is enormous.[2, 3] Both men and women have similar risk factors for stroke, such as hypertension, diabetes mellitus, and smoking; however, women have an increased predisposition toward stroke because of female conditions such as pregnancy and hormonal changes and because certain diseases preferentially affect women. Migraines, rheumatologic disorders, antiphospholipid antibody syndrome, and choriocarcinoma all place women at increased risk for stroke.[3] In this chapter we outline the major risk factors associated with stroke. The major stroke syndromes and women's options for treatment are also discussed.

Recently, more attention has been focused on the influence of gender on health and disease. Women have been underrepresented in previous studies and clinical trials, but efforts are now being made to obtain useful data on health and disease in women.[4]

EPIDEMIOLOGY OF STROKE IN WOMEN

Stroke is the third leading cause of death in the United States and the most common cause of major disability. In women, stroke is the second leading cause of death. In the United States, more than 200,000 women will suffer new strokes each year and more than 90,000 will die of them, accounting for 60% of all stroke fatalities.[5] Although the lifetime risk of having a stroke is higher in men, the risk of dying of a stroke is higher in women. The incidence of stroke has been decreasing in most industrialized countries over the past several decades.[6] Data from the World Health Organization collected from 27 population groups aged 55, 65, and 75 indicate that women have a greater relative reduction of stroke mortality with increasing age than in men.[6] When various risk factors are analyzed, such as consumption of animal fat, alcohol, and cigarettes, regional differences exist for these factors, although smoking is a clear risk for both women and men everywhere.[6] Although data reporting a steeper relative decline in stroke mortality for women may be positively interpreted as reflecting a lesser vulnerability to strokes, the negative aspect is that the magnitude of the problem makes the relative changes in stroke frequency less significant. In fact, other less global studies on stroke epidemiology have reported the same high mortality from strokes in women and men, with the exception of stroke due to subarachnoid hemorrhage (SAH).[7] Furthermore, other studies suggest that the incidence of stroke is similar in women and men, but the numbers are partly offset because the incidence of stroke in women increases substantially after age 75.[8] Whether the increased longevity of women may skew some of these data is arguable, but the important message is that risk factors contribute to stroke and therefore must be minimized.

The most frequent type of stroke, atherothrombotic brain infarction, accounts for 44 percent of strokes. This type of stroke includes infarction secondary to large vessel atherothrombosis and lacunar infarction. Cerebral embolism, which represents about 21% of strokes, has a slightly higher incidence in women (23%) than in men (18%). Transient ischemic attack (TIA) accounts for 20% of strokes and is more frequent in men.[9]

Several large cooperative studies indicate that TIAs may have a more benign natural course in women than in men. However, the European Stroke Prevention Trial found that the number of men and women who had TIAs and subsequent strokes was similar.[10] The risk of ischemic stroke after TIA increases 13% per year.[11] Asymptomatic carotid bifurcation bruits may be a significant risk factor for stroke and coronary death in men but not in women.[12]

Intracerebral hemorrhage accounts for approximately 11% of all strokes in both men and women. The incidence of aneurysmal SAH may be as much as 50% higher in women.[13] In addition, women have a higher rate of recurrent hemorrhage. However, gender does not influence overall outcome after SAH.

RISK FACTORS

Factors that significantly increase the risk for cerebrovascular disease are hypertension, hypercholesterolemia, diabetes mellitus, cigarette smoking, and cardiac disease, particularly atrial fibrillation.[14] Hypertension is the single most important risk factor for both ischemic and hemorrhagic strokes. Isolated systolic hypertension, which is present in 20% of men and 30% of women older than the age of 75, correlates with an increased risk of stroke, particularly in the elderly.[9]

Cardiac Diseases

Cardiac diseases are independent risk factors because they cause cardioembolic strokes. Unfortunately, women are evaluated less frequently for cardiac disease than are men, particularly when chest pain is the presenting symptom. Furthermore, women generally have a worse prognosis for coronary artery disease with both medical and surgical therapies. These two remediable aspects of cardiac disease in women have implications in stroke occurrence.[11]

Nonrheumatic atrial fibrillation increases the risk of stroke 5- to 25-fold depending on the associated risk factors.[14] In the elderly, the proportion of strokes associated with atrial fibrillation increases steadily with age, rising from 6.7% for patients 50 to 59 years old to 36.2% for patients 80 to 89 years old.[5] The Copenhagen Heart Study, which enrolled a high proportion of elderly women, showed that the presence of atrial fibrillation increases stroke risk for women 10 times more than it does for men. Furthermore, the mechanism by which atrial fibrillation causes stroke shows a gender differential: women are more likely to suffer cardioembolic strokes and men are more likely to suffer noncardioembolic strokes.[15]

Serum Cholesterol

Cholesterol and triglyceride levels are independent risk factors for coronary heart disease and carotid artery atherosclerosis, although the causal relationship is debated. However, the relation of total serum cholesterol and lipoprotein cholesterol fractions to stroke is inconsistent. Lipoprotein(a) and intermediate-density lipoproteins have recently been associated with significant risk for cerebrovascular disease in men.[16] Lipid metabolism appears to be different in men and women. In one study, dietary fat increased high-density lipoprotein-2 (HDL_2) levels in women, whereas men transported excess cholesterol preferentially in low-density lipoprotein (LDL).[17] Gender differences in lipid metabolism and the effect of these differences on cerebrovascular disease are not fully understood. Several studies have shown that the incidence of occlusive disease of the extracranial arteries is higher in men. In a study of 5033 consecutive autopsies from patients in the fourth to sixth decades of life, the percentage of women with no cerebral atherosclerosis was higher than that of men but the frequency of atherosclerotic lesions was the same in both sexes after the age of 65.[18] The Scandinavian Simvastatin Survival Study showed a significantly reduced risk of both cardiovascular and cerebrovascular events in women. Total cholesterol was reduced 25% and LDL was reduced 35%, whereas HDL was increased 8%.[19]

Diabetes Mellitus

Diabetes mellitus increases the risk of stroke fourfold. The effect of glucose intolerance on stroke is greater in women than in men.[5] This increased susceptibility is caused by accelerated atherosclerosis. Optimizing control of blood glucose as monitored in part by glycosylated hemoglobin (hemoglobin A_{1c}) may minimize vascular complications.

Smoking

Smoking is a significant independent risk factor for cerebrovascular disease and has been associated with an increase in overall risk of approximately 50% for smokers compared with nonsmokers. Over the past 25 years, more men than women have quit smoking. Furthermore, more young and disadvantaged women are smoking and the prevalence among adolescent girls has increased. Women who smoke have more than twice the risk of stroke compared with nonsmokers, and the risk of stroke correlates positively with quantity smoked.[19] In a study of middle-aged women smokers, the risk of ischemic and hemorrhagic stroke increased in a dose-dependent fashion. For women who smoked more than 25 cigarettes a day, the relative risk for stroke was 3.7 and for SAH 9.8, independent of other risk factors.[20] In the Copenhagen City Heart Study the quantity of cigarettes smoked correlated with the risk of stroke. In this prospective analysis, 7060 women aged 35 or older without stroke symptoms or TIAs were followed from their first examination between 1976 and 1978 to the first of two 5-year follow-up examinations or hospitalizations or death, until 1988. A Cox regression model was used to estimate the influence of risk factors on strokes. They found the relative risk of smoking to be 1.40 and the relative risk of lack of physical activity 1.45. Postmenopausal women smokers who were treated with hormone replacement therapy had a statistically significant reduction of 28% in the incidence of stroke.[15] This study, as well as others such as the Nurses' Health Study of 121,700 female registered nurses, reinforces the causative role of smoking in strokes in women and the apparent protective role of hormone replacement therapy in postmenopausal women.[21, 22]

In the Framingham Heart Study smoking was a risk factor for SAH, independent of age and sex. This dose-dependent risk disappeared with smoking cessation.[23] Smoking increases stroke risk by increasing platelet aggregability, inhibiting prostacyclin, and increasing fibrinogen levels.[24] In addition, the carbon monoxide in cigarette smoke reduces the oxygen-carrying capacity of blood and nicotine constricts arteries. The amount of smoking is also independently associated with the severity of carotid artery atherosclerosis.

Stopping smoking significantly reduces the occurrence of stroke. The Nurses' Health Study involved a cohort of 121,700 female registered nurses (89% white) who were 35 to 55 years of age at the start of the study in 1976.[23] The relative risk of stroke after a 12-year follow-up showed an age-adjusted relative risk in smokers of 2.58 (95% confidence interval of 2.08 to 3.19), whereas the risk in nonsmokers was 1.34 (95% confidence interval of 1.04 to 1.73). This increased risk of stroke disappeared 2 to 4 years after stopping smoking regardless of other risk factors, including the number of cigarettes smoked, the age smoking was started, and other known risk factors for stroke.[23]

Alcohol

For alcohol consumption, women have a more variable risk profile for stroke than that of men.[25] In a study of alcohol intake and strokes in 15,077 middle-aged and older women and men over a 20-year period, men were clearly more vulnerable to the effects of alcohol. For example, men who drank infrequently or who drank heavily had a significantly increased risk for ischemic strokes.[25] In women only ex-drinkers were at increased risk for ischemic strokes. Thus, for women, alcohol appears to have a beneficial effect in preventing strokes.

Oral Contraceptives

In an older study in the United States, women who used oral contraceptives had a significant eightfold increase in ischemic (not hemorrhagic) strokes, and estrogen in the range of 50 to 100 μg/d appeared to be thrombogenic.[26] However, when the dose of estrogen was reduced to 30 to 35 μg/d, no increase in the incidence of strokes was noted in women who had no other risk factors for stroke.[27]

The results of previous studies have varied depending on whether they were population- or cohort-based studies. In population-based studies, an entire population of women, both those who use and those who do not use oral contraceptives, is followed prospectively to record the incidence of stroke. In these studies, the incidence of stroke is not usually increased in women who use oral contraceptives. In contrast, cohort or case-control studies usually show an increased risk for stroke in oral contraceptive users; however, use of oral contraceptives with low-dose estrogen is not usually associated with an increased risk.[27]

In the Royal College of General Practitioners' Oral Contraceptive Study,[28] 253 women with first strokes or amaurosis fugax were compared with 759 female controls. In addition to smoking, social class, and hypertension, the use of oral contraceptives was a risk factor for stroke (odds ratio of 1.5 with a 95% confidence interval of 1.1 to 2.0). The risk of stroke was doubled for women who used oral contraceptives, whether or not they were smokers. Former users of oral contraceptives were also at increased risk, particularly if they smoked.[28]

In a case-control study of women younger than 40 years of age who suffered strokes during the years 1986 to 1988, the use of oral contraceptives was associated with a substantial increase in the risk of ischemic stroke (adjusted relative risk of 28.4).[29] A slight increase in the risk of SAH was also noted. The danger of SAH and smoking in women older than 35 has been reported.[30] A slightly increased risk of strokes associated with the use of oral contraceptives was reported in a prospective analysis of 300 young stroke patients aged 14 to 44 years.[31]

In a recent, large case-control study on the use of low-dose estrogen (30 to 35 μg estrogen), Petitti and colleagues[27] concluded that low-dose estrogen in oral contraceptives does not appear to increase the incidence of stroke. In their study from the California Kaiser Permanente Medical Care Program in Los Angeles, women between the ages of 15 and 44 were screened for fatal and nonfatal strokes during the 3-year period between 1991 and 1994. A total of 408 confirmed cases of stroke were identified from 1.1 million women during this 3.6 million woman-years observation, resulting in an incidence of 11.3 per 100,000 woman-years. For each stroke patient identified, three control women were interviewed. Information was obtained from 90% of the stroke patients. A total of 295 women who had had strokes were studied: 62 women were excluded for venous strokes (n = 6); stroke of unknown type (n = 3); pregnancy (n = 11); hysterectomy, bilateral oophorectomy, or both (n = 35); or no controls or inadequate information on oral contraceptive use (n = 7).

When compared with women who had previously or never used oral contraceptives, women on low-dose estrogen had an odds ratio for ischemic strokes of 1.18 (95% confidence interval, 0.54 to 2.59) after adjusting for other known risk factors for stroke. The odds ratio for hemorrhagic strokes was 1.14 (95% confidence interval, 0.60 to 2.16); but for hemorrhagic strokes, the odds ratio for women who smoked and used oral contraceptives showed a positive correlation of 3.64 (95% confidence interval, 0.95 to 13.87). This study again reinforces the association of smoking with stroke.

Although the exclusion of patients with certain types of strokes such as venous stroke could have biased results against an association between stroke and oral contraceptives, the inclusion of patients who had strokes caused by cardioembolic sources and arterial dissection could have biased results in favor of an association. The inclusion of patients with the latter two stroke types, for example, may be questioned because such strokes can occur without the use of oral contraceptives. Nonetheless, in a large, carefully conducted case-control study, Petitti and colleagues[27] have concluded that the use of oral contraceptives does not increase the risk of stroke in women who do not have other risk factors such as smoking.

Because the data from case-control and population-based studies are conflicting, the results found by Petitti and colleagues in their large low-estrogen oral contraceptive study are reassuring.[27] Nevertheless, patients should be informed of the results of various studies, and the decision on whether to take oral contraceptives should be a shared one between physician and patient.

The mechanism of oral contraceptives in causing thromboembolic events is uncertain, but reducing the dose of estrogen of 50 to 100 μg to the lower dose of 30 to 50 μg substantially reduced the incidence of thromoboembolic events.[32] In addition, reducing the dosage of progestin decreased the incidence of stroke and myocardial infarction.[32] The androgenic activity of progestins may negatively affect the risk of stroke and coronary heart disease. The adverse effects of oral contraceptives may relate to their effects on blood cholesterol, particularly on low- and high-density lipoproteins (LDL and HDL), which play a role in atherosclerosis. In a simplified view, LDL is considered a "bad" cholesterol because it delivers cholesterol to cells such as those in arteries, whereas HDL is a "good" cholesterol because it takes cholesterol away from cells to the liver for bile conversion. Development of atherosclerosis is a highly complicated, multifactorial, and incompletely understood process that involves not only cholesterol but also smooth muscle cell proliferation, connective tissue deposition, macrophage activation, and an inflammatory response. In a study comparing 1 mg ethynodiol diacetate (Demulen), 0.5 mg DL-norgestrel (Ovral), and 1 mg norethindrone acetate (Norlestrin), all three types of oral contraceptives increased cholesterol levels; however, DL-norgestrel (Ovral) caused the most significant increase in LDL.[33]

Hormone Replacement Therapy

The first National Health and Nutrition Survey from the United States reports the protective role of hormone replacement therapy against strokes in postmenopausal women. In a national sampling, 1910 postmenopausal white women between the ages of 55 and 74 years with no history of stroke symptoms were identified between 1971 and 1975. In the follow-up through 1987, 250 cases of stroke were identified. Using Cox proportional hazards regression models, the authors reported that women who used hormone replacement therapy had significantly fewer strokes than women who did not. The age-adjusted incidence rate of stroke was 82 per 10,000 woman-years in women who used hormone replacement therapy and 124 per 10,000 woman-years in women who did not. Relative risk reduction with hormone replacement against strokes was 0.69 with a 95% confidence interval (CI) of 0.47 to 1.00. For stroke mortality the relative risk was 0.37 with a CI of 0.14 to 0.92. These relative risk reductions have been adjusted for various risk factors such as age, blood pressure, diabetes mellitus, body mass index, smoking, hypertension, coronary artery disease, and socioeconomic status.[34] Other studies, including a meta-analysis of published data on the effects of hormones on other conditions, have shown that hormone replacement therapy protects women against strokes.[35]

In a study from Sweden, more than 23,000 women who were prescribed noncontraceptive estrogens between 1977 and 1983 were followed for a mean period of 6 years and women who had first strokes were analyzed. During the follow-up, 361 strokes occurred, compared with an expected 403, which indicated a stroke risk reduction to 0.90 with a 95% CI of 0.81 to 0.99. In women younger than 60 at study entry who were prescribed estradiol (1 to 2 mg) or conjugated equine estrogens (0.625 to 1.25 mg), the risk of any stroke was reduced by nearly 30% and the risk of acute strokes was reduced by 40%.[32] Women treated with combined estradiol-levonorgestrel had a lower risk of stroke. However, weaker compounds, particularly estriol, provided no protection against stroke. Thus, estrogens alone or cyclically combined with progestins can reduce the risk of stroke in postmenopausal women.[36]

RACIAL DIFFERENCES IN STROKE FOR WOMEN

In the United States, African-American women are particularly prone to hypertension, a major predisposing factor for strokes resulting from atherosclerosis and intracerebral hemorrhage. Data from the U.S. National Center for Health Statistics, from other multicenter studies by the National Heart, Lung, and Blood Institute, and from various population-based studies found that between 1988 and 1991, 3 million African-American women had hypertension. This incidence is higher than that in white women. Furthermore, hypertension in African-American women has an earlier onset and longer duration and is associated with greater rates of hypertension-related morbidity and mortality. Obesity is a major factor contributing to hypertension.[37] Aggressive interventional strategies are necessary for treating obese, hypertensive African-American women.[37]

DIAGNOSIS, CLASSIFICATION, AND DIFFERENTIAL DIAGNOSIS OF STROKES

As a first step in diagnosis, strokes should be defined as either ischemic or hemorrhagic. Ischemic strokes can be caused by large vessel atherosclerotic disease, cardioembolic events, small vessel disease (lacunar), or miscellaneous conditions (Table 22–1). Spontaneous intracerebral hemorrhages result from chronic hypertensive disease in 85% of cases. Other causes include occult vascular malformation, drug intake (e.g., sympathomimetic drugs, cocaine), arteritis, and coagulopathy. In most patients, SAH results from the rupture of an intracranial aneurysm.

Table 22–1. CLASSIFICATION OF STROKES

- I. Ischemic Strokes
  - A. Atherothrombotic (ABI) or thrombotic strokes
  - B. Cardioembolic strokes
    - 1. Arrhythmias
    - 2. Valvular pathologies
    - 3. Cardiomyopathies
    - 4. Anatomic or neoplastic strokes
  - C. Lacunar syndromes
  - D. Miscellaneous
    - 1. Arterial abnormalities other than atherosclerosis
    - 2. Venous (cortical) diseases with thrombosis
    - 3. Erythrocytes
    - 4. Platelets
    - 5. Serum proteins
- II. Hemorrhagic Strokes
  - A. Subarachnoid hemorrhage
  - B. Intracerebral hemorrhage

Computed tomography (CT) of the brain will indicate whether the stroke was ischemic or hemorrhagic. If an ischemic stroke is suspected, a complete laboratory investigation (complete blood cell count with differential, platelet count, and chemistry profile), Doppler studies of the carotid vessels, echocardiography, and a 24-hour Holter electrocardiogram are mandatory. Combined with the clinical data, these studies can indicate large artery disease, cardiogenic embolism, a lacunar ischemic lesion, or a stroke from miscellaneous causes. A magnetic resonance imaging (MRI) study with a normalization ratio angiogram can yield additional information if the initial CT is normal or inconclusive. An MRI enables noninvasive study of the intracranial circulation and provides a view of the posterior fossa, which may not be seen on CT.

If Doppler studies of the carotid vessels reveal moderate to severe stenosis or occlusion in a symptomatic carotid artery, a four-vessel cerebral angiogram should be performed to define the extent of the stenosis and the degree of collateral circulation. If vascular malformation or arteritis is suspected, angiography is the gold standard for diagnosis. If the diagnosis is inconclusive, physicians should consider conditions that cause the hematologic changes that can lead to stroke. The following tests should be considered: antinuclear antibodies, lupus anticoagulant, anticardiolipin antibodies, antithrombin III, protein C and protein S, serum homocysteine, cryoglobulin, hemoglobin electrophoresis, and human immunodeficiency virus assay.

CONDITIONS RELATED TO ISCHEMIC STROKE IN WOMEN

Mitral Valve Prolapse

Mitral valve prolapse (MVP) is more common in women (5% to 15% of women) than men and may become apparent during pregnancy. A recent study indicated that older women with MVP may have recurrent strokes.[38] Because embolization and bacterial endocarditis can occur on these prolapsed and redundant valves, physicians should routinely listen for a midsystolic click and a late systolic murmur on auscultation in pregnant women. Suspicious cases require study with echocardiography.[38, 39] Barnett was the first to postulate the relationship between cerebral ischemia and MVP.[40] The cerebral hemispheres are the most common site of ischemia in patients with MVP. Posterior circulation events are less frequent, occurring in about 20% of reported cases. In 8.5% of cases, multiple areas and both hemispheres are affected. Furthermore, a relationship exists between MVP and cerebroretinal ischemic events in young people. Retinal lesions have included amaurosis fugax, central retinal artery and retinal arteriolar branch occlusions with persistent defects of retinal or optic nerve origin, atypical Eales' disease, and central retinal vein thrombosis.[41, 42]

Noninfective thrombi from the prolapsing mitral valve leaflet are the most likely cause of ischemic events. Several studies have reported abnormalities in platelet activity in patients with MVP.[43, 44] Prophylactic therapy is unnecessary because the risk of stroke associated with MVP without valvular redundancy is low. If ischemic events occur in a patient with MVP and other possible causes of ischemia have been excluded, antiplatelet therapy is recommended before considering long-term anticoagulation.

Fibromuscular Dysplasia

Fibromuscular dysplasia is an uncommon angiopathy characterized by nonatherosclerotic dysplastic deformities in the walls of small- and medium-sized arteries. The angiopathy may affect the tunica intima, media, and adventitia and is often associated with hypertension. Fibromuscular dysplasia, a multifocal condition, most commonly affects the renal arteries. Cephalic vessels are the second most common site, with a high frequency of associated intracranial aneurysms. Of those patients with cerebrovascular fibromuscular dysplasia, 85% are women between the ages of 40 and 60.[45]

Clinical manifestations may be related to ischemic and hemorrhagic lesions. Fibromuscular dysplasia has been associated with many signs and symptoms, such as headache, tinnitus, vertigo, arrhythmia, hypertension, TIA, and syncope.[46, 47] Diagnosis is made via angiography with characteristic location and appearance of lesions. One large study showed that intracranial aneurysms associated with fibromuscular dysplasia were more prevalent in women.[48] Aneurysms of the internal carotid artery and middle cerebral artery occur almost twice as frequently in women as in men, whereas anterior cerebral artery aneurysms are more common in men.

Because of the low incidence of stroke or TIA and the prolonged course in patients in whom fibromuscular dysplasia is incidentally discovered, a conservative approach is recommended. In patients with stroke or TIA attributed to fibromuscular dysplasia, antiplatelet therapy should be instituted.

Collagen Vascular Diseases

Collagen vascular diseases are a diverse group of disorders that may affect the cerebral vasculature. Although uncommon, ischemic or hemorrhagic stroke has been documented as a complication of collagen vascular disease. More women than men are affected by giant cell arteritis, Takayasu's arteritis, systemic lupus erythematosus, rheumatoid arthritis, and Sjögren's syndrome. Furthermore, systemic lupus erythematosus and Takayasu's arteritis may be exacerbated during pregnancy and the puerperium.[49, 50]

Migraine

Migraine attacks commonly affect young women. In fact, 23% to 29% of women have migraines.[51] Various forms of migraine attacks are accompanied by transient neurologic deficits, which may persist and resemble conventional cerebrovascular syndromes. The incidence of migrainous infarction has been estimated at 3.36 per 100,000 per year. However, this estimate decreases to 1.44 per 100,000 population per year in the absence of other risk factors for stroke.[52] Despite the lack of an epidemiologic association, clinical reports suggest that migraine-related strokes may involve the retina, brainstem, or cerebral hemispheres. In any case, the specific stroke risk from migraine seems to be low, but certain subpopulations of migraine patients could be at higher risk.

In a study by Tzourio and coworkers,[53] the prevalence of migraine was the same for patients with stroke and for matched controls, except among women younger than 45 years of age, in whom migraine and stroke were significantly associated. Their risk was increased fourfold and became even greater when migraine patients smoked. Similarly, oral contraceptives have been implicated as a possible risk factor associated with migrainous stroke. In a case-control study, the Cooperative Study Group in Young Women evaluated the risk of cerebrovascular disease in women who used oral contraceptives. The use of oral contraceptives in patients with migraines increased the relative risk for thrombotic stroke from 2.0 to 5.9.[54] In other studies, however, migraines have not been linked with use of oral contraceptives in younger women.[55–57]

A few studies have suggested an association between migraine and MVP. The prevalence of MVP can actually increase twofold to threefold in young women with migraine as compared with young men. In two reports, the prevalence of MVP in patients with migraines was 20%.[58, 59] The frequency of MVP in patients with migraine exceeds by threefold the frequency of MVP in the general population (6%). Centonze and colleagues[60] reported on 10 patients with migraine and transient focal deficits, all of whom had echocardiographic evidence of MVP, suggesting that migraine patients with MVP may be prone to stroke. Platelet disorders in migraine patients have been well documented[61, 62] and could be a prominent feature in patients with MVP. Patients with migraine in association with antiphospholipid syndrome also have a higher risk for ischemic episodes.[63]

In conclusion, the risk of stroke associated with migraine is not significant; however, women with migraines who are younger than 45 years of age and who smoke or use oral contraceptives may be at higher risk for stroke. In addition, the coexistence of MVP or antiphospholipid syndrome with migraine should also be considered a higher-risk factor for stroke.

Susac's Syndrome

In 1979 Susac described two young women who developed paranoid psychosis, progressive neurologic dysfunction, hearing loss, and multiple branch retinal artery occlusions.[64] Since then, several additional cases of Sucac's syndrome have been reported. Susac's syndrome, a distinct clinical entity consisting of encephalopathy, branch retinal artery occlusions, and hearing loss,[65] almost exclusively affects young women between the ages of 21 and 41; only one man with this disorder has been reported. Branch retinal artery occlusions can present late in the course of the disease and can range widely in severity. Encephalopathy, which usually evolves subacutely, is frequently associated with psychiatric features, bilateral extensor plantar responses, and pseudobulbar speech. Hearing loss, usually bilateral, is almost always associated with tinnitus. Electroencephalography shows diffuse slowing, and MRI reveals numerous small infarcts in the white and gray matter that resemble those seen in multiple sclerosis. Cerebrospinal fluid analysis shows elevated protein levels and minimal or no pleocytosis. Although the pathogenesis is unknown, biopsy studies have shown arteriolar changes consistent with sclerosis and thickening, as well as multiple microinfarctions throughout the gray matter. In about 50% of patients, the disease goes into remission in 1 to 2 years, and most of these patients return to normal. Those patients who do not fully recover are usually left with mild to moderate dementia. Treatment is widely empirical, but good results have recently been reported with the use of aspirin and nimodipine.[65] High-dose steroids, anticoagulation, and immunosuppressants have been used with varied responses.

Pregnancy and the Puerperium

For many years women were thought to be at increased risk for stroke during pregnancy and the puerperium. Numerous reports published in the 1950s and 1960s estimated that the risk of stroke was increased approximately 13-fold in pregnant women compared with nonpregnant women of the same age.[66] However, most of these studies were conducted at one hospital with a limited sample size, and appropriate imaging techniques were not available to confirm the nature of the stroke and to separate hemorrhage from infarction. Grosset and associates[67] contend that previous studies are flawed by diagnostic inaccuracies because of earlier, less precise neuroimaging techniques.[68] Recent reports demonstrate that the increased risk of ischemic stroke in pregnancy is not as high as was previously thought. In a 10-year review from Saudi Arabia of 946 stroke patients, only 12 (1.3%) were pregnant or postpartum at the onset of stroke. Of the 12 cases of stroke in pregnant women, 9 were ischemic cerebral infarctions and 3 were hemorrhagic. On computing the relative risks to nonpregnant women of the same childbearing age, the authors found a slightly increased risk of 1.5.[68] Further data supporting the infrequency of strokes during pregnancy are provided by two recent large studies. Sharshar and coworkers[69] identified 31 cases of stroke (excluding cerebral venous thrombosis) in women during pregnancy and 2 weeks after delivery; 15 cases were ischemic (4.3 per 100,000 deliveries), and 16 were hemorrhagic (4.6 per 100,000 deliveries). Because of the similar rates of cerebral infarction and intracerebral hemorrhage in their study, which contrasts with the preponderance of ischemic stroke over intracerebral hemorrhage in studies of the overall incidence of stroke in young women, the authors inferred an increased risk of intracerebral hemorrhage during pregnancy and the postpartum period. Similarly, Kittner and colleagues[70] found that the risk of intracerebral hemorrhage and ischemic stroke per day was higher during the postpartum period than during any trimester of pregnancy. In both studies eclampsia was an important factor associated with hemorrhagic stroke.

Several mechanisms are postulated for the slight increased risk of ischemic stroke during pregnancy. The concentrations of plasma fibrinogen and factors VII and X increase in late pregnancy, and factor VIII activity also increases[71] whether antithrombin III and protein S decrease in the second or third trimester.[72] These changes in the coagulation and fibrinolytic system lead to a mild hypercoagulable state with increased blood viscosity and stasis, which predisposes the patient to cerebral ischemia. In the early puerperium, a secondary increase occurs in the level of fibrinogen, factor VIII activity remains well above nonpregnant levels, and the platelet count substantially increases. These changes, together with the limited physical activity of the mother immediately after childbirth, may explain thrombosis during the puerperium.[71] In addition, these changes may partly explain why arterial infarctions occur primarily in the second and third trimesters, whereas venous thrombosis most often occurs in the immediate postpartum period.

Arterial Infarctions in Pregnancy

Arterial occlusions cause 60% to 80% of ischemic strokes in pregnant women.[73] Of these, roughly 25% are related to atherosclerosis. Those patients with long-standing hypertension, hyperlipidemia, or diabetes mellitus or those who smoke or whose pre-existing arterial disease is prone to become symptomatic during pregnancy are at higher risk of stroke. Embolic events are an important cause of strokes during pregnancy. Patients with established cardiac conditions such as rheumatic heart disease, patent foramen ovale, and prosthetic valves may experience decompensation and may have an increased risk of cardiac emboli resulting from the increase in procoagulant activity in the blood.

Pregnancy can also trigger de novo maternal heart disease, as exemplified by peripartum cardiomyopathy. This syndrome of unknown origin is more prevalent in multiparous black women older than 30 years of age and, like other congestive cardiopathies, predisposes patients to formation of mural thrombi. In most cases, the heart returns to normal soon after delivery, but occasionally congestive heart failure persists. The treatment of peripartum cardiomyopathy is similar to that of other congestive cardiomyopathies; cautious anticoagulation with heparin is suggested if embolic complications occur or if mural thrombi are detected by echocardiography.[74]

Cardiac arrhythmias are another source of emboli during pregnancy. Atrial fibrillation can develop for the first time during pregnancy and can increase the risk of symptomatic brain embolism by up to 10%. Conventional treatment with digitalis, verapamil, and β-adrenergic blockers is safe. In drug-resistant cases, cardioversion may be used to restore sinus rhythm once the patient has received heparin for anticoagulation. If sinus rhythm is not restored, heparin should be continued during pregnancy before switching to oral long-term anticoagulation with warfarin.[75]

Other miscellaneous causes of emboli include fat, air, and amniotic fluid as well as metastatic choriocarcinoma, which presumably originates as arterial emboli. Arterial dissection, although uncommon, may cause stroke during pregnancy. Arterial dissections can occur spontaneously or with minor trauma; therefore, straining during vaginal delivery may be a contributing factor.[76] Heparin therapy is recommended to avoid embolic complications. Anticoagulation should be continued for at least 3 months.

In cases of transient or permanent deficits caused by arterial occlusive disease, a thorough physical examination is required and should include a complete laboratory profile, a CT examination of the head, Doppler studies of the carotid arteries, an echocardiogram, and an MRI study to visualize the circle of Willis if there is no evidence for extracranial arterial disease or cardiac abnormalities. Patients with proven cardioembolic sources should probably receive heparin therapy until at least the second trimester of pregnancy; warfarin should be avoided at this stage because of increased risk of teratogenic complications and fetal wastage. Those patients with significant extracranial stenosis of the carotid arteries should undergo endarterectomy. In patients with no identifiable causes, 325 mg of aspirin daily is recommended.

Venous occlusive disease may cause stroke during pregnancy or, more commonly, in the postpartum period. The incidence of cerebral venous thrombosis (CVT) is slightly higher in women than in men. Of the cases of CVT in women, 60% occur in women between 20 and 35 years of age, which reflects the association of CVT with oral contraceptives and pregnancy. The most frequently postulated pathophysiologic mechanism for CVT in obstetric patients is a hypercoagulable state associated with dehydration and anemia, but other factors such as protein S deficiency, which is common during pregnancy and puerperium, may also play an important role. CVT occurs 13 times more often during puerperium than during pregnancy, with symptoms usually appearing in the first 3 weeks after delivery.[77] In general, CVT is indicated by a wide spectrum of symptoms and signs. The most frequent presenting symptom is headache, followed by papilledema, motor deficits, seizures, and changes in mental status.[78] Clinical diagnosis is confirmed by radiologic investigation. MRI is the diagnostic method of choice; angiography should be used only in difficult or doubtful cases. In a study of pregnant women, Cantu and colleagues[77] reported that most patients presented acutely with parenchymal lesions (venous infarctions and intracerebral hemorrhages). The course was progressive but tended to subside or become stable in a short time (5 to 10 days) with a favorable outcome. These findings indicate that venous occlusion develops faster in pregnant women but is usually self-limited and resolves in a shorter time. Resolution may occur concomitantly with a return of the hypercoagulable state to normal. Evidence indicates that intravenous heparin is beneficial in patients with CVT who have no contraindication for its use. Treatment should be continued for at least 3 months.

Intracranial Hemorrhage in Pregnancy

The incidence of intracranial hemorrhage complicating pregnancy and the puerperium is similar, if not higher, than that of cerebral infarction. Nontraumatic intracranial hemorrhage may arise from a ruptured aneurysm, an arteriovenous malformation (AVM), or hypertension, particularly in patients with eclampsia. Rarely, primary bleeding may be related to hematologic disease or may have no obvious etiology. Of the various types of nontraumatic intracranial hemorrhage, SAH is most commonly associated with pregnancy and results from rupture of an intracranial aneurysm or an AVM. Clinically, SAH is associated with the sudden onset of a severe headache accompanied by nausea, vomiting, signs of meningeal irritation, and alterations in sensorium, which vary from somnolence to deep coma, depending on the volume of blood. The incidence of aneurysmal rupture during pregnancy is controversial but has been estimated to be between 1 in 2,000 and 1 in 10,000 pregnancies (a fivefold increase over that in nonpregnant women of the same age).[79] The risk of bleeding increases with each trimester.[80] If SAH is suspected during pregnancy, CT should be performed as soon as possible; and if the presence of subarachnoid blood is confirmed, angiography is mandatory. Once the aneurysm has been identified, early clipping is recommended; craniotomy and clipping have been successfully conducted in all stages of pregnancy.[81] Although cesarean section may be appropriate in women near term who have an acute hemorrhage, a risk of rebleeding during delivery exists in unclipped cases. Furthermore, pregnancy does not allow optimal medical management to prevent complications from SAH because possible interventions such as hypervolemic-hypertensive therapy may be hazardous. The management of patients with a known unruptured intracranial aneurysm who become pregnant is uncertain, but Hunt and colleagues[80] estimate that between 20,000 and 40,000 women with intracranial aneurysms successfully undergo childbirth each year in the United States. Unruptured, asymptomatic aneurysms, particularly those less than 8 mm in diameter, should probably be left untreated in pregnant women. Interventional considerations can be deferred until after delivery.

Traditionally, the risk of hemorrhage from an AVM was thought to increase significantly during pregnancy. Robinson and associates[82] reported that pregnancy carried an 87% risk of hemorrhage, which is much higher than that in the general population. In a more recent study, however, the risk of a nonfatal hemorrhage during pregnancy for patients with untreated AVMs was 3.5%, which is similar to that in nonpregnant women of a comparable age. However, in women with a history of cerebral hemorrhage, the risk of bleeding during a subsequent pregnancy was increased (5.8%).[83] These conflicting data reflect the lack of adequate studies. A population-based study of prospectively identified patients with AVMs should clarify this issue.

Hemorrhage from an AVM is most common during early pregnancy (16 to 20 weeks) and delivery.[82] These types of hemorrhages occur more frequently in younger, primiparous women than do aneurysmal hemorrhages. Pregnant women who bleed from an AVM should undergo a four-vessel cerebral angiogram. When feasible, surgical excision, proton beam therapy, or embolization should be attempted. If the malformation is not amenable to treatment, has been only partially resected, or has bled during the present pregnancy, elective cesarean section should be performed at 38 weeks of gestation.

Pregnancy-induced hypertension encompasses the hypertensive disorders of gestation including pre-eclampsia and eclampsia. The classic central nervous system manifestations of pre-eclampsia include severe headache, visual disturbances, excitability, nausea, vomiting, and hyperreflexia. Eclampsia is defined as the occurrence of convulsions or coma in patients with signs and symptoms of pre-eclampsia. Although the pathophysiologic mechanisms that underlie this uniquely reversible form of hypertension are unknown, pre-eclampsia is characterized by a marked increase in peripheral vascular resistance resulting from sympathetic vasoconstrictor overactivity.[84] When blood pressure rises to levels in which autoregulation is impaired, the endothelial tight junctions open and plasma and red blood cells leak into the extravascular space, which may result in petechial or gross intracranial hemorrhage. The main postmortem lesions in the brains of women who have died with eclampsia are edema, hyperemia, thrombosis, and hemorrhage. Sheehan[85] examined the brains of 48 eclamptic women shortly after their deaths and found hemorrhages ranging from petechiae to gross bleeding in 56% of the cases. Similarly, Govan[86] investigated the cause of death in 110 fatal cases of eclampsia and concluded that cerebral hemorrhage was responsible in 39 cases.

Eclampsia is treated with aggressive antihypertensive and anticonvulsant therapy. Agents such as hydralazine and nitroprusside can be used to lower blood pressure because they decrease peripheral resistance. Although a standard practice has been to use conventional anticonvulsants for seizure management, the choice of agent is controversial. The Eclampsia Trial Collaborative Group Study[87] provided strong support for the use of magnesium sulfate to control seizures rather than diazepam or phenytoin. Patients who develop focal cerebral lesions should have their pregnancies terminated and should be treated as described earlier. In addition, neuroimaging studies should be obtained and cerebral edema should be treated with hyperventilation or mannitol if the infant has already been delivered.

Miscellaneous Conditions in Pregnancy

Antiphospholipid Syndrome

Antiphospholipid antibodies (APAs) comprise a family of immunoglobulins characterized by their pattern of reactivity in a number of laboratory tests. Lupus anticoagulant (LA) and anticardiolipin antibodies (ACAs), two important APAs, are involved in the antiphospholipid syndrome, which is characterized by the triad of fetal loss, thromboembolic disease, and thrombocytopenia. Other clinical manifestations of this syndrome are heart valve disease, cutaneous necrosis, chorea, migraine, and obstetric problems such as fetal growth retardation, pre-eclampsia, postpartum serositis, and neonatal thrombosis. In women with a history of recurrent fetal loss, treatment during pregnancy is mandatory. Results of the most recent trials demonstrate that in patients with a history of pre-eclampsia, intrauterine growth retardation, a pathologic result on Doppler examination of the uterus, an abnormal angiotensin test result, or antiphospholipid syndrome, aspirin (100 mg/d) can prevent recurrence or development of pre-eclampsia or intrauterine growth retardation. Treatment should begin as soon as possible during pregnancy and should be continued until 36 weeks of gestation,[88] at which time, most obstetricians recommend that aspirin should be discontinued because of potential risk of hemorrhage during delivery. However, several studies of women with antiphospholipid syndrome who had strokes during the postpartum period after discontinuing aspirin indicate that such practice can be hazardous.[89] Thus, if aspirin has to be stopped for obstetric reasons, efficient anticoagulation therapy should begin as soon as possible. Anticoagulant therapy may be appropriate because recent data suggest that warfarin is superior to antiplatelet therapy in preventing recurrent thromboembolism.[90] Asymptomatic patients should not be treated because only 10% to 15% of patients with APAs develop symptoms.

Postpartum Cerebral Angiopathy

First described in 1980 by Rascol and colleagues,[91] postpartum cerebral angiopathy has not been well studied. Signs and symptoms, which usually begin within 1 month after delivery, include headache, seizures, vomiting, and, less often, focal neurologic signs. Angiography reveals multiple segmental constrictions involving large- and medium-sized intracranial vessels. Cerebrospinal fluid examination may be normal or may show a mild to moderate pleocytosis. Symptoms usually resolve in a few days, and the angiographic pattern reverses to normal in a few weeks. The etiology is unknown, but vasoconstriction in response to acute, transient hypertension may be a possible cause.[92] In most cases a severe and rapid rise in blood pressure occurs before the onset of symptoms; in half of the patients the rise was concomitant with the administration of ergot derivatives. A similar angiopathy has been described with pheochromocytoma or experimental hypertension, in which disappearance of segmental narrowing and dilation correlates with a return of blood pressure to normal levels. Because postpartum cerebral angiopathy is benign and self-limiting, it must be distinguished from isolated angiitis of the central nervous system, an often fatal disease with identical angiographic findings that usually affects older people. The angiographic appearance suggestive of arteritis is not specific for postpartum cerebral angiopathy. Awareness that acute elevation in blood pressure can mimic the angiographic appearance of angiitis will help avoid misdiagnosis and dangerous therapies for vasculitis.[93] Postpartum cerebral angiopathy has been linked with the use of ergot alkaloid derivatives such as ergonovine or bromocriptine. Barinagarrementeria and coworkers[94] reported a case of acute symptomatic vasospasm of the posterior circulation after intravenous administration of ergonovine without an associated increase in blood pressure, documenting a direct adverse drug effect. Similar results have been described with the use of bromocriptine,[95] which is a hydrogenated, semisynthetic ergot alkaloid derivative. Hydrogenation minimizes its vasopressor activity while increasing its vasodilating properties. Usually bromocriptine is a vasodilating drug, but the mechanism of vasospasm in some patients could result from a genetically determined error in metabolism: an inability to distinguish between the hydrogenated and nonhydrogenated ergot alkaloid compounds. Approximately 20 paradoxical responses to bromocriptine have been reported to the U.S. Food and Drug Administration. Some of these reactions include myocardial infarction, hypertension alone (mean onset about 6 days post partum), seizures with and without hypertension, and cerebrovascular accident with hypertension.[96] The use of bromocriptine to suppress lactation has been discontinued.

In rare cases, severe vasospasm may occur unrelated to migraine and may be devastating. A 27-year-old gravida 1, para 0 woman, 13 days post partum, developed a left hemiparesis and hypertension (170/100 mm Hg); her clinical course deteriorated, with severe cerebral vasospasm, bilateral cerebral infarctions, and death.[97] There is no clear explanation for the severe vasospasm except that her mild hypertension may have triggered a cascade of events starting with vascular injury and vasospasm in hormonally sensitized vessels.

PREVENTION AND MEDICAL AND SURGICAL TREATMENT OF STROKES

Reduction of risk factors, such as hypertension, cardiac disease, smoking, hypercholesterolemia, and diabetes mellitus, is the most important aspect of primary stroke prevention. The severe neurologic hazards of smoking while using oral contraceptives should be emphasized.

Brain infarction or TIAs resulting from atherothrombotic carotid disease should be treated surgically for secondary prevention if the degree of ipsilateral carotid stenosis is equal to or greater than 70%.[98, 99] With asymptomatic high-grade carotid stenosis (≥60% occlusion), the results of surgery are less compelling.[100] Although no gender differences were seen in the response of symptomatic patients to surgery, in asymptomatic patients the 5-year reduction in stroke risk was 66% in men and only 17% in women. The higher perioperative complication rate in women may have contributed to the lower rate.[100] The decision to use carotid endarterectomy for asymptomatic patents with stenosis greater than or equal to 60% should be made on an individual basis.[101]

For secondary prevention of strokes in patients with large-vessel atherothrombosis who are not surgical candidates, pharmacologic therapy should be instituted and risk factors should be controlled. Antiplatelet (i.e., aspirin or ticlopidine) and anticoagulant (i.e., warfarin) agents are the most widely used forms of pharmacologic therapy. No evidence indicates that one agent is superior to the other; however, most physicians start patients on an antiplatelet aggregate agent.

Aspirin is a cyclooxygenase inhibitor that blocks the production of thromboxane A_2 in platelets, thus preventing aggregation. Several studies have shown that aspirin reduces the recurrence of stroke by 25% to 30%. Whether aspirin has this effect in women is still being debated. Several studies have reported that the beneficial effects of aspirin are seen primarily in men,[102–105] whereas other studies have found no sex difference.[106, 107] Neither the UK-TIA aspirin trial[102] nor the Canadian Cooperative Study[103] showed efficacy of aspirin in women, but only one third of the patients were women. In contrast, French and Swedish trials[106, 107] reported no gender differences in aspirin efficacy. This sex difference may result from the small number of women enrolled in trials or may indeed reflect a true gender-specific response in platelet aggregability.[108] The dose of aspirin currently used is 325 mg/d.

An alternative antiplatelet aggregate agent is ticlopidine, which blocks the adenosine diphosphate–mediated pathway of platelet aggregation. Two double-blind, randomized clinical trials have confirmed the efficacy of ticlopidine in preventing stroke recurrence. The Canadian-American Ticlopidine Study (CATS) compared the effect of 500 mg/d of ticlopidine with that of placebo in 1053 patients who had recently had a stroke and found a 30% reduction in risk of stroke at 2 years in the ticlopidine group.[109] Similarly, the Ticlopidine Aspirin Strokes Study (TASS) compared the effect of 500 mg/d of ticlopidine with that of 1300 mg/d of aspirin in 3069 patients who had recently had a TIA or minor stroke. Fatal and nonfatal strokes were reduced by 21% at 3 years in the ticlopidine group compared with the aspirin group.[110] In both trials, the effect of ticlopidine on risk reduction was greater in women than in men, but this difference did not reach statistical significance.[111] Ticlopidine, given at a dose of 250 mg twice daily, has an incidence of side effects similar to that reported for aspirin; however, severe but reversible neutropenia has been documented with the use of ticlopidine in 2.4% of patients. Because this potentially serious side effect almost always occurs within the first 3 months of therapy, complete blood cell counts should be obtained every 2 weeks during that time.

In summary, ticlopidine is more effective than aspirin in preventing recurrent atherothrombotic stroke. Because of cost issues and side effects, aspirin is still recommended as the first drug of choice. However, certain groups such as women and patients with diabetes, renal failure, brainstem strokes, and diffuse intracranial atherosclerotic disease may benefit more from ticlopidine.[112]

Anticoagulation with warfarin is usually recommended for preventing strokes of cardioembolic origin. Primary prevention with warfarin is indicated in patients with atrial fibrillation, sick sinus syndrome, prosthetic cardiac valve replacement, certain cardiomyopathies, or recent myocardial infarction with left ventricular thrombus. Atrial fibrillation is one of the major causes of ischemic stroke, underlying approximately half of all cardioembolic events. The rate of ischemic stroke among people with atrial fibrillation averages 5% per year. Warfarin is particularly effective for preventing strokes in selected high-risk patients (history of hypertension, left ventricular systolic dysfunction, or TIA/stroke) whose rate of stroke would otherwise be greater than 7% per year. For high-risk atrial fibrillation patients younger than 75 years, an international normalized ratio (INR) of 2.0 to 3.0 is recommended; those older than 75 years should receive anticoagulation to achieve a target INR of 1.5 to 2.5 because the bleeding complication rate increases as patients get older. For secondary prevention, a higher target INR may be advisable (2.5 to 4.0). Those patients considered low-risk or those with a single episode of atrial fibrillation who are younger than 60 years of age may receive aspirin (325 mg/d) for prophylaxis.[113–116] Women with atrial fibrillation may be at increased risk for cardioembolic stroke compared with men, which suggests that female gender may be an independent risk factor for stroke in atrial fibrillation. In the Copenhagen Heart Study, atrial fibrillation increased the risk of stroke 10-fold in women but not in men.[15] Furthermore, in the Stroke Prevention in Atrial Fibrillation study, the benefits of aspirin were greater in men than in women.[116] Although these differences need to be confirmed, they suggest that the mechanisms for stroke may be different in men and women.[117]

Other conditions in which warfarin therapy may be useful include congenital deficiencies of coagulation inhibitors such as protein C, protein S, and antithrombin III. Evidence from retrospective studies suggests that patients with antiphospholipid syndrome may also benefit from anticoagulation, but this has not been proved. Patent foramen ovale has been associated with TIA or stroke in young adults. When an isolated patent foramen ovale is found in a patient who has had a recent ischemic stroke with no apparent cause, the best prophylactic regimen is unknown. Some physicians would recommend warfarin, especially for high-risk patients with coexistent systemic venous thrombosis or a sustained elevation of right atrial pressure.[118]

CONCLUSION

Patients need to be informed that certain drugs increase stroke risk and that special precautions and interventions are necessary for women with predisposing medical disorders, including cardiac and hematologic disorders such as antiphospholipid syndrome. Recent data indicate that the use of oral contraceptives with low-dose estrogen does not increase the risk of stroke in women who do not smoke. Strokes from other causes are numerous and can be unrelated to pregnancy or delivery. For these patients, specialized neurologic assessment by stroke specialists is warranted. Patients who should be seen by specialists include those with arterial dissection, moyamoya syndrome, aneurysms, hemorrhages, cardioembolism, and hematologic disorders. Finally, patients with certain risk factors for stroke, such as hypertension, diabetes mellitus, smoking, and elevated lipids, may benefit from advice on modifying their risk factors.

References

1. Castelli WP: Cardiovascular disease in women. Am J Obstet Gynecol 158:1553, 1988.
2. Kafrissen ME: Prevention of cardiovascular risk in women: A new concern for the obstetrician/gynecologist. Acta Obstet Gynecol Scand Suppl 152:13, 1990.
3. Knepper LE, Giuliani MJ: Cerebrovascular disease in women. Cardiology 86:339, 1995.
4. Merkatz RB, Temple R, Sobel S, et al: Working Group on Women in Clinical Trials. Women in clinical trials of new drugs—a change in Food and Drug Administration policy. N Engl J Med 329:292, 1993.
5. Kannel WB, Gordon T: Evaluation of cardiovascular risk factors in the elderly: The Framingham Study. Stroke 3:409, 1972.
6. Zhang XH, Sasaki S, Kesteloot H: Changes in the sex ratio of stroke mortality in the period of 1955 through 1990. Stroke 26:1774, 1995.
7. Davis P: Stroke in women. Curr Opin Neurol 7:36, 1994.
8. Vike J: Stroke and its effect in women. J Am Med Womens Assoc 49: 198, 1994.
9. Bonita R: Epidemiology of stroke. Lancet 339:342, 1992.
10. Sivenius J, Laakso M, Penttila IM, et al: The European Stroke Prevention Study—results according to sex. Neurology 41:1189, 1991.
11. American Heart Association: Heart and Stroke Facts. Dallas, American Heart Association, 1992.
12. Flora GC, Baker AB, Loewenson RB, et al: A comparative study of cerebral atherosclerosis in males and females. Circulation 38:859, 1968.
13. Wong MC, Giuliani MA, D'Agostino RB, et al: Cerebrovascular disease and stroke in women. Cardiology 77(Suppl 2):80, 1990.
14. Wolf PA, Belanger MA, D'Agostino RB: Management of risk factors. Neurol Clin 10:177, 1992.
15. Boysen G, Nyboe J, Appleyard M, et al: Stroke incidence and risk factors for stroke in Copenhagen, Denmark. Stroke 19:1345, 1988.
16. Scandinavian Simvastatin Survival Study Group: Randomized trial of cholesterol lowering in 4444 patients with coronary heart disease: The Scandinavian Simvastatin Survival Study. Lancet 344:1383, 1994.
17. Clifton PM, Nestel PJ: Influence of gender, body mass index and age on response of plasma lipids to dietary fat plus cholesterol. Arterioscl Thromb 12:955, 1992.
18. Pedro-Botet JP, Senti M, Nogues X, et al: Lipoprotein and apolipoprotein profiles in men with ischemic stroke: Role of lipoprotein(a), triglyceride-rich lipoproteins, and apolipoprotein E polymorphism. Stroke 23:1556, 1992.
19. Shinton R, Beevers G: Meta-analysis of relation between cigarette smoking and stroke. BMJ 298:789, 1989.
20. Colditz GA, Bonita R, Stampfer MJ, et al: Cigarette smoking and risk of stroke in middle-aged women. N Engl J Med 318:937, 1988.
21. Lindenstrom E, Boysen G, Nyboe J: Lifestyle factors and risk of cerebrovascular disease in women. Stroke 24:1468, 1993.
22. Jawachi I, Colditz GA, Stampfer MJ, et al: Smoking cessation and decreased risk of stroke in women. JAMA 269:232, 1993.
23. Sacco RL, Wolf PA, Bharucha NE, et al: Subarachnoid and intracerebral hemorrhage: Natural history, prognosis and precursive factors in the Framingham Study. Neurology 34:847, 1984.
24. Belch JJ, McArdle BM, Burns P, et al: The effects of acute smoking on platelet behavior, fibrinolysis and haemorheology in habitual smokers. Thromb Haemost 51:6, 1984.
25. Hansagi H, Romelsjö A, Gerhardsson de Verdier M, et al: Alcohol consumption and stroke mortality: 20-year followup of 15,077 men and women. Stroke 26:1768, 1995.
26. Collaborative Group for the Study of Stroke in Young Women: Oral contraception and increased risk of cerebral ischemia or thrombosis. N Engl J Med 288:871, 1973.
27. Petitti DB, Sidney S, Bernstein A, et al: Stroke in users of low-dose oral contraceptives. N Engl J Med 335:8, 1996.
28. Hannaford PC, Croft PR, Kay CR: Oral contraception and stroke: Evidence from the Royal College of General Practitioners' Oral Contraception Study. Stroke 25:935, 1994.
29. Thorogood M, Mann J, Murphy M, et al: Fatal stroke and use of oral contraceptives: Finding from a case-control study. Am J Epidemiol 136:35, 1992.
30. Longstreth WT, Nelson LM, Koepsell TD, et al: Cigarette smoking, alcohol use and subarachnoid hemorrhage. Stroke 23:1242, 1992.
31. Carolei A, Marini C, Ferranti E, et al: A prospective study of cerebral ischemia in the young: Analysis of pathogenic determinants. The National Research Council Study Group. Stroke 24:362, 1993.
32. Hedon B: The evolution of oral contraceptives: Maximizing efficacy, minimizing risk. Acta Obstet Gynecol Scand Suppl 152:7, 1990.
33. Lipson A, Stoy DB, LaRosa JC, et al: Progestins and oral contraceptive-induced lipoprotein changes: A prospective study. Contraception 34:121, 1986.
34. Finucane FF, Madans JH, Bush TL, et al: Decreased risk of stroke among postmenopausal hormone users: Results from a national cohort. Arch Intern Med 153:73, 1993.
35. Grady D, Rubin SM, Petitti DB, et al: Hormone therapy to prevent disease and prolong life in postmenopausal women. Ann Intern Med 117:1016, 1992.
36. Falkeborn M, Persson I, Terent A, et al: Hormone replacement therapy and the risk of stroke: Follow-up of population-based cohort in Sweden. Arch Intern Med 153:1201, 1993.
37. Gillum RF: Epidemiology of hypertension in African American women. Am Heart J 131:385, 1996.

38. Orencia AJ, Petty GW, Khandheria BK, et al: Mitral valve prolapse and the risk of stroke after initial cerebral ischemia. Neurology 45: 1083, 1995.
39. Nishimura RA, McGoon MD, Shub C, et al: Echocardiographically documented mitral valve prolapse: Long-term follow-up of 237 patients. N Engl J Med 313:1305, 1985.
40. Barnett HJM: Transient cerebral ischemia—pathogenesis, prognosis and management. Ann R Coll Phys Surg Can 7:153, 1974.
41. Barnett HJM, Bougher DR, Taylor DW, et al: Further evidence relating mitral valve prolapse to cerebral ischemic events. N Engl J Med 302:139, 1980.
42. Wolf PA, Sila CA: Cerebral ischemia with mitral valve prolapse. Am Heart J 113:1308, 1987.
43. Walsh PN, Kansu TA, Corbett JJ, et al: Platelets, thromboembolism and mitral valve prolapse. Circulation 63:552, 1981.
44. Fisher M, Weiner B, et al: Platelet activation and mitral valve prolapse. Neurology 33:384, 1983.
45. Luscher TF, Lie JT, Stanson AW, et al: Arterial fibromuscular dysplasia. Mayo Clin Proc 62:931, 1987.
46. Mettinger KL, Ericson K: Fibromuscular dysplasia and the brain: I. observations on angiographic, clinical and genetic characteristics. Stroke 13:46, 1982.
47. Sandok BA: Fibromuscular dysplasia of the internal carotid artery. Neurol Clin 1:17, 1983.
48. Osborn AG, Anderson RE: Angiographic spectrum of cervical and intracranial fibromuscular dysplasia. Stroke 8:617, 1977.
49. Machado EBV, Michet CJ, Ballard DJ, et al: Trends in clinical presentation of temporal arteritis in Olmsted County, Minnesota 1950–1985. Arthritis Rheum 31:745, 1988.
50. Sigal LH: The neurologic presentation of vasculitis and rheumatologic syndromes—a review. Medicine 66:157, 1987.
51. Waters WE, O'Connor PJ: Prevalence of migraine. J Neurol Neurosurg Psychiatry 38:613, 1975.
52. Henrich JB, Sandercock PAG, Warlow CP, et al: Stroke and migraine in the Oxfordshire Community Stroke Project. J Neurol 233:257, 1986.
53. Tzourio C, Iglesias S, Hubert JB, et al: Migraine and risk of ischemic stroke: A case-control study. BMJ 307:289, 1993.
54. Collaborative Group for the Study of Stroke in Young Women: Oral contraceptives and stroke in young women: Associated risk factors. JAMA 231:718, 1975.
55. Tzourio C, Markush RE, Karp HR, et al: Epidemiologic study of migraine symptoms in young women. Neurology 25:430, 1975.
56. Rothrock J, North J, Madden K, et al: Migraine and migrainous stroke: Risk factors and prognosis. Neurology 43:2473, 1993.
57. Bougousslavsky J, Regli F, Van Melle G, et al: Migraine stroke. Neurology 38:223, 1988.
58. Amat G, Jean Louis P, Loisy C, et al: Migraine and the mitral valve prolapse syndrome. Adv Neurol 33:27, 1982.
59. Gamberini G, D'Alessandro R, Labriola E, et al: Further evidence on the association of mitral valve prolapse and migraine. Headache 24: 39, 1984.
60. Centonze V, Amat G, Loisy C: Considerations sur les accidents vasculaires cerebraux chez les migraineux. Semin Hop Paris 56:1908, 1980.
61. Jones RJ, Forsythe AM, Amess JAL: Platelet aggregation in migraine patients during the headache-free interval. Adv Neurol 33:275, 1982.
62. D'Andrea G, Toldo M, Cortelazzo S, et al: Platelet activity in migraine. Headache 22:207, 1982.
63. Tietjen GE, Levine SR, Brown E, et al: Factors which predict antiphospholipid immunoreactivity in young people with transient focal neurologic events. Arch Neurol 50:833, 1993.
64. Susac JO, Hardimann JM, Selhorst JB: Microangiopathy of the brain and retina. Neurology 29:313, 1979.
65. Susac JO: Susac's syndrome. Neurology 44:591, 1994.
66. Wiebers DO. Ischemic cerebrovascular complications of pregnancy. Arch Neurol 42:1106, 1985.
67. Grosset DG, Ebrahim S, Bone I, et al: Stroke in pregnancy and puerperium: What magnitude of risk? J Neurol Neurosurg Psychiatry 58:129, 1995.
68. Awada A, Rajeh A, Duarte R, et al: Stroke and pregnancy. Int J Gynecol Obstet 48:157, 1995.
69. Sharshar T, Lamy C, Mas JL: Incidence and causes of strokes in pregnancy and the puerperium: A study in public hospitals of Ile de France. Stroke in Pregnancy Study Group. Stroke 26:930, 1995.
70. Kittner SJ, Stern BJ, Feeser BR, et al: Pregnancy and the risk of stroke. N Engl J Med 335:768, 1996.
71. Bonnar J, McNicol GP, Douglas AS: Coagulation and fibrinolytic mechanisms during and after normal childbirth. BMJ 2:200, 1970.
72. Comp PC, Thurnau GR, Welsh J, et al: Functional and immunologic protein S levels are decreased during pregnancy. Blood 68:881, 1986.
73. Cross JN, Castro PO, Jennett WB: Cerebral strokes associated with pregnancy and the puerperium. BMJ 3:214, 1968.
74. Cruishank DP: Cardiovascular, pulmonary, renal and hematologic diseases in pregnancy. In Scott JR, DiSaia PJ, Hammond CB, et al (eds): Danforth's Obstetrics and Gynecology. JB Lippincott, Philadelphia, 1990, p 433.
75. Stavem K, Steen T: Atrial fibrillation during pregnancy. Tidsskr Nor Laegeforen 113:2405, 1993.
76. Wiebers DO, Mokri B: Internal carotid artery dissection after childbirth. Stroke 16:956, 1985.
77. Cantu C, Barinagarrementeria F: Cerebral venous thrombosis associated with pregnancy and puerperium: Review of 67 cases. Stroke 24: 1880, 1993.
78. Ameri A, Bousser M: Cerebral venous thrombosis. Neurol Clin 10: 87, 1992.
79. Wiebers DO: Subarachnoid hemorrhage in pregnancy. Semin Neurol 8:226, 1988.
80. Hunt HB, Schifrin BS, Suzuki K: Ruptured berry aneurysms and pregnancy. Obstet Gynecol 43:827, 1974.
81. Minielly R, Yuzpe AA, Drake CG: Subarachnoid hemorrhage secondary to ruptured cerebral aneurysm in pregnancy. Obstet Gynecol 53: 64, 1979.
82. Robinson JL, Hall CS, Sedzimir CB: Arteriovenous malformations, aneurysms and pregnancy. J Neurosurg 41:63, 1974.
83. Horton JC, Chambers WA, Lyons SL, et al: Pregnancy and the risk of hemorrhage from cerebral arteriovenous malformations. Neurosurgery 27:867, 1990.
84. Schobel HP, Fischer T, Heuszer K, et al: Pre-eclampsia—a state of sympathetic overactivity. N Engl Med 335:1480, 1996.
85. Sheehan HL: Pathological lesions in the hypertensive toxemias of pregnancy. In Hommond J, Browne FJ, Wolstenholme GEW (eds): Toxemias of Pregnancy: Human and Veterinary. Blakiston, Philadelphia, 1950.
86. Govan ADT: The pathogenesis of eclamptic lesions. Pathol Microbiol (Basel) 24:561, 1961.
87. Which anticonvulsant for women with eclampsia? Evidence from the Collaborative Eclampsia Trial. Lancet 345:1455, 1995.
88. Uzan S, Merviel P, Beaufils M, et al: Aspirin during pregnancy: Indications and modalities of prescription after the publication of the later trials. Presse Med 25:31, 1996.
89. Huong DLT, Wechsler B, Edelman P, et al: Postpartum cerebral infarction associated with aspirin withdrawal in the antiphospholipid antibody syndrome. J Rheumatol 20:1229, 1993.
90. Khamashta MA, Cuadrado MJ, Mujic F, et al: The management of thrombosis in the antiphospholipid-antibody syndrome. N Engl J Med 332:993, 1995.
91. Rascol A, Guiraud B, Manelfe C, et al: Accidents vasculaires cérébraux de la grassesse et du post partum. In 2e Conference de la Salpetrière sur les Maladies Vasculaires Cérébrales, 1979. Baillière, Paris, 1980, p 84.
92. Bougousslavsky J, Despland PA, Regli F, et al: Postpartum cerebral angiopathy: Reversible vasoconstriction assessed by transcranial Doppler ultrasound. Eur Neurol 29:102, 1989.
93. Garner BF, Burns P, Bunning RD, et al: Acute blood pressure elevation can mimic arteriographic appearance of cerebral vasculitis (a postpartum case with relative hypertension). J Rheumatol 17:93, 1990.
94. Barinagarrementeria F, Cantu C, Balderrama J: Postpartum cerebral angiopathy with cerebral infarction due to ergonovine use. Stroke 23: 1364, 1992.
95. Janssens E, Hommel M, Mounier-Vehier F, et al: Postpartum cerebral angiopathy possible due to bromocriptine therapy. Stroke 26:128, 1995.
96. Postpartum hypertension, seizures, strokes reported with bromocriptine. FDA Drug Bull 14(1):3, 1984.
97. Geraghty JJ, Hoch DB, Roberts MR, et al: Fatal puerperal cerebral vasospasm and stroke in a young woman. Neurology 41:1145, 1991.
98. European Carotid Surgery Trialists' Collaborative Group: European Carotid Surgery Trial: Interim results for symptomatic patients with severe (70–99%) or with mild (0–29%) carotid stenosis. Lancet 337: 1235, 1991.
99. North American Symptomatic Carotid Endarterectomy Trial Collabo-

rators: Beneficial effect of carotid endarterectomy in symptomatic patients with high-grade stenosis. N Engl J Med 325:445, 1991.
100. Endarterectomy for Asymptomatic Carotid Artery Stenosis—Executive Committee for ACAS Study. JAMA 273:1421, 1995.
101. Brott T, Toole JF: Medical compared with surgical treatment of asymptomatic carotid stenosis. Ann Intern Med 123:720, 1995.
102. UK-TIA Study Group: United Kingdom Transient Ischemic Attack (UK-TIA) aspirin trial: Interim results. BMJ 269:316, 1988.
103. Canadian Cooperative Study Group: A randomized trial of aspirin and sulfinpyrazone in threatened stroke. N Engl J Med 299:53, 1978.
104. Candelise L, Landi G, Perrone P, et al: A randomized trial of aspirin and sulfinpyrazone in patients with TIA. Stroke 13:175, 1982.
105. Fields WS, Lemak NA, Frankowski RF, et al: Controlled trial of aspirin in cerebral ischemia. Stroke 8:301, 1977.
106. Bousser MG, Eschwege E, Haguenau M, et al: "AICLA" controlled trial of aspirin and dipyridamole in the secondary prevention of atherothrombotic cerebral ischemia. Stroke 14:5, 1983.
107. Britton M, Helmers C, Samuelsson K: High-dose acetylsalicylic acid after cerebral infarction. A Swedish Cooperative Study. Stroke 18: 325, 1987.
108. Spranger M, Aspey B, Harrison M: Sex difference in antithrombotic effect of aspirin. Stroke 20:34, 1989.
109. Gent M, Blakely JA, Easton JD, et al: The Canadian American Ticlopidine Study (CATS) in thromboembolic stroke. Lancet 1:1215, 1989.
110. Hass WK, Easton JD, Adams HP, et al: A randomized trial comparing ticlopidine hydrochloride with aspirin for the prevention of stroke in high-risk patients. N Engl J Med 321:501, 1989.
111. Hershey LA: Stroke prevention in women: Role of aspirin versus ticlopidine. Am J Med 91:288, 1991.
112. Grotta JC: Prevention of stroke with ticlopidine: Who benefits most? Neurology 42:111, 1992.
113. Boston Area Anticoagulation Trial for Atrial Fibrillation Investigators: The effect of low-dose warfarin on the risk of stroke in non-rheumatic atrial fibrillation. N Engl J Med 323:1505, 1990.
114. Stroke Prevention in Atrial Fibrillation Investigators: Warfarin versus aspirin for prevention of thromboembolism in atrial fibrillation. Lancet 343:687, 1994.
115. European Atrial Fibrillation Trial Study Group: Optimal oral anticoagulant therapy in patients with non-rheumatic atrial fibrillation and recent cerebral ischemia. N Engl J Med 333:5, 1995.
116. Stroke Prevention in Atrial Fibrillation Investigators: Superiority of adjusted-dose warfarin over low-intensity, fixed-dose warfarin plus aspirin for high-risk patients with atrial fibrillation. Lancet 348:633, 1996.
117. Miller VT, Rothrock JF, Pearce LA, et al: Ischemic stroke in patients with atrial fibrillation: Effects of aspirin according to stroke mechanism. Neurology 43:32, 1993.
118. Gautier JC, Durr A, Koussa J, et al: Paradoxal cerebral embolism: Role of patent oval foramen. Bull Acad Natl Med 174:1031, 1990.

22.2 The Surgical Perspective

Thomas J. Takach and James J. Livesay

Stroke is the third leading cause of death in the United States after heart disease and cancer and is the leading cause of severe disability for both women and men in the United States. Approximately 500,000 new strokes occur annually in the United States, resulting in more than 200,000 deaths per year. Two thirds of stroke survivors have some disability, and one third require prolonged institutional care.[1–3] In 1993, it was estimated that the annual direct and indirect cost of stroke in the United States was more than $18 billion.[4]

Despite being an issue of importance to both genders, early information concerning treatment and prevention of stroke was biased toward men. An evolving body of literature, however, has documented significant gender-based differences in the natural history and epidemiology of stroke. This, in turn, has led to current and evolving changes in the methods of detection, prevention, and treatment of cerebrovascular disease in women.

NATURAL HISTORY

Thromboembolic strokes associated with cerebrovascular disease are a major source of morbidity in women in the United States. Each year, approximately 87,000 women die of a stroke, of which thromboembolism is the most common cause.[5, 6] There are significant ethnic and gender differences in stroke rates in the United States (Figs. 22–1 and 22–2). Stroke mortality for black women is almost twice that for white women (45 vs. 26 per 100,000 population).[7–9] The death rate from stroke is 30% higher in men than in women.[10, 11] Although an earlier mortality is documented in men, stroke may be a more important entity for women given their greater longevity and, thus, the need for prolonged care and rehabilitation for surviving women.[11]

Recurrent strokes occur with twice the frequency in men

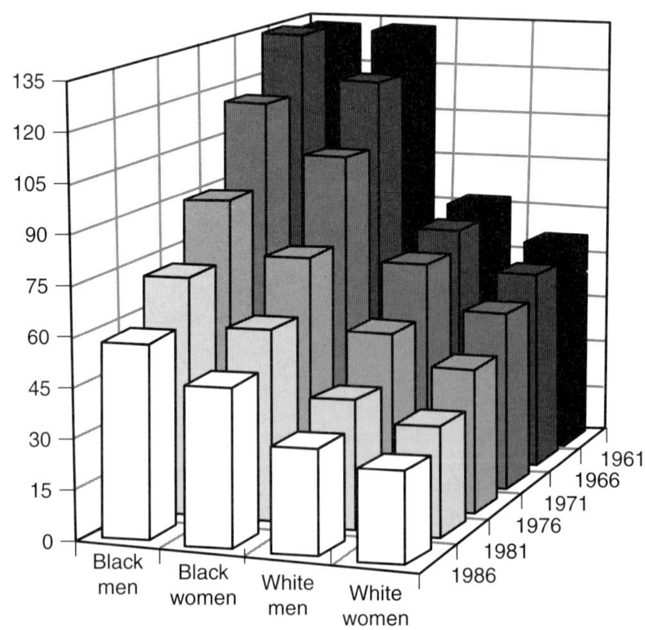

FIGURE 22–1. United States stroke rates per 100,000 population by sex and race, 1961–1986. (From United States Public Health Service, Centers for Disease Control and Prevention: Health United States 1990. Washington, DC, U.S. Government Printing Office, 1991, pp 85–148.)

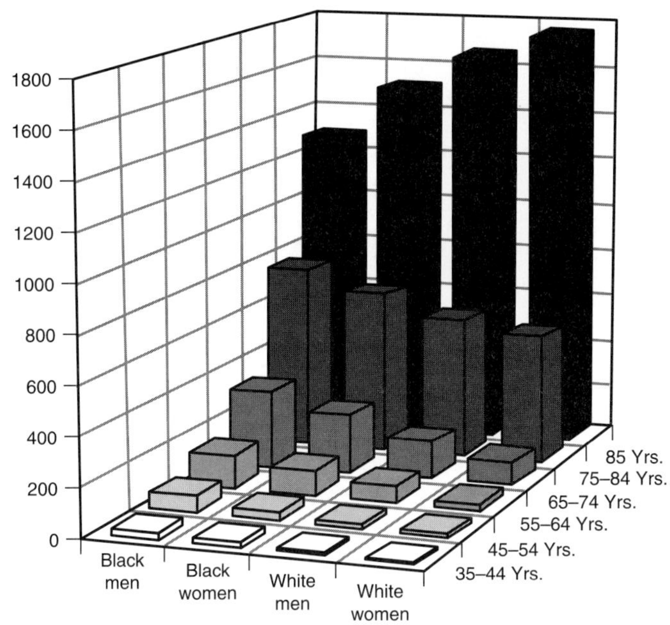

FIGURE 22–2. United States stroke rates per 100,000 population by sex, race, and age, 1988. (From United States Public Health Service, Centers for Disease Control and Prevention: Health United States 1990. Washington, DC, U.S. Government Printing Office, 1991, pp 85–148.)

compared with women.[2, 6, 11] Women also experience fewer transient ischemic attacks (TIAs) than men, and at least twice as many men will experience a stroke after a TIA.[6, 10–12] Because women have a better prognosis after TIAs and after the occurrence of a stroke, any study in which stroke or death is an endpoint requires a larger population of women to find statistically significant differences in treatment strategy.

Women are at increased risk for the development of stroke from multiple causes. Internal carotid artery dissections with the occurrence of stroke have been reported both during childbirth[10] and secondary to fibromuscular dysplasia.[13] Pregnancy is associated with a 3- to 13-fold increased risk of stroke, primarily because of intracranial etiology such as small vessel thrombosis.[12] SAH occurs more frequently in women than in men and has been associated with hypertension, cigarette smoking, and the use of estrogen.[6, 14] Mitral valve prolapse occurs more frequently in women than in men and predisposes to stroke via an atheroembolic mechanism.[6]

Stroke in the United States accounts for a higher percentage of deaths in women than in men in all decades of life. Since mortality rates increase with age, the largest difference occurs in the very old, those aged 85 years or older; in that age group, stroke accounts for 12% of the mortality rate in women compared with 9% in men.[15] By the year 2000, 38% of all women in the United States will be 45 years of age or older. By the year 2015, this proportion will be 45%.[15–17] With the increase in the population of older women, cerebrovascular disease is likely to be an issue of increasing importance in the health care of the United States.

RISK FACTORS

Several well-known factors have been associated with the risk of stroke in women. Hypertension is the strongest and most consistent risk factor for stroke. Other consistent and powerful risk factors include cigarette smoking, diabetes mellitus, elevated serum cholesterol, and a history of previous myocardial infarction or stroke.[10] Besides these well-known factors, several gender-specific factors have also been associated with ischemic stroke. These include pregnancy (toxemia, postpartum cerebral thrombosis, and hypercoagulability), autoimmune diseases, mitral valve prolapse, oral contraceptive use, and migraine headaches.[6, 10] Chronic atrial fibrillation may be the single most important risk factor in the aged.[18] Heavy alcohol use has also been shown to be a significant risk factor for hemorrhagic stroke, along with elevated blood pressure.[6, 10]

The issue of oral contraceptive use as a risk factor for stroke has generated significant controversy.[6, 10] Both ischemic stroke and hemorrhagic stroke have been documented to follow oral contraceptive use in both cohort and case-control studies.[6, 10] Furthermore, the variables of cigarette smoking and oral contraceptive use appear to be additive with regard to risk for development of stroke.[6, 11]

The body of literature establishing the above association was obtained before the evolution of oral contraceptive development in the 1980s. The data, which were analyzed and published, involved the use of high-dose estrogen rather than the low-dose compounds in favor today. Many authors suggest that the lower estrogen doses produce less risk of stroke than the previously used high-dose compounds.[6, 10, 12] Currently, an ongoing large prospective trial of low-dose estrogen oral contraceptives in England has yet to report any strokes in the patients being studied.[19] However, follow-up has been short-term, and resolution of the issue will depend on the long-term findings.

The use of replacement estrogen in postmenopausal women has also generated significant controversy. This mode of therapy has been reported to reduce the risk of coronary artery disease by one half.[16] However, the information regarding its impact on ischemic stroke has been conflicting. Framingham Heart Study data revealed an increased risk of stroke in women being treated with postmenopausal estrogen replacement, which was further increased with tobacco smoking.[20] In contrast, several large cohort studies have documented a decreased risk of cerebrovascular disease in women treated with postmenopausal estrogen replacement. Paganini-Hill and colleagues[21] demonstrated a 50% decrease in ischemic stroke in more than 5000 postmenopausal women receiving estrogen compared with those who did not. Although no prospective, randomized trials have been completed, epidemiologic findings have led to the consensus that postmenopausal estrogen use does confer some protection against ischemic stroke.

Stroke prevention may take the form of risk factor modification, medical therapy, or surgical therapy. Risk factor modification is accepted as state-of-practice therapy.[22–24] However, medical therapy for stroke prevention is controversial for women. Stroke prevention can occur both before (primary prevention) and after (secondary prevention) a neurologic event. This controversy regarding medical therapy as a mode of stroke prevention centers on the use of aspirin. In several studies, aspirin has had a beneficial effect in reducing primary myocardial infarction rates in men.[25, 26] These same studies, as well as a large observational study involving 87,000 female nurses, did not reveal any beneficial effect of aspirin in preventing stroke in men or women.[25–27]

When aspirin therapy was evaluated in a role of secondary prevention of stroke after TIAs or minor completed stroke, the results have been mixed.[28–34] Most trials report a benefit for men but not women. Only the AICLA trial from France[30] and the European Stroke Prevention Study[33] showed aspirin to have a significant benefit in the secondary prevention of stroke in women. Both of these studies combined aspirin and dipyridamole therapy. In a recent meta-analysis, aspirin was not shown to be beneficial in the secondary prevention of stroke in women.[35]

Various explanations have been provided regarding this discrepancy of the differing response to aspirin between men and women. Less than 30% of the population of any of the seven major series were females. Because women have a lower stroke rate and a better prognosis than in men after a stroke or TIA, the number of females in these studies may have been insufficient to detect a difference in the outcome between the aspirin and non-aspirin groups. Additionally, women may not have the same pharmacologic response to aspirin as that of men. This is supported by evidence that aspirin does not inhibit platelet aggregation in women as it does in men.[36–38] This may be secondary to the influence of testosterone.[38]

Although the data do not support the use of aspirin for primary or secondary stroke prevention in women at this time, promising data have emerged from randomized ticlopidine trials. Ticlopidine interferes with platelet aggregation by inhibiting the adenosine phosphate pathway. Two separate trials with the use of ticlopidine have demonstrated a beneficial effect by preventing secondary stroke in men and women.[39, 40] Of note was a greater benefit in men than in women. A major drawback associated with ticlopidine, however, is that some patients are intolerant of the drug. Greater than 50% of patients in each trial experienced adverse pharmacologic effects secondary to ticlopidine. Currently, there does not appear to be an acceptable medical agent that can decrease the risk of stroke in women either before or after an initial ischemic event.

ATHEROSCLEROSIS

After its first description by Cooley and associates in 1956,[41] carotid endarterectomy (CEA) became one of the most commonly performed procedures in the United States (Fig. 22–3).[42] In the 1980s, however, concerns were raised regarding the efficacy of CEA in preventing stroke and death compared with that of medical therapy alone for the treatment of atherosclerotic, extracranial cerebrovascular disease.[43–46] Randomized prospective trials were instituted in both symptomatic and asymptomatic patients for the purpose of establishing the efficacy, or lack thereof, of treatment with CEA.[47–61]

The results of these studies, whether completed or terminated early because of compelling preliminary data, have changed and clarified the indications for CEA. In addition, reviews of institutional results (perioperative morbidity and mortality) by multidisciplinary councils of the American Heart Association have led to strict practice guidelines and operative standards.[62]

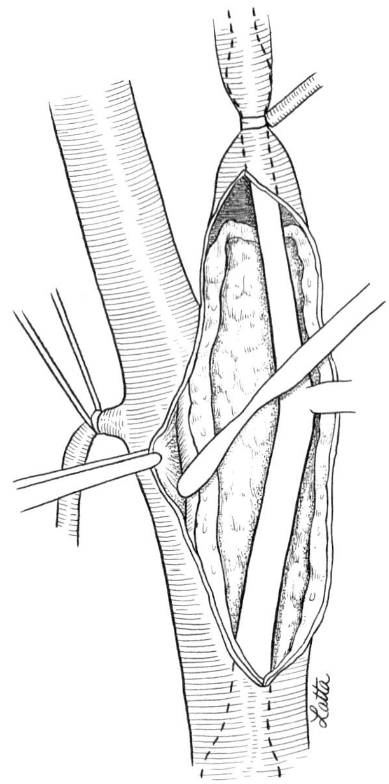

FIGURE 22–3. Carotid endarterectomy is initiated following placement of an indwelling shunt to maintain continuous cerebral perfusion.

For the first time, evidence was provided that CEA reduced the incidence of stroke and mortality in patients with both symptomatic and asymptomatic, high-grade carotid artery stenosis. Results of these studies show that symptomatic patients (i.e., those experiencing transient ischemic attack, amaurosis, or completed mild stroke) with a 70% ipsilateral carotid stenosis have an absolute risk reduction of 39% to 65% for stroke or death when treated with CEA as opposed to medical therapy alone.[48, 50, 51]

Of the three major symptomatic trials, the Veterans Administration Symptomatic Carotid Stenosis Trial was composed entirely of men, whereas the North American Symptomatic Carotid Endarterectomy Trial (NASCET) and European Carotid Surgery Trial (ECST) each included approximately 30% women in their study populations. No specific gender differences in outcome were noted by either study.

The long-awaited results of the Asymptomatic Carotid Atherosclerosis Study (ACAS) have been reported for the severe (60%) stenosis subgroup.[52] The trial was designed to test the hypothesis that the incidence of TIAs, stroke, and death in patients with asymptomatic carotid stenosis (minimum 60%) would be lower after CEA plus aspirin than after medical therapy (aspirin) alone.[52]

The executive committee of the ACAS invoked the National Institutes of Health "stopping rules" on preliminary review of the data. The ACAS authors issued a preliminary medical alert in October 1994. In addition, they published a review in May 1995 noting that, after a median follow-up of 2.7 years, the projected aggregate risk over 5 years for ipsilateral stroke, perioperative stroke, or death was 5.1%

for patients treated surgically and 11.0% for patients treated medically; the difference was statistically significant ($p < .004$). The aggregate risk reduction was 53% for patients treated surgically.[54]

In the ACAS study, initial plans called for 1500 patients in each group.[52] The dramatic results leading to early termination of the study led to enrollment of only 825 patients in the surgical group and 854 patients in the medical treatment group. In each group, 34% were women. In women, the stroke or death rate was reduced by only 17%, as opposed to 66% in men.[54] Although the difference between men and women was not statistically significant ($p = 0.10$), the outcome suggests that women experienced less benefit than did men after CEA. The percentage of women with perioperative complications was 3.6% compared with 1.7% for men ($p = .12$).

The results of the trials just discussed suggest that both men and women benefit from CEA in treating both symptomatic and asymptomatic, high-grade carotid artery stenosis. However, the benefit (decreased stroke and death) appears to be greater in men than in women. These trials are ongoing, and results of surgical versus medical therapy in men and women with moderate (30% to 60%) stenosis will be forthcoming.

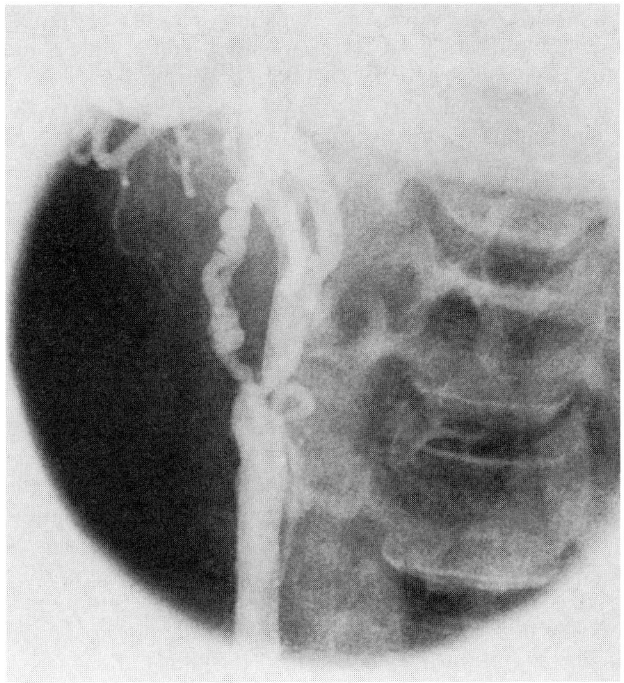

FIGURE 22–4. Angiogram demonstrating the concomitant presence of fibrodysplasia in the distal internal carotid artery and atherosclerotic plaque at the carotid bifurcation. The patient was successfully treated with carotid endarterectomy and intraoperative dilatation of the distal vessel.

FIBROMUSCULAR DYSPLASIA

Fibromuscular dysplasia (FMD) of the carotid artery is an important nonatherosclerotic cause of stroke in women. The role of feminizing hormones in influencing the development and progression of the disease is believed to be responsible for the predominance of the disease in women. Approximately 90% of patients with clinically and angiographically documented FMD are women.[63, 64]

Stanley and colleagues[13] have described four distinct histologic types of FMD: intimal fibroplasia, medial fibroplasia, medial hyperplasia, and perimedial dysplasia. In the carotid artery, medial fibroplasia is the most common histologic type.[13] Fibrous connective tissue replaces smooth muscle in the media of the arterial wall, leading to a series of stenoses and aneurysms that produce the classic "string of beads" appearance noted on arteriograms (Fig. 22–4).[13] The proposed model of pathogenesis involves medium-sized arteries that are relatively longer than normal. As a result of the vessel's length, a portion of the artery has a deficient medial blood supply from its vasa vasorum. The combined inadequate blood supply and normal arterial wall tension lead to disruption of the internal elastic lamina and medial damage. The hormonal environment may modify the physical stresses and repair mechanisms present within the arterial wall.[65–67]

Because many patients with FMD are without symptoms and the natural history of FMD is uncertain, the true incidence of FMD is unknown. However, several reviews utilizing arteriographic evaluations have noted that evidence of FMD is present in 0.25% to 0.5% of all carotid studies.[64, 68–70] The majority of patients with FMD of the carotid artery lesions will remain asymptomatic. However, one third of carotid lesions will progress with time and 10% will eventually produce symptoms.[68] Series of asymptomatic patients have been followed clinically for 2 to 8 years without developing neurologic manifestations of the disease. In patients who develop neurologic sequelae, TIAs are the most frequent symptom.[64] After the onset of neurologic symptoms, it is generally believed that more serious neurologic problems, including stroke, will follow.[64, 68]

In patients with documented carotid artery FMD, 25% to 50% will have associated renal artery FMD, 50% will have bilateral carotid artery disease, 20% will have concomitant intracranial aneurysms, and 7% to 19% will have vertebral artery FMD.[64, 68, 69] In patients who present with a spontaneous carotid dissection, 12% have evidence of FMD in the contralateral internal carotid artery. Despite occurring at a mean age of almost 10 years younger than in similar cohorts of patients with atherosclerotic disease, 18% to 20% of these patients have significant atherosclerosis of the carotid bulb.[63–65]

In view of the incompletely defined natural history of carotid artery FMD, several investigators have strongly suggested that operative intervention in the asymptomatic patient is unwarranted.[64, 68] Effeney and colleagues,[64, 65] however, have pointed to the potential first manifestation of FMD as a completed stroke and suggest consideration of the severity of the individual lesion, the relative age of the patient, and associated clinical problems. Several investigators agree that surgical intervention is warranted in patients with focal ischemic events or those with "critical" stenosis.[68–71]

The operative intervention required to treat carotid artery FMD differs substantially from that required to treat carotid artery atherosclerosis. The FMD lesion is amenable to dilatation and does not require an endarterectomy. The operation involves standard exposure of the carotid bifurcation with complete mobilization from the surrounding tissue to facilitate straightening of the vessel. After systemic anticoagulation, and with the vessel completely straight, increasingly larger dilators are used to progressively enlarge the lumen up to 3.5 to 4.0 mm. A few seconds of vigorous backbleeding from the internal carotid artery is used to flush out any intimal fragments or small thrombi. Forceps are used (without clamps) to occlude the vessel as the arteriotomy is closed.[72, 73]

Alternatively, surgical arterial dilatation may be accomplished by using angioplasty balloon catheters under direct vision with additional information provided by intraoperative fluoroscopy and arteriography.[74] This method, in theory, reduces the longitudinal shear forces produced by forcing a dilatator across the stenosis and will result in less trauma to the intima of the artery.

The largest operative experience has been reported by Effeney and colleagues[63–65] at the University of California at San Francisco. In an experience that included more than 150 operative procedures, only three early strokes, one perforation, no deaths, and one late occlusion were reported.[63–65] Hurlbert and Krupski[75] have argued that percutaneous transluminal angioplasty is contraindicated for the treatment of carotid artery FMD. They believe that without the ability to backbleed and flush away potential thromboembolic debris, the potential risk for development of neurologic sequelae secondary to thromboembolism is high.

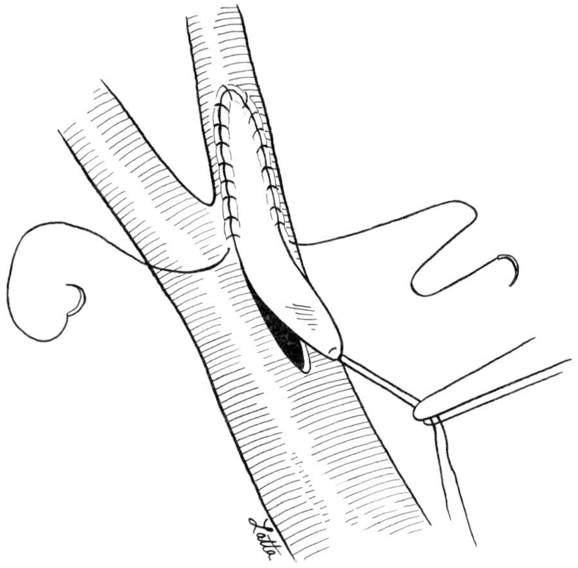

FIGURE 22–5. Closure of the carotid artery incision using patch angioplasty in order to minimize the potential for carotid restenosis.

POSTOPERATIVE STENOSIS

Of particular importance in women is the issue of postoperative outcome related to postoperative stenosis. Postoperative stenosis can result in recurrent carotid disease, which, in turn, can lead to neurologic symptoms and stroke. The documented benefits of CEA in reducing the risk of stroke and death in asymptomatic and symptomatic patients can be negated by excessively high perioperative complications.[61, 62] Carotid restenosis is a common postoperative complication whose incidence can effectively be decreased by modifying operative technique.

Carotid restenosis does not appear to be a result of recurrent or progressive atherosclerosis but rather is due to myointimal hyperplasia.[76] Women have been noted to develop myointimal hyperplasia more frequently than do men after CEA. This has been seen in both clinical and animal studies and is believed to be caused by differences in platelet aggregation between genders.[77, 78] Platelets are an important mediator of smooth muscle cell hyperplasia, and more reactive platelets in women may be responsible for more aggressive myointimal hyperplasia. In addition, gender-based differential responses to platelet-derived growth factors have also been demonstrated.[79, 80]

The combination of an increased incidence of aggressive myointimal hyperplasia and smaller arteries in women may account for an increased incidence of postoperative stenosis, as shown in a number of clinical studies.[81–92]

Carotid restenosis appears to have a different natural history than does primary atherosclerotic narrowing of the vessel secondary to plaque formation. Myointimal hyperplasia generally is manifested as smooth lesions that, in contrast to atherosclerotic plaque, do not tend to ulcerate or produce thromboemboli. Most clinical studies demonstrate that postoperative restenoses only infrequently (0.5% to 20%) result in neurologic symptoms.[76, 79, 80, 85, 88, 89, 93–96] Regression has been shown in myointimal hyperplasia.[76, 79, 88] Because of the relatively benign effects of myointimal hyperplasia and the significant morbidity associated with reoperation from carotid disease, most authors advise observation until myointimal restenosis becomes symptomatic or a critical stenosis develops.[76, 79, 80, 82, 88–93]

The postoperative use of aspirin to decrease carotid restenosis has not been successful in men or women.[76, 79, 81, 82] It has been suggested that patch angioplasty using either prosthetic material (polytetrafluoroethylene [PTFE] or Dacron) or saphenous vein at the time of surgery may decrease the incidence of postoperative carotid restenosis (Fig. 22–5).[81, 97, 98] Furthermore, some authors suggest that the strategy may be more important in women, specifically those with small-diameter carotid arteries.

Analysis of data produced by series using patch angioplasty generally supports the method as being effective in decreasing postoperative carotid restenosis.[81, 97, 98] However, a smaller number of series have failed to demonstrate a benefit of patching, and all series have noted complications associated with the patch material itself. Saphenous vein has been associated with patch rupture rates between zero and 1.4%.[85, 93, 97–104] The incidence of this complication has been decreased by using upper thigh vein rather than ankle vein. Archie and Green[101] demonstrated in vitro that smaller veins, such as ankle veins, have lower hoop strength than larger veins and are more susceptible to rupture. PTFE and Dacron have been acceptable alternatives to vein grafts in many studies.[99] However, PTFE and Dacron represent foreign material, which theoretically may cause greater susceptibility to infection.

Currently, many surgeons electively use patch angioplasty at the time of initial operation in all women, specifically those with small carotid vessels, in an attempt to minimize the potential for development of postoperative carotid artery restenosis.[105]

CONCLUSION

Stroke is the third leading cause of death in the United States after heart disease and cancer and is a leading cause of severe disability in women. However, because women generally have a better prognosis than that for men after stroke, any study in which stroke or death is an endpoint requires enrollment of a larger population of women so that differences in the efficacy of specific interventions or therapy can be statistically confirmed.

Compared with medical therapy alone, CEA has resulted in fewer strokes and death in both asymptomatic and symptomatic patients with severe carotid artery stenosis. The benefit in women, however, appears to be less than that in men. Fibrodysplasia predominantly affects the female gender and can effectively be treated with operative dilatation. In women, the frequent occurrence of postoperative stenosis secondary to myointimal hyperplasia and small-diameter arteries may be diminished by patch angioplasty of the carotid artery after endarterectomy.

Surgery appears to be an effective treatment option for carotid stenosis in symptomatic and asymptomatic women. The efficacy of any treatment option introduced in the future will need to be measured against the success and morbidity and mortality outcomes associated with CEA.

References

1. Mohr JP, Caplan LR, Melski JW, et al: The Harvard Cooperative Stroke Registry: A prospective registry. Neurology 28:754, 1978.
2. Sacco RL, Wolf PA, Kannel WB, et al: Survival and recurrence following stroke: The Framingham Study. Stroke 13:290, 1982.
3. Soltero I, Lieu K, Cooper R, et al: Trends in mortality from cerebrovascular diseases in the United States, 1960 to 1975. Stroke 9:549, 1978.
4. 1993 Heart and Stroke Facts Statistics. American Heart Association, Dallas, TX, 1992.
5. Bonita R, Stewart A, Beaglehole R: International trends in stroke mortality: 1970–1985. Stroke 21:989, 1990.
6. Barnett HJM: Stroke in women. Can J Cardiol 6(Suppl B):11B, 1990.
7. Cooper R, Sempos C, Hsieh SC, et al: Slowdown in the decline of stroke mortality in the United States, 1978–1986. Stroke 21:1274, 1990.
8. Kittner SJ, White LR, Losonczy KG, et al: Black-white differences in stroke incidence in a national sample: The contribution of hypertension and diabetes mellitus. JAMA 264:1267, 1990.
9. Public Health Service, Centers for Disease Control and Prevention. Health United States 1990. U.S. Public Health Service, Washington, DC, 1991, p 85.
10. Wong MCW, Giuliani MJ, Haley EC Jr: Cerebrovascular disease and stroke in women. Cardiology 77(Suppl 2):80, 1990.
11. Caplan LR, Gorelick PB, Hier DG: Race, sex, and occlusive cerebrovascular disease: A review. Stroke 17:648, 1986.
12. Davis P: Stroke in women. Curr Opin Neurol 7:36, 1994.
13. Stanley JC, Gewertz BL, Bove EL, et al: Arterial fibrodysplasia: Histopathologic character and current etiologic concepts. Arch Surg 110:561, 1975.
14. Marmot MG, Poulter NR: Primary prevention of stroke. Lancet 339: 344, 1992.
15. Wenger NK, Speroff L, Packard B: Cardiovascular health and disease in women. N Engl J Med 329:247, 1993.
16. Eaker ED, Chesebro JH, Sacks FM, et al: Cardiovascular disease in women. Circulation 88:1999, 1993.
17. Soldo BJ, Manton KG: Health status and service needs of the oldest old: Current patterns and future trends. Milbank Mem Fund Q Health Soc 63:286, 1985.
18. Wolf PA, Abbott RD, Kannel WB: Atrial fibrillation: A major contributor to stroke in the elderly. The Framingham Study. Arch Intern Med 147:1561, 1987.
19. Vessey MP, Lawless M, Yeates D: Oral contraceptives and stroke: Findings in a large prospective study. BMJ (Clin Res Ed) 289:530, 1984.
20. Wilson PW, Garrison RJ, Castelli WP: Postmenopausal estrogen use, cigarette smoking, and cardiovascular morbidity in women over 50. The Framingham Study. N Engl J Med 313:1038, 1985.
21. Paganini-Hill A, Ross RK, Henderson BE: Postmenopausal oestrogen treatment and stroke: A prospective study. BMJ 297:519, 1988
22. Thompson SG, Greenberg G, Meade TW: Risk factors for stroke and myocardial infarction in women in the United Kingdom as assessed in general practice: A case-control study. Br Heart J 61:403, 1989.
23. Colditz GA, Bonita R, Stampfer MJ, et al: Cigarette smoking and risk of stroke in middle-aged women. N Engl J Med 318:937, 1988.
24. Iso H, Jacobs DR Jr, Wentworth D, et al: Serum cholesterol levels and six-year mortality from stroke in 350,977 men screened in the Multiple Risk Factor Intervention Trial. N Engl J Med 320(14): 904, 1989.
25. Peto R, Gray R, Collins R, et al: Randomised trial of prophylactic daily aspirin in British male doctors. BMJ (Clin Res Ed) 296:313, 1988.
26. Physicians' Health Study Group: Preliminary report: Findings from the aspirin component of the ongoing Physicians' Health Study. N Engl J Med 318:262, 1988.
27. Manson JE, Stampfer MJ, Colditz GA, et al: A prospective study of aspirin use and primary prevention of cardiovascular disease in women. JAMA 266:521, 1991.
28. Fields WS, Lemak NA, Frankowski RF, et al: Controlled trial of aspirin in cerebral ischemia. Stroke 8:301, 1977.
29. The Canadian Cooperative Study Group: A randomized trial of aspirin and sulfinpyrazone in threatened stroke. N Engl J Med 299:53, 1978.
30. Bousser MG, Eschwege E, Haguenau M, et al: "AICLA" controlled trial of aspirin and dipyridamole in the secondary prevention of atherothrombotic cerebral ischemia. Stroke 14:5, 1983.
31. Sorensen PS, Pedersen H, Marquardsen J, et al: Acetylsalicylic acid in the prevention of stroke in patients with reversible cerebral ischemic attacks: A Danish cooperative study. Stroke 14:15, 1983.
32. Swedish Cooperative Study: High-dose acetylsalicylic acid after cerebral infarction. Stroke 18:325, 1987.
33. Sivenius J, Laakso M, Penttila IM, et al: The European Stroke Prevention Study: Results according to sex. Neurology 41:1189, 1991.
34. UK-TIA Study Group: United Kingdom Transient Ischaemic Attack (UK-TIA) Aspirin Trial: Interim results. BMJ (Clin Res Ed) 296: 316, 1988.
35. Sze PC, Reitman D, Pincus MM, et al: Antiplatelet agents in the secondary prevention of stroke: Meta-analysis of the randomized control trials. Stroke 19:436, 1988.
36. Kelton JG, Hirsh J, Carter CJ, et al: Sex differences in the antithrombotic effects of aspirin. Blood 52:1073, 1978.
37. Escolar G, Bastida E, Garrido M: Sex related differences in the effects of aspirin on the interaction of platelets with subendothelium. Thromb Res 44:837, 1986.
38. Spranger M, Aspey GS, Harrison MJ: Sex difference in antithrombotic effect of aspirin. Stroke 20:34, 1989.
39. Gent M, Blakely JA, Easton JD, et al: The Canadian American Ticlopidine Study (CATS) in thromboembolic stroke. Lancet 1:1215, 1989.
40. Hass WK, Easton JD, Adams HP Jr, et al: A randomized trial comparing ticlopidine hydrochloride with aspirin for the prevention of stroke in high-risk patients. Ticlopidine Aspirin Stroke Study Group. N Engl J Med 321:501, 1989.
41. Cooley DA, Al-Naaman YD, Carton CA: Surgical treatment of arteriosclerotic occlusion of common carotid artery. J Neurosurg 13:500, 1956.
42. Feinleib M, Ingster L, Rosenberg H, et al: Time trends, cohort effects, and geographic patterns in stroke mortality—United States. Ann Epidemiol 3:458, 1993.
43. Warlow C: Carotid endarterectomy: Does it work? Stroke 15:1068, 1984.
44. Plum F: Introduction: Should the efficacy of carotid endarterectomy in symptomatic patients be examined in a controlled clinical trial? In Powers WJ, Raichle ME (eds): Cerebrovascular Diseases: Fifteenth Research Conference/Princeton. Raven Press, New York, 1987, p 205.
45. Committee on Health Care Issues, American Neurological Association: Does carotid endarterectomy decrease stroke and death in patients with transient ischemic attacks? Ann Neurol 22:72, 1987.

46. Barnett JH, Plum F, Walton JN: Carotid endarterectomy—an expression of concern [editorial]. Stroke 15:941, 1984.
47. North American Symptomatic Carotid Endarterectomy Trial: Methods, patient characteristics, and progress. Stroke 22:711, 1991.
48. North American Symptomatic Carotid Endarterectomy Trial Collaborators: Beneficial effect of carotid endarterectomy in symptomatic patients with high-grade carotid stenoses. N Engl J Med 325:445, 1991.
49. Moneta GL, Edwards JM, Chitwood RW, et al: Correlation of North American Symptomatic Carotid Endarterectomy Trial (NASCET) angiographic definition of 70% to 99% internal carotid artery stenosis with duplex scanning. J Vasc Surg 17:152, 1993.
50. European Carotid Surgery Trialists' Collaborative Group: MRC European Carotid Surgery Trial: Interim results for symptomatic patients with severe (70–99%) or with mild (0–29%) carotid stenosis. Lancet 337:1235, 1991.
51. Mayberg MR, Wilson SE, Yatsu F, et al: Carotid endarterectomy and prevention of cerebral ischemia in symptomatic carotid stenosis. Veterans Affairs Cooperative Studies Program 309 Trialist Group. JAMA 266:3289, 1991.
52. The Asymptomatic Carotid Atherosclerosis Study Group: Study design for randomized prospective trial of carotid endarterectomy for asymptomatic atherosclerosis. Stroke 20:844, 1989.
53. Moore WS, Vescera CI, Robertson JT, et al: Selection process for surgeons in the Asymptomatic Carotid Atherosclerosis Study. Stroke 22:1353, 1991.
54. Executive Committee for the Asymptomatic Carotid Atherosclerosis Study. Endarterectomy for asymptomatic carotid artery stenosis. JAMA 273:1421, 1995.
55. The CASANOVA Study Group: Carotid surgery versus medical therapy in asymptomatic carotid stenosis. Stroke 22:1229, 1991.
56. Solis MM, Ranval TJ, Barone GW, et al: The CASANOVA Study: Immediate surgery versus delayed surgery for moderate carotid artery stenosis? [letter]. Stroke 23:917, 1992.
57. Diener HC: Comment on Solis MM et al [letter]. Stroke 23:917, 1992.
58. A Veterans Administration Cooperative Study: Role of carotid endarterectomy in asymptomatic carotid stenosis. Stroke 17:534, 1986.
59. Towne JB, Weiss DG, Hobson RW II: First phase report of Cooperative Veterans Administration Asymptomatic Carotid Stenosis Study: Operative morbidity and mortality. J Vasc Surg 11:252, 1990.
60. Hobson RW II, Weiss DG, Fields WS, et al: Efficacy of carotid endarterectomy for asymptomatic carotid stenosis. The Veterans Affairs Cooperative Study Group. N Engl J Med 328:221, 1993.
61. Takach TJ, Ott DA, Reul GJ, et al: Critical decision analysis for extracranial cerebrovascular disease. Tex Heart Inst J 23:45, 1996.
62. Moore WS, Barnett HJ, Beebe HG, et al: Guidelines for carotid endarterectomy: A multidisciplinary consensus statement from the Ad Hoc Committee of the American Heart Association. Stroke 26: 188, 1995.
63. Effeney DJ, Krupski WC, Stoney RJ, et al: Fibromuscular dysplasia of the carotid artery. Aust NZ J Surg 53:527, 1983.
64. Effeney DJ, Ehrenfeld WK, Stoney RJ, et al: Why operate on carotid fibromuscular dysplasia? 115:1261, 1980.
65. Effeney DJ, Ehrenfeld WK, Stoney RJ, et al: Fibromuscular dysplasia of the internal carotid artery. World J Surg 3:179, 1979.
66. Stanley JC, Fry WJ, Seeger JF, et al: Extracranial internal carotid and vertebral artery fibrodysplasia. Arch Surg 109:215, 1974.
67. Starr DS, Lawrie GM, Morris GC Jr: Fibromuscular disease of carotid arteries: Long-term results of graduated internal dilatation. Stroke 12: 196, 1981.
68. Rutherford RB: Fibromuscular dysplasia of the carotid artery. Semin Vasc Surg 4:167, 1991.
69. Stanley JC, Wakefield TW: Arterial fibrodysplasia. In Rutherford RB (ed): Vascular Surgery, 4th ed. WB Saunders, Philadelphia, 1995.
70. Collins GJ Jr, Rich NM, Clagett GP, et al: Fibromuscular dysplasia of the internal carotid arteries: Clinical experience and follow-up. Ann Surg 194:89, 1981.
71. Stewart MT, Moritz MW, Smith RB III, et al: The natural history of carotid fibromuscular dysplasia. J Vasc Surg 3:305, 1986.
72. Ehrenfeld WK, Stoney RJ, Wylie EJ: Fibromuscular hyperplasia of the internal carotid artery. Arch Surg 95:284, 1967.
73. Ehrenfeld WK, Wylie EJ: Fibromuscular dysplasia of the internal carotid artery. Arch Surg 109:676, 1974.
74. Lord RS, Graham AR, Benn IV: Radiologic control of operative carotid dilation: Aneurysm formation following balloon dilatation. J Cardiovasc Surg 27:158, 1986.
75. Hurlbert SN, Krupski WC: Carotid disease in women. Semin Vasc Surg 8:268, 1995.
76. Bernstein EF, Torem S, Dilley RB: Does carotid restenosis predict an increased risk of late symptoms, stroke, or death? Ann Surg 212: 629, 1990.
77. Johnson M, Ramwell PW: Androgen mediated sex differences in platelet aggregation. Physiology 17:256, 1974.
78. Johnson M, Ramey E, Ramwell PW: Sex and age differences in human platelet aggregation. Nature 253:355, 1975.
79. Nicholls SC, Phillips DJ, Bergelin RO, et al: Carotid endarterectomy: Relationship of outcome to early restenosis. J Vasc Surg 2:375, 1985.
80. Thomas M, Otis SM, Rush M, et al: Recurrent carotid artery stenosis following endarterectomy. Ann Surg 200:74, 1984.
81. Ten Holter JB, Ackerstaff RG, Thoe-Schwartzenberg GS, et al: The impact of vein patch angioplasty on long-term surgical outcome after carotid endarterectomy: A prospective follow-up study with serial duplex scanning. J Cardiovasc Surg 31:58, 1990.
82. Hansen F, Lindblad B, Persson NH, et al: Can recurrent stenosis after carotid endarterectomy be prevented by low-dose acetylsalicylic acid? A double-blind, randomised, and placebo controlled study. Eur J Vasc Surg 7:380, 1993.
83. Sanders EA, Hoeneveld H, Eikelboom BC, et al: Residual lesions and early recurrent stenosis after carotid endarterectomy: A serial follow-up study with duplex scanning and intravenous digital subtraction angiography. J Vasc Surg 5:731, 1987.
84. Cossman D, Callow AD, Stein A, et al: Early restenosis after carotid endarterectomy. Arch Surg 113:275, 1978.
85. Eikelboom BC, Ackerstaff RGA, Hoeneveld H, et al: Benefits of carotid patching: A randomized study. J Vasc Surg 7:240, 1988.
86. Ranaboldo CJ, Barros D'Sa AA, Bell PR, et al: Randomized controlled trial of patch angioplasty for carotid endarterectomy: The Joint Vascular Research Group. Br J Surg 80:1528, 1993.
87. Hans SS: Late follow-up of carotid endarterectomy with venous patch angioplasty. Am J Surg 162:50, 1991.
88. Healy DA, Zierler RE, Nicholls SC, et al: Long-term follow-up and clinical outcome of carotid restenosis. J Vasc Surg 10:662, 1989.
89. Ouriel K, Green RM: Clinical and technical factors influencing recurrent carotid stenosis and occlusion after endarterectomy. J Vasc Surg 5:702, 1987.
90. Cuming R, Worrell P, Woolcock NE, et al: The influence of smoking and lipids on restenosis after carotid endarterectomy. Eur J Vasc Surg 7:572, 1993.
91. Gelabert HA, el-Massry S, Moore WS: Carotid endarterectomy with primary closure does not adversely affect the rate of recurrent stenosis. Arch Surg 129:648, 1994.
92. Stoney RJ, String ST: Recurrent carotid stenosis. Surgery 80:705, 1976.
93. Rosenthal D, Archie JP Jr, Garcia-Rinaldi R, et al: Carotid patch angioplasty: Immediate and long-term results. J Vasc Surg 12:326, 1990.
94. Zbornikova V, Elfstrom J, Lassvik C: Restenosis and occlusion after carotid surgery assessed by duplex scanning and digital subtraction angiography. Stroke 17:1137, 1986.
95. DeGroote RD, Lynch TG, Jamil Z, et al: Carotid restenosis: Long-term noninvasive follow-up after carotid endarterectomy. Stroke 18: 1031, 1987.
96. Salvian A, Baker JD, Machleder HI, et al: Cause and noninvasive detection of restenosis after carotid endarterectomy. Am J Surg 146: 29, 1983.
97. Hertzer NR, Beven EG, O'Hara PJ, et al: A prospective study of vein patch angioplasty during carotid endarterectomy. Ann Surg 206: 628, 1987.
98. Katz MM, Jones GT, Degenhardt J, et al: The use of patch angioplasty to alter the incidence of carotid restenosis following thromboendarterectomy. J Cardiovasc Surg 28:2, 1987.
99. Katz D, Snyder SO, Gandhi RH, et al: Long-term follow-up for recurrent stenosis: A prospective randomized study of expanded polytetrafluoroethylene patch angioplasty versus primary closure after carotid endarterectomy. J Vasc Surg 19:198, 1994.
100. O'Hara PJ, Hertzer NR, Krajewski LP, et al: Saphenous vein patch rupture after carotid endarterectomy. J Vasc Surg 15:504, 1992.
101. Tawes RL Jr, Treiman RL: Vein patch rupture after carotid endarterectomy: A survey of the Western Vascular Society members. Ann Vasc Surg 5:71, 1991.
102. Archie JP Jr, Green JJ Jr: Saphenous vein rupture pressure, rupture stress, and carotid endarterectomy vein patch reconstruction. Surgery 107:389, 1990.

103. Myers SI, Valentine RJ, Chervu A, et al: Saphenous vein patch versus primary closure for carotid endarterectomy: Long-term assessment of a randomized prospective study. J Vasc Surg 19:15, 1994.
104. Riles TS, Lamparello PJ, Giangola G, Imparato AM: Rupture of the vein patch: A rare complication of carotid endarterectomy. Surgery 107:10, 1990.
105. Takach TJ, Ott DA, Reul GJ, et al: Carotid endarterectomy: Results in asymptomatic and symptomatic patients. Tex Heart Inst J 23:42, 1996.

SECTION

VIII

PREGNANCY

CHAPTER

23

Pregnancy, Hemodynamic Alterations, and the Cardiovascular System

James T. Willerson and Susan D. Mueller

Pregnancy causes marked and usually reversible changes in the female cardiovascular system. Maternal heart disease occurs in approximately 2% of pregnancies and is the most important nonobstetric cause of death during pregnancy.[1] During or soon after pregnancy, serious disorders may develop, including pulmonary hypertension, peripartum cardiomyopathy, and aortic, carotid, or coronary artery dissection. Cardiac and vascular diseases may occur in association with pregnancy, and some more common conditions are associated with a greater risk for morbidity and mortality. Underlying cardiovascular or endocrine problems may not allow normal physiologic adaptations, resulting in danger to the mother and fetus.

The marked adaptations in cardiac and vascular function during pregnancy protect the mother from stress, such as changes in blood pressure, sudden decreases in venous return to the heart, blood loss, and the higher oxygen and workload demands of pregnancy, labor, and delivery. Blood must be pumped through three (or more in the case of multiple conceptions) interconnected circulations: maternal, placental, and fetal. Normally, the blood volume increases by 130% to 150% of nonpregnancy values and cardiac output increases by up to 50% soon after conception. Uterine arterial blood flow increases substantially during pregnancy to meet the needs of the growing fetus. The maternal system returns to nonpregnancy conditions within weeks after delivery. The physical examination, hemodynamics, exercise response, and respiratory physiology adjust to pregnancy; and bedside findings must be interpreted in the context of the patient's baseline state and the stage of pregnancy.

The fetus and placenta themselves are associated with unique risks to the mother, such as placental vascular thrombosis or ischemia causing pregnancy-induced hypertension and, also, amniotic fluid embolism. Drugs administered to the mother may pose a hazard for the fetus. This may also be useful in treating fetal cardiac disease, such as selected arrhythmias, in utero. The ability to perform certain diagnostic tests in the mother is also limited because of concerns about radiation exposure to the fetus.

Severe cardiac valvular defects in the mother are best managed by correction before pregnancy. However, surgical repair during pregnancy may be necessary, because fetal mortality may exceed 50% in women with severe, untreated congenital heart disease.[2] Cardiopulmonary bypass has been successfully performed in pregnant patients since 1958, when Leyse and associates[3] performed the first (or one of the first) such procedures. The effects of anesthesia, mechanical ventilation, and hypothermia require special monitoring and management to minimize fetal mortality.

Emergencies may occur, including myocardial infarction (MI), aortic dissection, pulmonary or amniotic fluid embolism, and arrhythmias. Evaluation and treatment are special challenges. Cardiopulmonary resuscitation, when necessary, is performed with standard resuscitative measures, but with two critical differences. Special efforts must be made to displace the gravid uterus from abdominal vessels that may be compressed, thus lowering cardiac output, and there must be urgent consideration of emergency cesarean section to salvage the fetus.

The demographics of pregnant women are changing, as more women are delaying pregnancy. This may increase the risk for existing atherosclerosis or hypertension in the mother. There is an increased use by women of cocaine, intravenous drugs, alcohol, and cigarettes, placing the cardiovascular systems at risk for related diseases. In addition, more women who have undergone corrective surgery for valvular or congenital heart conditions are now surviving to puberty and becoming pregnant. Women once believed to be at too high a risk to tolerate pregnancy have safely been delivered of infants.

MATERNAL CARDIOVASCULAR PHYSIOLOGY

Pregnancy simulates three simultaneous stressors on the maternal cardiovascular system, including (1) an internal workload similar to that of endurance exercise, (2) an altered vasculature similar to that associated with a large arteriovenous fistula, and (3) a hemodynamic state similar to that found with high-output cardiac failure. In response, anatomic changes occur, such as enlargement of the heart, expansion of intravascular volume, and the opening of new vascular beds, which result in alterations in the pattern of blood flow. There may be changes in responsiveness of the vascular beds and of endothelium-derived factors on vasoactive eicosanoids during pregnancy.[4, 5] These changes represent an attempt to meet the increased end-organ demands of the mother and developing fetus for oxygen, nutrients, and waste product removal. In addition, there is a shift of the oxygen-hemoglobin dissociation curve that facilitates dissociation and placental transfer of oxygen.[6]

Hematologic and Blood Volume Changes

Normally, hematologic and body water changes occur in response to hormonal and other mediator signals (Fig. 23–1).

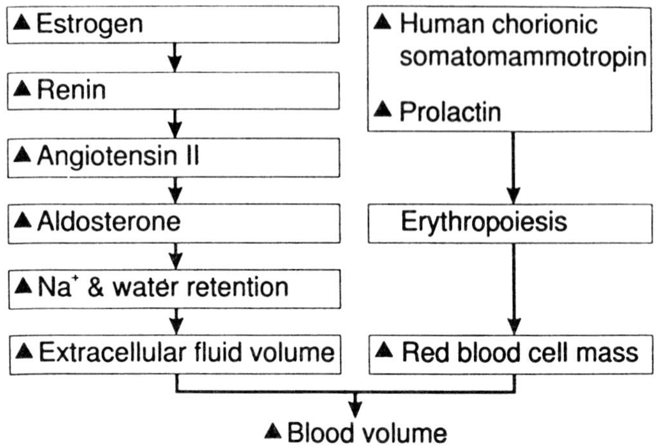

FIGURE 23–1. Mechanisms leading to hypervolemia during pregnancy are multiple, including increased levels of steroid hormones of pregnancy and volume mediators. Plasma renin levels are elevated, and production of renin is expanded to include the kidneys, uterus, and liver. The placenta may produce growth hormone-like substances, and in addition, atrial natriuretic factor is increased in the last trimester of pregnancy in some patients. (From Elkayam U, Gleicher N (eds): Cardiac Problems in Pregnancy, 2nd ed. Alan R. Liss, New York, 1990, pp 5–24, with permission.)

Estrogen may stimulate sodium reabsorption, and progesterone has a relaxing effect on venous smooth muscle, affecting venomotor tone and elasticity of venous walls. Maternal blood volume is increased by approximately 40% at term, with the most rapid increase taking place during the first half of pregnancy. This is initially due to plasma volume increases followed by an increase in red cell mass (Fig. 23–2).[7, 8] There is an accumulation of sodium (500–900 mEq) and total body water (6–8 L), most of which is extracellular, owing to a reduced colloid osmotic pressure and lower albumin concentrations.[9] An increase in atrial natriuretic factor has been found even in normotensive pregnancies, with rises in the first few days after delivery promoting fluid diuresis.[10, 11] Despite increased erythropoiesis, hemoglobin, hematocrit, and blood viscosity decrease slightly during pregnancy.[12] Serum levels of several coagulation factors are increased, including fibrinogen and plasminogen, and a slight shortening of the prothrombin time and partial thromboplastin time occurs as pregnancy progresses.[13] There have been reports of decreases in platelet levels during pregnancy, and platelets may also have a shorter half-life.[14, 15]

Cardiac Output

Cardiac output increases markedly during pregnancy, eventually reaching a level 30% to 50% higher than during the nonpregnant state. The increase in cardiac output begins around the fifth week of gestation and peaks between the mid-second (weeks 20 to 24) or third trimester. Cardiac output is maintained at that level until parturition (see Fig. 23–2). Initially, stroke volume is the major factor causing the increase in cardiac output, but as pregnancy progresses, an increased heart rate becomes the more predominant factor (Table 23–1).[16]

Redistribution of the greatly expanded blood volume occurs. Uterine blood flow increases by about 20% as the uterine muscle enlarges, and peripheral vascular resistance varies to change flow patterns (Fig. 23–3). If hypoxia, hypotension, or toxemia occurs, the maternal cardiovascular system is sensitive to the vasoconstrictive effects of systemic catecholamines.[17, 18]

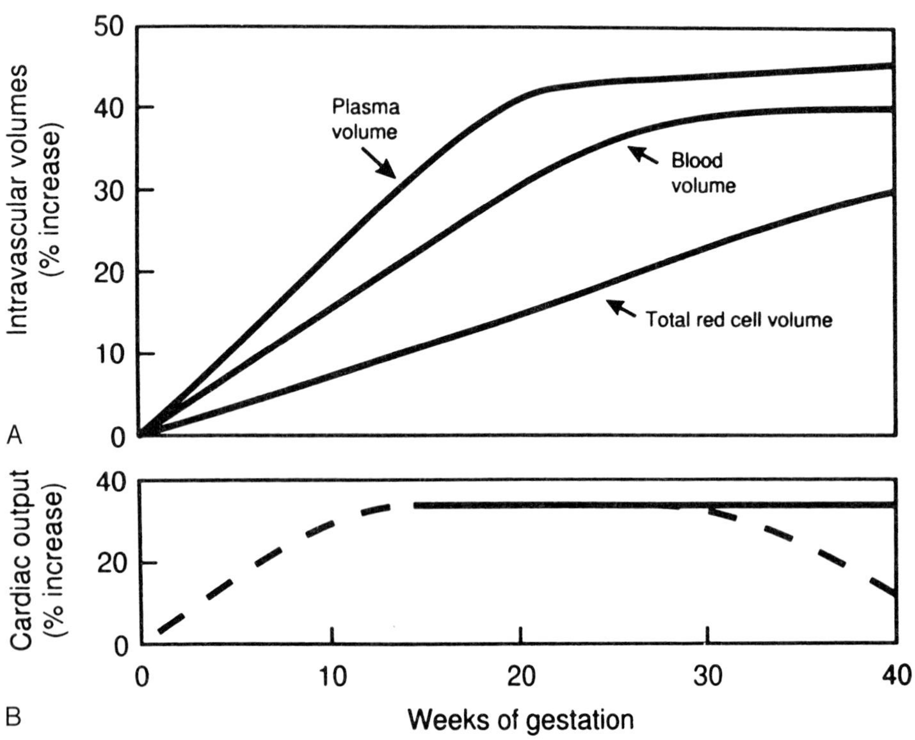

FIGURE 23–2. Timing of the 40% to 50% increase in blood volume during pregnancy, peaking at about week 30. *A*, Blood volume rises early in pregnancy owing to an increase in plasma volume, followed by an increase in red blood cell mass. *B*, These increases are shown in relation to the rise in cardiac output, which reaches values of 40% above nonpregnant levels by week 20 of pregnancy. Dashed line represents the decrease in cardiac output possible due to decreased venous return in the supine position after week 30 of gestation. (From Chatterjee K, et al (eds): Cardiology: An Illustrated Text-Reference. Gower Medical Publishing, Philadelphia, 1991, with permission.)

Table 23–1. CARDIOCIRCULATORY CHANGES DURING NORMAL PREGNANCY

	TRIMESTER		
PARAMETER	1st	2nd	3rd
Blood volume	↑	↑ ↑	↑ ↑ ↑
Cardiac output	↑	↑ ↑ ↑	↑ ↑
Stroke volume	↑	↑ ↑ ↑	↔ or ↓
Heart rate	↑	↑ ↑	↑ ↑ ↑
Systolic blood pressure	↔	↓	↔
Diastolic blood pressure	↓	↓ ↓	↔
Pulse pressure	↑	↑ ↑	↔
Systemic vascular resistance	↓	↓ ↓ ↓	↓ ↓
Oxygen consumption	↔ or ↑	↑ ↑	↑ ↑ ↑
Left ventricular volume	↔	↑	↑
Left ventricular systolic function	↔	↔	↔

↔, no change compared with nonpregnant level; ↑, small increase; ↑ ↑, moderate increase; ↑ ↑ ↑, large increase; ↓, small decrease; ↓ ↓, moderate decrease; ↓ ↓ ↓, large decrease.

From Elkayam U, Gleicher N (eds): Cardiac Problems in Pregnancy, 2nd ed. Alan R. Liss, New York, 1990.

Heart Rate

Heart rate, measured in the sitting, standing, or supine position, increases progressively during pregnancy, peaking and become stable during the third trimester, usually by about week 32. There is an average rise of 10 to 20 beats per minute, with mean values ranging from 78 to 89 beats per minute.[19] By the third trimester, the supine heart rate is greater than that in the left lateral recumbent position. This increased heart rate is beneficial in maintaining cardiac output. The stroke volume returns to nonpregnant values near the end of pregnancy.[19] Twin pregnancies lead to an earlier rise in maternal heart rate, with increases of as much as 40% above baseline near term.[20]

Blood Pressure

Blood pressure normally remains unchanged or may even decrease slightly despite the increased cardiac output (Fig. 23–4).[21] Peripheral vascular resistance and blood pressure fall during the second trimester when uteroplacental mass is growing most rapidly. Systemic arterial pressure falls during the first trimester, reaches a low in midpregnancy, and ordinarily returns to normal prepregnancy levels before term. Pulse pressure widens, since diastolic blood pressure falls more dramatically than systolic pressure.[22] Systemic vasodila-

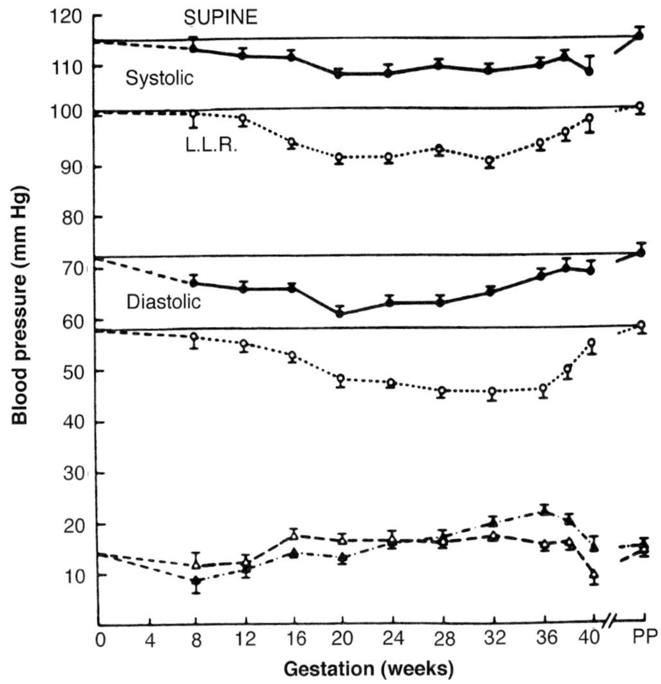

FIGURE 23–4. Systolic and diastolic pressure readings in the supine and left lateral recumbent (LLR) position from 8 weeks of pregnancy to the postpartum (PP) period. The lowest panel shows systolic pressure readings in open triangles and diastolic pressures in darkened triangles when the pregnant woman changes position from the LLF to the supine position. The systolic pressures show a greater change in the first 24 weeks of pregnancy, whereas the diastolic pressures are more dramatically affected after this period. (From Creasy RK, Resnik R (eds): Maternal-Fetal Medicine: Principles and Practice, 2nd ed. WB Saunders, Philadelphia, 1989, with permission.)

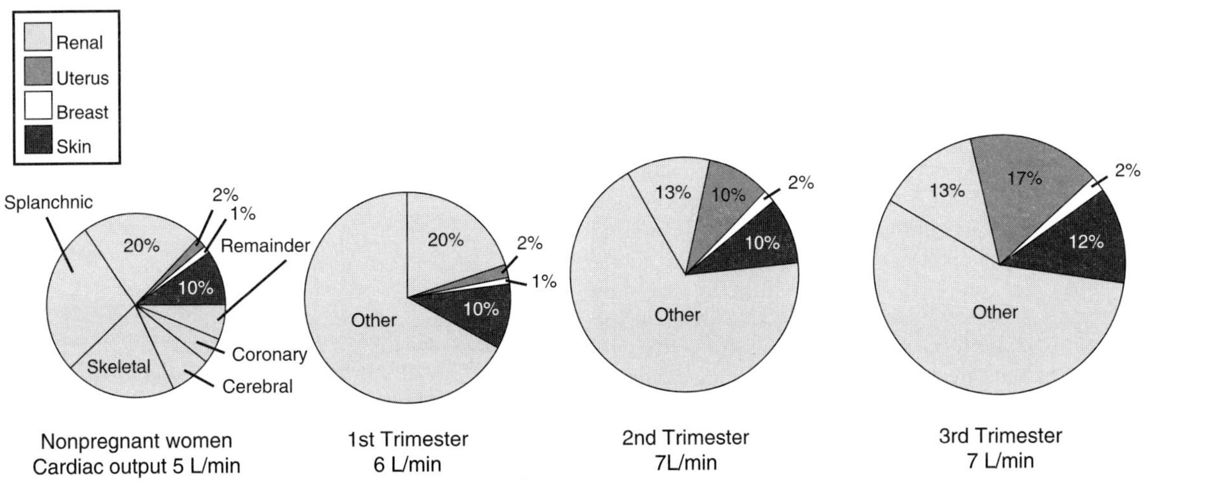

FIGURE 23–3. Percentage of total cardiac output flowing to organs in the nonpregnant and pregnant woman in each trimester of pregnancy. The increases in blood flow to the skin and breast may be responsible for the malar flush of pregnancy and a mammary souffle heard on auscultation. (From Burrow GN, Ferris TF (eds): Medical Complications During Pregnancy, 3rd ed. WB Saunders, Philadelphia, 1988, with permission).

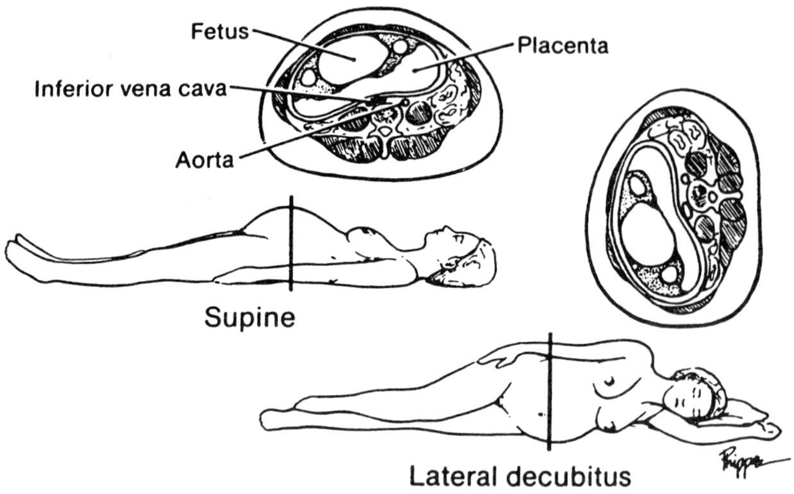

FIGURE 23–5. The gravid uterus may cause compression of abdominal vessels in the supine position. The inferior vena cava may be compressed, decreasing venous return to the heart. Aortic compression may be severe enough to cause a supine hypotensive syndrome and a decrease in uteroplacental perfusion. (From Lee RV, Mezzadri FC: Cardiopulmonary resuscitation of pregnant women. In Elkayam U, Gleicher N (eds): Cardiac Problems in Pregnancy, 2nd ed. Alan R. Liss, New York, 1990, pp 307–319, with permission.)

tation occurs, probably as a result of increased levels of gestational hormones, including progesterone, circulating prostaglandins, and atrial natriuretic factor, that foster relaxation of tubular structures, all in an environment of more heat production from the developing fetus and an enlarged uterus with a low-resistance circulation.[23, 24]

Hemodynamic Influence of a Gravid Uterus

Body position substantially affects cardiac output and thus uteroplacental blood flow, particularly in the supine position, during the third trimester.[25] The effect is so significant that a hypotensive pregnant patient should not be left supine. During the second half of pregnancy, the uterus expands beyond the pelvis. Mechanical compression of the iliac veins and arteries and the inferior vena cava against the spine decreases venous return to the heart and results in development of collateral paravertebral circulation to drain the lower extremities (Fig. 23–5).[26] There is also aortoiliac artery compression late in pregnancy that may have significant effects on uteroplacental perfusion, especially during low-flow states.[27] Uterine blood flow is about 3% of cardiac output during the first trimester and increases to between 10% and 20% by the third trimester.[23] At term, when a supine patient changes position to the lateral recumbent position, a 25% increase in cardiac output may occur. A supine hypotensive syndrome may develop, owing to compression of the inferior vena cava and pelvic veins, which can cause sequestration of up to 30% of blood volume.[28] During resuscitation and operative procedures, the supine position must be avoided by placing a wedge or blanket beneath the right hip to rotate the body slightly to the left; this may help to maintain uterine blood flow. There is also a mechanical effect on the diaphragm and lungs, with compression of the thoracic cavity causing changes in the chest x-ray and the cardiac examination (Fig. 23–6).[29]

Exercise Response

At rest, the pregnant patient usually has a sinus tachycardia, which helps to maintain the higher cardiac output at any given workload.[30] There is an increase in maternal oxygen consumption to approximately 20% above that in the nonpregnant state.[31] During the third trimester, the effect of the enlarged heart and the gravid uterus in decreasing venous return in certain positions limits the normal stroke volume response to exercise.[32] The maximal cardiac output is reached at lower levels of exercise during pregnancy, and increases in output in response to exercise are limited as pregnancy progresses.[32]

During the third trimester, normal subjects may experience a 25% decrease in uterine blood flow during mild exercise, which may cause fetal hypoxia and episodic bradycardia.[33] Strenuous exercise during pregnancy is not recommended. The usual effect of training is not seen during pregnancy but returns within weeks after delivery (Fig. 23–7).[34]

Hemodynamics of Labor and Delivery

Delivery has been described as a state of physiologic hemorrhage, with an average blood loss of approximately 500 ml.

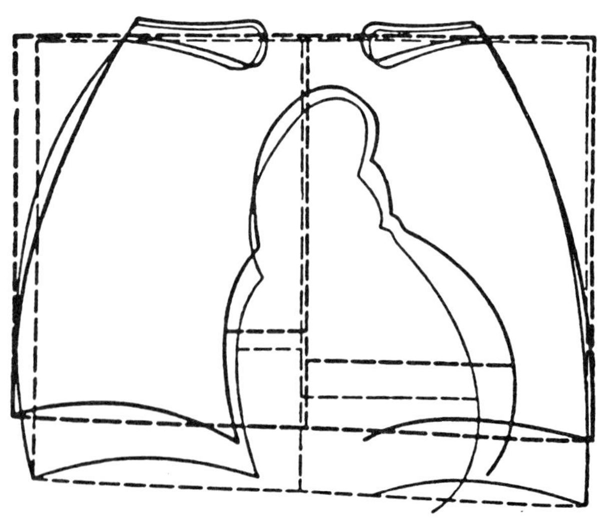

FIGURE 23–6. During pregnancy, there is an elevation of the diaphragm, causing a change in the cardiac outline seen on chest x-ray study and on physical examination. The heavy lines represent the pregnant state; the lighter lines represent the nonpregnant state. (From Klaften E, Palugyay J: Arch Gynaekol 131:347, 1927, with permission.)

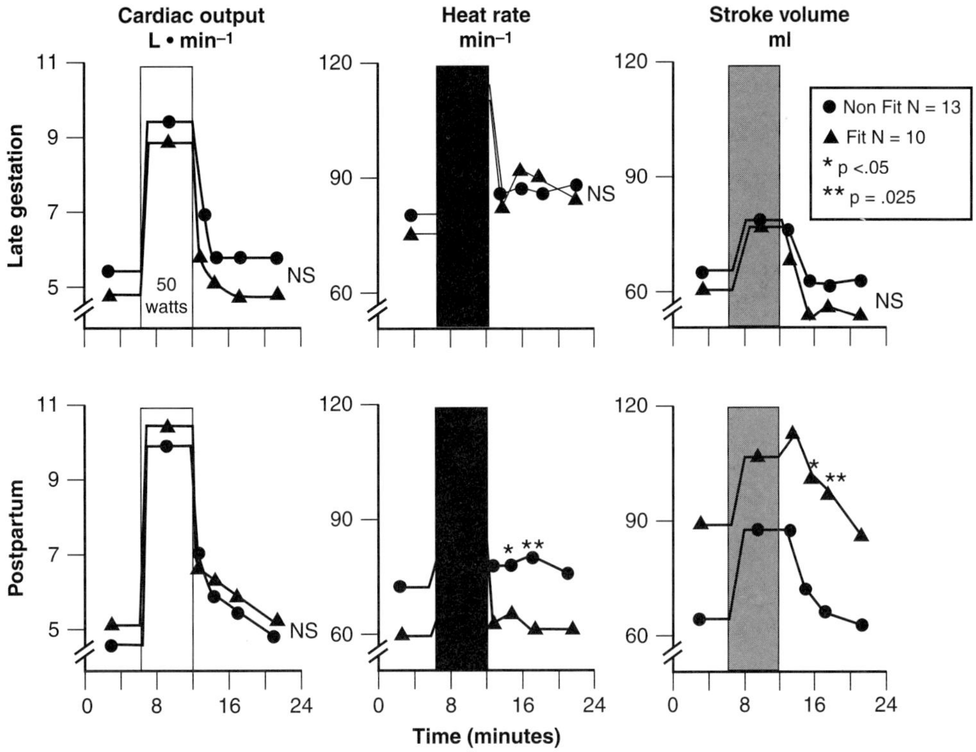

FIGURE 23–7. The usual effect of training is not seen during pregnancy but returns after delivery. This is shown by heart rate, cardiac output, and stroke volume measurements. Nonpregnant, physically trained individuals usually respond to exercise with a greater stroke volume and a smaller increase in heart rate than untrained individuals. Pregnancy causes an increase in cardiac ouput at any given level of exercise, and the maximum is reached at lower levels of exercise during pregnancy. Stroke volume response may be limited by a decrease in venous return from vena caval obstruction by the gravid uterus in late gestation. (From Burrow GN, Ferris TF (eds): Medical Complications During Pregnancy, 3rd ed. WB Saunders, Philadelphia, 1988, with permission.)

During labor, heart rate and blood pressure rise; cardiac output may increase by 30% to 60% during uterine contractions, with a cumulative increase between contractions, probably resulting from increased venous return of blood squeezed from the uterus (Table 23–2).[35] The rise in blood pressure is most marked during the second stage of labor. There is an increase in oxygen consumption of up to three times the normal level.

Hemodynamic changes are less pronounced in the left lateral recumbent position and are affected by the type of anesthesia and analgesia used. Caudal and local types of anesthesia usually do not alter hemodynamic variables and may be safer in patients with heart disease.[36] There is a less dramatic change in patients who undergo cesarean section, depending on the type of anesthesia used. Marked fluctuations are seen with subarachnoid block anesthesia; smaller fluctuations occur with thiopental, nitrous oxide, and succinylcholine and with epidural anesthesia without epinephrine.[37–39]

Table 23–2. CARDIOCIRCULATORY EFFECTS OF UTERINE CONTRACTION*

PARAMETER	CHANGE	COMMENTS
Blood volume	↑	300–500 ml
Cardiac output	↑	30–60% with cumulative increase between contractions
Heart rate	↑ ↓	Variable responses
Blood pressure	↑	Significant rise of both systolic and diastolic blood pressures; return to baseline between contractions
Peripheral resistance	↔	
Oxygen consumption	↑	Gradual increase to average of 100%

*Hemodynamic effects of uterine contractions are less pronounced in lateral recumbency than in the supine position.

↑, increase; ↓, decrease; ↔, no significant change.

From Elkayam U, Gleicher N (eds): Cardiac Problems in Pregnancy, 2nd ed. Alan R. Liss, New York, 1990.

Postpartum Changes

Immediately after delivery, cardiac output may be increased by 60% to 80%, depending on the type of anesthesia used, but it decreases soon thereafter. There is an increase in venous return as soon as the fetus is delivered, thus relieving caval compression. Autotransfusion of blood from the uterus into the systemic circulation occurs, increasing cardiac preload. There is a reduction in heart rate within hours after delivery, causing a decrease in cardiac output. Cardiac output usually falls to pre-pregnancy levels within 24 hours after delivery, but it may remain elevated for a few weeks.[35]

Physiology of Multiple Fetuses

More widespread use of fertility agents has raised the incidence of multiple fetuses. The uterus is larger in a multiple pregnancy, causing more mechanical effects, including compression and displacement of thoracic and abdominal contents. There are greater alterations in maternal physiology with multiple fetuses, including a more pronounced increase in heart rate. Blood volume increases by 50% to 60%, or 500 ml more with twin fetuses than with a single fetus.[40] Average blood loss is 935 ml with twins, almost 500 ml more than with a single fetus.[41] Cardiac output is increased over that in single pregnancies, whereas the end-diastolic dimensions are approximately the same.[42] During the third trimester, the increased cardiac output is due to increases in heart rate and stroke volume, whereas in a single pregnancy it is due to heart rate effects primarily by term. The risk for serious maternal complications is greater because of the increased stress. Pregnancy-induced hypertension is more prevalent and is associated with more frequent complications.

CARDIAC EVALUATION

The normal adaptations to pregnancy lead to subjective symptoms, changes in the physical examination, and altered diagnostic test results that may mimic or mask cardiac disease. Anatomic alterations occur, such as heart enlargement with an increase in left ventricular end-diastolic volume and a structural alteration in the heart muscle itself. Dynamics also change, with a constant variation in preload and afterload. Despite these changes, the ejection fraction is usually not changed during pregnancy.[43] Even women with normal pregnancies often have symptoms of fatigue, decreased exercise capacity, palpitations, orthopnea, dyspnea, lightheadedness, and hyperventilation (Table 23–3).[44] It is important to be aware both of the signs and symptoms of normal pregnancy and of those that may herald underlying heart or vascular disease (Table 23–4).

Table 23–3. CARDIAC SYMPTOMS AND FINDINGS DURING NORMAL PREGNANCY

Symptoms

Decreased exercise capacity
Tiredness
Dyspnea
Orthopnea
Lightheadedness
Syncope

Physical Findings

Inspection
- Hyperventilation
- Peripheral edema
- Distended neck veins with prominent A and V waves and brisk X and Y descents
- Capillary pulsation

Precordial palpation
- Brisk, diffuse, and displaced left ventricular impulse
- Palpable right ventricular impulse
- Palpable pulmonary trunk impulse

Auscultation
- Pulmonary rales
- Increased first heart sound with exaggerated splitting
- Persistent splitting of second heart sound
- Early and midsystolic ejection-type murmurs at the lower left sternal edge and/or over the pulmonary area
- Continuous murmurs (cervical venous hum, mammary souffle)
- Diastolic murmurs

From Elkayam U, Gleicher N (eds): Cardiac Problems in Pregnancy, 2nd ed. Alan R. Liss, New York, 1990.

Table 23–4. INDICATORS OF HEART DISEASE DURING PREGNANCY

Symptoms

Severe or progressive dyspnea
Progressive orthopnea
Paroxysmal nocturnal dyspnea
Hemoptysis
Syncope with exertion
Chest pain related to effort or emotion

Signs

Cyanosis
Clubbing
Persistent neck vein distention
Systolic murmur greater than grade I/VI in intensity
Diastolic murmur
Cardiomegaly, general or localized
A split second sound, persisting unchanged during expiration
Criteria for pulmonary hypertension
- Left parasternal lift
- Loud P_2

From Burrow GN, Ferris TF (eds): Medical Complications During Pregnancy, 3rd ed. WB Saunders, Philadelphia, 1988.

Cardiac Examination

Vasculature

The jugular veins are often distended by an increase in blood volume. Venous vascular beds are more prominent, especially in the lower extremities, even during the first trimester, before caval compression by the enlarged uterus occurs (Fig. 23–8). Venous distensibility increases in the legs, with compliance being highest in the second trimester; this is similar to the effects seen in women who are taking progestin-based oral contraceptives. The antecubital venous pressure remains unchanged (see Fig. 23–8). Arterial pulsations are usually full and rapidly collapsing.

Precordium

The precordium is usually active, with a palpable left ventricular impulse that is usually displaced to the left in later pregnancy. A palpable pulmonary artery and right ventricular impulse are usually present. On auscultation, an increased first sound with exaggerated splitting is sometimes noted. The second heart sound may be increased in intensity late in pregnancy and widely split in the left lateral position. Third and fourth heart sounds have been noted in some normal pregnant women, but they are usually considered abnormal.[45, 46]

Murmurs

Systolic murmurs are usually innocent and are caused by the hyperkinetic circulation of pregnancy. A systolic murmur

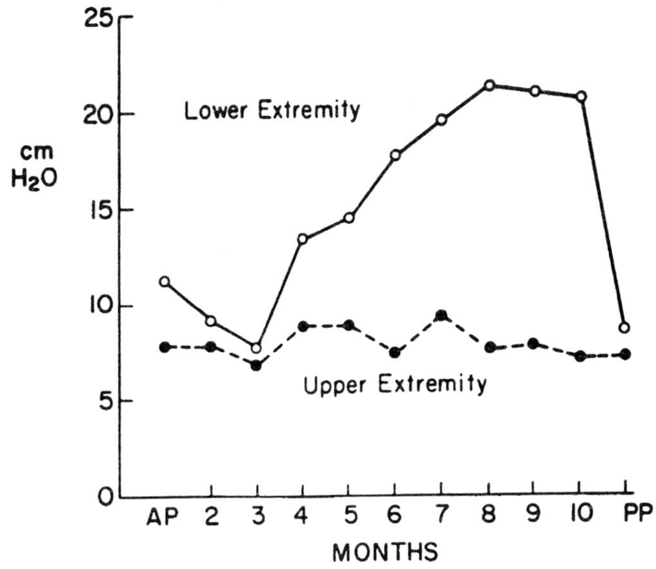

FIGURE 23–8. Upper and lower extremity venous pressures are shown in cm H_2O in relation to months of pregnancy (AP, antepartum measurement; PP, postpregnancy.) Venous distensibility in the calf is always greater than in the forearm and this widens as pregnancy progresses. (From Creasy R, Resnik R (eds): Maternal-Fetal Medicine: Principles and Practice, 2nd ed. WB Saunders, Philadelphia, 1989, with permission.)

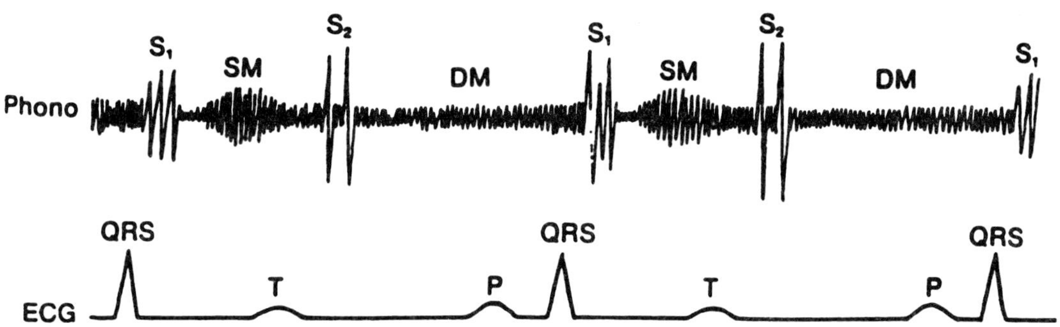

FIGURE 23–9. Phonocardiographic and electrocardiographic tracing of mammary souffle, a continuous murmur found in 15% of pregnant women near term or during lactation. (From Tilkian AG, Conover MB: Understanding Heart Sounds and Murmurs, 2nd ed. WB Saunders, Philadelphia, 1984, with permission.)

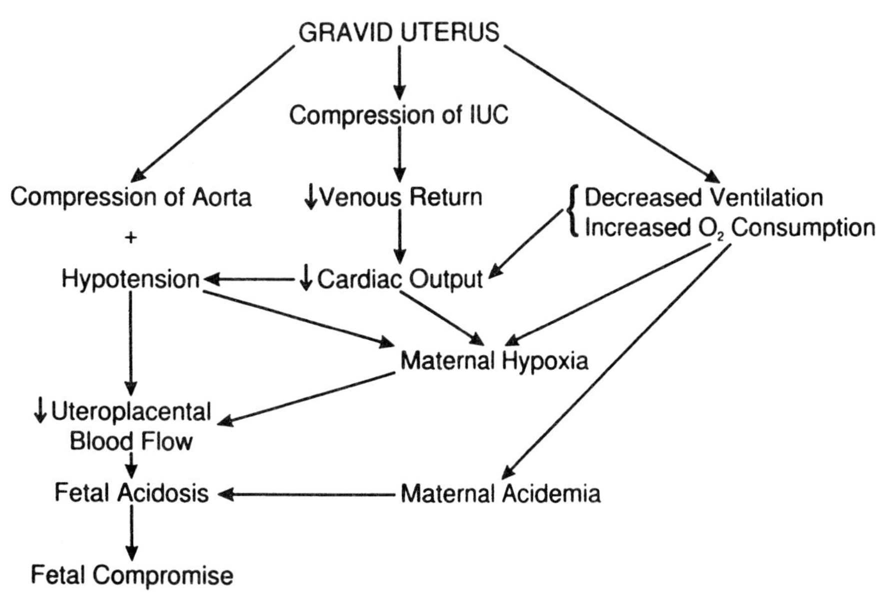

FIGURE 23–10. The effects of pregnancy and the gravid uterus on the cardiovascular system's response to cardiac arrest and resuscitation. (From Lee RV, Mezzadri FC: Cardiopulmonary resuscitation of pregnant women. In Elkayam U, Gleicher N (eds): Cardiac Problems in Pregnancy, 2nd ed. Alan R. Liss, New York, 1990, pp 307–319, with permission.)

Table 23–5. CAUSES OF MATERNAL CARDIOPULMONARY COMPROMISE

Cardiovascular
Decreased cardiac output
Arrhythmia
Critical valvular obstruction
Pericardial tamponade
Hypertrophic obstructive cardiomyopathy
Myocardial dysfunction
Ischemia/infarction
Coronary artery dissection
Peripartum cardiomyopathy
Myocarditis
Congestive heart failure
Trauma: cardiac contusion/perforation
Vascular
Aortic dissection/rupture
Pulmonary
Pulmonary embolism
Amniotic fluid embolism
Pneumothorax
Aspiration pneumonitis
Angioedema
Status asthmaticus
Obstetric Complications
Amniotic fluid embolism
Hemorrhage/hypovolemia
Tocolytic (contraction suppression) therapy
Shock
Hypovolemia
Sepsis
Anaphylaxis
Neurogenic causes
Trauma
Miscellaneous
Drugs: cocaine, poisoning, overdose
Electrolyte imbalance
Anesthetic complication

occurs in virtually every pregnant woman, beginning late in the first or early in the second trimester, and persists for the duration of the pregnancy. Innocent murmurs are usually grade I to III/VI, soft, and short and have a systolic ejection quality, usually peaking in midsystole. They are commonly heard over the entire precordium. Systolic murmurs should be evaluated further when there is a change in the character of the murmur, an associated fever, accompanying symptoms or signs of congestive heart failure, a change in cardiac rhythm, and when there is a history of intravenous drug use, rheumatic fever, mitral valve prolapse, or congenital heart disease.[47]

A cervical venous hum may be heard over the right supraclavicular fossa, which usually vanishes with pressure applied by the stethoscope at the site where the venous hum is heard or when the patient assumes the upright position.[45] A "mammary souffle," due to the increased blood flow in mammary vessels, may be detected either as a systolic or a continuous murmur (Fig. 23–9).[48, 49]

Any diastolic murmur should be carefully evaluated to rule out organic disease, even though some soft, medium- to high-pitched diastolic murmurs have been reported in normal pregnancies. Diastolic murmurs may be due to increased flow through the tricuspid or mitral valve or to physiologic dilatation of the pulmonary artery during pregnancy.[50]

Underlying systolic murmurs from aortic or pulmonic stenosis or diastolic murmurs from mitral stenosis may be louder because of the increased blood volume during pregnancy. Murmurs associated with regurgitation across the mitral and aortic valves often decrease in intensity secondary to a reduction in systemic vascular resistance during pregnancy.[45–47] In fact, these murmurs are sometimes inaudible during pregnancy. The increase in intravascular volume may also cause the systolic click and murmur of mitral valve prolapse and the systolic murmur of hypertrophic cardiomyopathy to become inaudible or shorter during the late stages of pregnancy.[50–52]

APPROACH TO CLINICAL PROBLEMS

Hypotension

Most unstable situations are handled by placing the patient in the left lateral decubitus position with fetal monitoring, administration of oxygen, maintenance of fluid, and removal of any agents that may be contributing to the hypotension. Hypotensive patients must not be left supine because of potential deleterious mechanical effects (see Figs. 23–5 and 23–10). If uteroplacental blood flow is reduced owing to reduced volume, this must be corrected.[53] In sepsis or low-flow states, there is a greater risk of intravascular coagulopathy because of the enhanced clotting factors associated with pregnancy.[13, 14] There is some danger in administration of large amounts of fluids because of the reduced colloid oncotic pressure and the resulting greater tendency for capillary leakage and even precipitation of pulmonary edema.[51]

Cardiac Arrest

The changes in cardiovascular physiology render pregnant women more susceptible to, and less tolerant of, cardiovas-

Table 23–6. RESUSCITATION STRATEGY FOR PREGNANT PATIENTS

TIME (min)	STRATEGY
0	Initiate CPR Intubate mother; control pH, PCO_2 Monitor fetal studies at least every 60 sec
1	Unwitnessed arrest, no maternal response: deliver and continue maternal resuscitation
4	Witnessed arrest, patient past 32 weeks, no maternal response: deliver and continue maternal resuscitation
	Witnessed arrest, patient 24–32 weeks, no maternal response: open-chest massage, if no response in 60–90 sec: deliver, surfactant for infant as needed, continue maternal resuscitation
	Witnessed arrest, patient past 24 weeks, maternal response: continue life support, deliver for fetal indications
15	Witnessed arrest, patient past 24 weeks, infant viable but still requires cardiac massage: deliver, continue maternal resuscitation

From Lee RV, Mezzadri FC: Cardiopulmonary resuscitation of pregnant women. In Elkayam U, Gleicher N (eds): Cardiac Problems in Pregnancy, 2nd ed. Alan R. Liss, New York, 1990, pp 307–319.

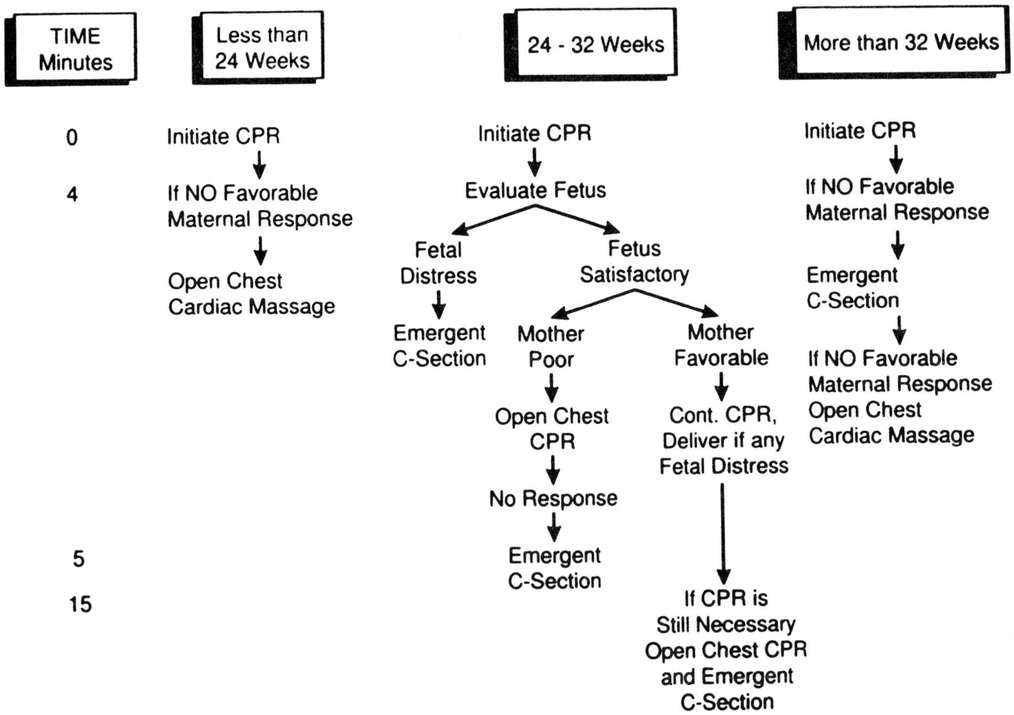

FIGURE 23–11. Approach to consideration of emergent cesarean section to salvage the fetus, considered in relation to age of gestation and duration of cardiopulmonary arrest. (From Lee RV, Mezzadri FC: Cardiopulmonary resuscitation of pregnant women. In Elkayam U, Gleicher N (eds): Cardiac Problems in Pregnancy, 2nd ed. Alan R. Liss, New York, 1990, pp 307–319, with permission.)

cular insult.[54] Precipitators of cardiac arrest (Table 23–5) include cardiovascular, pulmonary, and obstetric complications, as well as shock, surgery, or drug effects.[53–55]

In the supine position, the gravid uterus compresses iliac vessels, the inferior vena cava, and the abdominal aorta, which may cause hypotension with a reduction in cardiac output of up to 25% (see Fig. 23–10). To minimize the pressure from the gravid uterus during resuscitation, a pillow or wedge is placed under the right abdominal flank area and hip to displace the uterus slightly to the left, or continuous manual displacement to the left can be performed by an assistant.[53, 55] Standard resuscitative measures should be used, including defibrillation for ventricular fibrillation and standard pharmacologic therapy, including vasopressors (Table 23–6.[55]

If the initiation of resuscitative measures, fluid restoration, or the release of uterine mass effect does not produce immediate stability, emergent cesarean section should be considered (Fig. 23–11).[56, 57] This decision should be made and delivery performed within 4 to 5 minutes of cardiac arrest to maximize the chances of survival of mother and fetus, although there have been reports of infant survival after more than 20 minutes of cardiac arrest.

References

1. McAnulty JH, Metcalfe J, Ueland K: Heart disease and pregnancy. In Hurst JW, Schlant RC, Rackley CE, et al (eds): The Heart: Arteries and Veins, 7th ed. McGraw-Hill Information Services, New York, 1990, pp 1465–1478.
2. Otterson WN, Dunnihoo DR: Cardiac disease. In Pauerstein CJ (ed): Clinical Obstetrics. John Wiley & Sons, New York, 1987, pp 627–647.
3. Leyse R, Ofstun M, Dillard DH, et al: Congenital aortic stenosis in pregnancy, corrected by extracorporeal circulation, offering a viable male infant at term but with anomalies eventuating in his death at four months of age—report of a case. JAMA 176:1009, 1961.
4. Gant NF, Daley GL, Chand S, et al: A study of angiotensin II pressor response throughout primigravid pregnancy. J Clin Invest 52:2682, 1973.
5. Walsh SW, Parisi VM: Eicosanoids and hypertension in pregnancy. In Mitchell MD (ed): Eicosanoids in Reproduction. CRC Press, Orlando, FL, 1990, pp 249–272.
6. Guyton AC: Textbook of Medical Physiology, 5th ed. WB Saunders, Philadelphia, 1976.
7. Lund CJ, Donovan JC: Blood volume during pregnancy. Am J Obstet Gynecol 98:393, 1967.
8. Chesley LC: Plasma and red cell volumes during pregnancy. Am J Obstet Gynecol 112:440, 1972.
9. Lindheimer MD, Katz AI: Sodium and diuretics in pregnancy. N Engl J Med 288:891, 1973.
10. Cusson JR, Gutkowska J, Rey E, et al: Plasma concentration of atrial natriuretic factor in normal pregnancy. N Engl J Med 313:1230, 1985.
11. Rutherford AJ, Anderson JV, Elder MG, et al: Release of atrial natriuretic peptide during pregnancy and immediate puerperium. Lancet 1: 928, 1987.
12. Huisman A, Aarnoudse JG, Heuvelmans JHA, et al: Whole blood viscosity during normal pregnancy. Br J Obstet Gynaecol 94:1143, 1987.
13. Ozanne P, Linderkamp O, Miller FC, et al: Erythrocyte aggregation during normal pregnancy. Am J Obstet Gynecol 147:576, 1983.
14. Pitkin RM, Witte DL: Platelet and leukocyte counts in pregnancy. JAMA 242:2696, 1980.
15. Rakoczi F, Tallian F, Bagdany S, et al: Platelet life-span in normal pregnancy and pre-eclampsia as determined by nonradioisotope technique. Thromb Res 15:553, 1979.
16. Katz R, Karliner JS, Resnik R: Effects of a natural volume overload state (pregnancy) on left ventricular performance in normal human subjects. Circulation 58:434, 1978.
17. Dilts PV, Brinkman CR, Kirschbaum TH, et al: Uterine and systemic hemodynamic interrelationships and their response to hypoxia. Am J Obstet Gynecol 103:138, 1969.
18. Karlsson K: The influence of hypoxia on uterine and maternal placental

blood flow and the effect of alpha-adrenergic blockade. J Perinatol Med 2:176, 1974.
19. Metcalfe J, Ueland K: Maternal cardiovascular adjustments to pregnancy. Prog Cardiovasc Dis 16:363, 1974.
20. Rovinsky JJ, Jaffin H: Cardiovascular hemodynamics in pregnancy: III. Cardiac rate, stroke volume, total peripheral resistance, and central blood volume in multiple pregnancy: Synthesis of results. Am J Obstet Gynecol 95:787, 1966.
21. Christianson RE: Studies on blood pressure during pregnancy: I. Influence of parity and age. Am J Obstet Gynecol 125:509, 1976.
22. Rovinsky JJ: Blood volume and the hemodynamics of pregnancy. In Philipp EE, Parnes J, Newton M (eds): Scientific Foundation of Obstetrics and Gynaecology. FA Davis, Philadelphia, 1970, pp 332–340.
23. Metcalfe J, Romney SL, Ramsey LH, et al: Estimation of uterine blood flow in normal human pregnancy at term. J Clin Invest 34:1632, 1955.
24. Wood JE: The cardiovascular effects of oral contraceptives. Mod Concepts Cardiovasc Dis 4:37, 1972.
25. Ueland K, Novy MJ, Peterson EN, et al: Maternal cardiovascular dynamics: IV. The influence of gestational age on the maternal cardiovascular response to posture and exercise. Am J Obstet Gynecol 104: 856, 1969.
26. Kerr MG, Scott DB, Samuel E: Studies of the inferior vena cava in late pregnancy. BMJ 1:532, 1964.
27. Bieniarz J, Crottongini JJ, Curuchet E, et al: Aortocaval compression by the uterus in late human pregnancy: II. An angiographic study. Am J Obstet Gynecol 100:203, 1968.
28. Howard BK, Goodson JH, Mengert WF: Supine hypotensive syndrome in late pregnancy. Obstet Gynecol 1:371, 1953.
29. Kerr MG: The mechanical effects of the gravid uterus in late pregnancy. J Obstet Gynaecol Br Commonw 72:513, 1965.
30. Artal R, Wiswell R: Exercise in Pregnancy. Williams & Wilkins, Baltimore, 1986.
31. Prowse CM, Gaensler EA: Respiratory and acid-base changes during pregnancy. Anesthesiology 26:381, 1965.
32. Morton MJ, Metcalfe J: Changes in maternal hemodynamics during pregnancy. In Artal R, Wiswell R (eds): Exercise in Pregnancy. Williams & Wilkins, Baltimore, 1986.
33. Morris N, Osborn SB, Wright HP, et al: Effective uterine blood flow during exercise in normal and pre-eclamptic pregnancies. Lancet 2: 481, 1956.
34. Morton MJ, Paul MS, Campos GR, et al: Exercise dynamics in late gestation: Effects of physical training. Am J Obstet Gynecol 152:91, 1985.
35. Adams JG, Alexander AM: Alterations in cardiovascular physiology during labor. Am J Obstet Gynecol 12:542, 1958.
36. Ueland K, Hansen JM: Maternal cardiovascular dynamics: III. Labor and delivery under local and caudal analgesia. Am J Obstet Gynecol 103:8, 1969.
37. Ueland K, Gills RE, Hansen J: Maternal cardiovascular dynamics: I. Cesarean section under subarachnoid block anesthesia. Am J Obstet Gynecol 42:100, 1968.
38. Ueland K, Hansen J, Eng M, et al: Maternal cardiovascular dynamics: V. Cesarean section under thiopental, nitrous oxide and succinyl choline anesthesia. Am J Obstet Gynecol 108:615, 1970.
39. Ueland K, Akamatsu TJ, Eng M, et al: Cardiovascular dynamics: VI. Cesarean section under epidural anesthesia without epinephrine. Am J Obstet Gynecol 114:775, 1972.
40. Veille JC, Morton MJ, Burry KJ: Maternal cardiovascular adaptations to twin pregnancy. Am J Obstet Gynecol 153:261, 1985.
41. Long PA, Oats JN: Preeclampsia in twin pregnancy—severity and pathogenesis. Aust NZ J Obstet Gynaecol 27:1, 1987.
42. Quinley MM, Cruikshank DP: Polyhydramnios and acute renal failure. J Reprod Med 19:92, 1977.
43. Rubler S, Prabodhkumar MD, Pinto ER: Cardiac size and performance during pregnancy estimated with echocardiography. Clin Obstet Gynecol 40:534, 1977.
44. Milne JA, Howie AD, Pack AI: Dyspnea during normal pregnancy. Br J Obstet Gynaecol 85:260, 1978.
45. Cutforth R, MacDonald MB: Heart sounds and murmurs in pregnancy. Am Heart J 71:741, 1966.
46. O'Rourke RA, Ewy GA, Marcus FI: Cardiac auscultation in pregnancy. Med Ann DC 39:92, 1970.
47. Hurst JW, Staton J, Hubbard D: Precordial murmurs during pregnancy and lactation. N Engl J Med 259:515, 1958.
48. Grant RP: A precordial systolic murmur of extracardiac origin during pregnancy. Am Heart J 52:944, 1956.
49. Tabatznik B, Randall TW, Hersch C: The mammary souffle of pregnancy and lactation. Circulation 22:1069, 1960.
50. Perloff JK: The clinical recognition of congenital heart disease. In Braunwald E (ed): Heart Disease, 3rd ed. WB Saunders, Philadelphia, 1988, pp 990–991.
51. Hytten EF, Thomson AM, Taggart N: Total body water in normal pregnancy. J Obstet Gynaecol Br Commonw 73:553, 1966.
52. Sullivan JM, Ramanathan KB: Management of medical problems in pregnancy: Severe cardiac disease. N Engl J Med 313:304, 1985.
53. Lee RV, Mezzadri FC: Cardiopulmonary resuscitation of pregnant women. In Elkayam U, Gleicher N: Cardiac Problems in Pregnancy, 2nd ed. Alan R. Liss, New York, 1990, pp 307–319.
54. Sachs BP, Brown DAJ, Driscoll SG, et al: Maternal mortality in Massachusetts. N Engl J Med 316:667, 1987.
55. American Heart Association: Special resuscitation situations. JAMA 268:2249, 1992.
56. Songster GS, Clark SL: Cardiac arrest in pregnancy: What to do? Contemp Obstet Gynecol 27:141, 1985.
57. Lee RV, Rodgers BD, White LM, et al: Cardiopulmonary resuscitation of pregnant women. Am J Med 81:311, 1986.

CHAPTER 24

Congenital Heart Disease in Pregnancy: Pathophysiology, Clinical Recognition, Diagnosis, and Management

Jack M. Colman, Mathew Sermer, Gareth Seaward, and Samuel C. Siu

Remarkable advances have been made recently in the diagnosis and treatment of congenital heart disease (CHD), especially in the area of surgical repair. Because of these advances, 90% of patients with CHD now survive to adulthood.[1] The population is heterogeneous, and many of the conditions are rare. To manage effectively a pregnant patient with CHD, the effect of the normal physiologic changes of pregnancy (see Chapter 23) on the abnormal physiology of the congenital lesion must be anticipated. Therefore, the physician must understand the specific congenital anomaly, the type of prior surgical correction, and the residua and sequelae[2] after treatment. Few systematic studies of the natural history of CHD in pregnancy are available. Moreover, no controlled clinical trials have been conducted and broad experience in managing these cases is rare.[3] Seemingly contradictory or arbitrary statements and recommendations are often found in the literature. Time, experience, and data are necessary to define guidelines for treating pregnant women with CHD. Fortunately, the outcome of pregnancy is favorable in many women with CHD. If an unfavorable outcome is likely, appropriate preconception counseling should be offered. If the effect of pregnancy is unknown, the uncertainty should be acknowledged and advice should be tentative.

PATHOPHYSIOLOGY

Despite the variability of individual congenital lesions and the various types of surgical procedures used to treat them, certain pathophysiologic processes are common to different anomalies, and some generalizations can be applied.

Pressure Loading

Increased pressure load is imposed by outflow tract obstruction below, at, or above the level of the semilunar valves, or by an increase in resistance at the arteriolar level. The usual increases in stroke volume and cardiac output that occur in pregnancy[4] pose a major challenge to a pressure-overloaded ventricle. These increases may result in ventricular failure, arrhythmias, or myocardial ischemia. When a systemic-to-pulmonary shunt is present, offloading occurs across the shunt, which, in the case of right-sided obstruction, causes an increase in the right-to-left shunt and further systemic desaturation.

Volume Loading

Volume overload results from valvular insufficiency or left-to-right shunting. Pregnancy amplifies the volume challenge, but adverse consequences are attenuated by a reduction in peripheral vascular resistance that reduces systemic ventricular afterload, thereby lessening aortic or mitral regurgitation and limiting the increase in the left-to-right shunt. Notwithstanding, the incremental changes of pregnancy may cause congestive heart failure in patients with underlying ventricular dysfunction.

Cyanosis

Cyanosis in CHD is a surrogate measure of arterial hypoxemia. (Cyanosis resulting from increased peripheral extraction is not considered here.) No agreement has been reached on what constitutes a significant reduction in arterial oxygen saturation, but in one study most patients with clinical cyanosis had SaO_2 less than 0.85.[5] Arterial hypoxemia in CHD results when desaturated venous blood is not exposed to pulmonary alveolar oxygen before reaching the systemic circulation. This situation results from obligatory mixing (in a common atrium or ventricle), intrapulmonary arteriovenous malformations, or right-to-left shunting.

Maternal consequences of cyanosis include hyperviscosity caused by erythrocytosis, abnormal hemostasis, intravascular thrombosis, hyperuricemia, renal dysfunction, and gallstones. Severely cyanotic women are rarely encountered in pregnancy because those who have not undergone surgical correction or a palliative procedure are often advised to avoid conception; these patients have a high spontaneous abortion rate.[5] Patients who have undergone palliative procedures or those with milder lesions, even those without overt cyanosis who have good functional capacity, are also at risk because right-to-left shunting will increase during pregnancy as a consequence of the fall in peripheral vascular resistance.

Fetal outcome in cyanotic mothers is poor and relates

directly to maternal oxygen saturation.[5] In series reported by Presbitero and associates[5] and by Whittemore and colleagues,[6] the live birth rate was low (43% to 55%) and premature births (35%) and intrauterine growth restriction were common.[6]

When cyanosis results from reversed shunting in patients with the Eisenmenger reaction (obstructive pulmonary vascular disease that develops when a congenital left-to-right shunt is not corrected in a timely fashion), the prognosis for the mother is even worse and is determined primarily by the severity of the pulmonary vascular disease itself (see discussion of Eisenmenger's syndrome).

Myocardial Dysfunction

Chronic hypoxemia in early life, long-standing pressure or volume overload, and delayed or multiple surgical procedures may be precursors to chronic ventricular dysfunction. If the right ventricle is functioning as the systemic ventricle, the patient is at a further disadvantage. Women with ventricular dysfunction may be asymptomatic or minimally symptomatic before pregnancy (New York Heart Association [NYHA] class I or II). However, discrepancies between subjective functional class and aerobic capacity[7] are often seen. The conditions of these patients may deteriorate, and they may develop overt congenital heart failure in response to the increased cardiac output requirements of pregnancy. Fetal effects include low birth weight and prematurity.

Arrhythmias and Conduction Defects

Chamber dilatation, myocardial hypertrophy, and myocardial fibrosis are substrates for arrhythmias. After congenital cardiac surgery, additional myocardial scarring or damage to sinus or atrioventricular (AV) nodes may occur. Heart block may occur in congenitally corrected transposition of the great arteries because of abnormal development of the AV conducting pathways. Lateral AV nodal bypass tracts, which predispose to the Wolff-Parkinson-White type of AV reentrant tachyarrhythmias, are found in Ebstein's anomaly. Sinus node dysfunction is a common late consequence of a Mustard or Senning atrial switch procedure for classic transposition of the great arteries.

Pregnancy may exacerbate supraventricular tachyarrhythmias such as atrial flutter or fibrillation, which are likely to be poorly tolerated in patients with right-ventricle–dependent systemic circulations, univentricular connections, or severe ventricular hypertrophy.

Aortopathy

In Marfan's syndrome, cystic medial necrosis predisposes to dilatation and dissection. In coarctation, the aorta is abnormal at the coarctation site and may be abnormal at other sites in the arterial tree. Bicuspid aortic valve may also be associated with an ascending aortopathy.[8, 9] In pregnancy, hormonally mediated weakening of the elastic fibers in the aortic wall and the hemodynamic stress of a volume-loaded hyperdynamic circulation further predispose women to enlargement, dissection, or rupture of the aorta.

Unoperated or residual coarctation increases the risk of pregnancy-induced hypertension. Antihypertensive therapy is more complex because control of maternal upper-body blood pressure may excessively reduce pressure in the uterine artery distal to the coarctation and thus cause placental insufficiency.

Prosthetic Materials, Valves, and Conduits

Xenograft valves do not require anticoagulation, but they degenerate more rapidly in women of child-bearing age. It has been claimed that pregnancy may accelerate this process,[10] but this has not been substantiated by more recent studies.[11, 12] Mechanical valves do require anticoagulation, which introduces certain hazards. Conduits narrow through pseudointimal proliferation, or they may be intrinsically small (especially if implanted in childhood); narrowing results in obstruction, the effects of which are magnified by increased cardiac output during pregnancy. Any prosthetic material in the heart increases the risk of endocarditis.

CLINICAL RECOGNITION AND DIAGNOSIS

Atrial Septal Defect

The most common type of atrial septal defect (ASD) is of the ostium secundum and is located at the fossa ovalis; other less common ASDs include sinus venosus and coronary sinus types and the so-called ostium primum ASD. Mitral valve prolapse is often associated with secundum ASD.[13] Because symptoms may be absent, the diagnosis is sometimes made only when the increased cardiac output of pregnancy enhances the previously subtle systolic murmur and parasternal lift. The diagnosis is most easily confirmed by echocardiography, which shows volume overload of the right-sided heart chambers and a left-to-right shunt across the defect, and provides an estimate of pulmonary artery pressure.

The effect of increase in cardiac output of pregnancy on left-to-right shunting may be counterbalanced by the decrease in peripheral vascular resistance, which attenuates the net increase in the left-to-right shunt. Pregnancy is well tolerated in the absence of pulmonary hypertension[14, 15]; maternal mortality is less than 1%.[14, 15]

Labor and delivery are usually uncomplicated. Arrhythmias, right ventricular dysfunction, and progression of pulmonary hypertension are more likely in older patients, in patients with a large shunt, and in patients with pre-existing pulmonary hypertension. Paradoxical embolization may be occasionally encountered when systemic vasodilatation and elevation of pulmonary resistance combine to produce transient right-to-left shunting.

Pregnancy is usually uneventful in a woman with a closed ASD and no residual defect; however, atrial arrhythmias may occur, especially if the defect was closed later in life.[16]

Ventricular Septal Defect

A ventricular septal defect (VSD) is the most common congenital cardiac anomaly at birth. Uncorrected VSDs are uncommon in adults because small defects often close spontaneously in childhood[17] and most larger defects will have been corrected surgically. Defects are most common in the membranous interventricular septum ("perimembranous VSD"), but they are also found in the muscular trabecular septum and in the outlet septum, where they may be associated with aortic cusp prolapse and regurgitation. The most common VSD in an adult is small and "restrictive," and causes a small left-to-right shunt, no significant left ventricular volume overload, and no increase in pulmonary pressure. A moderate VSD causes enlargement of the left ventricle resulting from volume overload and mild to moderate pulmonary hypertension, which may reverse after closure of the defect. A large VSD in an adult is seen only in association with right ventricular outflow tract obstruction or with Eisenmenger's syndrome.[18]

The extent of chamber enlargement and the presence of associated aortic valvular defects and pulmonary hypertension can be assessed by clinical examination and transthoracic echocardiography.

Pregnancy and delivery are well tolerated in patients with a small VSD.[19] A moderate VSD without significant pulmonary hypertension does not substantially increase the risks associated with pregnancy; however, increased left atrial and ventricular volume overload may lead to atrial arrhythmias or to progressive left ventricular dysfunction. With an increase in obstruction of pulmonary flow, the hemodynamic fluctuations of pregnancy and labor may cause shunt reversal, which can lead to hypoxemia, cyanosis, and possibly paradoxical emboli.[20, 21] In patients who have an uncorrected VSD associated with Eisenmenger physiology,[21, 22] the risks associated with pregnancy are very high. In a patient with a closed VSD, pregnancy should be normal unless pulmonary hypertension persists or other residua are present.

Atrioventricular Septal Defect

Atrioventricular septal defect (AVSD) results from abnormal development of the AV junction, which in turn leads to abnormal AV valves. The "ostium primum ASD," which is a partial AVSD, is managed like other ASDs; this defect may be associated with mitral regurgitation through a "cleft mitral valve." A complete AVSD includes a VSD and a common AV valve that may be regurgitant; if unrepaired in childhood, an AVSD will be associated with severe pulmonary vascular disease. If an AVSD has been repaired in infancy, the nature of the residual defects and surgical sequelae determines pregnancy risk and management.

Patent Ductus Arteriosus

Persistent patent ductus arteriosus (PDA) accounts for 5% to 10% of congenital cardiac defects. Small defects are indicated by a continuous systolic-diastolic murmur lateral to the upper left sternal border that peaks at S_2. Moderate defects will have a similar murmur, evidence of left ventricular volume overload, and wide systemic pulse pressure resulting from rapid runoff into the low pressure pulmonary artery. In addition, mild pulmonary hypertension may be present. A large defect may be associated with substantial left atrial and left ventricular volume overload, but progressive pulmonary vascular disease reduces the degree of left-to-right shunting as the Eisenmenger reaction develops. Because the physical findings of left ventricular volume overload overlap those usually seen in pregnancy, echocardiography is used to define chamber size and function and to estimate the degree of pulmonary hypertension.

Occasionally, a clinically silent PDA may be found on echocardiography; these patients have an excellent prognosis and do not need prophylaxis for endocarditis or other interventions.[23] Pregnancy is well tolerated in patients with a small PDA. Furthermore, pregnancy is well tolerated in patients with moderate to large defects who do not have significant pulmonary hypertension as long as ventricular function is not depressed. In these patients, the main stress is volume overload, and the increase in pulmonary flow and pressure expected as a result of increased cardiac output is mitigated by the pregnancy-mediated fall in systemic vascular resistance. If pulmonary vascular resistance is increased, patients should be treated the same as those with large VSDs. Ductal aneurysms may be present and may rupture during pregnancy.[24, 25] Again, Eisenmenger physiology is associated with a significant increase in unfavorable outcomes.[20]

Pregnancy, labor, and delivery are normal in patients with a closed PDA, unless there is residual pulmonary hypertension.

Left Ventricular Outflow Tract Obstruction; Bicuspid Aortic Valve

Left ventricular outflow tract obstruction (LVOTO) can occur at the supravalvular, valvular, and/or subvalvular levels. The hemodynamic consequences are similar at all three levels.

Bicuspid aortic valve, the most common congenital cardiac lesion in adults, has an incidence of 1% to 2%[26]; however, only 20% of those affected are women. A bicuspid aortic valve often functions normally.[27] Even so, in pregnant patients, a bicuspid aortic valve should remind physicians to exclude the uncommon but important association with aortic coarctation and to consider prophylaxis against endocarditis. In addition, a bicuspid aortic valve may be associated with an ascending aortopathy.[8]

Aortic stenosis usually complicates pregnancy because of the presence of a congenital bicuspid aortic valve; other causes of aortic stenosis include subvalvular fibromuscular ridge, tunnel-like hypoplasia of the LVOTO, and supravalvular aortic stenosis. Women with symptomatic aortic stenosis should delay pregnancy until after surgical correction. However, the absence of symptoms before pregnancy does not always indicate that pregnancy will be well tolerated. Any patient who may have significant aortic stenosis should be assessed by transthoracic echocardiography to define the level and severity of the obstruction and the degree of left ventricular dysfunction.[28]

In severe aortic stenosis during pregnancy, the ability of the heart to increase stroke volume and cardiac output may be limited, filling pressures may be abnormally elevated, and left ventricular systolic pressure may be high, which may hasten or exacerbate left ventricular dysfunction. In addition, the noncompliant hypertrophied ventricle is very sensitive to decreases in preload, which may lead to a profound drop in cardiac output and thus hypotension. There are many potential causes of a decrease in preload during pregnancy, labor, and delivery: compression of the inferior vena cava in late pregnancy, the vasodilating effects of anesthetic agents, peripartum blood loss, the Valsalva maneuver, and others.

This adverse pathophysiology places pregnant women at risk. In older studies, high maternal mortality rates[29] suggested that pregnancy was contraindicated in women with aortic stenosis. Even pregnancy termination was thought to be associated with increased risks.[29] More recent studies have used echocardiographic assessment, maternal monitoring, and intervention when required and have shown less severe consequences. The cumulative maternal mortality in congenital aortic stenosis from 12 series involving 65 patients and 106 pregnancies (including the early series) was 11%, and the perinatal mortality was 4%.[28] In our own recent (1986 to 1992) experience with 25 pregnancies in 13 women, 23 percent of the patients had severe aortic stenosis (aortic valve area ≤ 0.7 cm^2), and we found no maternal or perinatal loss.[28] The risk of therapeutic abortion has not been substantiated, so it may be a viable option in severe cases of aortic stenosis. Recent data do not support the recommendation that all women with aortic stenosis should avoid pregnancy; however, overall experience suggests that aortic stenosis is a serious hazard in pregnancy.

When aortic regurgitation is the primary hemodynamic aberration, a favorable outcome is anticipated unless the lesion is so severe that significant left ventricular dysfunction occurs.

Coarctation of the Aorta

Coarctation of the aorta often occurs as a discrete stenosis at the level of the ligamentum arteriosum, but it may be associated with proximal aortic hypoplasia. Usually associated with a bicuspid aortic valve (85% of cases), coarctation of the aorta may also be associated with aneurysm of the circle of Willis, VSD, and Turner's syndrome. In most patients, the coarctation will have been repaired before pregnancy. However, some patients will have residual aortic hypoplasia, which is suggested by the presence of differences in arm and leg blood pressures or a murmur over the back. Doppler echocardiography may overestimate coarctation gradients in the presence of tunnel stenosis.[30]

Coarctation should be repaired before pregnancy. Correction reduces the risk of dissection and rupture and facilitates the management of hypertension. Maternal mortality in patients with uncorrected coarctation is 3% to 4%[14, 19, 20, 31] and is higher in the presence of associated cardiac defects, aortopathy, or chronic hypertension.[32] Aortic rupture is a risk in the third trimester and during labor.[33, 34] The management of hypertension in pregnant patients with an uncorrected coarctation is problematic because reducing upper body hypertension may lead to excessive hypotension below the coarctation site, which may affect the fetus.[34] Intrauterine growth restriction and premature labor and delivery are more common.

Even after coarctation repair, pregnancy can be complicated by hypertension that requires treatment. If there is residual hypoplasia of the aortic arch, upper-body systolic hypertension may occur with exercise. The risk of dissection and aortic rupture is reduced in patients with a repaired coarctation but not eliminated. Connolly and coworkers[35] described maternal and fetal outcomes in 87 pregnancies in 39 patients with repaired or unrepaired coarctation. They reported no maternal deaths and one early neonatal death; maternal hypertension was common.

Right Ventricular Outflow Tract Obstruction; Pulmonary Stenosis

Right ventricular outflow tract obstruction (RVOTO) may occur at the supravalvular, valvular, and/or subvalvular level. Subvalvular obstruction usually occurs in conjunction with a VSD (see later section on tetralogy of Fallot).

Valvular pulmonic stenosis is a relatively common form of CHD in adults.[36] A midsystolic murmur high along the left sternal edge that increases with inspiration is longer and is associated with a palpable right ventricular impulse in cases of severe pulmonic stenosis. These findings overlap normal physiologic signs in pregnancy. Echocardiography may be used to estimate the pressure gradient and to classify the stenosis as mild (< 49 mm Hg), moderate (50 to 79 mm Hg), or severe ($\geq$ 80 mm Hg). Gradients increase with cardiac output during pregnancy; therefore, the severity of pulmonic stenosis may be overestimated if no pre-pregnancy studies are available.

Mild pulmonic stenosis and pulmonic stenosis that has been alleviated by valvuloplasty or surgery are well tolerated during pregnancy.[19, 37]

A patient with severe pulmonic stenosis can be asymptomatic before pregnancy. Nevertheless, the increased hemodynamic load of pregnancy may result in right-sided heart failure, atrial arrhythmias, or tricuspid regurgitation. Severe pulmonic stenosis should be corrected (usually by balloon valvuloplasty) before pregnancy.[19] Women with uncorrected moderate to severe pulmonary stenosis require close surveillance during pregnancy. If symptoms progress, balloon valvuloplasty during pregnancy should be considered. Fetal outcome in a pregnancy complicated by pulmonic stenosis is favorable.[38]

Pulmonary regurgitation, rare as an isolated lesion, is a frequent sequela of previous pulmonary valve repair. Generally well tolerated, pulmonary regurgitation should be corrected before pregnancy if symptomatic right ventricular dilatation and dysfunction with tricuspid regurgitation are noted.

Tetralogy of Fallot

Tetralogy of Fallot is the most common cause of cyanotic CHD. Essential features are RVOTO at the infundibular level and a large nonrestrictive VSD; a large aortic root that overrides the interventricular septum and right ventricular hypertrophy are also always found. Valvular pulmonary stenosis is often present. Aortic regurgitation, common in adults, may occasionally be progressive despite surgical correction of the tetralogy.

The degree of RVOTO determines the clinical presentation and severity. Occasionally, RVOTO is mild with a net left-to-right shunt and no cyanosis. These patients, with acyanotic or "pink" tetralogy, may present as adults without surgical correction. Usually RVOTO is more severe, with a right-to-left shunt, reduced pulmonary blood flow, cyanosis, clubbing, and symptoms. Some patients present in pregnancy who have had only a palliative systemic-to-pulmonary shunt in early life to increase pulmonary blood flow (usually the Blalock-Taussig subclavian-artery-to-pulmonary-artery anastomosis).

In patients with uncorrected tetralogy of Fallot, physical findings depend on the nature of the palliative procedure and the associated abnormalities; a long midsystolic murmur along the left sternal border, right ventricular hypertrophy, a soft or absent pulmonary second sound, cyanosis, and clubbing may be present. A continuous murmur is expected with a functioning palliative shunt.

In pregnant patients with uncorrected tetralogy of Fallot who have undergone palliative procedures, the usual fall in systemic vascular resistance and rise in cardiac output exacerbate the right-to-left shunt, leading to increased maternal hypoxemia and cyanosis. Fetal loss in uncorrected cyanotic heart disease is as high as 43%, and maternal mortality is 4% to 15%; risk increases proportionally with hematocrit levels.[5, 19, 32, 39, 40]

In most women who have undergone surgical correction of tetralogy, the risks associated with pregnancy are low and approach that of the general population.[37, 39, 41] However, residua and sequelae include residual shunt, RVOTO, arrhythmias, pulmonary regurgitation, right ventricular dysfunction, pulmonary hypertension (because of a previous palliative shunt), or left ventricular dysfunction (due to previous volume overload); these conditions may increase the likelihood of complications and should be considered independently.

In complex pulmonary atresia, that is, pulmonary atresia with VSD and congenital systemic to pulmonary collateral vessels, management and outcome depend on the success of prior palliative or corrective procedures and the degree of cyanosis. In two studies of 66 pregnancies in 30 women, most of whom were cyanotic, there was one late maternal death and there were 11 major maternal complications. Fetal loss was high.[42, 43]

Ebstein's Anomaly

In patients with Ebstein's anomaly, the tricuspid valve is morphologically abnormal and is apically displaced into the right ventricle. Tricuspid regurgitation is often present. In 50% of cases, there is a right-to-left shunt through an ASD or patent foramen ovale, which causes cyanosis. Re-entrant tachyarrhythmias resulting from accessory lateral conduction pathways (Wolff-Parkinson-White syndrome) are found in 25% of patients. Severity varies widely. Patients with mild disease may present with only mild tricuspid regurgitation, no shunt, and normal function. Patients with severe disease may have such diminutive right ventricles or such severe outflow tract obstruction that they manifest univentricular physiology. In one report, Connolly and Warnes described 111 pregnancies in 44 women; no maternal mortality or morbidity was noted in 85 live births, but the incidence of fetal loss and premature births was increased. Birth weight was lower in cyanotic mothers.[44] Other reports show similar outcomes.[5, 45]

Complete Transposition of the Great Arteries

In this congenital anomaly the aorta arises from the right ventricle whereas the pulmonary artery arises from the left ventricle (AV concordance and ventriculoarterial discordance). One third of patients have significant associated anomalies. The most common are VSD and pulmonic stenosis. Because transposition of the great arteries is lethal without intervention, all adults will have had corrective surgery.

Most adults will have undergone an atrial switch procedure, which redirects systemic venous return to the left ventricle and then to the pulmonary artery and channels pulmonary venous return to the right ventricle and then to the aorta. The Mustard operation uses a pericardial baffle[46] to accomplish this redirection; the similar Senning operation uses atrial flaps.[47] After an atrial switch operation, the anatomic right ventricle supports the systemic circulation. Occasionally, patients with the combination of complete transposition, VSD, and pulmonic stenosis will have had a Rastelli operation.[48] This procedure directs left ventricular output to the aorta via the VSD and a baffle within the right ventricle and connects the right ventricle to the pulmonary artery with a valved conduit. In these patients, the anatomic left ventricle supports the systemic circulation. The Mustard and Senning operations have been replaced in most cases by an arterial switch procedure, which establishes the left ventricle as the systemic ventricle.[49] Few recipients of the arterial switch procedure have yet reached adulthood.

Limited information is available on outcome of pregnancy after the Mustard or Senning atrial switch repairs. Complications anticipated in such patients include sinus node dysfunction, atrial arrhythmias, and dysfunction of the systemic right ventricle. Pre-existing obstruction of systemic or pulmonary limbs of the atrial baffle may become manifest during pregnancy. In 30 pregnancies in 20 women described in five reports,[50–54] no maternal deaths were noted. However, a 23% rate of premature births and a 17% incidence of maternal heart failure, arrhythmias, or cardiac deterioration were reported.

Lao and coworkers reported a good outcome of pregnancy after the Rastelli operation.[53] Because the left ventricle supports the systemic circulation, heart failure is not anticipated, but stenosis of the valved conduit and arrhythmias are potential complications.

Congenitally Corrected Transposition of the Great Arteries

In patients with this anomaly, the aorta arises from the right ventricle and receives blood from the left atrium and the pulmonary artery arises from the left ventricle and receives blood from the right atrium (AV discordance and ventriculoarterial discordance). The circulation is correct physiologically but the systemic circulation is supported by the morphologic right ventricle. Associated anomalies, usually VSD (75%), pulmonary or subpulmonary stenosis (75%), and myxomatous changes of the systemic tricuspid valve (33%), are often present.

Limited information is available on pregnancy outcome. Anticipated problems include dysfunction of the systemic right ventricle and increased systemic AV valve regurgitation with heart failure.[55] Atrial arrhythmias and AV block are also seen in corrected transposition and could complicate the course of pregnancy. Many adult patients will have had surgical interventions, primarily VSD closure and relief of pulmonic stenosis, often with a valved conduit from the left ventricle to the pulmonary artery.[55] In two reports including 41 patients, there were 105 pregnancies, with 73% live births and no maternal mortality, although 7 patients developed important cardiac complications during pregnancy.[56, 57]

Marfan's Syndrome

Marfan's syndrome is a heritable autosomal dominant connective tissue disorder with ocular, skeletal, pulmonary, and cardiovascular manifestations.[58] The cardiovascular manifestations include mitral valve prolapse with variable mitral regurgitation and medial aortopathy with aortic dilatation and/or dissection as well as aortic regurgitation. The aortic complications are particularly life threatening and reduce life expectancy by as much as 40%.[58]

Hemodynamic stress and possibly hormonal effects during pregnancy increase the risk of aortic dissection. In older studies, pregnant women with Marfan's syndrome had a very high risk (30%) of death. More recent data from Pyeritz and McKusick[58] suggest an overall maternal mortality of 4% and fetal mortality of 21%; patients with the highest risk are those with moderate or severe aortic regurgitation, aortic root dilatation greater than 40 mm, a history of dissection, or significant mitral regurgitation. In 1995, Rossiter and associates[59] published a prospective evaluation of 45 pregnancies in 21 patients and reported no increase in obstetric complications or significant change in aortic root size, except in 3 patients; 2 had pre-existing aortic root involvement, and 1 experienced rapid aortic root dilatation during pregnancy. Thus, a patient with aortic root involvement or who is otherwise at high risk should receive preconception counseling. If early in pregnancy, she should be offered termination of the pregnancy. In contrast, women with little cardiovascular involvement and with an aortic root diameter less than 40 mm as shown by echocardiography may tolerate pregnancy well.[59]

During preconception counseling, the patient should be informed of the long-term maternal risk and of the 50% chance the fetus has of inheriting Marfan's syndrome. Pregnancy should occur before aortic root or valve involvement develops. Serial echocardiography during pregnancy may identify progressive aortic root dilatation that will require intervention, but dissection can occur with a normal-sized aortic root.[60]

Tricuspid Atresia, Univentricular Hearts, and the Fontan Operation

Women with tricuspid atresia and other forms of univentricular circulation occasionally reach the reproductive years without surgical intervention or only with palliative shunts. These women are invariably cyanotic. In older studies, maternal risk was high,[38] but patients with Eisenmenger's syndrome were included in those reports.[6] A more recent retrospective review of 26 pregnancies in 10 patients described no maternal mortality and a 4% incidence of treatable cardiovascular complications. Fetal outcome was poor (only 31% live births) and was inversely related to the level of maternal oxygen saturation; levels less than 0.85 were associated with the worst outcomes.[5]

The Fontan operation[61, 62] is a more definitive palliative procedure for patients with univentricular circulation. In this operation, systemic venous return is diverted to the pulmonary artery, usually without interposition of a subpulmonary ventricle. This procedure returns systemic oxygen saturation to normal levels and eliminates volume overload of the functioning ventricle. These patients have a limited ability to increase cardiac output in response to demands of exercise[7] and (presumably) pregnancy. Published experience with pregnancy is limited. A review by Canobbio and colleagues of 33 pregnancies in 21 women reported 15 (45%) term pregnancies.[63] No maternal mortality was reported, but two women (14%) had cardiac complications. The incidence of first-trimester abortion was high (39%). No data are available on the long-term effects of pregnancy on the mother. After the "ideal" Fontan operation, the 10-year survival rate is 80% and survival is only 60% in less favorable groups[64]; therefore, long-term maternal prognosis should be discussed during preconception counseling for a woman contemplating pregnancy after Fontan's operation.

Eisenmenger's Syndrome and Pulmonary Vascular Obstructive Disease

Eisenmenger's syndrome is an extreme form of pulmonary vascular obstructive disease that develops as a consequence of a pre-existing left-to-right shunt at the atrial, ventricular, or systemic arterial level. Pulmonary vascular resistance increases so much that pulmonary pressures approach systemic levels and the direction of shunt flow becomes bi-directional or reversed (i.e., right-to-left).[18] Once established, the pulmonary vascular disease may progress even after closure of the shunt.

Maternal mortality is around 30% in each pregnancy, and a previous successful pregnancy does not predict a favorable outcome in a subsequent one. Most complications occur at term and during the first postpartum week.[22] Thus, preconception counseling should stress the extreme pregnancy-associated risks and advise patients against pregnancy. Termination of pregnancy and permanent birth control should always be offered to patients with Eisenmenger's syndrome.[65–67]

Fetal outcome is also poor. Spontaneous abortion is common, and intrauterine growth restriction is seen in 50% of pregnancies. Preterm labor is frequent.[20] Perinatal mortality, which usually results from premature birth, is seen in 13% to 28% of pregnancies.[68, 69]

MANAGEMENT

Counseling

The most appropriate time to counsel women with CHD about pregnancy-associated risks is before conception; however, many women are first seen after conception. In counseling patients about the potential maternal and fetal outcomes, we consider the following six factors: (1) the nature of the underlying cardiac lesion, (2) maternal functional status, (3) the availability of further palliative or corrective surgery, (4) the presence of additional associated risk factors, (5) maternal life expectancy and ability to care for a child, and (6) the risk of CHD in offspring. Table 24–1 is a guide to the relative risk of various maternal cardiac conditions.

Because it is an important part of stratifying risk and developing management plans, the nature of the underlying cardiac lesion, including associated lesions, must be identified clearly. A detailed history, physical examination, electrocardiogram, and comprehensive echocardiographic study are necessary. Pediatric catheterization and operative reports are often helpful and should be obtained. Recent studies should be reviewed to clarify the nature of residua and sequelae, especially ventricular function, the level of pulmonary pressure, the severity of obstructive lesions, the persistence of shunts, and the presence of hypoxemia. If necessary, cardiac anatomy and function should be clarified by further investigations. These tests are more easily accomplished before pregnancy when issues of ionizing radiation are of less concern; however, many studies can be conducted at no risk to the fetus. Echocardiography often clarifies the important questions. Holter monitoring and an oxygen saturation test are easily performed. Exercise testing may be helpful before conception, but its safety and role in risk stratification during pregnancy are unknown. Radiation exposure of less than 10 rads is not associated with an increased risk of congenital abnormalities[70, 71]; cardiac catheterization, which delivers about 2 rads to the fetus,[72] may be considered if necessary. Magnetic resonance imaging is probably safe during pregnancy, but studies have involved only small numbers of women and follow-up has been short. Thus, magnetic resonance imaging should be used only when the perceived advantage outweighs the theoretic risk.

Table 24–1. RISK CLASSIFICATION OF CONDITIONS IN PATIENTS WITH CONGENITAL HEART DISEASE

High-Risk Conditions
New York Heart Association classes III and IV
Significant pulmonary hypertension (pulmonary vascular obstructive disease)
Marfan's syndrome with significant aortic root or aortic valve involvement
Severe aortic stenosis
Intermediate-Risk Conditions
Uncorrected cyanosis
Large left-to-right shunt
Uncorrected coarctation of the aorta
Mitral stenosis
Aortic stenosis
Prosthetic valves
Severe pulmonic stenosis
Low-Risk Conditions
Repaired lesions without residual cardiac dysfunction
Small left-to-right shunts
Mitral valve prolapse
Functionally normal bicuspid aortic valve
Mild-to-moderate pulmonic stenosis
Aortic or mitral regurgitation with good ventricular function

Adapted from Sermer M, Siu S, Seaward PGR: Pregnancy complicated by congenital heart disease. In Lee RV, Garner PR (eds): Current Obstetric Medicine, vol 3. Mosby–Year Book, Chicago, 1995, p 117.

Some women who present for pregnancy counseling may not understand the nature of their underlying cardiac lesion, the extent of corrective or palliative procedures, and the associated prognosis. Some patients may have assumed they were cured, until the prospect of pregnancy brings up issues of cardiac residua and limitations. In other cases, the cardiac condition may be minor, or the correction was satisfactory, and the patient can be assured that a normal pregnancy is anticipated.

Maternal functional status is widely used as a predictor of outcome. The NYHA functional classification has been most widely applied even though the data relating functional class to outcome of pregnancy were derived from a population with acquired (mainly rheumatic) heart disease. In a study of 482 pregnancies in 233 women with CHD, Whittemore and associates[6] compared patients with "excellent to good" status (NYHA class IA with no cardiac compromise and no residual structural defect) with those of "fair to poor" status (all the others). No maternal mortality was reported. Cardiovascular morbidity was less in mothers with excellent to good status compared with the others (Fig. 24–1). In addition, the rate of live birth was higher in mothers with good NYHA status (80%) than in mothers with fair to poor status (68%). In our retrospective study of 276 pregnancies in 221 women, we showed that poor functional class (NYHA class >2) or cyanosis, myocardial dysfunction, left-sided heart obstruction, prior arrhythmia, and prior cardiac events were independent predictors of maternal cardiac complications. Poor maternal functional class or cyanosis was also predictive of adverse neonatal events.[73]

Cardiac status should be optimized before conception. Both maternal and fetal outcomes are improved by surgery to correct cyanosis and relieve obstruction.[6] In patients who have not undergone operation to correct tetralogy of Fallot, the maternal mortality risk is 4% and the incidence of fetal death is 30%[74]; in patients who have undergone surgical repair, the outcomes are similar to those seen in a normal population.[75]

Preconception valve replacement requires weighing the need for ongoing anticoagulation with a mechanical valve against the likelihood of early reoperation if a xenograft tissue valve is used. Other alternatives include homografts or the use of a pulmonary autograft (Ross procedure). We prefer to use the Ross procedure for aortic stenosis in women of childbearing age; favorable maternal and fetal outcomes have been reported.[76]

Additional associated risk factors include a history of arrhythmia or congestive heart failure because either condition may recur with the added hemodynamic stress of pregnancy. Patients with prosthetic valves are at increased risk of thromboemboli, endocarditis, and hemorrhage if on anticoagulants. In addition, teratogenic drugs such as warfarin[77] or angiotensin-converting enzyme inhibitors[78] increase fetal risk.

A patient with limited physical capacity or with a condition that may result in premature death should be advised of her potential inability to care for her child. On the other hand, many pregnant women with CHD are unnecessarily concerned about their ability to safely complete a pregnancy. Reassurance should be given when appropriate.

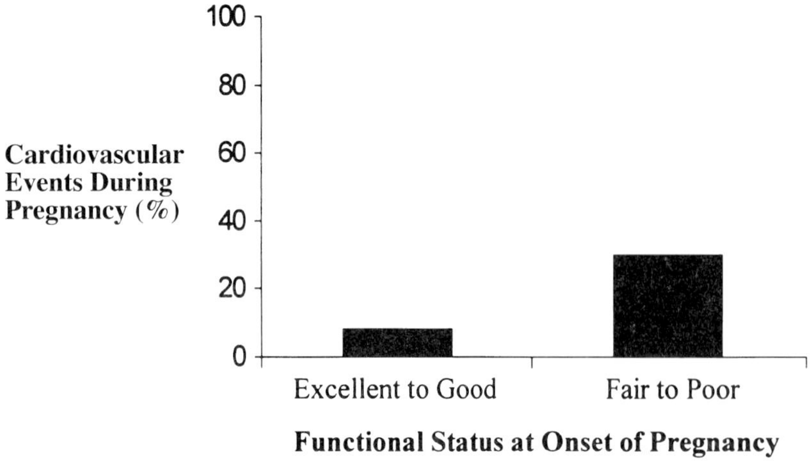

FIGURE 24–1. Proportion of pregnancies complicated by cardiovascular events in women with excellent-to-good versus fair-to-poor functional status at the onset of pregnancy. Women with excellent-to-good function included those who were in NYHA class IA and without postoperative cardiac residuas. Women with fair-to-poor status included those with abnormal electrocardiograms, cardiomegaly, postoperative residuas, or cardiac symptoms. (Reprinted from Whittemore R, Hobbins JC, Engle MA: Pregnancy and its outcome in women with and without surgical treatment of congenital heart disease. Am J Cardiol 50:641, 1982, with permission from Excerpta Medica, Inc.)

The desire to have children is sometimes so strong that information provided about significant maternal risk may not be assimilated. In such circumstances the mother should be made aware of the potential for fetal complications. For example, the likelihood of fetal loss, intrauterine growth restriction, and premature birth seen with maternal cyanotic heart disease and poor maternal functional class is high. In addition, fetal morbidity is significant when women with mechanical heart valves require anticoagulation during pregnancy.

The risk of recurrence of CHD in offspring should be addressed. In the general population, the risk is 0.4% to 0.6%; the risk with one offspring affected averages 2.3% (range, 1.5% to 5%) depending on the lesion. With two affected siblings, the risk is 7.3% (range, 5% to 10%); with mother affected, the risk is 6.7% (range, 2.5% to 18%); and with father affected, 2.1% (range, 1.5% to 3%).[23, 79, 80] Left-sided obstructive lesions have a higher recurrence rate. The defect in a sibling or offspring may differ from that in a previously affected individual. Certain conditions such as Marfan's syndrome[58] and velocardiofacial syndrome[81] are autosomal dominant, so the risk of recurrence in an offspring is 50%.

Antepartum Management

Pregnant women with CHD may be at particular risk for congestive heart failure, arrhythmias, thrombosis, emboli, adverse effects of anticoagulants, or the consequences of pulmonary hypertension. Specific risks in each patient vary according to the pathoanatomy and pathophysiology of the defect, so management recommendations should be applied selectively.

When ventricular dysfunction or congestive heart failure is possible, the patient's activity should be limited. For example, the patient may quit work, increase rest periods, or hire help with homemaking and child care. Severely affected women with class III or IV symptoms should be hospitalized by the middle of the second trimester. Pregnancy-induced hypertension, hyperthyroidism, infection, and anemia should be identified early and treated vigorously. The combination of betamethasone (which induces fetal lung maturity) and tocolytics (which suppress preterm labor) can induce or exacerbate congestive heart failure in patients with normal or reduced cardiac function.[82]

Patients with obstructive lesions such as aortic stenosis with ventricular hypertrophy are at risk not only from the effects of high filling pressure that is manifested as congestive heart failure but also from the effects of low filling pressure, which may lead to low cardiac output and possibly hypotension. Thus, both dehydration and overhydration should be avoided. Adequate filling pressures must be maintained; in late pregnancy, pressures may be maintained by assuming the left lateral decubitus position when recumbent. Diuretics should be used with extreme caution in such patients.

Arrhythmias may be poorly tolerated in the presence of ventricular hypertrophy, ventricular dysfunction, and in patients with right-ventricle–dependent systemic circulation or univentricular circulation. Occasional extra systoles do not require therapy, but sustained tachyarrhythmias such as atrial flutter or atrial fibrillation may lead to cardiovascular decompensation unless promptly treated. Treatment modalities are similar to those used in nonpregnant patients, but potential teratogens should be avoided. Cardioversion is safe in pregnancy.[83, 84]

Pregnancy is a hypercoagulable state because of increased levels of circulating clotting factors, faster platelet turnover, and reduced fibrinolytic activity[85]; therefore, thrombosis and thromboembolism are possible complications. When a pregnant woman requires anticoagulation, careful adjustment of drug and dose is required to maximize maternal safety and fetal well-being. Heparin and oral anticoagulants (most commonly warfarin) are used, but controversy continues as to which is better at different stages of pregnancy. Oral anticoagulation with warfarin, which is more acceptable to patients, is effective. Maternal safety is similar in pregnant and nonpregnant women; however, teratogenicity occurs during organogenesis (6 to 12 weeks' gestation), producing warfarin embryopathy.[77] The frequency of embryopathy is related to maternal warfarin dose and is low when the warfarin dose is 5 mg or less per day.[86–88] Uteroplacental bleeding can occur with warfarin[89] and may increase fetal loss. Fetal intracranial hemorrhage during vaginal delivery is a risk with warfarin even if the maternal warfarin effect is acutely neutralized. Hemorrhage occurs because of the enhanced effect of transplacental warfarin on fetal coagulation parameters and the reduced response of the fetal liver to vitamin K. Therefore, warfarin, if used during pregnancy, should be stopped at least 2 weeks before labor and replaced with heparin. The use of warfarin throughout pregnancy is recommended in Europe but historically not in North America (Table 24–2). Adjusted-dose subcutaneous heparin has no teratogenic effects because the drug does not cross the placenta. Maternal thrombocytopenia is a risk, and maternal osteoporosis may be seen when the drug is used for more than 3 months.[90, 91] Claims of inadequate effectiveness of heparin in patients with mechanical heart valves[92] have been countered by arguments that inadequate doses were used.[93, 94] Recent U.S.-based practice guidelines have suggested a policy similar to the earlier European recommendations.[95] Low-molecular-weight heparin has been suggested as an alternative to adjusted-dose unfractionated heparin.[96] Clinical trials examining optimal anticoagulation strategy are needed.[69]

If a woman with Eisenmenger's syndrome does not accept counseling to terminate the pregnancy or presents late in pregnancy, meticulous antepartum management is necessary. Hospitalization at 20 weeks' gestation should be considered. Continuous supplemental oxygen, although not of proven benefit, may be given to lower pulmonary pressure and maintain systemic oxygenation. Peripheral vascular resistance should be maintained by using support stockings, resting in the left lateral decubitus position, and avoiding dehydration and infection. Adequate iron replacement should be prescribed to avoid inappropriate drops in hemoglobin relative to the degree of hypoxemia[97] and to correct relative iron deficiency that may be associated with microcytosis (despite an elevated hematocrit). Anticoagulation with heparin, although not proved effective, may be used after 20 weeks to minimize in situ pulmonary thromboses and pulmonary thromboembolism.

Certain congenital lesions are associated with specific options for antepartum management that may be considered under appropriate circumstances. For example, in patients with severe symptomatic aortic stenosis and minimal regurgitation, palliative balloon valvuloplasty may allow successful completion of a pregnancy that otherwise would require early termination.[98] In patients with severe coarctation of the aorta, percutaneous transluminal dilatation and stent placement may be considered. In patients with Marfan's syndrome with aortopathy, activities that may raise blood pressure should be avoided. Long-term use of beta-adrenergic blockers is beneficial[99] and should be continued throughout pregnancy; teratogenicity has not been shown,[78, 100] but the incidence of intrauterine growth restriction may be increased.[101]

Fetal Considerations

Antepartum fetal management is directed toward detecting congenital cardiac anomalies[71, 79, 80, 102] and preventing and managing intrauterine growth restriction[103] and premature labor.[103, 104] Fetal echocardiography at 19 to 22 weeks will identify or exclude most forms of significant CHD. If the fetus is affected, plans should be made for early postnatal management. In a severely affected fetus, the possibility of pregnancy termination may be considered.

To minimize intrauterine growth restriction and premature labor, tobacco,[105–107] alcohol,[108] and potentially harmful drugs should be avoided. Reducing activity may be helpful.[109] Early hospitalization with rest and oxygen may be indicated for patients with cyanosis, pulmonary hypertension, or class III and IV symptoms. Fetal growth, amniotic fluid volume, and fetal well-being can be monitored with serial biophysical profiles beginning at 26 weeks' gestational age. Periodic examination for cervical effacement and dilatation should be considered. In cases of premature labor, intrauterine growth restriction, or a decrease in the volume of amniotic fluid, lung maturity should be hastened by administration of betamethasone[110] in patients less than 34 weeks' gestational age.

Multidisciplinary Approach and High-Risk Pregnancy Units

Many women with CHD should be managed in a high-risk pregnancy unit by a multidisciplinary team. The team should

Table 24–2. ANTICOAGULATION IN PREGNANCY

STAGE OF PREGNANCY	NORTH AMERICAN RECOMMENDATIONS*	EUROPEAN RECOMMENDATIONS†
First trimester	Warfarin is contraindicated in first trimester.	Oral anticoagulation with warfarin is preferred especially if the dose required to achieve therapeutic INR is low.
	Adjusted-dose subcutaneous heparin is indicated, with higher doses needed for patients with prosthetic heart valves.	Subcutaneous heparin is optional, but it increases maternal risk. Dose q12h with APTT twice control at midinterval.
Second trimester and first half of third trimester	Adjusted-dose subcutaneous heparin is preferred except for patients with high-risk prosthetic heart valves when warfarin may be used.	Warfarin is used, with target INR < 3.0. Heparin is not recommended.
Final month of pregnancy	Discontinue subcutaneous heparin at onset of labor.	Switch from warfarin to intravenous heparin in hospital. Withdraw heparin at onset of labor, and resume 6–12 h after delivery. Alternatively, continue warfarin and admit patient for planned cesarean section at 38 weeks' gestation.
Postpartum	Resume warfarin, which is safe during breast feeding. Continue heparin postpartum until target INR is achieved.	Resume warfarin, which is safe during breast feeding. Continue heparin postpartum until target INR is achieved.

*Ginsberg JS, Hirsh J: Use of antithrombotic agents during pregnancy. Chest Suppl 108:S305, 1995.

†Study Group of the Working Group on Valvular Heart Disease of the European Society of Cardiology: Guidelines for prevention of thromboembolic events in valvular heart disease. Eur Heart J 16:1320, 1995.

APTT, activated partial thromboplastin time; INR, international normalized ratio.

Table 24–3. CONDITIONS NOT REQUIRING DELIVERY IN A HIGH-RISK OBSTETRICS UNIT

- Repaired atrial septal defect
- Repaired ventricular septal defect, no residual shunt
- Closed patent ductus arteriosus
- Mild pulmonic stenosis
- Bicuspid aortic valve without stenosis
- Mild aortic stenosis
- Mild valvular regurgitation: aortic, mitral, tricuspid, pulmonic
- Small atrial septal defect, unrepaired, without right ventricular enlargement or symptoms
- Small restrictive ventricular septal defect without left ventricular enlargement or symptoms

include perinatologists, obstetricians, cardiologists knowledgeable in CHD, neonatologists, anesthesiologists, obstetric nurses, social workers, critical care physicians, and others. When dealing with a particularly complex problem, the team should meet early in the pregnancy to formulate a plan for antepartum management, labor and delivery, and postpartum care. The cardiac lesion, the anticipated effects of pregnancy, and the possible problems and emergencies should be defined early. Contingency management plans should be outlined. Because every member of the team cannot be available at all times, a clear written plan will minimize the likelihood of withholding appropriate treatment or instituting inappropriate treatment.

In contrast, many women with CHD do not require specialized units for obstetric care and can be managed in a community hospital setting (Table 24–3). The low-risk status of such patients should be clarified to avoid overtreatment. Initial consultation in a tertiary care facility may be helpful.

Labor and Delivery

Cesarean section is generally recommended only for obstetric indications and when warfarin anticoagulation has not been converted to heparin at least 2 weeks before the onset of labor, because of the risk of persisting fetal anticoagulation. In addition, cesarean section may be considered for a patient with Marfan's syndrome with dilated aortic root. Otherwise, vaginal delivery is preferred. Preterm induction is uncommon, but once fetal lung maturity is assured, carefully planned (weekday when possible) induction and delivery may be appropriate in high-risk situations. A planned delivery will ensure the availability of staff and equipment and the proper execution of the previously developed plan.

Invasive monitoring including use of an indwelling pulmonary artery catheter should be considered, if necessary. However, in many cases of complex CHD, invasive monitoring may not be necessary.

Heparin anticoagulation should be discontinued 4 to 6 hours before induction or reversed with protamine if spontaneous labor develops. Heparin can usually be resumed 6 to 12 hours post partum if there are no prolonged bleeding problems.

Prophylaxis for endocarditis should be initiated at the onset of active labor. The recommendations of the 1996 Consensus Conference on Adult Congenital Heart Disease of the Canadian Cardiovascular Society,[23] modified from the 1991 American Heart Association Guidelines,[111] state that cesarean section and vaginal delivery in the absence of infection do not require endocarditis prophylaxis except, perhaps, in patients at higher risk. However, many centers with extensive experience caring for women with CHD continue to advise prophylaxis for endocarditis in all deliveries in most patients with CHD. Prophylaxis for endocarditis is not recommended in patients with low-risk lesions such as repaired ASD, repaired PDA, repaired VSD with no residua, mild pulmonary stenosis, and uncorrected ASD in the absence of associated mitral valve prolapse.[111]

The anesthetic technique of choice is epidural anesthesia administered with care to avoid peripheral vasodilatation and with adequate volume preloading. Epidural fentanyl is particularly useful in patients with shunt lesions because it does not lower peripheral vascular resistance. In the presence of a shunt, air and particulate filters should be placed on all intravenous lines.

Labor is conducted in the left lateral decubitus position to attenuate hemodynamic fluctuations associated with contractions in the supine position.[112–115] The fetus is allowed to pass through the pelvis in response to uterine contractions, rendered painless by proper epidural anesthesia to lessen catecholamine enhancement of cardiac output, and unaugmented by maternal expulsive efforts. The latter part of the second stage of labor should be shortened, and delivery should be assisted by forceps or vacuum extraction.

After delivery, cardiac output increases further,[116] and hemodynamics do not return to baseline for many days; thus, patients should be monitored for a minimum of 72 hours post partum, sometimes in an intensive-care unit. Patients with Eisenmenger's syndrome require longer, close postpartum observation, because the risk of mortality persists for up to 7 days.[22] The neonate should be carefully examined for CHD.

Contraception

Advice on proper contraception should be provided.[117] The oral contraceptive pill is effective, with pregnancy rates less than 1% per year of use. Prothrombotic effects are associated with oral contraceptives[118, 119] and increase the risk of thromboembolism, especially in women already at higher risk, such as those with mechanical heart valves, severe ventricular dysfunction, slow flow through dilated chambers and conduits, or pulmonary vascular disease. If warfarin anticoagulation is being used, the prothrombotic effects of estrogen may be overridden and thus might not be relevant. Newer combined pills with low (20 μg) estrogen content may be safe and less thrombogenic; efficacy is adequate with strict patient compliance.[23] Levonorgestrel (Norplant) and medroxyprogesterone (Depo-Provera), both long-acting progesterone preparations, may be safe and effective even for women with cyanotic CHD and pulmonary vascular disease. Pills with progesterone only have a higher failure rate than combined estrogen and progesterone compounds, cause more fluid retention, and are associated with breakthrough bleeding in 30% of patients. Depression, especially in adolescents, can be seen.

Condoms in combination with spermicidal foam are safe and suitable if the 3% per year pregnancy rate in compliant users is acceptable. Other barrier methods have a considerably higher pregnancy rate. The intrauterine contraceptive device (IUD) is associated with a 3% per year pregnancy rate. Bacteremia may occur at insertion, and pelvic inflammatory disease is possible. Both of these conditions increase the risk of infective endocarditis. Cyanotic patients often experience increased uterine bleeding with such devices. In the presence of a shunt, a vasodepressor reaction at insertion may provoke or exacerbate a right-to-left shunt. Notwithstanding, if prophylactic antibiotics are used at insertion and if excessive bleeding does not mandate early removal, the IUD may be an option in selected patients otherwise at low risk for endocarditis. When a pregnancy is inadvisable because of high maternal risk (see Table 24–1), sterilization should be recommended. Tubal ligation or vasectomy of the partner are probably the most appropriate methods of sterilization; the choice depends on the particular circumstances.

The appropriateness and potential complications associated with various methods of birth control cannot be assessed in isolation. In each individual they must be balanced against the risks of alternative methods and the risk of undesired pregnancy.

References

1. Perloff JK: Medical center experiences. J Am Coll Cardiol 18:315, 1991.
2. Perloff JK: Residua and sequelae. In Perloff JK, Child JS (eds): Congenital Heart Disease in Adults, 2nd ed. WB Saunders, Philadelphia, 1998, p 303.
3. Webb GD, Harrison DA, Connelly MS: Challenges posed by the adult patient with congenital heart disease. In Steele JM (ed): Advances in Internal Medicine, vol 41. Mosby–Year Book, Chicago, 1996, p 437.
4. Elkayam U, Gleicher N: Hemodynamics and cardiac function during normal pregnancy and the puerperium. In Elkayam U, Gleicher N (eds): Cardiac Problems in Pregnancy, 3rd ed. Alan R. Liss, New York, 1998.
5. Presbitero P, Somerville J, Stone S, et al: Pregnancy in cyanotic congenital heart disease: Outcome of mother and fetus. Circulation 89:2673, 1994.
6. Whittemore R, Hobbins JC, Engle MA: Pregnancy and its outcome in women with and without surgical treatment of congenital heart disease. Am J Cardiol 50:641,1982.
7. Harrison DA, Liu P, Walters JE, et al: Cardiopulmonary function in adult patients late after Fontan repair. J Am Coll Cardiol 26: 1016, 1995.
8. Hahn RT, Roman MJ, Mogtader AH, et al: Association of aortic dilation with regurgitant, stenotic and functionally normal bicuspid aortic valves. J Am Coll Cardiol 19:283, 1992.
9. Roberts CS, Roberts WC: Dissection of the aorta associated with congenital malformation of the aortic valve. J Am Coll Cardiol 17: 712, 1991.
10. Oakley CM: Anticoagulants in pregnancy. Br Heart J 74:107, 1995.
11. North RA, Sadler L, Stewart AW, et al: Long-term survival and valve-related complications in young women with cardiac valve replacements. Circulation 99:2669, 1999.
12. Jamieson WRE, Miller DC, Akins CW, et al: Pregnancy and bioprostheses: Influence on structural valve deterioration. Ann Thorac Surg 60:5282, 1995.
13. Perloff JK: Congenital heart disease in adults. In Braunwald E (ed): Heart Disease: A Textbook of Cardiovascular Medicine, 4th ed. WB Saunders, Philadelphia, 1992, p 966.
14. Ueland K: Cardiac diseases. In Creasy RK, Resnik R (eds): Maternal Fetal Medicine, Principles and Practice. WB Saunders, Philadelphia, 1989, p 746.
15. Neilson G, Galea EG, Blunt A: Congenital heart disease and pregnancy. Med J Aust 1:1086, 1970.
16. Murphy JG, Gersh BJ, McGoon MD, et al: Long-term outcome after surgical repair of isolated atrial septal defect: Follow-up at 27 and 32 years. N Engl J Med 323:1645, 1990.
17. Corone P, Doyon F, Gaudeau S, et al: Natural history of ventricular septal defect: A study involving 790 cases. Circulation 55:908, 1977.
18. Wood P: The Eisenmenger syndrome: Or pulmonary hypertension with reversed central shunt. BMJ 2:701, 1958.
19. Clark SL: Structural cardiac disease in pregnancy. Curr Obstet Med 1:179, 1991.
20. Landon MB, Samuels P: Cardiac and pulmonary disease. In Gabbe SG, Niebyl JR, Simpson JL (eds): Obstetrics: Normal and Problem Pregnancies. Churchill Livingstone, New York, 1991, p 1057.
21. Schaefer G, Arditi LI, Solomon HA, et al: Congenital heart disease and pregnancy. Clin Obstet Gynecol 11:1048, 1968.
22. Gleicher N, Midwall J, Hochberger D, et al: Eisenmenger's syndrome and pregnancy. Obstet Gynecol Surv 34:721, 1979.
23. Connelly MS, Webb GD, Somerville J, et al: Canadian Consensus Conference on Adult Congenital Heart Disease 1996. Can J Cardiol 14:395, 1998.
24. Green NJ, Rollason PR: Pulmonary artery rupture in pregnancy complicating patent ductus arteriosus. Br Heart J 68:616, 1992.
25. Jayakrishnan AG, Loftus B, Kelly P, et al: Spontaneous postpartum rupture of a patent ductus arteriosus. Histopathology 21:383, 1992.
26. Roberts WC: The congenitally bicuspid aortic valve: A study of 85 autopsy cases. Am J Cardiol 26:72, 1970.
27. Fenoglio JJ Jr, McAllister HA Jr, DeCastro CM, et al: Congenital bicuspid aortic valve after age 20. Am J Cardiol 39:164, 1977.
28. Lao TT, Sermer M, MaGee L, et al: Congenital aortic stenosis and pregnancy—a reappraisal. Am J Obstet Gynecol 169:540, 1993.
29. Arias F, Pineda J: Aortic stenosis and pregnancy. J Reprod Med 20: 229, 1978.
30. Weyman AE, Griffin BP: Left ventricular outflow tract: The aortic valve, aorta, and subvalvular outflow tract. In Weyman AE (ed): Principles and Practice of Echocardiography, 2nd ed. Lea & Febiger, Philadelphia, 1994, p 498.
31. Deal K, Wooley CF: Coarctation of the aorta and pregnancy. Ann Intern Med 78:706, 1973.
32. Ramin SM, Maberry MC, Gilstrap LC III: Congenital heart disease. Clin Obstet Gynecol 32:41, 1989.
33. Hillestad L: Aortic coarctation and pregnancy. Acta Obstet Gynecol Scand 51:95, 1972.
34. Barash PG, Hobbins JC, Hook R, et al: Management of coarctation of the aorta during pregnancy. J Thorac Cardiovasc Surg 69:781, 1975.
35. Connolly HM, Ammash NM, Warnes CA: Pregnancy in women with coarctation of the aorta (abstract). J Am Coll Cardiol 27:43A, 1996.
36. Mahoney LT: Acyanotic congenital heart disease: Atrial and ventricular septal defects, atrioventricular canal, patent ductus arteriosus, pulmonic stenosis. Cardiol Clin North Am 11:603, 1993.
37. Hess DB, Hess LW: Management of cardiovascular disease in pregnancy. Obstet Gynecol Clin 19:679, 1992.
38. Shime J, Mocarski EJ, Hastings D, et al: Congenital heart disease in pregnancy: Short- and long-term implications. Am J Obstet Gynecol 156:313, 1987.
39. Batson GA: Cyanotic congenital heart disease and pregnancy. J Obstet Gynaecol Br Commonw 81:549, 1974.
40. Patton DE, Lee W, Cotton DB, et al: Cyanotic maternal heart disease in pregnancy. Obstet Gynecol Surv 45:594, 1990.
41. Lo TF, Tan NC: Fallot's tetralogy and pregnancy: A report of a successful pregnancy after complete correction. Med J Aust 2:141, 1971.
42. Connolly HM, Warnes CA: Outcome of pregnancy in patients with complex pulmonic valve atresia. J Am Coll Cardiol 79:519, 1997.
43. Neumayer U, Somerville J: Outcome of pregnancies in patients with complex pulmonary atresia. Heart 78:16, 1997.
44. Connolly HM, Warnes CA: Ebstein's anomaly: Outcome of pregnancy. J Am Coll Cardiol 23:1194, 1994.
45. Donnelly JE, Brown JM, Radford DJ: Pregnancy outcome and Ebstein's anomaly. Br Heart J 66:368, 1991.
46. Mustard WT: Successful two-stage correction of transposition of the great vessels. Surgery 55:469, 1964.
47. Senning A: Surgical correction of transposition of the great arteries. Surgery 45:966, 1959.
48. Rastelli GC, Wallace RB, Ongley PA: Complete repair of transposition of the great arteries with pulmonic stenosis: A review and report of a case corrected by using a new surgical technique. Circulation 39: 83, 1969.
49. Jatene AD, Fontes VF, Souza LC, et al: Anatomic correction of transposition of the great arteries. J Thorac Cardiovasc Surg 83: 20, 1982.

50. Nwosu UC: Pregnancy following Mustard operation for transposition of great arteries. J Tenn Med Assoc 85:509, 1992.
51. Lynch-Salamon DI, Maze SS, Combs CA: Pregnancy after mustard repair for transposition of the great arteries. Obstet Gynecol 82: 676, 1993.
52. Megerian G, Bell JG, Huhta JC, et al: Pregnancy outcome following Mustard procedure for transposition of the great arteries: A report of five cases and review of the literature. Obstet Gynecol 83:512, 1994.
53. Lao TT, Sermer M, Colman JM: Pregnancy following surgical correction for transposition of the great arteries. Obstet Gynecol 83:665, 1994.
54. Clarkson PM, Wilson NJ, Neutze JM, et al: Outcome of pregnancy after the Mustard operation for transposition of the great arteries with intact ventricular septum. J Am Coll Cardiol 24:190, 1994.
55. Connelly MS, Liu PP, Williams WG, et al: Congenitally corrected transposition of the great arteries in the adult: Functional status and complications. J Am Coll Cardiol 27:1238, 1996.
56. Connolly HM, Grogan M, Warnes CA: Pregnancy among women with congenitally corrected transposition of great arteries. J Am Coll Cardiol 33:1692, 1999.
57. Therrien J, Barnes I, Somerville J: Outcome of pregnancy in patients with congenitally corrected transposition of the great arteries. Am J Cardiol 84:820, 1999.
58. Pyeritz RE, McKusick VA: The Marfan syndrome: Diagnosis and management. N Engl J Med 300:772, 1979.
59. Rossiter JP, Repke JT, Morales AJ, et al: A prospective longitudinal evaluation of pregnancy in the Marfan syndrome. Am J Obstet Gynecol 173:1599, 1995.
60. Rosenblum NG, Grossman AR, Gabbe SG, et al: Failure of serial echocardiographic studies to predict aortic dissection in a pregnant patient with Marfan's syndrome. Am J Obstet Gynecol 146:470, 1983.
61. Fontan F, Baudet E: Surgical repair of tricuspid atresia. Thorax 26: 240, 1971.
62. Gale AW, Danielson GK, McGoon DC, et al: Modified Fontan operation for univentricular heart and complicated congenital lesions. J Thorac Cardiovasc Surg 78:831, 1979.
63. Canobbio MM, Mair DD, van derVelde M, et al: Pregnancy outcomes after the Fontan repair. J Am Coll Cardiol 28:763, 1996.
64. Fontan F, Kirklin JW, Fernandez G, et al: Outcome after a "perfect" Fontan operation. Circulation 81:1520, 1990.
65. Baum VC, Perloff JK: Anesthetic implications of adults with congenital heart disease. Anesth Analg 76:1342, 1993.
66. Jones P, Patel A: Eisenmenger's syndrome and problems with anaesthesia. Br J Hosp Med 54:214, 1995.
67. Weiss BM, Hess DM: Pulmonary vascular disease and pregnancy: Current controversies, management strategies, and perspectives. Eur Heart J 21:104, 2000.
68. Collins-Nakai RL, Rabinovitch M: Pulmonary vascular obstructive disease. Cardiol Clin 11:675, 1993.
69. Chan WS, Anand S, Ginsberg JS: Anticoagulation of pregnant women with mechanical heart valves: A systematic review of the literature. Arch Intern Med 160:191, 2000.
70. Barron WM: The pregnant surgical patient: Medical evaluation and management. Ann Intern Med 101:683, 1984.
71. Mossman KL, Hill LT: Radiation risks in pregnancy. Obstet Gynecol 60:237, 1982.
72. Metcalfe J, McAnulty JH, Ueland K: Heart Disease and Pregnancy. Physiology and Management, 2nd ed. Little, Brown & Co, Boston, 1986.
73. Siu S, Sermer M, Harrison D, et al: Risk and predictors for pregnancy-related complications in women with heart disease. Circulation 96: 2789, 1997.
74. Mendelson CL: Cardiac Disease in Pregnancy. FA Davis, Philadelphia, 1960.
75. Singh H, Bolton PJ, Oakley CM: Pregnancy after surgical correction of tetralogy of Fallot. BMJ 285:168, 1982.
76. Dore A, Somerville J: Pregnancy in patients with pulmonary autograft valve replacement. Eur Heart J 18:1659, 1997.
77. Hall JG, Pauli RM, Wilson KM: Maternal and fetal sequelae of anticoagulation during pregnancy. Am J Med 68:122, 1980.
78. Briggs GG, Freeman RK, Yaffe SJ: Drugs in Pregnancy and Lactation: A Reference Guide to Fetal and Neonatal Risk, 5th ed. Williams & Wilkins, Baltimore, 1998.
79. Nora JJ, Nora AH, Wexler P: Hereditary and environmental aspects as they affect the fetus and newborn. Clin Obstet Gynecol 24:851, 1981.
80. Morris CD, Menashe VD: Recurrence of congenital heart disease in offspring of parents with surgical correction. Clin Res 33:68A, 1985.
81. Young D, Shprintzen RJ, Goldberg RB: Cardiac malformations in the velocardiofacial syndrome. Am J Cardiol 46:643, 1980.
82. Van Iddekinge B, Gobetz L, Seaward PGR, et al: Pulmonary oedema after hexoprenaline administration in preterm labor: A report of 4 cases. S Afr Med J 79:620, 1991.
83. Finlay AY, Edmunds V: DC cardioversion in pregnancy. Br J Clin Pract 33:88, 1979.
84. Vogel JHK, Pryor R, Blount SG Jr: Direct-current defibrillation during pregnancy. JAMA 193:970, 1965.
85. Schafer AI: The hypercoagulable states. Ann Intern Med 102:814, 1985.
86. Iturbe-Alessio I, Fonseca MC, Mutchnik O, et al: Risks of anticoagulant therapy in pregnant women with artificial heart valves. N Engl J Med 315:1390, 1986.
87. Wong V, Cheng CH, Chan KC: Fetal and neonatal outcome of exposure to anticoagulants during pregnancy. Am J Med Genet 45:17, 1993.
88. Vitale N, DeFeo M, DeSanto LS, et al: Dose-dependent fetal complications of warfarin in pregnant women with mechanical heart valves. J Am Coll Cardiol 33:1637, 1999.
89. Bloomfield DK: Fetal deaths and malformations associated with the use of coumarin derivatives in pregnancy: A critical review. Am J Obstet Gynecol 107:883, 1970.
90. Barbour LA, Kick SD, Steiner JF, et al: A prospective study of heparin-induced osteoporosis in pregnancy using bone densitometry. Am J Obstet Gynecol 170:862, 1994.
91. Ginsberg JS, Kowalchuk G, Hirsh J, et al: Heparin effect on bone density. Thromb Haemost 64:286, 1990.
92. Salazar E, Izaguirre R, Verdejo J, et al: Failure of adjusted doses of subcutaneous heparin to prevent thromboembolic phenomena in pregnant patients with mechanical cardiac valve prostheses. J Am Coll Cardiol 27:1698, 1996.
93. Ginsberg JS, Hirsh J: Use of antithrombotic agents during pregnancy. Chest (Suppl) 108:S305, 1995.
94. Elkayam UR: Anticoagulation in pregnant women with prosthetic heart valves: A double jeopardy. J Am Coll Cardiol 27:1704, 1996.
95. Bonow RO, Carabello B, de Leon AC, et al: Guidelines for the management of patients with valvular heart disease: Executive summary. A report of the American College of Cardiology/American Heart Association task force on practice guidelines (committee on management of patients with valvular heart disease). Circulation 98:1949, 1998.
96. Ginsberg JS, Hirsh J: Use of antithrombotic agents during pregnancy. Chest 114:524S, 1998.
97. Perloff JK, Rosove MH, Child JS, et al: Adults with cyanotic congenital heart disease: Hematologic management. Ann Intern Med 109:406, 1988.
98. Lao TT, Adelman AG, Sermer M, et al: Balloon valvuloplasty for congenital aortic stenosis in pregnancy. Br J Obstet Gynaecol 100: 1141, 1993.
99. Shores J, Berger KR, Murphy EA, et al: Progression of aortic dilatation and the benefit of long-term beta-adrenergic blockade in Marfan's syndrome. N Engl J Med 330:1335, 1994.
100. Rubin PC: Current concepts: Beta blockers in pregnancy. N Engl J Med 305:1323, 1981.
101. Montan S, Ingemarsson I, Marsal K, et al: Randomised controlled trial of atenolol and pindolol in human pregnancy: Effects on fetal haemodynamics. BMJ 304:946, 1992.
102. Rose V, Gold RJ, Lindsay G, et al: Possible increase in the incidence of congenital heart defects among the offspring of affected parents. J Am Coll Cardiol 6:376, 1985.
103. Niswander KR, Berendes H, Deutschberger J, et al: Fetal morbidity following potentially anoxigenic obstetric conditions: V. Organic heart disease. Am J Obstet Gynecol 98:871, 1967.
104. Ueland K, Novy MJ, Metcalfe J: Hemodynamic responses of patients with heart disease to pregnancy and exercise. Am J Obstet Gynecol 113:47, 1972.
105. Abel EL: Smoking during pregnancy: A review of effects on growth and development of offspring. Hum Biol 52:593, 1980.
106. Elliot J: Maternal smoking and the fetus: One fear buried but others arise. JAMA 241:867, 1979.
107. Nieburg P, Marks JS, McLaren NM, et al: The fetal tobacco syndrome. JAMA 253:2998, 1985.
108. Eckhardt MJ, Harford TC, Kaelber CT, et al: Health hazards associated with alcohol consumption. JAMA 246:648, 1981.

109. Naeye RL, Peters EC: Working during pregnancy: Effects on the fetus. Pediatrics 69:724, 1982.
110. Effect of corticosteroids for fetal maturation on perinatal outcomes. NIH Consensus Development Conference Statement, May 27, 1994.
111. AHA Medical/Scientific Statement. Circulation 83:1174, 1991.
112. Ueland K, Hansen JM: Maternal cardiovascular dynamics. II. Posture and uterine contractions. Am J Obstet Gynecol 103:1, 1969.
113. Cunningham I: Cardiovascular physiology of labor and delivery. J Obstet Gynaecol Br Commonw 73:500, 1966.
114. Winner W, Romney SL: Cardiovascular responses to labor and delivery. Am J Obstet Gynecol 95:1104, 1966.
115. Knuttgen HG, Emerson K Jr: Physiological response to pregnancy at rest and during exercise. J Appl Physiol 36:549, 1974.
116. Ueland K, Hansen JM: Maternal cardiovascular dynamics: III. Labor and delivery under local and caudal analgesia. Am J Obstet Gynecol 103:8, 1969.
117. Leonard H, O'Sullivan JJ, Hunter S: Family planning requirements in the adult congenital heart disease clinic. Heart 76:60, 1996.
118. Beck WW Jr: Complications and contraindications of oral contraception. Clin Obstet Gynecol 24:893, 1981.
119. Brenner PF, Mishell DR Jr: Contraception for the woman with significant cardiac disease. Clin Obstet Gynecol 18:155, 1975.

CHAPTER 25

Valvular Heart Disease: Pathophysiology, Clinical Recognition, Diagnosis, and Management

Susan Wilansky

The incidence of heart disease in pregnancy ranges from 0.5% to 1.5%.[1] Managing pregnant patients with valvular heart disease requires continual interaction throughout the pregnancy among the patient, cardiologist, and obstetrician, with inclusion of the anesthesiologist at term. How well the pregnancy is tolerated depends on many factors: the hemodynamic abnormality of the valve disease (e.g., the regurgitant lesions are better tolerated than the stenotic ones), the severity of the lesion, the New York Heart Association (NYHA) functional status of the patient at the onset of pregnancy, the compliance of the patient, and the presence or absence of intervening complications (e.g., arrhythmias or febrile illnesses).

The NYHA functional status must be determined during the initial assessment of the pregnant patient with valvular heart disease because maternal mortality is, to some extent, predicted by the functional class at the beginning of pregnancy (Table 25–1).[2] Patients in functional class I to II usually fare well; the mortality is 0.4%.[3, 4] For patients in functional class III to IV, however, maternal morbidity (30%–50%) and mortality (7%–50%) are very high.[3, 4]

Mortality rates have been evaluated with respect to the nature and severity of specific valvular lesions. These include patients with mitral stenosis and NYHA class I to II status who have a mortality rate of less than 1% and patients with mitral stenosis and NYHA class III to IV status or associated atrial fibrillation (implying more advanced disease) who have mortality rates of 5% to 15%.[5]

DIAGNOSIS

The NYHA functional status of the patient should be determined on initial presentation. A careful physical examination to evaluate the severity of the lesion should then be conducted by Doppler echocardiography. The patient should be closely monitored throughout the pregnancy for the development of hypertension, infections, arrhythmias, and anemia—complications that may lead to serious hemodynamic compromise. Both obstetric and cardiac follow-up should intensify as the third trimester approaches, during which time the maximal volume load is being placed on the heart. In the last trimester, the patient should be evaluated on a very regular basis. The intermittent use of Doppler echocardiography throughout the pregnancy will allow the clinician to monitor the status of the left ventricle, the pulmonary artery pressure, and the course of the valvular lesion in question. Each of these is an important determinant of the outcome of the pregnancy and may influence the manner in which labor and delivery are approached.

Table 25–1. NEW YORK HEART ASSOCIATION FUNCTIONAL CLASS

CLASS	DEFINITION
I	No functional limitation
II	Mild functional limitation (angina, dyspnea, fatigue, palpitations) with ordinary activity
III	Marked functional limitation with minimal activity
IV	Severe limitations—symptoms occur at rest

Adapted from American Heart Association: 1994 revisions to Classification of Functional Capacity and Objective Assessment of Patients with Diseases of the Heart. Circulation 90:644, 1994. Reproduced, with permission, from the American Heart Association.

SPECIFIC CARDIAC LESIONS

Aortic Stenosis

The basic hemodynamic abnormality of aortic stenosis is fixed obstruction to left ventricular outflow, which limits cardiac output in advanced disease. The etiology is rheumatic or congenital (usually a bicuspid aortic valve) and is fortunately uncommon in women of childbearing age. Symptoms involving more significant disease include dyspnea, angina, and/or syncope. Physical findings pointing to severe aortic stenosis include a single or paradoxically split second heart sound (S_2), a late-peaking systolic ejection murmur at the second right interspace, and delayed carotid upstrokes. In the absence of systemic hypertension, electrocardiographic evidence of ventricular hypertrophy implies a significant gradient across the aortic valve.

The severity of aortic stenosis can be accurately quantitated by Doppler echocardiography. In a patient with normal ventricular function, a peak gradient of 70 mm Hg or greater and mean gradient of 50 mm Hg or greater across the aortic valve in early pregnancy denotes critical aortic stenosis. Gradients increase throughout the pregnancy in conjunction with the gradual doubling of the cardiac output by the third trimester. On the first visit, calculation of aortic valve area using the continuity equation will determine lesion severity (Table 25–2). Women with mild aortic stenosis should tolerate the pregnancy well. Patients with moderate to severe

Table 25–2. CALCULATION OF AORTIC VALVE AREA

AORTIC STENOSIS	AORTIC VALVE AREA (cm^2)
Mild	1.5–2.0
Moderate	1.0–1.5
Moderate to severe	0.75–1.0
Critical	<0.75

aortic stenosis should be cautioned against becoming pregnant until the condition has been surgically treated because high fetal and maternal mortality (32%[3] and 17%,[3, 4] respectively) has been reported in these patients. Those with more advanced disease will have a marked reduction in their activity levels and may even require complete bed rest. Should patients with significant aortic stenosis become pregnant, abortion should be discouraged. Maternal mortality is extremely high in such patients who terminate a pregnancy, reportedly up to 40%,[3–5] because of the high risk of hypotension due to blood loss, anemia, or placement in the supine position.[5]

Use of percutaneous balloon valvuloplasty has been reported in two patients with symptomatic critical aortic stenosis with successful maternal and fetal outcome.[6] Similar results have been shown in other single case reports.[6–8]

Aortic Insufficiency

Isolated aortic insufficiency is rare in pregnancy and is usually associated with rheumatic mitral stenosis (discussed in greater detail in the next section). This condition is characterized by volume loading of the left ventricle, but because diastolic filling time is reduced by the tachycardia of pregnancy, the regurgitant volume may be reduced to a lesser degree of severity as the pregnancy progresses.

A history of angina or dyspnea should alert the clinician to more advanced disease. Other signs include a widened pulse pressure, an absolute diastolic blood pressure of less than 40 mm Hg, and an Austin Flint diastolic rumble. Doppler echocardiography can help to semiquantitate the severity of the regurgitation as well as determine left ventricular size and function and pulmonary artery pressure. In the more advanced stages of disease, the patient may require sodium restriction, bed rest, diuretics, and even afterload reduction.

Mitral Stenosis

Mitral stenosis is the most common form of rheumatic heart disease in pregnancy.[3–5] As the mitral orifice becomes smaller, a higher left atrial pressure is required as the driving force to open up the valve. As the pregnancy progresses, the increased cardiac output and blood volume will increase the left atrial pressure. The increasing heart rate during pregnancy will lead to a shorter diastolic filling time and an increase in the gradient across the mitral valve. Any of these physiologic changes may raise the pulmonary capillary wedge pressure to the point of pulmonary edema. The increase in the pulmonary capillary wedge pressure will cause left atrial dilatation, and possible atrial arrhythmias (flutter and fibrillation), which can lead to the formation of left atrial thrombi and embolic phenomena.

Clinical symptoms of significant mitral stenosis include dyspnea, orthopnea, paroxysmal nocturnal dyspnea, and nocturnal cough. Hemoptysis is a worrisome symptom, indicating rupture of a connection between the bronchial and pulmonary veins.[9] Palpitations suggest the presence of either premature atrial contractions, atrial fibrillation, or atrial flutter.

Clinical signs of significant mitral stenosis include a right ventricular lift, elevated jugular venous pressure, a loud pulmonary component of S_2 indicative of pulmonary hypertension, a narrowed S_2–opening snap interval, a long diastolic rumble, and rales in the lung fields.

The severity of mitral stenosis can be quantitated with a high degree of accuracy by Doppler echocardiography (Table 25–3). Although the pressure half-time method for the calculation of mitral valve area is the usual echocardiographic technique, a study by Rokey and coworkers[10] has shown this method to be unreliable in pregnancy. Therefore, these authors recommend use of the continuity equation as the preferred method of calculation.

Medical management of the patient with mitral stenosis begins with very close clinical observation throughout the pregnancy. Impending pulmonary edema usually can be managed with bed rest and diuretics. Digitalis has been recommended for patients who are in NYHA functional class III to IV to achieve rate control should atrial fibrillation develop.[8] Cardioselective beta-adrenergic blocker therapy should be considered in patients with moderate to severe mitral stenosis to achieve slowing of the heart rate and allow for a longer diastolic filling period (and reduction of gradient across the mitral valve). New-onset atrial fibrillation can be managed with digoxin, β-adrenergic blockers, and anticoagulant therapy.[3]

Several studies have reported on the use of balloon mitral valvuloplasty during pregnancy. This technique is performed in the cardiac catheterization laboratory with total abdominal and pelvic shielding. Heparin is administered after a transseptal puncture, and the balloon is inflated across the mitral valve several times to reduce the mitral valve gradient. Complication rates of the procedure are low (Table 25–4).[11] Recently, balloon valvuloplasty with transesophageal echocardiographic guidance has been reported, thus obviating the need for fluoroscopy and radiation.[12]

Balloon mitral valvuloplasty should be reserved for the severely symptomatic patient with critical mitral stenosis who is refractory to medical management. It should not be performed during the period of organogenesis. Only the most experienced of invasive cardiologists should perform the procedure in pregnant patients in order to minimize fluoroscopy time and its potential risks. Table 25–5 includes a complete review of available literature of balloon mitral valvuloplasty in pregnancy.[13–17]

Table 25–3. DEGREES OF SEVERITY OF MITRAL STENOSIS

SEVERITY OF MITRAL STENOSIS	MITRAL VALVE AREA (cm^2)
Mild	>1.5
Moderate	1.0–1.5
Severe	<1.0

Table 25–4. COMPLICATIONS OF BALLOON MITRAL VALVULOPLASTY

COMPLICATION	%
Mortality	0–1
Tamponade	0–4
Thromboembolism	0.5–2
Severe mitral regurgitation	1–5
Perforation	0–4

Adapted from Berman AD, McKay RG, Grossman W: Balloon valvuloplasty. In Baim DW, Grossman W (eds): Cardiac Catheterization, Angiography, and Intervention, 5th ed. Williams & Wilkins, Baltimore, 1995, p 669.

Mitral Regurgitation

Mitral regurgitation, unless severe, is generally a well-tolerated lesion in pregnancy. Common causes include rheumatic fever, mitral valve prolapse, and previous endocarditis. The cause of the regurgitation can be readily established by two-dimensional echocardiography.

Clinical symptoms of significant mitral regurgitation include dyspnea and fatigue. Signs include the presence of a third heart sound, along with a holosystolic murmur and evidence of congestive heart failure.

Most authors recommend digitalis[5, 8] for severe mitral regurgitation in an attempt to control the heart rate should atrial fibrillation ensue. Anticoagulation is required should atrial fibrillation become established.

Mitral valve prolapse (MVP) is very frequent in women of childbearing years, with a reported incidence of 12% to 17%.[18, 19] The course of pregnancy is usually uneventful in women with MVP.[18–20] The typical auscultatory features of MVP (mid-to-late systolic click and murmur) may disappear as the pregnancy advances.[19] Because the tendency for the myxomatous leaflets to prolapse is reduced by increased preload and decreased afterload, the physiologic changes of pregnancy may decrease or abolish the typical clinical signs. The diagnosis can be firmly established by the use of two-dimensional echocardiography, which will typically show elongated or redundant mitral leaflet tissue with or without evidence of prolapse. Echocardiographic changes of MVP were studied by Rayburn and colleagues[21] in eight pregnant women with MVP early and late in pregnancy and again in the postpartum period. The prolapse disappeared on echocardiography in five of the women. The remaining three had echocardiographic evidence of prolapse at the end of pregnancy and post partum.

Some studies have reviewed the course of pregnancy in women with MVP. Rayburn reviewed his experience with 310 pregnant women, 75 of whom had MVP.[18] There were no differences in outcome between the two groups in terms of antepartum complications, postpartum outcome, and incidence of neonatal complications. Tang and coworkers confirmed this in a study of 37 patients with MVP.[22]

PREGNANCY AND PROSTHETIC VALVES

The pregnant woman with a prosthetic valve poses serious management issues for the obstetrician and cardiologist. In the scarce amount of literature on the subject, there is no agreement as to which valve is most appropriate in pregnancy.

In a large retrospective European study reported by Sbarouni and Oakley in 1994,[23] 214 pregnancies were reviewed in 182 women, most of whom had mechanical valves (133 of 182, 83%). The population was basically healthy, with 164 patients (90%) in NYHA functional class I to II, 144 (79%) in sinus rhythm, and 115 (63%) having a mitral valve prosthesis. Anticoagulation was used in 17% of women with biologic valves and in 99% of women with mechanical valves. Maternal and fetal outcomes from this study are summarized with a review of the literature in Tables 25–6,[23–25] 25–7,[23, 25] 25–8,[23, 24, 26–28] and 25–9.[23, 26, 27]

Several trends in maternal outcome may be noted from the retrospective studies of pregnant women with biologic valves. The chances of having a term infant and good maternal outcome are high. However, at 10 years, 50% or more of the patients with biologic valves, pregnant or not, will have structural deterioration requiring repeat valve surgery. Recommending a biologic valve to a woman of childbearing years, therefore, commits her to *at least* a second valve replacement during her lifetime.

The chances for having a healthy term infant in women with mechanical valves are highest if the mother is on anticoagulant therapy throughout the pregnancy. Current practice in North America includes the use of heparin in the first trimester (to avoid embryopathy), warfarin (Coumadin) until 36 weeks, and the reinstitution of heparin thereafter.

Table 25–5. COMPLICATIONS AND RESULTS OF BALLOON VALVULOPLASTY IN PREGNANCY

AUTHOR	YEAR	NO. OF PREGNANCIES	MVA (cm^2) PRE → POST	CARDIAC COMPLICATIONS (NO.)	FETAL/MATERNAL OUTCOME TO DELIVERY
Gangbar et al[13]	1992	2	0.7 → 2.3 1.1 → 3.3		2 normal term deliveries
Ribeiro et al[14]	1992	7	0.8 ± 0.2 → 1.9 ± 0.3	↑ MR, 1 grade (2) ASD (2)	7 term deliveries
Farhat et al[15]	1992	8	0.8 ± 0.15 → 2.4 ± 0.34	Trivial ASD (1)	8 term deliveries
Iung et al[16]	1994	13	1.0 ± 2.0 → 2.0 ± 0.02	Small ASD (8)	10 term deliveries 2 pregnant 1 C/S at 29 wks → PROM–fetal death
Kalra et al[17]	1994	27	0.78 ± 0.19 → 2.2 ± 0.12	↑ MR, 1 grade (7) Severe MR → MVR (1)	24 term deliveries 1 MVR, abortion at 6 mo 2 in 3rd trimester

ASD, atrial septal defect; C/S, cesarean section; MR, mitral regurgitation; MVA, mitral valve area; MVR, mitral valve replacement; PROM, premature rupture of membranes.

Table 25–6. FETAL OUTCOME: BIOLOGIC VALVES

AUTHOR	YEAR	NO. OF PREGNANCIES	OUTCOME	ANTICOAGULATION (%) Yes	No
Sbarouni and Oakley[23]	1994	63	Healthy	91	100
			Full-term	84	87.5
			Premature	7	12.5
			Stillbirths	4	0
			Therapeutic abortion	6	0
			Death	0	0
Lee et al[24]*	1994	95	Healthy		87.7
			Spontaneous abortion		12.3
Jamieson et al[25]†	1995	94	Healthy		74.5
			Full-term		84.2
			Premature		15.7
			Spontaneous abortion		10.6
			Therapeutic abortion		14.9
			Death		0

*No anticoagulation.
†Only three patients had anticoagulation in this study.

The maternal risk with mechanical valves, however, is extremely high. Sbarouni and Oakley[23] reported on 34 pregnancies in 29 women taking heparin (the level of anticoagulation was not reported). There was a 24% incidence of valve thrombosis, a 12% incidence of embolic events, and a 12% incidence of significant bleeding complications. Similar complications have also been reported in smaller patient groups. Therefore, the woman with valvular heart disease must be informed that, although mechanical valves are much more durable than biologic ones, the maternal risks are extremely high. Perhaps in the future the low-molecular-weight anticoagulants (enoxaparin and dalteparin) may play a role in the management of these patients, but whether they are efficacious or harmful in pregnant patients with prosthetic valves has yet to be determined.

Anticoagulation in Pregnancy

Oral anticoagulants can be potentially dangerous to the fetus in the first trimester of pregnancy. Fetal exposure is reported to result in so-called warfarin embryopathy (stippling of the bony epiphyses, nasal hypoplasia, and serious central nervous system disorders, including mental retardation, blindness, and deafness). Warfarin embryopathy causing serious malformation occurs in 3% to 5% of fetuses; a less serious form occurs in up to 25% of fetuses.[8] Furthermore, there is a higher incidence of miscarriage, stillbirth, and premature delivery.[24, 29–32]

Heparin, on the other hand, does not cross the placenta and has no effect on the fetus. However, the long-term effects carry the risk of valve thrombosis, premature delivery, and maternal osteoporosis. The Ad Hoc Committee of the Working Group on Valvular Heart Disease recommends two approaches[29]: (1) administer heparin in the first trimester, then change to warfarin until the 37th week, followed by reinstitution of heparin, or (2) use oral anticoagulation until the 37th week, then change to heparin a few weeks before delivery. As mentioned previously, the first option is more common in North America.

Endocarditis in Pregnancy

Endocarditis in pregnancy is extremely rare (0.0001%–1% of pregnancies).[8, 33] The predisposing conditions and events are similar to those of the nonpregnant patient. The clinical

Table 25–7. MATERNAL OUTCOME: BIOLOGIC VALVES

AUTHOR	YEAR	NO. OF VALVES	OUTCOME (%)		(Nonpregnant patients)
Sbarouni and Oakley[23]	1994	49	Valve deterioration	35	
			Elective surgery	31	
			Emergency surgery	4	
			Thromboembolism	0	
			Death	0	
Jamieson et al[25]	1995	255*	Valve deterioration	50.9	40.6
			Elective surgery	—	—
			Emergency surgery	—	—
			Thromboembolism	5.7	5.4
			Endocarditis	5.7	5.9
			Death	1.9	0

*Refers to total number of valves in 237 patients; 53 valves were placed in patients who were pregnant, and 202 valves were placed in patients who had never been pregnant.

Table 25–8. FETAL OUTCOME: METAL VALVES

AUTHOR	YEAR	NO. OF PREGNANCIES	OUTCOME	ANTICOAGULATION (%) Yes	ANTICOAGULATION (%) No
Chen et al[26]	1982	41	Healthy	67	91
			Spontaneous abortion	33	9
Vitali et al[27]	1986	98	Full-term	48	30
			Premature	9	30
			Spontaneous abortion	46	20
			Therapeutic abortion	17	
			Death	0	10
Pavankumar et al[28]	1988	37	Healthy	91	
			Full-term	85	
			Premature	6	
			Spontaneous abortion	6	
			Therapeutic abortion	0	
			Ectopic pregnancy	1	
			Death	9	
Lee et al[24]	1994	56	Healthy	72	
			Spontaneous abortion	28	
Sbarouni and Oakley[23]	1995	151	Healthy	92* 83† 73‡	91
			Full-term	64* 64† 57†	84
			Premature	29* 19† 17‡	6
			Stillbirths	1.5* 11† 13‡	4
			Therapeutic abortion	0* 3† 7‡	6
			Death	1.5* 3† 0‡	0

*Heparin, first trimester; then warfarin sodium.
†Warfarin during entire pregnancy.
‡Heparin during entire pregnancy.

presentation in pregnancy may be more subtle and be confused with more common infections, such as those of the urinary tract. The management principles of endocarditis are similar to those for nonpregnant patients (see Chapter 15). Serum drug levels may be reduced due to the expanded blood volume and increased glomerular filtration rate.[34] Penicillins and cephalosporins are safe in pregnancy. Data on aminoglycosides in pregnancy do not exist, and it is recommended that a child be monitored for hearing and kidney dysfunction if the mother received these medications.[35] Recommendations for chemoprophylaxis are similar to those discussed in the section on endocarditis.

SURGERY

Open heart surgery during pregnancy carries a maternal mortality risk of 2% and a fetal mortality risk of 20% to 30%.[36] The risk of spontaneous abortion is high in the first trimester, but if surgery occurs before 26 weeks' gestation, fetal mortality and morbidity (mostly neurologic) are unacceptably high. Furthermore, surgery should not be postponed until late in the third trimester because it may precipitate the onset of premature labor.

A review of open heart surgery at our institution from 1985 to 1996 revealed that four women underwent mitral valve surgery (three valve replacements, one commissurotomy) on an emergency basis immediately after cesarean section (gestation, 28–36 weeks). All mothers and infants were discharged in satisfactory condition. A fifth patient had resection of a large left ventricular mass with mitral valve replacement in the first trimester. She had a miscarriage 24 hours after surgery but was discharged in satisfactory condition. It should be noted that surgery is reserved for the critically ill patient whose condition is refractory to medical

Table 25–9. MATERNAL OUTCOME: MECHANICAL VALVES

AUTHOR	YEAR	NO. OF PREGNANCIES	OUTCOME (%)	
Chen et al[26]	1982	41	Embolism	7
			Hemorrhage	3
			Death	3
Vitali et al[27]	1986	98	Valve thrombosis	2
			Embolization	7
			Emergency surgery	1
			Death	2
Sbarouni and Oakley[23]	1994	151	Valve thrombosis	9
			Major embolic event	5
			Major bleeding	5
			Death	4

management and where there is no other option to save the woman's life.

References

1. Ueland K: Rheumatic heart disease and pregnancy. In Elkayam U, Gleicher N (eds): Cardiac Problems in Pregnancy: Diagnosis and Management of Maternal and Fetal Disease, 2nd ed. Alan R. Liss, New York, 1990, p 99.
2. American Heart Association: 1994 Revisions to Classification of Functional Capacity and Objective Assessment of Patients with Diseases of the Heart. Circulation 90:644, 1994.
3. Raymond R, Underwood DA, Moodie DS: Cardiovascular problems in pregnancy. Cleve Clin J Med 54:95–104, 1987.
4. Gianopoulos JG: Cardiac disease in pregnancy. Med Clin North Am 73:639, 1989.
5. Clark SL: Cardiac disease in pregnancy. Crit Care Obstet 18:237, 1991.
6. Banning AP, Pearson JF, Hall RJC: Role of balloon dilatation of the aortic valve in pregnant patients with severe aortic stenosis. Br Heart J 70:544, 1993.
7. Lao TT, Adelman AG, Sermer M, Colman JM: Balloon valvuloplasty for congenital aortic stenosis in pregnancy. Br J Obstet Gynaecol 100: 1141, 1993.
8. Elkayam U: Anticoagulation in pregnant women with prosthetic heart valves: A double jeopardy. J Am Coll Cardiol 27:1704, 1996.
9. Brady K, Duff P: Rheumatic heart disease in pregnancy. Clin Obstet Gynecol 32:21, 1989.
10. Rokey R, Hsu HW, Moise KJ Jr, et al: Inaccurate noninvasive mitral valve area calculation during pregnancy. Obstet Gynecol 84:950, 1994.
11. Berman AD, McKay RG, Grossman W: Balloon valvuloplasty. In Baim DW, Grossman W (eds): Cardiac Catheterization, Angiography, and Intervention, 5th ed. Williams & Wilkins, Baltimore, 1995, p 669.
12. Kültürsay H, Türkoglu C, Akin M, et al: Mitral balloon valvuloplasty with transesophageal echocardiography without using fluoroscopy. Cathet Cardiovasc Diagn 27:317, 1992.
13. Gangbar EW, Watson KR, Howard RJ, Chisholm RJ: Mitral balloon valvuloplasty in pregnancy: Advantages of a unique balloon. Cathet Cardiovasc Diagn 25:313, 1992.
14. Ribeiro PA, Mohamed EF, Awad M, et al: Balloon valvotomy for pregnant patients with severe pliable mitral stenosis using the Inoue technique with total abdominal and pelvic shielding. Am Heart J 124: 1558, 1992.
15. Farhat MB, Maatouk F, Betbout F, et al: Percutaneous balloon mitral valvuloplasty in eight pregnant women with severe mitral stenosis. Eur Heart J 13:1658, 1992.
16. Iung B, Cormier B, Elias J, et al: Usefulness of percutaneous balloon commissurotomy for mitral stenosis during pregnancy. Am J Cardiol 73:398, 1994.
17. Kalra GS, Arora R, Khan JA, et al: Percutaneous mitral commissurotomy for severe mitral stenosis during pregnancy. Cathet Cardiovasc Diagn 33:28, 1994.
18. Rayburn WF: Mitral valve prolapse and pregnancy. In Elkayam U, Gleicher N (eds): Cardiac Problems in Pregnancy: Diagnosis and Management of Maternal and Fetal Disease, 2nd ed. Alan R. Liss, New York, 1990, p 181.
19. Cowles T, Gonik B: Mitral valve prolapse in pregnancy. Semin Perinatol 14:34, 1990.
20. Degani S, Abinader G, Scharf M: Mitral valve prolapse and pregnancy: A review. Obstet Gynecol Surv 44:642, 1989.
21. Rayburn WF, LeMire MS, Bird JL, Buda AJ: Mitral valve prolapse: Echocardiographic changes during pregnancy. J Reprod Med 32:185, 1987.
22. Tang LCH, Chan SYW, Wong VCW, et al: Pregnancy in patients with mitral valve prolapse. Br J Obstet Gynaecol 23:217, 1985.
23. Sbarouni E, Oakley CM: Outcome of pregnancy in women with valve prostheses. Br Heart J 71:196, 1994.
24. Lee CN, Wu CC, Lin PY, et al: Pregnancy following cardiac prosthetic valve replacement. Obstet Gynecol 83:353, 1994.
25. Jamieson WRE, Miller C, Akins CW, et al: Pregnancy and bioprostheses: Influence on structural valve deterioration. Ann Thorac Surg 60:S282, 1995.
26. Chen WWC, Chan C, Lee PK, et al: Pregnancy in patients with prosthetic heart valves: An experience with 45 pregnancies. Q J Med (New Series) 51:358, 1982.
27. Vitali E, Donatelli F, Quaini E, et al: Pregnancy in patients with mechanical prosthetic heart valves: Our experience regarding 98 pregnancies in 57 patients. J Cardiovasc Surg 27:221, 1986.
28. Pavankumar P, Venugopal P, Kaul U, et al: Pregnancy in patients with prosthetic cardiac valves: A 10-year experience. Scand J Thorac Cardiovasc Surg 22:19, 1988.
29. Gohlik-Bärwolf C, Acar J, Burckhardt D, et al, Ad Hoc Committee of the Working Group on Valvular Heart Disease, European Society of Cardiology: Guidelines for prevention of thromboembolic events in valvular heart disease. J Heart Valve Dis 2:398, 1993.
30. Born D, Martinez EE, Almeida AM, et al: Pregnancy in patients with prosthetic heart valves: The effects of anticoagulation on mother, fetus, and neonate. Am Heart J 124:413, 1992.
31. Wong V, Cheng CH, Chan KC: Fetal and neonatal outcome of exposure to anticoagulants during pregnancy. Am J Med Genet 45:17, 1993.
32. Sareli P, England MJ, Berk MR, et al: Maternal and fetal sequelae of anticoagulation during pregnancy in patients with mechanical heart valve prostheses. Am J Cardiol 63:1462, 1989.
33. Cox SM, Leveno KJ: Pregnancy complicated by bacterial endocarditis. Clin Obstet Gynecol 32:48, 1989.
34. Jeyamalar R, Sivanesaratnam V: Management of infective endocarditis in pregnancy. Aust N Z J Obstet Gynaecol 31:123, 1991.
35. Cesario TC: Antibiotic therapy in pregnancy. In Elkayam U, Gleicher N (eds): Cardiac Problems in Pregnancy: Diagnosis and Management of Maternal and Fetal Disease, 2nd ed. Alan R. Liss, New York, 1990, p 437.
36. Paulus DA, Layon AJ, Mayfield WR: Intrauterine pregnancy and aortic valve replacement. J Clin Anesth 7:338, 1995.

CHAPTER

26 Management of Valvular Heart Disease

26.1 Obstetric Management

Brian Kirshon and Karolina Adam

The physiologic changes that occur in the cardiovascular system during pregnancy are usually well tolerated in a normal heart. However, when structural cardiac pathology (e.g., valvular heart disease) is present, it can be extremely hazardous, with implications for both maternal and fetal health. Women who have structural cardiac pathology usually have either rheumatic or congenital heart disease. With the declining incidence of rheumatic fever, however, congenital heart disease is now the more frequent cause of structural cardiac pathology.

Many obstetricians use the New York Heart Association (NYHA) functional classification system for their patients, although the system is not the best prognosticator for the outcome of pregnancy. Patients in NYHA functional class I should have negligible maternal mortality with proper prenatal management; these patients are generally asymptomatic with a cardiac lesion. Patients in functional class II are those who experience symptoms with moderate exertion. Functional class III includes patients who are symptomatic with mild exertion. Patients in functional class IV are symptomatic at rest. Patients in classes II and III have a 5% to 15% risk of maternal death, while those in class IV may have a mortality rate in excess of 25%.

Ideally, women with severe, symptomatic valvular heart disease should be diagnosed early and should be receiving treatment before pregnancy. However, valvular heart disease can be effectively managed during labor, delivery, and the postpartum stage through medical therapy and, in some cases, surgery.

SPECIFIC CARDIAC LESIONS

Pulmonary Valve Disease

Significant abnormalities of the pulmonary valve are rare. Congenital stenosis is usually mild and hemodynamically insignificant. The degree of obstruction, rather than its size, is the principal determinant of clinical performance. When the gradient exceeds 80 mm Hg, percutaneous or surgical correction is warranted. Upon review of the literature (including 106 pregnancies), there were no maternal deaths due to pulmonary stenosis.[1–3] There were no reported maternal deaths associated with isolated right ventricular lesions in 77 maternal cardiac deaths.

Mitral Stenosis

Mitral stenosis is the most common rheumatic valvular heart disease seen in pregnancy.[4] The hemodynamic defect is obstruction of left atrial outflow, resulting in decreased cardiac output and elevated pressure in the left atrium, pulmonary veins, and pulmonary capillaries. The sluggish flow in the distended left atrium increases the likelihood of thrombus formation. Pregnant women with mitral stenosis have a predisposition toward atrial fibrillation; pulmonary edema also may occur. The greatest risk to these patients—namely, heart failure and death—occurs late in pregnancy and in the early puerperium. Cardiac output is primarily dependent upon adequate diastolic filling and secondarily upon ventricular preload.

Tachycardia may be an early clinical sign of cardiac decompensation. Tachycardia may occur due to the exertion of pushing during delivery, or it may be secondary to the pain or anxiety associated with labor. Patients with tachycardia and mitral stenosis may have a rapid and dramatic decline in cardiac output and blood pressure. Therefore, it is appropriate to administer an oral beta-adrenergic blocker to women with severe mitral stenosis who enter labor with a pulse exceeding 90 beats per minute.[4] It is also important to remember that in the presence of mitral stenosis, pulmonary capillary wedge pressure is not an adequate reflection of left ventricular filling pressures. Therefore, it is important to avoid preload reduction (i.e., diuresis), which may result in a reduction in cardiac output.[4] Also, epidural anesthesia may result in dangerous intrapartum fluctuations in cardiac output.[4–7]

The most hazardous time for women with mitral stenosis appears to be in the immediate postpartum period.[4] Wedge pressure may increase 16 mm Hg immediately postpartum. Because frank pulmonary edema does not generally occur until wedge pressure reaches 28 to 30 mm Hg, it is wise to keep wedge pressure for such patients at 14 mm Hg or lower before delivery.[3–5] Pulmonary artery catheterization and attention to wedge pressure are, therefore, important parts of the intrapartum management of these patients. The second stage of labor should be shortened with the use of forceps. Some authorities recommend a cesarean section delivery; however, with the aggressive management outlined here, it appears that vaginal delivery is safe, even for women who have severe disease and pulmonary hypertension.[4]

Mitral Insufficiency

Mitral insufficiency of rheumatic origin is usually associated with other valvular lesions. The condition is usually well tolerated during pregnancy. If atrial fibrillation occurs, administration of digitalis is often necessary. Some authors have recommended prophylactic digitalis during pregnancy for women with significant mitral insufficiency. However, in Hibbard's review, in 28 maternal deaths, no maternal deaths were associated with mitral insufficiency unless there was coexisting mitral stenosis.[3] Congenital mitral valve prolapse (MVP) is the more common condition; and using strict criteria for diagnosis, the prevalence of mitral valve prolapse is approximately 2%.[8, 9]

The issue of antibiotic prophylaxis during uncomplicated vaginal delivery is controversial. In a study of over 2000 uncomplicated pregnancies, Sugrue et al.[10] noted that the incidence of positive blood cultures in noncardiac patients (drawn at placental separation and 5, 10, and 30 minutes later) was 1%. It is not known whether this low incidence of bacteremia occurs in pregnant women with cardiac disease.

The American Heart Association recommends prophylaxis in the setting of MVP in patients who have a click and murmur (with evidence for mitral regurgitation) (Table 26–1).[11] There is good evidence that patients with morphologically abnormal valves, that is, elongated, redundant, and thickened leaflet tissue on two-dimensional echocardiography, are at higher risk for developing endocarditis.[12]

Guidelines on antibiotic prophylaxis proposed by the Committee on Rheumatic Fever and Infective Endocarditis in the Young[11] specifically state that prophylaxis should be used for MVP with mitral insufficiency. They also state that uncomplicated vaginal delivery and cesarean section do not require prophylaxis. Whether a complication will develop is difficult to determine in advance. Should a complication occur, it may then be too late to administer antibiotics.

It seems prudent to advise antibiotic prophylaxis for delivery in women with known preexisting MVP and mitral insufficiency or evidence of the typical myxomatous mitral valve on two-dimensional echocardiography. Antibiotics should also be administered to women in whom a complicated delivery is expected. It is probably safe to withhold antibiotic therapy in the low-risk group with morphologically normal leaflets on echocardiography and no mitral insufficiency, although in current practice, prophylaxis is used in all patients with MVP.

Aortic Stenosis

Aortic stenosis is commonly of rheumatic origin and is usually associated with other lesions. However, in patients of childbearing age, congenital bicuspid aortic stenosis is becoming more prevalent than rheumatic aortic stenosis. In contrast to mitral stenosis, aortic stenosis usually does not become hemodynamically significant until the valve is one third or less of its normal size. The times of greatest risk for women with aortic stenosis appear to be during termination of a pregnancy or during delivery.[13] Maintaining cardiac output is crucial, and any factor leading to diminished venous return will result in an increased valvular gradient and a diminished cardiac output. Termination of pregnancy may be especially hazardous in this regard and carries a mortality rate of up to 40%.[13] Epidural anesthesia can result in hypotension and should be avoided. It is important to look for ischemic heart disease because this may accompany aortic stenosis. Death associated with aortic stenosis can occur secondary to myocardial infarction rather than as a direct complication of the valvular lesion.[9] Overall maternal mortality with aortic stenosis during pregnancy has been said to be as high as 17%, but other data suggest a lower mortality.[14] It appears that if the aortic valve gradient is in excess of 100 mm Hg, the risk of death is increased. Pulmonary artery catheterization should be used during labor and delivery, and the pulmonary wedge pressure should be maintained at or near 16 mm Hg in case of unexpected peripartum blood loss.[13]

Aortic Regurgitation

The most common cause of aortic regurgitation is rheumatic fever. Women with chronic insufficiency usually remain

Table 26–1. AHA RECOMMENDATIONS FOR ANTIBIOTIC PROPHYLAXIS: GASTROINTESTINAL/GENITOURINARY PROCEDURES

PROCEDURES REQUIRING PROPHYLAXIS	STANDARD REGIMEN	SPECIAL REGIMENS
Vaginal hysterectomy	Ampicillin 2.0 g IM or IV plus gentamicin 1.5 mg/kg IM or IV, given ½ to 1 h before procedure; one follow-up dose may be given 8 h later	Oral regimen for minor or repetitive procedures in low-risk patients
Urethral catheterization (especially in the presence of infection)		Amoxicillin 3.0 g orally 1 h before preocedure and 1.5 g 6 h later
Cytoscopy		Penicillin-allergic patients: vancomycin 1.0 g IV slowly over 1 h, plus gentamicin 1.5 mg/kg IM or IV given 1 h before procedure; may be repeated once 8–12 h later
Colonic surgery		
Esophageal dilatation		
Urinary tract surgery		
Gallbladder surgery		
Colonoscopy		
Upper GI endoscopy with biopsy		
Proctosigmoidoscopy		

Abbreviations: GI, gastrointestinal; IM, intramuscular; IV, intravenous.

From Shulman ST, Amren DP, Bisno AL, et al: Prevention of bacterial endocarditis: A statement for health professionals by the Committee on Rheumatic Fever and Infective Endocarditis of the Council on Cardiovascular Disease in the Young. Circulation 70:1123A, 1984. With permission.

asymptomatic until later in life. Aortic regurgitation is usually well tolerated during pregnancy. Antibiotic prophylaxis is advised during delivery. If pulmonary congestion develops, restriction of activity is important and treatment with digitalis, diuretics, and afterload reduction is indicated. If aortic regurgitation results from active endocarditis, early surgery should be considered, regardless of the stage of pregnancy. The mortality rate for such patients is very high with medical therapy alone.

Tricuspid Valve Disease

Although lesions of the tricuspid valve are uncommon, the incidence of tricuspid insufficiency is increasing due to cases of bacterial endocarditis that result from intravenous drug use.[15, 16] Tricuspid regurgitation is usually well tolerated during pregnancy, and women usually remain asymptomatic. Use of antibiotic prophylaxis at delivery is suggested.

VALVULAR PROSTHESES

All women with prosthetic heart valves are at higher risk during pregnancy. Full anticoagulation is necessary and administration of heparin is recommended (warfarin can cross the placenta and may result in adverse fetal effects). Antibiotic prophylaxis is mandatory; if infection occurs on the valve, surgery may be necessary. In women with heterograft prostheses, the risk of bacterial endocarditis is the same as in those with mechanical prostheses; however, in the former group, patients are less susceptible to thrombosis and thromboembolic events. Young women who are contemplating pregnancy should receive a tissue valve replacement, with the understanding that they may require reoperation in the future.

FETAL CONSIDERATIONS

Perinatal outcome in patients with cyanotic congenital cardiac disease correlates best with hematocrit. Successful outcome in patients with hematocrit exceeding 65% seems unlikely. The incidence of intrauterine growth restriction, stillbirth, and spontaneous abortion is increased in these women. One should also strive to keep maternal PO_2 above 70%.

Fetal echocardiography is indicated for prenatal diagnosis of congenital cardiac defects. Women should be counseled on the risk of fetal congenital anomalies. It has been previously stated that there is up to a 5% risk of a fetal cardiac abnormality in the face of a maternal defect, and some authors think that the risk may be as high as 10%.[17]

References

1. Neilson, G, Galea EG, Blunt A: Congenital heart disease and pregnancy. Med J Aust 30:1086, 1970.
2. Schaefer G, Arditi LI, Solomon HA, et al: Congenital heart disease and pregnancy. Clin Obstet Gynecol 11:1048, 1968.
3. Hibbard LT: Maternal mortality due to cardiac disease. Clin Obstet Gynecol 18:27, 1975.
4. Clark SL, Phelan JP, Greenspoon J, et al: Labor and delivery in the presence of mitral stenosis: Central hemodynamic observations. Am J Obstet Gynecol 152:986, 1985.
5. Clark SL: Critical Care Obstetrics, 2nd ed. Blackwell Scientific Publications, London, 1991, p 125.
6. Ueland K, Akamatsu TJ, Eng M, et al: Maternal cardiovascular dynamics. VI. Cesarean section under epidural anesthesia without epinephrine. Am J Obstet Gynecol 114:775, 1972.
7. Ueland K: Rheumatic heart disease and pregnancy. In Elkayam Y, Gleicher N (eds): Cardiac Problems in Pregnancy. Alan R. Liss, New York, 1982, p 82.
8. Wann LS, Grove JR, Hess TR, et al: Prevalence of mitral valve prolapse by two-dimensional echocardiography in healthy young women. Br Heart J 49:334, 1983.
9. Perloff JK, Child JS, Edwards JE: New guidelines for the clinical diagnosis of mitral valve prolapse. Am J Cardiol 57:1124, 1986.
10. Sugrue D, Blake S, Troy P, et al: Antibiotic prophylaxis against infective endocarditis after normal delivery: Is it necessary? Br Heart J 44: 499, 1980.
11. Shulman ST, Amren DP, Bisno AL, et al: Prevention of bacterial endocarditis: A statement for health professionals by the Committee on Rheumatic Fever and Infective Endocarditis of the Council on Cardiovascular Disease in the Young. Circulation 70:1123A, 1984.
12. Marks AR, Chong CY, Sanfilippo AJ, Ferre M, Weyman AE: Identification of high-risk and low-risk subgroups of patients with mitral valve prolapse. N Engl J Med 320:1031, 1989.
13. Arias F, Pineda J. Aortic stenosis and pregnancy. J Reprod Med 20: 229, 1978.
14. Easterline TR, Chadwick HS, Otto CM, et al: Aortic stenosis in pregnancy. Obstet Gynecol 72:113, 1988.
15. Banks T, Fletcher R, Ali N: Infective endocarditis in heroin addicts. Am J Med 55:448, 1973.
16. Dreyer NP, Fields BN: Heroin associated infective endocarditis: A report of 28 cases. Ann Intern Med 78:699, 1973.
17. Whittmore R, Hobbins JC, Engle MA: Pregnancy and its outcome in women with and without surgical treatment of congenital heart disease. Am J Cardiol 50:641, 1982.

26.2 Anesthetic Management

Lisa M. Hollier, Larry C. Gilstrap III, and Ezzat I. Abouleish

Heart disease currently complicates approximately 1.6% of pregnancies. The majority of cases are secondary to rheumatic valvular disease; however, as the incidence of rheumatic fever declines in this country, congenital lesions are increasingly more common. The incidence of maternal death during pregnancy ranges from 1% to 17% depending upon the severity of the maternal disease[1] (Table 26–2) and accounts for up to 25% of all maternal deaths.[2–6]

Because of these significant risks, optimal anesthetic management of the pregnant woman with significant complications of pregnancy, such as valvular heart disease, requires a team approach. Included in this team are the obstetrician or

Table 26–2. RISK FACTORS, BY RISK CATEGORY, FOR MATERNAL DEATH FROM VALVULAR CARDIAC DISEASE ASSOCIATED WITH PREGNANCY

Group I—Minimal Risk
Bioprosthetic valve
Mitral stenosis, NYHA classes I and II
Group II—Moderate Risk
Mitral stenosis with atrial fibrillation
Artificial valve
Mitral stenosis, NYHA classes III and IV
Aortic stenosis

Modified from Clark SL: Structural cardiac disease in pregnancy. In Clark SL, Cotton DB, Hankins GDV, Phelan JP (eds): Critical Care Obstetrics, 3rd ed. Blackwell Scientific Publications, Malden, MA, 1997, p 291.

maternal-fetal medicine specialist, the internist or cardiologist, and the anesthesiologist. The anesthesiologist should have a clear understanding of both the physiologic changes occurring in pregnancy and the differences that occur in women with cardiac disease. Appropriate selection of anesthesia is of paramount importance because of the complexity of these changes and the risk of maternal death.

This chapter outlines the physiologic changes of pregnancy with special relevance to women with cardiac disease. General considerations applying to all cardiac patients are then reviewed. Last, the pathophysiology and anesthetic considerations for the specific valvular lesions are addressed.

PHYSIOLOGIC ADAPTATIONS

The spectrum of physiologic changes that take place throughout pregnancy is profound. Some of the numerous changes that must be taken into consideration from an anesthetic standpoint are summarized in Table 26–3. Blood volume increases in singleton pregnancy by 40 to 45%.[7] The increase is even greater in women with multifetal gestations.[8] The change begins as early as 4 weeks of gestation and reaches a maximum near 32 weeks, after which the blood volume is relatively constant until delivery. The increased volume results from increases in both plasma and erythrocytes.

This normal increase in preload is important to consider during hydration prior to regional anesthesia, especially with certain types of valvular heart lesions (e.g., mitral stenosis). The increase in blood volume may also affect the serum levels of certain medications utilized during anesthetic procedures.

Table 26–3. PHYSIOLOGIC CHANGES THAT OCCUR DURING PREGNANCY

Cardiovascular
Increase in blood volume
Increase in cardiac output
Increase in heart rate
Decrease in systemic vascular resistance
Decrease in blood pressure in second trimester
Pulmonary
Increase in tidal volume
Decrease in residual volume
Other
Prolongation of gastric emptying time during labor
Increase in coagulation factors

Resting cardiac output also increases appreciably during early gestation, ranging from 20% to 50% over baseline values by 20 to 24 weeks. The increase is due to elevations in both heart rate and stroke volume. The output is further increased during each successive stage of labor and even more immediately postpartum (Fig. 26–1). Posture exerts a profound effect upon hemodynamics, especially in late pregnancy. Cardiac output may decline by as much as 30% from term levels when the gravida is in the supine position. The heart rate during normal pregnancy rises slowly and progressively during gestation. By term, it reaches a peak of 15 beats per minute over baseline. In singleton gestations, the changes in stroke volume are directly proportional to end-diastolic volume.[9] In multifetal pregnancies, however, cardiac output is increased predominantly by increased inotropic effect.[10]

Blood pressure normally declines in the midsecond trimester, rising again near term. Systemic vascular resistance is also noted to decrease during pregnancy. These changes are generally well tolerated in normal patients. However, additional attention must be paid to these changes in cardiac patients with preload-dependent disease, such as aortic stenosis.

Pulmonary changes in pregnancy include increases in tidal volume and minute ventilatory volume. The functional residual capacity and residual volume of air are decreased secondary to the elevation of the diaphragm. Lung compliance, however, is not altered by pregnancy.

Studies comparing pregnant women in each trimester with nonpregnant control subjects found no difference in gastric emptying time.[11] In contrast, during labor, especially after the administration of opioids, gastric emptying time is appreciably prolonged. This dramatically increases the risk of aspiration with general anesthesia.

The levels of several blood coagulation factors are increased during pregnancy. Fibrinogen increases by approximately 50%. Factors VII, VIII, IX, and X all have increased activity. In contrast, activities of factors XI and XIII are somewhat decreased.

GENERAL CONSIDERATIONS

A woman's functional status prior to or early in pregnancy is a useful indicator of her prognosis. The New York Heart Association (NYHA) classification subdivides women into four categories, as outlined in Table 26–4. In general, women who are in classes I and II prior to pregnancy do well. Unfortunately, the functional status of women may deteriorate in pregnancy. Nearly 50% of patients with cardiac disease will first develop pulmonary edema in pregnancy.

Two pregnancy complications of special relevance to women with valvular heart disease are pre-eclampsia and infection. Pre-eclampsia complicates approximately 5% of pregnancies, and the risk is increased in women with pre-existing cardiovascular disease. Women with pre-eclampsia do not have the normal volume expansion of pregnancy. However, because vasospasm has contracted the available space, the intravascular compartment is usually not underfilled. Thus, these patients are especially sensitive to attempts to expand the contracted blood volume and to blood loss at surgery or delivery. The severe hypertension that can accompany this disease also poses a significant risk

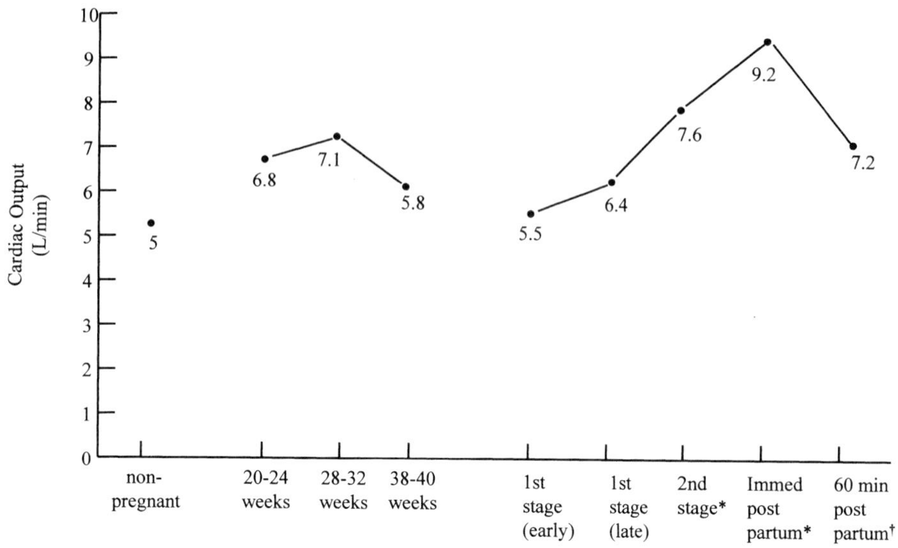

FIGURE 26–1. Cardiac output during gestation, labor, and postpartum period. †, supine; *, lithotomy. (Adapted from Ueland K, Metcalfe J: Circulatory changes in pregnancy. Clin Obstet Gynecol 18:41, 1975; and Ueland K, Hansen JM: Maternal cardiovascular dynamics: II. Posture and uterine contractions. Am J Obstet Gynecol 103:1, 1969.)

with intubation and extubation. Finally, edema in the tissues surrounding the airway makes "failed intubation" a concern with general anesthesia.

Chorioamnionitis develops during labor in 0.5 to 2% of parturients. The resultant fever and tachycardia can place additional stress on a patient with compromised function due to valvular heart disease.

Another general issue for consideration is the use of anticoagulants. Women with a mechanical valve prosthesis must be maintained on anticoagulant therapy. There are numerous reports in the literature regarding therapeutic options for these women.[12–15] Warfarin, regular heparin, and low-molecular-weight heparin have been used to prevent thromboembolism. Regional anesthesia in these women may be contraindicated, and should be used only after the return of a safe level of coagulation.

The need for antimicrobial prophylaxis against bacterial endocarditis in patients with valvular heart disease remains controversial. At present there have been no controlled trials in humans, and the American Heart Association (AHA) does not recommend routine prophylaxis for vaginal delivery. Because of the safety of the antibiotic regimens and the morbidity of endocarditis, one reasonable approach would be using the standard regimen recommended by the AHA for patients at highest risk (those with prosthetic heart valves, a previous history of endocarditis, or surgically constructed systemic pulmonary shunts or conduits) and using the alternative low-risk regimen in other pregnant cardiac patients (Table 26–5).

The use of invasive hemodynamic monitoring should be individualized, depending upon the clinical status of the patient. Women with NYHA class III or class IV disease may benefit from the additional information provided.[16] Central hemodynamic parameters during normal pregnancy are outlined in Table 26–6.

Table 26–4. NEW YORK HEART ASSOCIATION CLASSIFICATION SYSTEM

CLASS	DEFINITION
I	No functional limitation
II	Mild functional limitation (angina, dyspnea, fatigue, palpitations) with ordinary activity
III	Marked functional limitation with minimal activity
IV	Severe limitations—symptoms occur at rest

Adapted from American Heart Association: 1994 revisions to Classification of Functional Capacity and Objective Assessment of Patients with Diseases of the Heart. Circulation 90:644, 1994. With permission from the American Heart Assocation.

SPECIFIC VALVULAR LESIONS

Aortic Stenosis

Aortic stenosis is one of the most significant cardiac lesions, based on level of risk. These lesions may be congenital or

Table 26–5. REGIMENS FOR ENDOCARDITIS PROPHYLAXIS FOR GENITOURINARY/GASTROINTESTINAL PROCEDURES

DRUG	REGIMENS
	Standard Regimen
Ampicillin, gentamicin, and amoxicillin	Intravenous or intramuscular administration of ampicillin, 2 g, plus gentamicin, 1.5 mg/kg (not to exceed 80 mg), 30 min before procedure followed by amoxicillin, 1.5 g, orally 6 h after initial dose; alternatively, the parenteral regimen may be repeated once, 8 h after initial dose
	Penicillin-Allergic Regimens
Vancomycin and gentamicin	Intravenous administration of vancomycin, 1 g over 1 h; plus intravenous or intramuscular administration of gentamicin, 1.5 mg/kg (not to exceed 80 mg), 1 h before procedure; may be repeated once, 8 h after initial dose
	Alternative Low-Risk Regimen
Amoxicillin	3 g orally 1 h before procedure; then 1.5 g 6 h after initial dose

Adapted from Dajani AS, Bisno AL, Chung KJ, et al: Prevention of bacterial endocarditis: Recommendations by the American Heart Association. JAMA 264:2919, 1990. Copyrighted 1990, American Medical Association.

Table 26–6. CENTRAL HEMODYNAMIC CHANGES THAT OCCUR IN NORMAL NULLIPAROUS WOMEN BETWEEN 35 AND 38 WEEKS OF GESTATION AND 11 TO 13 WEEKS POSTPARTUM

HEMODYNAMIC PARAMETER	PREGNANT	POSTPARTUM	CHANGE
Mean arterial pressure (mm Hg)	90 ± 6	86 ± 8	No change
Pulmonary capillary wedge pressure (mm Hg)	8 ± 2	6 ± 2	No change
Central venous pressure (mm Hg)	4 ± 3	4 ± 3	No change
Heart rate (beats/min)	83 ± 10	71 ± 10	+17%
Cardiac output (L/min)	6.2 ± 1.0	4.3 ± 0.9	+43%
Systemic vascular resistance (dyne•sec•cm^{-5})	1210 ± 266	1530 ± 520	−21%
Pulmonary vascular resistance (dyne•sec•cm^{-5})	78 ± 22	119 ± 47	−34%
Serum colloid osmotic pressure (mm Hg)	18.0 ± 1.5	20.8 ± 1.0	−14%
COP-PCWP gradient (mm Hg)	10.5 ± 2.7	14.5 ± 2.5	−28%
Left ventricular stroke work index (g/m/m^{-2})	48 ± 6	41 ± 8	No change

Adapted from Clark SL, Cotton DB, Lee W, et al: Central hemodynamic assessment of normal term pregnancy. Am J Obstet Gynecol 161:1439, 1989. With permission.

may result from rheumatic fever. With stenosis, the normal valve opening of 2 to 3 cm^2 is narrowed. A systolic pressure gradient develops across the valve, and concentric left ventricular hypertrophy results. The cardiac output is fixed, and therefore, the sympathetic tone is increased to maintain the arterial blood pressure. The ventricle requires a greater time to eject the blood through the stenotic valve into the systemic circulation. During pregnancy, the transvalvular gradient increases progressively as a result of the increasing blood volume and decreasing systemic vascular resistance (SVR).[17]

The optimal anesthetic technique should be discussed during the antenatal care. The obstetric anesthesiologist ideally should be involved in the continuing progress of the patient during pregnancy. The plans for pain control during labor and anesthesia for delivery should be amended as needed during the course of pregnancy.

The goals of anesthesia in these patients are to avoid tachycardia, to maintain an adequate preload, and to prevent significant decrease in SVR. Patients with symptoms or transvalvular gradients greater than 50 mm Hg are best managed with pulmonary artery catheterization, which allows continuous hemodynamic assessment.[18] The optimal pulmonary capillary wedge pressure during labor is 15 mm Hg or greater. This provides protection against peripartum blood loss.

The optimal anesthetic/analgesic for parturients with significant aortic stenosis is a subject of considerable debate.[19, 20] Relatively common complications of regional techniques can result in death in women with severe heart disease. Rapid onset of sympathetic blockade accompanied by peripheral vasodilatation may cause a sudden decrease in cardiac output resulting in cardiogenic shock. In order to prevent the precipitous declines in preload and afterload, an incremental technique must be utilized to gradually bring up the level of the blockade. If hypotension occurs, it should be promptly and aggressively treated with lateral displacement of the uterus, judicious use of fluids, and the administration of vasopressors. Ephedrine is commonly used. However, it has both α and β sympathomimetic effects that can result in undesirable tachycardia. Phenylephrine, a pure alpha agonist, may be a better agent. In a study of left ventricular filling dynamics in nonpregnant patients with aortic stenosis, administration of a bolus of phenylephrine improved left ventricular filling.[21] A narcotic epidural with avoidance of hypotension may be a reasonable option for pain relief during labor, as would intravenous analgesics administered by PCA pump.[22]

General anesthesia eliminates the risk of hypotension due to the decrease in SVR accompanying the sympathetic blockade. One disadvantage of general anesthesia, however, is the sympathetic nervous system response to intubation, which can generate tachycardia and hypertension. One method of management involves induction with a cardiostable drug followed by a short-acting opioid.[23]

Mitral Stenosis

Mitral stenosis accounts for 90% of rheumatic heart disease in pregnancy, with 25% of patients first developing symptoms during pregnancy.[24] The normal mitral valve area is 4.0 cm^2. When valvular narrowing reaches 1–1.5 cm^2, the patient becomes symptomatic. The decreased mitral valve orifice causes obstruction to left ventricular filling and results in a fixed cardiac output. Initially, the left atrium can compensate; however, as the disease progresses, the left atrial volume will increase. Consequently, pulmonary hypertension and right-sided heart failure may occur.

Surgical therapy for the cardiac lesion is generally postponed until completion of the pregnancy; however, it may be lifesaving in some gestations (see Chapter 25).

Obstetric management for delivery may include either awaiting spontaneous labor or induction of labor to ensure an experienced team is available for monitoring. Cesarean delivery is reserved for obstetric indications.

The pain of labor and the resultant tachycardia can significantly compromise the patient with mitral stenosis. With a rapid ventricular rate, there is diminished filling of the coronary arteries, a reduction in ventricular filling, and a drop in cardiac output. Of the available options, the best pain relief for labor and delivery is provided by epidural techniques. Abrupt increases in preload can precipitate pulmonary edema in these patients. In preparing for administration of an epidural, strict attention must be given to avoid intravenous fluid overload. The hemodynamic effects of epidural anesthesia when patients are in the Trendelenburg position were studied by Ziskind and colleagues.[25] Marked reductions in heart rate, SVR, and pulmonary capillary wedge pressure occurred in all patients. When the patients were placed in Trendelenburg position, the PCWP could be increased and maintained at 25 mm Hg. This allowed the cardiac index to increase to baseline values.

If hypotension occurs, it should be corrected immediately. Infusion of ephedrine or phenylephrine should be used to increase blood pressure back to baseline using caution to ensure that this does not cause significant changes in heart rate.[26]

Attention to the principles previously discussed can prevent complications associated with general anesthesia. Drugs that can produce tachycardia (e.g., atropine, ketamine, pancuronium, meperidine) should be avoided. Use of a short-acting beta-adrenergic blocker (such as esmolol) may be beneficial in blunting the tachycardia and hypertension that can occur with intubation and extubation. Fluid balance must be carefully observed to minimize fluctuations in central venous pressure.

Women with severe mitral stenosis may have relatively high wedge pressures, and central hemodynamic monitoring is often necessary to maintain adequate preload without causing pulmonary edema.

Aortic Insufficiency

Aortic insufficiency is generally well tolerated during pregnancy.[27] As the incidence of rheumatic fever declines, other etiologies for aortic valvular incompetence such as connective tissue disease and congenital lesions are becoming important contributors. The pathophysiology involves regurgitation of blood from the aorta into the left ventricle during diastole. With longstanding disease, left ventricular hypertrophy may develop. Factors that lead to increased regurgitation are high afterload and bradycardia below 80 beats per minute.[26] During pregnancy, the falling SVR actually improves blood flow across the incompetent valve.[28, 29]

Epidural anesthesia can be beneficial for gravidas with aortic insufficiency. Not only does it provide adequate pain relief for labor and delivery, but it reduces afterload and does not cause bradycardia. When a general anesthetic is necessary, caution should be taken to prevent abrupt increases in SVR.

Mitral Insufficiency

The potential causes of mitral insufficiency include rheumatic disease, mitral valve prolapse, and dilated cardiomyopathies. The pathophysiology involves regurgitation of blood from the left ventricle across the mitral valve and into the left atrium during systole. The disease progresses to involve left ventricular hypertrophy. As with aortic insufficiency, bradycardia and increased SVR can contribute to decompensation.

This lesion is generally well tolerated during pregnancy, labor, and the postpartum period. Regional techniques provide adequate pain relief for labor and delivery. If general anesthesia is necessary, the same precautions that are used for patients with aortic insufficiency are used.

Mitral Valve Prolapse

Mitral valve prolapse (MVP) is diagnosed in as many as 15% of otherwise normal young women. Pathologic findings include myxomatous degeneration of the valve and redundancy of the valve leaflets. These changes in the mitral valve are seen with Marfan's syndrome, osteogenesis imperfecta, and occasionally coronary artery disease.

The majority of women with MVP are asymptomatic. Pregnancy, labor, and delivery are generally well tolerated. The choice of anesthesia is based on standard indications. Antimicrobial prophylaxis against endocarditis is often used, although it appears that only those patients with redundant mitral valve leaflets are at significantly increased risk of endocarditis.[30]

CONCLUSION

In summary, an understanding of the pathophysiology of pregnancy and its effect on the patient with valvular heart disease is essential. The collaboration of the anesthesiologist, cardiologist, and obstetrician can help to optimize outcomes for the gravida and her newborn.

References

1. Mangano DT: Anesthesia for the pregnant cardiac patient. In Shnider SM, Levinson G (eds): Anesthesia for Obstetrics, 3rd ed. Williams & Wilkins, Baltimore, 1993, p 486.
2. Koonin LM, Atrash HK, Lawson HW, Smith JC: Maternal mortality surveillance, United States 1979–1986. MMWR 40:551, 1991.
3. DeSwiet M: Maternal mortality from heart disease in pregnancy. Br Heart J 69:524, 1993.
4. Hogberg U, Innala E, Sandstrom A: Maternal mortality in Sweden, 1980–1988. Obstet Gynecol 84:240, 1994.
5. Berg CJ, Atrash HK, Koonin LM, Tucker M: Pregnancy related mortality in the United States, 1987–1990. Obstet Gynecol 88:161, 1996.
6. Jacob S, Bloebaum L, Shah G, Varner MW: Maternal mortality in Utah. Obstet Gynecol 91:187, 1998.
7. Pritchard JA: Changes in the blood volume during pregnancy and delivery. Anesthesiology 26:393, 1965.
8. Ueland K, Metcalfe J: Circulatory changes in pregnancy, Clin Obstet Gynecol 18:41, 1975.
9. Katz R, Kavliner JS, Resnik R: Effects of a natural volume overload state (pregnancy) on left ventricular performance in normal human subjects. Circulation 58:434, 1978.
10. Veille JC, Morton MJ, Burry KJ: Maternal cardiovascular adaptations to twin pregnancy. Am J Obstet Gynecol 153:261, 1985.
11. Macfie AG, Magides AP, Richmond MN, Reilly CS: Gastric emptying in pregnancy. Clin Sci 37:395, 1969.
12. Salazar E, Izaguirre R, Verdejo J, Mutchinick D: Failure of adjusted doses of subcutaneous heparin to prevent thromboembolic phenomena in pregnant patients with mechanical cardiac valve prostheses. J Am Coll Cardiol 27:1698, 1996.
13. Sareli P, England MJ, Berk MR, et al: Maternal and fetal sequelae of anticoagulation during pregnancy in patients with mechanical heart valve prostheses. Am J Cardiol 63:1462, 1989.
14. Pavankumar P, Venugopal P, Kaul U, et al: Pregnancy in patients with prosthetic cardiac valve: A 10-year experience. Scand J Thorac Cardiovasc Surg 22:19, 1988.
15. Ben Ismail M, Abid F, Trabelsi S, et al: Cardiac valve prostheses, anticoagulation, and pregnancy. Br Heart J 55:101, 1986.
16. American College of Obstetricians and Gynecologists: Invasive hemodynamic monitoring in obstetrics and gynecology. Educational Bulletin #175, December 1992.
17. Raymond R, Underwood DA, Moodie DS: Cardiovascular problems in pregnancy. Cleve Clin J Med 54:95, 1987.
18. Easterling TR, Chadwick HS, Otto CM, Benedetti TJ: Aortic stenosis in pregnancy. Obstet Gynecol 72:113, 1988.
19. Brighouse D: Anaesthesia for caesarean section in patients with aortic stenosis: The case for regional anesthesia. Anaesthesia 53:107, 1988.
20. Whitfield A, Holdcroft A: Anaesthesia for caesarean section in patients with aortic stenosis: The case for general anaesthesia. Anaesthesia 53(2): 109, 1998.
21. Goertz AW, Lindner KH, Schutz W, et al: Influence of phenylephrine bolus on left ventricular filling dynamics in patients with coronary artery disease and patients with valvular aortic stenosis. Anesthesiology 81:49, 1994.

22. Sharma SK, Sidawi JE, Ramin SM, et al: Cesarean delivery: A randomized trial of epidural vs patient-controlled meperidine analgesia during labor. Anesthesiology 87:487, 1997.
23. Redfern N, Bower S, Bullock RE, Hull CJ: Alfentanil for caesarean section complicated by severe aortic stenosis. Br J Anesth 59:1309, 1987.
24. Sugrue D, Blake S, MacDonald D: Pregnancy complicated by maternal heart disease at the National Maternity Hospital, Dublin, Ireland. 1969 to 1978. Am J Obstet Gynecol 139:1, 1981.
25. Ziskind Z, Etchin A, Frenkel Y, et al: Epidural anesthesia with the Trendelenburg position for cesarean section with or without a cardiac procedure in patients with severe mitral stenosis: A hemodynamic study. J Cardiothorac Anesth 4:354, 1990.
26. Abouleish EI: Obstetric anesthesia and the cardiac patient. Curr Rev Clin Anesth 11:105, 1991.
27. Cunningham FG, MacDonald PC, Gant NF, et al: Williams Obstetrics, 20th ed. Appleton & Lange, Stamford, 1997, p 1087.
28. McAnulty JH, Morton MJ, Ueland K: The heart and pregnancy. Curr Probl Cardiol 13:589, 1988.
29. Mendelson MA, Lang RM: Pregnancy and heart disease. In Barron WM, Lindheimer MD (eds): Medical Disorders During Pregnancy, 2nd ed. St. Louis, Mosby-Year Book, 1995, p 129.
30. Nishimura RA, McGoon MD, Shub C, et al: Echocardiographically documented mitral-valve prolapse: Long-term follow-up of 237 patients. N Engl J Med 313:1305, 1985.

CHAPTER 27

Hypertension

27.1 Pregnancy: Chronic Hypertension

Susan M. Ramin and Larry C. Gilstrap III

Until recently the classification of hypertension during pregnancy has been confusing. However, the National High Blood Pressure Education Program Working Group on High Blood Pressure in Pregnancy has recently reclassified hypertension in pregnancy as chronic hypertension, pre-eclampsia (hypertension with proteinuria), gestational hypertension (hypertension without proteinuria), and superimposed pre-eclampsia.[1] "Gestational hypertension" has replaced the older term pregnancy-induced hypertension. Gestational hypertension is pregnancy specific and includes hypertension without proteinuria or other signs and symptoms of pre-eclampsia. If it persists beyond 12 weeks postpartum, it becomes classified as "chronic hypertension." Chronic hypertension in pregnancy, although possibly made worse by pregnancy, is not pregnancy specific; this implies that the hypertension antedates the pregnancy and persists after the normal postpartum period. Hypertension in such women is usually manifested before 20 weeks' gestation.

The first part of this chapter will deal primarily with chronic hypertension. Gestational hypertension and pre-eclampsia are covered in detail in the second part of this chapter.

INCIDENCE AND EPIDEMIOLOGY

The exact incidence of chronic hypertension is unknown, owing to the lack of agreement on diagnostic criteria and classification. There is agreement, however, that hypertension is one of the most common medical complications encountered during pregnancy. Associated risk factors include maternal obesity, older age, and race. There is a higher incidence of hypertension in black and Hispanic populations.

The majority (90%) of cases of hypertension are essential hypertension.[1a] The remaining cases (10%) may be secondary to a variety of factors (Table 27–1).

DIAGNOSIS

As previously alluded to, the diagnosis of chronic hypertension is based on the presence of hypertension before the 20th week of pregnancy or on hypertension that antedates the pregnancy. Many women with chronic hypertension will have a past history of hypertension and/or will present on antihypertensive medication. Although there is no universally accepted blood pressure criteria, many clinicians use a blood pressure cutoff of 140/90 mm Hg.

The diagnosis of superimposed pre-eclampsia is often difficult to distinguish from simple worsening of the chronic vascular disease. However, criteria consistent with the diagnosis of chronic hypertension with superimposed pre-eclampsia include the following: (1) sudden acute and persistent elevation of blood pressure greater than or equal to 160/110 mm Hg; (2) development of persistent proteinuria; (3) development of symptoms such as headache, scotomata, or right upper quadrant pain; or (4) development of the HELLP syndrome (hemolysis, elevated liver enzymes, and low platelet levels). These are summarized in Table 27–2. Edema of the lower extremities is common to all pregnant women. The incidence of superimposed pre-eclampsia is probably related to the severity of the chronic hypertension and is estimated to be from 5% to 50%.[1a]

MATERNAL AND FETAL EFFECTS

Chronic hypertension may result in significant adverse maternal and fetal effects. Some maternal morbidity, such as cardiovascular decompensation or cerebrovascular accidents, is not particular to pregnancy but may be increased by the cardiovascular changes associated with pregnancy. Chronic hypertension may also increase the risk of renal decompensation or failure. Some of the adverse effects occurring during pregnancy and associated with chronic hypertension include superimposed pre-eclampsia, placental abruption, preterm delivery, intrauterine growth restriction, low birth weight, and increased perinatal mortality (Table 27–3).

MANAGEMENT

There is no unanimity regarding the efficacy of treatment of chronic hypertension during pregnancy with regard to both maternal and fetal outcomes. This is especially true comparing mild and moderate degrees of hypertension to severe disease. In one review of 593 women with chronic hyperten-

Table 27–1. ETIOLOGY OF CHRONIC HYPERTENSION DURING PREGNANCY

Essential—90%
Secondary—10%
• Renal disease
• Endocrine disorders
Diabetes
Pheochromocytoma
Thyrotoxicosis
• Connective tissue disorders
Lupus erythematosus
Scleroderma
• Arterial abnormalities
Coarctation
Renovascular hypertension

Adapted in part from Cunningham FG, MacDonald PC, Gant NF, et al: Hypertensive disorders in pregnancy. In Cunningham FG, et al (eds): Williams Obstetrics, 20th ed. Appleton & Lange, Norwalk, CT, 1997, pp 693–744.

Table 27–2. SIGNS AND SYMPTOMS OF SUPERIMPOSED PRE-ECLAMPSIA

- Acute persistent elevation of blood pressure ($\geq$160/110 mm Hg)
- Sudden development of proteinuria (usually $\geq$2+)
- Headache, scotomata, or epigastric or right upper quadrant pain
- Development of the HELLP syndrome (hemolysis, elevated liver enzymes, and low platelet levels)

sion who received no antihypertensives, the perinatal mortality was 32 per 1000 (deliveries between 1972–1974) and the incidence of superimposed pre-eclampsia was 6%.[2] Redman,[3] in a review of 184 women with chronic hypertension treated with methyldopa and/or hydralazine, reported that 1 in 4 women developed superimposed pre-eclampsia and the perinatal mortality was 1.6%.

Mabie and associates[4] reported on the course and outcome of 169 pregnancies in 156 women with chronic hypertension. Most women were seen before 20 weeks' gestation. Antihypertensive agents were given only if diastolic blood pressure was greater than 90 mm Hg. Methyldopa, 750 to 2000 mg, was the initial agent used if the woman was not taking an antihypertensive agent. Hydrochlorothiazide, 50 mg daily, was added if necessary to control the blood pressure. If the combination of methyldopa and hydrochlorothiazide was unsuccessful in achieving control, propranolol was added. Antihypertensive therapy was given to 82 women, whereas 82 women were given no treatment. Triple therapy was necessary in 5 women. There was no difference in perinatal mortality, but there was an increase in fetal growth restriction in the treatment group.

In another study of chronic hypertension during pregnancy, Sibai and colleagues[5] randomized 263 women with mild to moderate disease to methyldopa, to labetalol, or to no treatment at 6 to 13 weeks of pregnancy. The goal of therapy was to achieve a blood pressure of less than 140/90 mm Hg. All women in the control group were treated for a blood pressure of greater than 160/110 mm Hg. Somewhat surprising was that there was no significant difference in gestational age at delivery, premature delivery (i.e., <37 weeks), mean birth weight, superimposed pre-eclampsia, placental abruption, or perinatal mortality (1.1% for all three groups).

Although there is no clear-cut benefit to either mother or infant of antihypertensive therapy for pregnant women with chronic hypertension, there does appear to be a clear-cut association with outcome in whether superimposed pre-eclampsia develops. For example, Sibai and associates[6] reported a significant increase in the frequency of placental abruption (10% vs. 0.5%), intrauterine growth restriction (32% vs. 5%), and perinatal mortality (24% vs. 0.5%) and a difference in mean birth weight (2345 g vs. 3210 g) in the 21 women who developed superimposed pre-eclampsia compared with the 190 women with chronic hypertension who did not. In another study[7] of 44 women with severe chronic hypertension (i.e., blood pressure $\geq$ 170/110 mm Hg) between 6 to 11 weeks' gestation, 23 developed superimposed pre-eclampsia and 21 did not. All women received methyldopa and hydralazine to maintain blood pressure of $\leq$ 160/110 mm Hg and were hospitalized if blood pressure was $\geq$ 180/120 mm Hg. As with earlier reports, superimposed pre-eclampsia portended a worse outcome. There was an increase in preterm birth (100% vs. 38%), placental abruption (9% vs. 0%), and deterioration of renal function (65% vs. 24%). The mean gestational age at delivery was 28.6 versus 36.5 weeks, and the mean birth weight was 827 g versus 2632 g. Other factors besides antihypertensive therapy and the development of superimposed pre-eclampsia, which might affect outcome in pregnant women with chronic hypertension, include the presence of underlying renal disease, cardiovascular disease, and the degree and duration of hypertension.

In summary, treatment with antihypertensive medications appears to have little, if any, impact on pregnancy outcome, especially for women with mild disease.[1] The single best predictor is whether superimposed pre-eclampsia develops or not.

RECOMMENDATIONS FOR ANTIHYPERTENSIVE THERAPY

As previously mentioned, there are few, if any, data to support an improved pregnancy outcome with antihypertensive therapy. However, therapy may benefit the mother by the prevention of cardiac decompensation, renal decompensation, or cerebrovascular accidents. Although there are no clear-cut criteria for therapy during pregnancy, it would seem reasonable to utilize antihypertensive medications in the following situations[1, 8]: (1) diastolic blood pressure of 100 to 110 mm Hg; (2) left ventricular hypertrophy and diastolic blood pressure of greater than 95 mm Hg; and (3) presence of nephropathy and diastolic blood pressure of greater than 95 mm Hg. In addition, it would seem reasonable to continue antihypertensive therapy in pregnant women who are on medication before pregnancy and to use such therapy in women who have already had a cerebrovascular accident (Table 27–4).

ANTIHYPERTENSIVE MEDICATIONS

There are numerous antihypertensive medications available, the majority of which are relatively safe for use during

Table 27–3. POTENTIAL ADVERSE MATERNAL AND FETAL EFFECTS OF CHRONIC HYPERTENSION DURING PREGNANCY

Maternal Effects	Fetal Effects
• Cardiac decompensation	• Intrauterine growth restriction
• Cerebrovascular accident	• Low birth weight
• Placental abruption	• Prematurity
• Renal decompensation/failure	• Perinatal mortality

Table 27–4. RECOMMENDATIONS FOR ANTIHYPERTENSIVE THERAPY DURING PREGNANCY IN WOMEN WITH CHRONIC HYPERTENSION

- Antihypertensive agents before pregnancy
- Diastolic blood pressure of 100 to 110 mm Hg or more
- Left ventricular hypertrophy and diastolic blood pressure of >95 mm Hg
- Nephropathy and diastolic blood pressure of >95 mmHg
- Previous history or current risk of cerebrovascular accident

Table 27–5. ANTIHYPERTENSIVE MEDICATIONS* FOR TREATMENT OF CHRONIC HYPERTENSION DURING PREGNANCY

• Methyldopa	• Labetalol	• Nifedipine
• Hydralazine	• Verapamil	• Diuretics†

*Angiotensin-converting enzyme inhibitors are contraindicated during pregnancy.
† See text.

pregnancy (Table 27–5). The angiotensin-converting enzyme (ACE) inhibitors are contraindicated during pregnancy because they have been reported to be associated with fetal renal failure, oligohydramnios, pulmonary hypoplasia, hypocalvaria, and fetal death.[9–12] Examples of agents in this class include captopril, enalapril, and lisinopril.

Of all the antihypertensive medications available, methyldopa is probably the main drug used for treatment for chronic hypertension during pregnancy.[13] It has proven efficacy and safety, and the usual daily dose is 500 to 2000 mg total.

Hydralazine is used mainly for acute hypertension, such as with superimposed pre-eclampsia. It is not very effective when used orally for chronic hypertension.

The β-adrenergic blockers such as labetalol are also very effective (and safe) for use during pregnancy. The usual dose of labetalol is 200 to 400 mg twice daily up to 1200 mg (twice daily) for severe hypertension.

There are few data regarding the efficacy and safety of the calcium channel blockers for the treatment of chronic hypertension during pregnancy. In addition, the use of calcium channel blocking drugs may be associated with a decrease in uteroplacental blood flow.[14] However, they should be continued if severe hypertension is well controlled.

Diuretics should rarely, if ever, be used as primary therapy for control of hypertension during pregnancy. They may be associated with a decrease in uteroplacental blood flow and generally should not be initiated after 20 weeks' gestation except in conditions of fluid overload. Diuretic therapy to control blood pressure should be continued, however, in women who are on this medication before pregnancy or if initiated before 20 weeks' gestation.

BED REST, HOSPITALIZATION, AND LABORATORY EVALUATION

There are few data to support the use of bed rest as routine therapy for pregnant women with uncomplicated chronic hypertension. However, hospitalization may be used for women whose blood pressure is difficult to control as an outpatient, women who have questionable superimposed pre-eclampsia, or women who may need further evaluation for newly diagnosed chronic hypertension. Laboratory evaluation should generally include electrolytes, renal function tests, and cardiac evaluation (i.e., electrocardiogram and possibly echocardiogram). A chest radiograph may also be performed with an abdominal shield, although results may be difficult to interpret secondary to changes associated with pregnancy. Other laboratory evaluation for diabetes mellitus, systemic lupus erythematosus, or pheochromocytoma should be obtained as indicated.

Serial ultrasonography should be performed every 3 to 4 weeks to monitor fetal growth or more often if indicated. Some form of antepartum fetal testing should be used at least weekly to assess fetal well-being. Daily fetal movement monitoring along with either a weekly nonstress test or biophysical profile should be used beginning at 30 to 32 weeks' gestation, depending on the severity of blood pressure and other complications. The frequency of such monitoring may be increased (i.e., twice or three times weekly or even daily) as indicated. Unfortunately, scientific data are lacking as to which test is best and how often testing should be done.

TIMING AND METHOD OF DELIVERY

Women with well-controlled, but otherwise uncomplicated, essential hypertension and normal fetal testing may carry their infants to term. The majority of such women can undergo induction of labor at 38 to 40 weeks' gestation and can deliver vaginally. Women who develop superimposed severe pre-eclampsia should undergo delivery of the infant regardless of gestational age. Such women should receive magnesium sulfate for seizure prophylaxis and either intravenous hydralazine (initial dose of 5 to 10 mg and repeated every 10–20 minutes) or labetalol (initial dose of 10 mg, followed by subsequent doses of 20 mg, 40 mg, 40 mg, and 80 mg every 20 minutes until either the desired effect is achieved or a maximum dose of 300 mg is administered) to maintain diastolic blood pressure of less than 110 mm Hg and systolic blood pressure of less than 180 mm Hg.[1a] However, attempts should not be made to "normalize" blood pressure, because uteroplacental and renal blood flow may depend on a given blood pressure level.

Epidural analgesia/anesthesia is ideal for the management of pain during labor and for anesthesia if cesarean delivery or operative vaginal delivery is indicated. Cesarean delivery should be reserved for obstetric indications.

In women who have severe hypertension, renal disease, systemic lupus erythematosus, or intrauterine growth restriction of the fetus, the fetus most often is delivered prematurely for maternal and/or fetal indications.

CONCLUSION

Chronic hypertension is a common medical complication of pregnancy and may result in significant maternal and fetal morbidity and mortality. There are few data that antihypertensive therapy, per se, affects pregnancy outcome, but with severe disease such therapy may be of benefit to the mother in reducing the risk of cardiac or renal decompensation or cerebrovascular accidents. Superimposed pre-eclampsia, occurring in 5% to 50% of cases, is the single best predictor of pregnancy outcome.

References

1. Report of the National High Blood Pressure Education Program Working Group on High Blood Pressure. Am J Obstet Gynecol 183:S1–S22, 2000.

1a. Cunningham FG, MacDonald PC, Gant NF, et al: Hypertensive disorders in pregnancy. In Cunningham FG, et al (eds): Williams Obstetrics, 20th ed. Appleton & Lange, Norwalk, CT, 1997, pp 693–744.
2. Chesley LC: Superimposed preeclampsia or eclampsia. In Chesley LC (ed): Hypertensive Disorders in Pregnancy. Appleton-Century-Crofts, New York, 1978, pp 14, 302, and 482.
3. Redman CWG: Treatment of hypertension in pregnancy. Kidney Int 18:267, 1980.
4. Mabie WC, Pernoll ML, Biswas MK: Chronic hypertension in pregnancy. Obstet Gynecol 67:197, 1986.
5. Sibai BM, Mabie WC, Shamsa F, et al: A comparison of no medication versus methyldopa or labetalol in chronic hypertension during pregnancy. Am J Obstet Gynecol 162:960, 1990.
6. Sibai BM, Abdella TN, Anderson GD: Pregnancy outcome in 211 patients with mild chronic hypertension. Obstet Gynecol 61:571, 1983.
7. Sibai BM, Anderson GD: Pregnancy outcome of intensive therapy in severe hypertension in first trimester. Obstet Gynecol 67:517, 1986.
8. Rey E, Couturier A: The prognosis of pregnancy in women with chronic hypertension. Am J Obstet Gynecol 171:410, 1994.
9. Barr M, Cohen MM: ACE inhibitor fetopathy and hypocalvaria: The kidney-skull connection. Teratology 44:485, 1991.
10. Brent RL, Beckman DA: Angiotensin-converting enzyme inhibitors, an embryopathic class of drugs with unique properties: Information for clinical teratology counselors. Teratology 43:543, 1991.
11. Piper JM, Ray WA, Rosa FW: Pregnancy outcome following exposure to angiotensin-converting enzyme inhibitors. Obstet Gynecol 80:429, 1992.
12. Pryde PG, Sedman AB, Nugent CE, Barr M: Angiotensin-converting enzyme inhibitor fetopathy. J Am Soc Nephrol 3:1575, 1993.
13. Sibai BM: Treatment of hypertension in pregnant women. N Engl J Med 335:257, 1996.
14. Murad SHN, Tabsh KMA, Shilyanski G, et al: Effects of verapamil on uterine blood flow and maternal cardiovascular function in the awake pregnant ewe. Anesth Analg 64:7, 1985.

27.2 Pre-eclampsia and Eclampsia

Andrea G. Witlin and Michael Belfort

Pregnancy-induced hypertension (PIH) is described by the American College of Obstetricians and Gynecologists as a multiorgan disease process that may involve more than elevated blood pressure.[1] Several clinical subsets exist depending on the end-organ effects. For the purposes of this discussion the terms PIH, gestational hypertension, and pre-eclampsia will be used interchangeably unless otherwise specified. The differences between chronic hypertension, gestational hypertension, and pre-eclampsia are summarized in Table 27–6.

PRECONCEPTION COUNSELING RECOMMENDATIONS

Women with chronic hypertension contemplating pregnancy, or gravidas with hypertension seen at the first prenatal visit, should be counseled regarding management of the intended pregnancy. Periodic medical surveillance is the mainstay of management for evaluation and therapy for maternal disease.[2] Lifestyle modifications (e.g., weight reduction and exercise) as suggested by the Joint National Committee on Prevention, Detection, Evaluation, and Treatment of High Blood Pressure[3] for management of adult hypertension, differ from recommendations during pregnancy.[2] Weight reduction and vigorous exercise are not recommended for hypertensive gravidas.[2] Periodic bed rest and limitation of physical activity during pregnancy may optimize uteroplacental blood flow.[2] Salt restriction (as recommended for adult hypertensive patients)[3] is generally not recommended during gestation because gravidas with hypertension have decreased plasma volume relative to normotensive gravidas. However, a subset of gravidas with salt-sensitive hypertension, and select gravidas with renal disease, may benefit from sodium restriction during pregnancy.[2] As with ambulatory management of adult hypertensive patients,[3] home (self) blood pressure monitoring for hypertensive gravidas provides a realistic recording of blood pressure values.

OUTPATIENT MANAGEMENT OF HYPERTENSION

Hypertensive disorders are the most common medical complications of pregnancy and are a major cause of maternal and perinatal morbidity and mortality.[2] The only definitive

Table 27–6. HYPERTENSIVE DISORDERS OF PREGNANCY

CLINICAL FINDING	CHRONIC HYPERTENSION	GESTATIONAL HYPERTENSION	PRE-ECLAMPSIA
Time of onset of hypertension	<20 weeks' gestation	Usually in third trimester	≥20 weeks' gestation
Degree of hypertension	Mild or severe	Mild	Mild or severe
Proteinuria*	Absent	Absent	Usually present
Serum urate >5.5 mg/dl	Rare	Absent	Present in almost all cases
Hemoconcentration	Absent	Absent	Present in severe disease
Thrombocytopenia	Absent	Absent	Present in severe disease
Hepatic dysfunction	Absent	Absent	Present in severe disease

*Defined as ≥1+ by dipstick on two occasions or ≥300 mg in a 24-hour urine collection.
From Sibai BM: Treatment of hypertension in pregnant women. N Engl J Med 335:257–265, 1996. With permission from the Massachusetts Medical Society.

therapy for the maternal manifestations of pre-eclampsia is delivery. Unfortunately, immediate delivery is not always optimal from both a fetal and a maternal standpoint.[1] Pre-eclampsia presenting remotely from term without evidence of fetal compromise or maternal end-organ involvement may be managed expectantly to allow for fetal maturity. Historically, inpatient hospitalization is used for stabilization and evaluation of gravidas with gestational hypertension.[4] Recently, there has been a trend toward outpatient management of these women.[5]

Summary of Studies of Outpatient Management

Numerous studies have provided a rationale for ambulatory management of hypertension in pregnancy. We attempt here to incorporate their conclusions into current practice.

In a classic study of 346 nulliparous women with PIH monitored in the high-risk pregnancy unit at Parkland Hospital, the "gold standard" for comparison of inpatient management with ambulatory studies was established.[6] The time interval for study was 1971 to 1975. PIH was diagnosed as diastolic blood pressure greater than 90 mm Hg on two or more occasions at least 6 hours apart. If there was no clinical improvement after 24 hours of in-hospital observation, delivery was effected. If improvement was present, the patient was transferred to the high-risk unit for continued observation and management. The patients were allowed to ambulate as desired. Factors necessitating delivery included persistent or recurrent hypertension, rapid weight gain, decrease in creatinine clearance, significant proteinuria, clinical and/or ultrasound evidence of intrauterine growth restriction, and development of headache or visual symptoms. Eighty-five percent of the women became normotensive within 5 days after admission to the unit. Eleven percent of these women never had a recurrence of hypertension. Six percent of the women had severe hypertension that either persisted or worsened, thereby requiring delivery within 7 days of admission. The authors noted that many times the clinical changes suggestive of worsening disease were very subtle. Proteinuria was present in 47 women (13%) at some time during their hospitalization. Fifteen percent of the women required intravenous administration of hydralazine for blood pressure control during labor. This study was extended until a total of 545 nulliparas with PIH were followed on the high-risk unit.[4] The results were similar to the pilot study: 81% of women became normotensive after admission, 42% had recurrent hypertension before labor, 13% remained normotensive, and 6% had persistent hypertension.[4]

Crowther and colleagues[7] randomized 218 women with nonproteinuric hypertension to hospital admission or home care. The risk of developing severe hypertension was reduced by half in the hospitalized group, with a relative risk of 0.6 (95% CI 0.4–0.9). However, this did not translate into improved outcome. There was no significant difference in the development of severe proteinuria, intrauterine growth restriction, or admission to the neonatal intensive care unit.

Tuffnell and associates[8] randomized 54 women with mild hypertension (greater than 26 weeks' gestation) to either care in a day unit or standard care by their physician without benefit of the day unit. The control group was more likely to be admitted to the hospital (odds ratio 8.8 [95% CI 3.0–25.8]) and more likely to develop proteinuria (odds ratio 11.4 [95% CI 1.8–71.4]). Although the trend is definitely in favor of the day unit, these very wide confidence intervals preclude drawing strong conclusions. Proteinuria, preterm delivery, and perinatal death were not reduced by bed rest. The women preferred outpatient management. Twenty-eight percent of the women had deterioration in their status after their initial surveillance. This study suggests that the critical aspect is the mode of surveillance rather than the locale of service.

Barton and colleagues[5, 9, 10] reviewed the experience from the Healthdyne perinatal database in a series of three observational studies evaluating monitored outpatient management of mild hypertension in pregnancy. The first study[5] evaluated a prospective cohort of 592 women between 24 and 36 weeks' gestation undergoing monitored outpatient management. The outpatient management scheme included automated blood pressure and pulse measurement (four times per day), daily weight, fetal kick counts, duration of rest/sleep periods, and assessment of proteinuria. An automatic data recorder was provided by Healthdyne. Indications for hospitalization included worsening blood pressure, abnormal hematologic parameters, or fetal compromise. Indications for delivery included worsening maternal or fetal condition, spontaneous labor, or a favorable cervix at term. Pregnancy was prolonged 27.4 ± 3.3 days in the outpatient group. This compared favorably with previous reports of inpatient management.[4, 11] The mean number of inpatient antepartum days was reduced to 1.7 ± 5.8 days after intensive outpatient management. The gestational age at delivery was 36.7 ± 3.6 weeks. The cohort with proteinuria (defined as greater than or equal to 1+ on dipstick) yielded a greater incidence of antepartum hospitalization, decreased gestational age at delivery, shortened pregnancy prolongation, and lower birth weight. This adds to the information gained from previous studies suggesting increased morbidity associated with proteinuria.

The second study in the series[9] evaluated the feasibility of outpatient management in 60 teens (aged 13–19) matched with 120 adult controls. The mean pregnancy prolongation for the teen cohort was 23.5 ± 19.0 days, with a mean antepartum stay of 1.4 ± 2.8 days after ambulatory management. There were no maternal complications or neonatal deaths. The gestational age at delivery was 37.0 ± 2.0 weeks. Therefore, it was concluded that outpatient management was equally feasible in a teen population. Firm conclusions are limited by the small sample size.

The third series[10] evaluated a matched cohort of 379 mature gravidas (≥35 years) with 379 younger gravidas (≥20 to ≤30 years). The mean pregnancy prolongation was 23.5 ± 21.0 days with a gestational age at delivery of 37.2 ± 2.3 weeks. Again, the authors noted that the presence of proteinuria was associated with a lower gestational age at delivery, shorter pregnancy prolongation, and lower birth weight. The absence of proteinuria appeared to be protective for preterm delivery less than 37 weeks, with a relative risk of 0.6 (95% CI 0.5–0.8) in younger gravidas and a relative risk of 0.5 (95% CI 0.4–0.6) in the mature gravidas.

Although these studies by Barton and colleagues[5, 9, 10] favorably critiqued monitored outpatient management in a wide cohort of gravidas, these data must be evaluated in view of their possible selection bias, because the studies were not randomized. It is likely that only the most "ideal" candidates were selected for ambulatory management. Therefore, these results may not be generalizable to all gravidas. We need to be careful that managed care companies do not misinterpret these data to mean that all hypertension can be managed on an ambulatory basis.

THE RATIONALE FOR ANTIHYPERTENSIVE THERAPY DURING PREGNANCY

Medical intervention is usually recommended when the diastolic blood pressure exceeds 110 mm Hg,[1, 12, 13] given the risk of intracranial hemorrhage.[14] Cerebral autoregulation is operative between a mean arterial pressure (MAP) of 60 and 150 mm Hg.[15] This principle underlies the rationale for therapy for both acute and chronic hypertension during pregnancy. Furthermore, most women with pre-eclampsia/eclampsia will have an abnormal cerebral hemodynamic profile at a MAP of 110 to 150 mm Hg.[15]

The beneficial effects of antihypertensive therapy during pregnancy must be balanced against any potential adverse maternal, fetal, or neonatal effects. Adverse fetal effects may result indirectly from decreasing uteroplacental blood flow or by directly influencing the umbilical and fetal cardiovascular circulation. Randomized trials in nonpregnant women and retrospective studies in gravidas suggest that antihypertensive therapy decreases the incidence of stroke and cardiovascular complications in women with diastolic blood pressure exceeding 110 mm Hg. It is unknown whether lowering blood pressure in gravidas with mild uncomplicated hypertension (about 95% of all women with chronic hypertension) is beneficial. To improve perinatal outcomes, antihypertensive therapy in gravidas with mild hypertension must reduce the incidence of pre-eclampsia, abruptio placentae, preterm delivery, and fetal or neonatal death. In the past 30 years, at least seven studies have compared antihypertensive therapy with either no medication or a placebo in pregnant women with mild chronic hypertension.[16] There was no decrease in the frequency of superimposed pre-eclampsia or incidence of preterm delivery.

Sibai and associates[11] randomly allocated 200 primigravid women with mild pre-eclampsia at 26 to 35 weeks' gestation to treatment with either bed rest alone or bed rest in combination with labetalol. Labetalol reduced average systolic and diastolic blood pressure. However, there were no changes in renal function tests or proteinuria attributable to this beneficial effect on blood pressure.

Sibai and associates[17] also studied 300 women with a history of chronic hypertension before pregnancy who were randomized to receive initially either no medication or the antihypertensive medications methyldopa or labetalol. Antihypertensive therapy yielded no benefit in reducing the risk of superimposed pre-eclampsia, incidence of abruptio placentae, or cesarean delivery. Discontinuation of antihypertensive drugs at study entry did not increase the risk of either exacerbation of hypertension or development of superimposed pre-eclampsia.

Sibai and associates[18] performed a similar study to evaluate the effect of nifedipine on pregnancy outcome. All women had proteinuria (>300 mg/24 h) and/or elevated uric acid levels (≥6 mg/dl) at time of entry to the study. It appeared that nifedipine protected against development of severe hypertension (relative risk of 0.5 [95% CI 0.2–1.1]). However, this reduction in blood pressure did not translate into improved pregnancy prolongation or outcome. Also, the addition of nifedipine did not protect against the development of nephrotic range proteinuria (relative risk 1.6 [95% CI 0.8–3.4]).

ANTIHYPERTENSIVE MEDICATIONS

Various antihypertensive agents for both the outpatient therapy of chronic hypertension and parenteral therapy for acute life-threatening hypertension in pregnancy are reviewed. Outpatient antihypertensive therapy is applicable only to women with well-controlled, nonproteinuric, chronic hypertension. Gravidas with chronic hypertension who develop proteinuria, worsening hypertension, or superimposed pre-eclampsia should be managed as inpatients. Likewise, gravidas with pre-eclampsia remote from term, requiring antihypertensive agents, should have inpatient management (Table 27–7).

Table 27–7. ANTIHYPERTENSIVE DRUGS IN PREGNANCY

COMMON DRUGS FOR CHRONIC THERAPY OF HYPERTENSION			
Class	**Drug**	**Starting Dose**	**Maximum Dose**
Central α_2 agonist	Methyldopa	250 mg tid	4 g/d
Calcium channel blocker	Nifedipine	10 mg qid	120 mg/d
α/β Blocker	Labetalol	150 mg bid	2400 mg/d

COMMON DRUGS FOR ACUTE THERAPY OF SEVERE HYPERTENSION		
Class	**Drug**	**Dose**
Arteriolar dilator	Hydralazine	5–10 mg IV every 15–30 minutes
Calcium channel blocker	Nifedipine	10–20 mg PO every 30 minutes
	Nicardipine	1 mg/min IV to maximum of 5 mg IV every 15 minutes (maximum 15 mg/h)
α/β Blocker	Labetalol	20–40–80 mg IV every 20 minutes (up to 300 mg) or titrate IV dose (1–2 mg/min)
Arterial/venous dilator	Nitroprusside	0.2–0.5 μg/kg/min

Methyldopa (Aldomet) is the most commonly used drug to treat hypertension during pregnancy and is the standard against which other agents are compared. It is the only antihypertensive drug whose long-term safety for both mother and fetus has been assessed. Methyldopa lowers blood pressure by stimulation of the central α_2-receptors via α-methyl-norepinephrine (the active form of methyldopa). It might also act as an α_2 -peripheral blocker by means of a false neurotransmitter. Methyldopa reduces systemic vascular resistance (SVR) without causing physiologically significant changes in heart rate or cardiac output while maintaining renal blood flow. Neither acute fetal nor neonatal effects, nor long-term infant effects have been reported from chronic use of methyldopa during pregnancy. The dose of methyldopa is 1 to 2 g/d given in four divided doses up to a maximum of 4 g/d.

Calcium channel blockers such as nifedipine (Procardia, Adalat), nicardipine (Cardene), nimodipine, amlodipine, and nitrendipine lower blood pressure primarily by relaxing arterial smooth muscle. Calcium channel blockers act by inhibiting transmembrane calcium ion influx from the extracellular space into the cytoplasm. This blocks excitation-contraction coupling in smooth muscle fibers and results in vasodilatation and decreased peripheral resistance. Nifedipine has potent vasodilating properties without effecting any reduction in cardiac output. Nifedipine has been used both for treatment of chronic hypertension during pregnancy and for acute reduction in blood pressure. Neither adverse fetal effects nor change in uteroplacental flow or placental resistance has been reported after either short-term or long-term nifedipine therapy. Nifedipine has a rapid onset of action after oral administration. It has been used for both acute and chronic lowering of blood pressure during pregnancy. The decrease in blood pressure obtained from nifedipine therapy is proportional to the initial blood pressure level. The elimination half-life of nifedipine varies with drug formulation and appears to be accelerated during pregnancy as compared with the nongravid state.[19] The maximum daily dose is 120 mg. Common side effects include headache, flushing, tachycardia, and fatigue.

Theoretically, the concurrent use of nifedipine with magnesium sulfate may potentiate its antihypertensive effect and neuromuscular blockade, although clinically this has not been a significant problem. Recent reports of sudden death in patients receiving short-acting nifedipine should be interpreted with caution. The majority of these patients had underlying ischemic heart disease and cardiac dysfunction.[20] There have been no reported deaths related to nifedipine use in women with pre-eclampsia. An alternative to nifedipine use is nicardipine. Nicardipine may be used both orally for chronic therapy and parenterally for acute therapy. It is a more potent calcium channel blocker than nifedipine and is associated with increased peripheral and central vasodilation, a potential advantage for therapy of pre-eclampsia/eclampsia. Furthermore, it may prove to be a valuable alternative to nifedipine therapy, given the current controversy regarding the short-acting form of nifedipine as an antihypertensive agent.

Belfort and coworkers[21] have evaluated the calcium channel blocker, nimodipine, which has specific vasodilatory effects on human cerebral vessels, in the management of pre-eclampsia. Because of nimodipine's selective cerebrovasodilator effect and reduction of blood pressure, Belfort suggests that nimodipine may be useful in treating pre-eclampsia. Nimodipine deserves further investigation as an anti-seizure agent for the prevention of eclampsia associated with cerebral vasospasm and cerebral ischemia.

Labetalol (Normodyne, Trandate) is a combined α- and β-adrenoceptor antagonist that can induce a controlled, rapid decrease in blood pressure by means of decreased SVR in patients with severe hypertension.[22] The α-adrenergic blockade induces vasodilatation and improves the primary vasospasm present in pre-eclampsia. Unlike "pure" β-adrenergic blockers, labetalol maintains cardiac output, reduces total peripheral resistance, and does not decrease peripheral blood flow.[23] Mabie and associates compared bolus intravenous labetalol with intravenous hydralazine in the acute treatment of severe PIH. They found that labetalol had a more rapid onset of action without inducing reflex tachycardia.[24] For chronic therapy, an initial oral dose of 300 mg/d may be increased to a maximum daily dose of 1200 mg. Intravenous labetalol may be used for acute blood pressure reduction. The initial intravenous dosage is 20 mg, followed by subsequent doses every 20 minutes: 40 mg, 80 mg, 80 mg, 80 mg until either a desired effect or a maximum dose of 300 mg is reached. Alternatively, a constant intravenous infusion may be started at 1 to 2 mg/min until therapeutic goals are achieved, then decreased to 0.5 mg/min or discontinued as indicated clinically.[13] The maximum initial reduction (over the first 24 hours) of MAP in hypertensive emergencies during pregnancy should be limited to a decrease in MAP of 25%. Side effects of labetalol include scalp tingling, tremulousness, and headache.

Hydralazine (Apresoline) is a potent vasodilator that acts directly on smooth muscle. Hydralazine reduces vascular resistance through direct cyclic guanosine monophosphate–induced relaxation of arteriolar smooth muscle, affecting precapillary resistance vessels more than postcapillary capacitance vessels.[25] It is the most commonly used agent to control severe hypertension in pre-eclampsia and is given as an intravenous bolus injection. After intravenous administration, the hypotensive effect develops gradually over 15 to 30 minutes, peaking at 20 minutes. The usual bolus dose is 5 to 10 mg to be repeated every 20 to 30 minutes as needed. Maternal side-effects include headache, flushing, palpitations, nausea, and vomiting. Women with severe pre-eclampsia show a significant increase in maternal heart rate and cardiac index, with a decrease in MAP and SVR index after intravenous administration of hydralazine.[26, 27]

Sodium nitroprusside (Nitropress) is a potent arterial and venous dilator used for emergent therapy of hypertensive crisis. Sodium nitroprusside interferes with influx and intracellular activation of calcium. It is given as a continuous intravenous infusion due to its immediate onset and short duration of action. The initial infusion dose in gravid women should be 0.2 μg/kg/min rather than the usual dose of 0.5 μg/kg/min as is standard in nonpregnant patients. This drug should be reserved for extreme emergencies secondary to concerns of thiocyanate toxicity in the neonate. The solution is light sensitive and should be covered in foil and changed every 24 hours.[28] Arterial blood gases should be monitored to watch for developing metabolic acidosis, which may be an early sign of cyanide toxicity. Antepartum therapy should be limited because of the potential for fetal cyanide toxicity.[29]

The hemodynamic pattern associated with nitroprusside represents a cardiopulmonary baroreceptor reflex presumably related to the Bezold-Jarisch reflex and probably reflects nitroprusside's prominent venous dilator action on the relatively reduced blood volume characteristic of severe pre-eclampsia.

Nitroglycerin (Nitrostat IV, Nitro-Bid IV, Tridil) relaxes predominantly venous, but also arterial, vascular smooth muscle. It has been shown to decrease preload at low doses and afterload in high doses.[30] It is a rapid-acting potent antihypertensive agent with a very short hemodynamic half-life. Nitroglycerin is administered through an infusion pump at an initial rate of 5 μg/min and may be doubled every 5 minutes. Methemoglobinemia may result from high dose (>7 μg/kg/min) intravenous infusion. Because the vasospasm of pre-eclampsia is predominantly in the arterial vascular beds, nitroglycerin should be reserved for treatment of cases in which specific venodilation may be required, such as in pulmonary edema complicating hypertensive cardiomyopathy.

Clonidine (Catapres) is a powerful α_2 central stimulant. The usual oral dose in pregnancy is 0.1 to 0.3 g/d given in two divided doses to a maximum of 1.2 mg/d. Rebound hypertension has been reported after abrupt cessation of the drug. Horvath and colleagues compared clonidine and methyldopa in 100 pregnant women with hypertension at a mean gestation of 32 weeks.[31] There was no significant difference in perinatal outcome, and neither drug was associated with significant maternal or neonatal side effects. Horvath and colleagues concluded that clonidine was a safe and effective drug for treating hypertension in pregnancy.[31]

A variety of beta-blocking agents have been used to treat hypertension in pregnancy. These drugs have different actions, depending on their receptor selectivity and the presence of intrinsic sympathomimetic activity. Their use has been associated with neonatal bradycardia, hypoglycemia, fetal growth restriction, altered adaptation to perinatal asphyxia, and neonatal respiratory depression. However, there is no evidence to suggest an increase in fetal or neonatal mortality or severe morbidity, and it is likely that most of these reported side effects are due to maternal disease rather than to a drug effect.[32] Atenolol has adverse effects on uteroplacental and fetal hemodynamics[33] as well as on fetal growth; its use should be avoided in pregnancy.[34]

Although thiazide diuretics are generally the first drugs selected for antihypertensive therapy in nonpregnant patients, their continued use in pregnancy in women with chronic hypertension remains controversial. Gravid women with chronic hypertension treated with diuretics have a marked reduction in plasma volume when compared with a control group not receiving diuretics.[35] This may be detrimental to fetal growth. Our policy is to discontinue thiazide diuretics at the time of the first visit. Few chronic hypertensive women will require additional medications.[36] Likewise, diuretic therapy should not be initiated for antepartum control of hypertension in the woman with pre-eclampsia. We restrict diuretic therapy (loop diuretics) for those pregnancies complicated by pulmonary edema, renal disease, or cardiac disease. In view of their potential detrimental effects and no proven benefits, diuretics should be avoided in pregnancy.[32]

Chronic use of angiotensin-converting enzyme inhibitor (ACE-I) therapy in pregnancy is associated with fetal growth restriction, oligohydramnios, congenital malformation, neonatal renal failure, and death[37]; therefore, ACE-I therapy should be reserved for postpartum use.

Drug therapy for hypertension during pregnancy should be based on the severity of the hypertension, the potential risk for target organ damage, and the presence of pre-existing cardiovascular disease.[38, 39] The therapeutic objective in severe hypertension is to prevent maternal cerebrovascular accidents and congestive heart failure without compromising cerebral perfusion or jeopardizing uteroplacental blood flow. Therapeutic goals are thus for reduction of blood pressure to a level associated with decreased risk for loss of cerebral autoregulation, not normalization of blood pressure. For women with gestational hypertension or mild pre-eclampsia, the pregnancy outcome is usually favorable without drug therapy.

MATERNAL MANAGEMENT

Women presenting early in pregnancy with either a history of chronic hypertension or a history of pre-eclampsia in a prior pregnancy should have a baseline 24-hour urine test performed for total protein.

Guidelines for the ambulatory management of hypertension in pregnancy are as follows. Women with systolic blood pressure less than 150 mm Hg and diastolic blood pressure less than 100 mm Hg (with or without antihypertensive medication) are candidates for ambulatory management (Table 27–8). In accordance with previous studies suggesting increased morbidity associated with proteinuria, we have limited ambulatory management to women with less than 1000 mg urinary protein excretion per 24 hours. It was believed that there is an added risk of abruption and eclampsia associated with increasing proteinuria. However, a study by Witlin and associates[40] refuted that claim. In a series of 445 consecutively managed women with severe pre-eclampsia and eclampsia, proteinuria was not predictive of either eclampsia or abruption. To be considered for ambulatory management, renal and liver function tests should be reassuring, with no values suggesting severe pre-eclampsia. The patient must be compliant with restricted activity, instructions, and follow-up and must have a telephone and a readily available means of transportation to the doctor's office or hospital. Close communication between patient and physician is obligatory for the successful ambulatory management of mild pre-eclampsia.

Table 27–8. CANDIDATES FOR AMBULATORY MANAGEMENT

- Ability to comply with recommendations
- Diastolic blood pressure ≤ 100 mm Hg
- Systolic blood pressure ≤ 150 mm Hg
- 24-hour urine protein < 1000 mg or < 3+ dipstick
- Platelets > 120,000/mm^3
- Appropriate fetal growth
- Reassuring fetal testing
- Absent maternal symptoms (headache, visual change, epigastric or right upper quadrant pain)

SELECTED ASPECTS OF INPATIENT MEDICAL MANAGEMENT OF SEVERE PRE-ECLAMPSIA

Fluid Therapy

Fluid therapy for women with pre-eclampsia is controversial. Some authorities advocate fluid restriction, whereas others support volume expansion. Volume expansion may cause cerebral edema, seizures, pulmonary edema, and respiratory failure. In the United States, pulmonary edema and seizures are uncommonly seen secondary to the improved diagnostic and monitoring acumen. With the advent of continuous electrocardiographic monitoring, pulse oximetry, and echocardiography, the identification of a woman with incipient cardiac failure or borderline cardiac function has improved. Women with superimposed pre-eclampsia and/or a long-standing history of chronic hypertension are less likely to tolerate a fluid bolus. We recommend maintenance intravenous fluid (normal saline or lactated Ringer's solution) at a rate of 120 to 125 ml/h in pre-eclamptic women with a normal prepregnancy cardiac history. The development of cardiac failure or cerebral edema at these infusion rates is uncommon. Most untreated, severely pre-eclamptic women are volume depleted on presentation[26, 41] and respond well to a fluid bolus (500–1000 ml) of either crystalloid[41] or colloid.[26, 42] The fluid results in an increase in cardiac output, decrease in SVR, and an improvement in oxygen delivery and consumption. Pre-eclampsia is thought to be a fixed oxygen extraction state (similar to that seen in adult respiratory distress syndrome).[43] One of the few methods to improve oxygen consumption is to increase cardiac output.

Our approach is one of cautious volume expansion with 500 to 1000 ml of crystalloid in pre-eclamptic women without prior treatment. Repleting the intravascular space before instituting epidural anesthesia or using potent vasodilator drugs is advisable and may prevent ensuing fetal distress.[44–46]

Intravenous fluids cause decreased colloid osmotic pressure (COP) in laboring women.[47] Secondary to mobilization of interstitial fluids, COP also decreases in the puerperium. With a drop in COP and an increase in MAP, an imbalance may exist in the pulmonary circulation, thus predisposing the gravida to pulmonary edema. A smaller volume of colloid than crystalloid is required to achieve similar volume expansion, and colloids are believed to decrease COP less than crystalloids. Despite this, colloids have not demonstrated any significant clinical benefit over crystalloids during pregnancy.[48] Optimization of hemodynamic status should be achieved in women with severe pre-eclampsia.[27, 49] We recommend that initial fluid management be based on clinical and noninvasive hemodynamic parameters as outlined earlier.

Analgesia-Anesthesia

The use of conduction anesthesia in pre-eclampsia is controversial. Sympathetic blockade and peripheral vasodilatation resulting from the epidural anesthesia may precipitate hypotension and resultant fetal distress. This is relevant for women who are already volume contracted.[50–52] Alternatively, induction of general endotracheal anesthesia may result in significant rises in systemic arterial pressure in women with severe pre-eclampsia. This can increase cerebral perfusion pressure and may precipitate intracranial catastrophe. Hodgkinson and associates, using the pulmonary artery catheter, evaluated 10 severely pre-eclamptic/eclamptic women undergoing general anesthesia. They noted severe systemic and pulmonary hypertension during endotracheal intubation and extubation. In contrast, 10 women undergoing epidural anesthesia with 0.75% bupivacaine for cesarean section maintained stable systemic and pulmonary arterial pressures, with the exception of one woman who developed systemic hypotension that responded promptly to ephedrine.[53] Newsome demonstrated a drop in MAP and a slight but insignificant decrease in SVR without change in cardiac index, peripheral vascular resistance, central venous pressure (CVP), or pulmonary capillary wedge pressure (PCWP) in 11 women with severe pre-eclampsia undergoing lumbar epidural anesthesia.[54] Doppler ultrasound has been used to study fetal umbilical artery and maternal uterine artery blood velocity profiles, and there is evidence to suggest that regional anesthesia has a potential beneficial effect in pre-eclamptic women by reducing uterine artery vasospasm.[55] Hypotension can be prevented in most cases by left lateral displacement, thus preventing aortocaval occlusion and the supine hypotension syndrome.

Epidural anesthesia is safe in most pre-eclamptic women without coagulopathy and is usually the anesthesia of choice in women with severe pre-eclampsia.[54, 56, 57] Contraindications to epidural anesthesia include patient refusal, fetal distress requiring immediate delivery, local infection, septicemia, severe spinal deformities, and coagulopathy.[57] There is adequate evidence to suggest that if preceded by volume loading, epidural anesthesia is both beneficial and safe in women with severe pre-eclampsia.[46, 54, 56–60]

HEMODYNAMIC MONITORING FOR SEVERE PRE-ECLAMPSIA/ECLAMPSIA

Invasive Hemodynamic Monitoring

The pulmonary artery catheter, introduced nearly 30 years ago, has been very useful in the management of critically ill patients.[61] Clinicians have, however, obtained excellent results without invasive monitoring in women with severe pre-eclampsia.[62] Invasive hemodynamic monitoring was initially recommended for women with severe pre-eclampsia complicated by profound oliguria, pulmonary edema of uncertain etiology, hypertension unresponsive to conventional therapy, and medical conditions that would normally require such monitoring.[60] Early protocols developed to study the central hemodynamic parameters of severe pre-eclampsia revealed interesting data. There is considerable heterogeneity due to differences in clinical patient management before and at the time of catheterization.[46] Current indications for the use of pulmonary artery catheter in pre-eclampsia include (1) complications related to central volume status such as pulmonary edema of uncertain etiology, pulmonary edema unresponsive to conventional therapy, hypertension unresponsive to conventional therapy, and persistent oliguria despite aggressive volume expansion; (2) induction of conduction anesthesia in hemodynamically unstable patients; and (3) a medical complication that would otherwise require invasive monitoring.[60, 63, 64] The routine use of a pulmonary artery catheter in uncomplicated severe pre-eclampsia is not recommended.

Noninvasive Hemodynamic Monitoring

Most important hemodynamic information required for initial management of women with complicated severe pre-eclampsia can be acquired by the use of noninvasive monitoring methods such as two-dimensional echocardiography and Doppler ultrasound. Belfort and colleagues[65] prospectively studied 11 critically ill obstetric patients (4 patients with sepsis/adult respiratory distress syndrome, 2 patients with pre-eclampsia, 2 patients with cardiomyopathy, and 1 each with aortic valve disease, massive pulmonary embolus, and renal artery stenosis) requiring invasive monitoring for clinical management. The techniques employed in the measurement of cardiac output, left ventricular filling pressure, right atrial pressure, and ejection fraction have been reported in detail; the reader is referred elsewhere for further technical information and methodology.[65, 66] Simultaneous Doppler echocardiography and pulmonary artery catheterization readings of cardiac index, left ventricular filling pressure, pulmonary arterial systolic pressure, and right atrial pressure were compared using regression analysis. There was no significant difference between the two techniques in the estimation of cardiac index or intracardiac filling pressures. There was good correlation between the two methods for cardiac index ($R = 0.99$), left ventricular filling pressure ($R = 0.86$), pulmonary arterial systolic pressure ($R = 0.92$), and right atrial pressure ($R = 0.87$). These authors concluded that both two-dimensional and Doppler echocardiography allow rapid, reliable, noninvasive assessment of hemodynamic parameters in critically ill gravidas. They further tested their hypothesis in a group of 14 women with oliguria unresponsive to crystalloid boluses, hypertension unresponsive to hydralazine, and women at high risk for pulmonary edema.[67] All of these women were candidates for invasive monitoring. The women were studied with two-dimensional echocardiography and Doppler ultrasound without the need for a pulmonary artery catheter, and the study included women with intractable hypertension (1), pulmonary edema (2), complex cardiac lesions (2), oliguria (5), intractable hypertension and oliguria (1), and unexplained dyspnea with peripheral arterial oxygen desaturation (1). Although some women received up to 8 L of crystalloid, none developed pulmonary edema or left ventricular failure and none had seizures. Noninvasive management was successful in all 12 cases. These authors concluded that two-dimensional echocardiography and Doppler examination may be an effective monitoring alternative to invasive monitoring in the management of selected gravidas. A common indication for invasive monitoring includes the woman with oliguria who has failed to respond to an adequate fluid challenge. In many situations, two-dimensional echocardiography and Doppler assessment can provide reassurance to the physician that the woman has a good ejection fraction, is not in incipient cardiac failure, is centrally volume depleted, and could easily tolerate another 2 L of fluid.

Some women with severe pre-eclampsia have underlying chronic hypertension and are at risk for cardiomyopathy with systolic dysfunction. Some women will also manifest diastolic dysfunction or a combination of systolic and diastolic dysfunction. Echocardiography is essential for tailoring therapy in these women.[68] A knowledge of chamber dimensions, ejection fraction or fractional shortening, intracardiac pressures, and cardiac output allows a more informed decision regarding the choice of a preferential vasodilator (calcium channel blocker, arterial vasodilator) versus an agent with a predominantly negative inotropic effect (β-adrenergic blocker). Echocardiographic measurements allow the physician to estimate SVR and cardiac output after intervention. Thus, the hemodynamic consequences of volume expansion or antihypertensive therapy can be assessed immediately without the need for invasive monitoring.

Once it has been determined that cardiac function is normal, volume expansion can be carried out using evaluation of the CVP. Imaging of the inferior vena cava is easily accomplished using standard equipment, requires minimal training or special expertise, and is well accepted by the patients. This technique represents a practical way for the clinician to evaluate CVP without the need for sophisticated hemodynamic monitoring equipment and without exposing the patient to added risk. The ability to visualize right atrial and ventricular wall motion, and to simultaneously estimate right atrial pressure from the inferior vena cava, allows a more informed estimate of the state of filling of the central veins than the pulmonary artery catheter.

Additionally, noninvasive techniques can be performed on patients with a pulmonary artery catheter in situ for additional information. Such situations may include those in which there is disparity between left and right ventricular output, systolic or diastolic dysfunction, or impaired ventricular relaxation.

CARDIOPULMONARY COMPLICATIONS

During normal pregnancy there are significant increases in plasma volume (42%) and red blood cell volume (24%).[69] In pre-eclampsia there is a reduction in plasma volume, with hemoconcentration occurring in proportion to the severity of the disease.[69] Cardiac output is known to increase in normotensive pregnant subjects during the first trimester and then remain elevated until a slight fall at the end of the third trimester. In women who develop hypertension during pregnancy, a variable cardiac output and SVR pattern has been noted.[70]

Cotton and coworkers summarized the hemodynamic profile in 45 women with severe pre-eclampsia or eclampsia.[63] They observed a wide variety of hemodynamic measurements in these women; however, the majority were found to have an elevated systolic blood pressure, variably elevated SVR, hyperdynamic left ventricular function, normal to increased PCWP, and low CVP. These early studies using the pulmonary artery catheter were confounded by the fact that almost all women were treated (magnesium sulfate, volume expansion, hydralazine, oxytocin) before their catheterization, and thus the measurements reflected varying degrees of induced change. Thus, the early reports of very different cardiac output values for pre-eclampsia, varying from very low to hyperdynamic, may have been misleading in terms of the true hemodynamic profile in untreated women with severe pre-eclampsia.

The first to study untreated patients was Groenendijk, who showed that severe pre-eclampsia is associated with a low cardiac output, an elevated SVR, and low to normal PCWP.[41] Volume expansion resulted in an elevation of PCWP and cardiac index to normal pregnant values, a drop in SVR, and no change in systolic blood pressure. Vasodilatation using hydralazine then resulted in a further drop in SVR and systolic blood pressure, with a rise in cardiac index, and no change in PCWP. This work was supported by a similar study by Belfort and associates.[26] Using two-dimensional echocardiography and Doppler ultrasound, we showed reasonable correlation between CVP and PCWP in our severely ill patients (unpublished data) and believe that in most cases the CVP can be used to manage these women. In women who have isolated failure in either or both of their ventricles, a direct measure of left ventricular filling pressure is indicated.

Clark and associates documented the central hemodynamic parameters in normotensive late third-trimester pregnant women.[71] They demonstrated that most women with severe pre-eclampsia have SVR in the normal range for pregnancy and that left ventricular function in normal pregnancy as assessed by left ventricular stroke work index is not hyperdynamic. This supports the model of an initially hyperdynamic hypertension without vasospasm in pre-eclampsia.[72] This may be followed by the development of elevated SVR associated with vasospasm and a secondary decline in cardiac output and left ventricular stroke work index. Such a phenomenon has been documented in untreated nonpregnant patients with essential hypertension.[73]

Pulmonary Edema

Pulmonary edema is an occasional but severe complication in pregnancy and occurs in approximately 3% of women with severe pre-eclampsia/eclampsia.[74] Approximately 70% of cases occur post partum. Most (90%) antepartum cases are associated with underlying chronic hypertension. Benedetti and colleagues[75] studied 10 pre-eclamptic women with pulmonary edema and noted that in 8 of the 10 the condition developed in the postpartum period. Five patients had an abnormal COP-PCWP gradient, 3 demonstrated increased pulmonary capillary permeability, and 2 suffered left ventricular failure. The diagnosis of capillary leak was made when the ratio of the protein in the pulmonary edema fluid to the serum protein was greater than 0.4.[75] A decreased COP-PCWP gradient has been correlated with the development of pulmonary edema in nonpregnant patients.[76] Pregnancy is known to lower COP, and this is further lowered by pre-eclampsia. In the postpartum period, COP decreases further, owing to supine positioning, bleeding at the time of delivery, and intrapartum infusion of crystalloid solutions.[77] It is thus clear that nonhydrostatic factors (pulmonary capillary leak and decreased COP) may cause or contribute to pulmonary edema in women with pre-eclampsia. In other patients, highly elevated SVR may lead to cardiac dysfunction and secondary cardiogenic pulmonary edema. Occasionally, cardiac arrhythmias may contribute.[78] Finally, pulmonary edema may also be seen with normal left ventricular function if there has been iatrogenic fluid overload. In our experience, the development of pulmonary edema in an otherwise uncomplicated case of pre-eclampsia is usually not the result of cardiac decompensation but rather excess fluid infusion in a patient who is already mobilizing large amounts of extracellular edema fluid. Appropriate diuresis for these hemodynamically complex patients may be better defined after hemodynamic evaluation, using parameters derived from either noninvasive[79] or invasive methodologies. Afterload reduction with arterial vasodilators may be necessary in cases in which left ventricular failure results from increased afterload.[29] Continuous arterial blood pressure monitoring is often required to adequately manage these patients. When hypoxemia persists despite initial treatment, mechanical ventilation may be required for respiratory support pending correction of the underlying problem.

Renal Complications of Severe Pre-eclampsia

Renal biopsy in pre-eclamptic women frequently demonstrates a distinctive and specific glomerular capillary endothelial-cell change called glomerular endotheliosis.[80] Damage to the glomerular membrane results in renal dysfunction,[81, 82] and renal plasma flow and glomerular filtration rate are significantly diminished in pre-eclamptic women.[83] Urinary sediment changes (granular, hyaline, red cell, and tubular cell casts) are common in severe pre-eclampsia and reflect renal parenchymal damage but do not correlate with or predict the clinical course of disease.[84] Acute renal failure in pre-eclamptic pregnancies is uncommon.[85] This usually results from acute tubular necrosis, but occasionally bilateral cortical necrosis is seen.[18] In women with pre-eclampsia alone (i.e., without prior chronic hypertension), acute renal failure usually occurs in the postpartum period. In women with chronic hypertension and underlying renal disease, the condition may present ante partum. The mortality rate is high (10%), and there is significant morbidity. In cases of acute renal failure associated with "pure" pre-eclampsia, about 50% of women (9/18) reported by Sibai and Ramadan[86] needed short-term dialysis; all recovered fully within 6 weeks. The prognosis is worse when acute renal failure is associated with chronic hypertension and prior renal disease. In the same series, 42% (5/12) needed dialysis in the acute event and 82% (9/11) of survivors needed chronic dialysis.

Oliguria

Initial renal dysfunction in women with pre-eclampsia is most commonly manifested as oliguria, defined as urinary output less than 25 to 30 ml/h over 2 consecutive hours. This often parallels a rise in serum creatinine and blood urea nitrogen and a fall in creatinine clearance. Reversible hyperuricemia is a common feature of pre-eclampsia and usually precedes the development of uremia and proteinuria.[87]

Three different hemodynamic subsets of pre-eclamptic-eclamptic patients with persistent oliguria have been described using invasive monitoring parameters[88]:

1. A low PCWP, hyperdynamic left ventricular function, and mild to moderately increased SVR. These women responded to further volume replacement. This is the most common clinical scenario, and it is secondary to intravascular volume depletion.
2. Normal or increased PCWP, normal cardiac output, and normal SVR, accompanied by intense uroconcentration. The pathophysiologic basis of oliguria in this group is thought to be secondary to intrinsic renal arterial spasm out of proportion to any degree of systemic vasospasm. Low-dose dopamine (1–5 μg/kg/min) has been shown to produce a significant rise in urine output in severe pre-eclamptic women in this hemodynamic subgroup.[89]
3. Markedly elevated PCWP and SVR, with depressed ventricular function. These women respond to volume restriction and aggressive afterload reduction and to forced diuresis with furosemide. Oliguria in this subgroup is frequently associated with incipient pulmonary edema.

Noninvasive assessment may be useful in differentiating between these women. Often patients are noted to have urinary diagnostic indices consistent with prerenal dehydration but PCWP consistent with euvolemia.[90] The finding of normal PCWP in oliguric pre-eclamptic women supports the hypothesis that oliguria is often secondary to severe regional vasospasm.[62, 90]

Close monitoring of fluid intake and output is of paramount importance in all women diagnosed with pre-eclampsia. If urine output falls below 25 and 30 ml/h over 2 consecutive hours, a management plan should be instituted. Given the fact that plasma volume is diminished in pre-eclamptic gravidas, the cause of oliguria may be considered prerenal in most instances.[70, 88, 91] A fluid challenge of 500 to 1000 ml of normal saline or lactated Ringer's solution may be administered over 30 minutes. If urine output does not respond to an initial fluid challenge, additional challenges may be given as long as oxygen saturation remains greater than 95%. Before repetitive fluid challenges, however, we recommend that cardiac function and volume status be assessed using noninvasive methods. Oliguric patients with good left ventricular function and low right atrial pressure may be given a 500-ml bolus infusion of crystalloid every 30 minutes until urine output is noted to be greater than 30 ml in 1 hour. When left ventricular function is poor or right atrial pressure is between 10 and 15 mm Hg, smaller boluses (100–200 ml) should be given. Good left ventricular function may be defined by (1) an ejection fraction greater than 60%, (2) no evidence of diastolic or systolic dysfunction, (3) cardiac output greater than 6 L/min, and (4) normal chamber size. In cases in which repeated crystalloid boluses are given, the frequency of the ultrasound examination of the right atrial pressure should be based on the findings at the initial examination and amount of fluid given. If the initial examination shows good left ventricular function (as defined earlier), fluid boluses may be given every 30 minutes until urine output is greater than 30 ml/h or 3 L has been given. If after 3 L of volume expansion the urine output is still suboptimal, the right atrial pressure should be reassessed and further volume expansion must be based on this measurement. Repeat estimation of the right atrial pressure should be performed after each further liter of crystalloid is administered. At the time of the initial examination an attempt can be made to calculate the left ventricular end-diastolic pressure. If this can be calculated, initial fluid management decisions may based on this parameter. In those cases in which the heart rate is too rapid to allow adequate assessment of left ventricular end diastolic pressure, fluid management decisions can be based on the right atrial pressure measurement. Follow-up fluid management decisions may be predicated on the bedside right atrial pressure measurement, provided that left ventricular function is normal. In cases in which there is a discrepancy between the left ventricular end-diastolic pressure and the right atrial pressure and any degree of left ventricular dysfunction is suggested, the management should proceed under the guidance of a pulmonary artery catheter.

Expectant Management of Severe Pre-eclampsia

Either severe pre-eclampsia or superimposed pre-eclampsia developing early in pregnancy presents an obstetric dilemma. Delivery is the ultimate cure for maternal disease.[1, 2] However, delivery of infants younger than 34 weeks' gestation with immature fetal pulmonary profiles results in intensive and prolonged neonatal care and is associated with significant neonatal morbidity and mortality. We have not been able to demonstrate accelerated fetal lung maturity, improved neonatal outcome, or accelerated fetal neurologic and physical development in preterm infants born after indicated delivery for severe pre-eclampsia.[92–94] Given the ultimate goal of maternal safety first, collaborators at the University of Tennessee, Memphis[93, 94] developed a management program including maternal surveillance and daily fetal testing for expectant management of the gravida with severe pre-eclampsia remote from term.

Prompt delivery is indicated for the presence of imminent eclampsia, multiorgan dysfunction, or fetal distress or if severe pre-eclampsia develops after 34 weeks.[93] As reviewed earlier, pregnancy prolongation with intensive surveillance at a tertiary perinatal center may be indicated to improve neonatal survival and to reduce neonatal morbidity.[93] The University of Tennessee, Memphis, guidelines for conservative management of severe pre-eclampsia are described in Table 27–9.

After admission, all women are observed in the Labor and Delivery Unit for 12 to 24 hours to determine their eligibility for conservative management. Intravenous magnesium sulfate therapy is administered for seizure prophylaxis, glucocorticoid therapy is given for fetal lung maturation, and antihypertensive drug therapy is administered as indicated. Baseline laboratory studies (complete blood cell count with platelets, serum levels of creatinine, uric acid, aspartate aminotransferase, and lactate dehydrogenase, and 24-hour urine collection for total protein and creatinine clearance) are obtained.

Once the woman and fetus are judged to be suitable candidates for expectant management, the magnesium sulfate therapy is discontinued and the patient is managed on the antepartum ward. Blood pressure is measured every 4 to 6 hours, platelets are measured every day, and serum aspartate aminotransferase is checked every other day. Oral antihypertensive therapy is administered as needed to main-

Table 27–9. GUIDELINES FOR EXPECTANT MANAGEMENT OF SEVERE PRE-ECLAMPSIA REMOTE FROM TERM

MANAGEMENT PLAN	CLINICAL FINDINGS
Expedited delivery (within 72 hours)	*One or more of the following:* • Uncontrolled severe hypertension* • Eclampsia • Platelet count < 100,000/µl • AST or ALT level > 2 times upper limit of normal with epigastric pain or right upper quadrant tenderness • Pulmonary edema • Compromised renal function† • Persistent severe headache or visual changes
Expectant management	*One or more of the following:* • Controlled hypertension • Urinary protein > 5000 mg/24 h • Oliguria (<0.5 ml/kg/h) which resolves with routine fluid/food intake • AST or ALT level > 2 times upper limit of normal without epigastric pain or right upper quadrant tenderness

*Blood pressure persistently ≥ 160 mm Hg systolic or ≥ 110 mm Hg diastolic despite maximum recommended doses of two antihypertensive medications.

†Persistent oliguria (<0.5 ml/kg/h) or rise in serum creatinine of 1 mg/dl over baseline values.

AST, aspartate aminotransferase; ALT, alanine aminotransferase.

With permission from the Annual Review of Medicine, Volume 48, ©1997, by Annual Reviews.

tain blood pressure in the 130–150/80–100 mm Hg range. Hospitalization is continued until delivery.

Results[94] of a randomized controlled trial of aggressive versus expectant management in 95 women with severe pre-eclampsia at 28 to 32 weeks' gestation yielded the following results. Pregnancy was prolonged by an average of 15.4 days (range, 4 to 36 days) in the expectant management group. This pregnancy prolongation was associated with significant improvement in neonatal morbidity (respiratory distress syndrome and necrotizing enterocolitis) without significant increase in maternal morbidity. There was an associated reduction in incidence of admission to the neonatal intensive care unit and a lower average number of days spent in this unit.[94]

In summary, expectant/conservative management of severe pre-eclampsia is beneficial in a select group of women. This management should be practiced only at a tertiary care center. Development of severe pre-eclampsia beyond 34 weeks' gestation demands prompt delivery. One review of neonatal outcomes in 195 neonates born to mothers with severe pre-eclampsia and eclampsia suggests that the gestational age for terminating expectant management may be decreased to 32 weeks with an estimated fetal weight greater than 1200 g.[95]

Mild pre-eclampsia or controlled hypertension before term (<37 weeks) should be managed with close maternal surveillance and antepartum testing, because the disorder may worsen suddenly. Women with mild pre-eclampsia at term with a favorable cervix should undergo delivery to avoid further maternal or neonatal complications (Table 27–10).

Future Medical Risks and Screening

Those women with superimposed pre-eclampsia are likely to be at increased risk for development of chronic hypertension and its sequelae and should be followed at least annually for development of chronic hypertension, in a fashion analogous to that for annual surveillance for women with gestational diabetes.

Table 27–10. MATERNAL INDICATIONS FOR DELIVERY IN WOMEN WITH MILD PRE-ECLAMPSIA OR CONTROLLED HYPERTENSION

Progression to severe pre-eclampsia
Gestational age ≥ 37 weeks
• Bishop score ≥ 6
Gestational age ≥ 34 weeks
• Labor
• Premature rupture of membranes
• Vaginal bleeding

Women with complicated hypertension (associated with medical diseases such as type I diabetes, renal disease, collagen vascular disease, or cardiovascular disease) require more frequent surveillance for determination of disease progression.

Limited experience suggests that oral contraceptive use is safe for women with a history of pre-eclampsia or eclampsia. Progestin-only methods may be a satisfactory alternative for women with a history of thrombophilia.

CONCLUSION

Ambulatory or home care of mild hypertension in pregnancy appears safe in the well-selected patient. However, it is difficult to justify that ambulatory/home care is equivalent to in-hospital care for all women with pre-eclampsia. Most women enrolled in ambulatory studies represent those women with milder, better-controlled disease and those who are well motivated and more compliant.

References

1. American College of Obstetricians and Gynecologists: Technical Bulletin No. 219. Hypertension in Pregnancy. ACOG, Washington, DC, 1996.
2. Working Group on High Blood Pressure in Pregnancy: National High Blood Pressure Education Program Working Group report on high blood pressure in pregnancy. Am J Obstet Gynecol 163:1689–1712, 1990.
3. Joint National Committee on Prevention, Detection, Evaluation, and Treatment of High Blood Pressure: The sixth report of the joint national committee on prevention, detection, evaluation, and treatment of high blood pressure (JNC VI). Arch Intern Med 157:2413–2446, 1997.
4. Nathan L, Gilstrap LC: Management of mild pregnancy-induced hypertension remote from term. Semin Perinatol 18:79–93, 1994.
5. Barton JR, Stanziano GJ, Sibai BM: Monitored outpatient management of mild gestational hypertension remote from term. Am J Obstet Gynecol 170:765–769, 1994.
6. Hauth JC, Cunningham FG, Whalley PJ: Management of pregnancy-induced hypertension in the nullipara. Obstet Gynecol 48:253–259, 1976.
7. Crowther CA, Bouwmeester AM, Ashurst HM: Does admission to hospital for bed rest prevent disease progression or improve fetal outcome in pregnancy complicated by non-proteinuric hypertension? Br J Obstet Gynecol 99:13–17, 1992.
8. Tuffnell DJ, Lilford RJ, Buchan PC, et al: Randomized controlled trial of day care for hypertension in pregnancy. Lancet 339:224–227, 1992.
9. Barton JR, Stanziano GJ, Jacques DL, et al: Monitored outpatient

management of mild gestational hypertension remote from term in teenage pregnancies. Am J Obstet Gynecol 173:1865–1868, 1995.
10. Barton JR, Bergauer NK, Jacques DL, et al: Does advanced maternal age affect pregnancy outcome in women with mild hypertension remote from term? Am J Obstet Gynecol 176:1236–1243, 1997.
11. Sibai BM, Barton JR, Akl S, et al: A randomized prospective comparison of nifedipine and bed rest versus bed rest alone in the management of preeclampsia remote from term. Am J Obstet Gynecol 167:879–884, 1992.
12. Lubbe WF: Hypertension in pregnancy: Whom and how to treat. Br J Clin Pharmacol 24:15S–20S, 1987.
13. Naden RP, Redman CWG: Antihypertensive drugs in pregnancy. Clin Perinatol 12:521–538, 1985.
14. Goldby FS, Beilin LJ: Relationship between arterial pressure and the permeability of arterioles to carbon particles in acute hypertension in the rat. Cardiovasc Res 6:384–390, 1972.
15. Witlin AG, Friedman SA, Egerman RS, et al: Cerebrovascular disorders complicating pregnancy—Beyond eclampsia. Am J Obstet Gynecol 176: 1139–1148, 1997.
16. Sibai BM: Treatment of hypertension in pregnant women. N Engl J Med 335:257–265, 1996.
17. Sibai BM, Mabie WC, Shamsa F, et al: A comparison of no medication versus methyldopa or labetalol in chronic hypertension during pregnancy. Am J Obstet Gynecol 62:960–967, 1990.
18. Sibai BM, Gonzalez AR, Mabie WC, Moretti M: A comparison of labetalol plus hospitalization versus hospitalization alone in the management of preeclampsia remote from term. Obstet Gynecol 70:323–327, 1987.
19. Prevost RR, Akl SA, Whybrew WD, Sibai BM: Oral nifedipine pharmacokinetics in pregnancy-induced hypertension. Pharmacotherapy 2:174–177, 1992.
20. Dougall HT, McLay J: A comparative review of the adverse effects of calcium antagonists. Drug Saf 15:91–106, 1996.
21. Belfort MA, Saade GR, Moise K, et al: Nimodipine in the management of preeclampsia: Maternal and fetal effects. Am J Obstet Gynecol 171: 417–424, 1994.
22. Lund-Johnson P: Short- and long-term (six year) hemodynamic effects of labetalol in essential hypertension. Am J Med 75:24–31, 1983.
23. Pearce CJ, Wallin JD: Labetalol and other agents that block both alpha- and beta-adrenergic receptors. Cleve Clin J Med 61:59–69, 1994.
24. Mabie WC, Gonzalez AR, Sibai BM, Amon E: A comparative trial of labetalol and hydralazine in the acute management of severe hypertension complicating pregnancy. Obstet Gynecol 70:328–333, 1987.
25. Koch-Weser J: Hydralazine. N Engl J Med 295:320–323, 1976.
26. Belfort MA, Uys P, Dommissee J, Davey DA: Rapid volume expansion in severe gestational proteinuric hypertension: A haemodynamic study. Br J Obstet Gynaecol 96:634–641, 1989.
27. Visser W, Wallenburg HC: A comparison between the haemodynamic effects of oral nifedipine and intravenous dihydralazine in patients with severe pre-eclampsia. J Hypertens 13:791–795, 1995.
28. Pasch T, Schulz V, Hoppelshauser G: Nitroprusside-induced formation of cyanide and its detoxification with thiosulfate during deliberate hypotension. J Cardiovasc Pharmacol 5:77–85, 1983.
29. Strauss RG, Keefer JR, Burke T, Civetta JM: Hemodynamic monitoring of cardiogenic pulmonary edema complicating toxemia of pregnancy. Obstet Gynecol 55:170–174, 1980.
30. Herling IM: Intravenous nitroglycerin: Clinical pharmacology and therapeutic considerations. Am Heart J 108:141–149, 1984.
31. Horvath JS, Phippard A, Korda A, et al: Clonidine hydrochloride—a safe and effective antihypertensive agent in pregnancy. Obstet Gynecol 6:634–638, 1985.
32. Witlin AG, Sibai BM: Hypertensive diseases in pregnancy. In Reece AE, Hobbins J (eds): Medicine of the Fetus and Mother. Lippincott-Raven, Philadelphia, 1998.
33. Montan S, Ingermarsson I, Marsal K, Sjoberg NO: Randomized controlled trial of atenolol and pindolol in hymen pregnancy: Effects on fetal haemodynamics. BMJ 304:946–949, 1992.
34. Butters L, Kennedy S, Rubin PC: Atenolol in essential hypertension during pregnancy. BMJ 301:587–589, 1990.
35. Sibai BM, Grossman RA, Grossman HE: Effects of diuretics on plasma volume in pregnancies with long-term hypertension. Am J Obstet Gynecol 150:831, 1984.
36. Sibai BM, Abdella TN, Anderson GD, et al: Plasma volume findings in pregnant women with mild hypertension: Therapeutic considerations. Am J Obstet Gynecol 190:17, 1985.
37. Rosa FW, Bosco LA, Graham CF, et al: Neonatal anuria with maternal angiotensin-converting enzyme inhibition. Obstet Gynecol 74:371–374, 1989.
38. Sibai BM: Diagnosis and management of chronic hypertension in pregnancy. Obstet Gynecol 78:451–461, 1991.
39. Weber MA, Laragh JH: Hypertension: Steps forward and steps backward. The Joint National Committee's Fifth Report on Detection and Treatment of High Blood Pressure. Arch Intern Med 153:154–183, 1993.
40. Witlin AG, Saade GR, Mattar F, Sibai BM: Risk factors for abruptio placentae and eclampsia: Analysis of 445 consecutively managed women with severe preeclampsia and eclampsia. Am J Obstet Gynecol 180: 1322–1329, 1999.
41. Groenendijk R, Trimbos JBMJ, Wallenburg HCS: Hemodynamic measurements in preeclampsia: Preliminary observations. Am Obstet Gynecol 150:232–236, 1984.
42. Belfort MA, Anthony J, Kirshon B: Respiratory function in severe gestational proteinuric hypertension: The effects of rapid volume expansion and subsequent vasodilatation with verapamil. Br J Obstet Gynaecol 98:964–972, 1991.
43. Belfort MA, Anthony J, Saade GR, et al: The oxygen consumption: oxygen delivery (VO2:DO2) curve in severe preeclampsia: Evidence for a fixed oxygen extraction state. Am J Obstet Gynecol 169:1448–1455, 1993.
44. Spinnato JA, Sibai BM, Anderson GD: Fetal distress after hydralazine therapy for severe pregnancy-induced hypertension. South Med J 79: 559–562, 1986.
45. Wasserstrum N, Kirshon B, Willis RS, et al: Quantitive hemodynamic effects of acute volume expansion in severe preeclampsia. Obstet Gynecol 73:546–550, 1989.
46. Wasserstrum N, Cotton DB: Hemodynamic monitoring in severe pregnancy-induced hypertension. Clin Perinatol 13:781–799, 1986.
47. Gonik B, Cotton DB: Peripartum colloid osmotic pressure changes: Influence of intravenous hydration. Am J Obstet Gynecol 150:90–100, 1984.
48. Jones MM, Longmire S, Cotton DB, et al: Influence of crystalloid versus colloid infusion on peripartum colloid osmotic pressure changes. Obstet Gynecol 68:659–661, 1986.
49. Kirshon B, Cotton DB: Invasive hemodynamic monitoring in the obstetric patient. Clin Obstet Gynecol 30:579–590, 1987.
50. Pritchard JA, MacDonald PC, Grant NF: Williams Obstetrics, 17th ed. Appleton-Century-Crofts, Norwalk, CT, 1985, p 525.
51. Pritchard JA, Pritchard SA: Standardized treatment of 154 consecutive cases of eclampsia. Am J Obstet 123:543–552, 1975.
52. Lindheimer MD, Katz AI: Current concepts: Hypertension in pregnancy. N Engl J Med 313:675–680, 1985.
53. Hodgkinson R, Husain FJ, Hayashi RH: Systemic and pulmonary blood pressure during cesarean section in parturients with gestational hypertension. Can Anaesth Soc J 27:389–394, 1980.
54. Newsome LR, Bramwell RS, Curling PE: Severe preeclampsia: Hemodynamic effects of lumbar epidural anesthesia. Anesth Analg 65:31–36, 1986.
55. Ramos-Santos E, Devoe LD, Wakefield ML, et al: The effects of epidural anesthesia on the Doppler velocimetry of umbilical and uterine arteries in normal and hypertensive patients during active term labor. Obstet Gynecol 77:20–26, 1991.
56. Jouppila P, Jouppila R, Hollman A, Koivula A: Lumbar epidural analgesia to improve intervillous blood flow during labor in severe preeclampsia. Obstet Gynecol 59:158–161, 1982.
57. Gutsche B: The experts opine: Is epidural block for labor and delivery and for cesarean section a safe form of analgesia in severe preeclampsia or eclampsia? Surv Anesth 30:304–311, 1986.
58. Graham C, Goldstein A: Epidural analgesia and cardiac output in severe preeclamptics. Anesthesia 35:709–712, 1980.
59. Joyce TH, Debnath KS, Baker EA: Preeclampsia: Relationship of central venous pressure and epidural anesthesia. Anesthesiology 51:S297, 1979.
60. Clark SL, Cotton DB: Clinical indications for pulmonary artery catheterization in the patient with severe preeclampsia. Am J Obstet Gynecol 158:453–458, 1988.
61. Swan HJC, Ganz W, Forrester JS, et al: Catheterization of the heart in man with the use of flow-directed balloon-tipped catheter. N Engl J Med 283:447–451, 1970.
62. Pritchard JA, Cunningham FG, Pritchard SA: The Parkland Memorial Hospital protocol for the treatment of eclampsia: Evaluation of 245 cases. Am J Obstet Gynecol 148:951–963, 1984.

63. Cotton DB, Lee W, Huhta JC, Dorman KF: Hemodynamic profile of severe pregnancy-induced hypertension. Am J Obstet Gynecol 158: 523–529, 1988.
64. Clark SL, Divon MY, Phelan JP: Preeclampsia/eclampsia: Hemodynamic and neurologic correlations. Obstet Gynecol 66:337–340, 1985.
65. Belfort MA, Saade GR, Moise K, et al: Nimodipine in the management of preeclampsia: Maternal and fetal effects. Am J Obstet Gynecol 171: 417–424, 1994.
66. Rokey R, Belfort MA, Saade GR: Quantitative echocardiographic assessment of left ventricular function in critically ill obstetrics patients: A comparative study. Am J Obstet Gynecol 173:1148–1152, 1995.
67. Belfort MA, Mares A, Saade GR, et al: The use of two-dimensional echocardiography and Doppler ultrasound in managing obstetric patients. Obstet Gynecol 90:326–330, 1997.
68. Mabie WC, Hackman BB, Sibai BM: Pulmonary edema associated with pregnancy: Echocardiographic insights and implications for treatment. Obstet Gynecol 81:227–234, 1993.
69. Chesley LC: Plasma and red cell volumes during pregnancy. Am J Obstet Gynecol 112:440–450, 1972.
70. Lees MM: Central circulatory response to normotensive and hypertensive pregnancy. Postgrad Med J 55:311–314, 1979.
71. Clark SL, Cotton DB, Lee W, et al: Central hemodynamic observations in normal third trimester pregnancy. Am J Obstet Gynecol 161:1439–1442, 1989.
72. Easterling TR, Benedetti TJ: Preeclampsia: A hyperdynamic disease model. Am J Obstet Gynecol 160:1447–1453, 1989.
73. Lund-Johansen P: The haemodynamic pattern in mild and borderline hypertension. Acta Med Scand [Suppl] 686:15, 1983.
74. Sibai BM, Mabie BC, Harvey CJ, Gonzalez AR: Pulmonary edema in severe preeclampsia-eclampsia: Analysis of thirty-seven consecutive cases. Am J Obstet Gynecol 156:1174–1179, 1987.
75. Benedetti TJ, Kates R, Williams V: Hemodynamic observations in severe preeclampsia complicated by pulmonary edema. Am J Obstet Gynecol 152:330–334, 1985.
76. Fein A, Grossman RF, Jones JG, et al: The value of edema fluid protein measurement in patients with pulmonary edema. Am J Med 67:32–38, 1979.
77. Weil MH, Henning RJ, Puri VK: Colloid osmotic pressure: Clinical significance. Crit Care Med 7:113–116, 1979.
78. Naidoo DP, Bhorat I, Moodley J, et al: Continuous electrocardiographic monitoring in hypertensive crises in pregnancy. Am J Obstet Gynecol 164:530–533, 1991.
79. Desai DK, Moodley J, Naidoo DP, Bhorat I: Cardiac abnormalities in pulmonary edema associated with hypertensive crisis in pregnancy. Br J Obstet Gynaecol 103:523–528, 1996.
80. Spargo B, McCartney CP, Winemiller R: Glomerular capillary endotheliosis in toxemia of pregnancy. Arch Pathol 68:593–599, 1959.
81. Morris RH, Vassalli P, Beller PK, McCluskey RT: Immunofluorescent studies of renal biopsies in the diagnosis of toxemia of pregnancy. Obstet Gynecol 24:32–46, 1964.
82. Sheehan HL: Renal morphology in preeclampsia. Kidney Int 18:241–252, 1980.
83. Chesley LC, Duffus GM: Preeclampsia, posture, and renal function. Obstet Gynecol 38:1–5, 1971.
84. Leduc L, Lederer E, Lee W, Cotton DB: Urinary sediment changes in severe preeclampsia. Obstet Gynecol 77:186–189, 1991.
85. Krane NK: Acute renal failure in pregnancy. Arch Intern Med 148: 2347–2357, 1988.
86. Sibai BM, Ramadan MK: Acute renal failure in pregnancies complicated by hemolysis, elevated liver enzymes, and low platelets. Am J Obstet Gynecol 168:1682–1690, 1993.
87. Redman CWG, Beilin LJ, Bonner J: Renal function in preeclampsia. J Clin Pathol 10:94–96, 1976.
88. Clark SL, Greenspoon JS, Aldahl D, Phelan JP: Severe preeclampsia with persistent oliguria: Management of hemodynamic subsets. Am J Obstet Gynecol 154:490–494, 1986.
89. Kirshon B, Lee W, Mauer MB, Cotton DB: Effects of low-dose dopamine therapy in the oliguric patient with preeclampsia. Am J Obstet Gynecol 159:604–607, 1988.
90. Lee W, Gonik B, Cotton DB: Urinary diagnostic indices in preeclampsia-associated oliguria: Correlation with invasive hemodynamic monitoring. Am J Obstet Gynecol 156:100–103, 1987.
91. Gallery EDM, Hunyor SN, Gyory AZ: Plasma volume contraction: A significant factor in both pregnancy-associated hypertension (preeclampsia) and chronic hypertension in pregnancy. Q J Med 48:593–602, 1979.
92. Chari RS, Friedman SA, Schiff E, et al: Is fetal neurologic and physical development accelerated in preeclampsia? Am J Obstet Gynecol 174: 829–832, 1996.
93. Schiff E, Friedman SA, Sibai BM: Conservative management of severe preeclampsia remote from term. Obstet Gynecol 84:626–630, 1994.
94. Sibai BM, Mercer BM, Schiff E, Friedman SA: Aggressive versus expectant management of severe preeclampsia at 28 to 32 weeks' gestation: A randomized controlled trial. Am J Obstet Gynecol 171: 818–822, 1994.
95. Witlin AG, Saade GR, Mattar F, Sibai BM: Predictors of neonatal outcome in women with severe preeclampsia or eclampsia between 24 and 33 weeks. Am J Obstet Gynecol 182:607–611, 2000.

CHAPTER 28

Peripartum Cardiomyopathy

Roxann Rokey and Michael Belfort

Peripartum cardiomyopathy is an uncommon cause of heart failure. Although its clinical features have only been characterized in the 20th century, peripartum cardiomyopathy was initially described in ancient times. The cause of peripartum cardiomyopathy and how to prevent it are unknown. Nevertheless, effective treatment in most women is possible because of advances in our knowledge of the physiologic and pathologic changes that occur during pregnancy and the postpartum period. In addition, modern cardiovascular technologies and current therapeutic agents can be used to treat this potentially life-threatening illness.

Because peripartum cardiomyopathy is extremely rare, most physicians will see only a few women with this problem. Most women initially present with symptoms in the postpartum period; therefore, diagnosis and treatment affect only the mother. However, if symptoms of heart failure occur during pregnancy, the well-being of both mother and child must be considered. The purpose of this discussion is to aid the physician in the clinical recognition and effective treatment of women with peripartum cardiomyopathy.

DEFINITION

The term *peripartum cardiomyopathy* is used to describe idiopathic heart failure that develops in women during pregnancy or the early postpartum period. Diagnostic criteria of peripartum cardiomyopathy initially proposed by Demakis and associates in 1971 include (1) development of cardiac failure in the last month of pregnancy or within 5 months of delivery, (2) absence of a determinable etiology for cardiac failure, and (3) absence of demonstrable heart disease before the last month of pregnancy.[1] Amendments to this definition have been proposed,[2] and we believe the definition should be further amended.

Development of cardiac failure during or shortly after pregnancy is a critical diagnostic feature in the definition of peripartum cardiomyopathy. Diagnosis implies a primary cardiomyopathic process with depression in ventricular function of unknown etiology. As diagnostic techniques become more sophisticated and knowledge of pathophysiologic techniques expands, fewer cases of cardiomyopathy are diagnosed as idiopathic. Previous studies reporting the incidence of peripartum cardiomyopathy were based exclusively on clinical grounds and may have included patients with definable etiologic cardiovascular factors that were not diagnosed at the time.[1, 3]

A normal cardiovascular response to pregnancy includes decreased peripheral vascular resistance, left ventricular dilation with compensatory cardiac hypertrophy, and increased cardiac output, stroke volume, and heart rate. Cardiovascular disorders, subtle or explicit, are exacerbated by these adaptive changes. Superimposed on chronic cardiac disorders, symptoms consistent with heart failure would not be unexpected. Pregnant patients may have a subjective feeling of dyspnea, which may be mistaken for symptoms of heart failure, because of the normal pulmonary and hemodynamic responses and anatomic changes associated with pregnancy. The additional hemodynamic burden of pregnancy may unmask previously asymptomatic valvular lesions or abnormalities in left ventricular diastolic or systolic function. Toxic, metabolic, or infectious abnormalities produce symptoms of heart failure primarily or secondarily resulting in high or low cardiac output states. Symptoms of right-sided heart failure and shortness of breath can be caused by pulmonary emboli, amniotic fluid emboli, and primary pulmonary hypertension. Chronic hypertension, eclampsia, and pre-eclampsia may be important causes of impaired systolic and diastolic left ventricular function.

Because of technologic progress, noninvasive and, to a lesser degree, invasive cardiac evaluation now allow more thorough delineation of cardiovascular anatomy and function in pregnant or postpartum women with suspected heart failure. Echocardiography, an important tool in defining the anatomy and assessing hemodynamic abnormalities in pregnant women, can be used to study cardiac output, chamber size, and left ventricular systolic function. In addition, congenital disease and abnormalities in cardiac valves, the pericardium, the pulmonary vasculature, and diastolic function can be readily diagnosed. Thus, an echocardiographic finding of depressed left ventricular systolic function without an obvious etiologic cause is integral to the diagnosis of peripartum cardiomyopathy. Left ventricular dilation may or may not occur as an adaptive response to left ventricular systolic dysfunction, and this finding should not be required for a diagnosis of peripartum cardiomyopathy.

The reported timing of the presentation of peripartum cardiomyopathy varies. Demakis and colleagues limited the range from the last month of pregnancy to within 5 months after delivery.[1] Others have reported that symptoms may occur from the end of the last trimester to 6 months postpartum.[4–6] Many cases of peripartum cardiomyopathy previously described may not have been heart failure of a true idiopathic nature. If some of these cases were not idiopathic, the combination of idiopathic and nonidiopathic cases in these studies may have affected the reported timing of presentation. Furthermore, the severity of symptoms may have been a confounding variable in determining the diagnosis. Symptoms of heart failure can be viewed as a continuum ranging from extremely mild to very severe. Because cardiovascular disorders are fairly well tolerated in young patients and because peripheral vascular resistance decreases during pregnancy, impaired ventricular function during pregnancy may produce no symptoms or create symptoms so mild they are only detected by vigorous study. Onset of overt symptoms may be the culmination of a progressive process that began with subtle signs. Confining the diagnosis of peripartum cardiomyopathy to women with overt symptoms of heart failure during the last month of pregnancy may result in significant underreporting and, more importantly, withholding of appropriate treatment. Thus, we believe that the diagnosis of peripartum cardiomyopathy during pregnancy should include the third trimester. For the postpartum patient, the diagnosis should be limited to 6 months after delivery because most cases occur within this period.

In summary, our criteria for the diagnosis of peripartum cardiomyopathy are as follows: (1) development of heart failure in the last trimester of pregnancy or within the first 6 months of delivery, (2) echocardiographic documentation of impaired left ventricular systolic function with or without left ventricular dilation, and (3) lack of a conclusive cause for heart failure.

RISK FACTORS AND INCIDENCE

An accurate demographic description of risk factors for and the incidence of peripartum cardiomyopathy is problematic. Many reports in the past may have included patients with symptoms of heart failure related to a subsequently well-defined etiology.[1, 3, 6, 7] In addition, geographic location, the experience of specific medical centers, and referral patterns may have affected demographic descriptions.[8, 9]

In Nigeria, a postpartum practice of high salt intake combined with lying on heated mud beds may lead to symptoms of heart failure from volume overload in up to 10% of women.[8] Heart failure in these women is secondary to a definable exogenous cause, and a diagnosis of peripartum cardiomyopathy may not be appropriate in this setting. Whether an underlying cardiac abnormality predisposes these women to a more severe form of heart failure has not been studied.

Similar difficulties arise when evaluating the reported risk factors and incidence in the United States. Initial data suggested an incidence of 1 in 3000 to 4000 women. Reports assessing risk factors and incidence in the United States came from inner-city county hospitals in the south where women generally were multiparous, received less prenatal care, and had more comorbid problems, including hypertension. Many of these patients had symptoms postpartum. In other studies of similarly aged middle-class women who received prenatal care, parity was not a significant factor. Furthermore, in these patients, the onset of symptoms occurred more frequently during pregnancy.[7]

Our perceptions of the incidence of and risk factors for peripartum cardiomyopathy have changed as we have gained knowledge and technologic advances in this field. Often, disease previously considered idiopathic can now be attributed to an identifiable cause. A retrospective review of patients initially diagnosed over a 12-year period with peripartum cardiomyopathy indicated that several factors could have caused the development of congestive heart failure. Adjustments made for this apparent overestimation yielded an incidence of approximately 1 in 15,000 women.[3] This low incidence is generally accepted for patients with postpartum cardiomyopathy who present with overt symptoms. The incidence may increase if more aggressive efforts were made to detect subtle signs of heart failure during pregnancy or postpartum.

The previous discussion emphasizes that the demographic characterization of a disease process is inexorably linked to the prevailing definition of that process. A definition containing the terms "idiopathic" or "unknown etiology" is destined to change. As systematic efforts are made to establish risk factors, the incidence, the demographics, and the profile of risk factors may change. Thus, the diagnosis of peripartum cardiomyopathy should be based primarily on clinical symptoms and should not be dismissed because of demographic data.

CLINICAL PRESENTATION

The presenting symptoms in peripartum cardiomyopathy are similar to those of left ventricular systolic dysfunction from any cause and include dyspnea, orthopnea, fatigue, leg edema, and palpitations. These symptoms are common in normal pregnancies and are not specific to the diagnosis of peripartum cardiomyopathy. Indeed, interpretation of the New York Heart Association (NYHA) functional classification is limited during pregnancy because these symptoms are so common in routine uncomplicated pregnancies. Although nonspecific, these symptoms may increase clinical suspicion of impaired left ventricular systolic function. When symptoms are combined with physical findings of overt failure such as cardiomegaly, pulmonary rales, tachycardia, and elevated jugular venous pressure, heart failure is present. Echocardiography can provide definitive confirmation of depressed left ventricular systolic function. Tachycardia in the absence of other physical findings should alert physicians that cardiac abnormalities may exist. Persistent resting tachycardia is rare in uncomplicated pregnancy and postpartum periods. We have found that resting tachycardia frequently heralds the presence of peripartum cardiomyopathy both in overtly and in minimally symptomatic patients.

ETIOLOGY AND PATHOGENESIS

The diagnosis of peripartum cardiomyopathy is one of exclusion. A history of prior pregnancies and the type and timing of delivery must be obtained. Any familial history of peripartum or dilated cardiomyopathy or a personal history of cardiac disorders or systemic illness is significant.[10] A travel history should be obtained; any exposure to infectious agents is important. Drug use (both prescription and illicit) and alcohol abuse is important in determining a cause of congestive heart failure. Potentially reversible secondary causes of cardiomyopathy should be evaluated with biochemical tests such as a complete blood cell count, thyroid function tests, serum levels of urea nitrogen, and creatinine, phosphorus, iron, and calcium determinations. Patients should be evaluated for exposure to heavy metals, cobalt, or excessive quantities of iron (hemochromatosis) if the history and clinical situation are suggestive. In addition, patients should be assessed for systemic inflammatory illnesses. A myocarditis panel with acute and convalescent titers may also be appropriate.

Echocardiography, an important noninvasive tool for establishing the diagnosis of depressed left ventricular function, is valuable in confirming the presence of significant secondary causes of heart failure including valvular, congenital, and/or infiltrative abnormalities. Echocardiography may also be useful in assessing the presence of primary or secondary pulmonary disease.

Volume overload, toxemia, pre-eclampsia, hypertension, nutritional factors, tocolytic therapy, and other factors have been implicated in the genesis of peripartum cardiomyopathy.[2, 11] These factors are likely to be contributory and not causative because most patients with these conditions do not develop peripartum cardiomyopathy. Instead, a viral or autoimmune mechanism may be responsible for development of this condition, which is made worse by the additional hemodynamic burden of pregnancy. Whether peripartum cardiomyopathy is a separate entity unrelated to idiopathic cardiomyopathy is controversial. However, we, and others, believe they are separate conditions because of the clustering of cases of peripartum cardiomyopathy from the last trimester of pregnancy to 6 months after delivery and because improvement is expected in approximately 50% of women.

If the cause of peripartum cardiomyopathy is eventually shown to be a viral or autoimmune one, rapid strides in cardiovascular pathophysiology and molecular processes should increase our understanding of this disorder. Viral genetic material is found in roughly one third of patients with idiopathic dilated cardiomyopathy, which suggests a viral etiology. The incidence of myocarditis in peripartum cardiomyopathy is probably similar to that in patients with idiopathic cardiomyopathy.[12] Coxsackievirus B causes more than 50% of all viral myocarditis. Coxsackievirus A, echovirus, and influenza are other common cardiotropic viruses.[13] In the general population, exposure to one of these viruses may cause systemic illness but rarely clinically evident myocarditis; thus, once exposed, an individual's immune response to viral infection may be crucial in the development of myocarditis. Some animal studies support this theory; certain strains of pregnant mice infected with coxsackievirus or encephalomyocarditis (EMC) virus are susceptible to myocarditis.[14, 15] Increased suppressor cell activity, passage of fetal suppressor cells, other suppressor factor activity, and alterations in T4/T8 ratios have been described in pregnant women.[16, 17] Modification in suppressor cell activity could affect crucial processing of a viral agent. Genetically linked abnormalities in the immune response may predispose patients to myocarditis. In idiopathic cardiomyopathy, the HLA-DR4/HLA-DQWL antigen association is well known and may indicate a genetically linked risk for development of this disease with an appropriate inciting event.[18, 19] The known familial occurrence of peripartum cardiomyopathy supports a possible genetic link for this disorder.[10] Furthermore, cardiomyopathy has been described in infants of women with peripartum cardiomyopathy.

In addition to the initial response to viremia, autoimmune reactions may affect the severity of inflammatory response. Viral antigens, which have been found in myocytes, may stimulate an immune response directed at the myocardium. In addition, the absence of immunologic suppression may result in a stronger autoimmune response.

If a viral etiology is the inciting event in the development of idiopathic cardiomyopathy or peripartum cardiomyopathy, then a combination of genetic factors and immune response may ultimately contribute to the expression of the disease. Thus, variability in clinical response would be expected, with some patients developing overt and severe symptoms and others developing only subclinical to mild signs. Regardless of the underlying mechanism, myocarditis generally leads to contractile dysfunction and cell death. Any action that intensifies this process could cause earlier onset of clinical symptoms. The additional cardiovascular and hemodynamic burden of pregnancy could potentially impair myocardial function and intensify symptoms. However, the cardiovascular dynamics of pregnancy are constantly changing and may affect the timing of the onset of disease.

Cardiac output increases by 30% to 50% during pregnancy and peaks between the 20th and 24th week of pregnancy. The cause of this increase in cardiac output is controversial. Some investigators believe it results from an increase in stroke volume and, to a lesser extent, heart rate, which is only 10 to 20 beats per minute higher at term than in the nonpregnant state. However, others have reported that stroke volume does not significantly increase and that the increase results from an increased heart rate. Because of the increased cardiac output, maximal exercise-induced cardiac output will be achieved at a lower work level. Systemic vascular resistance reaches its lowest point by the 8th week of pregnancy. Both systolic and diastolic blood pressure decline slightly through the second trimester. Blood pressure gradually increases until term. Hemodynamic factors during birth are affected by the method of delivery, the type of sedation and anesthesia, and maternal posture. Catecholamines increase during labor and delivery. Mean arterial pressure and systolic and diastolic blood pressure also increase during labor. Major uterine contractions expel approximately 500 ml of blood into the circulation, which increases venous return, stroke volume, cardiac output, and blood pressure in the normal patient. Oxygen consumption doubles by the second stage of labor. In the postpartum period, hemodynamic factors depend on the type of delivery, the amount of blood loss, and the type of sedation and anesthesia. After delivery, there is an immediate influx of blood into the maternal circulation and cardiac output because the inferior vena cava is no longer obstructed. This autotransfusion is tempered by a preload reduction, which occurs in the form of blood loss (approximately 1000 ml with abdominal delivery and 500 ml with vaginal delivery). Heart rate decreases by 10 to 20 beats per minute after delivery. Hemodynamic factors gradually return to pre-pregnancy levels over a 4- to 12-week period after delivery.

Ventricular mechanics during and after pregnancy are variably affected by the hemodynamic state in normal pregnancy. Left ventricular dimension, wall thickness, and mass increase slightly during pregnancy. This increase parallels the increase in body surface area. After delivery these increases return to baseline levels. Stress changes in the left ventricular wall depend on ventricular dimension, cardiac index, and wall thickness. Relative global systolic ventricular function is preserved throughout pregnancy by a decrease in afterload. However, a recent report suggests that load-independent indices of ventricular contractility may diminish late in pregnancy and decrease markedly early after delivery compared with values in early pregnancy.[20] The significance of this finding is unknown because pre-pregnancy values were not measured.

In the nonpregnant state, left ventricular remodeling occurs in response to myocardial injury in an effort to preserve stroke volume and cardiac output. Left ventricular dilation with compensatory hypertrophy is expected in order to maintain normal wall stress. As left ventricular systolic performance deteriorates, a "normal" afterload becomes relatively increased. Progressive ventricular dilation occurs, and the hypertrophic response may be unable to compensate. Increasing catecholamine levels and angiotensin II affect not only cardiac myocyte function but also left ventricular end-diastolic pressure. These changes act in concert to produce the clinical picture seen in dilated cardiomyopathy. Progressive deterioration in stroke volume and ejection fraction, with or without compensatory hypertrophy, in the presence of normal or near-normal left ventricular size is an abnormal response to injury. This abnormal response has been well described, but the mechanism has not been identified.

Similar findings may be present in women who develop peripartum cardiomyopathy. Previous reports have indicated that most cases are diagnosed immediately postpartum or within the first few months.[1, 4, 5] Despite the well-known increase in cardiac output and heart rate, peripartum cardiomyopathy is not frequently described before delivery. Thus, if depressed left ventricular systolic function and impaired cardiac reserve were present antepartum, the marked afterload reduction caused by decreased systemic vascular resistance may delay frank symptomatic expression of disease. Additional impairment of contractility (as reported by Mone and associates[20]) may reduce contractile reserve further, but this reduction may not be sufficient to override the beneficial effect of afterload reduction. After delivery, however, the marginally compensated heart is further challenged by an increase in preload and an elevation of systemic vascular resistance caused by the loss of the low-resistance placental circuit. In addition to depressed contractility that already may be present, contractility may progressively deteriorate after the normal postpartum cardiovascular changes. Under these circumstances, it is not surprising that symptoms of heart failure are most frequently seen after delivery in women with peripartum cardiomyopathy.

PROGNOSIS

Prognosis cannot be predicted by initial clinical, hemodynamic, or laboratory data. Approximately 50% of women will recover cardiac function, usually within 6 months of the initial onset of symptoms and diagnosis. The other 50% will remain the same or experience progressive deterioration. The classic study of Demakis and associates in 1971 describing the outcome of women with peripartum cardiomyopathy showed clinical improvement in 14 of 25 patients (56%) at 6-month follow-up. Twelve of these women had a normal-sized heart, and the remaining 2 had persistent cardiomegaly at the 6-month evaluation. These 14 women did well and had good long-term survival. Women who had normal cardiac size and NYHA classification I or II tolerated subsequent pregnancies well; 8 of these women had 21 subsequent pregnancies without recurrence of heart failure. Unfortunately, 2 others had postpartum cardiac failure with subsequent pregnancies. Women with cardiomegaly at 6 months were sicker. In 11 of the 13 women with persistent cardiomegaly, the survival rate was 4 years. Six of the 13 women with cardiomegaly had a subsequent pregnancy; in 3 women permanent deterioration resulted in death. Only clinical criteria were used to diagnose peripartum cardiomyopathy in this study; some women who may have had etiologic factors that could be identified with modern technology may have been included in this study. Nevertheless, subsequent reports confirm that women who recover ventricular function do so within 6 months of the initial diagnosis.[21] Such patients should do well over the long term.

Until recently, women with progressive deterioration in cardiac function that was unresponsive to conservative and aggressive measures had a poor prognosis. Although successful treatment with immunosuppressive agents has been observed in women with active myocarditis, many women presenting with postpartum myocardiopathy have nonspecific biopsy findings, and the risk posed by using immunosuppressive agents is not warranted. Cardiac transplantation should be considered in these women. Controversy exists regarding short-term prognosis after transplantation.[22, 23] In general, younger transplant recipients have a higher frequency of rejection and rejection rates are higher in women than in men. Active myocarditis increases the risk of rejection. In addition to these potential problems, there are other concerns about the risk of rejection in women who have peripartum cardiomyopathy. Exposure to fetal cells during childbirth may sensitize the recipient to donor antigens. In two studies, outcome after heart transplantation was compared in women with peripartum cardiomyopathy and in an age-matched group with idiopathic cardiomyopathy. Rickenbacher and associates found no significant difference in the rate of rejection between the two groups, although infection rates tended to be higher in the group with peripartum cardiomypathy.[22] Keogh and associates found that the linearized rate of rejection in the first 6 months after transplantation was 31% to 33% higher in the peripartum cardiomyopathy group.[23] This finding could not be explained on the basis of underlying myocarditis because none of the women had active myocarditis on biopsy or on examination of the explanted heart. Panel-reactive antibody formation was less than 5%, and evaluation of the serologic crossmatch indicated no overt immunologic abnormalities. However, on clinical examination, these women appeared to be more immunologically active. Women with peripartum cardiomyopathy had more severe episodes of rejection that required cytolytic therapy or lymphoid irradiation (in over half of the patients). Furthermore, infection rates were higher in the peripartum cardiomyopathy group.

Despite the short-term concern of rejection, medium- to long-term survival after transplant in women with peripartum cardiomyopathy is favorable and is comparable to that in other groups. Thus, cardiac transplantation should be considered in a woman with peripartum cardiomyopathy who does not respond to aggressive measures.

Fetal prognosis in mothers with peripartum cardiomyopathy has not been adequately addressed. Increased rates of fetal death, fetal anomalies, and premature birth are not prominent features of peripartum cardiomyopathy. However, the potential for unplanned early delivery is a concern. Premature labor may be precipitated by decreased placental blood flow as a result of depressed cardiac output. A planned early delivery may be scheduled in an effort to minimize the duration of the hemodynamic burden in pregnant women with depressed ventricular function. In these instances, fetal lung maturity should be hastened, or the patient should be stabilized until fetal lungs mature.

The success of subsequent pregnancies in women who have had peripartum cardiomyopathy depends in part on family history, ventricular function, and cardiac size. Although a familial pattern of peripartum cardiomyopathy is rare, a patient with a strong family history should be advised to consider alternate forms of family growth. Most physicians agree that pregnancy is not advised in women with persistent left ventricular dysfunction resulting from peripartum cardiomyopathy because they are at high risk for symptomatic deterioration, complications, and death. For women who have normal left ventricular size and normal left ventricular systolic function, the risk of recurrent peripartum cardiomyopathy appears to be very low. However, myocardial contractile reserve may be diminished in these women with normal left ventricular systolic function and chamber size.[24] Whether this finding has a direct association with a risk of peripartum cardiomyopathy in subsequent pregnancies is unknown.

TREATMENT

Appropriate treatment of peripartum cardiomyopathy is mandated by the timing of onset of symptoms. Most cases occur directly after or within the first few weeks after delivery. Although comparatively rare, antepartum and intrapartum presentations also occur. Maternal management focuses primarily on treating heart failure and improving cardiac function. If heart failure occurs during pregnancy, management will include both the mother and the fetus. Treatment must be tailored to secure a successful outcome for both. Because peripartum cardiomyopathy is infrequent, we believe that a multidisciplinary approach with perinatologists, cardiologists, anesthesiologists, and neonatologists is crucial.

Antepartum Management

Women who present with peripartum cardiomyopathy during pregnancy should be advised that in most cases heart failure improves or stabilizes. However, deterioration is possible and careful monitoring before, during, and after birth is essential.

Antepartum management involves treating cardiac failure; treating and preventing thromboembolism; monitoring fetal growth and well-being; observing for preterm labor; determining the timing, location, and type of delivery; and evaluating the necessity of invasive hemodynamic monitoring in the peripartum period. Treatment of cardiac failure will be dictated primarily by the clinical status of the patient, who should be assessed frequently. Antepartum hospitalization of patients with cardiomyopathy and moderate to severe heart failure is recommended because of the potential for sudden deterioration in both maternal and fetal condition. In addition, hospitalization allows frequent fetal and maternal assessment and ensures close proximity to obstetric and pediatric services. Once the patient's condition has been stabilized, outpatient management can be considered.

Treatment of Heart Failure

Maternal hemodynamics should be optimized in the treatment of peripartum cardiomyopathy. Although treatment is similar to that for women with idiopathic cardiomyopathy, special considerations are necessary when heart failure occurs during pregnancy. Because afterload reduction occurs naturally during pregnancy because of the low-resistance placental circuit, increasing myocardial contractility and reducing preload is initially emphasized. When the diagnosis of cardiomyopathy is confirmed by echocardiography during pregnancy, activity should be limited according to symptoms. Complete bed rest is not advised because of deconditioning and the potential for thromboembolic events. Fluid and sodium restriction may be necessary if symptoms are moderate to severe. The type of medical therapy used depends on the severity of heart failure and the response to therapeutic measures. If mild failure is present, oral medications can be used. If failure is moderate to severe, intravenous medications should be considered to ensure complete absorption and to allow more accurate assessment of clinical response.

Initial conservative medical therapy includes the use of digoxin to enhance myocardial contractility and vagal influence on the heart. Increased clearance of digoxin occurs as pregnancy progresses. In fact, doses of 0.375 to 0.5 mg/day may be needed to achieve a therapeutic level. Thus, digoxin levels should be monitored and adjusted as necessary. Digoxin crosses the placenta but does not appear to have a deleterious effect on a fetus with a normal heart. Because a significant reduction in circulating blood volume has the potential for reducing placental perfusion and gas exchange, diuretics should be used judiciously. Diuretics should be used only when there is objective evidence of rales or hypoxemia; their administration should be flexible and tailored to individual clinical response.

Beta-adrenergic blockade therapy is important in the treatment of both idiopathic and peripartum cardiomyopathy. The beneficial effects of beta-adrenergic blockers include reduction of heart rate and consequent enhancement of diastolic filling, which may lead to an increase in stroke volume. However, beta-adrenergic blockers may reduce maternal myocardial contractility; therefore, relatively low doses should be used with close, regular monitoring. When prescribing these drugs during pregnancy, the physician should consider the specific properties of each beta-adrenergic blocker rather than thinking of them as a class. Uterine activity can be stimulated by $beta_2$ antagonists, which may lead to increased uterine tone and a possible reduction in uterine perfusion. Butters and coworkers showed that women receiving atenolol were delivered of infants weighing 500 g less than controls.[25] Propranolol has been associated with a depression in the neonatal respiratory center and sinus node activity and neonatal hypoglycemia.[26] Although initially thought to be safe for the fetus, intravenous administration of esmolol may be associated with fetal acidosis and bradycardia. When a cardioselective beta-adrenergic blocker is used at lower doses, fetal risk is reduced and substantial maternal cardiac benefits are attained.

Afterload reduction during pregnancy is rarely needed even in cases of peripartum cardiomyopathy. Occasionally, however, systemic vascular resistance may increase substantially as a compensatory response to moderate or severe heart failure. In such instances, afterload reduction is needed to improve maternal cardiovascular hemodynamics. Hydralazine, which reduces afterload by direct arteriolar smooth muscle cell dilation (cyclic guanosine monophosphate mediated), effectively controls hypertension during pregnancy. Initial enthusiasm for the long-term antenatal use of oral hydralazine has been tempered by reports of tachyphylaxis, lupus-like side effects, and the development of IgG class antiphospholipid antibodies. Intravenous hydralazine, however, is the first-line therapy for severe hypertension in patients with pre-eclampsia. Reflex tachycardia, a well-known side effect of hydralazine, can be blunted by pretreatment with beta-adrenergic blocking agents.

Angiotensin-converting enzyme (ACE) inhibitors are extremely beneficial in nonpregnant patients with heart failure caused by impaired left ventricular relaxation. However, routine use in pregnancy is contraindicated because ACE inhibitors cross the placenta and may cause serious fetal complications, including renal failure and death. Nevertheless, in pregnant women with severe cardiovascular deterioration unresponsive to more aggressive measures, the use of ACE inhibitors may be warranted. In such situations the patient should be fully informed of the potential fetal side effects, including permanent renal dysfunction and death.[27] If the patient chooses to continue the pregnancy, antenatal testing and ultrasound should be used to follow the amniotic fluid index and the fetal biophysical profile, and regular fetal biometry should be used to monitor fetal growth.

Women who do not respond appropriately to the just-mentioned measures require more aggressive intervention. Noninvasive methods can be used to assess cardiovascular dynamics; however, if heart failure does not rapidly respond, intracardiac hemodynamics should be assessed with a right-sided heart catheter to allow minute-to-minute titration of drugs. Intravenous inotropic agents such as dopamine and dobutamine may be necessary to manage symptoms of severe heart failure. In our experience, pregnant women are very sensitive to these agents, and low doses should be used initially to avoid overstimulation and tachycardia. High doses of dopamine and other sympathomimetic agents may decrease uterine perfusion and can compromise the fetus.

Treatment and Prevention of Thromboembolism

The hypercoagulable state of pregnancy results from increased circulating levels of all of the coagulation factors (except for factors XI and XIII); an increase in pregnancy-associated plasma-protein A, which neutralizes antithrombin III; and the placental production of fibrinolysis inhibitors. The risk of thromboembolic events is greatest in the early postpartum period (first 4 weeks), because of the additional procoagulants (tissue thromboplastins) released at the time of placental separation. Left ventricular dysfunction, relative immobility, and venous stasis further predispose the pregnant woman with peripartum cardiomyopathy to thromboembolic events. Indeed, clinically significant embolic episodes have been reported in a substantial number of pregnant women with clinically overt heart failure. For this reason, anticoagulation should be considered. Heparin is the anticoagulant of choice because it does not cross the placenta and its effects may be reversed if necessary. Fresh-frozen plasma and vitamin K are recommended for the reversal of heparin-induced anticoagulation in pregnancy. The use of protamine sulfate is discouraged in pregnant women unless rapid reversal of anticoagulation is absolutely essential, because fetal acidosis and distress have been reported after protamine injection.

When a thromboembolic episode occurs, full systemic heparin therapy should be instituted. Usually, heparin is administered as an intravenous load followed by a continuous infusion titrated to an activated partial thromboplastin time (aPTT) that is 1.5 to 2.0 times the normal value. Once the initial episode has been treated, subcutaneous injections of heparin should be used for the remainder of the pregnancy. The dose of heparin may vary widely (for example, 8,000 to 14,000 units twice a day) depending on the stage of pregnancy and should be titrated to an aPTT value obtained 6 hours after the injection. The use of warfarin (Coumadin) is contraindicated during certain times in pregnant women because of its teratogenic effects (in the first trimester, epiphyseal stippling and nasal hypoplasia) and the increased risk of fetal bleeding (intracranial and intraocular) in the second and third trimesters and during delivery. Warfarin may be started soon after delivery and should overlap heparin therapy for at least 3 days. Breast feeding is not contraindicated in women receiving warfarin.

For women with cardiomyopathy who have not had any thromboembolic events, we suggest intermittent subcutaneous administration of low-dose heparin (5,000 units twice per day). Heparin dosages in pregnant women may be 2.0 to 2.5 times higher than in nonpregnant women, and the use of the aPTT is recommended to determine the correct dose. In addition, as pregnancy progresses, dosage requirements increase. Complications of long-term heparin therapy include osteoporosis (vertebral collapse, femoral neck fractures), thrombocytopenia, and bleeding problems. We recommend that pregnant women on heparin should receive supplemental calcium (2 g/day total intake), refrain from vigorous exercise, and have a platelet count on a weekly basis. Dulitzki and colleagues[28] have reported on the use of low-molecular-weight heparin (enoxaparin) in pregnant women with cardiac disease. Enoxaparin was used in 41 pregnancies and was not associated with excessive bleeding after vaginal delivery or cesarean section. Furthermore, epidural anesthesia was uncomplicated by hemorrhagic events.[28] Advantages associated with the use of enoxaparin include lower risks of bleeding, thrombocytopenia, and osteoporosis. Moreover, enoxaparin does not cross the placenta in any trimester.[29] In addition, repeated testing of the aPTT and platelet count is not required. This therapy has been increasingly used in pregnancy. Initial results indicate that it is safe for thromboprophylaxis and treatment during pregnancy.

Timing, Location, and Type of Delivery

We advocate a scheduled delivery, which will allow careful orchestration and attendance of all services necessary to care for the mother and infant. Fetal lung maturity should be assessed in cases of preterm delivery if the gestational age is less than 39 weeks. A normal aPTT is recommended before amniocentesis. Amniotic fluid should be rapidly evaluated for fetal lung maturity, and if the fetus' lungs are mature, labor can be induced. If the fetus' lungs are immature, delivery can be postponed and heparin therapy reinitiated. Steroids can be given to enhance lung maturity. In patients in whom preterm delivery (24 to 34 weeks) is essential, steroids should be given before delivery if possible. At our institution we administer betamethasone (12 mg intramuscularly) 12 or 24 hours apart depending on the time available. The use of steroids has been associated with noncardiogenic pulmonary edema in some patients with preterm labor; patients with cardiomyopathy who are receiving steroids should be carefully observed for symptoms of this complication.

Delivery should be scheduled at an institution with physicians experienced in the management of women with peripartum cardiomyopathy. An appropriate team of physicians should include a maternal-fetal specialist, a cardiologist, an obstetric anesthesiologist, a neonatologist, and a nursing staff trained to handle high-risk cases.

Intrapartum Management

Induction of labor in stable pregnant women with peripartum cardiomyopathy is not contraindicated. Prostaglandin E_2 gel (dinoprostone [Prepidil]), vaginal inserts (dinoprostone [Cervidil]), or misoprostol (Cytotec), although not absolutely contraindicated, should be used with caution because of their potential for uterine hyperstimulation and subsequent fetal distress. If hyperstimulation does occur, administration of a uterine relaxant (a $beta_2$ stimulant such as terbutaline) is frequently required; however, this practice may be dangerous because of the cardiac stimulatory effect of terbutaline. The use of manual cervical dilators (Dilapan, Laminaria, Foley catheter) may be preferred if cervical dilation is required. Ideally, labor should be induced with oxytocin (Pitocin) once the Bishop score is greater than 7, and amniotomy should be performed once contractions are established. We do not use high-dose oxytocin and active management of labor regimens in patients with cardiac abnormalities. We prefer a low-dose, stepwise oxytocin protocol. A scheduled cesarean section should be performed for obstetric indications.

Anesthesia for patients in labor can be tailored to the patient's medical condition and the degree of pain control required. Epidural and spinal anesthesia (or a combination of the two) is not contraindicated. Combinations of intrathecal and spinal narcotic and local anesthetic can be skillfully administered by obstetric anesthesiologists with minimal risk for hypotension or decreases in cardiac output. Pain control is a very important aspect of intrapartum management in patients with limited cardiac reserve because tachycardia can quickly precipitate decompensation. Most anesthesiologists require that the aPTT be normal before administering a regional anesthetic, so coordinating the cessation of heparin therapy is important. In a patient undergoing a scheduled delivery, heparin therapy can be stopped on the evening before induction and the aPTT can be checked in the morning before induction of regional anesthesia. In some cases, once the epidural catheter is placed, low-dose heparin therapy (5000 units subcutaneously every 12 hours) can be restarted during labor if required. Heparin therapy may need to be continued throughout labor in some patients (e.g., one who had a recent embolic event). In these patients, regional anesthesia is precluded and patient-controlled analgesia pump therapy with narcotic analgesics may be more appropriate.

Women with peripartum cardiomyopathy should be watched closely during labor. Continuous electrocardiography and arterial pressure and peripheral oxygen saturation should be monitored. Not every woman with peripartum cardiomyopathy requires invasive hemodynamic monitoring during labor and delivery. Right-sided heart catheterization is recommended in women with peripartum cardiomyopathy who have one or more of the following conditions: (1) current congestive heart failure or pulmonary edema, (2) ejection fraction less than 30%, (3) hypotension of unknown cause, and (4) pulmonary hypertension. If catheterization is indicated in a woman undergoing a scheduled delivery, the right-sided heart catheter and arterial line should be inserted a few hours before the induction of labor to evaluate and optimize the hemodynamic status of the patient. During labor, patients should be placed in a semi-Fowler's position with a left lateral tilt to prevent aortocaval compression syndrome, which can reduce venous return and increase afterload. Particular attention should be paid to intravenous volume infusion. Central venous pressure or pulmonary capillary wedge pressure readings should be used judiciously. Tachycardia should be avoided by optimizing volume, controlling pain, preventing reduction in preload (aortocaval compression, blood loss, dehydration), and avoiding chorioamnionitis and maternal fever (prophylactic antibiotics, decreased number of vaginal examinations). Prolonged attempts to induce labor and lengthy latent and active stages of labor should be avoided because the risks of thromboembolism and hemodynamic fluctuation outweigh the potential benefit of a vaginal delivery. Heart rate should be maintained below 100 beats per minute. Although anesthesia is usually sufficient to control heart rate, short-acting beta-adrenergic blockers may be required.

During vaginal delivery the patient should be in a modified semi-Fowler's position, which entails placing her feet on stools below the level of her heart and delivering the infant in a sitting position. The lithotomy position should be discouraged because of the autotransfusion associated with elevation of the legs. Forceps or a vacuum extractor should be used to limit maternal straining efforts and Valsalva's maneuver and to shorten the second stage of labor.

Immediately after delivery of the infant, cardiac output can increase dramatically during and after the third stage of labor (delivery of the placenta); this period is the most common time for patients to decompensate. Methergine should be avoided because it induces a tonic contraction that can significantly increase uteroplacental transfusion and because it may result in severe hypertension. In addition, intravenous bolus doses of oxytocin should be avoided because of the potential for peripheral vasodilation and reduction in preload. Usually, the uterus will adequately contract in response to 20 units of oxytocin in 1 L of crystalloid infused at 125 ml/h. In cases in which volume infusion must be limited, the concentration of oxytocin can be doubled or tripled to reduce the flow rate. In the case of massive vaginal bleeding and uncontrolled postpartum hemorrhage, 15-methyl prostaglandin $F_{2\alpha}$ (Hemabate) (250 μg) may be used either intramuscularly or intramyometrially, or misoprostol may be used rectally.

Postpartum Management

After delivery, the risk of heart failure increases because of increasing preload and afterload. Placental delivery and uterine contractions can be associated with a substantial autotransfusion, which increases preload, and the loss of the low resistance placental "arteriovenous fistula" leads to a sudden increase in afterload. An epidural catheter may be helpful in this situation because controlled sympathectomy can be used to incrementally adjust afterload while oral or intravenous afterload reducing medications are titrated. Hydralazine and ACE inhibitors may be used alone or in combination to decrease afterload. Preload can be adjusted by patient positioning, diuretics, and fluid restriction.

Anticoagulants may be restarted within 4 hours after a vaginal delivery as long as lochia is normal; the uterus is well contracted; and no evidence of vaginal, vulval, or retroperitoneal bleeding is found. After cesarean section, anticoagulants may be restarted 6 hours after delivery if no evidence of bleeding is noted. Warfarin may be started at the same time as heparin, and use of the two agents should overlap for 3 days before discontinuing heparin. Systemic anticoagulation should be continued for 6 weeks post partum. In the absence of pregnancy, a known hypercoagulable state (protein C deficiency, protein S deficiency, antithrombin III deficiency, antiphospholipid syndrome, factor V Leiden mutation), or atrial fibrillation, routine long-term anticoagulation is no longer recommended.

Postpartum fever in women with peripartum cardiomyopathy should be investigated thoroughly because microthrombi, infarction, and subsequent abscess formation are often complications. The lungs and kidneys are the two most frequently affected organs, and any involvement should be aggressively treated. Changes in level of consciousness and lateralizing features noted on physical examination may herald cerebral embolization and should be immediately evaluated.

Patients should be evaluated 6 weeks after delivery when most pregnancy-induced hemodynamic changes have resolved. After delivery, drug dosages may need to be adjusted. The high dose of digoxin required during pregnancy and immediately postpartum should be decreased. If continued evidence of left ventricular failure is present, additional β-adrenergic blockade therapy, afterload reduction, and diuretics can be given. The clinically stable or mildly symptomatic woman should be evaluated 3, 6, and 12 months after delivery. Prognosis can be obtained from echocardiograms conducted at 6 and 12 months. Women in poor clinical condition who do not respond to conservative measures may be candidates for transplantation.

Breast feeding has reportedly been associated with increased cardiac output and in the past has been contraindicated.[30] The current view is that breast feeding is safe unless the patient is using ACE inhibitors.

The question of future pregnancies is important because it affects several areas of management. Options for contraception should be discussed with the patient. For women with persistently depressed left ventricular systolic function, estrogen-containing oral contraceptives are contraindicated because of the thromboembolic risk. Progesterone-containing pills, injections, and implants may be considered. The use of an intrauterine contraceptive device is not absolutely contraindicated and may be considered for patients in a stable monogamous relationship. Tubal ligation is another important option. Barrier and other methods are not recommended for long-term contraception because of their high failure rates.

References

1. Demakis JG, Rahimtoola SH, Sutton GC, et al: Natural course of peripartum cardiomyopathy. Circulation 44:1053, 1971.
2. Lampert MB, Lang RM: Peripartum cardiomyopathy. Am Heart J 130: 860, 1995.
3. Cunningham FG, Pritchard JA, Hankins GD, et al: Peripartum heart failure: Idiopathic cardiomyopathy or compounding cardiovascular events? Obstet Gynecol 67:157, 1986.
4. Carvalho A, Brandao A, Martinez EE, et al: Prognosis in peripartum cardiomyopathy. Am J Cardiol 64:540, 1989.
5. Davidson NM, Parry EH: Peri-partum cardiac failure. Q J Med 47: 431, 1978.
6. Adesanya CO, Anjorin FI, Adeoshun IO, et al: Peripartum cardiac failure: A ten year follow-up. Trop Geogr Med 41:190, 1989.
7. O'Connell JB, Costanzo-Nordin MR, Subramanian R, et al: Peripartum cardiomyopathy: Clinical, hemodynamic, histologic and prognostic characteristics. J Am Coll Cardiol 8:52, 1986.
8. Sanderson JE, Adesanya CO, Anjorin FI, et al: Postpartum cardiac failure—heart failure due to volume overload? Am Heart J 97:613, 1979.
9. Midei MG, DeMent SH, Feldman AM, et al: Peripartum myocarditis and cardiomyopathy. Circulation 81:922, 1990.
10. Pierce JA, Price BO, Joyce JW: Familial occurrence of postpartal heart failure. Arch Intern Med 111:651, 1963.
11. Lee W, Cotton DB: Peripartum cardiomyopathy: Current concepts and clinical management. Clin Obstet Gynecol 32:54, 1989.
12. Rizeq MN, Rickenbacher PR, Fowler MB, et al: Incidence of myocarditis in peripartum cardiomyopathy. Am J Cardiol 74:474, 1994.
13. Elstein E, Sole MJ: Frontiers in the diagnosis of viral myocarditis. Heart Failure 8:16, 1992.
14. Yokoyama T, Kanda T, Suzuki T, et al: Enhancement of myocardial damage and alteration of lymphocyte subsets in murine model of postpartum myocarditis. Am J Cardiovasc Pathol 4:343, 1993.
15. Dalldorf G, Gifford R: Susceptibility of gravid mice to coxsackievirus infection. J Exp Med 99:21, 1954.
16. Sanderson JE, Olsen EG, Gatei D: Peripartum heart disease: An endomyocardial biopsy study. Br Heart J 56:285, 1986.
17. Kovithavongs T, Dossetor JB: Suppressor cells in human pregnancy. Transplant Proc 10:911, 1978.
18. Carlquist JF, Menlove RL, Murray MB, et al: HLA Class II (DR and DQ) antigen associations in idiopathic dilated cardiomyopathy: Validation study and meta-analysis of published HLA association studies. Circulation 83:515, 1991.
19. Bender JR: Idiopathic dilated cardiomyopathy: An immunologic, genetic, or infectious disease, or all of the above? Circulation 83:704, 1991.
20. Mone SM, Sanders SP, Colan SD: Control mechanisms for physiological hypertrophy of pregnancy. Circulation 94:667, 1996.
21. Sutton MS, Cole P, Plappert M, et al: Effects of subsequent pregnancy on left ventricular function in peripartum cardiomyopathy. Am Heart J 121:1776, 1991.
22. Rickenbacher PR, Rizeq MN, Hunt SA, et al: Long-term outcome after heart transplantation for peripartum cardiomyopathy. Am Heart J 127: 1318, 1994.

23. Keogh A, Macdonald P, Spratt P, et al: Outcome in peripartum cardiomyopathy after heart transplantation. J Heart Lung Transplant 13: 202, 1994.
24. Lampert MB, Weinert L, Hibbard J, et al: Contractile reserve in patients with peripartum cardiomyopathy and recovered left ventricular function. Am J Obstet Gynecol 176:189, 1997.
25. Butters L, Kennedy S, Rubin P: Atenolol in essential hypertension during pregnancy. BMJ 301:587, 1990.
26. Habib A, McCarthy JS: Effects on the neonate of propranolol administered during pregnancy. J Pediatr 91:808, 1977.
27. Rosa FW, Bosco LA, Graham CF, et al: Neonatal anuria with maternal angiotensin-converting enzyme inhibition. Obstet Gynecol 74(3Pt1): 371, 1989.
28. Dulitzki M, Pauzner R, Langevitz P, et al: Low molecular weight heparin during pregnancy and delivery: Preliminary experience with 41 pregnancies. Obstet Gynecol 87:380, 1996.
29. Fejgin MD, Lourwood DL: Low molecular weight heparins and their use in obstetrics and gynecology. Obstet Gynecol Surv 49:424, 1994.
30. Seftel H, Susser M: Maternity and myocardial failure in African women. Br Heart J 23:43, 1961.

CHAPTER 29

Arrhythmias in Pregnancy

Susanna Mak and Louise Harris

Arrhythmias in pregnancy can be alarming to both the physician and the patient, even though most cases have a benign course. This chapter discusses the possible pathophysiologic mechanisms that affect the incidence of arrhythmias in pregnancy, the clinical diagnosis and management of patients with arrhythmias, and the more commonly used antiarrhythmic drugs. We will stress the importance of determining whether patients have underlying structural heart disease or metabolic abnormalities. Arrhythmias detected in the absence of structural heart disease generally follow a benign course; physicians should avoid unnecessary therapy and limit drug exposure of the unborn child.

MECHANISMS OF ARRHYTHMOGENESIS IN PREGNANCY

There are gender differences in cardiac electrophysiology and in the incidence of certain arrhythmias.[1] The mechanisms for these differences have not been well studied. It is unclear whether the differences result from morphologic variation in body size and exercise capacity, or the hormonal environment and the influence of the menstrual cycle, pregnancy, and menopause.[1] Pregnancy uniquely alters hormonal and hemodynamic factors. The hormonal milieu is dominated by high levels of sex steroid hormones including beta-human chorionic gonadotropin (beta-hCG) and estrogen. The hemodynamic alterations are profound and include an increase in circulating volume that doubles the cardiac output. These changes may alter electrophysiologic properties and thus the incidence of certain arrhythmias during pregnancy. The mechanisms by which these changes can occur include the following: (1) gender differences and hormonal effects on ion channels, (2) gender differences and hormonal effects on autonomic tone, and (3) electrophysiologic changes resulting from the change in hemodynamic profile.

Gender Differences and Hormonal Effects on Ion Channels

It has been observed that women with paroxysmal supraventricular tachycardia (PSVT) may exhibit a cyclical variation in the occurrence of their arrhythmia related to the menstrual cycle.[2] This suggests that hormonal milieu may influence cardiac electrophysiology. Few data have been published on the effect of gender or hormones on the expression of cardiac ion channels. Animal studies have demonstrated that estradiol may downregulate cardiac potassium channel expression[3] and influence L-type Ca^{2+} channel function.[4] Estrogen can influence ion channels in other tissues such as the uterus. Experiments in rat uteri have demonstrated that estrogen can induce a slowly activating, voltage-dependent potassium channel that requires approximately 4 seconds to reach its peak current.[5, 6] In these experiments, potassium channels were expressed over a 3-hour period; thus, estrogen rapidly affected ion channel expression. The mRNA for this channel was rapidly and reversibly induced, depending on the presence of estrogen. In these experiments, the presence or absence of the mRNA was influenced by the menstrual cycle, the phases of pregnancy, and the treatment with hormones. Marked hyperpolarization of membrane potentials in vascular smooth muscle has previously been observed after estrogen treatment[7]; the expression of the potassium channel may be the mechanism by which this hyperpolarization is achieved. Thus, it is possible that rapid, transient fluctuations in levels of circulating sex steroid hormones such as estrogen may alter cardiac electrophysiologic properties via an effect on cardiac ion channels. The effect of beta-hCG and prolactin on ion channels is unknown.

Gender Differences and Hormonal Effects on Autonomic Tone

Few studies on gender differences in autonomic tone in humans have been reported.[1] Estrogen can alter responses to sympathetic stimulation in many tissues. In studies of the urinary bladder, urethral, and uterine tissues of rabbits, estrogen affected adrenoceptor density and increased responses to noradrenaline and phenylephrine.[8–12] In studies of the effects of estrogen on cardiovascular physiology in humans, estrogen modulated cardiac autonomic nervous activity; it suppressed sympathetic activity while potentiating parasympathetic control of the cardiovascular system.[13] This finding suggests that the lower incidence of sudden death in women may result from an antifibrillatory effect of estrogen.[14–19]

Pregnancy, however, may have a separate influence on autonomic tone. Ekholm and associates[20] studied the effects of Valsalva's maneuver, orthostatic changes, quiet and deep breathing, and isometric handgrip on cardiovascular responses in midpregnancy. They concluded that although both parasympathetic and sympathetic cardiovascular responses are attenuated, parasympathetic responses are more greatly affected. Cohen and colleagues[21] demonstrated increased sympathetic nervous activity in rat hearts during pregnancy, as evidenced by higher cardiac turnover of injected ^{3}H-labeled norepinephrine. Further support for the idea that pregnancy may increase sympathetic tone comes from the observation that cocaine cardiotoxicity may be increased in pregnancy.[22] Cocaine acts by blocking extraneuronal catecholamine uptake.[23] Pregnancy-enhanced, cocaine-mediated cardiotoxicity has been studied in Langendorff preparations of whole hearts from pregnant and nonpregnant rats pretreated with progesterone, estrogen, or both.[24] The results suggest that the cardiotoxicity of cocaine in pregnancy (as manifested by cocaine-induced myocardial depression) is mediated by estrogen. In a study of noradrenaline infusions in pregnant women admitted for pregnancy termination, heart rate responses differed from those in nonpregnant women. This finding suggests differences in the uptake and metabolism of catecholamines during pregnancy.[25]

Enhanced sympathetic tone has long been recognized as arrhythmogenic. Numerous studies have reported the usefulness of adrenergic stimulation with isoproterenol, upright posture, and muscarinic receptor blockade with atropine as a means of inducing PSVT during electrophysiologic testing.[26] Waxman and coworkers[27–31] have demonstrated that PSVT is usually initiated by premature atrial beats that either occur spontaneously or are triggered by programmed stimulation. Furthermore, in patients with PSVT, the arrhythmia can be induced without programmed stimulation when adrenergic tone is increased by exercise or by isoproterenol. These authors have also demonstrated that maneuvers that reflexly increase vagal tone will terminate PSVT. Thus, although the data are limited, potentiation of sympathetic tone of the cardiovascular system during pregnancy or attenuation of parasympathetic responses may cause arrhythmogenesis.

Hemodynamic Changes and Electrophysiologic Properties

The hemodynamic changes of pregnancy have been well documented. The plasma volume increases as early as the sixth week of pregnancy and peaks at approximately 50% above nonpregnant levels by 32 to 34 weeks' gestation. After this time, plasma volume changes little. The red blood cell mass continues to rise throughout pregnancy. Cardiac output increases by the tenth week of gestation; it reaches a level of 40% above nonpregnant levels by 20 to 24 weeks, after which little change occurs. Cardiac output peaks while blood volume is still increasing and reflects increases in both stroke volume and heart rate.[32] Increases in left ventricular end-diastolic volume during pregnancy have been demonstrated with systolic time intervals and two-dimensional echocardiography.[33, 34] Left atrial dimension progressively increases throughout pregnancy and returns to baseline levels postpartum.[35] The gravid uterus has mechanical circulatory effects as pregnancy progresses, and it can compress the iliac veins and inferior vena cavae with marked effects on venous return and hence cardiac volume and output.[32] Venous return can fluctuate widely with changing position of the mother, thus resulting in variations of cardiac size.

In pregnancy, the resultant myocardial stretch from increases in circulating volume may contribute to arrhythmogenesis. Mechanical stretch can induce alterations in electrophysiologic properties. Animal studies using monophasic action potential electrodes and isolated heart preparations have shown that mechanical stretch can shorten action potential duration and decrease the refractory period in the ventricle.[36–38] In addition, animal studies have shown that both acute and chronic stretch is associated with depolarization of the membrane and a reduction in amplitude of resting and action potential. These changes are accompanied by a slowing in conduction velocity.[39] In isolated rabbit hearts, rapid volume pulses of progressively increasing amplitude induced transient diastolic membrane depolarizations that, above a certain amplitude, were associated with a premature ventricular response. Thus, abrupt distension of the myocardium can elicit premature depolarizations and subsequent premature propagated excitations.[40] Furthermore, volume changes and stretch can cause electrophysiologic changes in atrial myocardium.[39] In humans, although mechanoelectrical feedback effects have clearly been observed, the characteristics of stretch-induced electrophysiologic alterations have not been consistently reported.

However, the electrophysiologic changes caused by stretch are probably clinically significant in humans. Clinical observations such as termination of ventricular tachycardia with Valsalva's maneuver, despite pretreatment with atropine or coughing, indirectly support the clinical significance of myocardial stretch.[41, 42] Waxman and coworkers[41] demonstrated that the Valsalva strain phase, passive upright tilting, and the expiratory phase of respiration shorten the cycle length of atrial flutter in humans; this effect was unaffected by combined adrenergic receptor and muscarinic receptor blockade. This clinical observation supports contraction excitation coupling in the atria in humans. The authors concluded that the effect on atrial flutter cycle length was independent of autonomic tone and was, instead, mediated by the decrease in cardiac volume induced by all three maneuvers.[43] The increase in circulating volume during pregnancy with resulting changes in cardiac dimension and the potential for rapid variation in cardiac volume (because of the effects of the uterus on venous return) may be mechanisms for exacerbating arrhythmias such as extrasystoles and supraventricular tachycardias in pregnant patients.

SPECIFIC ARRHYTHMIAS AND THE PREGNANT PATIENT

Symptoms traditionally referable to the cardiovascular system, such as decreased exercise capacity, fatigue, dyspnea, orthopnea, and presyncope, are common complaints during normal pregnancy and may be attributed to many factors.[44] Palpitations may be reported by pregnant patients, and the incidence of arrhythmias may be increased by pregnancy. However, investigation of patients who report palpitations frequently fails to document evidence of arrhythmia. Ostrzega and associates[45] reported on 104 pregnant women referred for symptoms of palpitations and dizziness who were followed with Holter monitoring during pregnancy and the postpartum period. They found that 24% of patients had frequent arrhythmias, mostly premature ventricular and atrial complexes, PSVT, and nonsustained ventricular tachycardia. In nine patients, the number of premature complexes were compared during pregnancy and the postpartum period; atrial and ventricular irritability were significantly increased during pregnancy (Table 29–1). Most arrhythmias were benign, and, although some patients had increased electrical irritability during pregnancy (manifested as extrasystoles), 76% of patients with palpitations had no detectable arrhythmias.

Table 29–1. COMPARISON OF PREMATURE COMPLEXES DURING PREGNANCY AND THE POSTPARTUM PERIOD IN NINE PATIENTS

	Pregnancy	Postpartum
Premature complexes (per hour)	459 ± 474	70 ± 133*
Premature complexes (per 24 hours)	9073 ± 9210	1345 ± 1997†

*$p = .04$, compared with premature complexes during pregnancy.
†$p = .03$, compared with premature complexes during pregnancy.
From Ostrzega, et al: Evidence for increased incidence of arrhythmias during pregnancy: A study of 104 pregnant women with symptoms of palpitations, dizziness, or syncope. J Am Coll Cardiol 19:125A, 1992. Reprinted with permission from the American College of Cardiology.

Supraventricular Tachyarrhythmias

Although extrasystoles are common even in healthy, nonpregnant women, PSVT is the most common sustained arrhythmia reported in pregnancy by patients with normal hearts. Most patients have a reentrant tachycardia or, more rarely, atrial tachycardia secondary to enhanced automaticity. Atrial flutter and fibrillation are very uncommon in the absence of structural heart disease.[46]

Paroxysmal Supraventricular Tachycardia Caused by Reentry

This term is used to describe a tachycardia that is caused either by reentry within the atrioventricular (AV) node (approximately two thirds of patients) or by use of an accessory pathway, either overt or concealed, the so-called Wolff-Parkinson-White syndrome (approximately one third of patients) (Fig. 29–1). The predominant mechanism for PSVT is reentry within the AV node, which in most cases allows antegrade conduction to the ventricle over a "slow" pathway and retrograde conduction over a "fast" pathway. Also called AV nodal reentrant tachycardia (AVNRT), this PSVT is characterized on electrocardiogram (ECG) by a regular tachycardia with a QRS of supraventricular origin, sudden onset and termination, and rates between 150 and 250 bpm. The onset usually follows a premature atrial complex. Unless functional aberrant ventricular conduction or a previous conduction defect exists, the QRS complex is normal in contour and duration. P waves are generally buried in the QRS complex. Narrow QRS complex tachycardia may also occur because of a macroreentrant circuit that uses the AV node–His bundle as the antegrade limb and an extranodal accessory pathway as the retrograde or return limb, the so-called Wolff-Parkinson-White syndrome. This tachyarrhythmia, also called AV reciprocating tachycardia (AVRT), is often difficult to differentiate from AVNRT because the rates are very similar, the arrhythmia is regular, and the QRS complex in AVRT is narrow. The retrograde P wave is often inscribed after completion of the QRS complex, rather than being obscured within the QRS as in AVNRT.[47] The ECG in sinus rhythm of patients with AVRT may have either a normal QRS complex (i.e., the pathway is concealed) or the delta wave of Wolff-Parkinson-White syndrome (i.e., the pathway is overt). Wolff-Parkinson-White syndrome is characterized on ECG by (1) a PR interval less than 120 msec in sinus rhythm, (2) the presence of a delta wave (a slurred, slowly rising onset of the QRS in some leads), and (3) duration of QRS complex greater than 120 msec. The most common sustained arrhythmia associated with Wolff-Parkinson-White syndrome is the narrow complex AVRT described earlier. However, the accessory pathway, when overt, may be capable of rapid anterograde conduction during atrial fibrillation and atrial flutter.

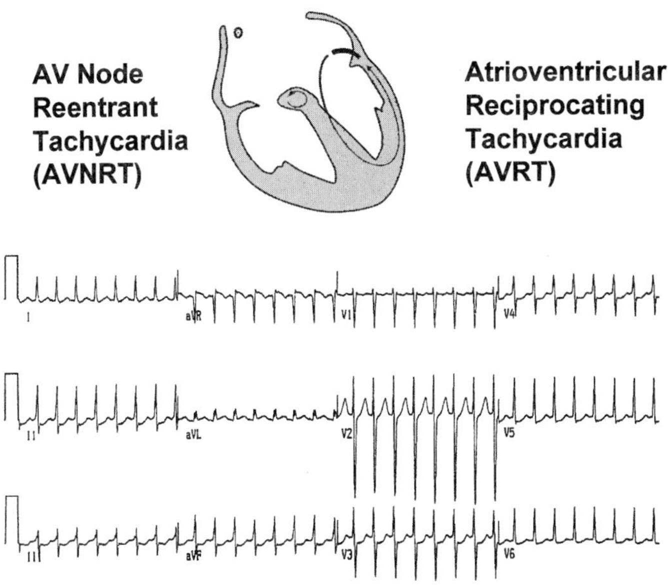

FIGURE 29–1. Typical electrocardiographic (ECG) findings in paroxysmal atrial tachycardia. This ECG appearance is most consistent with reentry over the atrioventricular node or an accessory pathway. (Adapted from Waugh RA, Wagner GS: Cardiac Arrhythmias: Practical Guide for the Clinician, 2nd ed. F.A. Davis, Philadelphia, 1994.)

The incidence of PSVT in pregnancy is unclear. The incidence of first onset of supraventricular tachyarrhythmia may be increased in pregnancy, and pregnancy can exacerbate symptoms in patients with pre-existing supraventricular tachyarrhythmias. In patients with pre-existing asymptomatic preexcitation and delta waves on the surface ECG, pregnancy increases the risk of onset of symptomatic tachyarrhythmias.[45, 48–50] However, most data have been derived from anecdotal reports and small case series,[46, 48–51] many of which do not contain electrophysiologic information to distinguish between mechanisms of narrow QRS complex tachycardia. More recently, the incidence of pregnancy-associated PSVT has been systematically assessed. Tawam and colleagues[52] retrospectively reviewed the presentation and course of PSVT and details of previous pregnancies of 60 women with PSVT who made hospital or emergency room visits over a 2-year period. Of the 60 women, 38 had previously been pregnant, 13 (34%) of whom had onset of PSVT during pregnancy. Using a person-year method of follow-up during the pregnant and nonpregnant period, the investigators reported that the relative risk of initial onset of PSVT during pregnancy was 5.1 (95% CI 2.8 to 9.2, $p < .001$). In an additional 11 patients (29%), pre-existing PSVT was exacerbated. The authors concluded that the initial onset of PSVT was more likely to occur during pregnancy and that pregnancy exacerbated the symptoms of pre-existing PSVT. In another series by Lee and associates,[53] 207 patients referred for electrophysiologic study and ablation of either AVNRT (n = 100) or accessory pathway physiology (n = 107) were evaluated. Only 8 (3.9%) of the 173 patients who had previously been pregnant recalled first onset of PSVT during pregnancy. Using a method similar to that of Tawam and colleagues,[52] Lee and associates reported that the relative risk of first onset of PSVT during pregnancy was 0.86 (95% CI 0.4 to 1.9, p = .35). However, 22% of patients who had PSVT during the nonpregnant state reported that PSVT attacks were exacerbated during pregnancy. In addition, patients were more symptomatic with episodes of PSVT that occurred during pregnancy than those in the nonpregnant state.

Thus, controversy exists as to whether the risk of the first episode of PSVT is increased during pregnancy. Both of the above-mentioned studies were retrospective and subject to recall bias. In the larger study by Lee and associates, patients were older and were referred for ablation (presumably more symptomatic). If patients were symptomatic with PSVT only at the time of pregnancy, it is unlikely they would be referred for ablation during pregnancy because of the exposure to fluoroscopy. The evidence does indicate that pregnancy exacerbates pre-existing PSVT or the symptoms associated with attacks. Exacerbations were previously thought to occur in the third trimester, which is the time of greatest hemodynamic burden[48, 49, 54]; however, more recent, larger studies show that periods of exacerbation are equally distributed throughout pregnancy.

Management—Acute Attack

The patient with an acute episode of PSVT usually presents to the emergency room with palpitations, which are often associated with dizziness, dyspnea, syncope, and chest pain. In patients without structural heart disease, episodes of tachycardia are generally well tolerated by both mother and fetus.[46, 48–51, 55–59] If hemodynamic compromise is evident, electrical cardioversion should be performed (see the section on cardioversion in pregnancy). Pharmacologic agents used to convert patients back to sinus rhythm include beta blockers, verapamil, and adenosine. For acute episodes of PSVT, vagal maneuvers such as carotid sinus massage should be attempted first. If they are unsuccessful, the drug of choice, especially in the second and third trimesters, is adenosine.

Adenosine is a purine-based nucleoside that depresses sinoatrial nodal automaticity, slows AV nodal conduction time, and terminates reciprocating and nodal reentrant tachycardia.[60] Multiple case reports confirm the effectiveness and safety of adenosine in pregnant patients.[61–65] Adenosine had little effect on fetal heart rate, and in one case, fetal heart rate recovered after deep variable decelerations had been noted during tachycardia.[64] Adenosine has a much shorter half-life (10 seconds) than esmolol (10 minutes) and verapamil (5.3 hours) and is preferred over both.[60, 66, 67] Animal studies have shown that placental exposure to adenosine is minimal because its half-life is shorter than the normal time required for blood circulation. In one study in guinea pigs, placental exposure to adenosine was controlled by uterine artery perfusion; only 12% of the perfused dose of adenosine was recovered from the fetal circulation, which suggests that only minimal amounts of adenosine cross the maternal-placental barrier.[68] In an in utero, chronically instrumented sheep model, adenosine (0.25 mg/kg/min) infused directly into the fetal carotid artery produced no significant effect on fetal blood gases or mean arterial pressure. However, a 30% increase in heart rate was observed after 1 hour of infusion.[69] In pregnant women, serum concentration of adenosine deaminase, the enzyme responsible for the nucleoside's rapid degradation, is approximately 75% of that in nonpregnant women.[70] The potential need for decreasing the dose of adenosine for PSVT in pregnancy may be attenuated by the normal increase in vascular volume during pregnancy.[71] Indeed, the reported experience has demonstrated that conventional doses of 6 mg and 12 mg are required for termination of the arrhythmia.[61–65]

In a retrospective survey of the use of adenosine in pregnant patients with an episode of PSVT, Elkayam and Goodwin[54] identified 38 episodes in 33 patients. Fetal bradycardia was noted in two patients after administration of multiple drugs, and fetal bradycardia persisted after successful termination of PSVT with adenosine in one patient. Therefore, fetal heart rate should be monitored during the acute treatment of maternal arrhythmias. Otherwise, no unfavorable acute effects on the fetus have been reported. Fetal outcomes were excellent; the live birth rate was 100%, and no evidence for fetal growth retardation was noted. However, premature births were seen in 20% of patients, although only one patient delivered earlier than the 34th gestational week. In four patients, concomitant conditions such as chronic hypertension, diabetes mellitus, and renal dysfunction may have contributed to premature birth. Congenital malformations were not seen in any newborns. Most of the patients in this study received adenosine during the second and third trimesters; the authors concluded that further study was necessary to determine the safety of adenosine use during the first trimester of pregnancy.

The reported experience with verapamil is more limited.[72–74] Although verapamil is useful in treating PSVT, adenosine is the preferred agent. The longer half-life of verapamil (5.3 hours) can cause significant hypotension, especially when it is given as a rapid intravenous bolus injection.[75] Furthermore, verapamil crosses the placenta in sufficient amounts that it is used to terminate susceptible supraventricular fetal arrhythmias.[76–78]

Management—Chronic/Suppressive

Patients with PSVT caused by reentry generally have structurally normal hearts and tolerate episodes of tachycardia well. No adverse fetal or maternal outcomes have been reported from otherwise healthy patients with paroxysmal tachycardia who may require occasional pharmacoconversion during the acute episodes. The decision to initiate chronic suppressive drug therapy must by weighed against the potential adverse side effects of beta blockers, calcium channel blockers, and class 1 agents (see section on drug therapy). Chronic drug therapy is *not* recommended unless the patient has intolerable symptoms or has frequent episodes of tachycardia.

Atrial Tachycardia

Atrial tachycardia, which is uncommon in both pregnant and nonpregnant women, is a regular tachycardia that has an atrial activation sequence that differs from that of normal sinus rhythm. Unlike PSVT, this arrhythmia does not require participation of the AV node in the reentrant circuit and can persist despite the induction of a high-grade AV block. This arrhythmia is characterized by atrial rates of between 100 to 240 bpm, a P wave morphology distinctly different from that in sinus rhythm, and persistence of the atrial tachycardia even with the induction of AV block. Differentiated from atrial flutter by the slower atrial rate,[79] this arrhythmia is usually seen in nonpregnant women who have structural heart disease. Haines and Dimarco[79] followed 19 patients with this arrhythmia long term; 17 patients (89%) had structural heart disease, 70% had left atrial enlargement, and 27% had severe left ventricular impairment and an ejection fraction less than 40%. In this series, the arrhythmia was difficult to treat; patients received an average of 2.5 ± 1.5 unsuccessful therapeutic trials with various drugs including digoxin, verapamil, beta blockers, and type 1a antiarrhythmic agents. Administration of adenosine to 14 patients and verapamil to 9 patients induced high-grade AV block, but the tachycardia was not eliminated in any patient. In 11 patients, amiodarone was required to suppress the arrhythmia. Long-term follow-up showed high mortality, probably caused by the degree of structural heart disease.

In pregnancy, this arrhythmia is rare. Although no electrophysiologic information is available from published reports,[55–57, 59, 80, 81] ECG has shown a clearly inscribed P wave in all patients, heart rates ranging from 135 to 215 bpm, and a diurnal variation in heart rate. This arrhythmia is often associated with organic heart disease in nonpregnant patients; however, in pregnant patients it usually occurs without structural heart disease[55–57, 59, 81] The arrhythmia may present between 15 and 38 weeks' gestation. As in nonpregnant patients, this arrhythmia in pregnant patients often persists and is refractory to treatment, including cardioversion.[55–57, 59, 81] Furthermore, the arrhythmia is unresponsive to vagal maneuvers, intravenous verapamil,[55–57] beta blockers,[55–57] digoxin,[55–57] adenosine,[57] disopyramide,[56] and procainamide.[57] Flecainide,[55–57] with and without beta blockers and amiodarone,[55] has successfully controlled the tachycardia rate. In all cases, delivery was successful with no adverse fetal sequelae, and the arrhythmia spontaneously terminated in the postpartum period. Favorable fetal and maternal outcomes have been reported despite continuous tachycardia at heart rates of 160 to 180 bpm from 15 weeks' gestation to delivery at 38 weeks' gestation. In all reported cases, the arrhythmia subsided and terminated shortly after delivery, which suggests that pregnancy may contribute to the initiation and maintenance of this tachyarrhythmia. Interestingly, in 70% of nonpregnant patients, left atrial enlargement has been associated with this arrhythmia.[79] Progressive enlargement of the left atrium, which occurs during pregnancy, may be a mechanism for sustaining this arrhythmia.

Management—Acute Attack

This specific arrhythmia in pregnancy is generally well tolerated by the mother and the fetus. Characteristically, the ventricular rate is slower than that observed in AVNRT or AVRT, and the atrial rate is slower than that observed in atrial flutter. However, because of sufficient overlap between the arrhythmias, diagnosis may be difficult to determine by surface ECG. With appropriate maternal and fetal monitoring, the administration of adenosine is safe in pregnancy and is useful as a therapeutic and diagnostic tool. If the tachycardia is dependent on the AV node as part of the reentrant circuit, then adenosine should terminate the arrhythmia and sinus rhythm should emerge for at least a brief period. If the tachycardia is not dependent on the AV node, then adenosine will block AV node conduction and allow analysis of the atrial activity. In atrial flutter, the hallmark sawtooth flutter waves at a rate of 250 to 350 bpm should emerge. In the case of atrial tachycardia, the atrial activity will again be organized but generally at slower rates (100 to 240 bpm) than those observed in atrial flutter. If an ECG in sinus rhythm is available, the sinus P wave morphology should be compared with the P wave in tachycardia to demonstrate that a clear difference exists and to confirm the diagnosis of atrial tachycardia. If an ECG in sinus rhythm is not available, the patient should be fully evaluated to ensure that the tachycardia is truly inappropriate and not sinus in origin in response to some stressor (e.g., labor, fever and infection, blood loss, marked anemia, or thyrotoxicosis).

When the diagnosis of atrial tachycardia is confirmed and if the patient is hemodynamically stable, experience suggests that emergent intervention, such as cardioversion, is not required and is not likely to be effective. Because this arrhythmia is difficult to treat, urgent cardioversion or administration of multiple intravenous AV nodal conduction blockers or antiarrhythmic agents is not recommended.

Management—Chronic/Suppressive

A cardiologist with a specific interest in electrophysiology should be consulted. Although pregnant women with atrial tachycardia usually have no evidence of structural heart disease, this arrhythmia is often associated with structural heart disease in the general population. Thus, a complete assessment including echocardiography is required. The decision to initiate chronic drug therapy depends on the patient's symptoms, the rate of the tachycardia, and whether the tachycardia is incessant. The hazards of pharmacologic therapy in pregnancy should be considered. Although conversion to sinus rhythm is ideal, the goal of therapy should be to achieve adequate rate control because the arrhythmia is often refractory to treatment. A trial of digoxin or beta blocker therapy is reasonable, but if the therapy is unsuccessful, amiodarone usually controls the rate of the tachycardia.[79] The risk of not treating an incessant tachycardia in asymptomatic patients is the development of a tachycardia-induced cardiomyopathy, which is reversible with control of the tachyarrhythmia.[82–84]

Atrial Flutter and Atrial Fibrillation

Atrial flutter is characterized by organized, fast atrial activity that has a sawtooth pattern on ECG. The atrial rate ranges from 250 to 350 bpm; however, conduction is usually 2:1 such that the ventricular rate is classically 150 bpm. Paroxysmal atrial flutter can occur in patients without structural heart disease, whereas chronic atrial flutter is usually associated with underlying heart disease such as rheumatic, ischemic, or dilated cardiomyopathy.[47] Atrial flutter, although rarely seen in pregnancy, has been associated with Graves' disease,[46] rheumatic heart disease,[85] and peripartum cardiomyopathy.[86] Of 482 pregnancies in 233 women with congenital heart disease who were followed prospectively, atrial flutter was identified in only two patients.[87] The pregnant patient with atrial flutter should be carefully evaluated with a history, physical examination, laboratory tests, and two-dimensional echocardiography to rule out endocrine abnormalities and structural heart disease.

Atrial fibrillation is an arrhythmia characterized by chaotic disorganized atrial activity with a depolarization rate of 350 to 600 bpm but without effective atrial contraction. Because of concealed conduction within the AV node, the ventricular rate is slower (usually 100 to 200 bpm) and irregular. Atrial fibrillation may be paroxysmal or chronic. Although the prevalence of atrial fibrillation is significant in the elderly population, chronic atrial fibrillation in women of childbearing age who do not have structural heart disease (so-called lone fibrillators) is rare. The arrhythmia is more common in patients with structural heart disease such as coronary artery disease, rheumatic heart disease, hypertensive heart disease, thyrotoxicosis, and congenital heart disease such as atrial septal defect.[47]

In most reports of atrial fibrillation in pregnancy, most patients had underlying rheumatic heart disease.[46, 88, 89] As the incidence of rheumatic heart disease declines, the number of pregnant patients with congenital heart disease has increased because more of these patients survive to childbearing age. Atrial fibrillation is common in these patients and can complicate atrial septal defects (both repaired and unrepaired) and Ebstein's anomaly. Furthermore, atrial fibrillation can be a postoperative complication of Mustard, Fontan, or Senning repairs.[90] Clinical presentation and hemodynamic consequences of atrial fibrillation depend on the ventricular rate and the underlying degree of heart disease. Patients with mitral stenosis are dependent on the length of diastole and the atrial systolic contribution for adequate left ventricular filling; these patients tolerate atrial fibrillation poorly in pregnancy with onset of dyspnea and pulmonary edema.[89]

Management

Atrial flutter or fibrillation during pregnancy in the absence of cardiac or systemic disease is rare, so all patients should be evaluated thoroughly with a history, physical examination, baseline biochemistry tests including thyroid function tests, and a two-dimensional echocardiogram to rule out hyperthyroidism, pulmonary pathology, unrecognized valvular or congenital heart disease, and cardiomyopathy. Initial treatment for both atrial flutter and fibrillation is dictated by the hemodynamic stability of the patient. If hemodynamic stability is threatened, continuous ECG monitoring, intravenous access, and oxygen and fetal monitoring are required; direct current cardioversion can be performed safely in pregnancy (see the section on cardioversion) with the appropriate support from an anesthetist. If the patient is hemodynamically stable, the general principles of treatment are similar to those of the nonpregnant patient with atrial fibrillation. Rate control can be accomplished with oral digoxin, beta blockers, or verapamil. If antiarrhythmic therapy is necessary to maintain sinus rhythm, group 1 agents and amiodarone are effective (see the section on pharmacotherapy). Anticoagulation should be considered, especially if patients have valvular pathology, cardiomegaly, or impaired ventricular function. Warfarin is contraindicated during the first trimester of pregnancy because it is teratogenic. In addition, warfarin is contraindicated within 2 weeks of delivery because it can produce a coagulopathy in the fetus, thereby creating the risk of severe bleeding during delivery. Although warfarin is fetopathic after the first trimester, the incidence of fetopathic effects in the second and third trimester is likely to be very low. The use of warfarin may be considered in high-risk situations if heparin cannot be used; however, if anticoagulants are indicated during pregnancy, heparin should be the first-line therapy. Long-term use of heparin can be complicated by osteopenia and osteoporosis; therefore, low-molecular-weight heparin, a fraction of heparin that does not produce the same side effects, may be used.[91]

Ventricular Tachycardia

Ventricular tachycardia arises distal to the bifurcation of the His bundle in the specialized conduction system, in ventricular muscle, or in combinations of both tissue types. A series of three or more bizarrely shaped premature ventricular complexes on ECG whose duration exceeds 120 msec suggests ventricular tachycardia. The R-R interval may be regular or it may vary, and the rate ranges from 70 to 250 bpm depending on the type of ventricular tachycardia. Ventricular tachycardia is arbitrarily defined as nonsustained when it stops spontaneously in less than 30 seconds; sustained ventricular tachycardia lasts more than 30 seconds or requires termination because of hemodynamic collapse. In most cases, atrioventricular dissociation occurs, although occasionally, retrograde conduction of ventricular impulses to the atria may be observed.[47]

All pregnant patients with ventricular tachyarrhythmias should be evaluated by a high-risk obstetric service in consultation with a cardiologist accustomed to managing patients with electrophysiologic problems. Ventricular tachycardia is rare in pregnancy. Patients can be categorized into two groups—those with underlying structural cardiac disease and those with primary electrical disease. In the general population, the most common cardiac abnormalities associated with ventricular arrhythmia are ischemic heart disease and cardiomyopathy. Because women of childbearing potential are younger, the associated cardiac lesions may differ from those seen in the general population. Ischemic heart disease presenting as myocardial infarction is rare[92] and can manifest as a catastrophic ventricular arrhythmia.[93, 94] Ventricular tachycardia may occur with peripartum cardiomyopathy,[86] congenital heart disease,[87, 95] mitral valve prolapse,[96, 97] valvular heart disease,[98, 99] myocardial fibrosis,[100] and both obstructive and nonobstructive hypertrophic cardiomyopathy.[101, 102] Metabolic conditions may predispose patients with otherwise normal hearts to ventricular arrhythmias. Hyperthyroidism[103] and hypomagnesemia[104] have been reported as systemic conditions associated with ventricular tachycardia in pregnancy.

Many case reports describe ventricular tachycardia in pregnant patients who have no evidence of underlying cardiac or systemic disease,[105–117] so-called idiopathic ventricular tachycardia, or primary electrical disease. Nonpregnant patients with ventricular tachycardia in the absence of structural cardiac disease have an excellent long-term prognosis, although there are reports of sudden death. Many patients with ventricular tachycardia in pregnancy have a form of catecholamine-sensitive ventricular tachycardia (Table 29–2). Brodsky and associates[118] published the largest series of patients presenting with symptomatic ventricular tachycardia that was first detected during pregnancy; seven patients had ventricular tachycardia, six of whom had normal ventricular function as determined by echocardiography. The relationship between adrenergic tone and arrhythmia was assessed by using the history, mean heart rate, and the effects of sleep and exercise on the arrhythmia. Their findings suggested a relationship between adrenergic tone and ventricular tachycardia in four patients. The arrhythmia was suppressed in five of six patients given large doses of beta blockers; the remaining patient required additional drug therapy. Maternal outcome was good, and no deaths were reported. In two of the mothers, ventricular arrhythmias continued after delivery. Fetal outcomes were good; no major abnormalities were noted despite high-dose beta blocker therapy. Other reports in the literature are isolated case reports or very small series of patients. However, most patients had primary electrical disease, and several of the patient histories suggested a possible role for catecholamine sensitivity. Fetal outcomes were very good. One sudden death was reported in a mother without associated cardiac disease.[110]

Management—Acute

Although symptoms of dyspnea, palpitations, presyncope, and syncope are reported, cardiac arrest is rare in patients without associated heart disease. Nevertheless, the initial presentation of ventricular tachycardia in pregnancy requires urgent evaluation. Patients should be immediately evaluated for hemodynamic stability, preferably in a setting in which cardiovascular collapse can be managed. Maternal and fetal monitoring is mandatory. Electrical cardioversion should be conducted immediately in cases of hemodynamic compromise. Agents that have been used successfully to terminate ventricular tachycardia include intravenous lidocaine, flecainide, quinidine, procainamide, and amiodarone. These drugs are usually administered at the same doses used in the nonpregnant patient.[119]

Table 29–2. FEATURES OF CATECHOLAMINE-SENSITIVE VENTRICULAR TACHYCARDIA

1. Normal coronary arteries
2. Normal or abnormal left ventricular contractility
3. Affects both sexes
4. Affects all ages
5. Usually responds to beta blocker therapy
6. May respond to some type 1 antiarrhythmic drugs
7. Usually not inducible by programmed electrical stimulation
8. Reproduced by exercise and by isoproterenol infusion
9. Usually relatively well tolerated by patients
10. Prognosis is usually benign but is determined by the underlying heart disease

From Vlay SC: Catecholamine-sensitive ventricular tachycardia. Am Heart J 114; 2:455, 1987.

Management—Chronic

Prompt assessment by a high-risk obstetric service and a cardiologist is advised. Patients should be fully evaluated with history, physical examination, and two-dimensional echocardiography to determine the presence or absence of structural heart disease (valvular disease, dilated cardiomyopathy, congenital heart disease, and hypertrophic cardiomyopathy) and systemic disease (electrolyte derangement or hyperthyroidism). Three conditions require special mention. (1) Idiopathic left ventricular tachycardia, or verapamil-sensitive ventricular tachycardia, has the morphology of right bundle branch block with a leftward axis and may respond to verapamil but not to beta blockers.[120] Usually found in patients with structurally normal hearts, this type of ventricular tachycardia has a benign prognosis and is amenable to catheter ablation. (2) Congenital long QT syndrome is a familial form of primary electrical disease characterized by a QT interval of more than 440 msec and is associated with the malignant ventricular arrhythmia known as torsades de pointes. Unlike many patients with other forms of primary electrical disease, these patients are at high risk for sudden death. Management of these patients is a therapeutic challenge during pregnancy[121]; ventricular arrhythmias may complicate the intrapartum course.[122, 123] Rashba and coworkers[124] reported on 111 women with congenital long QT syndrome who had one or more pregnancies. In a multivariate analysis, the postpartum interval was independently associated with cardiac events among these patients. Furthermore, treatment with beta-adrenergic blockers was independently associated with a decrease in the risk of cardiac events. These investigators concluded that treatment with beta blockers is indicated for these patients during pregnancy and should be continued during the postpartum interval. (3) Arrhythmogenic right ventricular dysplasia (ARVD), which may be difficult to distinguish from primary electrical disease, is an anatomic abnormality of the right ventricle characterized by fibrosis and fatty infiltration of the myocardium. ARVD can be difficult to diagnose with conventional cardiac imaging techniques.[125] Furthermore, it may be more difficult to treat than primary electrical disease and may have a worse prognosis.

Physicians should ascertain whether the patient had palpitations before pregnancy or a family history of arrhythmia or sudden death. In patients with no evidence of structural heart disease, the relationship between adrenergic tone and arrhythmia should be assessed. The setting in which the symptoms occur should be determined. Symptoms provoked by exertion or emotional upset suggest catecholamine-sensitive ventricular tachycardia; Holter monitoring with a detailed patient event record may be helpful. In addition, Holter monitoring may demonstrate sinus tachycardia and sleep suppression of arrhythmias.[118, 126] Ventricular tachycardia provoked by exercise testing may support a diagnosis of catecholamine-sensitive ventricular tachycardia and may predict response to therapy with beta blockers.[126–128]

Beta-adrenergic blockade can be used to suppress arrhythmias in patients who have evidence of catecholamine-sensitive ventricular tachycardia. Brodsky and associates[118] suggest titrating the dose to suppress symptoms and arrhythmias as determined by serial Holter monitoring or exercise testing. The authors reported that large doses of beta blockers were often required and generally well tolerated. Patients should be advised to avoid excessive exertion. Even in patients who have no structural heart disease and no evidence of increased adrenergic tone, beta-adrenergic blockade may be useful.[118, 129, 130] Therapy with beta blockers may be initiated in patients with structurally normal hearts during pregnancy even in the absence of a clear relationship to adrenergic tone. The decision to initiate chronic beta-blocker therapy depends on the patient's symptoms, a history of presyncope or syncope, and whether the arrhythmias are sustained. Because the prognosis is good for these patients, it is unclear if beta-adrenergic therapy influences the natural history.

In contrast, patients with structural heart disease who present with symptomatic sustained ventricular tachycardia have a worse prognosis, especially if ventricular dysfunction exists. The prognosis depends, in part, on the degree of functional and physiologic impairment. The risk of sudden death may be significant, and the benefits of therapy for the mother outweigh the risk of drug exposure to the fetus. Mexilitine, flecainide, procainamide, and quinidine have been reported as useful in pregnancy; however, their use was based on case series and isolated reports (see the section on antiarrhythmic therapy). Furthermore, these drugs have not improved survival in the nonpregnant population with structural heart disease, presumably because of proarrhythmic effects.[131, 132] Besides beta-adrenergic blockade, amiodarone is the only pharmacologic agent that may have some benefit in preventing sudden death.[133, 134] Despite the anecdotal evidence supporting the use of other antiarrhythmic agents, amiodarone should be used if antiarrhythmic therapy is required in pregnant patients with underlying structural heart disease and ventricular arrhythmias. Amiodarone has significant side effects for the mother and the fetus that should be discussed with the patient. In patients with a long-standing history of sustained ventricular arrhythmias before pregnancy, an alternative to drug therapy is the automatic implantable defibrillator,[135] which can be implanted before pregnancy. Reports suggest that the use of implantable defibrillators and shock discharge during pregnancy is safe.[136, 137] Echocardiographically guided electrophysiologic tests have been conducted in pregnant women to study the conduction system and the inducibility of malignant ventricular arrhythmias,[138] but the use of echocardiographically guided catheter ablation in pregnant women has not been reported.

Bradyarrhythmias

Symptomatic bradyarrhythmias in pregnancy are uncommon.[46] Sinus bradycardia is common in healthy young adults, in athletes, and during sleep[47]; however, during normal pregnancy, the heart rate gradually increases to achieve a peak rate of 10 to 20 bpm above baseline.[139] Significant conduction abnormalities are also uncommon.

First-Degree Atrioventricular Block

The normal PR interval, which represents the time for an impulse to travel from the sinus node to the ventricle, is 0.12 to 0.20 seconds. In first-degree AV block, the PR interval is prolonged beyond 0.20 seconds. First-degree AV block, which does not require treatment, may be observed in otherwise healthy individuals or may occur secondary to increased vagal tone, drug administration, ischemia, or rheumatic heart disease.

Second-Degree Atrioventricular Block

Second-degree AV block is diagnosed when atrial impulses intermittently fail to conduct to the ventricles. Two types of second degree AV block are seen: Mobitz type 1 (Wenkebach) and Mobitz type 2. Type 1 second-degree AV block is typically characterized on ECG by progressive PR prolongation that culminates in a nonconducted P wave. In type 2 second-degree block, the PR interval remains constant before the blocked P wave.[47] Mobitz type 1 AV block, which is generally benign, usually represents proximal block at the AV node. Type 1 AV block may occur in healthy individuals who have increased vagal tone, an excess of digitalis, congenital lupus, and other conditions. Mobitz type 2 AV block, often more serious, may precede a Stokes-Adams attack and complete heart block.[47] This type of block usually represents infra-Hisian conduction block and is associated with organic disease such as rheumatic heart disease, ischemia, or infarction. A permanent pacemaker is often required for treatment. During pregnancy, the incidence of type 2 second-degree heart block, which is usually acquired and associated with structural heart disease, is rare.

Third-Degree Atrioventricular Block

Complete AV block occurs when atrial activity is not conducted to the ventricles and a junctional or ventricular escape rhythm prevails. The ventricular rate in acquired complete heart block is less than 40 bpm but may be faster in congenital complete heart block. In adults, drug toxicity, coronary disease, and degenerative processes are the most common causes of complete heart block.[47] However, in otherwise healthy women of childbearing age, the cause of complete heart block is usually congenital. Congenital complete heart block results from an anatomic disruption between the atrial musculature and the AV node or bundle of His. Although complete AV block usually occurs in isolation, it may be associated with congenital heart disease such as ventricular septal defect and congenitally corrected transposition of the great vessels.

Unlike tachyarrhythmias, pregnancy has no effect on the incidence or severity of heart block. In fact, the course of heart block, which is usually established before pregnancy, is independent of pregnancy. In previous reviews of cardiac rhythm disorders in pregnancy, pre-existing acquired heart block was always associated with organic heart disease, most commonly rheumatic disease. The outcome of pregnancy in these patients related directly to the severity of the underlying heart disease. Congenital complete heart block usually has a favorable prognosis in adults, although sudden death can occur.[140–143] Patients with symptomatic congenital complete heart block, a prolonged QT interval, or a wide QRS complex on the surface ECG usually have received a pacemaker; whether asymptomatic patients should have pacemakers to prevent sudden death is under debate. In a series of 102 patients with congenital complete heart block who were prospectively followed,[143] 24 women without a pacemaker gave birth to 45 children. Of the 24 women, three had syncope during pregnancy, and a pacemaker was implanted in two. Eight women who had received a pacemaker before pregnancy had 14 uneventful pregnancies. Despite the recommendation of some investigators that all patients with congenital complete heart block have either temporary or permanent pacemaker support during labor,[144] pregnancy can be uneventfully completed without a pacemaker in asymptomatic patients in whom congenital complete heart block was diagnosed during pregnancy.[145, 146] Patients who develop symptoms of syncope or presyncope during pregnancy can safely undergo pacemaker implantation in late pregnancy (see later).

Pacemaker Therapy

Most patients with symptomatic complete heart block have received a pacemaker before pregnancy. Since 1964 when the first report of a patient who underwent a normal pregnancy and delivery with an artificial pacemaker was published,[147] the technology and ease of insertion has improved. Several reports have now been published of women who became pregnant with a permanent pacemaker in place. Pregnancy is uncomplicated in most cases.[148] Although complications during pregnancy are rare, pain or ulceration at the insertion site, usually caused by the increase in breast size and stretching of the skin over a supramammary insertion site, has been reported. An abdominal site of insertion should be avoided for similar reasons. A subpectoral site has been suggested for implantation of permanent pacemakers in women of childbearing age.[148] The smaller-sized, lower-profile, newer pulse generators may present less of a problem in this setting. In those patients in whom asymptomatic bradycardia or congenital complete heart block was not detected or was not treated before conception, pregnancy is generally well tolerated.[46, 143, 149] Implanting a permanent pacemaker early during the course of pregnancy is not necessary; therefore, the fetus is spared the accompanying radiologic exposure during the period of organogenesis. If it is necessary during the first trimester, insertion of the pacemaker can be performed under ECG and echocardiographic control[150, 151]; if fluoroscopic guidance is required, the teratogenic effects of radiation may necessitate medical termination of the pregnancy.[144] In patients with heart block, labor may be complicated by syncope, which is caused by slowing of the heart rate during Valsalva maneuvers performed at the time of the forceful contractions of the final stage of labor. Transvenous and external pacemakers have been used successfully in this situation.[144, 152–155]

Cardiac Arrest in Pregnancy

Cardiac arrest is defined as an abrupt cessation of cardiac pump function that may be reversed by prompt intervention but will inevitably lead to death without intervention.[156] Cardiac arrest in pregnancy, although rare, is devastating

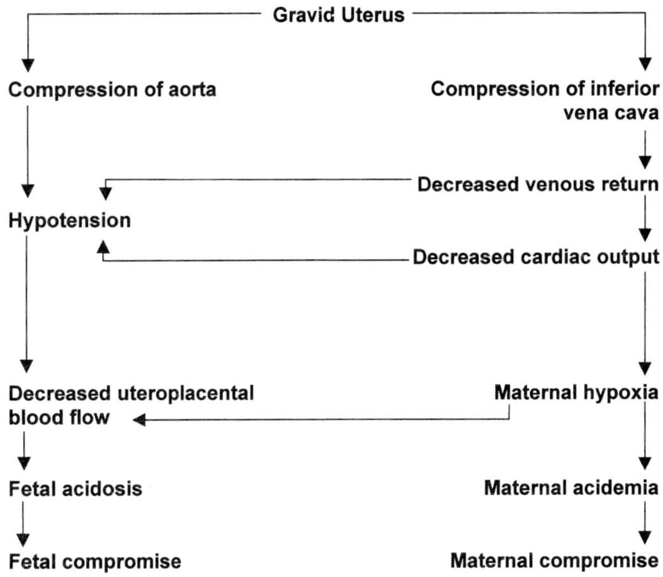

FIGURE 29–2. Pathophysiology of cardiopulmonary arrest during pregnancy. (Adapted from Lee RV, Rodgers BD, White LM, Harvey RC: Cardiopulmonary resuscitation of pregnant women. Am J Med 81:311, 1986. Copyright 1986 by Excerpta Medica, Inc.)

(Fig. 29–2); the survival of both the mother and the fetus depends on timely intervention. Over the past 100 years, the causes of maternal death have changed and the number of women who die during childbirth has decreased dramatically. In the past, a significant proportion of maternal deaths resulted from infection and obstetric causes, whereas now most maternal deaths result from acute catastrophic events such as pulmonary embolism, complications of anesthesia, and cerebrovascular accidents.[157, 158] Some causes of cardiopulmonary arrest are listed in Table 29–3.

Cardiopulmonary Resuscitation in Pregnancy

The alterations of physiology in pregnant women and the presence of the fetus significantly affect some principles of

Table 29–3. CAUSES OF CARDIOPULMONARY ARREST DURING PREGNANCY

Pulmonary and amniotic fluid embolus
Trauma
Hemorrhage and hypovolemia
Preexisting heart disease
Congenital heart disease
Acquired valvular disease
Arrhythmia
Idiopathic
Drug-induced
Myocardial infarction
Pregnancy-associated cardiomyopathy
Pregnancy-induced hypertension
Cerebrovascular accident
Angioedema of larynx/anaphylaxis
Asthma
Aspiration pneumonia
Septicemia
Iatrogenic
Complications of anesthesia
Complications of tocolytic treatment
Cardiac tamponade from central venous instrumentation

cardiopulmonary resuscitation (CPR). As discussed, maternal blood volume and cardiac output increase, peripheral vascular resistance falls, and the proportion of cardiac output that flows to the uterus increases from less than 2% in the nonpregnant state to 20% to 30% in pregnancy. By the second trimester, the perfusion of the uteroplacental vascular bed, which is maximally dilated, is passive and is determined by the perfusion pressure rather than by any component of autoregulation. The compression of the enlarging uterus on the inferior vena cava and the abdominal aorta can cause hypotension and can decrease cardiac output by as much as 25%.[159, 160] Respiratory changes include an increase in minute ventilation, an increase in oxygen consumption to meet the demands of the growing uteroplacental-fetal unit, and a decrease in functional residual capacity secondary to the upward displacement of the diaphragm by the gravid uterus. Thus, pregnant women have less reserve and are predisposed to more rapid decreases in arterial and venous oxygen tension during periods of hypoxia than are nonpregnant women.[161] In animal studies, maternal hypoxia reduces uteroplacental perfusion.[162] Fetal hemoglobin binds oxygen more avidly than does adult hemoglobin, and the fetal oxygen dissociation curve is shifted to the left of the maternal oxygen dissociation curve. Thus, fetal oxygen saturation is normally in the steep middle portion of the dissociation curve, and small changes in fetal PO_2 significantly change oxygen saturation. In addition, pregnant women are predisposed to aspirate gastric contents because of a decrease in gastrointestinal motility and esophageal sphincter tone.[163]

During cardiac arrest, aggressive airway control with early intubation is recommended to optimize oxygenation and to prevent aspiration. Standard closed chest compressions should be performed; however, this procedure should be modified to minimize the effects of the gravid uterus on venous return and cardiac output. A wedge such as a pillow, or a preformed wedge such as the Cardiff wedge, should be placed under the right abdominal flank and hip to displace the uterus to the left side of the abdomen. Alternatively, continuous manual displacement of the uterus off the midline can be attempted.[164, 165] Otherwise, standard defibrillation and pharmacologic therapy should be used without modification in pregnant patients with cardiac arrest.[164]

If the fetus is near term, a perimortem cesarean section must be considered. Prolonged attempts at resuscitation using closed chest compressions are difficult because of the mechanical constraints on venous return and cardiac output imposed by the gravid uterus and the awkward modifications required to relieve this compression. The uteroplacental-fetal unit depends on perfusion pressure within the vascular bed of the placenta; however, therapeutic doses of vasopressors may produce uteroplacental vasoconstriction.[162] For these reasons, perimortem cesarean section may maximize the chances of both maternal and infant survival[157, 162, 163, 166–169] Delivery of the fetus may alleviate the effects of aortocaval compression and allow recovery of venous return to the heart. Case reports have documented successful maternal resuscitation and response to CPR by emergent cesarean section.[169, 170] Marx[168] reported on five women who had cardiac arrest after inadvertent intravascular bupivacaine injection during attempted extradural block. All five patients required closed chest compression; cesarean section was performed immediately in three women with good neurologic outcomes. Cesarean section was delayed by several minutes in the other two patients, both of whom had irreversible neurologic injury. For the fetus, expedient delivery is vital. In a review of the literature by Katz and coworkers,[157] most fetal survivors were delivered within 5 minutes of maternal cardiac arrest. Cases of surviving healthy infants delivered more than 10 minutes after cardiopulmonary arrest were rare. In one case report, postmortem cesarean section performed 22 minutes after documented maternal cardiopulmonary arrest and 47 minutes after the fatal injury resulted in the birth of a clinically normal child when assessed at 18 months of age.[167]

In summary, in late pregnancy, an immediate perimortem cesarean section should be considered if initial attempts at CPR, leftward displacement of the gravid uterus, fluid volume restoration, and standard application of the advanced cardiac life support (ACLS) algorithms have failed to restore effective circulation. A perimortem cesarean section should be performed within 4 to 5 minutes of the arrest.[164]

Antiarrhythmic Drugs in Pregnancy

Adenosine

Adenosine is the agent of choice for the acute termination of PSVT (see section on acute treatment of PSVT).

Digoxin

Digoxin, the most widely used cardiac glycoside, has been used in pregnancy for a variety of indications. It is used for supraventricular arrhythmias, including tachycardias in which part of the reentrant circuit requires the AV node, and for rate control of atrial fibrillation and atrial flutter. Digoxin crosses the placenta easily and quickly[171–174] and appears in human breast milk.[171, 175] Although digoxin use in pregnancy has been associated with premature labor or low birth weight,[176] most antenatal studies have shown that therapeutic doses of digoxin do not adversely affect the fetus; no reports of teratogenicity have been published.[44, 119, 177] Two reports of adverse fetal outcome were associated with digoxin overdose in the mother.[178, 179] Thus, digoxin is considered safe for pregnant and lactating women. Serum concentrations of digoxin in pregnant women are lower than those in nonpregnant women, possibly because of increased renal elimination during pregnancy.[172] The dose of digoxin is the same for pregnant and nonpregnant women.[119, 177] Although digoxin concentrations during gestation may be below the standard therapeutic range, the dosage should be increased only if the desired therapeutic effect has not been obtained; the dosage should be reduced again after delivery.

Beta-Adrenergic Antagonists

Beta blockers have been used extensively in pregnancy for various conditions including pregnancy-associated hypertension,[180–182] hypertrophic cardiomyopathy,[183] and hyperthyroidism.[184, 185] Beta blockers are useful for PSVT, rate control in atrial fibrillation and flutter, as well as ventricular tachycardia, especially in the setting of catecholamine sensitivity and absence of structural heart disease. They cross the placenta easily,[119] and they increase myometrial activity, although beta blockers have not clearly been implicated in premature labor.[186] Despite reports of fetal bradycardia, birth apnea, hypoglycemia, polycythemia, hyperbilirubinemia, intrauterine growth retardation, and prolonged labor, beta blockers are widely used in pregnancy.[119, 177] No fetal malformations have been attributed to beta blockers. Although it is the most widely used beta blocker in pregnancy, propranolol has been associated with adverse reactions such as decreased fetal tone, hypoglycemia, and low birth weight.[119] Theoretically, a selective beta-1 antagonist such as metoprolol should not affect extracardiac tissues such as the uterus; thus, metoprolol is preferred over propranolol. Data from prospective trials have shown that metoprolol is safe in pregnancy, and it is the preferred beta blocker for use in pregnancy. Full doses of up to 400 mg per day have been administered without evidence of teratogenic or other adverse effects on the fetus.[187, 188] In a series of patients with ventricular tachycardia, large doses of metoprolol had no adverse effects.[118] Metoprolol is excreted in breast milk in concentrations that are higher than concentrations in maternal plasma.[189, 190] However, given the amount of breast milk consumed, the daily infant dose is very small and the resultant concentration of drug in the infant's serum is negligible.[191, 192] Atenolol has also been used in pregnancy with favorable results[193–195]; however, atenolol has been associated with low birth weights.[196] Experience with other beta blockers, including the short-acting intravenous agent esmolol, is limited. Esmolol has been used in one pregnant patient to manage maternal thyrotoxicosis; fetal and maternal outcomes were good.[197]

Calcium Channel Blockers

These agents block the slow calcium channel. For arrhythmias in the nonpregnant population, verapamil and diltiazem are useful for prophylaxis against PSVT and for controlling the ventricular rate in atrial fibrillation and atrial flutter.

Verapamil

In a limited number of case reports, intravenous verapamil has been used successfully to manage acute attacks of PSVT; however, because of the hypotension associated with bolus intravenous injection, adenosine is preferred in this setting. Oral verapamil crosses the placenta and is excreted in breast milk. Oral verapamil has been used for hypertension in pregnancy and for preventing premature labor, with few adverse effects. However, maternal or fetal bradycardia, heart block, depression of contractility, and hypotension have been observed when verapamil has been used to treat fetal supraventricular tachycardia. Although verapamil can be used in pregnancy, caution is advised. Little information is available regarding the use of diltiazem in pregnancy.[119]

Class 1a Antiarrhythmic Agents

There has been much historical experience with this class of agents in pregnancy. However, recent studies of the use of some class 1 agents in the nonpregnant population[131] have shown an increase in mortality and have raised concerns about the safety and proarrhythmic effects of these drugs.

Quinidine

Quinidine has been used effectively to suppress atrial premature beats, ventricular premature beats, atrial fibrillation and flutter, tachyarrhythmias associated with Wolff-Parkinson-White syndrome, and malignant ventricular arrhythmias.[198] Quinidine, which has been used for over half a century in pregnant patients,[105, 199] is largely protein bound and metabolized by the liver.[200] Because of changes in plasma protein concentrations during pregnancy, total plasma quinidine concentrations may fall, and the circulating level of free drug may be underestimated.[177] Quinidine crosses the placenta readily and is used to treat fetal arrhythmias.[77, 201] The concentration of quinidine excreted in breast milk is lower than that found in maternal serum.[202] Although most reports of quinidine use in pregnancy are case reports, no teratogenic effects or adverse fetal outcomes have been documented, even when large doses have been used throughout pregnancy.[46, 119, 177, 202, 203] Rarely, quinidine may cause minimal uterine contractions but usually not until spontaneous uterine contractions have begun.[199] Premature labor may be precipitated at therapeutic doses, and spontaneous abortion has been reported with toxic doses of the related drug quinine.[204] Because of its safety record in pregnancy, quinidine previously has been recommended as the drug of choice to control supraventricular arrhythmias such as atrial fibrillation.[205] However, quinidine does have adverse cardiovascular effects, including prolongation of the QT interval, and it may cause potentially lethal ventricular arrhythmias (e.g., torsades de pointes). The results of a recent meta-analysis suggest that nonpregnant patients on chronic therapy with quinidine may be at greater risk of sudden cardiac death.[206] Although it has been an acceptable antiarrhythmic medication in pregnancy, quinidine should not be used in patients with underlying structural heart disease and in patients predisposed to electrolyte imbalances (e.g., hyperemesis). If quinidine is used in these patients, serial determinations of the QT interval and of electrolyte and quinidine levels are advised. If quinidine is used with warfarin (Coumadin) or digoxin, the dose may need to be adjusted because of drug interactions.

Procainamide

Procainamide, which can be used for the same indications as quinidine, is often used to terminate ventricular arrhythmias.[207, 208] Procainamide crosses the placenta and has been used to treat fetal arrhythmias.[209, 210] Although it is excreted in breast milk, the daily dose of procainamide for the nursing infant is negligible.[211] No adverse fetal and maternal effects have been noted; however, the evidence is anecdotal.[212] The intravenous form is used for conversion of ventricular arrhythmias and tachyarrhythmias associated with Wolff-Parkinson-White syndrome. The long-term use of procainamide in pregnancy is not recommended because of its relatively slow elimination rate and the development of antinuclear antibodies and a lupus-like syndrome.[119, 137, 177]

Disopyramide

Effective for the same indications as quinidine or procainamide, disopyramide also has marked negatively inotropic effects, which make it useful in hypertrophic obstructive cardiomyopathy. The experience with disopyramide in pregnancy is limited. Disopyramide crosses the placenta and is secreted in breast milk.[213, 214] Results of case reports are conflicting. In one report, pregnancy was uneventful despite disopyramide use throughout the third trimester.[213] In another case report, the induction of uterine contractions coincided with disopyramide dosing.[215] In a placebo-controlled trial of labor induction in pregnant women, disopyramide induced uterine contractions when compared with placebo.[216] The authors suggested that disopyramide may be used to induce labor. Because of the limited experience with disopyramide in pregnancy and the potential for uterine contractions, we do not recommend disopyramide as a first-line agent for treating arrhythmias in pregnant women.

Class 1b Antiarrhythmic Agents

Lidocaine

Lidocaine, the most widely used type 1b agent, is used to treat ventricular tachycardia or fibrillation. Much of the experience with lidocaine in pregnancy has been gained through its use as a local anesthetic. Lidocaine can cross the placenta after both epidural and intravenous administration to the mother.[217–219] Lidocaine has been thought to be safe in pregnancy, with no evidence of teratogenic effects.[137, 220] However, fetal bradycardia can be precipitated,[221, 222] and elevated plasma levels of lidocaine may cause a low Apgar score initially, although the effect is transient.[223] Neonatal lidocaine toxicity has been reported after local administration of lidocaine for episiotomy.[224, 225] When lidocaine is administered in the presence of fetal acidosis, toxicity of both the central nervous system and the cardiac system may occur in the fetus and newborn.[226, 227] Lidocaine is usually used as an antiarrhythmic in patients with serious ventricular arrhythmias. The smallest effective doses should be used.[119, 177]

Mexiletine

The experience with mexiletine in pregnancy is too limited to recommend it as a first-line antiarrhythmic agent in pregnancy.[96, 228–230] In all cases, pregnancy and delivery were uncomplicated. One neonate was small for gestational age,[96] and transient bradycardia was reported in one newborn.[228]

Class 1c Antiarrhythmic Agents

These agents have been used to treat both ventricular and supraventricular arrhythmias. Since the publication of the CAST trial,[131] in which mortality was increased in patients treated with flecainide for suppression of ventricular arrhythmias after myocardial infarction, these agents have not been recommended for ventricular arrhythmias. However, both flecainide and propafenone are used for supraventricular tachycardias such as atrial fibrillation, especially in patients with no evidence of structural heart disease.

Flecainide

The experience with flecainide in pregnancy is anecdotal. Flecainide readily crosses the placenta and is excreted in breast milk.[231, 232] No adverse or teratogenic effects have been reported when flecainide has been used to treat fetal, infant, and childhood arrhythmias.[231, 233–235] Successful maternal administration of flecainide has also been reported. Flecainide, which is safe in the third trimester of pregnancy,[55–57, 231, 232] has been used to treat refractory incessant atrial tachycardia in pregnant women.[55–57]

Propafenone

The use of propafenone in pregnancy from 19 and 25 weeks to delivery has been presented in two case reports.[99, 236] Although both fetal and maternal outcomes were good, the information is insufficient to recommend the use of propafenone as a first-line agent for arrhythmias in pregnancy.

Class 3 Antiarrhythmic Agents

The most widely used type 3 antiarrhythmic agents are amiodarone and sotalol. These potent antiarrhythmic agents are useful for treating supraventricular and ventricular tachyarrhythmias.

Amiodarone

The use of amiodarone has increased, especially since the proarrhythmic effects of type 1 antiarrhythmics have become evident. Once used only for refractory ventricular arrhythmias, amiodarone has gained acceptance for treating both supraventricular and ventricular tachyarrhythmias. Because of its prolonged half-life of up to 40 days with long-term therapy and its side effects of hepatic inflammation, hyperthyroidism and hypothyroidism, and pulmonary fibrosis,[237] amiodarone was not initially used in pregnancy. However, its use in pregnancy has been unavoidable in some circumstances and inadvertent in other cases. The transplacental passage of amiodarone and its active metabolite is limited[238, 239]; however, the drug contains high amounts of iodine (75 mg per 200-g dose).[237] Iodine, which rapidly crosses the placenta and concentrates in the fetal thyroid as early as 14 weeks, is associated with neonatal goiter. Amiodarone is excreted in the breast milk at concentrations high enough to expose the nursing infant to therapeutic doses.[240–242] Amiodarone has been used during pregnancy, even during the first trimester, with no adverse outcomes.[100, 240–245] However, bradycardia,[240, 246] transient prolongation of the QT interval,[241, 245] hypothyroidism,[246–249] low birth weight,[241, 246, 249–251] premature birth,[246, 248, 251, 252] and one infant death have been reported.[253] In two larger compiled series of patients, the incidence of hypothyroidism was 9%, and 21% and 35% of babies in the two studies, respectively, had low birth weight for gestational age.[246, 254] One infant exposed to amiodarone from the time of conception had a large ventricular septal defect; another had congenital jerk nystagmus and synchronous head titubation. One infant exposed to amiodarone from 20 weeks' gestation had hypotonia, hypertelorism, and micrognathia and was developmentally delayed.[246] Magee and coworkers[255] studied the neurodevelopment of children exposed to amiodarone in utero. Although social and cognitive development was generally acceptable, some difficulties with language and arithmetic skills were detected. Therefore, amiodarone should be used in pregnancy only for potentially life-threatening ventricular arrhythmias. Patients should be followed closely, and maternal and neonatal thyroid function should be monitored. Breast feeding is discouraged because of significant amiodarone exposure to the infant.

Sotalol

Sotalol has class 3 antiarrhythmic properties and is a noncardioselective beta blocker. Sotalol readily crosses the human placenta[256, 257] and is excreted into breast milk.[257, 258] The experience with sotalol comes largely from its use as an antihypertensive agent, although it has been used safely to treat arrhythmias in pregnancy.[232] No adverse maternal or fetal consequences were observed in 12 pregnant patients who received large doses of sotalol.[256] The experience with sotalol in pregnancy is limited, and caution must be advised despite the favorable outcomes reported so far.

Electrical Cardioversion

Electrical cardioversion may become necessary in pregnant patients with cardiac arrhythmias. Experience shows that cardioversion is safe in all stages of pregnancy, even at high energy.[58, 59, 81, 93, 106, 112, 259–263] A theoretical risk of inducing fetal arrhythmia exists, but it is remote because the energy that reaches the fetal heart is small. Furthermore, young mammalian hearts have a high fibrillatory threshold. Nevertheless, cardioversion should be reserved for emergent situations, and the fetal heart rate should be monitored.

Implantable Cardioverter-Defibrillators

The clinical use of implantable cardioverter-defibrillators (ICDs) increased significantly in the 1990s. Several clinical trials have demonstrated improved survival with these devices compared with antiarrhythmic therapy in nonpregnant patients who have survived malignant ventricular arrhythmias or who are at high risk of such arrhythmias.[264–266] The prevalence of women of childbearing age with ICDs will also increase as these devices allow survival into the reproductive years. Natale and coworkers[267] performed a retrospective multicenter analysis of 44 women who had ICDs and became pregnant. Although device discharge was documented in 11 patients, maternal and fetal outcome was good. Pregnancy did not appear to increase the risk of major ICD-related complications, nor did labor or delivery precipitate any inappropriate shocks. The authors concluded that the presence of an ICD should not deter women from becoming pregnant if no other cardiac contraindications to pregnancy exist. Implantation of an ICD before a woman becomes pregnant is a therapeutic consideration for those contemplating pregnancy and who have a history of ventricular arrhythmia. Avoidance of pharmacologic therapy is an obvious advantage for fetal development; however, device therapy does not always preclude the need for antiarrhythmic drugs.[267]

References

1. Kadish AH: The effects of gender on cardiac electrophysiology and arrhythmias. In Zipes DP and Jalife J (eds): Cardiac Electrophysiology: From Cell to Bedside. W.B. Saunders, Philadelphia, 1994, p 1268.
2. Rosano GMC, Leonardo F, Sarrel PM: Cyclical variation in paroxysmal supraventricular tachycardia. Lancet 347:786, 1996.
3. Drici MD, Burklow TR, Haridasse V, et al: Sex hormones prolong the QT interval and downregulate potassium channel expression in the rabbit heart. Circulation 94:1471, 1996.
4. Nakajima T, Iwasawa K, Oonuma H, et al: Antiarrhythmic effect and its underlying ionic mechanism of 17beta-estradiol in cardiac myocytes. Br J Pharmacol 127:429, 1999.
5. Pragnell M, Snay KJ, Trimmer JS, et al: Estrogen induction of a small, putative K^+ channel mRNA in rat uterus. Neuron 4:807, 1990.
6. Boyle MB, MacLusky NJ, Naftolin F, Kaczmarek LK: Hormonal regulation of K^+-channel messenger RNA in rat myometrium during oestrus cycle and in pregnancy. Nature 330:373, 1987.
7. Harder DR, Coulson PB: Estrogen receptor and effects of estrogen on membrane electrical properties of coronary vascular smooth muscle. J Cell Physiol 100:375, 1979.
8. Ekstrom J, Iosif CS, Malmberg L: Effects of long-term treatment with estrogen and progesterone on in vitro muscle responses of the female rabbit urinary bladder and urethra to autonomic drugs and nerve stimulation. J Urol 150:1284, 1993.
9. Batra S, Andersson KE: Oestrogen-induced changes in muscarinic receptor density and contractile responses in the female rabbit urinary bladder. Acta Physiol Scand 137:135, 1989.
10. Levin RM, Shofer FS, Wein AJ: Estrogen-induced alterations in the autonomic responses of the rabbit urinary bladder. J Pharmacol Exp Ther 215:614, 1980.
11. Batra S, Owman C, Rydstrom H, Sjoberg NO: Modulation by continuous oestrogen treatment and by progesterone of oestrogen receptors in the rabbit uterus. J Endocrinol 115:199, 1987.
12. Larsson B, Andersson KE, Batra S, et al: Effects of estradiol on norepinephrine-induced contraction, alpha adrenoceptor number and norepinephrine content in the female rabbit urethra. J Pharmacol Exp Ther 229:557, 1984.
13. Du XJ, Riemersma RA, Dart AM: Cardiovascular protection by oestrogen is partly mediated through modulation of autonomic nervous function. Cardiovasc Res 30:161, 1995.
14. Dahlberg ST: Gender difference in the risk factors for sudden cardiac death. Cardiology 77 (suppl 2):31, 1990.
15. Kannel WB, Schatzkin A: Sudden death: Lessons from subsets in population studies. J Am Coll Cardiol 5(Suppl 6):141B, 1985.
16. Romo M, Salomaa V: FINMONICA Study Group, Coronary heart disease deaths outside hospital, abstracted. Eur Heart J 11:172, 1990.
17. Gillum RF: Sudden cardiac death in the United States: 1980–1985. Circulation 79:756, 1989.
18. Freedman RA, Swerdlow CD, Soderholm-Difatte V, Mason JW: Clinical predictors of arrhythmia inducibility in survivors of cardiac arrest: Importance of gender and prior myocardial infarction. J Am Coll Cardiol 12:973, 1988.
19. Vaitkus PT, Kindwall KE, Miller JM, et al: Influence of gender on inducibility of ventricular arrhythmias in survivors of cardiac arrest with coronary artery disease. Am J Cardiol 67:537, 1991.
20. Ekholm EMK, Piha SJ, Antila KJ, Erkkola RU: Cardiovascular autonomic reflexes in mid pregnancy. Br J Obstet Gynaecol 100:177, 1993.

21. Cohen WR, Galen LH, Vega-Rich M, Young JB: Cardiac sympathetic activity during rat pregnancy. Metabolism 37:771, 1988.
22. Slutsker L: Risks associated with cocaine use during pregnancy (review). Obstet Gynecol 79:778, 1992.
23. Bayorh MA, Zukowska-Grojec Z, Kopin IJ: Effect of desipramine and cocaine on plasma norepinephrine and pressor responses to adrenergic stimulation in pithed rats. J Clin Pharm 23:24, 1983.
24. Kurtzman JT, Thorp JM Jr, Spielman FJ, et al: Estrogen mediates the pregnancy-enhanced cardiotoxicity of cocaine in the isolated perfused rat heart. Obstet Gynecol 83:613, 1994.
25. Ramsay MM, Broughton Pipkin F, Rubin PC: Pressor, heart rate and plasma catecholamine responses to noradrenaline in pregnant and nonpregnant women. Br J Obstet Gynaecol 100:170, 1993.
26. Waxman MB, Wald RW, Cameron DA: The effects of autonomic tone on supraventricular tachycardias. In Zipes DP and Jalife J (eds): Cardiac Electrophysiology: From Cell to Bedside, 2nd Ed. W.B. Saunders, Philadelphia, 1994, p 699.
27. Waxman MB, Bonet JF, Finley JP Wald RW: Effects of respiration and posture in paroxysmal supraventricular tachycardia. Circulation 62:1011, 1980.
28. Waxman MB, Cameron DA, Wald RW: Interactions between the autonomic nervous system and tachycardias in man. In Zipes DP (ed): Cardiology Clinics, Arrhythmias-II. W.B. Saunders, Philadelphia, 1983, p 143.
29. Waxman MB, Cameron DA, Wald RW, Lascault GR: The use of autonomic maneuvers for diagnosis and treatment of cardiac arrhythmias. In Wagner GS, Waugh RA, Ramo BW (eds): Cardiac arrhythmias. Churchill Livingstone, New York, 1983, p 675.
30. Waxman MB, Wald RW, Sharma AD, et al: Vagal techniques for termination of paroxysmal supraventricular tachycardia. Am J Cardiol 46:655, 1980.
31. Waxman MB, Sharma AD, Cameron DA, et al: Reflex mechanisms responsible for early spontaneous termination of paroxysmal supraventricular tachycardia. Am J Cardiol 49:259, 1982.
32. Wasserstrum N: Maternal physiology. In Hacker NF, Moore JG (ed): Essentials of Obstetrics and Gynecology. W.B. Saunders, Philadelphia, 1986, pp 34–46.
33. Liebson PR, Mann LI, Evans MI, et al: Cardiac performance during pregnancy: Serial evaluation using external systolic time intervals. Am J Obstet Gynecol 122:1, 1975.
34. Rubler S, Danami PM, Pinto ER: Cardiac size and performance during pregnancy estimated with echocardiography. Am J Cardiol 40: 534, 1977.
35. Katz R, Karliner JS, Resnick R: Effects of a natural volume overload state (pregnancy) on left ventricular performance in normal human subjects. Circulation 58:434, 1978.
36. Franz MR, Burkhoff D, Yue DT, Sagawa K: Mechanically induced action potential changes and arrhythmia in isolated and in situ canine hearts. Cardiovasc Res 23:213, 1989.
37. Calkins J, Maughan WL, Kass DA, et al: Electrophysiological effect of volume load in isolated canine hearts. Am J Physiol 256:H1697, 1989.
38. Reiter MJ, Synhorst DP, Mann DE: Electrophysiological effects of acute ventricular dilatation in the isolated rabbit heart. Circ Research 62:554, 1988.
39. Franz MR: Stretch activated arrhythmias. In Zipes DP and Jalife J (eds): Cardiac Electrophysiology: From Cell to Bedside. W.B. Saunders, Philadelphia, 1994.
40. Franz MR, Cima R, Wang D, et al: Electrophysiological effects of myocardial stretch and mechanical determinants of stretch-activated arrhythmias. Circulation 86:968, 1992.
41. Waxman MB, Wald RW, Finley JP, et al: Valsalva termination of ventricular tachycardia. Circulation 62:843, 1980.
42. Wei JY, Greene HL, Weisfeldt ML: Cough-facilitated conversion of ventricular tachycardia. Am J Cardiol 45:174, 1980.
43. Waxman MB, Yao L, Cameron DA, Kirsh JA: Effects of posture, Valsalva maneuver and respiration on atrial flutter rate: An effect mediated through cardiac volume. J Am Coll Cardiol 17:1545, 1991.
44. Elkayam U: Pregnancy and cardiovascular disease. In Braunwald E (ed): Heart Disease. 4th ed. W.B. Saunders, Philadelphia, 1992.
45. Ostrzega E, Mehra A, Widerhorn J, et al: Evidence for increased incidence of arrhythmias during pregnancy: A study of 104 pregnant women with symptoms of palpitations, dizziness or syncope, abstracted. J Am Coll Cardiol 19:125, 1992.
46. Mendelson CL: Disorders of the heartbeat during pregnancy. Am J Obstet Gyne 72:1271, 1956.
47. Zipes DP: Specific arrhythmias: Diagnosis and treatment. In Braunwald E (ed): Heart Disease, 4th ed. W.B. Saunders, Philadelphia, 1992, p 667.
48. Widerhorn J, Widerhorn ALM, Rahimtoola SH, Elkayam U: WPW syndrome during pregnancy: Increased incidence of supraventricular arrhythmias. Am Heart J 123:796, 1992.
49. Gleicher N, Meller J, Sandler RZ, Sullum S: Wolff-Parkinson-White syndrome in pregnancy. Obstet Gynecol 58:748, 1981.
50. Kounis NG, Zavras GM, Papadaki PJ, et al: Pregnancy-induced increase of supraventricular arrhythmias in Wolff-Parkinson-White syndrome. Clin Cardiol 18:137, 1995.
51. Szekely P, Snaith L: Paroxysmal tachycardia in pregnancy. Br Heart J 15:195, 1953.
52. Tawam M, Levine J, Mendelson M, et al: Effect of pregnancy on paroxysmal supraventricular tachycardia. Am J Cardiol 72:838, 1993.
53. Lee SH, Chen SA, Wu TJ, et al: Effects of pregnancy on first onset and symptoms of paroxysmal supraventricular tachycardia. Am J Cardiol 76:675, 1995.
54. Elkayam U, Goodwin TM: Adenosine therapy for supraventricular tachycardia during pregnancy. Am J Cardiol 75:521, 1995.
55. Doig JC, McComb JM, Reid DS: Incessant atrial tachycardia accelerated by pregnancy. Br Heart J 67:266, 1992.
56. Murphy JJ, Hutchon DJ: Incessant atrial tachycardia accelerated by pregnancy. (Letter) Br Heart J 68:342, 1992.
57. Treakle K, Kostic B, Hulkower S: Supraventricular tachycardia resistant to treatment in a pregnant woman. J Fam Pract 35:581, 1992.
58. Schroeder JS, Harrison DC: Repeated cardioversion during pregnancy. Treatment of refractory paroxysmal atrial tachycardia during 3 successive pregnancies Am J Cardiol 27:445, 1971.
59. Hubbard WN, Jenkins BA, Ward DE: Persistent atrial tachycardia in pregnancy. Br Med J 287:327, 1983.
60. Dimarco JP, Sellers TD, Berne RM, et al: Adenosine: Electrophysiologic effects and therapeutic use of terminating paroxysmal supraventricular tachycardia. Circulation 68:1254, 1983.
61. Harrison JK, Greenfield RA, Wharton JM: Acute termination of supraventricular tachycardia by adenosine during pregnancy. Am Heart J 123:1386, 1992.
62. Podolsky SM, Varon J: Adenosine use during pregnancy. Ann Emerg Med 20:1027, 1991.
63. Mason BA, Ricci-Goodman J, Koos BJ: Adenosine in the treatment of maternal paroxysmal supraventricular tachycardia. Obstet Gynecol 80:478, 1992.
64. Afridi I, Moise KJ Jr, Rokey R: Termination of supraventricular tachycardia with intravenous adenosine in a pregnant woman with Wolff-Parkinson-White syndrome. Obstet Gynecol 80:481, 1992.
65. Leffler S, Johnson DR: Adenosine use in pregnancy: Lack of effect on fetal heart rate. Am J Emerg Med 10:548, 1992.
66. Gorczynski RJ: Basic pharmacology of esmolol. Am J Cardiol 56: 3F, 1985.
67. McTavish D, Sorkin EM: Verapamil. An updated review of its pharmacodynamic and pharmacokinetic properties, and therapeutic use in hypertension. Drugs 38:19, 1989.
68. Wheeler C, Yudivevish DL: Transport and metabolism of adenosine in the perfused guinea-pig placenta. J Physiol (Lond) 405:511, 1988.
69. Koos BJ, Matsuda K: Fetal breathing, sleep state, and cardiovascular responses to adenosine in sheep. J Appl Physiol 68:489, 1990.
70. Jaqueti J, Martinez-Hernandez D, Hernandez-Garcia R, et al: Adenosine deaminase in pregnancy serum. Clin Chem 36:2144, 1990.
71. Mariani PJ: Pharmacotherapy of pregnancy-related SVT. Ann Emerg Med 21:229, 1992.
72. Klein V, Repke JT: Supraventricular tachycardia in pregnancy: Cardioversion with verapamil. Obstet Gynecol 63:16S, 1984.
73. Byerly WG, Hartmann A, Foster DE, Tannenbaum AK: Verapamil in the treatment of maternal paroxysmal supraventricular tachycardia. Ann Emerg Med 20:552, 1991.
74. Mariani PJ, Mitchell BK: The littlest cardiologist. JAMA 263:3258, 1990.
75. DiMarco JP, Miles W, Akhtar M, et al: Adenosine for paroxysmal supraventricular tachycardia: Dose ranging and comparison with verapamil. Assessment in placebo-controlled, multicenter trials. The Adenosine for PSVT Study Group. Ann Intern Med 113:104, 1990.
76. Wolff F, Breuker KH, Schlensker KH, Bolte A: Prenatal diagnosis and therapy of fetal heart rate anomalies: With a contribution on the placental transfer of verapamil. J Perinat Med 8:203, 1980.
77. Bergmans MG, Jonker GJ, Koch HC: Fetal supraventricular tachycardia. Review of the literature. Obstet Gynecol Surv 40:61, 1985.

78. Kleinman CS, Copel JA, Weinstein EM et al: Treatment of fetal supraventricular tachyarrhythmias. JCU J Clin Ultrasound 13:265, 1985.
79. Haines DE, DiMarco JP: Sustained intraatrial reentrant tachycardia: Clinical, electrocardiographic and electrophysiologic characteristics and long-term follow-up. J Am Coll Cardiol 15:1345, 1990.
80. Proclemer A, Feruglio GA: [Permanent idiopathic sinus tachycardia in pregnancy. Description of a case.] G Ital Cardiol 18:333, 1988.
81. Robards GJ, Saunders DM, Donnelly JM: Refractory supraventricular tachycardia complicating pregnancy. Med J Aust 2:278, 1973.
82. Packer DL, Bardy GH, Worley SJ, et al: Tachycardia-induced cardiomyopathy: A reversible form of left ventricular dysfunction. Am J Cardiol 57:563, 1986.
83. Lemery R, Brugada P, Cheriex E, Wellens HJJ: Reversibility of tachycardia-induced left ventricular dysfunction after closed-chest catheter ablation of the atrioventricular junction for intractable atrial fibrillation. Am J Cardiol 60:1406, 1987.
84. Cruz FE, Cheriex EC, Smeets JL, et al: Reversibility of tachycardia-induced cardiomyopathy after cure of incessant supraventricular tachycardia. J Am Coll Cardiol 16:739, 1990.
85. Panja M, Mitra K, Kar AK, et al: A clinical profile of heart disease in pregnancy. Indian Heart J 34:667, 1986.
86. Homans DC: Peripartum cardiomyopathy. N Engl J Med 312:1432, 1985.
87. Whittemore R, Hobbins JC, Engle MA: Pregnancy and its outcome in women with and without surgical treatment of congenital heart disease. Am J Cardiol 50:641, 1982.
88. Jensen J, Wegner C, Keys EH, Smith HR: Pregnancy and heart disease—an 8 year experience. Obstet Gynecol 39:443, 1940.
89. Szekely P, Snaith L: Atrial fibrillation and pregnancy. Br Med J 1: 1407, 1961.
90. Saxon LA, Perloff JK: Arrhythmias and conduction disturbances associated with pregnancy. In Podrid PJ, Kowey PR (eds): Cardiac Arrhythmia: Mechanisms, Diagnosis and Management. Williams & Wilkins, Baltimore, 1995.
91. Hirsh J: Guidelines for antithrombotic therapy—Recommendations from the American College of Chest Physicians, 2nd ed. B.C. Decker Inc., Hamilton, Ontario, 1996.
92. Hankins GD, Wendel GD Jr, Leveno KJ, et al: Myocardial infarction during pregnancy: A review. Obstet Gynecol 65:139, 1985.
93. Curry JJ, Quintana FJ: Myocardial infarction with ventricular fibrillation during pregnancy treated by direct current defibrillation with fetal survival. Chest 58:82, 1970.
94. O'Donnell M, Meecham J, Tosson SR, Ward S: Ventricular fibrillation and reinfarction in pregnancy. Postgrad Med J 63:1095, 1987.
95. Perloff JK: Pregnancy and congenital heart disease. J Am Coll Cardiol 18:340, 1991.
96. Lownes HE, Ives TJ: Mexiletine use during pregnancy and lactation. Am J Obstet Gynecol 157:446, 1987.
97. Braverman AC, Bromley AS, Rutherford JD: New onset ventricular tachycardia during pregnancy. Int J Cardiol 33:409, 1991.
98. Spritzer RC, Seldon M, Mattes LM, et al: Serious arrhythmias during labor and delivery in women with heart disease. JAMA 211:1005, 1970.
99. Brunozzi LT, Meniconi L, Chilcchi P, et al: Propafenone in the treatment of chronic ventricular arrhythmias in a pregnant patient. Br J Clin Pharmacol 26:489, 1988.
100. Rey E, Bachrach LD, Burrow GN: Effects of amiodarone during pregnancy. Can Med Assoc J 136:956, 1987.
101. Shah DM, Sunderji SG: Hypertrophic cardiomyopathy and pregnancy: Report of a maternal mortality and review of literature. Obstet Gynecol Surv 40:444, 1985.
102. Plomp TA, Vulsma T, de Vijlder JJ: Use of amiodarone during pregnancy. Eur J Obstet Gynecol Reprod Biol 43:201, 1992.
103. Kinugawa T, Fujimoto Y, Miyakoda H, et al: A case of paroxysmal ventricular tachycardia in pregnancy. Jpn Circ J 53:807, 1989.
104. Varon ME, Sherer KM, Abramowicz JS, Akiyama T: Maternal ventricular tachycardia associated with hypomagnesemia. Am J Obstet Gynecol 167:1352, 1992.
105. McMillan TM, Bellet S: Ventricular paroxysmal tachycardia: Report of a case in a pregnant girl of sixteen years with an apparently normal heart. Am Heart J 7:70, 1931.
106. Peters CM, Penner SL: Orthostatic paroxysmal ventricular tachycardia. Am Heart J 32:645, 1946.
107. Hair TE, Eagan JT, Orgain ES: Paroxysmal ventricular tachycardia in the absence of demonstrable heart disease. Am J Cardiol 9:209, 1962.
108. Adams CW: Functional paroxysmal ventricular tachycardia. Am J Cardiol 9:215, 1962.
109. Rally CR, Walters MB: Paroxysmal ventricular tachycardia without evident heart disease. Can Med Assoc J 15:732, 1962.
110. Pine JL, Fox L, Shook D: Paroxysmal ventricular tachycardia complicating pregnancy. Am J Cardiol 15:732, 1965.
111. Gettes LS, Surawicz B: Long-term prevention of paroxysmal arrhythmias with propranolol therapy. Am J Med Sci 254:257, 1967.
112. Russell RO Jr: Paroxysmal ventricular tachycardia associated with pregnancy. Ala J Med Sci 6:111, 1969.
113. Reed RL, Cheney CB, Fearon RE, et al: Propranolol therapy throughout pregnancy: A case report. Anesth Analg 53:214, 1974.
114. Menon KPS, Mahapatra RK: Paroxysmal ventricular tachycardia associated with Bell's palsy in a teenager at late pregnancy. Angiology 35: 534, 1984.
115. Brodsky MA, Sato DA, Oster PD, et al: Paroxysmal ventricular tachycardia with syncope during pregnancy. Am J Cardiol 58:563, 1986.
116. Vlay SC: Catecholamine-sensitive ventricular tachycardia. Am Heart J 114:455, 1987.
117. Juneja MM, Ackerman WE, Kaczorowski DM, et al: Continuous epidural lidocaine infusion in the parturient with paroxysmal ventricular tachycardia. Anesthesiology 71:305, 1989.
118. Brodsky M, Doria R, Allen B, et al: New-onset ventricular tachycardia during pregnancy. Am Heart J 123:933, 1992.
119. Cox JL, Gardner MJ: Treatment of cardiac arrhythmias during pregnancy. Prog Cardiovasc Dis 36:137, 1993.
120. Sung RJ, Shapiro WA, Shen EN, et al: Effects of verapamil on ventricular tachycardias possibly caused by reentry, automaticity and triggered activity. J Clin Invest 72:350, 1983.
121. Bruner JP, Barry MJ, Elliott JP: Pregnancy in a patient with idiopathic long QT syndrome. Am J Obstet Gynecol 149:690, 1984.
122. O'Callaghan AC, Normandale JP, Morgan M: The prolonged Q-T syndrome: A review with anaesthetic implications and a report of two cases. Anaesth Intensive Care 10:50, 1982.
123. Ledwich JR, Fay JE: Idiopathic recurrent ventricular fibrillation. Am J Cardiol 24:255, 1969.
124. Rashba EJ, Zareba W, Moss AJ, et al: Influence of pregnancy on the risk for cardiac events in patients with hereditary long QT syndrome. Circulation 97:451, 1998.
125. Chua GL, Iwanochko RM, Choi R, Liu P: Magnetic resonance imaging in the diagnosis of arrhythmogenic right ventricular dysplasia. Can J Cardiol 12E(Suppl):123E, 1996.
126. Wiesfeld AC, Crijns HJ, Tuininga YS, Lie KI: Beta adrenergic blockade in the treatment of sustained ventricular tachycardia or ventricular fibrillation. Pacing Clin Electrophysiol 19:1026, 1996.
127. Codini MA, Sommerfeldt L, Eybel CE, et al: Clinical significance and characteristics of exercise-induced ventricular tachycardia. Cathet Cardiovasc Diag 7:227, 1981.
128. Woelfet A, Foster JR, Simpson RJ Jr, et al: Reproducibility and treatment of exercise-induced ventricular tachycardia. Am J Cardiol 53:751, 1984.
129. Huikiri HV, Cox M, Interian A Jr, et al: Efficacy of intravenous propranolol for suppression of inducibility of ventricular tachyarrhythmias with different electrophysiologic characteristics in coronary artery disease. Am J Cardiol 64:1305, 1989.
130. Duff HJ, Mitchell LB, Wyse DG: Antiarrhythmic efficacy of propranolol: Comparison of low and high serum concentrations. J Am Coll Cardiol 8:959, 1986.
131. The Cardiac Arrhythmia Suppression Trial (CAST) Investigators: Preliminary report: Effect of encainide and flecainide on mortality in a randomized trial of arrhythmia suppression after myocardial infarction. N Engl J Med 321:406, 1989.
132. Teo KK, Yusuf S, Furberg CD: Effects of prophylactic antiarrhythmic drug treatment in acute myocardial infarction. JAMA 270:1589, 1993.
133. The CASCADE Investigators: Randomized antiarrhythmic drug therapy in survivors of cardiac arrest (the CASCADE Study). Am J Cardiol 72:280, 1993.
134. Doval HC, Nul DR, Grancelli HO, et al: Randomized trial of low-dose amiodarone in severe congestive heart failure: Grupo de Estudio de la Sobrevida en la Insuficiencia Cardiaca en Argentina [GESICA]. Lancet 344:493, 1994.
135. Lehmann MH, Saksena S: Implantable cardioverter defibrillators in cardiovascular practice: Report of the policy conference of the North American Society of Pacing and Electrophysiology. NASPE Policy Conference Committee. Pacing Clin Electrophysiol 14:969, 1991.

136. Piper JM, Berkus M, Ridgway LE III: Pregnancy complicated by chronic cardiomyopathy and an automatic implantable cardioverter defibrillator. Am J Obstet Gynecol 167:506, 1992.
137. Page RL: Treatment of arrhythmias during pregnancy. Am Heart J 130:871, 1995.
138. Lee MS, Evans SJ, Blumberg S, et al: Echocardiographically guided electrophysiologic testing in pregnancy. J Am Soc Echocardiogr 7: 182, 1994.
139. Elkayam U, Gleicher N: Hemodynamics and cardiac function during normal pregnancy and puerperium. In Elkayam U, Gleicher N (eds): Cardiac Problems in Pregnancy, 2nd ed. Alan R Liss, New York, 1990, p 5.
140. Campbell M, Emanuel R: Six cases of congenital complete heart block followed for 34–40 years. Br Heart J 29:577, 1967.
141. Pinsky WW, Gillette PC, Garson AJR, McNamara DG: Diagnosis, management, and long-term results of patients with congenital complete atrio-ventricular block. Pediatrics 69:728, 1982.
142. Pordon CM, Moodie DS: Adults with congenital complete heart block: 25-year follow-up. Cleve Clin J Med 59:587, 1992.
143. Michaelsson M, Jonzon A, Riesenfeld T: Isolated congenital complete atrioventricular block in adult life. A prospective study. Circulation 92:442, 1995.
144. Dalvi BV, Chaudhuri A, Kulkarni HL, Kale PA: Therapeutic guidelines for congenital complete heart block presenting in pregnancy. Obstet Gynecol 79:802, 1992.
145. Kenmure AC, Cameron AJ: Congenital complete heart block in pregnancy. Br Heart J 29:910, 1967.
146. Eddy WA, Frankenfeld RH: Congenital complete heart block in pregnancy. Am J Obstet Gynecol 128:223, 1977.
147. Shouse EE, Acker JE: Pregnancy and delivery in a patient with external-internal cardiac pacemaker. Obstet Gynecol 24:817, 1964.
148. Jaffe R, Gruber A, Fejgin M, et al: Pregnancy with an artificial pacemaker. Obstet Gynecol Surv 42:137, 1987.
149. Abramovici H, Faktor JH, Gonen Y, et al: Maternal permanent bradycardia: Pregnancy and delivery. Obstet Gynecol 63:381, 1984.
150. Gudal M, Kervancioglu C, Oral D, et al: Permanent pacemaker implantation in a pregnant woman with the guidance of ECG and two-dimensional echocardiography. Pacing Clin Electrophysiol 10:543, 1987.
151. Lau CP, Lee CP, Wong CK, et al: Rate responsive pacing with a minute ventilation sensing pacemaker during pregnancy and delivery. Pacing Clin Electrophysiol 13:158, 1990.
152. Giuffrida JG, Bizzarri DV, Lagman L, Grimaldi RD: Obstetrical anesthesia in myocardial infarction and complete heart block. JAMA 204: 617, 1968.
153. Schonbrun M, Rowland W, Quiroz AC: Complete heart block in pregnancy: Successful use of an intravenous pacemaker in 2 patients during labor. Obstet Gynecol 27:243, 1966.
154. Ginns HM, Hollinrake K: Complete heart block in pregnancy treated with an internal cardiac pacemaker. J Obstet Gynaecol Br Commonw 77:710, 1970.
155. Berestka SA, Spellacy WN: Complete heart block associated with pregnancy and treated with an internal pacemaker. Lancet 87:461, 1967.
156. Myerburg RJ, Castellanos A: Cardiac arrest and sudden cardiac death. In Braunwald E (ed): Heart Disease, 4th ed. W.B. Saunders, Philadelphia, 1992, pp. 756–789.
157. Katz VL, Dotters DJ, Droegemueller W: Perimortem caesarian delivery. Obstet Gynecol 68:571, 1986.
158. Kaunitz AM, Hughes JM, Grimes DA, et al: Causes of maternal mortality in the United States. Obstet Gynecol 65:605, 1985.
159. Kerr MG, Scott DB, Samuel E: Studies of the inferior vena cava in late pregnancy. Br Med J 1:532, 1964.
160. Kerr MG: The mechanical effects of the gravid uterus in late pregnancy. J Obstet Gyne Brit Commonw 72:513, 1965.
161. Archer GW Jr, Marx GF: Arterial oxygen tension during apnoea in parturient women. Br J Anaesth 46:358, 1974.
162. Lee RV, Rodgers BD, White LM, Harvey RC: Cardiopulmonary resuscitation of pregnant women. Am J Med 81:311, 1986.
163. Dildy GA, Clark SL: Cardiac arrest during pregnancy. Obstet Gynecol Clin North Am 22:303, 1995.
164. Cummins RO ed: Textbook of Advanced Cardiac Life Support. American Heart Association, 1994
165. Rees GA, Willis BA: Resuscitation in late pregnancy. Anaesthesia 43: 347, 1988.
166. Strong TH Jr, Lowe RA: Perimortem cesarean section. Am J Emerg Med 7:489, 1986.
167. Lopez-Zeno JA, Carlo WA, O'Grady JP, Fanaroff AA: Infant survival following delayed postmortem cesarian delivery. Obstet Gynecol 76: 991, 1989.
168. Marx GF: Cardiopulmonary resuscitation of late-pregnant women. [Letter.] Anesthesiology 56:156, 1982.
169. Lindsay SL, Hanson GC: Cardiac arrest in near-term pregnancy. Anaesthesia 42:1074, 1987.
170. DePace NL, Betesh SS, Kotter MN: "Postmortem" cesarean section with recovery of both mother and offspring. JAMA 248:971, 1982.
171. Chan V, Tse F, Wong V: Transfer of digoxin across the placenta and into breast milk. Br J Obstet Gynaecol 85:605, 1978.
172. Rogers MC, Willerson JT, Goldblatt A, Smith TW: Serum digoxin concentrations in the human fetus, neonate, and infant. N Engl J Med 287:1010, 1972.
173. Saarikoski S: Placental transfer and fetal uptake of normal ^{3}H-digoxin in humans. Br J Obstet Gynaecol 83:879, 1976.
174. Luxford AM, Kellaway GS: Pharmokinetics of digoxin in pregnancy. Eur J Clin Pharmacol 25:117, 1983.
175. Finley JP, Waxman MB, Wong PY et al: Digoxin excretion in human milk. J Pediatr 94:339, 1979.
176. Weaver JB, Pearson JF, Lickrish GM: Influence of digitalis on time of onset and duration of labour in women with cardiac disease. Br Med J 3:519, 1973.
177. Rotmensch HH, Rotmensch S, Elkayam U: Management of cardiac arrhythmias during pregnancy; current concepts. Drugs 33:623, 1987.
178. Potondi A: Congenital rhabdomyoma of the heart and intrauterine digitalis poisoning. J Forensic Sci 11:81, 1967.
179. Sherman JL, Locke RV: Transplacental neonatal digitalis intoxication. Am J Cardiol 6:834, 1966.
180. Tcherdakoff PH, Collard M, Berrard E, et al: Propranolol in hypertension during pregnancy. Br Med J 2:670, 1978.
181. Bott-Kanner G, Schweitzer A, Reisner SH et al: Propranolol and hydrallazinen [sic] in the management of essential hypertension in pregnancy. Br J Obstet Gynaecol 87:110, 1980.
182. Sandstrom B: Adrenergic beta receptor blockers in hypertension of pregnancy. Clin Exp Hypertens [B] 1:127, 1982.
183. Turner GM, Oakley CM, Dixon HG: Management of pregnancy complicated by hypertrophic obstructive cardiomyopathy. Br Med J 4: 281, 1968.
184. Bullock JL, Harris RE, Young R: Treatment of thyrotoxicosis during pregnancy with propranolol. Am J Obstet Gynecol 121:242, 1975.
185. Langer A, Hung CT, McAnulty JA, et al: Adrenergic blockade. A new approach to hyperthyroidism in pregnancy. Obstet Gynecol 44: 181, 1974.
186. Wansborough H, Hakanishi H, Wood C: The effect of adrenergic receptor blocking drugs on the human uterus. J Obstet Gynaecol Br Commonw 75:189, 1968.
187. Sandstrom B: Antihypertensive treatment with the adrenergic beta-receptor blocker metoprolol during pregnancy. Gynecol Invest 9:195, 1978.
188. Wichman K, Roden G, Karlberg BE: A placebo controlled trial of metoprolol in the treatment of hypertension in pregnancy. Scand J Clin Lab Invest 169(Suppl):90, 1984.
189. Sandstrom B, Regardh CG: Metoprolol excretion into breast milk. Br J Clin Pharmacol 9:518, 1980.
190. Kulas J, Lunell NO, Rosing U, et al: Atenolol and metoprolol: A comparison of their excretion into human breast milk. Acta Obstet Gynecol Scand 118:65, 1984.
191. Lindeberg S, Sandstrom B, Lundborg P, et al: Disposition of the adrenergic blocker metoprolol in the late pregnant woman, the amniotic fluid, the cord blood, and the neonate. Acta Obstet Gynecol Scand 118(Suppl):61, 1984.
192. Liedholm H, Melander A, Bitzen PO, et al: Accumulation of atenolol and metoprolol in human breast milk. Eur J Clin Pharmacol 20: 229, 1981.
193. Rubin PC, Butters L, Low RA, et al: Atenolol in the treatment of essential hypertension during pregnancy. Br J Clin Pharmacol 14: 279, 1982.
194. Fowler MB, Brudevell M, Mackson G, et al: Essential hypertension and pregnancy: Successful outcome with atenolol. Br J Clin Pract 38: 73, 1984.
195. Reynolds B, Butters L, Evans J, et al: First year of life after the use of atenolol in pregnancy associated hypertension. Arch Dis Child 59: 1061, 1984.

196. Butters L, Kennedy S, Rubin PC: Atenolol in essential hypertension during pregnancy. Br Med J 310:587, 1990.
197. Isley WL, Dahl S, Gibbs H: Use of esmolol in managing a thyrotoxic patient needing emergency surgery. Am J Med 89:122, 1990.
198. Anderson JL, Harrison DC, Meffin PJ, Winkle RA: Antiarrhythmic drugs: Clinical pharmacology and therapeutic uses. Drugs 15:271, 1978.
199. Meyer J, Lackner JE, Schochet SS: Paroxysmal tachycardia in pregnancy. JAMA 94:1901, 1930.
200. Mason JW, Hondeghem LM: Quinidine. Ann NY Acad Sci 432:162, 1984.
201. Spinnato JA, Shaver DC, Flynn GS, et al: Fetal supraventricular tachycardia: In utero therapy with digoxin and quinidine. Obstet Gynecol 64:730, 1984.
202. Hill LM, Malkasian GD: The use of quinidine sulfate throughout pregnancy. Obstet Gynecol 54:366, 1979.
203. Lesch M, Lewis E, Humphries JO: Paroxysmal ventricular tachycardia in the absence of organic heart disease: Report of a case and review of the literature. Ann Intern Med 66:950, 1967.
204. Webster LT: Drugs used in the chemotherapy of protozoal infections—malaria. In Gilman AG, Rall TW, Niew AS, et al (eds): Goodman and Gilman's The Pharmacological Basis of Therapeutics. Pergan, New York, 1990, p 978.
205. Widerhorn J, Rahimtoola SH, Elkayam U: Cardiac Rhythm Disorders. In Gleicher N (ed): Principles and Practice of Medical Therapy in Pregnancy, 2nd ed. Appleton and Lange, Norwalk, 1992, pp. 826–833.
206. Coplen SE, Antman EM, Berlin JA, et al: Efficacy and safety of quinidine therapy for maintenance of sinus rhythm after cardioversion: A meta-analysis of randomized control trials. Circulation 82:1106, 1990.
207. Hoffman BF, Rosen MR, Witt AL: Electrophysiology and pharmacology of cardiac arrhythmias. VII. Cardiac effects of quinidine and procainamide. Am Heart J 90:117, 1975.
208. Giardina EG: Procainamide: Clinical pharmacology and efficacy against ventricular arrhythmias. Ann NY Acad Sci 432:177, 1984.
209. Dumesic DA, Silverman NH, Tobias S, et al: Transplacental cardioversion of fetal supraventricular tachycardia with procainamide. N Engl J Med 307:1128, 1982.
210. Given BD, Phillippe M, Sanders SP et al: Procainamide cardioversion of fetal supraventricular tachyarrhythmia. Am J Cardiol 53:1460, 1984.
211. Pittard WB III, Glazier H: Procainamide excretion in human milk. J Pediatr 102:631, 1983.
212. Allen NM, Page RL: Administration of procainamide during pregnancy. Clin Pharm 12:58, 1993.
213. Shaxted EJ, Milton PH: Disopyramide in pregnancy: A case report. Curr Med Res Opinion 6:70, 1979.
214. Karim A, Cook C, Campion J: Placental and milk transfer of disopyramide and its metabolites in rats. Drug Metab Dispos 6:346, 1978.
215. Leonard RF, Braun TE, Levy AM: Initiation of uterine contractions by disopyramide during pregnancy. N Engl J Med 299:84, 1978.
216. Tadmor OP, Keren A, Rosenak D, Gal M, et al: The effect of disopyramide on uterine contractions during pregnancy. Am J Obstet Gynecol 162:482, 1990.
217. Reynolds F, Taylor G: Maternal and neonatal blood concentrations of bupivacaine: a comparison with lignocaine during continuous extradural analgesia. Anaesthesia 25:14, 1970.
218. Blankenbaker WL, Kifazio CA, Berry FA: Lidocaine and its metabolites in the newborn. Anesthesiology 42:325, 1975.
219. Brown WU, Bell GC, Lurie AO et al: Newborn blood levels of lidocaine and mepivacaine in the first postnatal day following maternal epidural anesthesia. Anesthesiology 42:698, 1976.
220. Heinonen OP, Slone D, Shapiro S: Birth Defects and Drugs in Pregnancy. PSG Pub Inc., Littleton, Mass, 1977.
221. Teram K, Benowitz N, Heymann MA, Kahanpaa K, et al: Effects of lidocaine on heart rate, blood pressure, and electrocardiogram in fetal sheep. Am J Obstet Gynecol 118:935, 1974.
222. Liston WA, Adjepon-Yamoah KK, Scott DB: Fetal and maternal lidocaine levels after paracervical block. Br J Anesth 45:750, 1973.
223. Shnider SM, Way EL: Plasma levels of lidocaine in mother and newborn following obstetrical conduction anesthesia: Clinical applications. Anesthesiology 29:951, 1968.
224. Kim WY, Pomerance JJ, Miller AA: Lidocaine intoxication in a newborn following local anesthesia for episiotomy. Pediatrics 64:634, 1979.
225. DePraeter C, Vanhaesebrouck P, DePraeter N, et al: Episiotomy and neonatal lidocaine intoxication. Eur J Pediatr 150:685, 1991.
226. Biehl D, Shnider SM, Levinson G, et al: Placental transfer of lidocaine: Effects of fetal acidosis. Anesthesiology 48:409, 1978.
227. Brown WU, Bell GC, Alper MH: Acidosis, local anesthetics and the newborn. Obstet Gynecol 48:27, 1976.
228. Timmis AD, Jackson G, Holt DW: Mexiletine for control of ventricular dysrhythmias in pregnancy. Lancet 2:647, 1980.
229. Lewis AM, Johnston A, Patel L, et al: Mexiletine in human blood and breast milk. Postgrad Med J 57:546, 1981.
230. Gregg AR, Tomich PG: Mexiletine use in pregnancy. J Perinat Med 8:33, 1988.
231. Palmer CM, Norris MC: Placental transfer of flecainide. Am J Dis Child 140:144, 1990.
232. Wagner X, Jouglard J, Moulin M, et al: Coadministration of flecainide acetate and sotalol during pregnancy: Lack of teratogenic effects, passage across the placenta, and excretion in human breast milk. Am Heart J 199:700, 1990.
233. Wren C, Hunter S: Maternal administration of flecainide to terminate and suppress fetal tachycardia. Br Med J 296:249, 1988.
234. Allan LD, Chita SK, Sharland GK, et al: Flecainide in the treatment of fetal tachycardias. Br Heart J 65:46, 1991.
235. Perry JC, Ayres NA, Carpenter RJ: Fetal supraventricular tachycardia treated with flecainide acetate. J Pediatr 118:303, 1991.
236. Libardoni M, Piovan D, Busato E, et al: Transfer of propafenone and 5-OH-propafenone to foetal plasma and maternal milk. Br J Clin Pharmacol 32:527, 1991.
237. Gill J, Heel RC, Fitton A: Amiodarone: An overview of its pharmacological properties and review of its therapeutic use in cardiac arrhythmias. Drugs 43:69, 1992.
238. Penn IM, Barrett PA, Pannikote V, et al: Amiodarone in pregnancy. Am J Cardiol 56:196, 1985.
239. Arnoux P, Seyral P, Llurens M, et al: Amiodarone and digoxin for refractory fetal tachycardia. Am J Cardiol 59:166, 1987
240. McKenna WJ, Harris L, Rowland E, et al: Amiodarone therapy during pregnancy. Am J Cardiol 51:1231, 1983.
241. Naccarelli GV, Rinkenberger RL, Dougherty A, et al: Amiodarone: Pharmacology and antiarrhythmic and adverse effects. Pharmacotherapy 5:298, 1985.
242. Strunge P, Frandsen J, Andreasen F: Amiodarone during pregnancy. Eur Heart J 9:106, 1988.
243. Pitcher D, Leather HM, Storey GC, et al: Amiodarone in pregnancy. Lancet 1:597,1983.
244. Robson DJ, Jeeva-Raj MV, Storey GC, et al: Use of amiodarone during pregnancy. Postgrad Med J 61:75, 1985.
245. Foster CJ, Love HG: Amiodarone in pregnancy: Case report and review of literature. Int J Cardiol 20:307, 1988.
246. Magee LA, Downar E, Sermer M, Boulton BC, et al: Pregnancy outcome after gestational exposure to amiodarone in Canada. Am J Obstet Gynecol 172:1307, 1995.
247. Dewolf D, De Schepper, Verharren H, et al: Congenital hypothyroid goiter and amiodarone. Acta Paediatr Scand 77:616, 1988.
248. Laurent M, Betremieux, P, Biron Y, Lellelloco A: Neonatal hypothyroidism after treatment by amiodarone during pregnancy. Am J Cardiol 61:142, 1987.
249. Haffajee CI: Amiodarone pharmacokinetics. Am Heart J 106:847, 1983.
250. Gembruch U, Manz M, Bald R et al: Repeated intravascular treatment with amiodarone in a fetus with refractory supraventricular tachycardia and hydrops fetalis. Am Heart J 118:1335, 1989.
251. Widerhorn J, Bhandari AK, Bughi S et al: Fetal and neonatal adverse effects profile of amiodarone treatment during pregnancy. Am Heart J 122:1162, 1991.
252. Rey E, Duperron L, Gauthier R et al: Transplacental treatment of tachycardia-induced fetal heart failure with verapamil and amiodarone. Am J Obstet Gynecol 153:311, 1985.
253. Wladimiroll JW, Stewart A: Treatment of fetal cardiac arrhythmias. Br J Hosp Med 34:134, 1985.
254. Ovadia M, Mitermayer B, Hoyer GL, Marcus F: Human experience with amiodarone in the embryonic period. Am J Cardiol 73:316, 1994.
255. Magee LA, Nulman I, Rovet JF, et al: Neurodevelopment after in utero amiodarone exposure. Neurotoxicol Teratol 21:261, 1999.
256. O'Hare MF, Murnaghan GA, Russell CJ et al: Sotalol as a hypotensive agent in pregnancy. Br J Obstet Gynecol 87:814, 1980.
257. Erkkola R, Lammintausta R, Liukko P et al: Transfer of propranolol and sotalol across the human placenta, their effect on maternal and fetal plasma renin activity. Acta Obstet Gynecol Scand 61:31, 1982.

258. Hackett LP, Wojnar-Horton RE, Dusci LJ et al: Excretion of sotalol in breast milk. Br J Clin Pharmacol 29:277, 1990.
259. Vogel JH, Pryor R, Blount SG JR: Direct current defibrillation during pregnancy. JAMA 193:970, 1965.
260. Desilva RA, Graboys TB, Podrid PJ et al: Cardioversion and defibrillation. Am Heart J 100:881, 1980.
261. Sussman HF, Duque D, Lesser ME: Atrial flutter with 1:1AV conduction: Report of a case in a pregnant woman successfully treated with DC countershock. Dis Chest 49:99, 1966.
262. Finlay AT, Edmunds V: DC cardioversion in pregnancy. Br J Clin Pract 33:88, 1979.
263. Klepper I: Cardioversion in late pregnancy: The anesthetic management of a case of Wolff-Parkinson-White syndrome. Anaesthesia 36: 611, 1981.
264. Antiarrhythmic Versus Implantable Defibrillators (AVID) Investigators: A comparison of antiarrhythmic drug therapy with defibrillators in patients resuscitated from near-fatal ventricular arrhythmias. N Engl J Med 337:1576, 1997.
265. Moss AJ, Hall WJ, Cannom DS, et al: Improved survival with an implanted defibrillator in patients with coronary disease at high risk for ventricular arrhythmias. N Engl J Med 335:1933, 1996.
266. Kuck KH, Cappato R, Siebels J, et al: Randomized comparison of antiarrhythmic drug therapy with implantable defibrillators in patients resuscitated from cardiac arrest: The Cardiac Arrest Study Hamburg (CASH). Circulation 102:748, 2000.
267. Natale A, Davidson T, Geiger MJ, et al: Implantable cardioverter-defibrillators and pregnancy. A safe combination? Circulation 96: 2808, 1997.

CHAPTER 30

Drugs and Pregnancy

Susan D. Mueller and James T. Willerson

FETAL EFFECTS

Cardiovascular drugs may affect uterine myometrial tone and uteroplacental blood flow (Table 30–1). The fetus may be affected by altered hemodynamics in the mother or by teratogenic effects of drugs. Placental transfer of drugs can be beneficial for the treatment of selected problems in utero.[1, 2] Medication levels in the mother must be monitored, because the levels of some medications may decrease by as much as 40% during pregnancy. Although many drugs have a potentially unfavorable effect on a developing fetus, when drug administration becomes necessary, the risk-benefit ratio should be evaluated and the smallest effective dose used.

LACTATION

Drugs may also be transferred to the neonate through breast milk during lactation. Usually, 1% to 2% of the maternal dose of any drug appears in the breast milk. Some drugs are clearly contraindicated during breast-feeding, but in most cases, not enough information is available to rule out this use definitively. If a mother requires medication during lactation, close monitoring of the infant's ingested dose and plasma levels are necessary, along with observation for adverse effects or toxicity.[3, 4]

CARDIAC GLYCOSIDES

Digoxin has been used extensively for the treatment of maternal congestive heart failure (CHF) and supraventricular tachycardias in the mother or fetus. There are no reports of teratogenicity with the use of this agent in humans, but excessive doses can be detrimental to the mother and may be lethal to the fetus.[5] Digoxin can be used alone or in combination with a second drug such as verapamil, sotalol, or flecainide in the treatment of supraventricular tachycardia or atrial flutter. Pregnancy itself may be associated with increased levels of digoxin-like substances, especially when systemic arterial hypertension is present. These substances interfere with the digoxin radioimmunoassay and may cause errors in measurement.[6]

Few adverse effects have been observed in fetuses and mothers who have been receiving long-term digoxin.[7] Because the fetal heart has only a limited capacity to bind digoxin during the first half of pregnancy and there is significant maternal protein binding, only small amounts of digoxin are available to the fetus. In some instances, low birth weights have been reported. This may also be due to the fact that mothers receiving digoxin usually have a shorter duration of pregnancy, with lower birth weights rather than intrauterine growth retardation. The total amount of digoxin ingested daily by an infant who is breast-feeding has been estimated to be approximately 1% of the pediatric recommended dose; adverse clinical effects are not usually seen. Digoxin can be continued in breast-feeding mothers.

TREATMENT OF ARRHYTHMIAS

The most extensive experience with antiarrhythmic drug therapy during pregnancy has been with digoxin, quinidine, and propranolol.[8] However, the choice of antiarrhythmic drugs depends on the specific arrhythmia being treated, the cardiac condition of the patient or fetus, and the known or anticipated actions of the antiarrhythmic drug being considered. For benign arrhythmias, a conservative approach starting initially with preventive measures is appropriate. In the case of more severe or symptomatic arrhythmias, pharmacologic therapy should be instituted using drugs with proven safety in the fetus. Electrical cardioversion of the patient

Table 30–1. EFFECTS OF α- AND β-ADRENERGIC RECEPTOR STIMULATION AND BLOCKADE ON MATERNAL-FETAL PHYSIOLOGY

	STIMULATION		BLOCKADE	
	Alpha-Receptor	Beta-Receptor	Alpha-Receptor	Beta-Receptor
Fetal heart rate	↔*	↑†	↔	↔‡
Maternal heart rate	↔	↑	↔	↓
Umbilical blood flow	↔	↑	↔	↓
Myometrial activity	↑	↓	↓	↑

*↔, no effect.
†↑, increase.
‡↓, decrease.
From Frishman WH, Chesner M: Use of beta-adrenergic blocking agents in pregnancy. In Elkayam U, Gleicher N (eds): Cardiac Problems in Pregnancy, 2nd ed. Alan R. Liss, New York 1990, pp 351–360. Reprinted by permission of Wiley-Liss, Inc., a subsidiary of John Wiley & Sons, Inc.

can usually be performed with relative safety in both mother and fetus.

In one recently completed study, 25 fetuses with the diagnosis of supraventricular tachycardia were reported from January 1989 to October 1997 among 3117 pregnant women referred for fetal cardiac evaluation.[8] There were 17 fetuses with the diagnosis of supraventricular tachycardia and eight with atrial flutter. Gestational ages ranged from 26 to 40 weeks. Twelve patients were hydropic at presentation: six with supraventricular tachycardia, and six with atrial flutter. Four fetuses with supraventricular tachycardia showed structural alterations, including two with Ebstein's anomaly and two with ventricular septal defects.

Patients were admitted to a Fetal Cardiology Unit for monitoring and treatment. Among 17 fetuses with supraventricular tachycardia, 12 showed a good response to digoxin administration, but this drug was not useful in any of the patients with atrial flutter. In two patients with supraventricular tachycardia and in six with atrial flutter, the pregnancy was interrupted to perform postnatal cardioversion. The mortality rate in this study was three of 17 fetuses in the supraventricular tachycardia group (including two patients with Ebstein's anomaly) and zero of eight in the atrial flutter group. From this study, it is apparent that fetal supraventricular tachyarrhythmias are uncommon in the general population of pregnant women. Nevertheless, the fetus may be subject to severe heart failure and death. Thus, accurate diagnosis and early treatment of these conditions are extremely important. Diagnosis of fetal arrhythmias may be made by fetal echocardiography; this technique may be used to examine the influence of the arrhythmia on the heart itself. It is generally conceded that digoxin is the treatment of choice for fetal supraventricular tachycardias. However, although administering digoxin to the mother is often effective in treating supraventricular tachycardia in the fetus, on occasion it may be ineffective secondary to poor transplacental drug transfer.

Recently, Parilla and colleagues treated eight pregnancies complicated by fetal supraventricular tachycardia (SVT) and hydrops fetalis with transplacental therapy or with combined maternal and direct fetal intramuscular therapy with digoxin.[9] These authors described the response to treatment following maternal intravenous administration of digoxin or a combination of fetal intramuscular digoxin plus maternal intravenous digoxin for eight hydropic fetuses during nine successful pharmacologic conversions. The maternal intravenous administration of digoxin was given using standard loading and maintenance protocols. Fetal intramuscular administration of digoxin was accomplished at a dose of 88 μg/kg per 12 to 24 hours to a maximum of three injections in the fetal buttock. Time to onset of the first 2 hours of sinus rhythm, time to onset of more than 90% of sinus rhythm, and time to resolution of hydrops fetalis were noted. The mean heart rate was 257 ± 36 beats per minutes, and the mean gestational age was 29 ± 4.8 weeks. Fetal SVT was the result of a reentrant mechanism in all cases. For the three fetuses that underwent successful cardioversion following maternal intravenous administration of digoxin, the time to onset of the first 2 hours of sinus rhythm was 145 ± 114 hours, the time to onset of more than 90% sinus rhythm was 176 ± 55 hours, and hydrops fetalis resolved in 41 ± 37 days. In each of the mothers treated in this manner, additional antiarrhythmic drugs were also given to the mother. In the four fetuses treated by fetal intramuscular digoxin administration and maternal intravenous therapy, the time to onset of the first 2 hours of sinus rhythm was 5.5 ± 4 hours, the time to onset of more than 90% sinus rhythm was 22 ± 14 hours, and resolution of hydrops fetalis occurred in 25 ± 21 days. In two failed cardioversions, with transplacental treatment alone, the time to onset of the first 2 hours of sinus rhythm was 203 ± 180 hours, and the time to onset of more than 90% sinus rhythm was 313 ± 270 hours. Once fetal intramuscular therapy was begun in these fetuses, the time to onset for the first 2 hours of sinus rhythm was 17 ± 7 hours and time to onset of more than 90% sinus rhythm was 60 ± 13 hours. Hydrops fetalis resolved in 45 days in one fetus; the other fetus never had resolution of hydrops despite 100 days of antiarrhythmic therapy. Thus, direct fetal intramuscular injection of digoxin combined with transplacental therapy appeared to shorten the time to initial conversion of SVT and to sustain sinus rhythm in the fetus with SVT complicated by hydrops fetalis.

Fetal tachyarrhythmias may be life-threatening conditions for the fetus; long-standing tachyarrhythmias may lead to fetal cardiac failure, hydrops, and death. Normalization of the fetal cardiac rhythm leads to resolution of fetal hydrops in most instances. Fetuses with a persistent heart rate over 180 beats per minute with a 1:1 atrioventricular conduction on M-mode echocardiography are defined as having SVT. Fetal hydrops is diagnosed if the following signs are seen: pleural or pericardial effusion, or ascites and skin edema, sometimes with right ventricular dysfunction and enlargement. Resolution of hydrops often requires 4 to 6 weeks after termination of the arrhythmia and usually occurs in the following sequence: diminution of ascites, pleural and pericardial effusions, and disappearance of skin and scalp edema.[10]

Another recent report suggests that rate-based management of fetal supraventricular tachycardia is important in the successful culmination of a pregnancy.[11] Guntheroth and colleagues have evaluated the clinical course of 22 fetuses with supraventricular tachycardia to determine whether heart rate alone might serve as a basis for conservative management. Hydrops was not encountered with heart rates under 230 beats per minute in this series of patients. The conditions of all 22 fetuses stabilized without invasive administration of medication. Eighteen were delivered vaginally and only four by cesarean section. No fetal or neonatal losses occurred. Regardless of the type of supraventricular tachycardia, reducing heart rate in these fetuses to levels preventing or resolving hydrops allowed vaginal term delivery. Digoxin, beta blockers, or verapamil might be used for purposes of reducing heart rate in the fetus with SVT.

NEONATAL VENTRICULAR TACHYCARDIA

Villain and associates[11a] undertook a retrospective study in two fetuses and eight neonates 1 to 20 days of age with ventricular tachycardia (VT). The VT was persistent in two patients, observed in runs of variable variation in the other eight patients, and incessant in seven of these patients. Only two patients were symptomatic: cardiac failure with shock 16 hours after birth and hydramnios at 16 weeks of gestation.

The arrhythmia was monomorphic nine times out of 10, with fixed rates (three cases) or variable rates (seven cases) that were greater than 150 beats per minute. Intravenous magnesium sulfate in the severe and permanent forms, oral beta blockers to treat VT associated with acceleration of the sinus rhythm, and oral amiodarone alone or with propranolol (in one case) were prescribed. Three neonates were not treated either from the outset or after the inefficacy of amiodarone. Nine patients had their VTs converted to sinus rhythm and were treatment free 12 to 24 months later. The other patient had a slow, well-tolerated VT. No etiology was detected in nine patients. In the remaining patient, there was a metabolic disease of beta oxidation of long-chain fatty acids. These authors concluded that isolated, idiopathic VT in the neonate usually carries a good prognosis and that relatively simple treatment with beta blockers or amiodarone is usually associated with restoration of sinus rhythm and definitive cure during the first year of life. However, VT may be associated with the presence of severe congenital heart disease, be persistent, and be the cause of fetal or later infant death.

DIURETIC AGENTS

Diuretics have been used to manage hypertension, heart failure, and fluid retention and to prevent pre-eclampsia.[12–17] Their efficacy to prevent or change the perinatal outcome of pre-eclampsia has not been proved, and they prevent the normal volume expansion of pregnancy. Diuretics may have deleterious effects, by decreasing placental perfusion due to volume restriction. Their administration does not alter amniotic fluid volume significantly. Furosemide crosses the placenta and increases fetal urine production. In fact, it can be used as a provocative test of kidney function.[13] Thiazides have not been reported to increase the risk and development of congenital defects but may confer a higher risk of hyperglycemia in the mother, resulting in fetal hypoglycemia.[14–16] There have been reports of thiazide-induced hemolytic anemia and thrombocytopenia in the newborn, as well as a possible relationship to an antiplatelet antibody, and of hyponatremia and bradycardia, with the bradycardia often related to hypokalemia.[17–19] Therefore, diuretics should be limited to treatment of severe CHF in the mother or fetus; the routine use of diuretics is not recommended because of electrolyte imbalances in the mother, fetus, and amniotic fluid and the potential for resulting deaths.[14, 15]

Furosemide is excreted in breast milk, but no adverse effects have been reported. Thiazides are excreted at 25% of the maternal blood concentration and may suppress lactation.[20]

ORGANIC NITRATES

Nitroglycerin is used to treat or prevent angina in the mother. Intravenous nitroglycerin has been used effectively and safely for pregnancy-induced hypertension.[21–23] Fetal heart rate deceleration and bradycardia have been reported in a few patients, along with attenuation of spontaneous beat-to-beat variability. Reports of small groups of patients showed a significant incidence of malformations, but this has not been proved to be a result of nitroglycerin or other vasodilators.[24] Nitrates may not be free of side effects, and further studies are needed to clarify their effects before they are recommended for routine use during pregnancy. No data are available on lactation.

ANGIOTENSIN-CONVERTING ENZYME INHIBITORS

Hypertension is often treated with angiotensin-converting enzyme (ACE) inhibitors, such as captopril and enalapril. In animals, exposure to ACE inhibitors during pregnancy has caused prolonged fetal hypotension and death. Renal perfusion and glomerular plasma flow are relatively low during gestation and require high levels of angiotensin II to maintain the glomerular filtration rate.[25, 26] ACE inhibitors prevent conversion of angiotensin I to angiotensin II and may lead to in utero renal failure.[27, 28] Enalapril use in early gestation has been associated with severe renal malformations, severe hypotension, and renal failure in the fetus.[29, 30] Captopril use has been associated with stillbirths and severe renal toxicity in newborns.[31] Multiple birth defects have been reported when fetuses were exposed to multiple drugs of which captopril was one. There are reports of a rare skull ossification defect in fetuses born to mothers treated with ACE inhibitors and an increased incidence of low-birth-weight infants, severe oligohydramnios, neonatal anuria, and renal failure, which may be fatal.[32–36]

Thus, the use of ACE inhibitors during the second and third trimester of pregnancy has been associated with a pattern of defects known as ACE inhibitor fetopathy.[37] The dominant feature of the fetopathy is renal tubular dysplasia. Other associated conditions include hypocalvaria, intrauterine growth retardation, and patent ductus arteriosus. These features may be related to fetal hypotension secondary to the ACE-induced decreases in fetal angiotensin or increased bradykinin. No adverse fetal effects have been linked to first-trimester use of ACE inhibitors, but there has been no systematic evaluation of births to women with such exposures. In a recent study[37] to determine whether features of ACE inhibitor fetopathy occurred after first trimester exposure, the Organization of Teratology Information Services in North American initiated the ACEI Registry, and two members of the European Network of Teratology Information Services participated. In a recent report from the ACEI Registry, infants of 66 women who self-reported first-trimester-only exposure to ACE inhibitors showed no evidence of renal tubular dysplasia. One would conclude that the use of the ACE inhibitors is contraindicated during the second and third trimesters of pregnancy.

SODIUM NITROPRUSSIDE

Nitroprusside has been used to control blood pressure and to treat CHF in patients who have aortic dissections or intracranial aneurysm, those who must undergo surgery, and those with severe hypertension. The drug crosses the placenta in animals and humans, but there are no reports of teratogenicity. Transient fetal bradycardia may occur.[38–42]

With significant doses and long-term use of nitroprusside,

there is a potential for cyanide accumulation in the mother or fetus, or both, which could lead to fetal death. In a limited number of pregnant patients, nitroprusside has been used without unfavorable effects on the fetus. Therefore, nitroprusside is effective but potentially toxic. It should be used only for short periods of time during pregnancy and only in very ill patients who have not responded to other medical therapies. When it is given for several days (which is not recommended), maternal serum pH, plasma cyanide, red blood cell cyanide, and methemoglobin levels should be monitored. Nitroprusside cannot be safely recommended for routine use during pregnancy. There is no reported information on its use in breast-feeding mothers.

CALCIUM CHANNEL ANTAGONISTS

Verapamil has been used during pregnancy to treat maternal or fetal supraventricular arrhythmias, premature labor, severe pre-eclampsia, and severe gestational proteinuric hypertension. This drug has no reported teratogenic effects.[43–45] Transplacental transfer allows the treatment of in utero fetal tachycardias.[43, 45] This drug is usually discontinued at the onset of labor. Long-term data are needed to establish its safety during pregnancy. Hypotension may occur in patients given verapamil by rapid intravenous bolus, with a drop in uteroplacental blood flow and fetal hypoxia. Verapamil is excreted in breast milk, but no pharmacologic effects have been observed in neonates. Its use is compatible with breast-feeding.

Nifedipine has been used during pregnancy as a tocolytic or uterine contraction blocking agent for the treatment of hypertensive emergencies and of chronic essential hypertension.[44–47] Severe adverse reactions, including fetal hypoxia and acidosis, have been reported in rhesus monkeys given intravenous magnesium and nifedipine. There have been reports of decreased blood pressure without a reduction in uteroplacental blood flow. In some studies using nifedipine with beta blockers for long-term treatment of pregnant hypertensive patients, there have been reports of premature delivery and small infants. More information is needed on the long-term use of this agent before it can be recommended for use in pregnancy. It is often used to treat severe hypertension in the mother. It is excreted in breast milk.[48]

BETA-ADRENERGIC BLOCKING AGENTS

Propranolol

Propranolol has been used to treat patients with mitral valve prolapse, cardiac arrhythmias, hypertrophic cardiomyopathy, and hyperthyroidism in pregnancy.[49–52] It readily crosses the placenta and may reach levels equal to or lower than the mother's blood levels.[53–56] It is not a teratogen and appears to be relatively safe if newborns are monitored for signs of extreme beta-blockade, such as bradycardia and hypoglycemia.[54, 55] The long-term effects of in utero exposure to this agent have not been studied. However, it may have possible adverse effects on the fetus and neonate, such as growth retardation, bradycardia, hyperbilirubinemia, delayed onset of respiration in the newborn, and hypoglycemia. Because blockade of myometrial $beta_2$-adrenergic receptors with beta blockers may stimulate uterine contractions, more selective $beta_1$-receptor blockers may be preferable for use during gestation. Propranolol is excreted in breast milk, but no adverse effects have been observed in infants.[20]

Metoprolol

Metoprolol is used to treat hypertensive patients and has not been shown to produce teratogenic or major side effects in the fetus. It is secreted in breast milk in small quantities and can be safely used unless hepatic function in the newborn is impaired.[20, 56–58]

Atenolol

Atenolol has been used to treat hypertension during pregnancy, with some adverse reactions reported. Low-birth-weight infants have been reported in mothers who have received this drug during pregnancy.[59] This effect has been noted more frequently with atenolol than with other antihypertensive agents and may make this beta blocker less than ideal for use in the pregnant woman.[59] It is secreted in breast milk, but no adverse effects have been seen in children. Therefore, breast-feeding should not be discontinued.[20, 56]

Labetalol

Labetalol has been used to treat hypertension and has been shown to be safe and effective. With this drug, there may be reductions in blood pressure without significant decreases in uterine blood flow. It is secreted in breast milk without adverse effects noted in infants.[20, 56]

D,L-Sotalol

A retrospective study by Sonesson and associates[60] in the period from 1991 to 1995 examined the experience with sotalol in the treatment of 14 fetuses with supraventricular tachycardias. The SVT was diagnosed in a structurally normal heart at a gestational age of 24 to 35 (median 28) weeks. In eight fetuses, hydrops was evident at presentation. In all patients, pharmacologic conversion with digoxin was tried before sotalol was started. Sotalol was given orally to the mothers in a dose of 80 to 160 mg twice a day. Cardioversion was obtained in 10 fetuses. After birth, reentry tachycardia could be documented in seven of these patients and preexcitation in five patients. In two fetuses not responding to sotalol, a long R and P tachycardia was demonstrated; even when using digoxin, sotalol, flecainide, or propafenone in different combinations after birth, complete suppression of the arrhythmia was not obtained. Two severely hydropic fetuses died after beginning sotalol. The 12 surviving infants were doing well, except for one infant with a cerebral lesion probably related to the arrhythmia. These findings show that sotalol can be useful in the treatment of fetal supraventricular tachycardia.

PREGNANCY AND PATIENTS WITH HEREDITARY LONG QT SYNDROME

Zareba and colleagues[61] evaluated the effects of pregnancy on women with hereditary long QT syndrome. The study was a retrospective analysis of 422 women, including 111 probands affected with the long QT syndrome and 311 first-degree relatives enrolled in a long QT syndrome registry who had one or more pregnancies. The first-degree relatives were classified as affected, with a QTc of more than 0.47; borderline, with a QTc equal to 0.45 to 0.47; and unaffected, with a QTc of less than 0.45. The incidence of cardiac events was defined as the combined incidence of long QT syndrome–related death, aborted cardiac arrest, and syncope. The frequency of cardiac events was compared during pregnancy and postpartum intervals of 40 weeks each. Multivariate logistic regression analysis was performed to identify independent predictors of cardiac events among the probands. The pregnancy and postpartum intervals were not associated with cardiac events among first-degree relatives. The postpartum interval was independently associated with cardiac events among probands; the pregnancy interval was not associated with cardiac events. Treatment with beta-adrenergic blockers was independently associated with a decrease in the risk for cardiac events among the probands. Thus, the postpartum interval is associated with a significant increase in risk for cardiac events among probands with the long QT syndrome but not among first-degree relatives. Prophylactic treatment with beta-adrenergic blockers should be continued during the pregnancy and at postpartum intervals in probands with the long QT syndrome.

One recent case report from Mache and colleagues[62] describes a neonate who presented with sustained irregular heart rate during labor and was found to have QT prolongation and repetitive polymorphic ventricular tachycardia (torsades de pointes) postnatally. Propranolol and propafenone successfully controlled the ventricular arrhythmias. Follow-up electrocardiograms and Holter records showed persistent QT prolongation and intermittent episodes of T-wave alternans. On propranolol monotherapy, the young child did well and during follow-up was free of ventricular arrhythmias.

OBSTETRIC DRUGS WITH CARDIAC EFFECTS

To reduce the incidence of premature delivery, tocolytics such as terbutaline are used to stop premature labor.[63] These agents may cause maternal tachycardia and are hazardous in patients with mitral stenosis and some other forms of cardiovascular disease.[57, 63] Terbutaline should not be used in patients with underlying heart disease or hypertension, because it has been associated with maternal pulmonary edema, especially when corticosteroids are used to promote fetal lung maturation.[58, 63] Synthetic oxytocin is preferable to the natural product because it is free of pressor agents. It can be given to minimize blood loss after delivery but should be administered slowly, because bolus injection may cause hypotension. Prostaglandins employed in small doses to induce abortion or labor do not usually produce significant hemodynamic effects, but maternal flushing, tachycardia, and hypotension occur when too large a dose is given. Injection of hypertonic solutions into the uterus to produce abortion may result in hypervolemia and, in some cases, hypernatremia, causing intravascular volume overload in the mother.

References

1. Lilja H, Karlsson K, Lindecranz K, et al: Treatment of intrauterine supraventricular tachycardia with digoxin and verapamil. J Perinat Med 12:151, 1984.
2. Spinnato JA, Shaver DC, Flinn GS, et al: Fetal supraventricular tachycardia: In utero therapy with digoxin and quinidine. Obstet Gynecol 64:730, 1984.
3. Rotmensch HH, Elkayam U, Frishman W: Antiarrhythmic drug therapy during pregnancy. Ann Intern Med 98:487, 1983.
4. Mitani GM, Steinberg I, Lien E, et al: The pharmacokinetics of antiarrhythmic agents in pregnancy and lactation. Clin Pharmacokinet 12: 253, 1987.
5. Mitani GM, Harrison EC, Steinberg I, et al: Digitalis glycosides in pregnancy. In Elkayam U, Gleicher N (eds): Cardiac Problems in Pregnancy, 2nd Ed. Alan R Liss, New York, 1990, pp 417–428.
6. Valdes R Jr: Endogenous digoxin-like immunoreactive factors: Impact on digoxin measurements and potential physiologic implications. Clin Chem 31:1525, 1985.
7. Given BD, Phillippe M, Sanders SP, et al: Procainamide cardioversion of fetal supraventricular tachyarrhythmia. Am J Cardiol 53:1460, 1984.
8. Zielinsky P, Dillenburg RF, de Lima GG, Zimmer LP: Fetal supraventricular tachyarrhythmias: Experience of a fetal cardiology referral center. Arq Bras Cardiol 79:337–340 1998.
9. Parilla BV, Strasburger JF, Socol ML: Fetal supraventricular tachycardia complicated by hydrops fetalis: A role for direct fetal intramuscular therapy. Am J Perinatol 13:483–486, 1996.
10. Petrikovsky B, Schneider E, Ovadia M: Natural history of hydrops resolution in fetuses with tachyarrhythmias diagnosed and treated in utero. Fetal Diagn Ther 11:292–295, 1996.
11. Guntheroth WG, Cyr DR, Shields LE, Nghim HV: Rate-based management of supraventricular tachycardia. J Ultrasound Med 15:453–458, 1996.
11a. Villain E, Butera G, Bonnet D, et al: Neonatal ventricular tachycardia. Arch Mal Coeur Vaiss 91:623–629, 1998.
12. Bocci A, Pupita F, Revelli E, et al: The water-salt metabolism in obstetrics and gynecology. Minerva Ginecol 17:103, 1965.
13. Barrett RJ, Rayburn WF, Barr M Jr: Furosemide (Lasix) challenge test in assessing bilateral fetal hydronephrosis. Am J Obstet Gynecol 147: 846, 1983.
14. Pulle C: Diuretic therapy in monosymptomatic edema of pregnancy. Minerva Med 56:1622, 1965.
15. DeCecco L: Furosemide in the treatment of edema in pregnancy. Minerva Med 56:1586, 1965.
16. Sibai BM, Grossman RA, Grossman HG: Effects of diuretics on plasma volume in pregnancies with long-term hypertension. Am J Obstet Gynecol 150:831, 1984.
17. Carswell W, Semple PF: The effect of furosemide on uric acid levels in maternal blood, fetal blood and amniotic fluid. J Obstet Gynaecol Br Commonw 81:472, 1974.
18. Jerkner K, Kutti J, Victorin L: Platelet counts in mothers and their newborn infants with respect to antepartum administration of oral diuretics. Acta Med Scand 194:473, 1973.
19. Rodriquez SU, Leikin SL, Hiller MC: Neonatal thrombocytopenia associated with ante-partum administration of thiazide drugs. N Engl J Med 270:881, 1964.
20. Committee on Drugs, American Academy of Pediatrics: Transfer of drugs and other chemicals into human milk. Pediatrics 84:924, 1989.
21. Peng ATC, Gorman RS, Shulman SM, et al: Intravenous nitroglycerin for uterine relaxation in the postpartum patient with retained placenta. Anesthesiology 71:172, 1989.
22. Snyder SW, Wheeler AS, James FM III: The use of nitroglycerin to control severe hypertension of pregnancy during cesarean section. Anesthesiology 51:563, 1979.
23. Snyder SW, Wheeler AS, James FM III: The use of nitroglycerin

to control severe hypertension of pregnancy during cesarean section. Anesthesiology 51:563, 1979.
24. Cotton DB, Longmire S, Jones MM, et al: Cardiovascular alterations in severe pregnancy-induced hypertension: Effects of intravenous nitroglycerin coupled with blood volume expansion. Am J Obstet Gynecol 154:1053, 1986.
25. Broughton Pipkin F, Turner SR, Symonds EM: Possible risk with captopril in pregnancy: Some animal data. Lancet 1:1256, 1980.
26. Duminy PC, Burger PT: Fetal abnormality associated with the use of captopril during pregnancy. S Afr Med J 60:805, 1981.
27. Broude AM: Fetal abnormality associated with captopril during pregnancy. S Afr Med J 61:68, 1982.
28. Guignard JP, Burgener F, Calame A: Persistent anuria in a neonate: A side effect of captopril? Int J Pediatr Nephrol 2:133, 1981.
29. Smith AM: Are ACE inhibitors safe in pregnancy? Lancet 2:750, 1989.
30. Kreft-Jais C, Plouin P-F, Tchobroutsky C, et al: Angiotensin-converting enzyme inhibitors during pregnancy: A survey of 22 patients given captopril and nine given enalapril. Br J Obstet Gynaecol 95:420, 1988.
31. Rothberg AD, Lorenz R: Can captopril cause fetal and neonatal renal failure? Pediatr Pharmacol 4:189, 1984.
32. Rosa FW, Bosco LA, Graham CF, et al: Neonatal anuria with maternal angiotensin-converting enzyme inhibition. Obstet Gynecol 74:371, 1989.
33. Millar JA, Wilson PD, Morrison N: Management of severe hypertension in pregnancy by a combined drug regimen including captopril: Case report. Aust NZ Med J 96:796, 1983.
34. Boutroy MJ, Vert P, Hurault de Ligny B, et al: Captopril administration in pregnancy impairs fetal angiotensin converting enzyme activity and neonatal adaptation. Lancet 2:935, 1984.
35. Knott PD, Thorpe SS, Lamont CAR: Congenital renal dysgenesis possibly due to captopril. Lancet 1:451, 1989.
36. Develin RG, Fleiss PM: Captopril in human blood and breast milk. J Clin Pharmacol 21:110, 1981.
37. Postmarketing surveillance for angiotensin-converting enzyme inhibitor use during the first trimester of pregnancy—United States, Canada, and Israel, 1987–1995. MMWR 46:240–242, 1997.
38. Rigg D, McDonogh A: Use of sodium nitroprusside for deliberate hypotension during pregnancy. Br J Anaesth 53:985, 1981.
39. Dochin Y, Amirav B, Sahar A, et al: Sodium nitroprusside for aneurysm surgery in pregnancy. Br J Anaesth 50:849, 1978.
40. Paul J: Clinical report of the use of sodium nitroprusside in severe preeclampsia. Anaesth Intensive Care 3:72, 1975.
41. Willoughby JS: Case reports: Sodium nitroprusside, pregnancy and multiple intracranial aneurysms. Anaesth Intensive Care 12:358, 1984.
42. Stempel JE, O'Grady JP, Morton MJ, et al: Use of sodium nitroprusside in complications of gestational hypertension. Obstet Gynecol 60:533, 1982.
43. Holbrook RH Jr: Effects of calcium antagonists during pregnancy. Am J Obstet Gynecol 160:1018, 1989.
44. Gilbert RD: Effects of calcium antagonists during pregnancy. Reply. Am J Obstet Gynecol 160:1018, 1989.
45. Klein V, Repke JT: Supraventricular tachycardia in pregnancy: Cardioversion with verapamil. Obstet Gynecol 63:165, 1984.
46. Read MD, Wellby DE: The use of calcium antagonist (nifedipine) to suppress preterm labour. Br J Obstet Gynaecol 93:933, 1986.
47. Lindow SW, Davies N, Davey DA, et al: The effect of sublingual nifedipine on uteroplacental blood flow in hypertensive pregnancy. Br J Obstet Gynaecol 95:1276, 1988.
48. Ehrenkranz RA, Ackerman BA, Hulse JD: Nifedipine transfer into human milk. J Pediatr 114:478, 1989.
49. Pruyn SC, Phelan JP, Buchanan GC: Long-term propranolol therapy in pregnancy: Maternal and fetal outcome. Am J Obstet Gynecol 135: 485, 1979.
50. Pyeritz RE: Propranolol retards aortic root dilatation in the Marfan syndrome. Circulation 68(Suppl III):365, 1983.
51. Sabom MB, Curry RC, Wise DE: Propranolol therapy during pregnancy in a patient with idiopathic hypertrophic subaortic stenosis: Is it safe? South Med J 71:328, 1978.
52. Datta S, Kitzmiller JL, Ostheimer GW, et al: Propranolol and parturition. Obstet Gynecol 51:577, 1978.
53. Eliahou HE, Silverberg DS, Reisin E, et al: Propranolol for the treatment of hypertension in pregnancy. Br J Obstet Gynaecol 85:431, 1978.
54. Habib A, McCarthy JS: Effects on the neonate of propranolol administered during pregnancy. J Pediatr 91:808, 1977.
55. Sabom M, Curry C, Wise D: Propranolol therapy during pregnancy in a patient with idiopathic hypertrophic subaortic stenosis: Is it safe? South Med J 71:328, 1978.
56. Rubin PC: Beta-blockers in pregnancy. N Engl J Med 305:1323, 1981.
57. Strigal R, Pfeiffer U, Aschenbrenner G, et al: Influence of the B-1 selective blocker, metoprolol, on the development of pulmonary edema in tocolytic therapy. Obstet Gynecol 67:537, 1986.
58. Ross MG, Strubblefield PG, Kitzmiller JL: Intravenous terbutaline and simultaneous B-1 blockage for advanced premature labor. Am J Obstet Gynecol 147:897, 1983.
59. Lip GY, Beevers M, Churchill D, Shaffer LM, Beevers DG: Effect of atenolol on birth weight. Am J Cardiol 79:1436, 1997.
60. Sonesson SE, Fouron JC, Wesslen-Eriksson E, et al: Foetal supraventricular tachycardia treated with sotalol. Acta Paediatr 87:584–587, 1998.
61. Rashba EJ, Zareba W, Moss AJ, et al: Influence of pregnancy on the risk for cardiac events in patients with hereditary long QT syndrome. LQTS Investigators. Circulation 97:451–456, 1998.
62. Mache CJ, Beitzke A, Haidvogl M Jr, et al: Perinatal manifestations of idiopathic long QT syndrome. Pediatr Cardiol 17:118–121, 1996.
63. Ingemarsson I: Cardiovascular complications of terbutaline for premature labor. Am J Obstet Gynecol 142:117, 1982.

CHAPTER 31

Primary Pulmonary Hypertension and Pregnancy

Adaani E. Frost

INTRODUCTION

Primary pulmonary hypertension (PPH), a rare disease, is usually seen in women of childbearing age. This chapter covers the potential impact of pregnancy on the onset of PPH, and the effects of pregnancy on mother and child in patients with established PPH.

ROLE OF PREGNANCY IN DISEASE ONSET

The impact of pregnancy on hemodynamic factors in healthy women and in those with congenital heart disease and valvular heart disease has been reviewed in other chapters. Given the physiologic and hemodynamic consequences of pregnancy, one might expect that pregnancy would frequently unmask pre-existing pulmonary hypertension, and that a significant association would exist between pregnancy and new-onset or newly diagnosed PPH. In addition, because thrombosis contributes to the progression of PPH, one might expect that the additional risks of thrombosis associated with pregnancy could accelerate or potentially initiate pulmonary hypertension in predisposed patients. However, in a review of 73 women of childbearing age (15 to 50 years old) who had PPH, the timing of disease onset or deterioration was related to pregnancy in only 8% of cases.[1]

According to data from the Patient Registry for the Characterization of Primary Pulmonary Hypertension commissioned by the National Heart, Lung, and Blood Institute of the National Institutes of Health and Prevention (NIH), the live birth rate per patient in the registry was 2.3, and 54% of the patients had taken oral contraceptives at some time. These data are similar to those in the general population.[2] Furthermore, previous reports suggest that neither pregnancy[3] nor oral contraceptive use[4] appears to cause PPH. These findings appear counterintuitive considering the contribution of thrombosis to the evolution of PPH; thus, as yet unrecognized factors (hormones, or endogenous vasodilators associated with pregnancy) may reduce the risk of thromboembolism in pregnant women.

THE IMPACT OF PREGNANCY ON PRIMARY PULMONARY HYPERTENSION

Pregnancy in association with established PPH is a lethal condition; mortality can be as high as 50%.[5] Primary pulmonary hypertension is considered a contraindication to pregnancy. In a review of English-language journals, only 34 cases of pregnancy in patients with PPH have been reported since 1963.[3, 6–19] In these reports, patient outcome was poor. Only 14 of the 34 (41%) patients survived. In addition, the likelihood of survival in pregnant patients with PPH was not greater in the recent articles. Although more sensitive diagnostic techniques allow for earlier diagnosis, and newer treatment options have increased survival in nonpregnant patients, the survival benefit for the pregnant patient has not improved. Thus, a clear plan for prenatal care, delivery, and postpartum care should be based on experience and general physiologic principles.

PRENATAL MANAGEMENT

Early recognition of PPH in a pregnant patient is critical to successful outcome of the pregnancy. Only inferences rather than verifiable conclusions can be drawn from a review of the literature because the number of patients studied has been small and information on patients has been incomplete.

Better prenatal care in this high-risk situation should have a beneficial effect on patient and infant survival. In the above-mentioned studies, most patients who survived presented earlier in the course of pregnancy than did nonsurvivors (13 to 27 weeks versus 24 to 38 weeks).

As expected, patients with more severe pulmonary hypertension at presentation and delivery had a significantly poorer outcome. All patients who died had enlarged, pulsatile livers on clinical examination or indirect evidence of passive congestion of the liver as shown on results of liver function tests. Similarly, significant lower limb edema was reported with greater frequency in nonsurvivors.

Cardiac output increases significantly during pregnancy. Therefore, a lower cardiac output should be a marker of worse right ventricular function and should be associated with an increased mortality. In pregnant patients with PPH, the likelihood of death was higher with a lower cardiac output as measured by thermodilution with a Swan-Ganz catheter. Cardiac output was 4.5 to 5.9 L/min in patients who underwent catheterization and survived.

An effective cardiac output supports an effective systemic blood pressure. Nonsurvivors tended to have lower mean and systolic blood pressures than did survivors. Acceptable blood pressure readings or modest hypertension was seen in survivors.

As in the general population of patients with PPH, pulmonary artery pressure (systolic, diastolic, or mean) did not predict survival.

During prenatal care, cardiac status should be carefully assessed by performing a diagnostic right-sided heart catheterization, and end-organ (liver and kidney) function should be evaluated.

Routine treatment of PPH should be optimized according to the principles outlined in Chapter 8. However, heparin should replace warfarin for routine anticoagulation. Whereas the use of calcium channel blockers in pregnancy is well established, the safety of continuous intravenous prostacyclin has not been evaluated. In patients in whom conventional therapy with calcium channel blockers has failed, continuous intravenous prostacyclin should be considered after discussing the risks and benefits. Data suggest that disturbances in the endogenous production of prostacyclin may play a role in the development of pregnancy-associated hypertension and pre-eclampsia. Although the potential impact of long-term infusions of prostacyclin on fetal development and uterine contractions is unknown, epoprostenol (a synthetic prostacyclin) should be used judiciously and with informed consent in patients in whom conventional therapy has failed. Although isoproterenol has been used as an alternative to epoprostenol, there are no data on the long-term use of isoproterenol as a vasodilator. Administration of oxygen, which is an effective vasodilator, should be considered. Digoxin is generally regarded as part of conventional therapy.

DELIVERY

Although maternal outcome is similar with vaginal delivery and cesarean section, cesarean section should be reserved for obstetric indications, such as arrested labor, cephalopelvic disproportion, and fetal distress. Vaginal delivery is probably less risky; however, active pushing during labor should be avoided in patients with PPH. A Valsalva maneuver, which is required during active pushing, significantly reduces venous return and raises intrapleural pressures. This maneuver is likely to precipitate acute right ventricular strain and decreased cardiac output, which will jeopardize mother and infant.

The benefits of using Swan-Ganz catheterization to monitor status during delivery have not been proved. Mortality does not seem to be affected by diligent monitoring during delivery. In fact, at least one death has been related to the removal of the Swan-Ganz catheter. However, therapeutic options were limited in earlier studies, and outcome probably reflected the limited treatment options and a lack of understanding of the disease rather than an adverse outcome of monitoring. Monitoring the patient during delivery and the postpartum period should include electrocardiogram, routine fetal monitoring, continuous pulse oximetry, blood pressure (either noninvasive cuff or arterial line), and a multilumen central line for the administration of inotropes, vasodilators, fluid, and blood. In addition, the following types of monitoring should also be available in case the patient requires respiratory or circulatory support: oximetric Swan-Ganz catheterization (preferably with continuous cardiac output capacity) and anesthesia support to manage analgesia.

Inhalation anesthesia can produce vasodilation with a reduction in pulmonary vascular resistance. The judicious use of epidural catheters is an alternative for managing pain in the second stage of labor. Hypotension in a patient with PPH can precipitate cardiac arrest because the patient has little or no ability to increase cardiac output in response to systemic hypotension. A peripheral vasoconstrictor should be used to counteract the peripheral vasodilating effect of the analgesia- and epidural-induced hypotension. Two vasoconstrictors that can be used are neosynephrine, which has no inotropic effect, and dopamine, which has some inotropic effect on the right and left sides of the heart. In cases of postpartum hypotension associated with a decrease in cardiac output, the use of a vasodilator with inotropic effect is preferable (e.g., amrinone). Long-acting narcotics or sedatives should be avoided because of the potential for hypotension. Although epidural, caudal, and pudendal blocks can pose problems, these may be the wisest choices for pain control during delivery.

Anticoagulation should be reversed before the onset of labor. In marginal patients or in those with a tendency for thrombosis (e.g., a history of deep venous thrombosis or questionable ventilation perfusion lung scans), placement of an inferior vena caval filter should be considered. Although there are no data on the use of caval filters in this high-risk population, reanticoagulation in the immediate postpartum period is associated with a risk of significant bleeding, and reversal of anticoagulation before a prolonged labor leaves a supine, relatively immobile patient at risk for deep venous thrombosis and pulmonary embolus.

Significant blood loss should be replaced expeditiously. However, precipitous volume loading of the right side can result in further right ventricular distension, compromise of the left ventricular cavity caused by septal shift, and a further decline in cardiac output. Thus, aggressive replacement of fluids is a poor choice for the same reasons and is unlikely to be beneficial in treating systemic hypotension. In patients with a patent foramen ovale (PFO), systemic hypotension or increasing pulmonary vascular resistance can result in significant oxygen desaturation caused by enhancement of the right-to-left shunt through the PFO. In these patients, systemic vascular resistance should be increased by administering vasoconstrictors with or without inotropic capacity, and pulmonary vasodilators such as oxygen, nitric oxide, prostacyclin, and alprostadil (synthetic prostaglandin E_1 [PGE_1]) should be used. These regional or short-acting vasodilators have little or no effect on the systemic vascular resistance. An alternative pulmonary vasodilator is amrinone, which has a powerful pulmonary vascular vasodilator effect and a positive inotropic action on the heart, but it can decrease systemic vascular resistance. No studies on the use of amrinone in this setting have been reported. Amrinone is often used for decreasing pulmonary vascular resistance in difficult cardiovascular surgical cases. In addition, amrinone has been used in a few cases of pulmonary hypertension. Dobutamine, which has a positive inotropic effect and is a vasodilator, is contraindicated during labor because it decreases uteroplacental flow.

POSTPARTUM CARE

The postpartum period is inexplicably associated with a high mortality in patients with PPH. Although the earliest case reports of pregnancy and delivery in patients with PPH frequently described death during the second stage of labor or immediately after delivery, recent case reports indicate that patients usually survive this hemodynamically challenging period. A pattern of late death from 1 to 14 days postpartum has emerged. The cause of death is usually sudden massive cardiovascular collapse.

Potential risks during the postpartum period include deep venous thrombosis, pulmonary embolus, bleeding, infection (endometritis, mastitis, urinary tract infection, pneumonia), fluid and electrolyte disturbances, arrhythmias (related to electrolyte disturbances), and atelectasis.

In these high-risk patients, sequelae of a common postpartum condition can be life threatening. Anticoagulation should be resumed as early after delivery as possible, even if the patient has had a caval filter, because in situ thrombosis appears to be part of the pathophysiology of PPH. Anticoagulation is not beneficial in patients with Eisenmenger's syndrome[20] and has contributed to postpartum bleeding. The physiology and the contribution of thrombosis to the disease is clearly different in patients with Eisenmenger's syndrome, and anticoagulation should be used cautiously because of concerns about bleeding.

Blood loss should be carefully assessed, and the patient should receive transfusions earlier than the usual patient. In addition, a higher hemoglobin level should be attained in patients with PPH, especially in patients with a significant right-to-left shunt caused by a PFO. These patients are usually cyanotic or have marginal oxygenation and require a hematocrit level of 55% to 60% to maintain adequate tissue oxygenation.

The differential diagnosis of sudden oxygen desaturation in the postpartum patient with PPH should include the development of a PFO or an increased shunt resulting from the above-mentioned mechanisms.

Another cause of oxygen desaturation in these patients is the development of an intrapulmonary shunt, which occurs when a supine patient with cardiomegaly develops basal atelectasis (usually in the left lower lobe). Under normal circumstances, hypoxic vasoconstriction to the area of atelectatic lung would shunt blood to normally ventilated areas of lung, thus preserving ventilation and perfusion matching. In patients with significant pre-existing pulmonary hypertension, such local vasoconstriction does not occur or (more likely) does not prevent ongoing perfusion of the unventilated lung. This situation creates an intrapulmonary shunt, with resulting hypoxemia that is unresponsive to increasing FiO_2. Rapid recognition of atelectasis on chest radiograph and physical examination and initiation of aggressive physiotherapy and incentive spirometry are essential. This condition is easier to prevent than to treat, and routine incentive spirometry should be part of both prenatal and postnatal care. Withholding physiotherapy in a patient with low oxygen saturation in this setting results in progression of the condition.

Early recognition of infection and appropriate treatment is warranted in patients with PPH. The febrile patient should be monitored in an intensive care setting. Early ambulation of these patients, including removal of indwelling bladder catheters, and careful attention to venous access lines will help minimize the likelihood of infection, deep venous thrombosis, and atelectasis. The Swan-Ganz catheter should be removed within 24 hours if the patient is hemodynamically stable. In addition, a clean central line should be maintained until the patient is hemodynamically stable, infection-free, and mobile. Routine intensive care unit recommendations for the care of central lines should be followed; lines where one or more ports are blocked should be removed and a new line inserted if it is clinically indicated. Furthermore, lines should be replaced in patients with fever.

In addition to routine care, late postpartum care should include re-evaluation of the pulmonary hypertension and noninvasive assessment of hemodynamic status.

IMPACT ON BABY

Although fetal mortality was high (40%) in early reports,[3] the deaths were associated with maternal death, elective and spontaneous abortion, and congenital cardiac disease (in one patient). Patients who carry the pregnancy successfully to term usually have a live, healthy baby.

CONCLUSION

Few data are available on the appropriate management of the patient with PPH before, during, and after birth. Maternal mortality is high. Patients should consider terminating the pregnancy in difficult situations, and appropriate contraception should be instituted.

References

1. Dawkins KD, Burke CM, Billingham ME, Jamieson SW: Primary pulmonary hypertension and pregnancy. Chest 89:383, 1986.
2. Rich S, Dantzker DR, Ayres SM, et al: Primary pulmonary hypertension. A national prospective study. Ann Intern Med 107: 216, 1987.
3. McCaffrey RM, Dunn LJ: Primary pulmonary hypertension in pregnancy. Obstet Gynecol Surv 19:567, 1964.
4. Kleiger RE, Boxer M, Ingham RE, Harrison DC: Pulmonary hypertension in patients using oral contraceptives. Chest 69:143, 1976.
5. Roberts NV, Keast PJ: Pulmonary hypertension and pregnancy—a lethal combination. Anaesth Intensive Care 18:366, 1990.
6. Sinnenberg RJ: Pulmonary hypertension in pregnancy. South Med J 73:1529, 1980.
7. Sorenssen MB, Korshin JD, Fernandes A, Secher O: The use of epidural analgesia for delivery in a patient with pulmonary hypertension. Acta Anaesth Scand 26:180, 1982.
8. Abboud TK, Raya J, Noueihed R, Daniel J: Intrathecal morphine for relief of labor pain in a parturient with severe pulmonary hypertension. Anesthesiology 59:477, 1983.
9. Feijen HWH, Hein PR, Van Lakwijk-Vondrovicova EL, Nijhuis GMM: Primary pulmonary hypertension and pregnancy. Eur J Obstet Gynecol Reprod Biol 15:159, 1983.
10. Nelson DM, Main E, Crafford W, Ahumada GG: Peripartum heart failure due to primary pulmonary hypertension. Obstet Gynecol 62: 58, 1983.
11. Tsou E, Waldhorn RE, Kerwin DM, et al: Pulmonary venoocclusive disease in pregnancy. Obstet Gynecol 64:281, 1984.
12. Roessler P, Lambert TF: Anaesthesia for caesarean section in the presence of primary pulmonary hypertension. Anaesth Intensive Care 14:317, 1986.
13. Takeuchi T, Nishii O, Okamura T, Yaginuma T: Primary pulmonary hypertension in pregnancy. Int J Gynecol Obstet 26:145, 1988.
14. Slomka F, Salmeron S, Zetlaoui P, et al: Primary pulmonary hypertension and pregnancy: Anesthetic management for delivery. Anesthesiology 69:959, 1988.
15. Robinson DE, Leicht CH: Epidural analgesia with low-dose bupivacaine and fentanyl for labor and delivery in a parturient with severe pulmonary hypertension. Anesthesiology 68:285, 1988.
16. Nootens M, Rich S: Successful management of labor and delivery in primary pulmonary hypertension. Am J Cardiol 71:1124, 1993.

17. Martinez JM, Comas C, Sala X, et al: Maternal primary pulmonary hypertension associated with pregnancy. Eur J Obstet Gynecol Reprod Biol 54:143, 1994.
18. Smedstad KG, Cramb R, Morison DH: Pulmonary hypertension and pregnancy: A series of eight cases. Can J Anaesth 41:502, 1994.
19. Kiss H, Egarter C, Asseryanis E, et al: Primary pulmonary hypertension in pregnancy: A case report. Am J Obstet Gynecol 172:1052, 1995.
20. Pitts JA, Crosby WM, Basta LL: Eisenmenger's syndrome in pregnancy: Does heparin prophylaxis improve the maternal mortality rate? Am Heart J 93:321, 1977.

SECTION

IX

VASCULAR DISEASE

CHAPTER

32 Deep Venous Thrombosis

32.1 Pathophysiology

Gerald S. Cyprus

PATHOPHYSIOLOGY

Venous thrombosis—the presence of a thrombosis in a vein—occurs primarily in the lower extremities[1] but may occur in any venous system. The basic mechanism is usually one of stasis or slowing of flow.[2–4] Thrombosis at sites outside the lower extremities usually signals (1) unusual mechanisms, such as paroxysmal nocturnal hemoglobinuria,[5] (2) myeloproliferative disorders, such as polycythemia vera, or (3) deficiencies of antithrombin III, protein C, or protein S. The thrombus that forms in the venous system, termed a "red thrombus," consists primarily of coagulated blood and only small amounts of platelets. A "white thrombus," usually seen in arterial thrombosis, contains few or no red cells and is usually composed chiefly of platelets and fibrin. These platelets have an integral role in the genesis of a thrombus in the arterial circulation.

The coagulation process can begin with disruption or injury of the venous endothelium, which frequently occurs in surgical procedures; stasis in the postoperative period, particularly after abdominal and orthopedic procedures, exacerbates the process. Stasis alone can also produce thrombosis, perhaps because of a lack of dilution or inactivation of activated clotting factors.

CAUSES OF THROMBOSIS

The origin of thrombosis may be hereditary or acquired; in some cases, the causative factor is unknown. Liver disease in which there is decreased production of clotting inhibitors, such as proteins C and S, antithrombin III, and plasminogen, can be associated with a greater thrombotic tendency. The nephrotic syndrome, with its loss of protein (including these inhibitors), is also associated with thrombogenic potential.

The cause of venous thrombosis depends in part on its particular location in the body. *Upper-extremity thrombosis* can be related to presence of a venous catheter. Such a thrombosis can also result from hyperextension of the arm, such as that done in weight lifting. In the *lower extremity,* there is a very strong association between venous thrombosis and *stasis* following orthopedic or abdominal surgery. Fractures of the lower back, pelvis, or lower extremities likewise confer a greater tendency toward thrombosis.

General immobilization after myocardial infarction or stroke or in the setting of congestive heart failure may predispose a patient to stasis and subsequent thrombosis. *Obesity* also has been considered a risk factor for increased thrombotic tendency, particularly in individuals who are immobile.

Often associated with thrombosis are deficiencies of normal inhibitors of the clotting process, which can be inherited or acquired. These include *deficiencies of antithrombin III, protein C, and protein S.*[6] There is in addition a *hereditary resistance to activated protein C,*[7,8] which seems to be linked to an abnormality of factor V (Leiden mutation). It should be noted that the cause of thrombosis may not be apparent. The incidence of inherited deficiencies such as those of proteins C and S in the setting of recurrent thromboembolism is only 15%, whereas other factors that predispose to thrombosis, such as a patient's postoperative state, obesity, and pregnancy, are more apparent.

When one considers the low frequency with which these inherited deficiencies of natural anticoagulants occur in the normal population, it is easy to appreciate why the actual rate of diagnosis is less than 15%. Antithrombin III deficiency occurs in 1 in 2000 to 5000 people, and protein C deficiency or protein S deficiency in 1 in 16,000.

Use of *oral contraceptives,* particularly high-dose estrogens, has been associated with an increased tendency to thrombosis. Pregnancy,[9] particularly in the third trimester, also can predispose a woman to venous thrombosis.[8] This is in part related to the stasis caused by the gravid uterus, often of the left iliac vein. There is also a higher rate of venous thrombosis in the postpartum period, suggesting the presence of a hypercoagulable state.

Trousseau's syndrome involves *malignancies,* particularly adenocarcinomas, that are associated with an increased tendency toward clotting, which is often migratory or in multiple sites. This syndrome was originally described in association with carcinoma of the pancreas but also can be seen with other malignancies, such as those of the gastrointestinal tract, breast, and lung.

The *antiphospholipid syndrome,* with the presence of lupus anticoagulant or anticardiolipin antibody, can cause a thrombotic tendency, including a higher incidence of miscarriage. "Lupus anticoagulant" is actually a misnomer, as it refers to prolongation of the partial thromboplastin time resembling or suggesting a possible bleeding diathesis, whereas in reality, there is a potential for thrombosis.

Certain *hematologic conditions,* such as polycythemia vera, primary thrombocytosis, and paroxysmal nocturnal hemoglobinuria, can raise the potential for thrombosis, often in exotic sites such as the hepatic, portal, and splenic veins. In addition, deficiency of antithrombin III or protein C or S can be associated with these more uncommon thromboses.[10] Disseminated intravascular coagulation can, of course, be associated with bleeding or with thrombosis.

Certain *chemotherapeutic agents* have been associated with a thrombotic syndrome, including thrombotic thrombocytopenic purpura (caused by mitomycin). Pulmonary veno-occlusive disease has been seen with administration of bleomycin. The high-dose conditioning regimens given in preparation for marrow transplantation have been associated with the development of hepatic veno-occlusive disease. Methotrexate has been associated with hepatic vein occlusion. In one series of patients with breast cancer who were receiving chemotherapy in an adjuvant setting, a 10% incidence of venous thrombosis during the chemotherapy was found.

Heparin-induced thrombocytopenia with thrombosis syndrome (HITTS) has been noted with growing frequency, presumably because of greater clinician awareness.[11–13] Often this syndrome is first noted in the context of worsening thrombosis in a patient receiving heparin. The early tendency was to raise the heparin dosage, until it was revealed that heparin not only induced thrombosis but also, paradoxically, caused the thrombocytopenia. This effect is seen both with unfractionated heparin and with the newer low-molecular-weight heparins, albeit less frequently with the latter.

SITE-SPECIFIC THROMBOSES

In patients with hypercoagulability, most sites of thrombosis are venous rather than arterial. Exceptions (in which there may be greater arterial thrombosis) include the antiphospholipid syndrome (associated with anticardiolipin antibody, lupus anticoagulant, or both), sickle cell anemia, and paroxysmal nocturnal hemoglobinuria, as well as myocardial infarctions or strokes.

Superior vena caval thrombosis occurs in relation to mechanical obstruction by tumors of the upper mediastinum, such as those of lung cancer or lymphoma.[14] Occasionally, thrombosis of the subclavian vein, for example, from an indwelling infusion catheter, may propagate to produce vena caval thrombosis.

Inferior vena caval thrombosis has been associated with tumors such as hypernephroma, hepatocellular carcinoma,[15] and adrenal cortical carcinomas.[16, 17] This occlusion may result in hepatic venous thrombosis, or the so-called Budd-Chiari syndrome. This particular area of the circulation is vulnerable to thrombosis in the setting of the various hematologic disorders previously noted, including polycythemia vera, primary thrombocytosis, and paroxysmal nocturnal hemoglobinuria. Oral contraceptives and pregnancy have also been associated with thrombosis of the hepatic vein. Approximately one third of cases of the Budd-Chiari syndrome are idiopathic.[18–20]

Portal vein and splenic vein thromboses are also associated with tumor invasion and primary hematologic disorders such as polycythemia vera. In addition, there has been an association with intra-abdominal infections, biliary surgery, pregnancy, and oral contraceptives.

Mesenteric vein thrombosis most commonly is due to intra-abdominal infection but also is associated with hematologic disorders such as polycythemia vera.[21] Deficiencies of antithrombin III and proteins C and S are also associated with mesenteric vein thrombosis.

Renal vein thrombosis can be seen as an extension of thrombosis in the inferior vena cava. It is also associated with the nephrotic syndrome, probably through the loss of protective anticoagulants such as proteins C and S.[22]

Retinal vein thrombosis has been seen rarely in association with the antiphospholipid syndrome, but no association is yet noted with deficiency of antithrombin III or protein C or S.[23, 34] This thrombosis has been associated with local tumors, raised intravascular pressure, leukostasis, polycythemia, dysproteinemias, and hemoglobinopathies.

Adrenal vein thrombosis is seen with severe systemic stress, antiphospholipid syndrome, and the heparin-induced thrombocytopenia thrombosis syndrome.[25, 26]

SUMMARY

The pathophysiology and causes of venous thrombosis of the lower extremities are straightforward; this condition is commonly attributed to stasis or surgery. Thrombosis in more exotic locations, such as the hepatic venous system or portal caval system, is much less common and has an unusual pathogenesis. The heritable causes of thrombosis, such as protein C deficiency, should be considered in a young patient with thrombosis or in any patient with recurrent thromboses.

References

1. Alving BM, Comp PC: Recent advances in understanding clotting and evaluating patients with recurrent thrombosis. Am J Obstet Gynecol 167:1184, 1992.
2. Rhee RY, Gloviczki P, Luthra HS, et al: Iliocaval complications of retroperitoneal fibrosis. Am J Surg 168:179, 1994.
3. John TG, Chalmers N, Redhead DN, et al: Inferior vena caval thrombosis following severe liver trauma and perihepatic packing. Br J Radiol 68:314, 1995.
4. Paolillo V, Sicuro M, Nejrotti A, et al: Pulmonary embolism due to compression of the inferior vena cava by a hepatic hemangioma. Tex Heart Inst J 20:66, 1993.
5. Ishiguchi T, Fukatsu H, Itoh S, et al: Budd-Chiari syndrome with long segmental inferior vena cava obstruction in a case of paroxysmal nocturnal hemoglobinuria. J Vasc Interv Radiol 3:421, 1992.
6. Clouse LH, Comp PC: The regulation of hemostasis: The protein C system. N Engl J Med 314:1298, 1986.
7. Dahlback B: Resistance to activated protein C caused by mutation in factor V as a pathogenic risk factor for venous thrombosis. Thromb Haemost 74:139, 1995.
8. Bertina RM, Reitsma PH, Rosendaal FR, et al: Resistance to activated protein C and factor V Leiden as risk factors for venous thrombosis. Thromb Haemost 74:449, 1995.
9. Toglia MR, Weg JG: Venous thromboembolism during pregnancy. N Engl J Med 335:108, 1996.
10. Dhiman RK, Saraswat VA, Radhakrishnan S, et al: Multiple venous thromboses and membranous obstruction of inferior vena cava in association with hereditary protein C deficiency. J Gastroenterol Hepatol 7:434, 1992.
11. Chong BH: Heparin-induced thrombocytopenia. Br J Haematol 89:431, 1995.
12. Fondu P: Heparin-associated thrombocytopenia: An update. Acta Clin Belg 50:343, 1995.
13. Magnani HN: Heparin-induced thrombocytopenia. Thromb Haemost 70:554, 1993.
14. Parish JM, Marschke RF, Dines DE, et al: Etiologic considerations in superior vena cava syndrome. Mayo Clin Proc 56:407, 1981.
15. Mitomo O, Nakajima T, Kado B, et al: Useful interventional thrombolytic and anticoagulant therapy for thrombosis due to embolization in Budd-Chiari syndrome. Radiat Med 10:246, 1992.
16. Martinez-Ibanez V, Sanchez de Toledo J, DeDiego M, et al: Wilms' tumors with intracaval involvement. Med Pediatr Oncol 26:268, 1996.
17. Oberholzer HF, Falkson G, DeJager LC: Successful management of inferior vena cava and right atrial nephroblastoma tumor thrombus with preoperative chemotherapy. Med Pediatr Oncol 20:61, 1992.

18. Lu CL, Chou YH, Hwang SJ, et al: Membranous obstruction of inferior vena cava with Budd-Chiari syndrome in Taiwan. J Gastroenterol Hepatol 10:287, 1995.
19. Mitchell MD, Boitnott JK, Kaufman S, et al: Budd-Chiari syndrome: Etiology, diagnosis, and management. Medicine 61:199, 1982.
20. Klein AS, Cameron JL: Diagnosis and management of the Budd-Chiari syndrome. Am J Surg 160:128, 1990.
21. DeStefano V, Leone G, Teofili L, et al: Mesenteric vein thrombosis in protein S congenital deficiency. Thromb Res 57:935, 1990.
22. Llach F, Arieff AI, Massry SG: Renal vein thrombosis and nephrotic syndrome. Ann Intern Med 83:8, 1975.
23. Asherson RA, Merry P, Acheson JF, et al: Antiphospholipid antibodies: A risk factor for occlusive ocular vascular disease. Ann Rheum Dis 48:358, 1989.
24. Heckerlin PS, Froelich CJ, Schade SG: Retinal vein thrombosis in a patient with pernicious anemia and anticardiolipin antibodies. J Rheumatol 16:1144, 1989.
25. Alperin N, Babu S, Weinstein A: Acute adrenal insufficiency and the antiphospholipid syndrome. Ann Intern Med 111:950, 1989.
26. Findling JW, Korducki JM, Lahiri PK, et al: Bilateral adrenal hemorrhage associated with heparin-induced thrombocytopenia. Wis Med J 86:27, 1987.

32.2 Clinical Recognition, Diagnosis, and Management

Vincenzo Pasceri and James T. Willerson

Thrombophlebitis or *venous thrombosis* indicates the presence of thrombus within a superficial or deep vein and the accompanying inflammatory response in the vessel wall. Thrombosis of a deep vein of the legs is a common and serious disorder, potentially lethal because of its most deadly complication, pulmonary embolism.[1] Although more than 250,000 cases of deep venous thrombosis (DVT) and pulmonary embolism are diagnosed each year in the United States, these conditions are still largely underdiagnosed. Possibly as many as 50% of cases are not diagnosed correctly and do not receive proper treatment.[2] DVT frequently occurs in hospitalized patients, but it may occur in apparently healthy individuals in whom proper diagnosis and treatment may be delayed. Patients with DVT who are not adequately treated are at high risk of complications, including pulmonary embolism and chronic venous insufficiency. Unfortunately, signs and symptoms suggestive of DVT are sometimes nonspecific and very subtle, making the diagnosis difficult.

EPIDEMIOLOGY AND RISK FACTORS

It is difficult to determine the true incidence of DVT. Studies assessing the diagnosis of DVT in hospitalized patients may underestimate the incidence because they do not take into account the incidence in outpatients, in whom the condition often is underdiagnosed. In addition, the diagnosis should be confirmed by the appropriate test (usually venography). A community study based on hospital diagnoses performed in the United States has found an incidence of DVT of 4.8 per 10,000 (and 2.3 per 10,000 for pulmonary embolism). However, a prospective population study performed in Sweden, in which a group of 850 men aged 50 to 80 years were monitored, found higher incidences of both DVT (about 18 per 10,000 per year) and pulmonary embolism (20 per 10,000 per year).[3] A large autopsy study, with an autopsy frequency of 80% of the deaths occurring in the town of Malmoe, Sweden, confirmed these data.[4] In the United States, approximately 260,000 cases of thromboembolism (including pulmonary embolism) are diagnosed each year; it is estimated, however, that at least 500,000 cases of thromboembolism occur each year.

The pathophysiology of thrombophlebitis was initially described by Virchow in 1856 as the classic triad of stasis, vascular damage, and increase in blood coagulability. Although the simultaneous presence of all three factors is not common, the value of the original Virchow's triad has been confirmed by the modern studies on the pathogenesis of DVT. Owing to its peculiar pathogenic mechanisms, the risk factors for venous thrombosis are often different from those for arterial diseases.

Nonheritable Risk Factors

A number of clinical conditions have been associated with increased risk of venous thrombosis (Table 32–1). These conditions may affect one or more of the components of

Table 32–1. RISK FACTORS FOR DEEP VENOUS THROMBOSIS

Nonheritable risk factors	Previous thromboembolism
	Age >40 yr
	Surgery (lower limb or pelvic surgery or anesthesia >30 min)
	Trauma
	Paralysis
	Immobility
	Low cardiac output
	Pregnancy
	Oral contraceptive
	Estrogen treatment (including tamoxifen and raloxifene)
	Varicose veins
	Sepsis
Heritable risk factors	Factor V Leiden
	Increased levels of factor VIII
	Prothrombin 2
	Protein C deficiency
	Protein S deficiency
	Dysfibrinogenemia

Virchow's triad and can be classified as nonheritable and heritable factors.[5, 6] Among nonheritable factors, surgery, especially pelvic and spinal surgery, and immobility are probably the most important risk factors. Without proper prevention strategies, venous thrombosis may occur in more than 50% of patients undergoing orthopedic surgical procedures involving the hip or knee. The prevalence of venous thrombosis is particularly high in patients with malignancies, most especially in those undergoing surgery or with immobility. The risk of occult malignancies in patients with primary DVT or pulmonary embolism appears to be low, and an aggressive search for occult cancer is not usually warranted in these patients,[5] although the risk of cancer is higher in patients with recurrent thromboembolism.[8] Trauma (especially involving the spine, pelvis, or legs) is also associated with DVT. Congestive heart failure is associated with DVT, probably as a result of the associated venous stasis as well as coagulation abnormalities. Acute myocardial infarction is a risk factor for DVT, although modern treatments, including anticoagulants, thrombolytics, and early mobilization of patients, have greatly reduced the incidence of venous thrombosis and pulmonary embolism. Advanced age is a risk factor and is associated with many other risk factors for DVT. The incidence of DVT may be as low as 1 per 100,000 per year in childhood, but it reaches about 1 per 100 per year in subjects older than 80 years.

The risk of DVT is also higher during pregnancy and in the first month after delivery. Estrogens present in oral contraceptives may alter the coagulation balance and raise the risk of DVT. The increase in risk seems to be proportional to the estrogen dose. Use of low-dose estrogen oral contraceptives may still cause a three- or fourfold increase in the risk of DVT, but the absolute risk is very low (about 4 cases per 10,000 per year). Oral contraceptives are contraindicated in high-risk women, that is, women with history of thromboembolic disease, smokers older than 35 years, and women with hereditary coagulation abnormalities. Epidemiologic studies have suggested a higher risk of DVT with oral contraceptives containing third-generation progestins than with second-generation products, but these findings are still debated.[9] Hormone replacement treatment is also associated with a two- to fourfold increase in DVT in postmenopausal women. Treatment with the estrogen agonist-antagonists tamoxifen and raloxifene is also associated with higher risk for DVT.

The antiphospholipid syndrome, systemic lupus erythematosus (SLE), myeloproliferative disease, dysfibrinogenemia, and disseminated intravenous coagulation may also cause venous thrombosis. Venulitis occurring in thromboangiitis obliterans, Behçet's disease, and homocysteinuria also may cause venous thrombosis. The role of obesity as a risk factor is not clear and is probably related to its relationship with relative immobility.

Heritable Risk Factors

A number of hereditary disorders that alter the hemostatic balance are associated with DVT (Table 32–1).[10, 11] The most common (3% to 5% of white population) is factor V Leiden, a mutation of factor V (Arg506Gln) resulting in resistance to activated protein C.[12] Factor V Leiden is less common in nonwhite populations (prevalence about 2.2% among Hispanic Americans, 1.2% in African Americans, and 0.5% in Asian Americans).[13] Estimates of the risk associated with this mutation vary from a threefold to a sixfold increase.[14] The absolute incidence of venous thrombosis in carriers of this mutation is low, only about 6 to 10 per 10,000 per year; thus, the value of population screening for factor V Leiden is uncertain.

Prothrombin 20210A is a factor II (prothrombin) mutation that has been associated with higher risk of thrombosis.[15] Prothrombin 20210A is common in white populations, with a prevalence of about 2% to 4%. This mutation is more common in southern Europe than in northern Europe, and it is rare in individuals of Asian and African descent.[16] Prothrombin 20210A is associated with an increase in the risk of DVT, but the increase is probably smaller than that for factor V Leiden (relative risk about 2 to 3).[17]

Rare hereditary disorders that produce systemic hypercoagulability include antithrombin III deficiency and protein C and protein S deficiencies. Because these hereditary disorders are uncommon (their pooled prevalence is less than 1% of the population), it is difficult to accurately assess the risk of DVT. A reasonable estimate is that these disorders may be associated with about a five- to 10-fold increase in the risk of DVT. Risk may be higher with antithrombin III deficiency.

Increased levels of factor VIII are common. Levels 50% higher than the average are present in about 10% of the population and have been associated with a six-fold increase in the risk of DVT. Levels of factor VIII are determined by several genes, including those for the von Willebrand factor, the ABO blood group (individuals with group O blood have lower levels of factor VIII), and as yet unknown genes.

Hyperhomocysteinemia is associated with a moderate increase in the risk of venous thrombosis, and approximately a 2.5-fold increase in risk for people with homocysteine concentration more than two standard deviations higher than the population average. This condition may be due to mutations in the genes regulating homocysteine metabolism or vitamin deficiency.

The presence of multiple risk factors is common among patients with DVT, and the combination of different risk factors may have synergic effects. For instance, presence of both hyperhomocysteinemia and factor V Leiden is associated with a 10-fold increase in the risk of thromboembolic events.[18] The value of prevention strategies in people with multiple risk factors is still unclear.

HISTORY AND PHYSICAL EXAMINATION

Usually, DVT begins in the veins of the calf, but it may also arise directly from the femoral or iliac veins. Although the risk of pulmonary embolism for thrombi localized in the calf is low, calf thrombi propagate to femoral and iliac veins in about one quarter of cases.[19, 20] Approximately 50% of patients have no symptoms or signs in the early phases.[21] Conversely, up to 75% of patients in whom venous thrombosis is suspected do not have this problem when the appropriate diagnostic tests are performed. It is important to underscore that a clinical diagnosis of DVT based only on history and physical examination is often inaccurate.

Typical symptoms of DVT are pain, warmth, redness, and swelling in the calf or leg. Usual findings are edema, distention of collateral veins, and the presence of a palpable cord.[22] Cyanosis may be present if venous obstruction is severe. Cough or sneezing may provoke pain along the course of a vein ("Louvel's sign"). Pain or discomfort (manifested as resistance to dorsiflexion) may be provoked by dorsiflexion of the ankle ("Homans' sign"). Inflation of a sphygmomanometer cuff may induce pain in the affected calf at a pressure lower than the unaffected one ("Lowenberg's sign"). The dorsal veins of the feet may remain distended even after elevation of the legs (the so-called sentinel veins). Extensive thrombosis of the iliofemoral veins may produce the clinical picture of *phlegmasia cerulea dolens,* with acute edema and cyanosis of the leg and severe pain. *Phlegmasia alba dolens,* characterized by edema, pain, and paleness, is caused by marked edema exceeding capillary perfusion pressure. Distal gangrene and pulmonary embolism are common complications of these serious conditions. Affected patients often need treatment with thrombolytics or embolectomy.

Symptomatic DVT in the axillary and subclavian veins is uncommon and is associated with presence of central venous catheters, thrombophilic states, and previous history of thromboembolism in the legs. Pulmonary embolism occurs in approximately 10% of cases.[23] Ultrasonography is an accurate diagnostic method for this rare form of venous thrombosis.[24]

The differential diagnosis of DVT consists of calf muscle contusion, cellulitis, compression of the iliac vein, lymphedema, arterial occlusion, ruptured Baker's cyst, superficial thrombophlebitis, and chronic venous insufficiency. Bilateral leg swelling is more often due to systemic diseases (heart, kidney, or liver diseases). Although some of these conditions can be easily diagnosed, DVT should be identified or excluded with the appropriate diagnostic tests.

In summary, none of the clinical signs has a good sensitivity or specificity for diagnosis of DVT. Diagnostic tests are able to confirm the diagnosis of DVT only in approximately half of patients with clinical suspicion of DVT.[21] However, a clinical score may be used to limit the use of invasive procedures to confirm the diagnosis of DVT.

Wells and associates[25, 26] have proposed an integrated clinical score to be used in association with ultrasonography (Table 32–2).[25, 26] In their model, patients with a score of 3 or more points (high risk) had a frequency of DVT of approximately 75%; patients with a score of 1 or 2 (moderate risk) had a DVT frequency of 17%; and patients with a score of zero (low risk) had a 3% frequency of DVT.[26] Patients with both normal ultrasonography results and a low clinical score were unlikely to have DVT, and further invasive tests were not required. In patients with discordance between clinical findings and ultrasonography results—either a high or moderate clinical risk but apparently normal ultrasonography, or abnormal ultrasonography results but low clinical score—the diagnosis was confirmed by venography. Patients with moderate clinical risk but normal ultrasonography results underwent ultrasonography again after 1 week.

Table 32–2. CLINICAL SCORE FOR DEEP VENOUS THROMBOSIS

1. Assign 1 point for presence of each of the following:
   - Cancer
   - Paralysis or immobility of a limb
   - Recent major surgery or immobilization
   - Tenderness along the course of deep veins
   - Swelling of the leg
   - Swelling of the calf (>3 cm in diameter compared with the unaffected calf)
   - Pitting edema
   - Collateral superficial veins
2. Determine the score by adding the points assigned. Subtract 2 points if an alternative diagnosis is likely.
3. Determine the patient's risk as follows:
   - ≥3 points: High risk
   - 1–2 points: Moderate risk
   - 0 points: Low risk

Adapted from Wells PS, Anderson DR, Bomaris J, et al: Value of assessment of pretest probability of deep-vein thrombosis in clinical management. Lancet 350:1795, 1997.

DIAGNOSIS

Laboratory Testing

Among the laboratory tests that help in the diagnosis of DVT, circulating D-dimer (a derivative of crosslinked fibrin) is the most promising.[1, 27] Elevated (higher than 500 μg/ml) plasma levels of D-dimers as detected on enzyme-linked immunosorbent assay (ELISA) are very sensitive in detecting venous thrombosis (sensitivity, 93% to 98%). However, this assay is not specific for this condition (specificity only 25% to 38%).[28, 29] Nevertheless, because of their high sensitivity, D-dimer measurements have strong potential as exclusionary tests in patients with suspected venous thrombosis.[30] Although standard ELISAs are often time-consuming, several rapid ELISA and latex assays are currently available[27] the sensitivity of each test should be confirmed.[31] Because D-dimers have a very low specificity, their measurement can be used to rule out the presence of DVT, but positive test results must be confirmed by other diagnostic tests. Perrier and colleagues[32] have used D-dimer levels in a diagnostic strategy that includes ultrasonography, clinical score, and lung scan.[32]

Ultrasonography

Currently, duplex Doppler ultrasonography is the most widely used diagnostic test for DVT detection.[33, 34] Acute thrombi are usually anechoid but may be identified from incompressibility of the vein with light pressure of the transducer and/or from the presence of abnormal Doppler signals (absence of flow, loss of respiratory variations in venous flow). Lack of compressibility is considered the most reliable sign of DVT.[35] Positive ultrasonography results can be considered diagnostic for DVT and call for anticoagulant therapy. Compression ultrasonography has good sensitivity and specificity (both greater than 90%) for proximal vein thrombosis (including the popliteal vein). Sensitivity and specificity for proximal vein thrombosis are both higher than 95%.[25, 36, 37] However, sensitivity for calf vein thrombosis is only 50% to 80%.[25, 37, 38] Thus, serial ultrasonography evaluations are recommended for detection of extension of a calf DVT. Although ultrasonography remains highly specific in all groups of patients, its sensitivity is lower in asymptomatic patients (about 76% in proximal DVT and only 11% for calf thrombosis in a review of seven published studies).[37] A cost-effective diagnostic approach is to test patients with negative ultrasonography results for D-dimer levels; patients with negative D-dimer results are unlikely to have DVT, whereas patients with positive D-dimer results should undergo ultrasonography examination after 1 week to rule out extension of thrombosis into the proximal veins.[1] This strategy appears safe and may limit the performance of invasive tests.

Impedance Plethysmography

Impedance plethysmography is a functional test assessing the volume changes that occur in the limb when venous flow is enhanced or reduced. This test assesses changes in blood volume by determining voltage change when an electric current is passed through the limb. The test has a good sensitivity for diagnosis of DVT in the proximal veins. Its sensitivity for calf DVT is low.[39] Other causes of impaired venous flow (e.g., congestive heart failure, venous compression) may produce false-positive results of impedance plethysmography. Thus, the test has a good specificity for proximal DVT when it is positive in only one leg. Abnormal results in both legs can be nonspecific and should be confirmed by further tests. Impedance plethysmography requires access to the calf and thigh and cannot be used in uncooperative subjects or in patients with severe edema or marked obesity. Plethysmography is an easy bedside diagnostic test in symptomatic patients, but ultrasonography is more accurate.[38, 40] Some studies have also suggested a low sensitivity for impedance plethysmography in patients with no or minor symptoms (sensitivity only 65%),[41] possibly because of a lower sensitivity for the detection of popliteal and small proximal thrombi.[41a]

Contrast Venography

Contrast venography is considered the standard for diagnosis of DVT.[42] Presence of intraluminal filling defects is highly specific for DVT. This invasive test is expensive and uncomfortable and has limited risks (superficial phlebitis, hypersensitivity, and, rarely, minor thrombosis).[43] Use of a non-ionic contrast medium can reduce the incidence of side effects.[44] Thus, this test is not practical for follow-up monitoring and should be limited to the conditions in which a confirmatory test is really needed. Venography is particularly useful in diagnosis of thrombosis of the calf veins and when noninvasive test results are inconclusive. This test has some limitations in patients with previous thromboplebitis, in whom it is often difficult to distinguish acute from chronic thrombosis.

Other Tests

Radiographic scanning with fibrinogen I 125 can detect active clot formation. Although this technique is very sensitive for detecting the development of calf thrombi, it requires several hours and has been largely supplanted by less complex tests.

Radionuclide angiography using labeled macroaggregates of albumin has a good predictive value for proximal DVT, but it is not a reliable method for detection of calf thrombosis. Magnetic resonance imaging (MRI) can also be used for diagnosis of DVT.[45, 46] Although more experience is needed, MRI appears to be a reliable noninvasive alternative to venography and may allow better imaging of the pelvic veins. MRI also seems to have a better sensitivity than echography for proximal vein thrombosis.[47] The possibility of visualizing both peripheral veins and the lung in the same session is also another advantage of this technique.

Compression ultrasonography is usually the initial test. Both plethysmography and ultrasonography have good specificity, and a positive result of either is diagnostic. However, when results are negative, follow-up with second tests at 7 days is required. Alternatively, it is possible to use a high-sensitivity test, such as measuring for the presence of D-dimers; patients with negative D-dimer results are at low risk and do not require further investigation, but in patients with positive D-dimer results, the diagnosis must be confirmed by venography. Venography is the most accurate test, but it is usually reserved for patients in whom results of noninvasive tests are inconclusive.

PREVENTION

There are no simple and reliable tests for effective screening of patients for DVT, and only prevention strategies can reduce the incidence of DVT and pulmonary embolism. Prevention is not required for patients younger than 40 years old with no risk factors who are undergoing uncomplicated general surgery (risk of proximal vein thrombosis is less than 0.5%).[48] Patients at moderate risk for DVT include those who are undergoing major surgery (more than 30 minutes of anesthesia), who are older than 40 years, or who have risk factors (risk of proximal vein thrombosis, 1% to 4%). High-risk patients include patients undergoing orthopedic surgery (knee/hip surgery) or abdominal or pelvic surgery for malignancies, those with previous venous thromboembolism, and those with stroke or spinal cord injury (risk of proximal vein thrombosis 5% to 10%; risk of fatal pulmonary embolism, 1% to 5%).[48] Prevention strategies include mechanical measures, such as early mobilization and the use of compression stockings and external pneumatic compression, and pharmacologic treatments, including low-dose heparin, low-molecular-weight heparins, and oral anticoagulants. Complete guidelines for prevention of DVT have been published.[48]

Low-dose heparin (5000 U subcutaneously every 8 to 12 hours beginning 2 hours before surgery) is safe and effective in preventing DVT in patients with moderate risk who are undergoing surgery, but it is relatively ineffective in high-risk patients, such as those undergoing major hip, knee, or pelvic surgery (Table 32–3).[49] Low-molecular-weight (LMW) heparins given subcutaneously or adjusted-dose heparin given intravenously should be used in such high-risk patients. LMW heparins are as effective as unfractionated heparin in DVT prevention after general surgery and are more effective than low-dose unfractionated heparin in high-risk patients (undergoing major hip, knee or pelvic operations). LMW heparins are effective in a once-daily dose, but often a twice-daily dose has been used in clinical trials in high-risk patients (see Table 32–3).[50] It is not clear whether LMW heparins should be started before or after surgery in high-risk patients; however, the results of a meta-analysis suggest that

Table 32–3. PREVENTION STRATEGIES FOR DEEP VENOUS THROMBOSIS (DVT)

For the patient at moderate risk (age >40 yr or prolonged surgery [>30 min anesthesia] or other risk factors):
- Low-dose heparin, 5000 U SC 2 h before surgery and q 8–12 h.
- Low-molecular-weight heparins (e.g. dalteparin, 2500 U 1–2 h before surgery and once daily thereafter, or enoxaparin, 2000 U 1–2 hours before surgery and once daily thereafter.)

For the patient at high risk (abdominal or pelvic surgery for cancer, previous DVT, hypercoagulable status, knee/hip surgery, stroke/spinal cord injury):
- Adjusted-dose heparin (usually 3500 U SC q 8 h with aPTT 1.0–1.5).
- Oral anticoagulants starting the day before surgery (INR, 2.0–3.0).
- Low-molecular-weight heparin (e.g., dalteparin, 5000 U once daily starting 10–12 h before surgery, or enoxaparin 3000 U twice daily).
- Intermittent-compression devices in combination with anticoagulants or alone when anticoagulants are contraindicated.

aPTT, activated partial thromboplastin time; DVT, deep venous thrombosis; INR, international normalized ratio.

preoperative treatment is associated with a lower incidence of DVT.[51] Oral anticoagulants, started the day before surgery and with a target International Normalized Ratio (INR) of 2.0 to 3.0, are also effective in preventing DVT. External pneumatic compression devices can prevent DVT, especially when all anticoagulant regimens are contraindicated (such as with neurosurgery). The effects of aspirin alone in prevention of DVT are being tested in a large trial,[52] but aspirin is not currently recommended for prevention of DVT. Placement of a prophylactic inferior vena cava filter has been used in high-risk patients in whom anticoagulation is contraindicated.

The frequency of recurrent DVT is approximately 25% at 5 years and recurrence is strongly associated with the presence of cancer or of coagulation abnormalities.[53] Aggressive prevention strategies are required in affected patients.

TREATMENT

The aim of the treatment of venous thrombosis is to limit the risk of its complications, pulmonary embolism and chronic venous insufficiency.[41] Anticoagulation is the cornerstone of treatment of DVT. Patients with proximal DVT should receive anticoagulation therapy for at least 3 months. Anticoagulation does not directly lyse thrombi in the veins of the legs or in the pulmonary arteries, but it can block thrombus extension and allows natural fibrinolysis to occur. Acute anticoagulation should be obtained with heparin. Heparin acts on the natural anticoagulant factor, antithrombin III, which in turn inactivates thrombin (factor IIa) and factors IXa and Xa. Heparin should be administered as an intravenous bolus, followed by either intravenous infusion with a target-activated partial thromboplastin time (aPTT) of 1.5 to 2.5 as the control value, or as subcutaneous LMW heparin (Table 32–4).[54, 54a] Risk of recurrent thromboembolism is high when heparin treatment is inadequate (aPTT less than 1.5). Coagulation tests should be performed before treatment is begun, every 6 hours (or before each subcutaneous dose of heparin) until the aPTT is stable within therapeutic range, and daily thereafter. Nomograms can be used to adjust heparin infusion according to the aPTT. Platelet counts should be checked on a daily basis. Heparin has a narrow therapeutic index and may cause several complications, including major bleeding and heparin-induced thrombocytemia.[55] The incidence of major bleeding with heparin treatment is usually less than 5%. Heparin-induced thrombocytopenia raises the risk of both arterial and venous thromboembolism. Heparin should be stopped if the platelet count falls below 100,000/μl; a direct-acting antithrombin, such as hirudin, can be substituted.

Because patients with thrombosis localized in the calf are at low risk of pulmonary embolism, they either can be monitored with serial ultrasonography examinations for 1 to 2 weeks without anticoagulation, in order to exclude extension of thrombosis in the proximal veins, or can receive standard anticoagulation therapy for 3 months.[41, 56] Patients with symptomatic calf vein thrombosis may be at higher risk of proximal extension. One small randomized trial in 51 symptomatic patients found a higher rate of thromboembolic complications in patients with calf thrombosis not treated with anticoagulants than in patients who received 3 months of anticoagulation therapy.[57] However, several studies have confirmed the safety of monitoring with serial ultrasonography or plethysmography without anticoagulation in such patients.

Anticoagulant treatment should be administered for at least 3 months, and treatment with oral anticoagulants is required. Oral anticoagulants inhibit the synthesis of the coagulation factors II, VII, IX, and X and of the natural anticoagulants protein C and protein S. Because protein C has a short plasma half-life, oral anticoagulants can induce a paradoxical hypercoagulative status in the 1 to 2 days of treatment. Treatment with oral anticoagulants alone (without

Table 32–4. ACUTE ANTICOAGULATION REGIMENS IN VENOUS THROMBOEMBOLISM*

Heparin: 5000 U IV bolus + 750–1500 U/h infusion (aPTT, 1.5–2.5)[54]

aPTT	BOLUS	INFUSION
<45 sec (<1.5 control)	5000 U	+240 U/hr
46–54 sec (1.5–1.7 control)	0	+120 U/h
55–85 sec (1.7–2.7 control)	0	0
86–110 sec (2.7–3.5 control)	0	STOP 1 hour and −120 U/h
>110 sec (>3.5 control)	0	STOP 1 hour and −240 U/h

Weight-adjusted heparin: 80 U/Kg IV bolus + 18/U/Kg/h[54a]

aPTT	BOLUS	INFUSION
<35 sec (<1.2 control)	80 U/Kg	+4 U/Kg/h
35–45 sec (1.2–1.5 control)	40 U/Kg	+2 U/Kg/h
46–70 sec (1.5–2.3 control)	0	0
71–90 sec (2.3–3.0 control)	0	−2 U/Kg/h
>90 (>3.0 control)	0	STOP 1 hour and −3 U/Kg/h

Subcutaneous treatment: heparin 5000 U IV bolus + 17,500 SC injection q 12 h (aPTT 1.5–2.5)

- Low-molecular-weight heparins:
  - †Enoxaparin, 100 U/Kg SC q 12 h
  - Dalteparin, 120 U/Kg SC q 12 h
  - Dalteparin, 200 U/Kg SC q 24 h
  - Nadroparin, 90 U/Kg SC q 12 h
  - Tinzaparin, 175 U/Kg SC q 24 h

*Superscript numbers indicate references.
†100 U = 1 mg
aPTT, activated partial thromboplastin time.

heparin) is associated with a higher rate of thromboembolic complications. Thus, oral anticoagulants should be started during heparin treatment, and heparin should be stopped only after an INR of 2.0 to 3.0 has been obtained for 3 consecutive days.[58] Use of oral anticoagulants is contraindicated in the first trimester and in the last few weeks of pregnancy. Two other therapeutic options include LMW heparin throughout pregnancy or in the first trimester and last month of gestation or warfarin in the second and most of the third trimester. Warfarin should be stopped 1 to 2 weeks before the anticipated delivery date.

LMW heparins have several potential advantages compared with unfractionated heparin. They have a longer half-life and can be given once or twice daily by subcutaneous injection without laboratory monitoring. They are also associated with a lower risk of thrombocytopenia. LMW heparins allow outpatient treatment of DVT.[59, 60] Several randomized trials have confirmed that LMW heparins are probably safer than and at least as effective as unfractionated heparin in treatment of DVT[59, 60] and of pulmonary embolism.[61, 62] Results of a meta-analysis also suggested a lower mortality in patients treated with LMW heparins, in particular in patients with cancer.[1]

Several regimens for LMW heparin therapy have been tested. Usually twice-daily injections are required, but even a single daily injection has been successfully tested.[63] However, twice-daily enoxaparin is currently the only LMW heparin approved by the U.S. Food and Drug Administration (FDA) for outpatient treatment of DVT. Given subcutaneously either once or twice daily, LMW heparin is also effective in treatment of submassive pulmonary embolism.[64, 65] However, it should be kept in mind that a bleeding risk exists for some 20 hours after its withdrawal. Thus, LMW heparins pose special risks in patients who will need a surgical procedure. They also cannot be used safely as an alternative to unfractionated heparin when thrombocytopenia develops as a complication of heparin therapy.

Although most trials have tested 7 to 10 days of treatment with LMW heparin followed by oral anticoagulants, LMW heparins may also be an alternative to oral anticoagulants in secondary prevention of DVT, in particular when monitoring of the therapeutic dose of oral anticoagulants is difficult.[66, 67]

Optimal duration of anticoagulation after the first episode of DVT is debated, and a 3-month period is widely used. Randomized trials have confirmed that 3 months of treatment is superior to 4 weeks,[68] and 6 months is superior to 6 weeks.[69] Subgroup analysis of these trials has shown that patients with reversible risk factors (e.g., immobility, surgery) are at low risk of recurrences and that 4 to 6 weeks of treatment may be sufficient. Patients with idiopathic DVT or with risk factors require longer anticoagulation.

A 1996 trial that randomly assigned 162 patients with idiopathic DVT to receive either 3 or 24 months of anticoagulant treatment was terminated because of a significantly higher incidence of new thromboembolic episodes in the short-term treatment group (27% versus 1% per year). The incidence of major bleeding in the treatment group was 4%.[70] Prevalence of factor V Leiden was 26%, of prothrombin G20210A 5%, and of lupus anticoagulant 3%, but only the lupus anticoagulant was significantly associated with recurrent thromboembolism in this study. Although a previous study found a high risk of recurrences in carriers of factor V Leiden, a later study found no increase in recurrences in patients with factor V Leiden or prothrombin mutation. Further studies are needed to determine the appropriate duration of anticoagulant treatment in such patients. In particular, the optimal treatment of patients with factor V Leiden or prothrombin mutation is not yet clear.

Long-term anticoagulant therapy is indicated in patients with metastatic malignancies and DVT, because they have a high risk of recurrences. In patients with recurrent episodes of DVT, permanent anticoagulation significantly reduces the risk of further thromboembolism.[71] Recurrent thromboembolism during anticoagulant treatment poses a difficult clinical problem. Patients can be treated with a more vigorous anticoagulation regimen (INR 3.0–4.5), with aspirin plus anticoagulants, or with a caval vein filter for prevention of pulmonary embolism.

Direct thrombin inhibitors, such as hirudin, napsagatran, and argatroban, have been used in animal models of venous thrombosis and have been tested in preliminary clinical trials for prevention of DVT.[72, 73] Thrombin inhibitors may have a role in the treatment of patients with heparin-induced thrombocytopenia.

Use of thrombolytic drugs in DVT is controversial. Thrombolytic treatment is associated with higher risk of bleeding but can reduce the incidence of postphlebitic syndrome. There is no evidence, however, that thrombolytic treatment reduces the risk of pulmonary embolism in patients with DVT.[74] Use of thrombolytics has been limited to cases of massive thrombophlebitis. Prolonged infusions of streptokinase also raise the risk of allergic reactions. Local catheter-delivered thrombolysis is an option. Venous thrombectomy is usually limited to use in patients with severe ischemia caused by massive edema due to DVT.

CHRONIC VENOUS INSUFFICIENCY

Chronic venous insufficiency is usually a complication of DVT (post-thrombotic syndrome), although almost half of patients with chronic venous insufficiency do not have a definite history of previous DVT. Prevalence of post-thrombotic syndrome after DVT was 23% in one study, although use of elastic stockings can significantly reduce the rate of this complication.[72] Post-thrombotic syndrome is also associated with high risk of recurrent ipsilateral DVT.[53] Manifestations of post-thrombotic syndrome are usually evident within 24 months after the DVT.[53, 72] Chronic venous insufficiency may also be a consequence of arteriovenous fistula or compression of a pelvic vein (usually by malignancy).[73]

Venous insufficiency is caused by deformation or destruction of the valves of the deep and perforating veins of the legs by the thrombotic and inflammatory process of thrombophlebitis.[74] Such anatomic and functional damage leads to chronic venous reflux and increased venous pressure in the deep vein system, from which it is transmitted to superficial skin and tissues by the perforating veins. Calf muscle contractions that increase antegrade venous flow if venous valves are competent worsen venous reflux and further raise venous pressure, resulting in an "ambulatory venous hypertension" when the valves are incompetent. Increased venous pressure causes edema, usually more marked in the ankle and calf.

Secondary changes of the skin and subcutaneous tissues, such as brownish pigmentation of the skin and fibrosis, are common. Recurrent ulcerations, usually localized in the lower medial leg, are also common and lead to fragile local scars. Eczematous eruptions can be present as well. Varicosities of the superficial veins also occur when significant reflux through the perforating veins is present. Simple superficial vein insufficiency, with normal function of the deep vein system, causes varicosities, but edema is usually less severe and secondary changes and complications (fibrosis, ulcerations) are less common. Systemic causes of leg edema, such as congestive heart failure, hypoalbuminemia, and renal disease, are usually easily detected. Lymphedema is associated with chronic edema (but usually without pitting in the chronic phase) and skin pigmentation; however, the edema is not responsive to elevation of the legs, and varicosities are not present.

Venous insufficiency is a chronic disease that can be controlled only with daily treatments requiring good patient compliance.[74] Control of edema is the cornerstone of treatment and may greatly reduce the incidence of ulceration. Use of elastic stockings during the day and leg elevation at night is often effective. Periodic elevation during the day is also required in many patients to prevent edema formation.

Treatment of ulceration and of eczematous eruption is often difficult. Because ulcers are secondary to venous hypertension, measures to reduce venous pressure and edema (such as bed rest and leg elevation) are essential. Treatment also includes compresses of saline solution, usually applied three times daily. When edema is reduced, it is possible to apply a paste or bandage venous boot, which provides compression of the leg and allows the patient to walk. Secondary infections (bacterial or fungal) are common and should be treated with the appropriate antibiotics after the organism is identified by culture of a specimen. Recurrent or nonhealing ulcerations often require surgical treatment, with ablation of incompetent deep veins and adjunctive ligation of perforating veins. Endoscopic techniques are also available and have reduced the morbidity associated with these interventions. Deep venous reconstruction is a possibility in selected cases.

VARICOSE VEINS

Varicosities of the superficial veins of the legs are extremely common in women and probably affect at least 20% to 25% of the adult population to some extent.[76] Patients often have a family history of the disorder. Although it is not clear whether the primary problem is incompetence of valves or dilatation of the vein lumen with secondary valve incompetence, valve leakage is the most important element in the pathogenesis of varicose veins. Superficial veins are not supported by muscle or connective tissue; thus, superficial vein incompetence produces the characteristic dilated and winding varicosities.[77, 78] Reflux due to incompetence of the communicating veins may also have a role in some patients.

Risk factors for varicose veins are family history, female sex, pregnancies, and obesity. Varicosities are more common in the greater saphenous system (medial and anterior thigh and calf) but may also occur in the lesser saphenous system (posterolateral calf).[79] Varicose veins are common during pregnancy, owing to relaxation of the venous wall and greater venous pressure in the legs. Partial or complete regression often occurs after delivery.

Competence of the great saphenous vein system can be assessed by the Trendelenburg test. After emptying of the venous system, a tourniquet is applied on the thigh to occlude the superficial veins, and the patient stands for 1 minute. The superficial veins should be slowly filled by the arterial flow, with no further filling at the release of the tourniquet. Incompetence of the great saphenous vein causes a sudden filling at the release of the tourniquet, whereas incompetence of the deep communicating veins causes a rapid filling of superficial veins even during tourniquet compression.

Presence of deep vein obstruction can be assessed by the Perthes test. While the patient stands, a tourniquet is applied on the thigh to occlude the superficial vein. The patient is then asked to walk for 5 minutes to drain the blood from the varicosities into the communicating veins. No reduction of varicosities during walking strongly suggests incompetence of both superficial and communicating veins; worsening of varicosities during walking, often associated with pain, indicates obstruction of the deep venous system.

The presence of limb symptoms in patients with varicose veins was assessed in a large study involving more than 1500 patients (860 women). In this study, limb symptoms, such as heaviness or tension, swelling, aching, restless legs, cramps, and pruritus, were significantly more common in women than in men. However, the correlation between symptoms and presence of trunk varices was low, suggesting that, in these patients, some lower limb symptoms probably have a nonvenous cause.[80] Symptoms are more common at the end of the day or during menstruation. Although mild swelling may occur, significant edema and ulceration are usually signs of obstruction of the deep vein system. A possible complication is superficial thrombophlebitis of the varicosities.

Management of varicose veins is usually conservative, consisting of general measures such as weight reduction, use of elastic stockings, avoidance of long periods of sitting or standing, and periodic elevation of the legs. Sclerotherapy has been used for treatment of small varicosities,[81] but its real value is controversial. Stripping and ligation of the long saphenous vein to the below-knee level, or of the lesser saphenous veins, or both, is indicated in symptomatic patients and in patients with recurrent episodes of superficial thrombophlebitis. Simple surgical saphenofemoral ligation can be an effective treatment, but it is associated with a relatively high incidence of reoperation (20%) within 5 years of the first procedure; only about 6% of patients who undergo stripping of the saphenous vein require reoperation.[82] In one large series of patients, the risk of major surgical complications was only 0.8% (mainly DVT).[83]

References

1. Lensing AW, Prandoni P, Prins MH, Buller HR: Deep-vein thrombosis. Lancet 353:479, 1999.
2. Albert JS, Dalen JE: Epidemiology and natural history of venous thromboembolism. Prog Cardiovasc Dis 36:417, 1994.
3. Hansson PO, Welin L, Tibblin G, Eriksson H: Deep vein thrombosis and pulmonary embolism in the general population: The Study of Men Born in 1913. Arch Intern Med 157:1665, 1997.

4. Nordstrom M, Lindblad B: Autopsy-verified venous thromboembolism within a defined urban population—the city of Malmo, Sweden. APMIS 106:378, 1998.
5. Phillips MD: Interrelated risk factors of venous thromboembolism. Circulation 95:1749, 1997.
6. Rosendaal FR: Venous thrombosis: A multicausal disease. Lancet 353: 1167, 1999.
7. Sorensen HT, Mellemkjaer L, Steffensen FH, et al: The risk of a diagnosis of cancer after primary deep venous thrombosis or pulmonary embolism. N Engl J Med 338:1169, 1998.
8. Prandoni P, Lensing AW, Buller HR, et al: Deep-vein thrombosis and the incidence of subsequent symptomatic cancer. N Engl J Med 327: 1128, 1992.
9. Vandenbroucke JP, Helmerhorst FM, Bloemenkamp KW, Rosendaal FR: Third-generation oral contraceptive and deep venous thrombosis: From epidemiologic controversy to new insight in coagulation [see comments]. Am J Obstet Gynecol 177:887, 1997.
10. Lane DA, Mannucci PM, Bauer KA, et al: Inherited thrombophilia: Part 1. Thromb Haemost 76:651, 1996.
11. Lane DA, Mannucci PM, Bauer KA, et al: Inherited thrombophilia: Part 2 [published erratum appears in Thromb Haemost 77:1047, 1997]. Thromb Haemost 76:824, 1996.
12. Bertina RM, Reitsma PH, Rosendaal FR, Vandenbroucke JP: Resistance to activated protein C and factor V Leiden as risk factors for venous thrombosis. Thromb Haemost 74:449, 1995.
13. Ridker PM, Miletich JP, Hennekens CH, Buring JE: Ethnic distribution of factor V Leiden in 4047 men and women: Implications for venous thromboembolism screening. JAMA 277:1305, 1997.
14. Price DT, Ridker PM: Factor V Leiden mutation and the risks for thromboembolic disease: A clinical perspective. Ann Intern Med 127: 895, 1997.
15. Poort SR, Rosendaal FR, Reitsma PH, Bertina RM: A common genetic variation in the 3′-untranslated region of the prothrombin gene is associated with elevated plasma prothrombin levels and an increase in venous thrombosis. Blood 88:3698, 1996.
16. Rosendaal FR, Doggen CJ, Zivelin A, et al: Geographic distribution of the 20210 G to A prothrombin variant. Thromb Haemost 79:706, 1998.
17. Ridker PM, Hennekens CH, Miletich JP: G20210A mutation in prothrombin gene and risk of myocardial infarction, stroke, and venous thrombosis in a large cohort of US men. Circulation 99:999, 1999.
18. Ridker PM, Hennekens CH, Selhub J, et al: Interrelation of hyperhomocyst(e)inemia, factor V Leiden, and risk of future venous thromboembolism. Circulation 95:1777, 1997.
19. Moser KM, LeMoine JR: Is embolic risk conditioned by location of deep venous thrombosis? Ann Intern Med 94:439, 1981.
20. Huisman MV, Buller HR, ten Cate JW, Vreeken J: Serial impedance plethysmography for suspected deep venous thrombosis in outpatients: The Amsterdam General Practitioner Study. N Engl J Med 314:823, 1986.
21. Barnes RW, Wu KK, Hoak JC: Fallibility of the clinical diagnosis of venous thrombosis. JAMA 234:605, 1975.
22. Kahn SR: The clinical diagnosis of deep venous thrombosis: Integrating incidence, risk factors, and symptoms and signs. Arch Intern Med 158: 2315, 1998.
23. Becker DM, Philbrick JT, Walker FB: Axillary and subclavian venous thrombosis: Prognosis and treatment. Arch Intern Med 151:1934, 1991.
24. Prandoni P, Polistena P, Bernardi E, et al: Upper-extremity deep vein thrombosis: Risk factors, diagnosis, and complications. Arch Intern Med 157:57, 1997.
25. Wells PS, Hirsh J, Anderson DR, et al: Accuracy of clinical assessment of deep-vein thrombosis [published erratum appears in Lancet 346: 516, 1995]. Lancet 345:1326, 1995.
26. Wells PS, Anderson DR, Bormanis J, et al: Value of assessment of pretest probability of deep-vein thrombosis in clinical management. Lancet 350:1795, 1997.
27. Janssen MC, Wollersheim H, Verbruggen B, Novakova IR: Rapid D-dimer assays to exclude deep venous thrombosis and pulmonary embolism: Current status and new developments. Semin Thromb Hemost 24:393, 1998.
28. Bounameaux H, Cirafici P, de Moerloose P, et al: Measurement of D-dimer in plasma as diagnostic aid in suspected pulmonary embolism [see comments]. Lancet 337:196, 1991.
29. Goldhaber SZ, Simons GR, Elliott CG, et al: Quantitative plasma D-dimer levels among patients undergoing pulmonary angiography for suspected pulmonary embolism. JAMA 270:2819, 1993.
30. Ginsberg JS, Wells PS, Kearon C, et al: Sensitivity and specificity of a rapid whole-blood assay for D-dimer in the diagnosis of pulmonary embolism. Ann Intern Med 129:1006, 1998.
31. Kutinsky I, Blakely S, Roche V: Normal D-dimer levels in patients with pulmonary embolism. Arch Intern Med 159:1569, 1999.
32. Perrier A, Desmarais S, Miron MJ, et al: Non-invasive diagnosis of venous thromboembolism in outpatients. Lancet 353:190, 1999.
33. Pearson SD, Polak JL, Cartwright S, et al: A critical pathway to evaluate suspected deep vein thrombosis. Arch Intern Med 155:1773, 1995.
34. Kearon C, Ginsberg JS, Hirsh J: The role of venous ultrasonography in the diagnosis of suspected deep venous thrombosis and pulmonary embolism. Ann Intern Med 129:1044, 1998.
35. Lensing AW, Prandoni P, Brandjes D, et al: Detection of deep-vein thrombosis by real-time B-mode ultrasonography. N Engl J Med 320: 342, 1989.
36. Becker DM, Philbrick JT, Abbitt PI: Real-time ultrasonography for the diagnosis of lower extremity deep venous thrombosis: The wave of the future? Arch Intern Med 149:1731, 1989.
37. Comerota AJ, Katz ML, Hashemi HA: Venous duplex imaging for the diagnosis of acute deep venous thrombosis. Haemostasis 23(Suppl 1): 61, 1993.
38. Heijboer H, Buller HR, Lensing AW, et al: A comparison of real-time compression ultrasonography with impedance plethysmography for the diagnosis of deep-vein thrombosis in symptomatic outpatients. N Engl J Med 329:1365, 1993.
39. Hull R, Taylor DW, Hirsh J, et al: Impedance plethymography: The relationship between venous filling and sensitivity and specificity for proximal vein thrombosis. Circulation 58:898, 1978.
40. Wells PS, Hirsh J, Anderson DR, et al: Comparison of the accuracy of impedance plethysmography and compression ultrasonography in outpatients with clinically suspected deep vein thrombosis: A two centre paired-design prospective trial. Thromb Haemost 74:1423, 1995.
41. Ginsberg JS: Management of venous thromboembolism. N Engl J Med 335:1816, 1996.
41a. Kearon C, Hirsh J: Factors influencing the reported sensitivity and specificity of impedance plethysmography for proximal deep vein thrombosis. Thromb Haemost 72:652, 1994.
42. Sandler DA, Martin JF, Duncan JS, et al: Diagnosis of deep-vein thrombosis: Comparison of clinical evaluation, ultrasound, plethysmography, and venoscan with X-ray venogram. Lancet 2:716, 1984.
43. Bettmann MA, Paulin S: Leg phlebography: The incidence, nature and modification of undesirable side effects. Radiology 122:101, 1977.
44. Lensing AW, Prandoni P, Buller HR, et al: Lower extremity venography with iohexol: Results and complications. Radiology 177:503, 1990.
45. Erdman WA, Jayson HT, Redman HC, et al: Deep venous thrombosis of extremities: Role of MR imaging in the diagnosis. Radiology 174: 425, 1990.
46. Spritzer CE, Norconk JJ Jr, Sostman HD, Coleman RE: Detection of deep venous thrombosis by magnetic resonance imaging. Chest 104: 54, 1993.
47. Evans AJ, Sostman HD, Witty LA, et al: Detection of deep venous thrombosis: Prospective comparison of MR imaging and sonography. J Magn Reson Imaging 6:44, 1996.
48. Clagett GP, Anderson FA Jr, Geerts W, et al: Prevention of venous thromboembolism. Chest 114:531S, 1998.
49. Collins R, Scrimgeour A, Yusuf S, Peto R: Reduction in fatal pulmonary embolism and venous thrombosis by perioperative administration of subcutaneous heparin: Overview of results of randomized trials in general, orthopedic, and urologic surgery. N Engl J Med 318:1162, 1988.
50. Weitz JL: Low-molecular-weight heparins [published erratum appears in N Engl J Med 337:1567, 1997]. N Engl J Med 337:668, 1997.
51. Hull RD, Brant RF, Pineo GF, et al: Preoperative vs postoperative initiation of low-molecular-weight heparin prophylaxis against venous thromboembolism in patients undergoing elective hip replacement. Arch Intern Med 159:137, 1999.
52. MacMahon S, Rodgers A, Collins R, Farrell B: Antiplatelet therapy to prevent thrombosis after hip fracture: Rationale for a randomised trial [see comments]. J Bone Surg Br 76:521, 1994.
53. Prandoni P, Lensing AW, Cogo A, et al: The long-term clinical course of acute deep venous thrombosis. Ann Intern Med 125:1, 1996.
54. Hull RD, Raskob GE, Rosenbloom D, et al: Optimal therapeutic level of heparin therapy in patients with venous thrombosis. Arch Intern Med 152:1589, 1992.
54a. Raschke RA, Reilly BM, Guidry JR, et al: The weight-based heparin

dosing nomogram compared with a "standard care" nomogram. A randomized controlled trial. Arch Intern Med 119:874, 1993.
55. Hirsh J, Fuster V: Guide to anticoagulant therapy. Part 1: Heparin. American Heart Association. Circulation 89:1449, 1994.
56. Hyers TM, Agnelli G, Hull RD, et al: Antithrombotic therapy for venous thromboembolic disease. Chest 114:561S, 1998.
57. Lagerstedt CI, Olsson CG, Fagher BO, et al: Need for long-term anticoagulant treatment in symptomatic calf-vein thrombosis. Lancet 2: 515, 1985.
58. Hirsh J, Fuster V: Guide to anticoagulant therapy. Part 2: Oral anticoagulants. American Heart Association [published erratum appears in Circulation 91:A55, 1995]. Circulation 89:1469, 1994.
59. Levine M, Gent M, Hirsh J, et al: A comparison of low-molecular-weight heparin administered primarily at home with unfractionated heparin administered in the hospital for proximal deep-vein thrombosis. N Engl J Med 334:677, 1996.
60. Koopman MMW, Prandoni P, Piovella F, et al: Treatment of venous thrombosis with intravenous unfractionated heparin administered in the hospital as compared with subcutaneous low-molecular-weight heparin administered at home. N Engl J Med 334:682, 1996.
61. Low-molecular-weight heparin in the treatment of patients with venous thromboembolism. The Columbus Investigators. N Engl J Med 337: 657, 1997.
62. Simonneau G, Sors H, Charbonnier B, et al: A comparison of low-molecular-weight heparin with unfractionated heparin for acute pulmonary embolism. The THESEE Study Group. Tinzaparine ou Heparine Standard: Evaluations dans l'Embolie Pulmonaire. N Engl J Med 337: 663, 1997.
63. Charbonnier BA, Fiessinger JN, Banga JD, et al: Comparison of a once daily with a twice daily subcutaneous low molecular weight heparin regimen in the treatment of deep vein thrombosis. FRAXODI group. Thromb Haemost 79:897, 1998.
64. Schulman S: Long-term prophylaxis in venous thromboembolism: LMWH or oral anticoagulation? Haemostasis 28(Suppl S3):17, 1998.
65. Lassen MR, Borris LC, Anderson BS, et al: Efficacy and safety of prolonged thromboprophylaxis with a low molecular weight heparin (dalteparin) after total hip arthroplasty—the Danish Prolonged Prophylaxis (DaPP) Study. Thromb Res 89:281, 1998.
66. Schulman S, Rhedin AS, Lindmarker P, et al: A comparison of six weeks with six months of oral anticoagulant therapy after a first episode of venous thromboembolism. Duration of Anticoagulation Trial Study Group. N Engl J Med 332:1661, 1995.
67. Kearon C, Gent M, Hirsh J, et al: A comparison of three months of anticoagulation with extended anticoagulation for a first episode of idiopathic venous thromboembolism. N Engl J Med 340:901, 1999.
68. Schulman S, Granqvist S, Holmstrom M, et al: The duration of oral anticoagulant therapy after a second episode of venous thromboembolism. The Duration of Anticoagulation Trial Study Group. N Engl J Med 336:393, 1997.
69. Ginsberg JS, Nurmohamed MT, Gent M, et al: Use of Hirulog in the prevention of venous thrombosis after major hip or knee surgery. Circulation 90:2385, 1994.
70. Eriksson BI, Ekman S, Kalebo P, et al: Prevention of deep-vein thrombosis after total hip replacement: Direct thrombin inhibition with recombinant hirudin, CGP 39393. Lancet 347:635, 1996.
71. Rogers LQ, Lutcher CL: Streptokinase therapy for deep vein thrombosis: A comprehensive review of the English literature. Am J Med 88: 389, 1990.
72. Brandjes DP, Buller HR, Heijboer H, et al: Randomised trial of effect of compression stockings in patients with symptomatic proximal-vein thrombosis. Lancet 349:759, 1997.
73. Angle N, Bergan JJ: Chronic venous ulcer. BMJ 314:1019, 1997.
74. Ibrahim S, MacPherson DR, Goldhaber SZ: Chronic venous insufficiency: Mechanisms and management. Am Heart J 132:856, 1996.
75. Padberg FT Jr: Surgical intervention in venous ulceration. Cardiovasc Surg 7:83, 1999.
76. Callam MJ: Epidemiology of varicose veins. Br J Surg 81:167, 1994.
77. Skudder PA, Farrington DT: Venous conditions associated with pregnancy. Semin Dermatol 12:72, 1993.
78. Somjen GM: Anatomy of the superficial venous system. Dermatol Surg 21:35, 1995.
79. Houghton AD, Panayiotopoulos Y, Taylor PR: Practical management of primary varicose veins. Br J Clin Pract 50:103, 1996.
80. Bradbury A, Evans C, Allan P, et al: What are the symptoms of varicose veins? Edinburgh vein study cross sectional population survey. BMJ 318:353, 1999.
81. Green D: Sclerotherapy for the permanent eradication of varicose veins: Theoretical and practical considerations. J Am Acad Dermatol 38:461, 1998.
82. Dwerryhouse S, Davies B, Harradine K, Earnshaw JJ: Stripping the long saphenous vein reduces the rate of reoperation for recurrent varicose veins: Five-year results of a randomized trial. J Vasc Surg 29: 589, 1999.
83. Critchley G, Handa A, Maw A, et al: Complications of varicose vein surgery. Ann R Coll Surg Engl 79:105, 1997.

CHAPTER 33

Pulmonary Emboli

Herbert L. Fred, Ramesh Hariharan, and James K. Alexander

Pulmonary embolism (PE)* is one of the few relatively common medical conditions for which the Bible contains no recognizable description.[1] In fact, the first clear case description of PE did not appear until 1837.[2] That patient was a short, fat laundry woman of 65 years who, while talking with neighbors, abruptly manifested swelling and violaceous discoloration of her face followed by redness and prominence of her eyes and loss of consciousness. She recovered rapidly but died soon thereafter during a similar attack. Postmortem examination showed a large heart with dark, organized clots in the right ventricle and pulmonary artery. Several years later, the first description of postpartal PE appeared.[3] The clots in that patient presumably originated in her left leg, where phlegmasia alba dolens had developed several days before death.

Since those early reports, the literature on PE has reached astronomic proportions. Yet, despite great progress in our recognition and management of PE, this disease continues to be a major problem for patient and physician alike.

INCIDENCE

Each year in this country, PE strikes an estimated 650,000 people,[4] killing about 200,000 of them.[5] It attacks both sexes with equal frequency.[6] All age groups are affected, but most of the victims are middle aged or older.[7] Although a concurrent illness is usually present, PE can strike seemingly healthy, active persons,[8] including children[9] and adolescents.[10]

PREDISPOSING FACTORS

PE characteristically appears in a setting of congestive heart failure, trauma (especially to the lower extremities and pelvis), immobility (resulting from medical illness, surgical procedures, or prolonged sitting), venous disease in the legs, malignancy,[10a] or any combination thereof. In approximately 50% of cases of deep vein thrombosis, activated protein C resistance may be the cause.[11–13] This entity results primarily from a point mutation in factor V (factor V Leiden) that involves the binding site of protein C.[14, 15]

Other factors predisposing to PE include obesity; polycythemia; indwelling venous catheters; deficiencies of protein C or S or antithrombin III; elevated levels of clotting factors VIII[15a] and XI[15b]; antiphospholipid antibodies[16]; hyperhomocysteinemia[17, 18]; mutations in the prothrombin gene[19, 19a, 19b]; postmenopausal therapy with estrogen plus progestin[19c]; and use of antipsychotic drugs.[19d, 19e]

Oral contraceptives increase the risk of venous thromboembolism 3- to 12-fold.[20, 21] This risk begins within 4 months of starting such contraception, is unrelated to its duration, and persists up to 3 months after stopping it.[20] Decreasing the estrogen content of these contraceptives reduces the risk only partially.[22] Although the pathogenesis of thrombosis in this setting is unclear, evidence now suggests that activated protein C resistance caused by factor V Leiden may be responsible.[21, 23–25] Factor V Leiden displays a strong interaction with all types of oral contraceptives and increases the risk of a thromboembolic event by 30- to 50-fold.[24]

Pregnancy sets up a hypercoagulable state that lasts about 11 months.[26, 26a] In addition to venous stasis from compression by the gravid uterus, pregnancy is associated with a marked increase in levels of coagulation factors II, VII, and X, and a decrease in fibrinolytic activity.[26] The level of protein C is unaffected, but the concentrations of antithrombin III and protein S decrease throughout gestation. Several studies have demonstrated a significant contribution of factor V Leiden to the hypercoagulability in these women.[25, 27, 28] Instrument-assisted or operative delivery, prolonged bed rest, multiparity, and advanced maternal age are additional risk factors.

PE occurs once in every 2000 pregnancies[29] and accounts for 12% to 15% of maternal deaths in the United States[30] and Europe.[31] Although deep venous thrombosis is equally common in all three trimesters, the risk of PE is greatest in the third trimester and in the immediate postpartal period.[32, 33]

SOURCE AND DISTRIBUTION OF EMBOLI

Statistics vary as to the sites from which pulmonary emboli originate. Finding thrombi in peripheral veins or in the right atrium or right ventricle does not prove that these sites are the source of emboli. In fact, thrombi sometimes exist in these areas when no pulmonary emboli are evident. And once a clot becomes detached from a vein, that vessel may be empty when examined by imaging techniques or at autopsy. Nevertheless, most pulmonary emboli arise from veins in the lower extremities[34] or pelvis.[35] Occasionally, the heart is the source.[36] Other sites of origin include the inferior vena cava, veins in the upper extremities,[37] renal veins,[38] and veins of the cerebral sinuses and nasopharynx.[8]

Once released into the venous circulation, emboli go to both lungs with about the same frequency. They affect the lower lobes (especially the right) four times more often than the upper lobes. And most of the emboli lodge in the

*PE as used here refers to the intravascular movement of a bland blood clot from its origin in a peripheral vein or the right side of the heart to lodgment in a pulmonary artery, with or without resultant infarction of the lung.

larger (elastic) or intermediate-sized (muscular) pulmonary arteries.[39]

PATHOPHYSIOLOGY

Pathology

Acute PE is a dynamic process. The emboli begin to lyse immediately after reaching the lung. In the absence of pre-existing cardiopulmonary disease, complete lysis usually takes place within several weeks. Occasionally, even large emboli lyse within a few days. The physiologic alterations lessen over hours or days as the pulmonary circulation improves. Yet, massive emboli may cause death within minutes or hours without sufficient time for infarction to develop. Infrequently, embolic events recur over months or years, causing progressive pulmonary arterial obstruction with consequent chronic pulmonary hypertension, increasing dyspnea, and cor pulmonale.

When the bronchial circulation is intact, pulmonary infarction rarely develops. Collateral circulation from the bronchial arteries keeps the lung tissue viable despite pulmonary arterial blockage. Pulmonary infarction is more likely in patients with pre-existing cardiopulmonary disease and compromised bronchial circulation.[40] The mechanism of infarction involves hemorrhage into the alveoli. Such hemorrhage results from rupture of pulmonary arterioles perfused by bronchial arteries at systemic pressure.[41] Infarcts may heal by absorption and fibrosis, leaving a linear scar.

Physiology

Pulmonary Hypertension

Pulmonary hypertension in association with acute PE correlates predominantly with the degree of vascular obstruction and, to some extent, with the elevated pulmonary vascular resistance that results from vasoconstriction.[42] In the normal lung, obstruction of 50% to 60% of the pulmonary vascular bed is necessary to increase the pulmonary vascular resistance.[43] Lesser degrees of obstruction, however, can lead to pulmonary hypertension if the patient has pre-embolic conditions such as obstructive lung disease or mitral stenosis.[44]

Vasoconstriction in acute PE is multifactorial in origin. Besides having a vasoconstrictive effect per se, thrombin in the embolus also activates platelets.[45] In turn, platelet activation causes release of serotonin, adenosine diphosphate, thromboxane A_2, and platelet growth factor, all of which are vasoconstrictors.[46, 47] Furthermore, injury from embolization impairs prostaglandin release by endothelium and favors vasoconstriction.[48] Although hypoxemia can induce vasoconstriction, oxygen administration has little effect on pulmonary vascular resistance.[49] In PE, therefore, hypoxemia is not a major factor in the pathogenesis of pulmonary hypertension.

Pulmonary arterial systolic pressure may rise to levels as high as 100 mm Hg with acute PE. Lesser degrees of elevation are more common, however, owing to the development of significant tricuspid regurgitation. The higher pressures tend to develop in patients with pre-existing cardiopulmonary disease.[44]

Pulmonary Function

Tachypnea, often with dyspnea, almost always occurs after an embolic episode. It appears to be of reflex origin, resulting most likely from stimulation of juxtacapillary receptors in the alveolocapillary membrane. This stimulation increases vagal afferent activity, which, in turn, stimulates medullary respiratory neurons.[50] Another important factor is ventilation of nonperfused lung, the physiologic hallmark of PE.[51]

In acute PE, ventilation perfusion (V_A/Q) mismatch occurs, varying with the size of vessels involved, the extent of reduction of the pulmonary vascular bed, and the patient's pre-embolic cardiopulmonary status.[52] Ventilation of poorly or nonperfused segments of lung results in a high V_A/Q. By contrast, a low V_A/Q reflects persistent perfusion of poorly ventilated areas. The diminished ventilation results from local bronchoconstriction, atelectasis, or reduced lung compliance.[53, 54]

Arterial blood gas analysis often shows hypoxemia, hypocarbia, respiratory alkalosis, and an increase in the alveolar-arterial PO_2 gradient [$P(A\text{-}a)O_2$].[55–57] But even when the arterial oxygen tension (PaO_2), arterial carbon dioxide tension ($PaCO_2$), and $P(A\text{-}a)O_2$ are all normal, PE may still be present in about 15% of patients with, and in about 30% of those without, pre-existing cardiopulmonary disease.[57] Furthermore, an increase in the $P(A\text{-}a)O_2$ can also occur in conditions other than PE.[57, 58] Therefore, the results of arterial blood gas measurements do not confirm or exclude the diagnosis of PE.

Cardiac Function

As the extent of pulmonary vascular obstruction increases in patients without pre-existing heart or lung disease, pulmonary artery and right heart pressures become elevated. At very high pressures, right ventricular dysfunction supervenes, leading to a fall in pulmonary artery pressure, low cardiac output, and shock.[59] Severe right ventricular hypokinesis and leftward shift of the interventricular septum characterize this preterminal phase.[60]

CLINICAL FEATURES

Manifestations of PE depend on the number and size of emboli, presence or absence of pulmonary infarction, duration of the thromboembolic process, and type and severity of associated diseases. The clinical picture, therefore, can vary considerably. Moreover, one cannot consistently judge the seriousness of PE by the nature of its presentation. A large embolus, for example, may be clinically silent, whereas a small embolus may produce an alarming set of findings. We believe that the best way to understand and remember the protean expressions of PE is to separate them into those occurring before and those appearing after pulmonary infarction develops.

Pulmonary Embolism Without Infarction

Dyspnea without orthopnea is the most common and important symptom.[7] It often is sudden in onset, progressing at times to gasping respirations. Frequently, however, the dyspnea is mild and fleeting. *Chest pain* is rare; when it is present, it is typically dull and retrosternal and usually reflects occlusion of major pulmonary arteries.[61] *Wheezing respirations,* ordinarily transient and occasionally recurrent, can be a heralding feature.[62] *Neurologic abnormalities,* such as syncope, convulsions, restlessness, anxiety, stupor, coma, and weakness or paralysis of limbs, predominate in about 5% of the cases and may be the first, the most prominent, or the only manifestation.[63] *Apprehension* and *a sense of impending doom* are common.[64] Rarely, the patient experiences a sudden strong urge to defecate and may faint or die during defecation.[65]

Tachycardia[64] is frequent, and *tachypnea*[66] is almost always present. *Signs of venous thrombosis in the legs,* such as pain, heat, discoloration, or enlargement, develop in less than half of the patients and may not appear for days or even months after the onset of pulmonary symptoms.[67] *Cyanosis* generally appears when embolism is massive or there is coexisting cardiopulmonary disease, shock, or both. *Hypotension* is relatively uncommon. Characteristically, it is of short duration, but if persistent, it indicates that the diagnosis is wrong or that the embolus is massive. In some cases, sudden, profound, or prolonged shock is the *only* indication of PE. *Acute cor pulmonale* can result from massive PE and may be accompanied by an accentuated pulmonic valve closure sound, right ventricular gallop rhythm, or increased jugular venous pressure.

One point merits special attention. Signs of PE without infarction may regress spontaneously just as dramatically as they appear. In these cases, the patient seems well one minute and moribund the next, only to recover rapidly.

Pulmonary Embolism with Infarction

Fewer than 10% of pulmonary emboli lead to infarction of the lung.[68] *Pleuritic pain* emerges in about half of the patients with infarction and may be sudden or gradual in onset and mild or severe.[69] *Hemoptysis* occurs in about a third of these patients.[7] At first, it is bright red; then it appears as dark clots, followed by dark brown, semiliquid material. *Fever* of varying duration and pattern is common.[70, 70a] Temperatures usually range between 100°F and 103°F but can reach 105°F in the absence of demonstrable infection.[71] *Cough* is uncommon and, when present, is intermittent and mild.[72] *Pleural friction rub,* which is audible in only about a fourth of the patients,[69] sometimes precedes radiographic evidence of pulmonary infarction. *Rales and signs of pleural effusion* are common, but classic signs of consolidation rarely, if ever, appear. *Jaundice* can develop when the infarction is extensive or when congestive heart failure, hepatic disease, or both, are present.[73]

RADIOGRAPHIC FINDINGS

The radiographic patterns of PE depend on the size, number, and distribution of the emboli; the pre-existing anatomic and functional status of the heart and lungs; and the frequency with which chest radiographs are obtained. Before frank infarction develops, the chest radiograph may show no abnormality.[74] In some cases, however, one or both main pulmonary arteries become enlarged with decreased peripheral vascular markings in the affected portions of lung (oligemia) and engorged vessels in the nonaffected areas (pleonemia). The hemidiaphragm on the involved side may become elevated consequent to atelectasis.

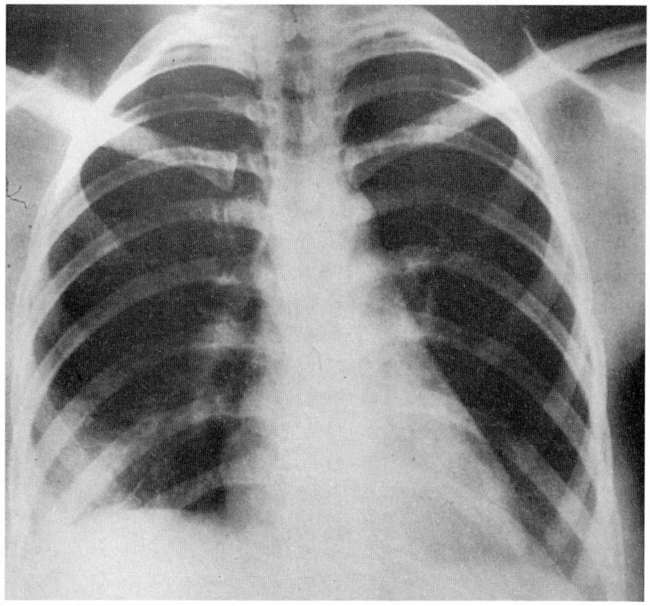

FIGURE 33–1. This 21-year-old woman experienced sudden right-sided pleuritic pain several days after a cross-country train ride. Her chest radiograph shows a hazy infiltrate at the base of the right lung. A pulmonary arteriogram demonstrated a large filling defect in the artery to the right lower lobe. With anticoagulant therapy, the patient's pleurisy and radiographic abnormality resolved.

After infarction develops, the chest radiograph almost always shows some abnormality, typically within 24 hours. Rarely, the abnormality takes approximately 5 days to appear.[74a] Any segment of lung may be involved, but the lower lobes, especially the right, are the usual sites (Figs. 33–1 and 33–2*A*).[75] Atelectasis and small pleural effusions are common; large pleural effusions may also occur. Parenchymal densities range in size from mere visibility to that of a completely opacified lobe. Their patterns are so diverse that no shape necessarily suggests or excludes pulmonary infarction.

The radiographic findings of pulmonary infarction can mimic those of many diseases, especially bacterial pneumonia.[71] Sometimes, the infarction simulates cancer,[76] and if cavitation occurs, the lesion can be mistaken for pulmonary abscess.

Chronic major vessel thromboembolic pulmonary hypertension usually results in clear lung fields. In some patients, however, the right atrium and right ventricle are dilated with enlargement or asymmetry of the central pulmonary arteries.[77]

ELECTROCARDIOGRAPHIC FINDINGS

In most cases of PE, the electrocardiogram provides little or no help. Even when the embolism is massive, electrocardio-

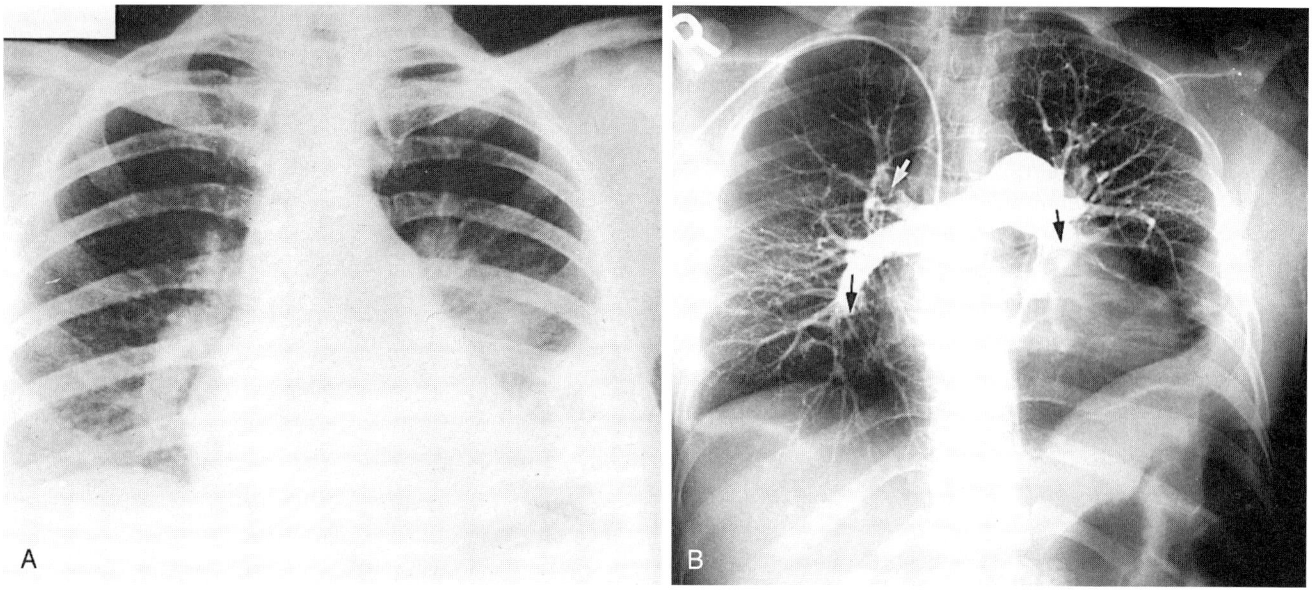

FIGURE 33–2. This 29-year-old woman complained of dyspnea and bloody sputum without fever or chest pain. On physical examination she had tachycardia, right ventricular gallop, and rales bilaterally. *A*, Chest radiograph shows cardiomegaly, infiltrates in both lower lobes, and prominence of the artery to the right lower lobe. *B*, Pulmonary arteriogram demonstrates obstructed pulmonary arteries *(black arrows)* and a large, right-sided filling defect *(white arrow)*. Subsequent investigations disclosed thrombosis of the right renal vein.

graphic signs of right ventricular strain may not evolve. Abnormalities that do appear are nonspecific and often fleeting, and may go undetected unless multiple tracings are obtained within a short time. The transient nature of these alterations is characteristic, however, and should suggest PE. Sinus and supraventricular tachycardias, S-T segment and T-wave changes in the right precordial leads, and right bundle branch block are the most frequent manifestations.

In patients with obliterative pulmonary hypertension from recurrent small pulmonary emboli[78] or from chronic major vessel pulmonary thromboemboli,[77] the electrocardiogram may be normal, or show right axis deviation, P-pulmonale, or a pattern of right ventricular hypertrophy and strain.

MISCELLANEOUS LABORATORY FINDINGS

Routine laboratory tests in patients with PE give nonspecific results. The total leukocyte count usually is normal or slightly elevated,[78a] but it may reach 40,000 per mm^3 in the presence of massive necrosis of pulmonary tissue.[71] Sputum, if examined soon after infarction develops, commonly shows many erythrocytes but few leukocytes or organisms. Pleural fluid, when present, is bloody in 50%[69] to 65%[79] of the cases and may be a transudate or exudate.[79]

Plasma levels of D-dimer, a degradation product of cross-linked fibrin, are nearly always increased,[80] but because of poor specificity, such increase has limited diagnostic usefulness. Conversely, a normal plasma level of D-dimer is strong evidence against PE.[80–82, 82a] Nevertheless, until D-dimer testing becomes standardized and more widely validated in prospective outcome studies, its widespread use is not recommended.[83]

DIAGNOSIS

Constant awareness of PE is the key to its early recognition. Important clues are fever of unknown origin and fever unaffected by antimicrobial agents (especially in patients who have congestive heart failure or who are postpartal or postsurgical); congestive heart failure that increases rapidly in severity or is unresponsive to the usual therapeutic measures; unexplained wheezing; sudden, profound, or prolonged shock; paroxysmal arrhythmias, especially sinus tachycardia; and bloody pleural effusion, pulmonary parenchymal infiltrates, or "lung abscess" of unknown cause. If one waits for hemoptysis, pleural friction rub, venous disease in the legs, abnormal chest radiograph or electrocardiographic changes to develop, most cases will escape recognition. By contrast, one should never reject the diagnosis because of high fever, normal jugular venous pressure, "atypical" pulmonary lesions, failure to uncover the source of emboli, or because the patient is young or appears otherwise healthy.

The *VA/Q lung scan* is a good way to screen for PE and to follow its course.[84–89] Perfusion scans image the distribution of intravenously injected macroaggregates of albumin labeled with technetium 99m (^{99m}Tc). These radioactive particles are 10 to 100 μm in diameter, and even the smallest of them has a cross-sectional area larger than the average pulmonary capillary. Consequently, most of these particles become trapped at the precapillary level during their initial transit through the lungs. Distribution of macroaggregated albumin in a segment of lung is proportional to the relative pulmonary blood flow to that segment. Thus, the radioactivity recorded from different regions of the lung is an index of the relative amounts of capillary perfusion in those sites.

Ventilation scans involve the inhalation and washout of a tracer, usually xenon 133 (^{133}Xe) gas. This technique determines regional pulmonary ventilation, and when performed in association with the perfusion scan, it may enhance recognition of PE. Ventilation without perfusion points to pulmonary vascular obstruction,[90] whereas reduction of both ventilation and perfusion generally implies parenchymal or bronchial disease.[91]

Abnormal scans show high, intermediate, or low probability for PE.[85, 87, 88, 90, 91] High-probability scans typically demonstrate large segmental perfusion defects without corresponding ventilatory or radiographic abnormalities. Low-probability scans demonstrate small segmental or nonsegmental perfusion defects with matching ventilatory and radiographic abnormalities. Intermediate scans fit neither of these patterns and are indeterminate.

Of the extensive literature on lung scanning,[84–97a] the Prospective Investigation of Pulmonary Embolism Diagnosis (PIOPED) merits particular attention.[88] It compared VA/Q scanning with pulmonary arteriography in 755 patients; of these patients, 251 had PE by arteriography but only 102 (41%) had a high-probability lung scan. Other smaller studies have shown similar results.[92, 93] Moreover, from 15% to 30% of patients with low-probability lung scans do, in fact, have PE.[88, 90–92, 95] These findings show that both high- and low-probability lung scans are limited in predicting the presence or absence of PE. On the other hand, a normal lung scan is as reliable as a normal pulmonary arteriogram in ruling out PE.[86, 94, 95]

Pulmonary arteriography is the most reliable means of establishing the presence of pulmonary emboli and determining their location and extent.[88, 90, 93] In experienced hands, it is relatively safe.[90, 96, 98] Arteriographic findings diagnostic of PE include completely obstructed pulmonary arteries (Figs. 33–2*B* and 33–3) and intra-arterial filling defects (Fig. 33–2*B*).[96, 99, 100] Changes in arterial caliber proximal or distal to the embolus may appear (Fig. 33–3), as well as a decrease in volume of affected lung segments. Intra-arterial webs, pouchlike filling defects, or intimal irregularities suggest previous thromboemboli.[101, 102]

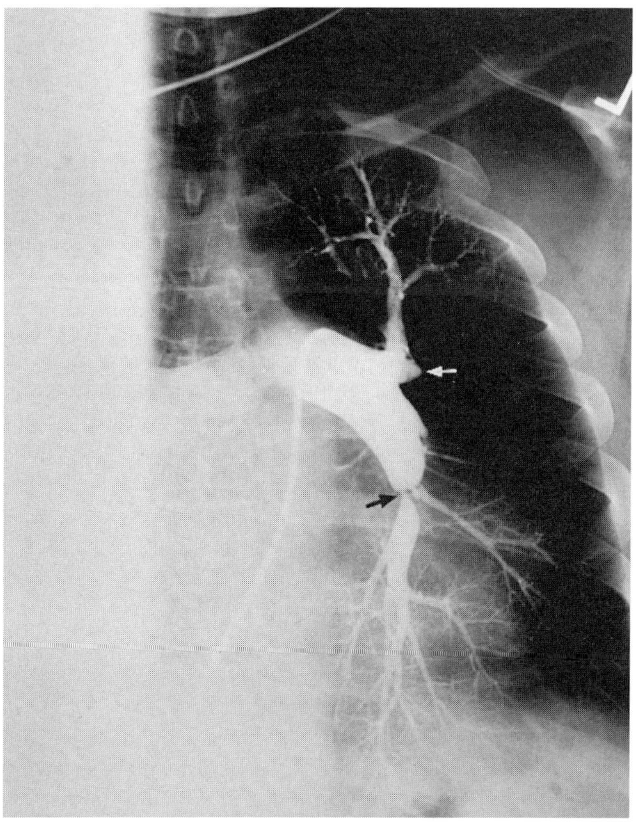

FIGURE 33–3. Selective pulmonary arteriogram of a 35-year-old woman with recurrent episodes of shortness of breath and blood-tinged sputum. Note complete obstruction of one artery *(white arrow)* and marked constriction of another artery *(black arrow)* with poststenotic dilatation.

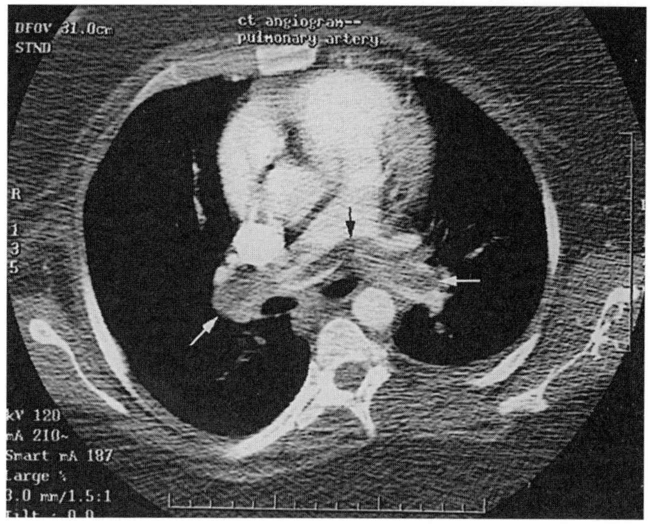

FIGURE 33–4. Contrast-enhanced spiral computed tomographic study shows a large filling defect *(arrows)* in the bifurcation of the pulmonary arterial trunk. The patient, a 31-year-old diabetic woman with a painful swollen right leg and sudden onset of dyspnea, died just as thrombolytic therapy was being initiated.

Echocardiography is valuable in detecting right ventricular dysfunction, particularly when the systemic arterial pressure remains normal.[103–105] Such testing is important because right ventricular dysfunction in patients with PE correlates with increased mortality.[106–107a] And because such dysfunction is not always clinically apparent, the echocardiogram becomes an excellent means of monitoring therapeutic efficacy.[108–109a] It can also identify diseases that masquerade as PE.

The echocardiographic signs of PE include dilated right atrium, dilated hypokinetic right ventricle, flattening or paradoxic motion of the interventricular septum, and Doppler evidence of tricuspid or pulmonary regurgitation.[109–112] Regional right ventricular dysfunction with normal motion of the apical wall is another strong clue.[113] Additionally, the echocardiogram may show clots in the right atrium or right ventricle[113a] and occasionally in the central pulmonary arteries.[112, 114]

Contrast-enhanced *spiral* or *electron-beam computed tomography* images the pulmonary vessels directly. Emboli appear as filling defects within the opacified arteries (Fig. 33–4). Compared with pulmonary arteriography, this technique has a mean sensitivity and specificity of about 90% for detecting emboli in the main, lobar, or segmental arteries but not beyond.[115–117c] In fact, because of its greater sensitivity and specificity, this technique is gradually replacing lung scanning to screen for PE.[117d, 118] It has the advantage of being minimally invasive and of demonstrating chest disease that can masquerade clinically as PE.[118, 119] Moreover, it provides an excellent means of monitoring the resolution of centrally located emboli.[116, 119]

Gadolinium-enhanced *magnetic resonance angiography* can also identify large thromboemboli in the central pulmonary arteries but is not reliable in detecting clots in arteries beyond the segmental level.[120] Although its sensitivity is slightly lower than that of spiral computed tomography, its specificity is the same.[121, 122] And it is a valid means of documenting venous thrombosis in the pelvis and lower limbs.[83, 122]

Venous ultrasonography,[123–127] *impedance plethysmography,*[128] and *contrast venography*[129–131] are standard means of establishing the diagnosis of deep vein thrombosis. Based on the concept that pulmonary embolism and lower extremity deep vein thrombosis are manifestations of the same disease process, these investigations, when positive, are frequently used as surrogate evidence of PE.[89, 90, 132, 133] Venous ultrasonography using compression is the most accurate noninvasive means of diagnosing the first episode of symptomatic proximal deep vein thrombosis.[127] When it is negative, however, this study is not conclusive and should be repeated 5 to 7 days later before excluding deep vein thrombosis.[126, 127] Venous ultrasonography and impedance plethysmography are especially useful screening tests in pregnant women suspected of having PE.[26, 127]

Contrast venography remains the gold standard for diagnosing deep vein thrombosis. Although it is invasive and associated with risks from the use of contrast media, this technique may become necessary in situations in which noninvasive studies typically yield inconclusive results.[127] These situations include asymptomatic postoperative patients suspected of having proximal deep vein thrombosis, patients thought to have calf vein thrombosis, and patients suspected of having recurrent deep vein thrombosis.[127, 130, 134]

Angioscopy[135–137] and *intravascular ultrasound*[138] have not been adequately tested as methods for diagnosing PE. Nevertheless, angioscopy may prove useful in assessing the resolution of pulmonary thromboemboli.

Many physicians are reluctant to perform imaging studies during pregnancy because they are fearful of the radiation effects on the fetus. Yet, the combination of chest radiography, ventilation-perfusion scanning, and pulmonary arteriography exposes the fetus to less than 10% of the radiation dose known to cause significant fetal injury.[139] Nevertheless, the pregnant woman with suspected PE should be investigated aggressively, because the diagnosis of PE carries major therapeutic implications: the need for prolonged heparin therapy during pregnancy, the potential need for prophylaxis during subsequent pregnancies, and concern about future use of oral contraceptives and estrogen-replacement therapy.[26]

DIFFERENTIAL DIAGNOSIS

The manifestations of PE are so protean that even experienced clinicians occasionally mistake the illness for some other disorder. Conversely, other disorders not infrequently masquerade as PE. The differential diagnosis, therefore, is much broader than generally appreciated (Table 33–1).[140]

In this section, we consider only conditions that occur commonly in or have special relevance to women, are unique to women, or can be rapidly fatal if misdiagnosed. We show how confusion in diagnosis arises, and we mention, when possible, simple means of resolving the issue. Additionally, we indicate when specialized diagnostic procedures are indispensable for proper management.

Table 33–1. DIFFERENTIAL DIAGNOSIS OF PULMONARY EMBOLISM

A. Respiratory disorders
  1. Parenchymatous
    a. Pneumonia
    b. Pyogenic abscess
    c. Neoplasm
    d. Granulomatous infection
    e. Amebiasis
    f. Obstructive pulmonary disease
    g. Atelectasis
    h. Asthma
  2. Pleural
    a. Viral (coxsackievirus)
    b. Tuberculosis
    c. Neoplasm
    d. Systemic lupus erythematosus
  3. Congenital
    a. Agenesis of pulmonary artery
B. Cardiovascular disorders
  1. Myocardial infarction
  2. Congestive heart failure
  3. Pericarditis
  4. Acute cardiac tamponade
  5. Dissecting hematoma of aorta
  6. Right-sided intracavitary cardiac lesions
C. Neurologic disorders
  1. Disturbances of consciousness
  2. Convulsive disorders
  3. Cerebrovascular disease
D. Psychiatric disorders
  1. Anxiety states
  2. Munchausen's syndrome
E. Abdominal disorders
  1. Acute cholecystitis
  2. Subdiaphragmatic abscess
  3. Ruptured viscus
  4. Pancreatitis
  5. Splenic infarction
F. Infectious disorders
  1. Bacteremia
  2. Peritonitis
G. Pulmonary-renal disorders
  1. Goodpasture's syndrome
  2. Wegener's granulomatosis
  3. Uremia
H. Hematologic disorders
  1. Acute blood loss
    a. Intraintestinal
    b. Intrathoracic
    c. Intraperitoneal and/or retroperitoneal
  2. Sickle cell disease
  3. Disseminated intravascular coagulation
I. Metabolic disorders
  1. Pheochromocytoma
  2. Lactic acidosis
J. Other particulate matter
  1. Fat
  2. Amniotic fluid
  3. Tumor
  4. Air

Infectious Disorders

Septic Pulmonary Embolism

Although both septic pulmonary embolism (SPE) and PE are thromboembolic processes that target the lung, they differ in their pathogenesis, clinical features, and treatment (Table 33–2). In SPE, the emboli originate in suppurative foci involving peripheral veins, the right side of the heart, or both. And because the emboli consist largely of microorganisms mixed with clot or other particulate matter, their pulmonary manifestations represent infection (see Color Plate 33–1) more than infarction. The spectrum of offending pathogens is broad and varies with the nature and location of the septic focus.

In previous years, SPE usually occurred in patients with suppurative disease in the head or neck,[141, 142] or in women with suppurative pelvic thrombophlebitis consequent to postabortal, postpartal, or other gynecologic manipulations.[143] Now, SPE occurs more commonly in intravenous drug users,[144] especially those with right-sided endocarditis.[145]

Radiographically demonstrable pulmonary changes provide the first clue to SPE and are a requisite for the diagnosis. The abnormalities are frequently subtle and their recognition and correct interpretation may require review of sequential films (Fig. 33–5*A* and *B*). In most cases, the lesions are multiple and involve both lungs. They vary in size from 0.3 cm to 7.0 cm in diameter and appear patchy

Table 33–2. RELATIVE DIFFERENCES BETWEEN SEPTIC AND BLAND PULMONARY EMBOLISM

	SEPTIC	BLAND
Major Predisposing Factors	Infected systemic veins; right-sided endocarditis; intravenous drug abuse	Congestive heart failure; fracture of pelvic or long bones; immobility; bland venous disease of legs
Embolic Material		
Size	Small	Large
Content	Microorganisms mixed with clot or other particulate matter	Thrombus alone
Incidence	Uncommon	Common
Patient's Age	Below 50 years	Above 50 years
Clinical Findings		
Shaking chills	Common	"Never"
High fever	Typical	Uncommon
Sputum (when present)	Purulent; occasionally bloody	Bloody
Blood cultures	Positive	Negative
Chest Radiograph		
Infiltrates		
Number	Many	Few
Size	Small	Large
Type	Nodular or patchy	Segmental
Location	Any lobe	Lower lobes
Cavities	Typical	Uncommon
Air-fluid level	Common	Rare
Pleural effusion	Infrequent	Common
Course (Untreated)		
Progressive deterioration	Typical	Uncommon
Abrupt and catastrophic worsening	Rare	Common
Spontaneous remission	Rare	Common
Treatment	Antibiotics	Anticoagulants
Predominant Pathologic Change	Pneumonia; microabscess formation; arteritis	Arterial obstruction; infarction

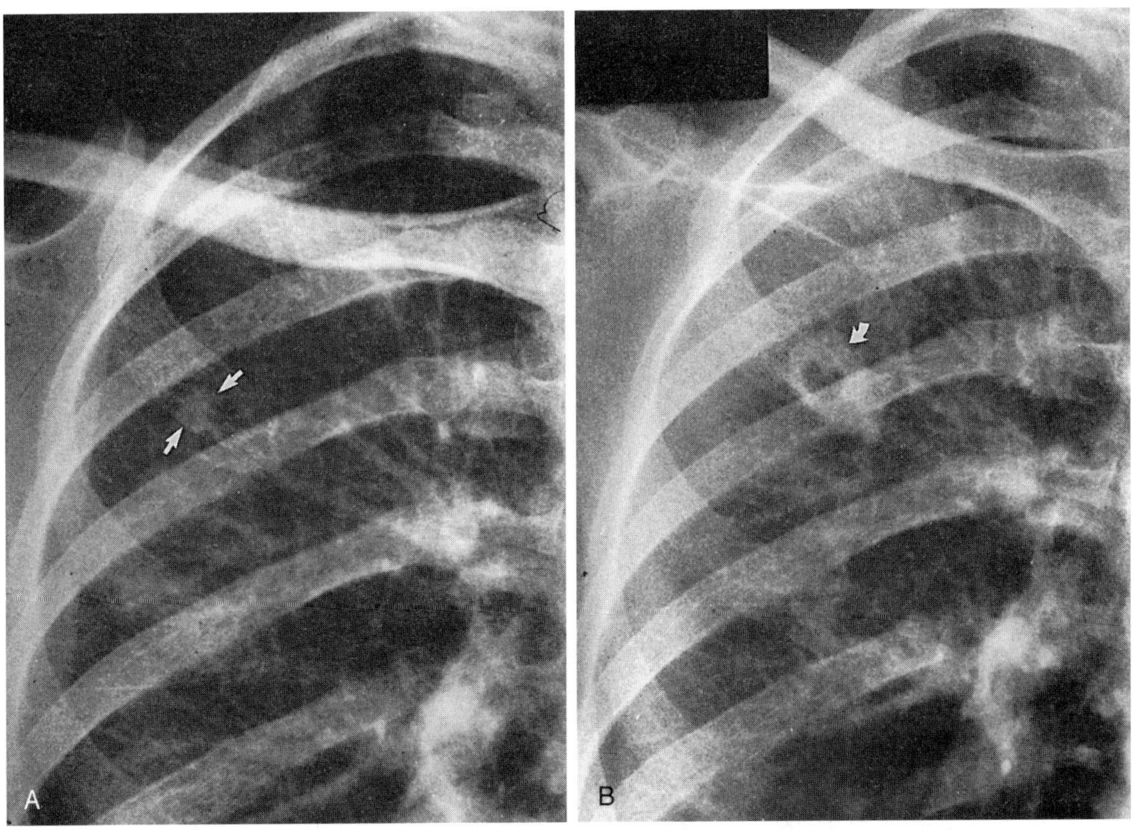

FIGURE 33–5. Views of right upper lung showing progressive enlargement and cavitation of an isolated, small infiltrate *(arrows)*. The patient was a 25-year-old woman with heroin addiction and staphylococcal tricuspid endocarditis. These radiographs were made at admission *(A)* and on day four *(B)*.

or nodular, hazy or dense, and confluent or ring-shaped. Cavitation, often with air-fluid levels, is the rule.[146] New lesions may appear and others may enlarge during the first week or so of appropriate therapy.

SPE can masquerade radiographically as pulmonary metastases,[147] tuberculosis,[141, 142] and other cavitary disorders of the lung.[148] In such cases, the finding of bacteremia or of rapid changes in size, number, and distribution of the parenchymal densities favors SPE.

Lung scanning and pulmonary arteriography are of limited usefulness in SPE. The scan may be normal in the presence of tiny septic emboli, and the arteriogram is unreliable as a means of assessing structural integrity of vessels beyond the subsegmental level. Computerized tomography may complement radiography by disclosing unsuspected or otherwise undetectable nodules in the lung.[149] Echocardiography may clinch the diagnosis if it demonstrates vegetations on the tricuspid or pulmonic valve.

Treatment consists of administering antibiotics, draining any associated abscess, removing indwelling venous catheters, and sometimes excising the infected venous segment.[146] If septic pelvic thrombophlebitis is the source, ligation of the inferior vena cava and both ovarian veins may become necessary.[150] Patients with right-sided endocarditis unresponsive to antibiotic therapy may require tricuspid valvulectomy.[151] The role of anticoagulants remains controversial.[152–154] We do not use these agents because of their potential to induce serious hemorrhage from infected pulmonary arteries.

Other Particulate Matter

Amniotic Fluid Embolism

Precipitous hypotension accompanied by cardiorespiratory embarrassment is characteristic of this illness and closely simulates some cases of PE. Representing a dramatic and potentially catastrophic complication of pregnancy, amniotic fluid embolism (AFE) occurs once in every 8000[155] to 80,000[156] confinements. It has a high mortality rate in clinically recognized cases and accounts for roughly 10% of all maternal deaths.[157] Half of these deaths take place within the first hour after onset of symptoms.[158] Nonlethal cases, however, are well documented,[159–161] and others undoubtedly escape detection. About half of the maternal fatalities result from cardiorespiratory failure and half from hemorrhagic complications consequent to disseminated intravascular coagulation.[161] Fetal mortality approaches 40%.[157] The pathogenesis of this syndrome remains speculative.

AFE occurs under a variety of circumstances: first-trimester curettage abortion; second-trimester abortion with saline, urea, or hysterectomy; abdominal trauma; amniocentesis; vaginal delivery or cesarean section; and postpartum.[158] It typically affects multigravidas, two thirds of whom are over 30 years of age. Ordinarily, the prenatal course is uneventful, but labor is prolonged. Symptoms usually begin during labor, delivery, or within a few hours postpartum; they are commonly preceded by rupture of the membranes. Hypotension is the rule, but cyanosis, dyspnea, shivering, and restlessness are frequent, too. Pulmonary edema appears in about a third of the patients and coagulation defects in about a half. The

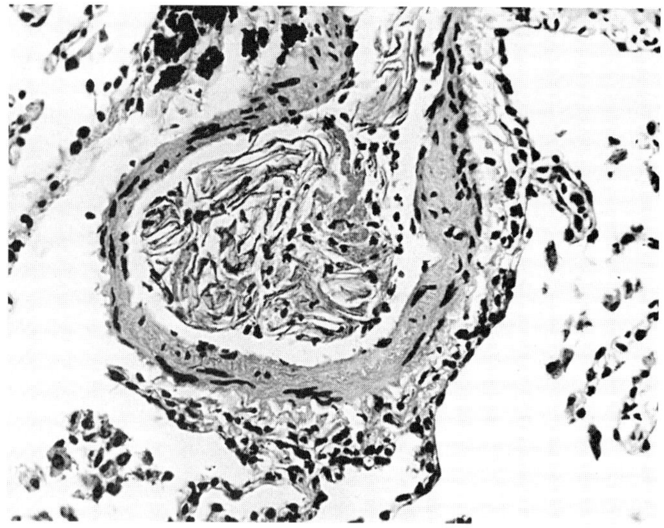

FIGURE 33–6. Small muscular pulmonary artery at its branching into an arteriole. The lumen contains amniotic debris characterized by squames that have clear slits between them and appear in parallel sheets. (Squames are sloughed epithelial cells from the skin of the fetus.) (Hematoxylin and eosin, × 310.)

chest radiograph may be normal or show varying degrees of perihilar edema.

An unequivocal diagnosis of AFE is possible only at necropsy. The characteristic histopathologic findings are pulmonary edema, alveolar hemorrhage, and multiple pulmonary emboli composed of mucin, amorphous debris, epithelial squames (Fig. 33–6), and occasionally, lanugo hair. Special stains, such as alcian blue or acid mucopolysaccharide to distinguish mucin, and Sudan Black or oil red O to document fat, help bring out the typical histologic pattern of AFE. Finding amniotic debris in the buffy coat of blood obtained from the pulmonary artery[159, 160, 162] or right atrium,[161] or finding lanugo hairs or squamous cells in the sputum[163–165] provides strong antemortem evidence of AFE.

Many catastrophic illnesses can simulate AFE. These illnesses include hypovolemic shock caused by placenta previa, abruptio placentae, or ruptured uterus; profuse bleeding associated with retained placental fragments or severe cervical or perineal lacerations; septic shock; and anaphylactic response to drugs.

Accurate clinical distinction between AFE and PE is difficult at best. In favor of AFE are multiparity, maternal age over 30 years, onset of symptoms late in labor, during delivery, or in the immediate postpartal period, difficult or prolonged labor, radiographic evidence of pulmonary edema, and coagulation defects such as thrombocytopenia, hypoprothrombinemia, and hypofibrinogenemia.

Perfusion lung scans in cases of presumed AFE have shown no characteristic pattern.[162, 166, 167] In at least two cases,[159, 166] however, pulmonary arteriography clarified the diagnosis by excluding PE.

Treatment of AFE is supportive. A few survivors of clinically diagnosed AFE have had uneventful subsequent pregnancies.[164, 166]

Fat Embolism

In a patient with recent fracture of the long bones, the sudden development of respiratory disability, pulmonary parenchymal infiltrates, central nervous system abnormalities, or combinations thereof, suggests fat embolism[158] as well as PE. In such cases, the best clue to fat embolism is the appearance of a petechial rash over the anterior part of the shoulders, the anterosuperior portion of the chest, the base of the neck, the axillae and conjunctivae, or occasionally, the abdomen and thighs.[168] When present, the petechiae typically emerge 24 to 36 hours after the injury, persist for 3 to 4 days, and then fade rapidly.

Additional features favoring fat embolism are onset of symptoms within hours to a few days after the injury; diffuse, bilateral, "snowstorm-like" densities on chest radiograph simulating pulmonary edema but without pleural effusion or cardiomegaly; a sharp drop in the hematocrit value consequent to intrapulmonary hemorrhage; increased erythrocyte aggregation and hemolysis; thrombocytopenia resulting from platelet aggregation; and demonstration of fat globules in the retinal arterioles, cerebrospinal fluid, or on the surface of the urine. Differentiating fat embolism from PE on clinical grounds alone can be difficult, and sometimes impossible. In such cases, pulmonary arteriography is the best means of clarifying the issue.

Respiratory Disorders

Pneumonia

Both pulmonary infarction and bacterial pneumonia can cause dyspnea, tachypnea, cough, pleuritic pain, fever, hemoptysis, leukocytosis, and similar abnormalities on chest radiograph.[71] To minimize diagnostic error, the physician should consider both disorders when making a tentative diagnosis of either, particularly when the process involves the lower lobes, especially the right. Because accurate clinical distinction often takes several days and is sometimes impossible, we treat for both conditions as long as the diagnosis remains unclear.

Certain features can be helpful in differentiating these two illnesses. Patients with pulmonary infarction seldom have a troublesome cough, manifest shaking chills only when the emboli are septic, and almost never have classic physical signs of consolidation or grossly purulent sputum. A pleural friction rub has no differential value unless it occurs in the absence of parenchymal infiltrates on chest radiograph. Then, pneumonia is unlikely.

Pulmonary arteriography is the most specific means of differentiating bacterial pneumonia from pulmonary infarction. In PE, the affected pulmonary arteries show filling defects or obstruction, or both; in pneumonia, they show tapering with poor distal flow but no intraluminal abnormalities (Fig. 33–7).[71]

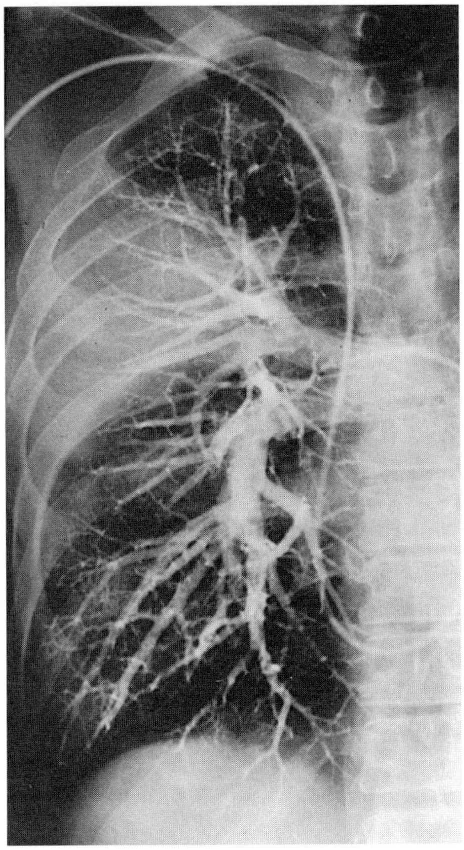

FIGURE 33–7. Selective pulmonary arteriogram of a 60-year-old patient with pneumococcal bacteremia and right upper lobe pneumonia. Arteries in the affected area show tapering with poor distal flow but no filling defects or obstruction.

Obstructive Pulmonary Disease

Like PE, obstructive pulmonary disease may cause wheezing, breathlessnesss, cough, hemoptysis, fever, and cyanosis. The chest radiograph in either disorder may show prominence of one or both main pulmonary arteries together with localized or diffuse zones of increased radiolucency in which the peripheral vascular markings are diminished or absent. Additionally, either disorder may manifest electrocardiographic evidence of supraventricular arrhythmias, right-axis deviation, or a pattern suggesting right ventricular overload. In such instances, purulent sputum and hypercapnia suggest obstructive pulmonary disease, whereas hypocapnia favors PE. Because perfusion defects occur in both conditions, lung scanning has limited usefulness, and spiral computed tomography[169, 170] or pulmonary arteriography may become necessary.

Asthma

Common to both PE and bronchial asthma are recurrent attacks of wheezing, dyspnea, and anxiety, associated with a normal-appearing chest radiograph or with scattered pulmonary parenchymal infiltrates, cyanosis, and signs of rapidly developing pulmonary hypertension. A long-standing history of atopy, elevated blood eosinophil count, tenacious and occasionally purulent sputum, or prompt therapeutic response to bronchodilators favors bronchial asthma. If, however, the patient is acutely ill, the diagnosis in doubt, and precise differentiation mandatory, pulmonary arteriography can settle the issue.

Cardiovascular Disorders

Myocardial Infarction

PE often mimics myocardial infarction, particularly in the first few hours after the embolic episode and before distinct clinical or radiographic signs of pulmonary infarction develop. To complicate matters, PE occasionally is a sequel of myocardial infarction,[171] and myocardial infarction occasionally results from the systemic hypotension and pulmonary hypertension brought about by PE. Nevertheless, certain features are helpful in distinguishing between these two entities.

One good way of differentiating these disorders is to correlate the patient's blood pressure with the electrocardiogram. If hypotension develops concomitant with or after the onset of chest pain, and the accompanying electrocardiogram does not show definite or strongly suggestive evidence of acute myocardial infarction, cardiac necrosis is most unlikely. In contrast, when PE causes hypotension, the electrocardiogram typically shows only sinus tachycardia and nonspecific T-wave changes or, sometimes, right-sided heart strain.

The duration of hypotension is another important diagnostic clue. Hypotension from myocardial infarction ordinarily persists and usually requires vasopressor therapy. By contrast, hypotension from PE ordinarily is transient, disappearing within minutes to a few hours, often without the aid of vasopressors. If prolonged, it indicates massive obstruction to pulmonary blood flow with consequent decrease in cardiac output.

Finally, two contrasting features of PE and myocardial infarction deserve emphasis. Patients with PE characteristically have dyspnea out of proportion to the degree of pain, hypotension, cyanosis, or radiographic changes. They may also appear moribund one minute and nearly well the next. Conversely, in patients with acute myocardial infarction, dyspnea frequently is absent and, when present, usually reflects the degree of associated pulmonary vascular congestion. And once patients with myocardial infarction appear moribund, they rarely recover spontaneously or rapidly.

Congestive Heart Failure

Among features common to both congestive heart failure and PE are dyspnea, wheezing, apprehension, cyanosis, tachycardia, rales in the lung, hypotension, pleural effusion, bright red sputum, elevated jugular venous pressure, hepatomegaly, and peripheral edema. To complicate the picture, congestive heart failure predisposes the patient to PE, and PE sometimes precipitates and is responsible for the persistence of congestive heart failure.

Clinical differentiation of these two disorders may be difficult. Points favoring PE are distinct clots of blood in the sputum, a normal heart size, and no pulmonary congestion on chest radiograph. Echocardiographic demonstration of contractile dysfunction predominantly of or limited to the left ventricle will usually establish a cardiac cause. Occasionally, pulmonary arteriography or direct measurement of pulmonary capillary pressure, or both, may be necessary for exact diagnosis.

Acute Cardiac Tamponade

When this illness presents with abrupt onset of dyspnea, tachypnea, tachycardia, cyanosis, distended neck veins, hepatomegaly, hypotension, and occasionally, chest pain, it closely simulates massive PE. Pulsus paradoxus, inspiratory distension of neck veins (Kussmaul's sign), and distant heart sounds also may occur in either disorder. Because small amounts of pericardial fluid accumulated rapidly can lead to significant hemodynamic alteration without significant cardiomegaly, chest radiographs may not be useful in separating these two processes. Correct diagnosis may require echocardiography, computed tomography, magnetic resonance angiography, cardiac catheterization, or pulmonary arteriography.

Dissecting Hematoma of the Aorta

Chest pain, usually severe and occasionally pleuritic, together with dyspnea, tachypnea, hypotension, neurologic manifestations, and even hemoptysis, are features of dissecting hematoma of the aorta that simulate PE. The diagnosis can be particularly confusing when the hematoma ruptures into the pericardial sac causing cardiac tamponade, or into the pleural space (usually the left), resulting in hemothorax. A hematocrit value of the pleural fluid approaching that of peripheral blood is evidence of a ruptured vessel and weighs heavily against pulmonary infarction. Widening of the aorta, mediastinum, or both, on chest radiograph is another sign of dissecting hematoma. Precise diagnosis ordinarily requires computed tomography, magnetic resonance angiography, echocardiography, pulmonary arteriography, or combinations thereof.

Neurologic Disorders

Because the neurologic manifestations of PE are usually abrupt in onset and often transient and recurrent, they commonly masquerade as those of cerebrovascular disease.[63] Conversely, cerebrovascular disease, such as hemorrhagic infarction and subdural hematoma, may be associated with labored respirations, pulmonary parenchymal infiltrates,[172] and electrocardiographic changes.[173] Consequently, differentiation of these two conditions can be difficult. Findings suggestive of PE are cardiorespiratory abnormalities or signs of phlebitis that occur in association with sudden, transient, or recurrent neurologic dysfunction. Another clue to PE is syncope at rest, especially in the elderly, bedridden, or cardiac patient.

TREATMENT

The ideal treatment of PE is prevention of the initial thrombus formation.[174–176] To accomplish this goal, several measures—used singly or in combination—are worthwhile: early full ambulation (especially for postpartal and postoperative patients), elastic stockings or intermittent pneumatic compression for bedridden persons and those undergoing major operative procedures,[177] and anticoagulant medication for patients at particular risk for PE.

Current methods for preventing PE in hospitalized patients,[175, 178–209] in patients discharged after lower extremity arthroplasty,[194, 195] and in pregnant women[26, 210] appear in Table 33–3. Whether pregnant women with a history of previous PE should receive anticoagulants prophylactically is not settled.[211, 211a] Because warfarin readily crosses the placenta, can cause fetal hemorrhage, and is teratogenic, it should be avoided throughout pregnancy.[26] Nevertheless, pregnant women with mechanical heart valves, those who suffer recurrent PE while receiving heparin, and those with contraindications to heparin therapy may require warfarin.[211b] In such cases, the potential adverse effects of warfarin on the fetus must be made clear to the patient. After delivery, warfarin therapy is safe and is not a contraindication to breast feeding.

Once PE has occurred, the type of therapy depends on the severity of the illness, the nature of any associated diseases, the skill and experience of the physician, and the available facilities. Even considering these factors, it may be difficult, at times, to decide on a fixed course of treatment, primarily because one cannot predict accurately in a given patient whether or when another embolus will occur, whether it will be clinically detectable, or how extensive it may be.

In addition to supportive measures, immediate anticoagulation with unfractionated heparin is standard (barring obvious contraindications). Heparin acts largely by binding to antithrombin III.[212] The resultant heparin-antithrombin III complex inactivates both thrombin and activated factor X. Because of the heterogeneous nature of unfractionated heparin, the response to therapy with this agent varies considerably.[213] Hence, frequent monitoring of the activated partial thromboplastin time (APTT) is necessary.

It is important to achieve a therapeutic threshold rapidly (i.e., an APTT ratio 1.5 times the control).[214–216] Failure to do so is associated with a high incidence of recurrent PE.[217] We favor an intravenous bolus of 5000 to 10,000 U heparin followed by a continuous infusion of 1200 to 1500 units/hour. Based on the APTT value, the dose is adjusted at intervals of 4 to 6 hours, and the infusion is continued for at least 5 days.[218]

Pregnant women with PE should receive heparin intravenously for 10 days followed by heparin subcutaneously throughout gestation.[26, 211] The intravenous regimen is the same as that mentioned earlier. The subcutaneous regimen consists of approximately 20,000 U every 12 hours, which is adjusted to maintain the APTT at 1.5 times the control. For patients in labor, heparin therapy should be discontinued at the onset of regular uterine contractions.

Low-molecular-weight heparin offers several therapeutic advantages over unfractionated heparin: longer half-life, more predictable anticoagulant activity, no need for laboratory monitoring, and lower incidence of thrombocytopenia.[196, 219–224a] It is also effective when administered subcutaneously. But since low-molecular-weight heparins are distinct compounds with different pharmacokinetic profiles and dosage regimens, the results with one preparation cannot be extended to those of another. Nevertheless, these agents are safe and effective in the treatment of proximal deep vein thrombosis[196, 220, 221] and may become the best option for treating PE.[83, 223, 225–227b]

For long-term anticoagulation in the nonpregnant patient, therapy with warfarin sodium is standard.[228] This drug inhibits the enzyme vitamin K epoxide reductase. As a consequence, body stores of vitamin K become depleted; the synthesis of coagulation factors II, VII, IX, and X becomes impaired; and the prothrombin time is prolonged.

Warfarin can be administered along with, or shortly after, the institution of heparin therapy.[229–231] The usual recommended therapeutic range is an International Normalized Ratio (INR) of 2.0 to 3.0.[232] But in patients with the antiphospholipid antibody syndrome, the target INR is 3.5.[233]

Levels of coagulation factor VII decrease within hours after the initiation of warfarin therapy. But it takes about 5 days for levels of the other coagulation factors to decrease.[228, 234] Therefore, heparin therapy should be continued for at least 2 to 3 days after the target INR has been reached.

The duration of anticoagulation varies.[235, 236] Two months may suffice in patients with a definable and reversible cause of PE (e.g., fractured pelvis, postoperative state, or postpartum). When the cause cannot be identified, therapy should be continued for at least 6 months.[232, 232a, 232b] For patients with recurrent PE and for those with the antiphospholipid antibody syndrome, lifelong anticoagulation is probably necessary. In patients with other underlying thrombophilic conditions, the duration of therapy remains unclear.[234, 236, 237]

Thrombolytic therapy deserves immediate consideration in patients who are hemodynamically unstable from massive PE. Such treatment promotes dissolution of clots much faster than that achieved with anticoagulants alone.[98, 108, 238–241] The resultant decrease in clot burden relieves strain on the right ventricle, allowing cardiac function to improve.[108, 111, 241a, 242] This therapy may also reduce the rate of recurrent PE by dissolving the initiating thrombi. Proof of such an effect, however, is lacking.[243]

Some patients with massive PE are hemodynamically stable but have echocardiographic evidence of right ventricular dysfunction. Experience to date, albeit observational, suggests that these patients may also benefit from thrombolytic therapy.[104, 105, 107, 107a] Although randomized clinical trials of thrombolytic therapy in PE demonstrate no reduction in mortality, the scintigraphic, echocardiographic, and angiographic findings do improve.[243–246]

One additional point deserves emphasis: If the patient is in shock and the clinical evidence points strongly to PE, thrombolytics can be lifesaving and should be administered without seeking absolute diagnostic confirmation.[104, 246a] The potential benefit from thrombolytics in such cases far outweighs the risk of significant hemorrhage.[241a, 246b] In this setting, bedside transthoracic echocardiography can be invaluable in demonstrating right ventricular pressure overload while excluding other diagnostic considerations such as cardiac tamponade, left ventricular failure, and aortic dissection.[104, 241a]

Whereas the window for thrombolytic therapy in acute myocardial infarction is but a few hours,[247–249] it is days to weeks in PE.[108, 250] The United States Food and Drug Administration has approved three thombolytic treatment protocols for PE (Table 33–4). All three lyse clots effectively, but recombinant tissue-type plasminogen activator acts most rapidly and produces the fewest systemic reactions. No laboratory monitoring or dose adjustment is necessary, and heparin is not used during the infusion. Anticoagulation is mandatory, however, on completion of thrombolytic therapy.

Table 33–3. PROPHYLAXIS OF VENOUS THROMBOEMBOLISM

1. Medical inpatients	Unfractionated heparin 5000 U twice daily[175, 178] (with or without GCS,† IPC,‡ or aspirin§[179, 180]) or Low-molecular-weight heparin Enoxaparin 40 mg daily[180a]
2. Intensive care unit	Same as 1.[181–183]
3. General surgery	Unfractionated heparin 5000 U twice daily[184–187] or Low-molecular-weight heparin[187, 188] Enoxaparin 40 mg daily or Dalteparin 2500 to 5000 U daily[189, 190] or Nadroparin‖ 3100 U daily or Tinzaparin‖ 3500 U daily (Each of the above with or without GCS, IPC, or aspirin)
4. Cardiothoracic surgery	Same as 1.[191]
5. Hip replacement	Low-molecular-weight heparin Enoxaparin 30 mg twice daily[192–195] or Heparinoid Danaparoid 750 U twice daily[196] or Recombinant Hirudin Desirudin‖ 15 U twice daily[197, 198] or Adjusted-dose unfractionated heparin to maintain APTT¶ ratio 1.5 times that of the control value[199] or Adjusted-dose warfarin (target INR°° 2.5)[200] (Each of the above with or without GCS[201] and IPC[202])
6. Knee replacement	Low-molecular-weight heparin Enoxaparin 30 mg twice daily[194, 195, 203] or Ardeparin 50 U/kg twice daily[204] (Each of the above with or without IPC)
7. Neurosurgery	GCS and IPC[205] or GCS with low-molecular-weight heparin Enoxaparin 40 mg daily[206]
8. Spinal surgery	GCS with or without IPC[207]
9. Trauma (excluding brain)	GCS and IPC with or without low-molecular-weight heparin Enoxaparin 30 mg twice daily[208] or Adjusted-dose unfractionated heparin to maintain APTT ratio 1.5 times that of the control value[209]
10. Pregnancy	Unfractionated heparin 7500 U to 10,000 U twice daily[26] or Adjusted-dose unfractionated heparin to maintain APTT ratio 1.5 times that of the control value[26] or Low-molecular-weight heparin Dalteparin 5000 U daily[210] or Enoxaparin 40 mg daily[26]

°All listed medications except aspirin and warfarin are administered subcutaneously.
†GCS, graduated compression stockings.
‡IPC, intermittent pneumatic compression.
§Dose varies from 80 to 325 mg daily.
‖Not approved by the United States Food and Drug Administration.
¶APTT, activated partial thromboplastin time.
°°INR, International Normalized Ratio.

Table 33–4. THROMBOLYTIC TREATMENT PROTOCOLS FOR PULMONARY EMBOLISM

	STREPTOKINASE	UROKINASE	RECOMBINANT TISSUE-TYPE PLASMINOGEN ACTIVATOR
Loading dose	250,000 U over 30 min	4400 IU/kg over 10 min	None
Maintenance dose	100,000 U/h for 24 h	4400 IU/kg/h for 12–24 h	50 mg/h for 2 h

Contraindications to thrombolytic therapy ordinarily include active internal bleeding, pregnancy, multiple trauma, and intracranial hemorrhage.[98] All contraindications become relative, however, when the patient is dying from massive PE.

Interruption of blood flow through the inferior vena cava, either totally (by ligation) or partially (by use of filters or various suturing techniques), merits serious consideration when anticoagulant therapy is contraindicated or when PE recurs despite optimal anticoagulation.[251–253] Caval interruption is mandatory following pulmonary embolectomy. Moreover, in women with suppurative pelvic thrombophlebitis and septic pulmonary emboli unresponsive to antibiotic or anticoagulant therapy, ligation of the inferior vena cava and both ovarian veins may be lifesaving.

Six caval filters are currently available in this country—three types of Greenfield filters, the Bird's nest filter, the Simon nitinol filter, and the Vena Tech filter.[253–256] In some European centers, caval filters specifically designed for temporary use are also available.[257–260] All of these devices are being used prophylactically with increasing frequency in a wide variety of clinical circumstances.[253, 261–264] In some cases, however, thrombi proximal to a filter, especially thrombi in the heart, can negate the filter's potential advantages.[265] When the patient is pregnant or premenopausal and requires a vena caval filter, the device should be placed in the suprarenal portion of the inferior vena cava to entrap emboli that traverse the ovarian veins.[26]

The role of pulmonary embolectomy remains controversial. Some authors suggest that this procedure should be considered more often,[266] even in patients with no hemodynamic compromise.[267] Others argue that the successful completion of pulmonary arteriography virtually precludes the need for embolectomy.[268] Still others say that there are no indications for pulmonary embolectomy.[269] We favor this operation when thrombolytic therapy is contraindicated or has failed and the patient is either moribund or shows steady deterioration despite vigorous medical management.[270] Arteriography is still the best means of establishing the presence and precise location of surgically accessible pulmonary thromboemboli.

Transvenous pulmonary embolectomy with catheter suction is another method of treating massive PE.[271–272a] Its in hospital mortality rate of about 30% is similar to that of open embolectomy.[273] Catheter embolectomy, however, is limited in its ability to remove thrombi that have already become adherent to the wall of the pulmonary artery. More recent catheter-based techniques attempt mechanical fragmentation of the clot with high-velocity jets of saline.[274, 275] These various techniques offer promise for patients who, from old age and coexisting disease, are particularly poor surgical risks, do not have access to cardiopulmonary bypass facilities, or have contraindications to heparin and thrombolytic therapy.

For patients with chronic thromboembolic pulmonary hypertension consequent to major vessel occlusion, pulmonary artery thromboendarterectomy is currently the only effective therapy.[276, 277] When the thromboemboli are surgically inaccessible, however, balloon pulmonary angioplasty can improve pulmonary blood flow distribution and increase pulmonary vascular capacitance, thereby decreasing right ventricular afterload.[277a]

COURSE AND PROGNOSIS

Pulmonary arteriograms performed serially have shown that major clots can resolve spontaneously and completely within 7 to 14 days.[278, 279] In one case, an embolus to a lobar artery resolved almost completely within 30 hours.[280] These observations help explain why most patients with PE survive the initial episode, irrespective of the type of treatment.

Deaths from PE usually occur in the first 2 weeks after diagnosis.[281] About 75% of the patients with fatal PE die within the first hour.[282] Most of them have serious underlying disease such as heart failure or cancer.

Recurrence is uncommon in patients who are properly diagnosed and treated.[243, 283] In a prospective study comprising 399 cases of PE diagnosed by lung scanning and arteriography, 33 patients (8.3%) had clinically apparent recurrence.[281] Other prospective therapeutic trials have shown rates of recurrence ranging from 4% to 19%.[238, 239]

The long-term outlook for patients with PE depends largely on the nature and severity of any underlying disease. For those without pre-existing heart disease, prognosis is good.[284] During a 9-year follow-up, 12 of 72 patients who had survived massive PE died; in no case, however, did death result from chronic pulmonary hypertension or from definite recurrence of PE.[285] Chronic cor pulmonale from PE is relatively rare,[284] but may arise in patients with repeated embolic episodes that go unrecognized and therefore untreated.

References

1. Bennett R: The Diseases of the Bible: The Religious Tract Society, London, 1887.
2. Hélie M: Inflammation de l'artère pulmonaire. Mort subite. Bull Soc Anat de Paris 8:254, 1837.
3. Gammeltoft SA: Case of embolism in puerpera described by Chr. August Egeberg, Norway in 1844. Acta Med Scand 266(Suppl):55, 1952.
4. Bell WR, Simon TL: Current status of pulmonary thromboembolic disease: Pathophysiology, diagnosis, prevention, and treatment. Am Heart J 103:239, 1982.

5. Lilienfeld DE, Chan E, Ehland J, et al: Mortality from pulmonary embolism in the United States: 1962 to 1984. Chest 98:1067, 1990.
6. Marshall R: Pulmonary Embolism: Mechanism and Management. Charles C Thomas, Springfield, IL, 1965, p 14.
7. Goyette EM: The diagnosis and management of pulmonary embolism and infarction. Dis Chest 25:15, 1954.
8. Rexrode WO: Massive pulmonary embolism in an otherwise healthy young patient. Respir Care 31:803, 1986.
9. Emery JL: Pulmonary embolism in children. Arch Dis Child 37: 591, 1962.
10. Ramirez LM: Thromboembolic disease in adolescence. JAMA 170: 1808, 1959.
10a. Sørensen HT, Mellemkjaer L, Olsen JH, et al: Prognosis of cancers associated with venous thromboembolism. N Engl J Med 343:1846, 2000.
11. Dahlback B, Carlsson M, Svensson PJ: Familial thrombophilia due to a previously unrecognized mechanism characterized by poor anticoagulant response to activated protein C: Prediction of a cofactor to activated protein C. Proc Natl Acad Sci USA 90:1004, 1993.
12. Zoller B, Svensson PJ, He X, et al: Identification of the same factor V mutation in 47 out of 50 thrombosis prone families with inherited resistance to activated protein C. J Clin Invest 94:2521, 1994.
13. Svensson PJ, Dahlback B: Resistance to activated protein C as a basis for venous thrombosis. N Engl J Med 330:517, 1994.
14. Bertina RM, Koeleman BPC, Koster T, et al: Mutation in factor V associated with resistance to activated protein C. Nature 369:64, 1994.
15. Greengard JS, Sun X, Xu X, et al: Activated protein C resistance caused by Arg506Gln mutation in factor Va. Lancet 343:1361, 1994.
15a. Kyrle PA, Minar E, Hirschl M, et al: High plasma levels of factor VIII and the risk of recurrent venous thromboembolism. N Engl J Med 343:457, 2000.
15b. Meijers JC, Tekelenburg WL, Bouma BN, et al: High levels of coagulation factor XI as a risk factor for venous thrombosis. N Engl J Med 342:696, 2000.
16. Hughes GRV: The antiphospholipid antibody syndrome: Ten years on. Lancet 342:341, 1993.
17. den Heijer M, Koster T, Blom HJ, et al: Hyperhomocysteinemia as a risk factor for deep-vein thrombosis. N Engl J Med 334:759, 1996.
18. Selhub J, D'Angelo A: Relationship between homocysteine and thrombotic disease. Am J Med Sci 316:129, 1998.
19. Margaglione M, Brancaccio V, Giuliani N, et al: Increased risk for venous thrombosis in carriers of the Prothrombin G→A^{20210} gene variant. Ann Intern Med 129:89, 1998.
19a. De Stefano V, Martinelli I, Mannucci PM, et al: The risk of recurrent deep venous thrombosis among heterozygous carriers of both factor V Leiden and the G20210A prothrombin mutation. N Engl J Med 341:801, 1999.
19b. Gerhardt A, Scharf RE, Beckmann MW, et al: Prothrombin and factor V mutations in women with a history of thrombosis during pregnancy and the puerperium. N Engl J Med 342:374, 2000.
19c. Grady D, Wenger NK, Herrington D, et al: Postmenopausal hormone therapy increases risk for venous thromboembolic disease. The Heart and Estrogen/Progestin Replacement Study. Ann Intern Med 132: 689, 2000.
19d. Zornberg GL, Jick H: Antipsychotic drug use and risk of first-time idiopathic venous thromboembolism: A case-control study. Lancet 356: 1219, 2000.
19e. Tapson VF: Risk of venous thromboembolism with use of antipsychotic drugs. Lancet 356:1206, 2000.
20. Venous thromboembolic disease and combined oral contraceptives: Results of international multicentre case-control study. World Health Organization Collaborative Study of Cardiovascular Disease and Steroid Hormone Contraception. Lancet 346:1575, 1995.
21. Effect of different progestagens in low oestrogen oral contraceptives on venous thromboembolic disease. Lancet 346:1582, 1995.
22. Bottiger LE, Boman G, Eklund G, et al: Oral contraceptives and thromboembolic disease: Effects of lowering estrogen content. Lancet 1:1097, 1980.
23. Vandenbroucke JP, Koster T, Briet E, et al: Increased risk of venous thrombosis in oral contraceptive users who are carriers of factor V Leiden mutation. Lancet 344:1453, 1994.
24. Bloemenkamp KWM, Rosendaal FR, Helmerhorst FM, et al: Enhancement by factor V Leiden mutation of risk of deep-vein thrombosis associated with oral contraceptives containing a third-generation progestagen. Lancet 346:1593, 1995.
25. Hirsch DR, Mikkola KM, Marks PW, et al: Pulmonary embolism and deep venous thrombosis during pregnancy or oral contraceptive use: Prevalence of factor V Leiden. Am Heart J 131:1145, 1996.
26. Toglia MR, Weg JG: Venous thromboembolism during pregnancy. N Engl J Med 335:108, 1996.
26a. Greer IA: The challenge of thrombophilia in maternal-fetal medicine. N Engl J Med 342:424, 2000.
27. Cumming AM, Tait RC, Fildes S et al: Development of resistance to activated protein C during pregnancy. Br J Haematol 90:725, 1995.
28. Hellgren M, Svensson PJ, Dahlback B: Resistance to activated protein C as a basis for venous thromboembolism associated with pregnancy. Am J Obstet Gynecol 173:210, 1995.
29. de Swiet M, Fidler J, Howell R, et al: Thromboembolism in pregnancy. In Jewell D (ed): Advanced Medicine. Pitman Medical, London, 1981, p 309.
30. Syverson CJ, Chavkin W, Atrash HK, et al: Pregnancy-related mortality in New York City, 1980 to 1984: Causes of death and associated risk factors. Am J Obstet Gynecol 164:603, 1991.
31. Hogberg U, Innala E, Sandstrom A: Maternal mortality in Sweden, 1980–1988. Obstet Gynecol 84:240, 1994.
32. Rutherford S, Montoro M, McGehee W, et al: Thromboembolic disease associated with pregnancy: An 11-year review. Am J Obstet Gynecol 164:286, 1991.
33. Ginsberg JS, Brill-Edwards P, Burrows RF: Venous thrombosis during pregnancy: Leg and trimester of presentation. Thromb Haemost 67: 519, 1992.
34. Gore I, Tanaka K: Phlebothrombosis, pulmonary embolization and pulmonary hypertension. Am J Med Sci 244:351, 1962.
35. Sevitt S, Gallagher N: Venous thrombosis and pulmonary embolism: A clinicopathological study in injured and burned patients. Br J Surg 48:475, 1961.
36. Chakko S, Richards F III: Right-sided cardiac thrombi and pulmonary embolism. Am J Cardiol 59:195, 1987.
37. Harley DP, White RA, Nelson RJ, et al: Pulmonary embolism secondary to venous thrombosis of the arm. Am J Surg 147:221, 1984.
38. Marks J, Truscott BM, Withycombe JFR: Treatment of venous thrombosis with anticoagulants: Review of 1,135 cases. Lancet 2:787, 1954.
39. Smith GT, Dexter L, Dammin GJ: Postmortem quantitative studies in pulmonary embolism. In Sasahara AA, Stein M (eds): Pulmonary Embolic Disease. Grune and Stratton, New York, 1965, p 120.
40. Ellis FH Jr, Grindlay JH, Edwards JE: The bronchial arteries. II. Their role in pulmonary embolism and infarction. Surgery 31:167, 1952.
41. Dalen JE, Haffajee CI, Alpert JS, et al: Pulmonary embolism, pulmonary hemorrhage, and pulmonary infarction. N Engl J Med 296: 1431, 1977.
42. Kelly MA, Fishman AP: Pulmonary thromboembolic disease. In Fishman AP (ed): Pulmonary Diseases and Disorders. McGraw-Hill, New York, 1988, p 1049.
43. Okhuda K, Nakahara K, Weidner J, et al: Lung fluid exchange after uneven pulmonary artery obstruction in sheep. Circ Res 43:152, 1978.
44. Sharma GVRK, McIntyre KM, Sharma S, et al: Clinical and hemodynamic correlates in pulmonary embolism. Clin Chest Med 5:421, 1984.
45. Haver VM, Namm DH: Characterization of the thrombin induced contraction of vascular smooth muscle. Blood Vessels 21:53, 1984.
46. Demling RH, Wong C, Fox R, et al: Relationship of increased lung serotonin levels to endotoxin induced pulmonary hypertension in sheep: Effects of a serotonin antagonist. Am Rev Respir Dis 152: 1257, 1985.
47. Duel TF, Huang JS: Platelet-derived growth factor. J Clin Invest 74: 669, 1984.
48. Znyda Am Dernbinska-Kiec A, Chytkowski A, Gryglewoki RJ: Experimental atherosclerosis in rabbits. Platelet aggregation, thromboxane A2 generation, and antiaggregatory potency. Prostaglandins 14:1035, 1977.
49. Manier G, Castaing Y: Influence of cardiac output on oxygen exchange in acute pulmonary embolism. Am Rev Respir Dis 145:130, 1992.
50. Stein M, Levy SE: Reflex and humoral responses to pulmonary embolism. Prog Cardiovasc Dis 17:167, 1974.
51. Burki NK: The dead space to tidal volume ratio in the diagnosis of pulmonary embolism. Am Rev Respir Dis 133:679, 1986.
52. Delcroix M, Melot C, Vanderhoeft P, et al: Embolus size affects gas exchange in canine autologous blood clot pulmonary embolism. J Appl Physiol 74:1140, 1993.
53. Colp CR, Williams MH: Pulmonary function following pulmonary embolization. Am Rev Respir Dis 85:799, 1962.

54. Wilson J, Pierce AK, Johnson RL, et al: Hypoxemia in pulmonary embolism. J Clin Invest 50:481, 1971.
55. Dantzker DR, Bower JS: Clinical significance of pulmonary function tests: Alterations in gas exchange following pulmonary thromboembolism. Chest 81:495, 1982.
56. Cvitanic O, Marino PL: Improved use of arterial blood gas analysis in suspected pulmonary embolism. Chest 95:48, 1989.
57. Stein PD, Goldhaber SZ, Henry JW, et al: Arterial blood gas analysis in the assessment of suspected acute pulmonary embolism. Chest 109:78, 1996.
58. Stein PD, Terrin ML, Hales CA, et al: Clinical, laboratory, roentgenographic and electrocardiographic findings in patients with acute pulmonary embolism and no pre-existing cardiac or pulmonary disease. Chest 100:598, 1991.
59. Alpert JS, Francis GS, Vieweg MD, et al: Left ventricular function in massive pulmonary embolism. Chest 71:108, 1977.
60. Lualdi JC, Goldhaber SZ: Right ventricular dysfunction after acute pulmonary embolism: Pathophysiologic factors, detection, and therapeutic implications. Am Heart J 130:1276, 1995.
61. Gorham LW: A study of pulmonary embolism. Arch Intern Med 108:189, 1961.
62. Olázabal FJ Jr, Román-Irizarry LA, Oms JD, et al: Pulmonary emboli masquerading as asthma. N Engl J Med 278:999, 1968.
63. Fred HL, Yang M: Sudden loss of consciousness, dyspnea, and hypoxemia in a previously healthy young man. Circulation 91:3017, 1995.
64. Miller R, Berry JB: Pulmonary infarction: A frequently missed diagnosis. Am J Med Sci 222:197, 1951.
65. Kollef MH, Schacter DT: Acute pulmonary embolism triggered by the act of defecation. Chest 99:373, 1991.
66. Sagall EL, Bornstein J, Wolff L: Clinical syndrome in patients with pulmonary embolism. Arch Intern Med 76:234, 1945.
67. Stevens AE: The late appearance of leg symptoms in pulmonary embolus. Lancet 2:1005, 1961.
68. Smith GT, Dammin GJ, Dexter L: Postmortem arteriographic studies of the human lung in pulmonary embolization. JAMA 188:143, 1964.
69. Israel HL, Goldstein F: The varied clinical manifestations of pulmonary embolism. Ann Intern Med 47:202, 1957.
70. Murray HW, Ellis GC, Blumenthal DS, et al: Fever and pulmonary thromboembolism. Am J Med 67:232, 1979.
70a. Stein PD, Afzal A, Henry JW, et al: Fever in acute pulmonary embolism. Chest 117:39, 2000.
71. Beall AC Jr, Fred HL, Cooley DA: Pulmonary embolism: Cause, consequences, prevention and treatment. Curr Prob Surg February 1964.
72. Parker BM, Smith JR: Pulmonary embolism and infarction: A review of the physiologic consequences of pulmonary arterial obstruction. Am J Med 24:402, 1958.
73. Kugel MA, Lichtman SS: Factors causing clinical jaundice in heart disease. Arch Intern Med 52:16, 1933.
74. Elliott CG, Goldhaber SZ, Visani L, et al: Chest radiographs in acute pulmonary embolism. Results from the International Cooperative Pulmonary Embolism Registry. Chest 118:33, 2000.
74a. Fleischner FG: Pulmonary embolism. Clin Radiol [Lond] 13:169, 1962.
75. Smith MJ: Roentgenographic aspects of complete and incomplete pulmonary infarction. Dis Chest 23:532, 1953.
76. Perkins RB, Bradshaw HH: Pulmonary infarction mistaken for bronchogenic carcinoma. JAMA 151:545, 1953.
77. Moser KM, Auger WR, Fedullo PF: Chronic major-vessel thromboembolic pulmonary hypertension. Circulation 81:1735, 1990.
78. Goodwin JF, Harrison CV, Wilcken DEL: Obliterative pulmonary hypertension and thromboembolism. Br Med J 701:777, 1963.
78a. Afzal A, Noor HA, Gill SA, et al: Leukocytosis in acute pulmonary embolism. Chest 115:1329, 1999.
79. Bynum LJ, Wison JE III: Characteristics of pleural effusions associated with pulmonary embolism. Arch Intern Med 136:159, 1976.
80. Perrier A, Desmarais S, Goehring C, et al: D-dimer testing for suspected pulmonary embolism in outpatients. Am J Respir Crit Care Med 156:492, 1997.
81. Oger E, Leroyer C, Bressollette L, et al: Evaluation of a new, rapid, and quantitative D-dimer test in patients with suspected pulmonary embolism. Am J Respir Crit Care Med 158:65, 1998.
82. Perrier A: Noninvasive diagnosis of pulmonary embolism. Hosp Pract 33:47, 1998.
82a. Ginsberg JS, Wells PS, Kearon C, et al: Sensitivity and specificity of a rapid whole-blood assay for D-dimer in the diagnosis of pulmonary embolism. Ann Intern Med 129:1006, 1998.
83. Opinions regarding the diagnosis and management of venous thromboembolic disease: ACCP Consensus Committee on Pulmonary Embolism. Chest 113:499, 1998.
84. Hull RD, Hirsch J, Carter CJ, et al: Diagnostic value of ventilation-perfusion lung scanning in patients with suspected pulmonary embolism. Circulation 88:819, 1985.
85. Alderson PO, Martin EC: Pulmonary embolism: Diagnosis with multiple imaging modalities. Radiology 164:297, 1987.
86. Hull RD, Raskob GE, Coates G, et al: Clinical validity of a normal perfusion lung scan in patients with suspected pulmonary embolism. Chest 97:23, 1990.
87. Webber MM, Gomes AS, Roe D, et al: Comparison of Biello, McNeil, and PIOPED criteria for the diagnosis of pulmonary emboli on lung scans. Am J Radiol 154:975, 1990.
88. Value of the ventilation/perfusion scan in acute pulmonary embolism: Results of the prospective investigation of pulmonary embolism diagnosis (PIOPED). JAMA 263:2753, 1990.
89. Moser KM, Fedullo PF, Littlejohn JK, et al: Frequent asymptomatic pulmonary embolism in patients with deep venous thrombosis. JAMA 271:223, 1994.
90. Hull RD, Hirsch J, Carter CJ, et al: Pulmonary angiography, ventilation lung scanning, and venography for clinically suspected pulmonary embolism with abnormal perfusion lung scan. Ann Intern Med 98:891, 1983.
91. McNiel BJ: Ventilation-perfusion studies and the diagnosis of pulmonary embolism: Concise communication. J Nucl Med 21:319, 1980.
92. Alderson PO, Rujanevech N, Seckler-Walker RH, et al: The role of Xe-133 ventilation studies in the radionuclide detection of pulmonary embolism. Radiology 120:633, 1976.
93. Cheeley R, McCartney WH, Perry JR: The role of noninvasive tests versus pulmonary angiography in the diagnosis of pulmonary embolism. Am J Med 70:17, 1981.
94. Kipper MS, Moser KM, Kortman KE, et al: Long-term follow-up of patients with suspected pulmonary embolism and a normal lung scan. Chest 82:411, 1982.
95. Kelley MA, Carson JL, Palevsky HI, et al: Diagnosing pulmonary embolism: New facts and strategies. Ann Intern Med 114:300, 1991.
96. Alexander JK, Gonzalez DA, Fred HL: Angiographic studies in cardiorespiratory diseases. JAMA 198:575, 1966.
97. Stein PD, Gottschalk A: Critical review of ventilation-perfusion lung scans in acute pulmonary embolism. Prog Cardiovasc Dis 37:13, 1994.
97a. Meyerovitz MF, Mannting F, Polak JF, et al: Frequency of pulmonary embolism in patients with low-probability lung scan and negative lower extremity venous ultrasound. Chest 115:980, 1999.
98. Stein PD, Hull R, Raskob G: Risks for major bleeding from thrombolytic therapy in patients with acute pulmonary embolism: Consideration of noninvasive management. Ann Intern Med 121:313, 1994.
99. Ferris EJ, Stanzler RM, Rourke JA, et al: Pulmonary angiography in pulmonary embolic disease. Am J Roentgenol Rad Ther Nucl Med 100:355, 1967.
100. Lowman RM, Reardon J, Hipona FA, et al: The role of pulmonary angiography in pulmonary embolism. Angiology 18:291, 1967.
101. Peterson KL, Fred HL, Alexander JK: Pulmonary arterial webs: A new angiographic sign of previous thromboembolism. N Engl J Med 277:33, 1967.
102. Auger WR, Fedullo PF, Moser KM, et al: Chronic major-vessel thromboembolic pulmonary artery obstruction: Appearance at angiography. Radiology 182:393, 1992.
103. Wolfe MW, Lee RT, Feldstein ML, et al: Prognostic significance of right ventricular hypokinesis and perfusion defects in pulmonary embolism. Am Heart J 127:1371, 1994.
104. Kasper W, Konstantinides S, Geibel A, et al: Management strategies and determinants of outcome in acute major pulmonary embolism: Results of a multicenter registry. J Am Coll Cardiol 30:1165, 1997.
105. Goldhaber SZ: Pulmonary embolism thrombolysis: Broadening the paradigm for its administration. Circulation 96:716, 1997.
106. Ribeiro A, Lindmarker P, Juhlin-Dannfelt A, et al: Echocardiography Doppler in pulmonary embolism: Right ventricular dysfunction as a predictor of mortality rate. Am Heart J 134:479, 1997.
107. Konstantinides S, Geibel A, Olschewski M, et al: Association between thrombolytic treatment and the prognosis of hemodynamically stable patients with major pulmonary embolism: Results of a multicenter registry. Circulation 96:882, 1997.

107a. Grifoni S, Olivotto I, Cecchini P, et al: Short-term clinical outcome of patients with acute pulmonary embolism, normal blood pressure, and echocardiographic right ventricular dysfunction. Circulation 101: 2817, 2000.
108. Goldhaber SZ, Haire WD, Feldstein ML, et al: Alteplase versus heparin in acute pulmonary embolism: Randomized trial assessing right ventricular function and pulmonary perfusion. Lancet 341:507, 1993.
109. Goldhaber SZ: Pulmonary embolism for cardiologists. J Am Coll Cardiol 30:1172, 1997.
109a. Ribeiro A, Lindmarker P, Johnsson H, et al: Pulmonary embolism: One-year follow-up with echocardiography Doppler and five-year survival analysis. Circulation 99:1325, 1999.
110. Kasper W, Meinertz T, Henkel B, et al: Echocardiographic findings in patients with proved pulmonary embolism. Am Heart J 112:1284, 1986.
111. Come PC: Echocardiographic evaluation of pulmonary embolism and its response to therapeutic interventions. Chest 101:151, 1992.
112. Ritoo D, Sutherland GR, Samuel L, et al: Role of transesophageal echocardiography in diagnosis and management of central pulmonary artery thromboembolism. Am J Cardiol 71:1115, 1993.
113. McConnell MV, Solomon SD, Rayan ME, et al: Regional right ventricular dysfunction detected by echocardiography in acute pulmonary embolism. Am J Cardiol 78:469, 1996.
113a. Chartier L, Béra J, Delomez M, et al: Free-floating thrombi in the right heart: Diagnosis, management, and prognostic indexes in 38 consecutive patients. Circulation 99:2779, 1999.
114. Pruszczyk P, Torbicki A, Pacho R, et al: Noninvasive diagnosis of suspected severe pulmonary embolism: Transesophageal echocardiography vs spiral CT. Chest 112:722, 1997.
115. Teigen CL, Maus TP, Sheedy PF II, et al: Pulmonary embolism: Diagnosis with contrast-enhanced electron-beam CT and comparison with pulmonary angiography. Radiology 194:313, 1995.
116. Remy-Jardin M, Remy J, Wattinne L, et al: Central pulmonary thromboembolism: Diagnosis with spiral volumetric CT with the single-breath-hold technique—comparison with pulmonary angiography. Radiology 185:381, 1992.
117. Remy-Jardin M, Remy J, Deschildre F, et al: Diagnosis of pulmonary embolism with spiral CT: Comparison with pulmonary angiography and scintigraphy. Radiology 200:699, 1996.
117a. Mullins MD, Becker DM, Hagspiel KD, et al: The role of spiral volumetric computed tomography in the diagnosis of pulmonary embolism. Arch Intern Med 160:293, 2000.
117b. Rathbun SW, Raskob GE, Whitsett TL: Sensitivity and specificity of helical computed tomography in the diagnosis of pulmonary emoblism: A systematic review. Ann Intern Med 132:227, 2000.
117c. Bates SM, Ginsberg JS: Helical computed tomography and the diagnosis of pulmonary embolism. Ann Intern Med 132:240, 2000.
117d. Groth ML, Hurewitz AN, Katz DS, et al: Conventional pulmonary angiography and CT pulmonary angiography (CTPA) for pulmonary embolism (PE): What are clinicians really doing? Chest 118:81S, 2000.
118. Goodman LR, Lipchik RJ: Diagnosis of acute pulmonary embolism: Time for a new approach. Radiology 199:25, 1996.
119. Ferretti GR, Bosson JL, Buffaz PD, et al: Acute pulmonary embolism: Role of helical CT in 164 patients with intermediate probability at ventilation-perfusion scintigraphy and normal results at duplex US of the legs. Radiology 205:453, 1997.
120. White RD, Winkler ML, Higgins CB: MR imaging of pulmonary arterial hypertension and pulmonary emboli. AJR Am J Roentgenol 149:15, 1987.
121. Meneveau N, Francois S, Metz D, et al: Comparative efficacy of a two-hour regimen of streptokinase versus alteplase in acute massive pulmonary embolism: Immediate clinical and hemodynamic outcome and one-year follow up. J Am Coll Cardiol 31:1057, 1998.
122. Ellis D: Acute pulmonary embolism: Advances in imaging. Br J Hosp Med 58:303, 1997.
123. Cronan JJ: Venous thromboembolic disease: The role of US. Radiology 186:619, 1993.
124. Turkstra F, Kuijer PMM, van Beek EJR, et al: Diagnostic utility of ultrasonography of leg veins in patients suspected of having pulmonary embolism. Ann Intern Med 126:775, 1997.
125. Lensing AWA, Doris CI, McGrath FP, et al: A comparison of compression ultrasound with color Doppler ultrasound for the diagnosis of symptomless postoperative deep vein thrombosis. Arch Intern Med 157:765, 1997.
126. Birdwell BG, Raskob GE, Whitsett TL, et al: The clinical validity of normal compression ultrasonography in outpatients suspected of having deep venous thrombosis. Ann Intern Med 128:1, 1998.
127. Kearon C, Julian JA, Math M, et al: Noninvasive diagnosis of deep venous thrombosis. Ann Intern Med 128:663, 1998.
128. Hull RD, Hirsh J, Carter CJ, et al: Diagnostic efficacy of impedance plethysmography for clinically suspected deep-vein thrombosis. Ann Intern Med 102:21, 1985.
129. Weinmann EE, Salzman EW: Deep-vein thrombosis. N Engl J Med 331:1630, 1994.
130. Hull R, Hirsh J, Sackett DL, et al: Clinical validity of a negative venogram in patients with clinically suspected venous thrombosis. Circulation 64:622, 1981.
131. Agnelli G, Ranucci V, Veschi F, et al: Clinical outcome of orthopedic patients with negative lower limb venography at discharge. Thromb Haemost 74:1042, 1995.
132. Bone RC: Ventilation/perfusion scan in pulmonary embolism: The emperor is incompletely attired. JAMA 263:2794, 1990.
133. Opinions regarding the diagnosis and management of venous thromboembolic disease. ACCP Consensus Committee on Pulmonary Embolism. Chest 109:233, 1996.
134. Anderson D, Gross M, Robinson S, et al: Ultrasonographic screening for deep vein thrombosis following arthroplasty fails to reduce posthospital thromboembolic complications: The Postarthroplasty Screening Study (PASS). Chest 114:119S, 1998.
135. Moser KM, Shure D, Harrell JH, et al: Angioscopic visualization of pulmonary emboli. Chest 2:198, 1980.
136. Beckman D, Solmos B, Herod G, et al: Intraoperative pulmonary angioscopy using the flexible fiberoptic choledochoscope. Ann Thorac Surg 41:563, 1986.
137. Uchida Y, Oshima T, Hirose J, et al: Angioscopic detection of residual pulmonary thrombi in the differential diagnosis of pulmonary embolism. Am Heart J 130:854, 1995.
138. Sagar KB, Rhyne TL, Greenfield LJ: Intravascular ultrasound. Circulation 67:365, 1983.
139. Ginsberg JS, Hirsh J, Rainbow AJ, et al: Risks to the fetus of radiologic procedures used in the diagnosis of maternal venous thromboembolic disease. Thromb Haemost 61:189, 1989.
140. Fred HL, Hariharan R: Pulmonary thromboembolism. In Willerson JT, Cohn JN (eds): Cardiovascular Medicine, 2nd ed. W.B. Saunders, New York, 2000, p 1835.
141. Hussey HH, Katz S: Septic pulmonary infarction: Report of 8 cases. Ann Intern Med 22:526, 1945.
142. Hussey HH: The pathogenesis of septic pulmonary embolism. Med Clin North Am 34:1751, 1950.
143. Collins CG, MacCallum EA, Nelson EW, et al: Suppurative pelvic thrombophlebitis: I. Incidence, pathology, and etiology: A study of 70 patients treated by ligation of the inferior vena cava and ovarian vessels. Surgery 30:298, 1951.
144. O'Donnell AE, Pappas LS: Pulmonary complications of intravenous drug abuse: Experience at an inner-city hospital. Chest 94:251, 1988.
145. Hecht SR, Berger M: Right-sided endocarditis in intravenous drug users: Prognostic features in 102 episodes. Ann Intern Med 117: 560, 1992.
146. Fred HL, Harle TS: Septic pulmonary embolism. Dis Chest 55: 483, 1969.
147. Dodd GD, Boyle JJ: Excavating pulmonary metastases. AJR Am J Roentgenol 85:277, 1961.
148. Lynch EC, Fred HL, Greenberg SD: Pulmonary cavitation in Wegener's granulomatosis. AJR Am J Roentgenol 92:521, 1964.
149. Huang R-M, Naidich DP, Lubtat E, et al: Septic pulmonary emboli: CT-radiographic correlation. Am J Radiol 153:41, 1989.
150. Collins CG: Suppurative pelvic thrombophlebitis: A study of 202 cases in which the disease was treated by ligation of the vena cava and ovarian vein. Am J Obstet Gynecol 108:681, 1970.
151. Arbulu A, Asfaw I: Tricuspid valvulectomy without prosthetic replacement. Ten years of clinical experience. J Thorac Cardiovasc Surg 82: 684, 1981.
152. Dunn LJ, Van Voorhis LW: Enigmatic fever and pelvic thrombophlebitis: Response to anticoagulants. N Engl J Med 276:262, 1967.
153. Lerner AM: Role of bacteroides (Letter). N Engl J Med 276:1267, 1967.
154. Josey WE, Staggers SR Jr: Heparin therapy in septic pelvic thrombophlebitis: A study of 46 cases. Am J Obstet Gynecol 120:228, 1974.
155. Steiner PE, Lushbaugh CC: Maternal pulmonary embolism by amni-

otic fluid as a cause of obstetric shock and unexpected deaths in obstetrics. JAMA 117:1245; 1341, 1941.
156. Lewis TLT: The changing practice of obstetrics. In Lewis TLT (ed): Progress in Clinical Obstetrics and Gynecology, 2nd ed. Churchill Livingstone, London, 1964, p 48.
157. Peterson EP, Taylor HB: Amniotic fluid embolism: An analysis of 40 cases. Obstet Gynecol 35:787, 1970.
158. Dudney TM, Elliott CG: Pulmonary embolism from amniotic fluid, fat, and air. Prog Cardiovasc Dis 36:447, 1994.
159. Dolyniuk M, Orfei E, Vania H, et al: Rapid diagnosis of amniotic fluid embolism. Obstet Gynecol 61:28S, 1983.
160. Masson RG, Ruggieri J, Siddiqui MH: Amniotic fluid embolism: Definitive diagnosis in a survivor. Am Rev Respir Dis 120:187, 1979.
161. Dashow EE, Cotterill R, Benedetti TJ, et al: Amniotic fluid embolus: A report of two cases resulting in maternal survival. J Reprod Med 34:660, 1989.
162. Agia G, Wyatt L, Re E: Pulmonary microvascular cytology: A new diagnostic application of the pulmonary artery catheter (Letter). Chest 90:627, 1986.
163. Tuck CS: Amniotic fluid embolus. Proc R Soc Med 65:94, 1972.
164. Clark SL: Successful pregnancy outcomes after amniotic fluid embolism. Am J Obstet Gynecol 167:511, 1992.
165. Stromme WB, Fromke VL: Amniotic fluid embolism and disseminated intravascular coagulation after evacuation of missed abortion. Obstet Gynecol 52:76S, 1978.
166. Lumley J, Owen R, Morgan M: Amniotic fluid embolism: A report of three cases. Anaesthesia 34:33, 1979.
167. Gregory MG, Clayton EMJ: Amniotic fluid embolism. Obstet Gynecol 42:236, 1973.
168. Stephens JH, Fred HL: Petechiae associated with systemic fat embolism. Arch Dermatol 86:515, 1962.
169. Mayo JR, Remy-Jardin M, Müller NL, et al: Pulmonary embolism: Prospective comparison of spiral CT with ventilation-perfusion scintigraphy. Radiology 205:447, 1997.
170. Cross JJL, Kemp PM, Walsh CG, et al: A randomized trial of spiral CT and ventilation perfusion scintigraphy for the diagnosis of pulmonary embolism. Clin Radiol 53:177, 1998.
171. Ahdout DJ, Damani P, Ultan LB: Recurrent acute pulmonary emboli in association with acute myocardial infarction. Chest 96:682, 1989.
172. Richards P: Pulmonary oedema and intracranial lesions. Br Med J 2: 83, 1963.
173. Surawicz B: Electrocardiographic pattern of cerebrovascular accident. JAMA 197:913, 1966.
174. Hirsh J: Antithrombotic therapy in deep vein thrombosis and pulmonary embolism. Am Heart J 123:1115, 1992.
175. Clagett GP, Anderson FA, Heit J, et al: Prevention of venous thromboembolism. Chest 108:312, 1995.
176. Prevention of venous thromboembolism: International Consensus Statement (guidelines according to scientific evidence). Int Angiol 16: 3, 1997.
177. Morehead RS, Tzouanakis AE, Berger R: Preventing VTE: A guide to nonpharmacologic therapies. J Crit Illness 13:486, 1998.
178. Halkin H, Goldberg J, Modan M, et al: Reduction of mortality in general medical in-patients by low-dose heparin prophylaxis. Ann Intern Med 96:561, 1982.
179. Collaborative overview of randomized trials of antiplatelet therapy—III: Reduction in venous thrombosis and pulmonary embolism by antiplatelet prophylaxis among surgical and medical patients. Antiplatelet Trialists' Collaboration. Br Med J 308:235, 1994.
180. Cohen AT, Skinner JA, Kakkar VV: Antiplatelet treatment for thromboprophylaxis: A step forward or backwards? Br Med J 308:1213, 1994.
180a. Samama MM, Cohen AT, Darmon JY, et al: A comparison of enoxaparin with placebo for the prevention of venous thromboembolism in acutely ill medical patients. N Engl J Med 341:793, 1999.
181. Hirsch DR, Ingenito EP, Goldhaber SZ: Prevalence of deep venous thrombosis among patients in medical intensive care. JAMA 274: 335, 1995.
182. Ryskamp RP, Trottier SJ: Utilization of venous thromboembolism prophylaxis in a medical-surgical ICU. Chest 113:162, 1998.
183. Goldhaber SZ: Venous thromboembolism in the intensive care unit: The last frontier for prophylaxis. Chest 113:5, 1998.
184. Abernathy EA, Hartsuck JM: Postoperative pulmonary embolism: A prospective study utilizing low dose heparin. Am J Surg 128:739, 1974.
185. Prevention of fatal postoperative pulmonary embolism by low doses of heparin. An international multicentre trial. Lancet 2:45, 1975.
186. Collins R, Scrimgeour A, Yusuf S, et al: Reduction in fatal pulmonary embolism and venous thrombosis by perioperative administration of subcutaneous heparin: Overview of results of randomized trials in general, orthopedic, and urologic surgery. N Engl J Med 318:1162, 1988.
187. Nurmohamed MT, Rosendaal FR, Büller HR, et al: Low-molecular-weight heparin versus standard heparin in general and orthopaedic surgery: A meta-analysis. Lancet 340:152, 1992.
188. Jørgensen LN, Wille-Jørgensen, Hauch O: Prophylaxis of postoperative thromboembolism with low molecular weight heparins. Br J Surg 80:689, 1993.
189. Bergqvist D, Benoni G, Bjorgell O, et al: Low-molecular-weight heparin (enoxaparin) as prophylaxis against venous thromboembolism after total hip replacement. N Engl J Med 335:696, 1996.
190. Caen JP: A randomized double-blind study between a low molecular weight heparin Kabi 2165 and standard heparin in the prevention of deep vein thrombosis in general surgery: A French multicenter trial. Thromb Haemost 59:216, 1988.
191. Ramos R, Salem BI, De Pawlikowski MP, et al: The efficacy of pneumatic compression stockings in the prevention of pulmonary embolism after cardiac surgery. Chest 109:82, 1996.
192. Turpie AGG, Levine MN, Hirsh J, et al: A randomized controlled trial of a low-molecular-weight heparin (Enoxaparin) to prevent deep-vein thrombosis in patients undergoing elective hip surgery. N Engl J Med 315:925, 1986.
193. Mohr DN, Silverstein MD, Murtaugh PA, et al: Prophylactic agents for venous thrombosis in elective hip surgery: Meta-analysis of studies using venographic assessment. Arch Intern Med 153:2221, 1993.
194. Leclerc JR, Gent M, Hirsh J, et al: The incidence of symptomatic venous thromboembolism during and after prophylaxis with enoxaparin: A multi-institutional cohort study of patients who underwent hip or knee arthroplasty. Arch Intern Med 158:873, 1998.
195. Hirsh J: Evidence for the needs of out-of-hospital thrombosis prophylaxis: Introduction. Chest 114:113S, 1998.
196. de Valk HW, Banga JD, Wester JWJ, et al: Comparing subcutaneous danaparoid with intravenous unfractionated heparin for the treatment of venous thromboembolism: A randomized controlled trial. Ann Intern Med 123:1, 1995.
197. Eriksson BI, Ekman S, Kälebo P, et al: Prevention of deep-vein thrombosis after total hip replacement: Direct thrombin inhibition with recombinant hirudin, CGP 39393. Lancet 347:635, 1996.
198. Eriksson BI, Wille-Jørgensen P, Kälebo P, et al: A comparison of recombinant hirudin with a low-molecular-weight heparin to prevent thromboembolic complications after total hip replacement. N Engl J Med 337:1329, 1997.
199. Leyvraz PF, Richard J, Bachman F, et al: Adjusted versus fixed-dose subcutaneous heparin in the prevention of deep-vein thrombosis after total hip replacement. N Engl J Med 309:954, 1983.
200. Hamilton HW, Crawford JS, Gardiner JH, et al: Venous thrombosis in patients with fracture of the upper end of the femur. J Bone Joint Surg 52:268, 1970.
201. Imperiale TF, Speroff T: A meta-analysis of methods to prevent venous thromboembolism following total hip replacement. JAMA 271:1780, 1994.
202. Hull RD, Raskob GE, Gent M, et al: Effectiveness of intermittent pneumatic leg compression for preventing deep vein thrombosis after total hip replacement. JAMA 263:2313, 1990.
203. Leclerc JR, Geerts WH, Desjardins L, et al: Prevention of venous thromboembolism after knee arthroplasty: A randomized, double-blind trial comparing enoxaparin with warfarin. Ann Intern Med 124: 619, 1996.
204. Levine MN, Gent M, Hirsh J, et al: Ardeparin (low-molecular-weight heparin) vs graduated compression stockings for the prevention of venous thromboembolism: A randomized trial in patients undergoing knee surgery. Arch Intern Med 156:851, 1996.
205. Turpie AGG, Hirsh J, Gent M, et al: Prevention of deep vein thrombosis in potential neurosurgical patients: A randomized trial comparing graduated compression stockings alone or graduated compression stockings plus intermittent pneumatic compression with control. Arch Intern Med 149:679, 1989.
206. Agnelli G, Piovella F, Buoncristiani P, et al: Enoxaparin plus compression stockings compared with compression stockings alone in the prevention of venous thromboembolism after elective neurosurgery. N Engl J Med 339:80, 1998.
207. Catre MG: Anticoagulation in spinal surgery: A critical review of the literature. Can J Surg 40:413, 1997.

208. Geerts WH, Jay RM, Code KI, et al: A comparison of low-dose heparin with low-molecular-weight heparin as prophylaxis against venous thromboembolism after major trauma. N Engl J Med 335: 701, 1996.
209. Green D, Lee MY, Ito VY, et al: Fixed- vs adjusted-dose heparin in the prophylaxis of thromboembolism in spinal cord injury. JAMA 260: 1255, 1988.
210. Hunt BJ, Doughty HA, Majumdar G, et al: Thromboprophylaxis with low molecular weight heparin (Fragmin) in high risk pregnancies. Thromb Haemost 77:39, 1997.
211. Ginsberg JS, Hirsh J: Use of antithrombotic agents during pregnancy. Chest 108:305S, 1995.
211a. Brill-Edwards P, Ginsberg JS, Gent M, et al: Safety of withholding heparin in pregnant women with a history of venous thromboembolism. N Engl J Med 343:1439, 2000.
211b. Ginsberg JS, Greer I, Hirsh J: Use of antithrombotic agents during pregnancy. Chest 119:122S, 2001.
212. Hirsh J, Dalen JE, Deykin D, et al: Heparin: Mechanism of action, pharmacokinetics, dosing considerations, monitoring, efficacy, and safety. Chest 102:337S, 1992.
213. Brill-Edwards P, Ginsberg S, Johnston M, et al: Establishing a therapeutic range for heparin therapy. Ann Intern Med 119:104, 1993.
214. Hull RD, Raskob GE, Hirsh J, et al: Continuous intravenous heparin compared with intermittent subcutaneous heparin in the initial treatment of proximal-vein thrombosis. N Engl J Med 315:1109, 1986.
215. Cruickshank MK, Levine MN, Hirsh J, et al: A standard heparin nomogram for the management of heparin therapy. Arch Intern Med 151:333, 1991.
216. Raschke RA, Reilly BM, Guidry JR, et al: The weight-based heparin dosing nomogram compared with a standard care nomogram: A randomized control trial. Ann Intern Med 119:874, 1993.
217. Hull RD, Raskob GE, Brant RF, et al: Relation between the time to achieve the lower limit of the APTT therapeutic range and recurrent venous thromboembolism during heparin treatment for deep vein thrombosis. Arch Intern Med 157:2562, 1997.
218. Hull RD, Raskob GE, Rosenbloom D, et al: Heparin for 5 days compared with 10 days in the initial treatment of proximal venous thrombosis. N Engl J Med 322:1260, 1990.
219. Tapson VF, Hull RD: Management of venous thromboembolic disease. The impact of low-molecular-weight heparin. Clin Chest Med 16: 281, 1995.
220. Levine M, Gent M, Hirsh J, et al: A comparison of low-molecular-weight heparin administered primarily at home with unfractionated heparin administered in the hospital for proximal deep-vein thrombosis. N Engl J Med 334:677, 1996.
221. Koopman MMW, Prandoni P, Piovella F, et al: Treatment of venous thrombosis with intravenous unfractionated heparin administered in the hospital as compared with subcutaneous low-molecular-weight heparin administered at home. N Engl J Med 334:682, 1996.
222. Weitz JI: Low-molecular-weight heparins. N Engl J Med 337:688, 1997.
223. Koopman MMW, Büller HR: Low-molecular-weight heparins in the treatment of venous thromboembolism. Ann Intern Med 128:1037, 1998.
224. Antman EM, Handin R: Low-molecular-weight heparins: An intriguing new twist with profound implications. Circulation 98:287, 1998.
224a. Aguilar D, Goldhaber SZ: Clinical uses of low-molecular-weight heparins. Chest 115:1418, 1999.
225. Schafer AI: Low-molecular-weight heparin: An opportunity for home treatment of venous thrombosis. N Engl J Med 334:724, 1996.
226. Simonneau G, Sors H, Charbonnier B, et al: A comparison of low-molecular-weight heparin with unfractionated heparin for acute pulmonary embolism. N Engl J Med 337:663, 1997.
227. The Columbus Investigators: Low-molecular-weight heparin in the treatment of patients with venous thromboembolism. N Engl J Med 337:657, 1997.
227a. Hull RD, Raskob GE, Brant RF, et al: Low-molecular-weight heparin vs heparin in the treatment of patients with pulmonary embolism. American-Canadian Thrombosis Study Group. Arch Intern Med 160: 229, 2000.
227b. Hull RD, Raskob GE, Brant RF, et al: Is there enough evidence that low-molecular-weight heparin is superior to unfractionated heparin in pulmonary embolism? Arch Intern Med 160:2065, 2000.
228. Hirsh J, Dalen JE, Deykin D, et al: Oral anticoagulants: Mechanism of action, clinical effectiveness, and optimal therapeutic range. Chest 102:312S, 1992.
229. Freedman MD: Clinical therapeutic conference: Recurrent venous thrombotic and thromboembolic disease. Am J Ther 5:51, 1998.
230. Gallus A, Jackaman J, Tillett H, et al: Safety and efficacy of warfarin started early after submassive thrombosis or pulmonary embolism. Lancet 2:1293, 1986.
231. Rosiello RA, Chan CK, Tencza F, et al: Timing of oral anticoagulation therapy in the treatment of angiographically proven acute pulmonary embolism. Arch Intern Med 147:1469, 1987.
232. Schulman S, Rhedin A-S, Lindmarker P, et al: A comparison of six weeks with six months of oral anticoagulant therapy after a first episode of venous thromboembolism. N Engl J Med 332:1661, 1995.
232a. Kearon C, Gent M, Hirsh J, et al: A comparison of three months of anticoagulation with extended anticoagulation for a first episode of idiopathic venous thromboembolism. N Engl J Med 340:901, 1999.
232b. Schafer AI: Venous thrombosis as a chronic disease. N Engl J Med 340:955, 1999.
233. Khamashta MA, Cuadrado MJ, Mujic F, et al: The management of thrombosis in the antiphospholipid-antibody syndrome. N Engl J Med 332:993, 1995.
234. Hull RD, Pineo GF: Current concepts of anticoagulation therapy. Clin Chest Med 16:269, 1995.
235. Research Committee of the British Thoracic Society: Optimum duration of anticoagulation for deep-vein thrombosis and pulmonary embolism. Lancet 340:873, 1992.
236. Hirsh J: The optimal duration of anticoagulant therapy for venous thrombosis. N Engl J Med 332:1710, 1995.
237. Goldhaber SZ: Pulmonary embolism. N Engl J Med 339:93, 1998.
238. Urokinase pulmonary embolism trial: Phase I results. A cooperative study. JAMA 214:2163, 1970.
239. Urokinase-streptokinase embolism trial: Phase 2 results. A cooperative study. JAMA 229:1606, 1974.
240. Goldhaber SZ, Kessler CM, Heit J, et al: A randomized controlled trial of recombinant tissue-type plasminogen activator versus urokinase in the treatment of acute pulmonary embolism. Lancet 2:293, 1988.
241. Meyer G, Sors H, Charbonnier B, et al: Effects of intravenous urokinase versus alteplase on total pulmonary resistance in acute massive pulmonary embolism: A European multicenter double-blind trial. J Am Coll Cardiol 19:239, 1992.
241a. Arcasoy SM, Kreit JW: Thrombolytic therapy of pulmonary embolism: A comprehensive review of current evidence. Chest 115:1695, 1999.
242. Come PC, Kim D, Parker JA, et al: Early reversal of right ventricular dysfunction in patients with acute pulmonary embolism after treatment with intravenous tissue plasminogen activator. J Am Coll Cardiol 10:971, 1987.
243. Dalen JE, Alpert JS, Hirsh J: Thrombolytic therapy for pulmonary embolism: Is it effective? Is it safe? When is it indicated? Arch Intern Med 157:2550, 1997.
244. PIOPED Investigators: Tissue plasminogen activator for the treatment of acute pulmonary embolism. Chest 97:528, 1990.
245. Levine M, Hirsh J, Weitz J, et al: A randomized trial of a single bolus dosage regimen of recombinant tissue plasminogen activator in patients with acute pulmonary embolism. Chest 98:1473, 1990.
246. Dalla-Volta S, Palla A, Santolicandro A, et al: PAIMS 2-alteplase combined with heparin versus heparin in the treatment of acute pulmonary embolism: Plasminogen Activator Italian Multicenter Study 2. J Am Coll Cardiol 20:520, 1992.
246a. Gulba DC, Schmid C, Borst HG, et al: Medical compared with surgical treatment for massive pulmonary embolism. Lancet 343:576, 1994.
246b. Ahearn GS, Hadjiliadis D, Tapson VF, et al: Thrombolytic therapy with tissue plasminogen activator (TPA) in the first trimester of pregnancy after massive pulmonary embolism (PE). Chest 116:405S, 1999.
247. Gruppo Italiano per lo Studio della Streptochinasi nell'Infarto Miocardico (GISSI): Effectiveness of intravenous thrombolytic treatment in acute myocardial infarction. Lancet 1:397, 1986.
248. Randomized trial of intravenous streptokinase, oral aspirin, both, or neither among 17,187 cases of suspected acute myocardial infarction: ISIS-2 (Second International Study of Infarct Survival) Collaborative Group. Lancet 2:349, 1988.
249. Bobbio M, Bergerone S, Maggioni AP, et al: Administration of thrombolytic therapy to 17,944 patients with acute myocardial infarction: The GISSI-3 database. Am Heart J 135:443, 1998.

250. Daniels LB, Parker JA, Patel SR, et al: Relation of duration of symptoms with response to thrombolytic therapy in pulmonary embolism. Am J Cardiol 80:184, 1997.
251. Donaldson MC, Wirthlin LS, Donaldson GA: Thirty-year experience with surgical interruption of the inferior vena cava for prevention of pulmonary embolism. Ann Surg 191:367, 1980.
252. Bomalski JS, Martin GJ, Hughes RL, et al: Inferior vena cava interruption in the management of pulmonary embolism. Chest 82:767, 1982.
253. Greenfield LJ, Proctor MC: Current indications for caval interruption: Should they be liberalized in view of improving technology? Semin Vasc Surg 9:50, 1996.
254. Dorfman G: Percutaneous inferior vena caval filters. Radiology 174: 987, 1990.
255. Grassi CJ: Inferior vena caval filters: Analysis of five currently available devices. AJR Am J Roentgenol 156:813, 1991.
256. Whitehill TA: Caval interruption methods: Comparison of options. Semin Vasc Surg 9:59, 1996.
257. Bovyn G, Gory P, Reynaud P, et al: The Tempofilter: A multicenter study of a new temporary caval filter implantable for up to six weeks. Ann Vasc Surg 11:520, 1997.
258. Neill AM, Appleton DS, Richards P: Retrievable inferior vena caval filter for thromboembolic disease in pregnancy. Br J Obstet Gynaecol 104:1416, 1997.
259. Vos LD, Tielbeek AV, Bom EP, et al: The Gunther temporary inferior vena cava filter for short-term protection against pulmonary embolism. Cardiovasc Intervent Radiol 20:91, 1997.
260. Neuerburg JM, Gunther RW, Vorwerk D, et al: Results of a multicenter study of the retrievable Tulip vena cava filter: Early clinical experience. Cardiovasc Intervent Radiol 20:10, 1997.
261. Mansour M, Chang AE, Sindelar WF: Interruption of the inferior vena cava for the prevention of recurrent pulmonary embolism. Am Surg 51:375, 1985.
262. Cohen JR, Tenenbaum N, Citron M: Greenfield filter as primary therapy for deep venous thrombosis and/or pulmonary embolism in patients with cancer. Surgery 109:12, 1991.
263. Arnold TE, Karabinis VD, Mehta V, et al: Potential for overuse of the inferior vena cava filter. Surg Gynecol Obstet 177:463, 1993.
264. Decousus H, Leizorovicz A, Parent F, et al: A clinical trial of vena caval filters in the prevention of pulmonary embolism in patients with proximal deep-vein thrombosis. N Engl J Med 338:409, 1998.
265. Alberts WM, Tonner JA, Goldman AL: Echocardiography in planned interruption of the inferior vena cava. South Med J 82:772, 1989.
266. Stoschitzky K, Stark G, Dacar D: Massive pulmonary embolism. N Engl J Med 337:1561, 1997.
267. Glassford DM Jr, Alford WC Jr, Burrus GR, et al: Pulmonary embolectomy. Ann Thorac Surg 32:28, 1981.
268. Crane C, Hartsuck J, Birtch A, et al: The management of major pulmonary embolism. Surg Gynecol Obstet 128:27, 1969.
269. Sautter RD, Myers WO, Ray JF III, et al: Pulmonary embolectomy: Review and current status. Prog Cardiovasc Dis 17:371, 1975.
270. Fred HL, Natelson EA: Selection of patients for pulmonary embolectomy. Dis Chest 56:139, 1969.
271. Timsit J-F, Reynaud P, Meyer G, et al: Pulmonary embolectomy by catheter device in massive pulmonary embolism. Chest 100:655, 1991.
272. Greenfield LJ, Proctor MC, Williams DM, et al: Long-term experience with transvenous catheter pulmonary embolectomy. J Vasc Surg 18: 450, 1993.
272a. Blaustein HS, Schur I, Shapiro JM: Acute massive pulmonary embolism in a Jehovah's witness: Successful treatment with catheter thrombectomy. Chest 117:594, 2000.
273. Gray HH, Miller GAH, Paneth M: Pulmonary embolectomy: Its place in the management of pulmonary embolism. Lancet 1:1441, 1988.
274. Koning R, Cribier AC, Gerber L, et al: A new treatment for severe pulmonary embolism: Percutaneous rheolytic thrombectomy. Circulation 96:2498, 1997.
275. Fava M, Loyola S, Flores P, et al: Mechanical fragmentation and pharmacologic thrombolysis in massive pulmonary embolism. J Vasc Interv Radiol 8:261, 1997.
276. Moser KM, Auger WR, Fedullo PF, et al: Chronic thromboembolic pulmonary hypertension: Clinical picture and surgical treatment. Eur Respir J 5:334, 1992.
277. Jamieson SW: Pulmonary thromboendarterectomy. Heart 79:118, 1998.
277a. Feinstein JA, Goldhaber SZ, Lock JE, et al: Balloon pulmonary angioplasty for treatment of chronic thromboembolic pulmonary hypertension. Circulation 103:10, 2001.
278. Fred HL, Axelrad MA, Lewis J, et al: Rapid resolution of pulmonary thromboemboli in man. An angiographic study. JAMA 196:1137, 1966.
279. Dalen JE, Banas JSJ, Brooks HL, et al: Resolution rate of acute pulmonary emboli in man. N Engl J Med 280:1194, 1969.
280. Sautter RD, Fletcher FW, Ousley JL, et al: Extremely rapid resolution of a pulmonary embolus. Report of a case. Dis Chest 52:825, 1967.
281. Carson JL, Kelley MA, Duff A, et al: The clinical course of pulmonary embolism. N Engl J Med 326:1240, 1992.
282. Donaldson GA, Williams C, Scannell JG, et al: A reappraisal of the application of the Trendelenburg operation to massive fatal embolism: Report of a successful pulmonary-artery thrombectomy using a cardiopulmonary bypass. N Engl J Med 268:171, 1963.
283. Douketis JD, Kearon C, Bates S, et al: Risk of fatal pulmonary embolism in patients with treated venous thromboembolism. JAMA 279:458, 1998.
284. Paraskos JA, Adelstein SJ, Smith RE, et al: Late prognosis of acute pulmonary embolism. N Engl J Med 289:55, 1973.
285. Hall RJC, Sutton GC, Kerr IH: Long-term prognosis of treated acute massive pulmonary embolism. Br Heart J 39:1128, 1977.

SECTION

X

PERICARDIAL DISEASE

CHAPTER 34

Pathophysiology, Clinical Recognition, Diagnosis, and Management

Ralph Shabetai and James T. Willerson

GENERAL CONSIDERATIONS

Pericardial heart disease is an abnormality of the heart and circulation secondary to an abnormality of the pericardium. In contrast, *pericardial disease* is limited to the pericardium and has no cardiovascular manifestations, so it is not discussed here.

The major forms of pericardial heart disease are acute pericarditis, pericardial effusion, cardiac tamponade, and constrictive pericarditis. Pericarditis tends to cause effusion, which in turn may progress to cardiac tamponade or constrictive pericarditis.

Because pericardial heart disease is so much rarer than other forms of heart disease, it may not be considered until late in its course, or it may be omitted altogether from the differential diagnosis. Therefore, the key to successful recognition and management lies in a high index of suspicion: When cardiovascular and hemodynamic abnormalities (particularly edema, dyspnea, chest pain, and cardiomegaly) are not readily explained otherwise, pericardial heart disease must be ruled out.

In general, the pathophysiology, diagnosis, and treatment of pericardial heart disease are the same in men and women. Nevertheless, a few forms of the disease are specific to women and are mentioned in the appropriate sections.

ACUTE PERICARDITIS

Pathophysiology

The term *acute pericarditis* is commonly reserved for what has been called "acute fibrinous," or "dry," pericarditis, a syndrome consisting of chest pain, a pericardial friction rub, and diffuse electrocardiographic (ECG) ST segment elevation. The pathology is that of acute inflammation. Edema causes a slight thickening of the pericardium. Acute fibrinous pericarditis owes its name to the widespread shaggy coat of fibrin observed at autopsy or surgical exploration. This feature is particularly noticeable in patients with hemodialysis-related acute pericarditis, which also tends to give the pericardium a hemorrhagic appearance.

Etiology

Acute pericarditis may be caused by a viral, bacterial, or fungal infection or by degenerative disease (such as amyloidosis), trauma (including iatrogenic injury), radiation, neoplasia, metabolic disorders, autoimmune disorders (especially systemic lupus erythematosus [SLE] and rheumatoid arthritis), drug therapy, or chylopericardium. Many cases of pericarditis are classified as idiopathic, although they may actually result from an undetected viral infection.

With or without effusion,[1, 2] pericarditis may occur during the course of an acute myocardial infarction (MI).[3] In such cases, it takes the form of acute contiguous pericarditis or a delayed pericardial effusion (Dressler's syndrome), which, along with the postpericardiotomy syndrome and traumatic pericardial disease, exemplifies the postpericardial injury syndrome.[4]

Symptoms

The most common major presenting complaint is retrosternal chest pain, which may resemble the pain of either myocardial ischemia or pleuritis. This pain is worsened by inspiration and coughing but is relieved by sitting up. Unlike myocardial ischemic pain, it rarely radiates to the left arm and the chest, but radiation to the trapezius ridge is characteristic. When the pain is crushing in nature, it can lead to an initial misdiagnosis of acute MI. Respiration may be shallow and rapid, causing the patient to complain of dyspnea. Symptoms of viremia and toxemia may also be present, along with symptoms of the underlying cause.

Diagnosis

Clinical Examination

Upon clinical examination, the patient commonly has fever, tachycardia, sweating, and flushing. The pathognomonic physical finding is the pericardial friction rub, which is heard on auscultation of the middle to lower left sternal edge, between the sternal edge and apex, or at the apex itself. Alternatively, the rub may be widespread and audible over the entire precordium. The classic pericardial friction rub has three components—atrial systolic, ventricular systolic, and diastolic; sometimes, however, only the systolic and diastolic components are present, or the rub is confined to systole.[5]

Usually the sound is fine and high-pitched, with a superficial scratching character, and it seems to originate closer to the patient's skin than do heart sounds and murmurs. It may vary in distribution and intensity, becoming louder during inspiration, and it may obscure any cardiac murmurs. Auscultation of the rub can be particularly difficult in pregnant women with acute viral pericarditis. In this setting, care should be taken not to confuse it with physiologic systolic murmur or venous hum of pregnancy.

When acute pericarditis follows an MI, the friction rub is often inconstant and may not be detected unless auscultation is performed frequently. A pericardial rub is almost routinely audible for the first several days after cardiac surgery.

Clinical Laboratory Findings

Laboratory findings usually include an elevated erythrocyte sedimentation rate and leukocytosis. If acute pericarditis is a manifestation of an MI or other systemic disease, the laboratory data will help determine the underlying cause. Levels of creatine kinase MB and troponins I and T may be mildly elevated even when no other evidence of myocarditis is present. Pericardial fluid abnormalities include elevated white blood cell counts with predominantly neutrophils in bacterial pericarditis, and mononuclear cells in viral, tuberculous, or malignant effusions. Protein concentrations are usually increased to levels equal to or greater than 3 gm/dl in infectious and neoplastic effusions; pH is low (less than 7.0) and lactate dehydrogenase (LDH) values are increased. Intrapericardial fluid glucose values are usually reduced in effusions of bacterial or neoplastic origin but are very low with pericardial effusions due to rheumatic arthritis. SLE cells may be found in pericardial fluids in patients in whom SLE is the cause of the pericarditis.

Radiographic Examination

The chest radiograph usually appears normal, but an associated parenchymal opacity or pleural effusion may be detected.

Electrocardiography

On ECG, acute pericarditis is characterized by diffuse elevation of the ST segment.[6] In contrast to the pattern of an evolving MI, the T wave usually remains upright during ST segment elevation. Depression of the PR segment is a specific, but insensitive, sign of acute pericarditis (Fig. 34–1).

Echocardiography

Echocardiography may be carried out to help confirm the clinical diagnosis of acute pericarditis or to establish it in doubtful cases. In some cases, echocardiography shows a small, clinically unsuspected pericardial effusion, which is a useful confirmatory finding. Patients with a small effusion are still considered to have "dry" pericarditis. Unless the effusion is enlarging or causing cardiac tamponade, the case should be managed as if an effusion were not present. The friction rub may persist even if the effusion is large.

The absence of a pericardial effusion by no means excludes the diagnosis of pericarditis, which may indeed be dry. In uncomplicated cases, the echocardiogram confirms the absence of myocardial or valvular disease and verifies the normal size and function of the cardiac chambers.

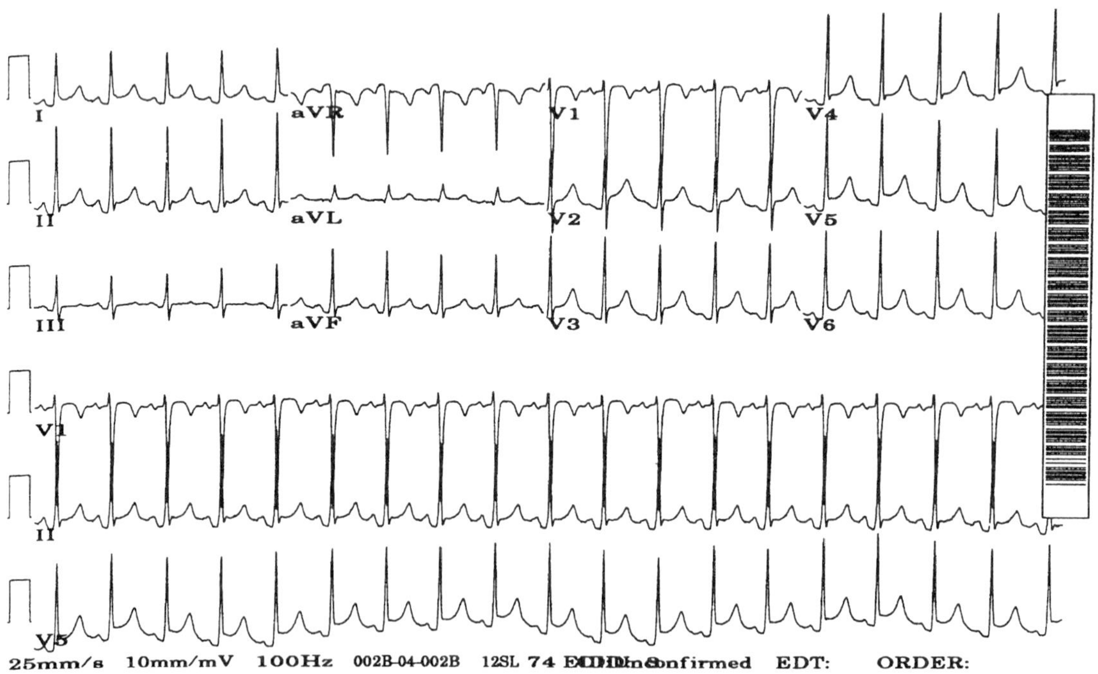

FIGURE 34–1. Electrocardiogram from a patient with acute viral or idiopathic pericarditis. Note ST-segment elevation in leads I, aVF, aVL, and V_4 through V_6 and PR-segment depression in leads I and II and in leads V_3 through V_6. The ST segment is depressed in lead aVR. (From Shabetai R: Etiology, pathophysiology, clinical recognition, and treatment. In Willerson JT, Cohn JN (eds): Cardiovascular Medicine, 2nd ed. Churchill Livingstone, New York, 2000, p 1245, with permission.)

Treatment

In most cases, acute pericarditis has a benign course. Although aspirin may suffice, the initial treatment often requires a nonsteroidal anti-inflammatory agent, most especially indomethacin. Once this therapy is begun, most patients are free of pain and fever within 24 to 48 hours. Treatment is usually continued for 3 or 4 weeks. In the few patients in whom this approach is unsuccessful, colchicine (1 to 2 mg/day) may be effective, with or without continuation of the other anti-inflammatory agent, the dosage of which can be increased if necessary. Only when these therapies fail should prednisone be used.

In some patients, acute pericarditis progresses to acute cardiac tamponade (see later) or, rarely, to constrictive pericarditis (see later).

Recurrent Pericarditis

The most important complication of acute pericarditis is recurrent pericarditis, which is an uncommon but extremely troublesome syndrome.[7] Relapses may occur for weeks, months, or even years. Treatment is similar to that for acute pericarditis, but the recurrent form may be resistant to nonsteroidal anti-inflammatory agents. Again, colchicine may lessen the need for prednisone treatment.[8] Because of the complications associated with high-dose prednisone, every effort should be made to avoid its use, especially because withdrawal from the drug can precipitate a recurrence of pericarditis.

When prednisone must be used, it should be initiated in a high dose (60 or 75 mg/day), ideally given as a single daily dose (at 7 to 8 AM), which should be maintained until all symptoms and signs of pericarditis, including the erythrocyte sedimentation rate, have returned to normal. After 1 or 2 weeks of total disease suppression, the dose should be slowly and progressively reduced. When this treatment is successful, prednisone can then be discontinued. If symptoms or signs recur, however, the lowest suppressing dose should be reinstituted and maintained for 3 or 4 weeks, probably with an appropriate dose of indomethacin, after which another attempt can be made to reduce the dose or to stop treatment. The same protocol should be continued until all evidence of pericarditis disappears.

Patients who require prednisone must be watched carefully for osteoporosis and other symptoms of prednisone toxicity. If these symptoms occur or if prednisone is clearly not having the desired effect, a pericardiectomy should be considered. Although this operation may be curative, relapses may still occur; nevertheless, they tend to be fewer and milder and to resolve faster than if surgery is not performed.

PERICARDIAL EFFUSION

Pathophysiology

Any type of pericarditis may result in a pericardial effusion. The effusion may be small or large, hemodynamically benign or life-threatening, and transudative, exudative, sanguineous, or chylous.

Etiology

Cardiac causes of pericardial effusion include rupture of an aortic aneurysm or dissection into the pericardial space and rupture related to a MI. Strictly speaking, these massive hemorrhages into the pericardium are not effusions, but they have the same pathophysiology as effusions and are potent causes of cardiac tamponade. Although congestive heart failure is considered the leading cause of pericardial effusion at autopsy, this finding is clinically uncommon. A silent pericardial effusion is fairly common in late pregnancy.[9] In these cases, the ECG is usually normal or may show nonspecific ST-T segment changes. The onset of a pericardial effusion during pregnancy is attributed to water and salt retention, because the incidence is greater in women who gain more weight.[9–11] A pericardial effusion may also be seen in women with breast cancer. In fact, one report concluded that small, clinically unsuspected pericardial effusions are common in women with metastatic breast cancer. In this series,[12] 50% of patients with known metastatic disease and a pericardial effusion had malignant pericardial disease; however, patients without metastatic breast cancer (but with clinical pericardial disease) did not experience malignant pericardial involvement. Rarely, cervical or ovarian carcinoma may metastasize to the pericardium and cause a malignant pericardial effusion.[13-16]

Diagnosis

Physical findings are nonspecific for diagnosis of a pericardial effusion and are generally inadequate to allow recognition of small pericardial effusions. Rather, the diagnosis is based on results of radiography, scintigraphy, or echocardiography.

Radiographic Examination

Pericardial effusion is strongly suggested when a patient experiences unexpected cardiomegaly with clear lung fields and previous radiographs show a normal-sized heart. In severe heart failure complicated by tricuspid regurgitation, however, the radiograph may also show massive cardiomegaly with clear lung fields. Moreover, massive cardiomegaly may accompany heart diseases that cause a large volume overload, such as severe aortic or mitral regurgitation. Whenever these abnormal loading conditions are present without heart failure, the heart appears large on the chest radiograph, but the lungs remain relatively clear.

Scintigraphy

Scintigraphy shows a clear zone of pericardial effusion that separates the radioactivity in the heart from that in the liver.

Echocardiography

When a pericardial effusion is suspected, it may be definitively diagnosed by means of echocardiography (Fig. 34–2), which not only can estimate the size of the effusion but also can suggest whether cardiac tamponade is present. In most cases, the effusion surrounds the heart. In other cases, particularly after cardiac surgery, the effusion is localized. When a pericardial effusion begins to deposit fibrin and to become organized, the change is often recognizable because of opacities within the pericardial fluid image.[17] Although smaller effusions may not be visible behind the left atrium, large ones in this area are well visualized because they surround the rest of the heart.

With an uncomplicated pericardial effusion, echocardiography can clarify the size of the cardiac chambers and the degree of systolic and diastolic function. With a particularly large pericardial effusion, the heart has a rocking or pendular motion within the motionless pericardial space.[18] (On the ECG, this pendular motion may be reflected as electrical alternans.)

During respiration, Doppler examination often shows increased variation in the velocity of inflow through the mitral and tricuspid valves and of ejection through the aortic and pulmonary valves. In the presence of cardiac tamponade, this finding becomes even more marked. If tamponade is suspected, a comprehensive echocardiographic Doppler examination should be performed, the extent being tailored to individual need.

When a pericardial effusion occurs in the presence of dilated heart failure, the extent of the heart failure can be determined by judging the size of the pericardial effusion, the extent of hypokinesis, and the dimensions of the cardiac chambers. In such cases, echocardiography should show serious regional wall motion abnormalities or evidence of valvular heart disease. With severe cardiac tamponade, the left ventricular wall may appear thickened; however, its greater size simply reflects a reduced cardiac volume.

Echocardiography may also show a clinically unsuspected benign pericardial effusion, as is common in pregnant women.[9] Likewise, after an acute MI, echocardiography may show a pericardial effusion in patients who lack a pericardial friction rub or other evidence of pericarditis. Silent pericardial effusion is often detected by serial echocardiograms after cardiac surgery but is of no clinical significance.

Treatment

Patients who have pericardial effusion without tamponade should be observed as outpatients for 1 to 3 weeks to allow the effusion to resolve. Aspirin, indomethacin, or both should be given to control pain and anxiety and to prevent further effusion. If the effusion is suspected of being purulent, pericardiocentesis is indicated to confirm the diagnosis. If infection is confirmed, specific antimicrobial drugs are given; the purulent effusion must be completely removed, often by an intrapericardial catheter.

If the effusion is malignant, pericardiectomy or creation of a pericardial "window" (i.e., removal of a wide segment of the pericardium) is generally indicated.[12] When the patient's general condition is such that thoracotomy and pericardial resection are inadvisable, an alternative strategy is catheter drainage of the pericardial fluid followed by intrapericardial instillation of tetracycline, thiotepa, or nitrogen mustard to obliterate the intrapericardial space through fibrosis.[19–22] Aggressive radiation or chemotherapy of the responsible tumor (usually breast, lung, or stomach) may also be advisable.

CARDIAC TAMPONADE

Cardiac tamponade is defined as compression of the heart by pericardial fluid under increased pressure. As such, and until the end stage, it is a disorder of impaired venous return and impedance to diastolic filling of the ventricles.

After cardiac surgery, tamponade is an ever-present danger.[23] Although it usually occurs in the recovery room or intensive care unit, cardiac tamponade can also occur after hospital discharge.[24] Therefore, it must be considered when

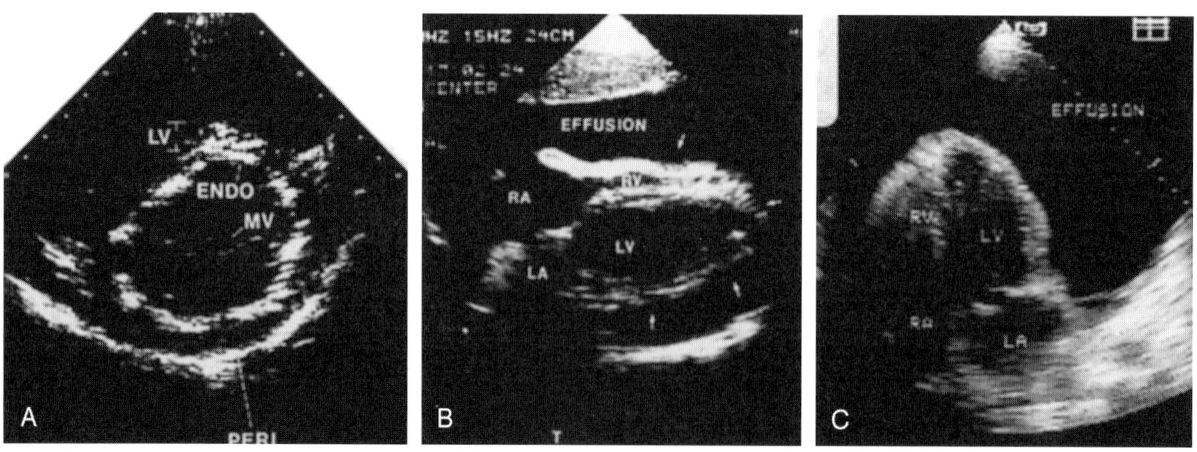

FIGURE 34–2. *A*, Short-axis view of the left ventricle (LV) in a patient with a moderate to large pericardial effusion. ENDO, endocardium; MV, mitral valve; PERI, pericardium. Note the echo-free space between the pericardium and the heart. *B*, Large pericardial effusion in the subcostal view. The effusion (labeled) is anterior to the right ventricle (RV), which is severely compressed. A copious effusion is also visible posterior to the left ventricle (LV). LA, left atrium; RA, right atrium. *C*, Massive pericardial effusion seen in the four-chamber view. The effusion is circumferential. (From Shabetai R: Etiology, pathophysiology, clinical recognition, and treatment. In Willerson JT, Cohn JN (eds): Cardiovascular Medicine, 2nd ed. Churchill Livingstone, New York, 2000, p 1245, with permission.)

any patient who has recently undergone cardiac surgery experiences unexplained dyspnea, cardiomegaly, increased jugular venous pressure, or other evidence of hemodynamic compromise. Cardiac tamponade may rarely occur in advanced-stage breast cancer, especially in pregnant women.[25]

Diagnosis

Physical Examination

The severity of cardiac tamponade can be determined at the bedside, and in some cases, the diagnosis can also be established in that setting. The key physical finding is the jugular venous pressure. When this pressure remains normal and there is no reason (such as a major hemorrhage) for profound hypovolemia, cardiac tamponade is not likely to be present. In these cases, the systemic arterial pressure, the peripheral pulses, and the heart rate remain normal.

When the intrapericardial pressure rises to 10 to 12 mm Hg, moderately severe tamponade is present. At this stage, a skilled observer can also detect an abnormality of the waveform of the jugular venous pulsations. In severe tamponade, the intrapericardial pressure reaches 15 mm Hg, and there is a corresponding rise in the venous pressures on both sides of the circulation (Fig. 34–3). The systemic arterial pressure may decrease, and pulsus paradoxus often appears. This phenomenon causes an abnormally large decrease (more than 10 mm Hg) in the systemic arterial pressure during inspiration; it is paradoxical because the peripheral pulse is apparently irregular in the presence of a regular heartbeat. In the most severe cases, the pulse may disappear altogether during inspiration.

If the pericardial and intracardiac pressures increase to more than 20 mm Hg, severe cardiac decompensation will occur, marked by a greatly decreased arterial pressure and cardiac output, leading to dyspnea, chest discomfort, and impaired renal function.

The physical examination should be complemented by echocardiography, especially in complex cases, in which tamponade may be hard to diagnose at the bedside.

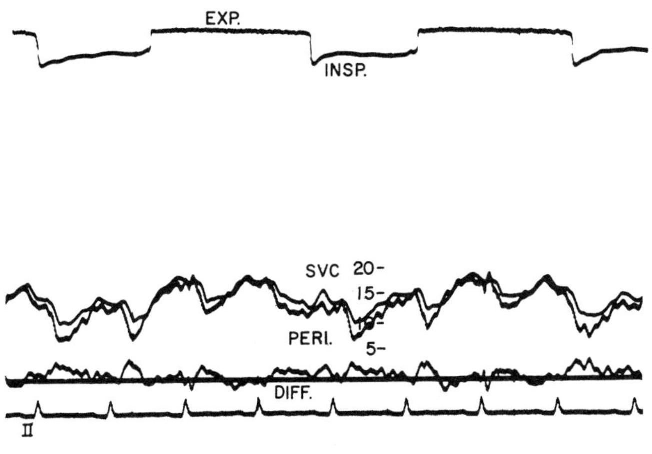

FIGURE 34–3. Pericardial (PERI) and superior vena caval (SVC) pressures recorded by means of a differential transducer during catheterization and pericardiocentesis in a patient with severe cardiac tamponade. The two pressures are virtually identical, and both are severely elevated. Pressure falls during inspiration (INSP). The waveform shows a dominant *x* but no *y* descent. The phase of respiration is indicated by a thermistor tracing at the top of the figure. The difference between the pressures (DIFF) is shown fluctuating around the zero baseline. EXP, expiration. (From Shabetai R: Etiology, pathophysiology, clinical recognition, and treatment. In Willerson JT, Cohn JN (eds): Cardiovascular Medicine, 2nd ed. Churchill Livingstone, New York, 2000, p 1245, with permission.)

Electrocardiography

ECG is seldom useful for diagnosing pericardial tamponade: Either the results are normal or, if abnormalities are present, they are not specific. Rarely, the tracing may show the characteristic abnormalities of acute pericarditis with widespread elevation of the ST segment and, sometimes, depression of the PR segment. Alternans of the P wave, QRS complex, and T waves (every other P, QRS, and T wave alternating to be similar in appearance) usually indicates a large pericardial effusion,[26] often caused by a malignant or tuberculous effusion. However, this form of alternans, although relatively specific, is not very sensitive.[27]

Echocardiography

Because the echocardiographic features of cardiac tamponade are highly characteristic, they are of great value in establishing the diagnosis and assessing its severity.[28] Tamponade is strongly suggested by greater respiratory variation in the atrioventricular inflow velocity and in the blood velocity through the semilunar valves.[29, 30] It is also suggested by compression of the right atrial border[31, 32] that results in its normal convexity being reversed and the atrium appearing to have a concave outer wall. Collapse of the right ventricle in early diastole[33] is another change suggestive but not pathognomonic of cardiac tamponade; the longer into diastole this collapse can be seen, the more severe the tamponade is likely to be (Fig. 34–4). Except in patients with severe hypovolemia, the inferior vena cava is dilated and is not compressed during inspiration. This finding is useful when the jugular pressure cannot easily be evaluated.

On the other hand, echocardiographic signs of cardiac tamponade may not be present, particularly if the tamponade is complicated by another cardiac condition. Furthermore, signs that are normally diagnostic of cardiac tamponade may be found on the echocardiograms of patients with pericardial effusion but not tamponade. Thus, the diagnosis may be made on clinical grounds, echocardiographic grounds, or both.

Whenever cardiac tamponade is suspected, the obvious question is whether the patient has a pericardial effusion. If an effusion is absent, tamponade cannot be present. When associated with tamponade, a pericardial effusion is usually moderate to large in size. On echocardiography, it appears as a motionless echo-free space around the heart.

Cardiac tamponade diminishes the volume of the ventricles, which therefore appear to have thicker walls on echocardiography. Not surprisingly, a decrease in ventricular volume creates the substrate for pseudoprolapse of the mitral valve, which is a minor echocardiographic sign of tamponade.

In some patients with cardiac tamponade and a very

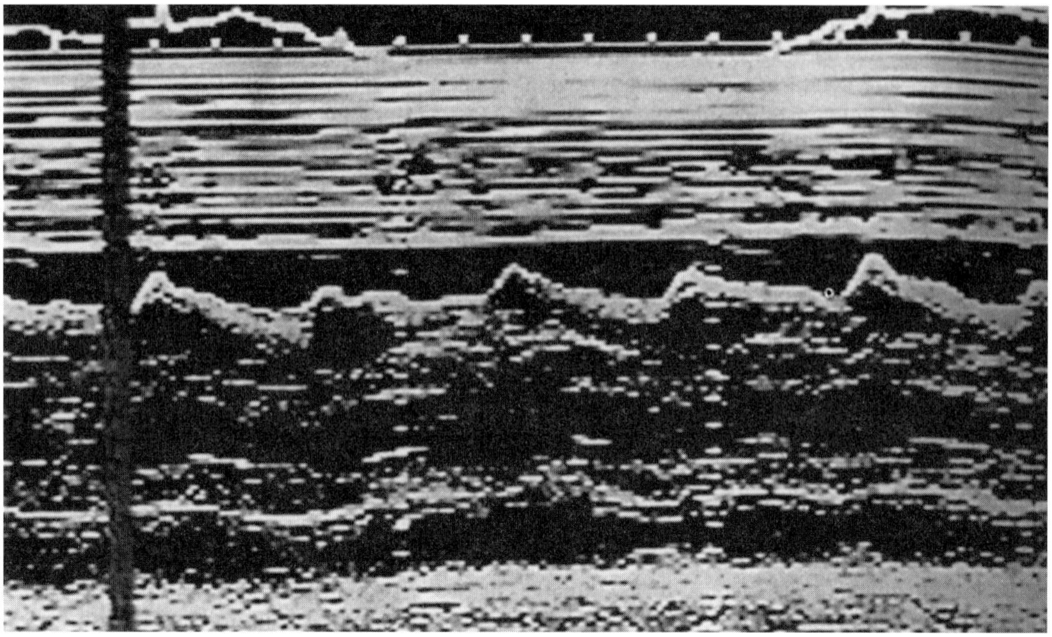

FIGURE 34–4. M-mode echocardiogram from a patient with cardiac tamponade. A large pericardial effusion is present anteriorly and posteriorly. The right ventricular free wall (topmost moving image) moves toward the interventricular septum during diastole, indicating right ventricular diastolic collapse, a difficult condition to assess by echocardiography. (From Shabetai R: Etiology, pathophysiology, clinical recognition, and treatment. In Willerson JT, Cohn JN (eds): Cardiovascular Medicine, 2nd ed. Churchill Livingstone, New York, 2000, p 1245, with permission.)

large, usually malignant, pericardial effusion, the whole heart appears to swing dramatically in the echo-free space. This motion influences the organ's electric axis, often causing electrical alternans on the ECG (see preceding section).

Cardiac Catheterization

In most cases, cardiac tamponade can be diagnosed without cardiac catheterization. If the diagnosis is in doubt or underlying heart disease is suspected, however, the patient should undergo catheterization, at least of the right side of the heart.

Treatment

Because cardiac tamponade presents a spectrum ranging from a slightly elevated pericardial pressure to a pressure of 25 to 30 mm Hg in extreme cases, treatment must be tailored to each patient. For successful management, the following principles should be borne in mind:

1. Cardiac compression can occur in the presence of a localized and relatively mild tamponade and can sometimes be managed conservatively.
2. False-positive compression can occur, for example, as a result of a massive pleural effusion.
3. Severe cardiac tamponade can exist in the absence of echocardiographic right-sided cardiac compression or pulsus paradoxus, especially (but not exclusively) in the presence of preexisting heart disease and after cardiac surgery.

The general goal of treatment is to evacuate pericardial fluid very rapidly, thereby lowering the pericardial pressure and, thus, the intracardiac atrial and ventricular diastolic pressures. This goal may be accomplished by means of pericardiocentesis, a surgical pericardiotomy, or (less commonly) a balloon pericardiostomy. Because of space constraints, this discussion considers pericardiocentesis alone. The details of this procedure have been described elsewhere and are not repeated here.[34]

In extreme cases, the need for pericardiocentesis may be so urgent that there is no time to obtain a diagnostic echocardiogram. Patients without clinical evidence of cardiovascular compromise (except an increase in the jugular venous pressure of 5 to 7 mm Hg), however, may simply be admitted to the hospital to see whether the hemodynamic situation deteriorates, indicating the need to remove pericardial fluid.

Pericardiocentesis may be performed in the cardiac catheterization laboratory or the operating room but is increasingly being done in the intensive care unit with echocardiographic monitoring.[35] With a multichannel pressure-recording system, right atrial and systemic arterial pressures can be recorded simultaneously with the mean pulmonary wedge pressure; the mean right atrial and mean pulmonary wedge pressures should not differ from the intrapericardial pressure by more than 2 or 3 mm Hg when tamponade is present.

Once the baseline pressures have been recorded, the measurements can be repeated while aliquots of pericardial fluid are removed. In uncomplicated cardiac tamponade, all the pressures return to normal, the pericardial pressure being lower than the right atrial and pulmonary wedge pressures throughout the cardiac and respiratory cycles.

After removal of the first 100 ml of pericardial fluid, the right atrial and pulmonary wedge pressures should diminish dramatically, and the systemic arterial pressure should rise substantially. The severity of pulsus paradoxus should diminish, and the heart rate may decrease. Withdrawal of intrapericardial fluid progressively lessens the severity of cardiac tamponade, so the pericardial pressure gradually declines. The decrease in the right atrial and pulmonary wedge pressures is identical to that in the pericardial pressure, so all three pressures remain in equilibrium.[36] After the pericardial pressure has fallen lower than the preexisting pulmonary wedge pressure (e.g., 10 mm Hg), further pericardiocentesis has no additional effect on the pulmonary wedge pressure, but the right atrial and pericardial pressures remain identical until the normal right atrial pressure is reached, at which point the pericardial pressure declines below right atrial pressure. The former becomes subatmospheric, and the latter levels off at around 5 mm Hg.[37]

The foregoing sequence of hemodynamic events applies to uncomplicated cardiac tamponade in patients without preexisting heart disease or constrictive pericarditis. If the right atrial pressure remains abnormal after pericardiocentesis, the clinician should consider effusive-constrictive pericarditis (whose characteristic hemodynamic findings are unmasked by pericardiocentesis), tricuspid regurgitation or right-sided heart failure (documented by right ventriculography or Doppler echocardiography), and tricuspid stenosis (documented by simultaneous pressure recordings of the right atrial and right ventricular pressures or by Doppler echocardiography). The ability to carry out these additional investigations is a major advantage of performing pericardiocentesis in the catheterization laboratory.

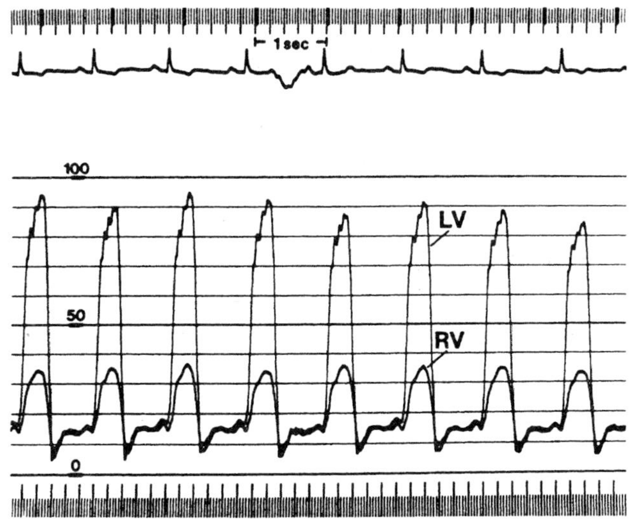

FIGURE 34–5. Pressures recorded simultaneously from right ventricle (RV) and left ventricle (LV) in a patient with constrictive pericarditis. Note the dip-and-plateau configuration of the diastolic pressures, which are elevated to 15 mm Hg and are equilibrated. Respiratory variation in left and right ventricular peak systolic pressures is neither in phase nor exactly 180 degrees out of phase. (From Shabetai R: Etiology, pathophysiology, clinical recognition, and treatment. In Willerson JT, Cohn JN (eds): Cardiovascular Medicine, 2nd ed. Churchill Livingstone, New York, 2000, p 1245, with permission.)

CONSTRICTIVE PERICARDITIS

As another major pericardial cause of cardiac compressive disease, constrictive pericarditis shares some important characteristics with cardiac tamponade, but the two conditions also have important clinical and pathophysiologic differences.[34] Constrictive pericarditis can be subacute or chronic, but it is seldom acute.

Pathophysiology

In constrictive pericarditis, the pericardium becomes scarred because of a previous insult and loses all or most of its normal compliance. Venous return to the heart and diastolic filling of the ventricles are therefore impeded. In the most severe cases, the heart is compressed so that the end-diastolic ventricular volume is appreciably decreased, limiting the stroke volume despite a normal or increased ventricular ejection fraction. As a result, the ventricular diastolic pressures are raised on both sides of the heart (Figs. 34–5 and 34–6), leading to elevated pulmonary venous and systemic venous pressures, which cause congestion of the lungs and systemic tissues. In most cases, systemic congestion is more profound than pulmonary congestion.

The clinical picture resembles that of congestive heart failure. However, because ventricular systolic function is normal[38] and ventricular diastolic dysfunction is due to increased pericardial, not myocardial, stiffness, constrictive pericarditis is not a form of congestive heart failure. The latter condition results from overload of the heart, whereas in constrictive pericarditis, the heart is underloaded and only the circulation is overloaded.[39] Diuretics should be used only when fluid retention has made the patient uncomfortable. It is a serious error to try to achieve a normal jugular pressure or "dry weight," because venous pressure must remain ele-

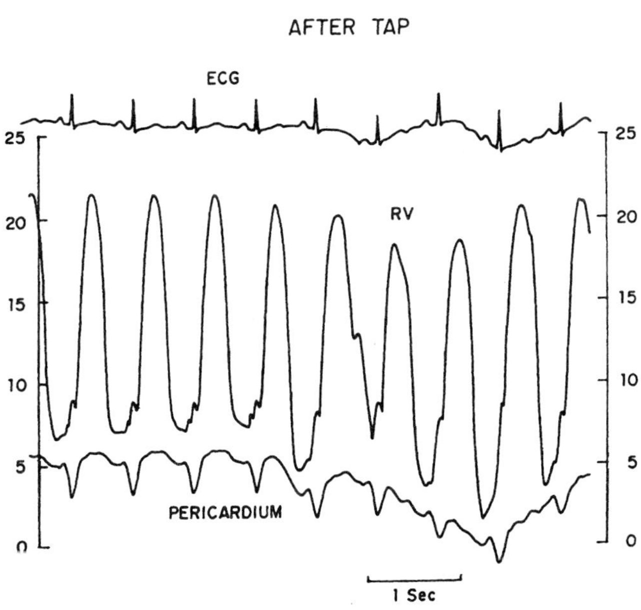

FIGURE 34–6. Simultaneous recording of right ventricular (RV) and pericardial pressures immediately after pericardiocentesis. Note that ventricular diastolic pressure exceeds pericardial pressure throughout the respiratory and cardiac cycles. Also, there is a fall in pericardial pressure coincident with ventricular ejection. ECG, electrocardiogram. (From Shabetai R: Etiology, pathophysiology, clinical recognition, and treatment. In Willerson JT, Cohn JN (eds): Cardiovascular Medicine, 2nd ed. Churchill Livingstone, New York, 2000, p 1245, with permission.)

vated to maintain cardiac output. Preload and afterload reduction therapies generally are not appropriate for patients with constrictive pericarditis.

Etiology

Almost any cause of pericarditis can eventually result in constrictive pericarditis.[40] Neoplastic pericardial disease and postradiation pericardiopathy are common causes of constrictive pericarditis, especially in patients who have received extensive radiation for lymphoma, breast, or lung cancer, or other malignant disease with metastatic thoracic involvement. Women who have undergone aggressive irradiation for breast cancer are particularly at risk. Constrictive pericarditis may also be iatrogenic, occurring (weeks to years) after 0.1% to 0.3% of cardiac operations,[41] or may follow blunt as well as sharp chest trauma.

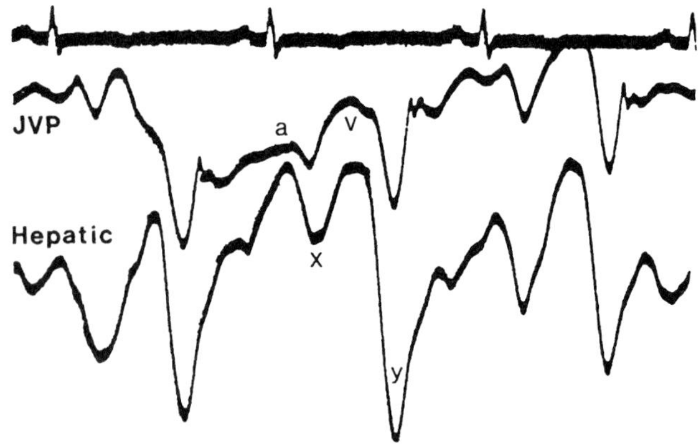

FIGURE 34–7. Noninvasive recordings of jugular venous pulsations (JVP) and hepatic pulsations in a patient with severe constrictive pericarditis. *Top*, Electrocardiogram. Displacement transducers were placed over the jugular and hepatic pulsations. Note the close correspondence in waveform. (From Manga P, Vythilingom S, Mitha A: Pulsatile hepatomegaly in constrictive pericarditis. Br Heart J 52:465, 1984, with permission.)

Diagnosis

Whenever a patient has unexplained fluid retention and a high jugular venous pressure, constrictive pericarditis should be considered. The differential diagnosis consists of constrictive pericarditis, restrictive cardiomyopathy, and cardiac tamponade.[29, 42-48] When the first two conditions are hard to distinguish, an endomyocardial biopsy should be considered at the time of the hemodynamic study.[42] Magnetic resonance imaging, rapid-speed CT imaging, or transesophageal echocardiography provides an accurate measurement of pericardial thickness and allows a correct diagnosis to be made. For a complete discussion of this subject, the reader is referred to a previous discussion by Shabetai.[34] Tricuspid valve disease and cirrhosis of the liver must also be ruled out. It has been established that plasma brain natriuretic peptide is elevated in diastolic dysfunction of myocardial origin; this elevation may not occur in constrictive pericarditis.

History

A history of any condition associated with pericarditis is important in establishing the diagnosis. The symptoms are similar to those of right-sided heart failure: edema, increased abdominal girth and weight, breathlessness, and fatigue. Right-sided congestion usually predominates over left. By the time the patient consults a physician, these symptoms may be far advanced.

Clinical Examination

Clinical findings depend on the severity and chronicity of constrictive pericarditis. The most important physical finding is an abnormal jugular venous pressure, which may be as high as 20 cm H_2O. For the examination, the patient must stand or sit upright, because jugular venous pulsations are otherwise damped. Even if the external jugular vein is distended and prominent, the jugular venous pulse should be evaluated. As described elsewhere, the dominant abnormality is the rapid deep y descent of the jugular venous pulse.[34] Whereas sinus rhythm is the rule in mild to moderate cases, atrial fibrillation almost always occurs in chronic cases.

With mild constrictive pericarditis, the jugular venous pressure is only about 7 or 8 cm H_2O. There may be no signs of ascites, pleural effusion, or even edema. However, in severe, chronic constrictive pericarditis, edema may extend to the thighs, and ascites can be diagnosed at the bedside. Dull, decreased breath sounds may indicate a pleural effusion, which is commonly present. Examination of the abdomen is particularly important to assess the possibility of ascites and to evaluate the liver, which in severe cases is enlarged and may pulsate (Fig. 34–7).

Constrictive pericarditis does not produce a characteristic murmur, but it may cause a loud third heart sound ("pericardial knock") that occurs approximately 100 msec after the second heart sound. With respect to timing, this third heart sound resembles the third heart sound of heart failure and the opening snap of mitral stenosis.

Clinical Laboratory Findings

In severe cases, the plasma concentrations of sodium chloride and potassium may be decreased, especially for patients receiving large doses of a diuretic. The blood urea nitrogen and serum creatinine concentrations are elevated, and creatinine clearance is markedly diminished. Liver function tests show increased levels of bilirubin and enzymes secondary to hepatic congestion, which also causes the serum albumin level to decrease. The underlying cause of constrictive pericarditis may result in additional laboratory abnormalities.

Chest Radiography

Although the heart often appears small on chest films, this finding is by no means universal. Sometimes, the heart size is hard to evaluate because of pleural effusion and a high diaphragm. In some cases, ringlike calcification of the pericardium is easily seen, especially in a lateral or oblique projection. Calcification is also easily recognized on fluoroscopy or computed tomography. Severe pulmonary hypertension does not develop, and the right ventricle is impaired to the same extent as the left ventricle.

Electrocardiography

Nonspecific ST-segment and T-wave changes are commonly seen on the ECG.[49] Rarely, ventricular-depolarization changes, such as bundle branch block, are present.[50] In longstanding constrictive pericarditis, atrial fibrillation often occurs. P mitrale is common for patients in whom sinus rhythm is preserved, and the QRS voltage is usually low, that is, less than 5 mm in leads I through aVF.

Echocardiography

Standard echocardiography is not particularly helpful for diagnosing constrictive pericarditis,[51] but Doppler echocardiography is an important tool, especially for differentiating between constrictive pericarditis and restrictive cardiomyopathy.

Other Imaging Modalities

The pericardium is satisfactorily imaged with computed tomography.[52, 53] In normal patients, this structure either is invisible or appears as a thin line. In constrictive pericarditis, however, the pericardial thickness may be increased to less than 1 cm. If present, calcification can be identified (Fig. 34–8). Unfortunately, in some cases, the scarred visceral pericardium forms a tight skin around the heart but is not particularly thickened. Thus, although increased pericardial thickness is a valuable diagnostic finding, false-negative results occur.

For imaging the pericardium, magnetic resonance imaging[54] (Fig. 34–9) may be superior even to computed tomography, and either of these techniques is indicated when constrictive pericarditis is suspected.

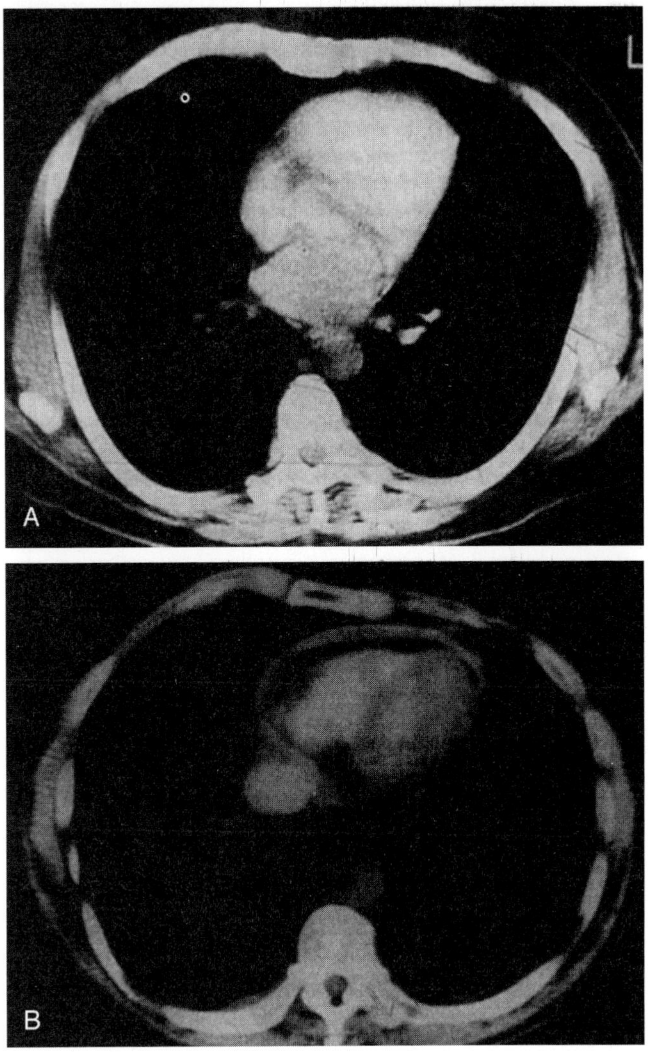

FIGURE 34–8. *A*, Computed tomogram from a patient without pericardial disease. *B*, Computed tomogram of a patient with calcified constrictive pericarditis. The calcification is clearly seen with use of this technique. (From Shabetai R: Etiology, pathophysiology, clinical recognition, and treatment. In Willerson JT, Cohn JN (eds): Cardiovascular Medicine, 2nd ed. Churchill Livingstone, New York, 2000, p 1245, with permission.)

Cardiac Catheterization

Cardiac catheterization is indicated if (1) the physician has trouble differentiating constrictive pericarditis from restrictive cardiomyopathy or (2) the patient is being evaluated for a possible pericardiectomy. In the former situation, an endomyocardial biopsy performed during cardiac catheterization may be critical[42]; in the latter situation, assessment of the coronary arteries is important. The characteristic findings have been described elsewhere[34] and are not repeated here.

Treatment

Mild constrictive pericarditis does not require specific treatment, but, largely for cosmetic reasons, patients with such a disorder are sometimes given a low-dose diuretic. Patients with moderate to severe symptoms are better served by pericardiectomy. The results are usually very gratifying, except in patients with postradiation constrictive pericarditis, who usually have concurrent myocardial damage.

CONCLUSION

Pericardial heart disease can take several forms. In order of increasing severity, they range from acute pericarditis (often with pericardial effusion) to cardiac tamponade or constrictive pericarditis. Conditions specific to women include pericardial effusion during late pregnancy (with SLE) and pericardial metastases from breast, ovarian, or cervical cancer. Otherwise, the pathophysiology, diagnosis, and treatment of pericardial heart disease are generally the same in men and women. The most important key to a successful outcome is a high index of suspicion, especially in patients who have recently undergone cardiac operations.

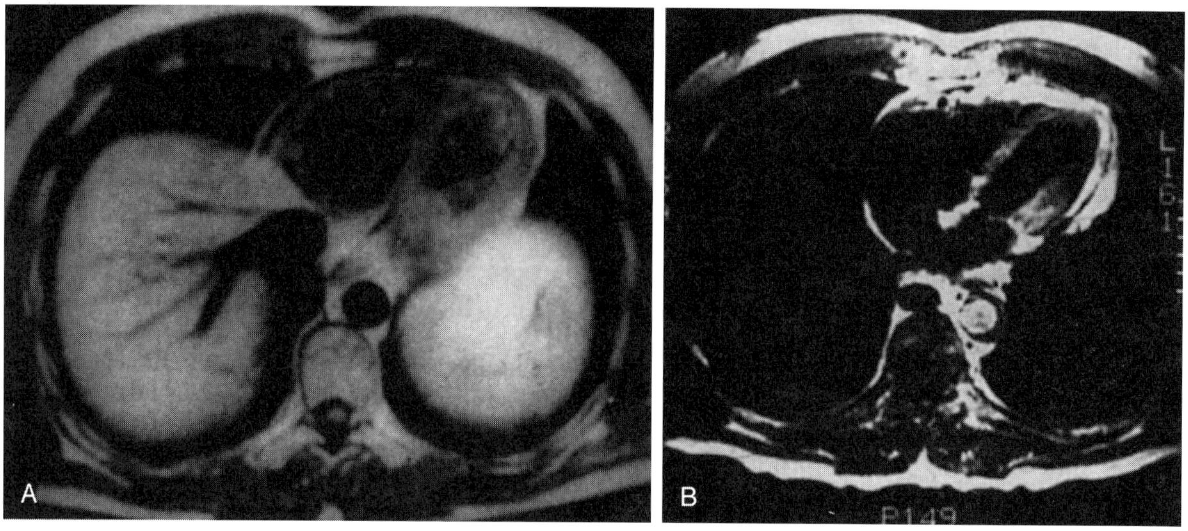

FIGURE 34–9. *A,* Magnetic resonance image of a patient without pericardial disease. The pericardium is visualized at the top of the image as a thin, dark, curved line. *B,* Magnetic resonance image from a patient with constrictive pericarditis secondary to tuberculosis. The dark area (*top right*) is a grossly thickened and calcified pericardium. The low-intensity line around the thick-walled left ventricle is pericardium with epicardial and pericardial fat. (From Shabetai R: Etiology, pathophysiology, clinical recognition, and treatment. In Willerson JT, Cohn JN: Cardiovascular Medicine, 2nd ed. Churchill Livingstone, New York, 2000, p 1245, with permission.)

References

1. Galve E, Garcia-Del-Castillo H, Evangelista A, et al: Pericardial effusion in the course of myocardial infarction: Incidence, natural history, and clinical relevance. Circulation 73:294, 1986.
2. Pierard LA, Albert A, Henrard L, et al: Incidence and significance of pericardial effusion in acute myocardial infarction as determined by two-dimensional echocardiography. J Am Coll Cardiol 8:517, 1986.
3. Marsa R, Mehta S, Willis N, et al: Constrictive pericarditis after myocardial revascularization: Report of three cases. Am J Cardiol 44:177, 1979.
4. Prabhu AS, Ross RD, Heinert MR, et al: Decreased incidence of postoperative pericardial effusions after cardiac surgery for congenital heart disease. Am J Cardiol 77:774, 1996.
5. Spodick DH: Acoustic phenomena in pericardial disease. Am Heart J 81:114, 1971.
6. Spodick DH: Diagnostic electrocardiographic sequences in acute pericarditis: Significance of PR segment and PR vector changes. Circulation 48:575, 1973.
7. Fowler NO, Harbin AD III: Recurrent acute pericarditis: Follow-up study of 31 patients. J Am Coll Cardiol 7:300, 1986.
8. Adler Y, Finkelstein Y, Guindo J, et al: Colchicine treatment for recurrent pericarditis: A decade of experience. Circulation 97:2183, 1998.
9. Haiat R, Halphen C: Silent pericardial effusion in late pregnancy: A new entity. Cardiovasc Intervent Radiol 7:267, 1984.
10. Halphen C, Haiat R, Clement F, Michelon B: Silent pericardial effusion in late pregnancy: Echocardiographic detection in the third trimester of pregnancy (author's transl). J Gynecol Obstet Biol Reprod (Paris) 11:245, 1982.
11. Abduljabbar HS, Marzouki KM, Zawawi TH, Khan AS: Pericardial effusion in normal pregnant women. Acta Obstet Gynecol Scand 70: 291, 1991.
12. Buck M, Ingle JN, Giuliani ER, et al: Pericardial effusion in women with breast cancer. Cancer 60:263, 1987.
13. Jamshed A, Khafaga Y, El-Husseiny G, et al: Pericardial metastasis in carcinoma of the uterine cervix. Gynecol Oncol 61:451, 1996.
14. Nelson BE, Rose PG: Malignant pericardial effusion from squamous cell cancer of the cervix. J Surg Oncol 52:203, 1993.
15. Malviya VK, Casselberry JM, Parekh N, Deppe G: Pericardial metastases in squamous cell cancer of the cervix: A report of two cases. J Reprod Med 35:49, 1990.
16. Rieke JW, Kapp DS: Successful management of malignant pericardial effusion in metastatic squamous cell carcinoma of the uterine cervix. Gynecol Oncol 31:338, 1988.
17. Sinha PR, Singh BP, Jaipuria N, et al: Intrapericardial echogenic images and development of constrictive pericarditis in patients with pericardial effusion. Am Heart J 132:1268, 1996.
18. Rigney DR, Goldberger AL: Nonlinear mechanics of the heart's swinging during pericardial effusion. Am J Physiol 257:H1292, 1989.
19. Hancock EW: Neoplastic pericardial disease. Cardiol Clin 8:673, 1990.
20. Kralstein J, Frishman WH: Malignant pericardial diseases: Diagnosis and treatment. Cardiol Clin 5:583, 1987.
21. Martinoni A, Cipolla CM, Civelli M, et al: Intrapericardial treatment of neoplastic pericardial effusions. Herz 25:787, 2000.
22. Bishiniotis TS, Antoniadou S, Katseas G, et al: Malignant cardiac tamponade in women with breast cancer treated by pericardiocentesis and intrapericardial administration of triethylenethiophosphoramide (thiotepa). Am J Cardiol 1:362, 2000.
23. D'Cruz IA, Overton DH, Ganesh MP: Pericardial complications of cardiac surgery: Emphasis on the diagnostic role of echocardiography. J Card Surg 7:257, 1992.
24. Nottestad SY, Mascette AM: Loculated pericardial effusion and cardiac tamponade late after cardiac surgery. Chest 101:852, 1992.
25. Khabele D, Chasen S: Cardiac tamponade as an unusual presentation of advanced breast cancer in pregnancy. J Reprod Med 44:989, 1999.
26. Littmann D, Spodick DH: Total electrical alternation in pericardial disease. Circulation 17:912, 1958.
27. Spodick DH: Electric alternation of the heart: Its relation to the kinetics and physiology of the heart during cardiac tamponade. Am J Cardiol 10:155, 1962.
28. D'Cruz IA, Cohen HC, Ravindra P, et al: Diagnosis of cardiac tamponade by echocardiography: Changes in mitral valve motion and ventricular dimensions, with special reference to paradoxical pulse. Circulation 52:460, 1975.
29. Appleton CP, Hatle LK, Popp RL: Cardiac tamponade and pericardial effusion: Respiratory variation in transvalvular flow velocities studied by Doppler echocardiography. J Am Coll Cardiol 11:1020, 1988.
30. Fowler NO: The significance of echocardiographic-Doppler studies in cardiac tamponade. J Am Coll Cardiol 11:1031, 1988.
31. Kronzon I, Cohen ML, Winer HE: Diastolic atrial compression: A sensitive echocardiographic sign of cardiac tamponade. J Am Coll Cardiol 2:770, 1983.
32. Gillam LD, Guyer DE, Gibson TC, et al: Hydrodynamic compression of the right atrium: A new echocardiographic sign of cardiac tamponade. Circulation 68:294, 1983.
33. Schiller NB, Botvinick EH: Right ventricular compression as a sign of cardiac tamponade: An analysis of echocardiographic ventricular dimensions and their clinical implications. Circulation 56:774, 1977.
34. Shabetai R: Etiology, pathophysiology, clinical recognition, and treatment of pericardial disease. In Willerson JT, Cohn JN (eds): Cardiovascular Medicine, 2nd ed. Churchill Livingstone, New York, 2000, p 1245.

35. Sohn DW, Shin GJ, Oh JK, et al: Role of transesophageal echocardiography in hemodynamically unstable patients. Mayo Clin Proc 70:925, 1995.
36. Holt JP, Rhode EA, Kines H: Pericardial and ventricular pressure. Circ Res 8:1171, 1960.
37. Reddy PS, Curtiss EI, O'Toole JD, et al: Cardiac tamponade: Hemodynamic observations in man. Circulation 58:265, 1978.
38. Lewis BS, Gotsman MS: Left ventricular function in systole and diastole in constrictive pericarditis. Am Heart J 86:23, 1973.
39. Klopfenstein HS, Schuchard GH, Wann LS, et al: The relative merits of pulsus paradoxus and right ventricular diastolic collapse in the early detection of cardiac tamponade: An experimental echocardiographic study. Circulation 71:829, 1985.
40. Fowler NO: Constrictive pericarditis: Its history and current status. Clin Cardiol 18:341, 1995.
41. Ribeiro P, Sapsford R, Evans T, et al: Constrictive pericarditis as a complication of coronary artery bypass surgery. Br Heart J 51:205, 1984.
42. Schoenfeld MH, Supple EW, Dec GW Jr, et al: Restrictive cardiomyopathy versus constrictive pericarditis: Role of endomyocardial biopsy in avoiding unnecessary thoracotomy. Circulation 75:1017, 1987.
43. Vaitkus PT, Kussmaul WG: Constrictive pericarditis versus restrictive cardiomyopathy: A reappraisal and update of diagnostic criteria. Am Heart J 122:1431, 1991.
44. Kushwaha SS, Fallon JT, Fuster V: Restrictive cardiomyopathy. N Engl Med J 336:267, 1997.
45. Hinkamp TJ, Sullivan HJ, Montoya A, et al: Chronic cardiac rejection masking as constrictive pericarditis. Ann Thorac Surg 57:1579, 1994.
46. Hatle LK, Appleton CP, Popp RL: Differentiation of constrictive pericarditis and restrictive cardiomyopathy by Doppler echocardiography. Circulation 79:357, 1989.
47. Santamore WP, Bartlett R, Van Buren SJ, et al: Ventricular coupling in constrictive pericarditis. Circulation 74:597, 1986.
48. Shabetai R, Fowler NO, Guntheroth WG: The hemodynamics of cardiac tamponade and constrictive pericarditis. Am J Cardiol 26:480, 1970.
49. Surawicz B, Lasseter KC: Electrocardiogram in pericarditis. Am J Cardiol 26:471, 1970.
50. Levine HD: Myocardial fibrosis in constrictive pericarditis: Electrocardiographic and pathologic observations. Circulation 48:1268, 1973.
51. Tei C, Child JS, Tanaka H, et al: Atrial systolic notch on the interventricular septal echogram: An echocardiographic sign of constrictive pericarditis. J Am Coll Cardiol 1:907, 1983.
52. Isner JM, Carter BL, Bankoff MS, et al: Differentiation of constrictive pericarditis from restrictive cardiomyopathy by computed tomographic imaging. Am Heart J 105:1019, 1983.
53. Silverman PM, Harell GS, Korobkin M: Computed tomography of the abnormal pericardium. AJR Am J Roentgenol 140:1125, 1983.
54. White CS: MR evaluation of the pericardium. Top Magn Reson Imaging 7:258, 1995.

SECTION XI

ARRHYTHMIAS

CHAPTER 35

Supraventricular Tachycardia

Rollo P. Villareal, Amy L. Woodruff, and Ali Massumi

Gender differences in the incidence of certain clinical arrhythmias have been reported (Table 35–1).[1–4] Some of these are related to known differences in the frequency of underlying organic heart disease, such as coronary artery disease (CAD) and associated ventricular arrhythmias. However, clinical and experimental observations suggest that true differences in electrophysiological properties between men and women do exist. Awareness of these differences has important clinical implications for and raises special therapeutic issues in the management of arrhythmias in women. The purposes of this chapter are to outline these differences and the potential mechanisms that may cause them and provide a brief review of the supraventricular tachycardias (SVTs) in which gender differences have been described. A separate chapter addresses rhythm disturbances of ventricular origin.

GENDER DIFFERENCES IN ELECTROCARDIOGRAPHIC AND ELECTROPHYSIOLOGIC PROPERTIES

The exact pathophysiologic mechanisms by which gender influences the occurrences of supraventricular tachyarrhythmias are far from being understood. The current state of understanding stems from clinical and electrocardiographic observations and from the surprisingly sparse experimental data on cellular electrophysiologic mechanisms yielded by studies that have focused mainly on repolarization in ventricular myocardium. Nevertheless, the available data support the following two general mechanisms: (1) direct or indirect hormonal effects on the expression or function of ion channels and (2) differences in autonomic tone, which may act alone or in concert (Table 35–2).

Clinical and Electrocardiographic Observations

Heart Rate

As early as 1920, Bazett[5] observed that women had a higher resting heart rate (HR) than did men. This observation was later corroborated by several other investigators.[6–10] In a large population-based study (n = 5116), the average HR of women was 3 to 5 bpm faster than that of men.[6] These observations may be explained partly by differences in body habitus and exercise tolerance, but certainly differences in intrinsic electrophysiologic properties of the sinus node (SN) and autonomic modulation could have a role. In a study of resting HR before and after double autonomic blockade, women had a significantly shorter sinus cycle length than men.[10] Although this finding detracts greatly from the autonomic hypothesis, it raises the possibility of intrinsic differences in SN automaticity. In a study of 100 consecutive patients without structural heart disease, both corrected and uncorrected SN recovery times were shorter in women.[1, 11] Inappropriate sinus tachycardia, a rare but increasingly recognized clinical entity, is significantly more common in women.[12–14]

Heart Rate Variability

Gender- and age-related differences in heart rate variability (HRV) and baroreceptor sensitivity have been reported by multiple researchers.[15–17] Specifically, women tend to have both a lower low-frequency (LF) power and a higher high-frequency (HF) power to LF power (HF:LF) ratio, suggesting a greater parasympathetic influence on their HRs than on those of men. In one study by Huikuri and associ-

Table 35–1. GENDER-RELATED PREDOMINANCE OF CLINICAL ARRHYTHMIAS

ARRHYTHMIA TYPE	MALE PREDOMINANCE	FEMALE PREDOMINANCE
Bradyarrhythmias	AV block Carotid sinus syndrome	Sinus node disease
Supraventricular tachyarrhythmias	Premature atrial contraction Atrial fibrillation AV reentrant tachycardia Wolff-Parkinson-White syndrome	Inappropriate sinus tachycardia AV node reentrant tachycardia
Ventricular tachyarrhythmias	Premature ventricular contraction Ventricular tachycardia Sudden cardiac death Sudden unexplained death syndrome Brugada's syndrome	Congenital LQTS Acquired LQTS

AV, atrioventricular; LQTS, long QT syndrome.
Adapted from Linde C: Women and arrhythmias. Pacing Clin Electrophysiol 23:1550, 2000, with permission from the author and publisher.

Table 35–2. POSTULATED MECHANISMS FOR GENDER DIFFERENCES IN CARDIAC ARRHYTHMIA

MECHANISM	SUPPORTIVE FINDINGS
Effects on cellular electrophysiology	Presence of estrogen receptors
	Modulation of L-type Ca^{2+} channels
	Modulation of potassium channels (I_{KR}, I_{KI})
Autonomic modulation	Basal heart rate disparity
	Heart rate variability
	Baroreceptor sensitivity
	Muscle sympathetic nerve activity
	Dispersion of repolarization
	Nitric oxide expression
Varying combinations of first two mechanisms	M-cell
	Long QT syndromes
	Dispersion of repolarization

I_{KR}, rapidly activating delayed rectifier potassium current; I_{KI}, inward rectifier potassium current.

ates,[17] postmenopausal women receiving estrogen replacement therapy demonstrated restoration of baroreceptor sensitivity and increased power of both HF and LF domains. These data strongly suggest that gender differences in autonomic modulation exist and may be explained at least in part by hormonal influences.

QT Interval

Differences between men and women in QT interval have also been described by Bazett and confirmed by others.[5, 8, 18] Women have a longer corrected QT interval (QTc) than men, and the difference becomes more pronounced at lower HRs. In a population-based Canadian study, the observation was made that the QT difference was due to a drop in the QTc that occurred in males after puberty (when androgen levels are highest) and that the QTc gradually increased with age until 50 years, at which point it paralleled that of women.[19] Similar observations on male QT shortening at puberty were made in families with genotypically characterized long QT syndrome.[20] These findings support the hypothesis that actions of the sex steroids may explain the gender differences in the QT interval.

Clinical Distribution of Arrhythmias

Gender differences in the epidemiology of arrhythmias have been described. Inappropriate sinus tachycardia is overwhelmingly a disease of women.[12–14] Intrinsic differences in SN physiology or some form of dysautonomia may partially account for this. In a population of 623 patients who underwent invasive electrophysiologic testing because of various tachycardias, atrioventricular (AV) node reentrant tachycardia (AVNRT) was twice as common in women, whereas atrial tachycardia affected the two sexes equally.[3] The reverse was true for AV reentrant (circus-movement) tachycardia (AVRT), atrial fibrillation (AF), and ventricular fibrillation (VF), which demonstrated a male predominance. Similar trends in the distribution of the SVTs, AF, VF, and sudden death have been seen in our hospital registry at the Texas Heart Institute and St. Luke's Hospital (except for AVRT, which occurred equally in men and women) (unpublished data) and in the Framingham cohort.[2]

Insulander and colleagues[21] reported that a significantly shorter slow-pathway refractory period existed in women with dual AV node physiology. A shorter refractory period increases the "window of opportunity" in which a premature atrial or ventricular stimulus may induce tachycardia. This finding may explain, at least in part, the propensity for AVNRT in women. The occurrence of CAD explains the male predominance of AF, ventricular tachyarrhythmias, and sudden death, although a molecular basis for some of these differences has emerged and may provide some insight (see later). The reasons for predominance of circus-movement tachycardia in men and the absence of any difference in atrial tachycardia are open to conjecture. To our knowledge, there has been no attempt to explain this in the literature.

Menstrual Cycle Changes

Burke and associates[22] reported that the average HR was lower during menses than during the follicular or luteal phases of the menstrual cycle and that the response to double autonomic blockade was identical. Myerburg and colleagues[23] reported that the chance of inducing SVT during electrophysiologic testing was greatest at the onset of menses or during the premenstrual phase. Rosano and coworkers[24] correlated the cyclic variation of spontaneous episodes of SVT to the temporal profile of ovarian hormones. There was significant direct correlation between progesterone levels and the frequency and duration of SVT episodes and an inverse correlation with beta-estradiol level. Increases in frequency and duration of episodes were noted on day 28 in comparison with day 7 of the menstrual cycle. These observations illustrate that estrogen hinders and progesterone enhances the SVT-prone state. Whether this effect is a result of modulation of autonomic tone, direct cellular electrophysiologic effects, a combination of both, or the effect of some yet to be described factor is unknown.

Pregnancy and the Postpartum Period

SVT is reported to be the most common arrhythmia during pregnancy and the postpartum period. This statement draws weak support from three studies, all of which are retrospective. Tawam and colleagues[25] studied 60 women with SVT and found higher risk (relative risk of 5.1) of onset or exacerbation during pregnancy, regardless of the mechanism or trimester. Lee and associates[26] reported contrary findings; in their cohort of 207 women, the incidence of first onset of SVT during pregnancy was 4%, which is exceedingly rare. If and when SVT did occur, it manifested in women with accessory pathways and was generally less well tolerated, regardless of the tachycardia mechanism. These findings are somewhat consistent with those of Widerhorn and associates,[27] who reported an increased incidence of SVT in women with Wolff-Parkinson-White (WPW) syndrome during pregnancy. These observations support the argument that the progesterone-rich gravid state facilitates SVT. Conversely, SVT is a very common arrhythmia in women in this age group. Other than a suggestion of a higher rate of episodes in women with known accessory pathways, it is unclear whether a true association exists.

Effects of Sex Hormones on Cellular Electrophysiology

One postulated mechanism of gender differences in cardiac arrhythmia is the effect of sex hormones on cellular electrophysiology (see Table 35–2). The notion that sex hormones can exert direct or indirect actions on the cardiovascular system is supported by the demonstration of cytoplasmic and nuclear receptors specific for these hormones in the various tissues of the cardiovascular system and its neuroregulatory system.[28] In a study by Johnson and colleagues,[29] ventricular myocytes from estrogen receptor–deficient mice showed greater expression of cardiac L-type calcium channels. The density of ion channels appears to be regulated by the estrogen receptor, with diminished estrogen receptor occupancy upregulating the number of functional L-type calcium channels. A higher level of functional calcium channels could explain a shorter sinus cycle on the basis of a more rapid phase 0 of the action potential. The relatively higher HR in women is present throughout the various age groups, however, and does not appear to widen further into menopause, if one were to invoke this mechanism. One would also expect that the QT interval would shorten because there is less opposition to the repolarizing currents during phase 3. This is clearly not what is observed clinically.[5, 8, 18] Hence, other mechanisms must be operational.

Drici and colleagues[30] demonstrated that administration of estradiol to ovariectomized rats decreases the messenger RNA (mRNA) for two distinct classes of delayed rectifier potassium channels and prolongs the QT. They also showed that dihydrotestosterone (DHT) has similar effects on mRNA levels and the QT interval, although administration of quinidine resulted in QT prolongation only in the estradiol-treated mice. These findings are consistent with those reported by Liu and associates,[31] who studied gender differences in the potassium currents and cycle length–dependent QT in rabbits. In female rabbits, two repolarizing potassium currents (I_{KR} and I_{KI}) were of significantly less magnitude. Moreover, there was significantly greater QT prolongation for corresponding increments in cycle length. Hara and coworkers[32] administered estradiol and DHT to ovariectomized rabbits and found that DHT actually shortened the early part of ventricular repolarization whereas estradiol prolonged the duration of the action potential by exerting its effects on the latter part of repolarization. The administration of an I_{KR} blocker resulted in a significantly greater action potential prolongation and even evidence of afterdepolarizations in the estradiol-treated subjects.

The differences in potassium channels and currents support the clinical observations of longer QT intervals, response to administration of class III agents, and predisposition to proarrhythmia in women (discussed at greater length in another chapter). The combined effect of reducing L-type calcium currents and prolonging repolarization via its effects on the potassium currents may partly explain the less frequent occurrence of AF in women. It is important to emphasize that although these observations were made in ventricular myocardium, it seems reasonable, given the paucity of data on atrial myocardium, to suggest that similar or related mechanisms may be operational in the atria.

Effects of Sex Hormones on Autonomic Tone

Another postulated mechanism of gender differences in cardiac arrhythmia is the effect of sex hormones on autonomic tone (see Table 35–2). In an elegant review of the subject, Larsen and Kadish[33] propose that sex steroid–induced changes in autonomic tone might have some role in the gender-related differences in cardiac arrhythmias. This theory arose from early observations that resting HR was consistently higher in women than in men.[5, 6] Subsequently, experiments employing double autonomic blockade demonstrated that intrinsic HR in women is higher than in men.[10] This finding suggests that the gender-related differences may be intrinsic to the SN, with minimal to no input from the sympathetic or parasympathetic nervous systems.

In the interim, other studies evaluating gender differences in HRV and baroreceptor sensitivity have been reported (see earlier) and strongly suggest that hormonal influence on autonomic tone does exist.[17] Ng and colleagues[34] evaluated the influence of age and gender on sympathetic tone by measuring muscle sympathetic nerve activity (MSNA). They reported significantly greater MSNA in men than in women and increasing MSNA with age. Both sympathetic and parasympathetic influences have been implicated in the genesis of arrhythmias in patients with both acquired and congenital long QT syndromes and the Brugada syndrome.[35–39] The recognition that an M-cell region and heterogeneity exist within the myocardium provides a mechanism by which differential responses of the various myocardial cell types to sympathetic or parasympathetic excess or withdrawal could lead to a greater transmural dispersion of repolarization and the genesis of cardiac arrhythmias.

Rubart and associates[40] suggest another potential mechanism by which sex steroids can affect autonomic tone, which is by way of nitric oxide (NO). Estradiol has been shown to augment NO release from endothelial cells, which in turn can modulate autonomic input by inhibiting neurotransmitter release or by antagonizing the actions of norepinephrine at the cellular level.[41] The net effect, as demonstrated in the canine model, is modulation of sinus discharge and AV nodal conduction by augmentation of vagal tone and inhibition of sympathetic neurotransmission.[42] These experimental findings may provide some additional explanation for the cyclic variation in paroxysmal SVT (PSVT).[24]

CLINICAL TACHYCARDIAS OF SUPRAVENTRICULAR ORIGIN

SVTs may be classified mechanistically according to their dependence on the AV node for maintenance of the tachycardia (Table 35–3). The AV node–dependent tachycardias include AVNRT, a permanent form of junctional reciprocating tachycardia (PJRT), and AVRT. The AV node–independent tachycardias include AF, atrial flutter, atrial

Table 35–3. SUPRAVENTRICULAR TACHYCARDIAS

AV node dependent
AV node reentrant tachycardia
Permanent junctional reciprocating tachycardia
AV reentrant tachycardia (Wolff-Parkinson-White syndrome)
AV node independent
Atrial fibrillation
Atrial flutter
Atrial tachycardias (reentry, automatic)
Inappropriate sinus tachycardia
Sinus node reentrant tachycardia

tachycardia (AT), inappropriate sinus tachycardia (IST), and sinus node reentrant tachycardia (SNRT). Detailed description of each of these arrhythmias is beyond the scope of this chapter; but AVNRT, AVRT, AF and IST, for which gender differences have been described, are dealt with individually. Table 35–4 summarizes the salient differences between and the treatment options for the various SVTs. It is important to emphasize that these treatment options are the same for both men and women. Special considerations exist, however, when antiarrhythmic therapy is being administered in the setting of pregnancy or lactation; this situation is discussed in a separate section.

Atrioventricular Node Reentrant Tachycardia

The most common type of AV node–dependent tachycardia is AVNRT. It accounts for approximately 60% of all narrow complex tachycardias seen in clinical practice.[43–45] A 2:1 female predominance has been reported in at least two large series.[3, 46] Reproducible initiation and termination of paroxysmal AVNRT with programmed stimulation support the mechanism of reentry, as does the common finding of longitudinal physiologic dissociation of the AV node (dual AV node physiology) in many patients with AVNRT.[43, 46, 47] A shorter refractory period of the slow pathway has been described in women and may partially explain the higher incidence.[21]

Two forms of AVNRT exist, the common (90%) and the uncommon (10%). In the common form, antegrade conduction is via the slow pathway and retrograde conduction is up the fast pathway (slow-fast). The reverse occurs in the uncommon form (fast-slow). In the common variant, because depolarization of the atria and ventricles is nearly simultaneous, patients may complain of a pounding or full sensation in the head or neck. An electrocardiogram (ECG) obtained during tachycardia will most likely reveal a narrow complex rhythm without discernible P waves. In the uncommon variant, because the retrograde limb of the circuit is slowly conducting, the retrograde P is usually visible after the T wave and before the next QRS complex. This has been described as a "long R-P" tachycardia and must be differentiated from AVRT, ST, SNRT, PJRT, and AT.[48] Short-term management, which is aimed at terminating the tachycardia, consists of vagal maneuvers, pharmacologic approaches (e.g., adenosine, class II and class IV antiarrhythmic agents) and nonpharmacologic approaches (e.g., atrial overdrive pacing or direct current [DC] cardioversion). Long-term therapy is aimed at preventing recurrences and can be pharmacologic (e.g., class I through IV agents and digoxin) or nonpharmacologic (radiofrequency [RF] ablation, which is the treatment of choice). Despite differences in epidemiology, RF ablation is equally successful (>95% success rate) in men and women.[46, 49] The experience at our institution mirrors that presented in the literature: Women constituted 64% of patients undergoing RF ablation for AVNRT (n = 371), and success rates were comparable (unpublished data).

Atrioventricular (Circus-Movement) Reentrant Tachycardia

The second most common mechanism of paroxysmal SVT is reentry using the AV node as the antegrade limb and an accessory atrioventricular pathway (AP) for the retrograde limb.[43–45, 50] These APs can either be concealed (i.e., not evident on the resting ECG) or, more commonly, manifest (i.e., demonstrating preexcitation or antegrade conduction on the resting ECG—the classic WPW syndrome).

AVRT is twice as common in men as in women.[3, 51] Although APs are more common in men, spontaneous orthodromic AVRT is seen more frequently in women. In contrast, APs are more likely to be manifest in men. In a study of 690 patients evaluated for APs, aborted sudden death due to AF and VF was less common in women, reflecting a less favorable natural history of WPW syndrome in men.[4] Our hospital registry mirrors this distribution of arrhythmias, with the exception that ablation for AP (n = 273) occurred with equal frequency in men and women (male/female ratio, 138: 135) (unpublished data).

Patients may have no symptoms or may experience palpitations, lightheadedness, presyncope, syncope, or sudden death. An ECG during the tachycardia most likely shows a narrow complex rhythm with a distinct retrograde P in the ST segment or T wave. If the AP is slowly conducting, the retrograde P may be seen after the T wave and before the next QRS complex (a long R-P tachycardia). The dependence of this SVT on the AV node lends itself to control in the acute and chronic settings with multiple AV node–active agents (e.g., class IA, IC, II, and III agents). Caution is warranted in the administration of digoxin and class IV agents in the presence of WPW syndrome. These agents exert no effect on the accessory pathway and, in the presence of AF, may facilitate disastrous rapid antegrade conduction down the AP. The procedure of choice is RF ablation, which is successful in more than 90% of cases, with little morbidity.[52–54] Outcomes are similar in women and men. Given the higher incidence of SVT in women with AP during pregnancy, RF ablation should be considered before such patients attempt pregnancy.

Atrial Fibrillation

AF is the most common SVT, affecting approximately 0.4% of the overall population.[2, 55, 56] Its incidence rises dramatically with age, and its development is associated not only with greater morbidity but also with an approximate doubling of all-cause mortality. Men are at greater risk for AF than women. In the Framingham Heart Study, men had a

Table 35–4. CHARACTERISTICS OF THE VARIOUS SUPRAVENTRICULAR TACHYCARDIAS

	AV NODE–DEPENDENT TACHYCARDIAS					AV NODE–INDEPENDENT TACHYCARDIAS							
	Common AVNRT	Uncommon AVNRT	Orthodromic AVRT	Antidromic AVRT	PJRT	Atrial Fibrillation	Typical Atrial Flutter	Atypical Atrial Flutter	MAT	Automatic AT	IART	IST	SNRT
Mechanism	Reentry using slow (antegrade) and fast (retrograde) pathways	Reentry using fast (antegrade) and slow (retrograde) pathways	Macro-reentry using the AV node antegrade and the AP retrograde	Macro-reentry using the AP antegrade and the AV node retrograde	Macro-reentry using the AV node antegrade and a very slow 1 AP retrograde	Multiple wavefronts of reentry in the atria	Macro-reentrant circuit in the RA using the TV-IVC isthmus	Macro-reentry circuit not utilizing TV-IVC isthmus	Abnormal automaticity or activity triggered from multiple foci in RA or LA	Abnormal automaticity or triggered activity from a focus in the RA or LA	Reentry around a scar or area of slow conduction in the RA or LA	Abnormal automaticity in the sinus node	Reentry within or around the area of the SN
P wave	Retrograde concentric	Retrograde concentric	Retrograde, depending on AP insertion	Retrograde concentric	Retrograde concentric	Coarse or fine	Flutter waves	Flutter waves	3 different P morphologies	Depends on location	Depends on location	Similar to NSR	Similar to NSR
R-P:P-R	<1	>1	Usually <1, unless slow AP, then >1	<1	>1	NA	NA	NA	Variable	>1	>1	>1	>1
Regularity*	Yes	Yes	Yes	Yes	Yes	No	Yes	Yes	No	Yes	Yes	Yes	Yes
Presentation	Paroxysmal	Paroxysmal	Paroxysmal	Paroxysmal	Incessant	Chronic paroxysmal	Chronic paroxysmal	Chronic paroxysmal	Paroxysmal	Incessant paroxysmal	Paroxysmal	Chronic incessant	Paroxysmal
Sudden initiation	Yes	Yes	Yes	Yes	Yes	Both	Yes	Yes	No	No	Yes	No	Yes
Sudden termination	Yes	Yes	Yes	Yes	Yes	Yes	Yes	Yes	No	No	Yes	No	Yes
Programmed stimulation	Inducible	Inducible	Inducible	Inducible	Inducible	Inducible	Inducible	Inducible	Noninducible	Noninducible	Inducible	Noninducible	Inducible
Vagal maneuvers	Terminate	Terminate	Terminate	Terminate	May terminate	No effect	No effect/rarely terminate	No effect	No effect	No effect	No effect/rarely terminate	No effect	Terminate
Adenosine	Terminates	Terminates	Terminates	Terminates	Terminates	Slows VR	Slows VR	Slows VR	Slows VR	Slows VR	May terminate	No effect	May terminate
Effect of AVB	Terminates	Terminates	Terminates	Terminates	Terminates	Persists	Persists	Persists	Persists	Persists	Persists	Persists	Persists
Coexisting organic heart disease	No	No	Usually no	Usually no	Secondary cardiomyopathy	Often	Often	Often	Usually COPD	Often	Sometimes	No	Sometimes
Nonpharmacologic therapy	RFA of slow pathway	RFA of slow pathway	RFA of AP	RFA of AP	RFA of slow pathway	AVN ablation + PPM	RFA of TV-IVC isthmus	RFA of flutter circuit, RFA of AV node + PPM, AVN modification	Treat underlying	RFA of site of earliest activation	RFA of site of earliest activation demonstrating concealed entrainment	RFA of site of earliest activation near SN or superior SN	RFA of site of earliest activation near SN
Pharmacologic therapy	Classes II, IV; digoxin	Classes II, IV; digoxin	Classes IA, IC	Classes I, II, III; avoid class IV and digoxin in WPW	Classes II, IV; digoxin	Classes IA, IC, II, III, IV; digoxin	Classes IA, IC, II, III, IV; digoxin	Classes IA, IC, II, III, IV; digoxin	Class II, class IV, digoxin for rate control	Classes IA, IC, II, III, IV; digoxin	Classes IA, IC, II, III, IV; digoxin	Classes II, III, IV; digoxin	Classes II, III, IV; digoxin

AVN, AV node; AP, accessory pathway; AT, atrial tachycardia; AV, atrioventricular; AVB, AV block; AVNRT, AV node reentrant tachycardia; AVRT, AV reentrant tachycardia; COPD, chronic obstructive pulmonary disease; IART, intra-atrial reentrant tachycardia; IST, inappropriate sinus tachycardia; LA, left atrium; MAT, multifocal atrial tachycardia; NSR, normal sinus rhythm; PJRT, permanent form of junctional reciprocating tachycardia; PPM, permanent pacemaker; RA, right atrium; R-P:P-R, ratio of R-P wave internal to P-R interval; RFA, radiofrequency ablation; SN, sinus node; SNRT, SN reentrant tachycardia; TV-IVC, tricuspid valve–inferior vena cava; VR, ventricular response; WPW, Wolff-Parkinson-White syndrome.

*Regularity of ventricular response.

1.5 times greater risk of experiencing the arrhythmia than women. When AF occurred in women, however, the female survival advantage was diminished and the risk of death was higher than in men.[2, 56] These differences remained true even after data were adjusted for other risk factors. Data from the Coronary Artery Surgery Study showed that in patients with CAD, men had a 5.4 times greater risk of AF than women.[57] The prevalence of AF is higher in men than in women in all age groups. However, because there are almost twice as many women than men older than 75 years in the general population, the absolute number of women with AF in older age groups exceeds that of men.[2, 56, 58, 59]

Men are also more likely to experience AF after cardiothoracic surgery.[60] Strong risk factors for postoperative AF are advanced age and male sex. It remains unclear why men are more susceptible than women to the development of this arrhythmia. Gender differences in prognosis for patients with AF exist. Women are more likely than men to experience recurrent AF after successful pharmacologic or electrical cardioversion.[61] Additionally, there is some evidence to suggest that, compared with men, women are at higher risk for systemic embolization in AF.[62] Other studies, however, show no significant difference in the risk.

The treatment of AF revolves around the following three issues[63]: (1) rate control, (2) prevention of thromboembolic complications, and (3) conversion to and maintenance of sinus rhythm. Rate control is best achieved with class II and class IV agents. Digoxin is best suited for this purpose in the setting of a depressed left ventricle. The risk of thromboembolic complications is reduced immediately with heparin and over the long term with warfarin. The decision to administer warfarin long term is based on the presence of any of the following risk factors: hypertension, age greater than 65 years, diabetes mellitus, prior embolic event, low ejection fraction, left ventricular hypertrophy, and increased left atrial size.[64–66] Otherwise, regular aspirin should suffice.

Conversion to sinus rhythm can be achieved by pharmacologic or DC cardioversion, both of which can be done safely if the duration of AF is known to be less than 48 hours.[63] If the duration is greater than 48 hours, acceptable options are either a transesophageal echocardiogram (TEE) followed by cardioversion if no clot is visible or anticoagulation for 3 weeks prior to cardioversion. Usually some pharmacologic agent is needed to maintain sinus rhythm. Use of flecainide and propafenone in the absence of structural heart disease has the most support in the literature.[67–72] Sotalol, quinidine, and procainamide may also be used. Amiodarone is very effective in restoring and maintaining sinus rhythm, but its routine use in this setting is limited by its side effect profile.[73–76] In the presence of organic heart disease, particularly in association with a depressed ejection fraction, amiodarone is probably the drug of choice, although dofetilide (which has now been approved for use) and azimilide (whose trial results are being awaited) show promise. If the ventricular response remains inordinately high in spite of maximal medical therapy, AV node ablation followed by implantation for a pacemaker may be a reasonable alternative.[77–79] The benefit of the various strategies is similar regardless of gender. However, caution must be exercised in the administration of antiarrhythmics to women, in whom QT prolongation and proarrhythmia occur more commonly.

Inappropriate Sinus Tachycardia

IST is an uncommon clinical syndrome characterized by an elevated resting HR accompanied by an exaggerated response to stress or exercise. It was previously called "nonparoxysmal sinus tachycardia." One of the hallmarks of IST is its chronic and persistent nature. The underlying mechanisms are not yet completely defined but seem to involve either enhanced automaticity or abnormal autonomic regulation of the SN (either excess sympathetic or reduced parasympathetic).[14, 80] Studies that have utilized autonomic blockade, autonomic maneuvers, and HRV analysis provide support for one or both mechanisms and suggest the possibility of a multifactorial etiology.

Patients with IST can present with the entire spectrum of symptoms ranging from infrequent palpitations to incessant tachycardia. Although this condition rarely causes hemodynamic embarrassment, of concern is the possibility of tachycardia-induced cardiomyopathy, which has been reported.[81] In the cases of IST reported to date, patients have been young (less than 40 years old) and overwhelmingly female (approximately 90%).[12–14, 80, 82] There seems to be a predilection for health care workers. The diagnosis of IST is one of exclusion and rests on demonstrating the following signs[12, 13, 83]:

- A resting HR of 100 bpm or higher or an HR increasing to 100 bpm or higher with minimal exertion (such as standing or walking slowly)
- P-wave morphology identical to that during sinus rhythm
- Endocardial atrial activation in a high-to-low and right-to-left pattern, supporting origin in the sinus node
- An inability to induce or terminate the tachycardia with standard programmed stimulation
- Chronic and nonparoxysmal duration of the tachycardia
- Exclusion of secondary causes (e.g., fever, anemia, hyperthyroidism).

Therapy for IST is empiric. Most published reports have identified beta blockers or verapamil as the initial therapeutic choice. There are no published reports on the experience with other antiarrhythmics, although agents known to affect sinus node automaticity or autonomic tone (i.e., amiodarone, propafenone) may warrant an empiric trial. The experience with RF ablation or modification of the SN is growing, and this modality shows great promise.[82, 84, 85] Ablation of the SN appears to be more effective when guided by intracardiac echocardiography to allow identification of more appropriate endocardial ablation sites.[86]

SPECIAL CONSIDERATIONS

A detailed description of the use of each of the antiarrhythmic drugs during pregnancy and lactation is beyond the scope of this chapter. Contained herein is a brief overview of the subject. The reader is referred to more comprehensive texts for additional information.[87–90]

Pregnancy

Arrhythmias that occur during pregnancy may put the lives of both the mother and the fetus at risk. When the arrhyth-

Table 35–5. ANTIARRHYTHMIC DRUG SAFETY PROFILES DURING PREGNANCY AND LACTATION

DRUG	TERATOGEN	FDA CATEGORY*	RECOMMENDATION DURING PREGNANCY	RECOMMENDATION DURING LACTATION
Class IA				
Quinidine	No	C	+ +	+
Procainamide	No	C	+ + †	+
Disopyramide	No	C	+ ‡	+
Class IB				
Lidocaine	No	B	+ +	+
Mexiletene	No	C	+ ‡	+
Class IC				
Flecainide	No	C	+ ‡	+
Propafenone	No	C	+ ‡	?
Class II				
Propranolol	No	C	+ +	+
Metoprolol	No	C	+ +	+
Class III				
Amiodarone	?	D	NR	—
Sotalol	No	B	+ ‡	+
Ibutilide	Yes§	C	NR	?
Class IV				
Verapamil	No	C	+ ‡	+
Diltiazem	?	C	NR	+
Other				
Digoxin	No	C	+ +	+
Adenosine	No	C	+ +	?

FDA, U.S. Food and Drug Administration; + +, recommended agent; +, acceptable agent; NR, agent not recommended; ?, lack of sufficient data.
*See Table 35–6.
†Procainamide is recommended during pregnancy for short-term administration only.
‡Note, however, that limited data exist.
§Ibutilide shown to be teratogenic when given in supraclinical doses to laboratory animals.
Modified from Page RL: Treatment of arrhythmias during pregnancy. Am Heart J 130:871, 1995, with permission.

mias are well tolerated and cause minimal symptoms, observation, rest, or vagal maneuvers can be used. When symptoms become debilitating or are recurrent and are associated with hemodynamic embarrassment, antiarrhythmic drug therapy becomes necessary. Table 35–5 summarizes the safety profiles of the various antiarrhythmic drugs during pregnancy and lactation; Table 35–6 presents the U.S. Food and Drug Administration (FDA) pregnancy risk classification for use of antiarrhythmic drugs.

In general, no antiarrhythmic agent is completely safe to use during pregnancy, but most pose low risk and are well tolerated. Unfortunately, as shown in Table 35–6, most drugs belong to category C; there are simply not enough data to make a firm recommendation. Hence, drug therapy should be avoided during the first trimester of pregnancy, if possible. If drugs are to be used, those with the longest safety record should be used (e.g., digoxin, quinidine, procainamide, lidocaine, adenosine, and beta blockers). Drugs to be avoided include amiodarone, ibutilide, and phenytoin.

Table 35–6. U.S. FOOD AND DRUG ADMINISTRATION PREGNANCY RISK DRUG CLASSIFICATION

CATEGORY	DESCRIPTION
Category A	Controlled studies show no risk.
Category B	No evidence of risk in pregnant women. Either (1) animal studies show risk but human studies do not or (2) animal studies do not show risk but no adequate studies in humans have been conducted.
Category C	Studies in pregnant women are lacking, and animal studies either show fetal risk or are lacking as well.
Category D	Positive evidence of risk. Investigational or postmarketing data show risk to the fetus.

Physiologic changes that occur with pregnancy may alter the pharmacokinetics (volume of distribution and protein binding) of certain drugs (i.e., digoxin). Thus, drug levels and patient response must be closely monitored. Exposure to fluoroscopy with the intent of RF ablation or device implantation poses a heavy fetal risk for congenital malformations, hematologic malignancies, and mental retardation, even with the use of lead shielding. These risks persist beyond the first trimester and should be avoided at all costs. Finally, DC cardioversion is safe, well tolerated, and effective. It should not be delayed if indicated.

Lactation

All of the antiarrhythmic drugs listed in Table 35–5 are excreted into breast milk to varying extents and generally pose no threat to the infant, with a few exceptions. Acebutolol, sotalol, and amiodarone are highly concentrated in breast milk and may have untoward effects on the nursing infant. Firm recommendations are limited by insufficient data in many instances.

Catheterization Laboratory Procedures and Electrophysiologic Testing in Women

As mentioned previously, exposure to ionizing radiation poses multiple risks to the fetus. Thus, in our practice, we routinely obtain pregnancy tests in women who are of childbearing age prior to planned procedures and, as an added precaution, provide pelvic shielding to all women. On a different note, in some patients, failure to induce SVT with programmed stimulation may reflect some hormonal influence, as evidenced by the cyclic variations in SVT occurrence and inducibility. Although this has not posed a problem to us, patients with recurrent suggestive symptoms whose SVT has not been inducible may benefit from a "timely" reevaluation.

SUMMARY AND CONCLUSION

There are clear gender differences in the incidence and prevalence of certain cardiac arrhythmias that suggest the existence of fundamental electrophysiologic differences as well. The exact mechanisms are unknown and remain to be fully elucidated. The scant evidence available suggests two general mechanisms: sex steroid hormone effects on ion channels and modulation of autonomic tone.

Many questions and avenues for investigation remain open. For instance, what are the physiologic effects of gonadal hormones (estrogens, androgens, and progesterone) on human atrial myocytes? How do the gonadal hormones affect the various ion channels that are increasingly being described? Are receptors to gonadal hormones distributed differently in men and women? Is the distribution of ion channels in the atrium the same as it is in the ventricle? Is there an M-cell equivalent in atrial myocardium? Does hormone replacement or antagonism have therapeutic or detrimental value in arrhythmia management?

The answers to these questions may clarify the basic mechanisms of these gender differences and facilitate the development of newer, more effective diagnostic and therapeutic modalities. Currently, although differences in the epidemiology of AVNRT, AVRT, AF, and IST have been described, therapeutic options (with the exception of the use of specific drugs during pregnancy and lactation) are broad and generally effective regardless of gender.

References

1. Linde C: Women and arrhythmias. Pacing Clin Electrophysiol 23: 1550, 2000.
2. Benjamin EJ, Levy D, Vaziri SM, et al: Independent risk factors for atrial fibrillation in a population-based cohort: The Framingham Heart Study. JAMA 271:840, 1994.
3. Rodriguez LM, de Chillou C, Schlapfer J, et al: Age at onset and gender of patients with different types of supraventricular tachycardias. Am J Cardiol 70:1213, 1992.
4. Timmermans C, Smeets JL, Rodriguez LM, et al: Aborted sudden death in the Wolff-Parkinson-White syndrome. Am J Cardiol 76:492, 1995.
5. Bazett H: An analysis of the time-relations of electrocardiograms. Heart 7:353, 1920.
6. Liu K, Ballew C, Jacobs DR Jr, et al: Ethnic differences in blood pressure, pulse rate, and related characteristics in young adults. The CARDIA study. Hypertension 14:218, 1989.
7. Levinson S, Liu K, Stamler J, et al: Ethnic differences in blood pressure and heart rate of Chicago school children. Am J Epidemiol 122:366, 1985.
8. Stramba-Badiale M, Locati EH, Martinelli A, et al: Gender and the relationship between ventricular repolarization and cardiac cycle length during 24-h Holter recordings. Eur Heart J 18:1000, 1997.
9. Bjerregaard P: Mean 24 hour heart rate, minimal heart rate and pauses in healthy subjects 40–79 years of age. Eur Heart J 4:44, 1983.
10. Burke JH, Goldberger JJ, Ehlert FA, et al: Gender differences in heart rate before and after autonomic blockade: Evidence against an intrinsic gender effect. Am J Med 100:537, 1996.
11. Kadish AH: The effect of gender on cardiac electrophysiology and arrhythmias. In Zipes DP (ed): Cardiac Electrophysiology from Cell to Bedside. WB Saunders, Philadelphia, 1995, p 1268.
12. Krahn AD, Yee R, Klein GJ, Morillo C: Inappropriate sinus tachycardia: Evaluation and therapy. J Cardiovasc Electrophysiol 6:1124, 1995.
13. Lee RJ, Shinbane JS: Inappropriate sinus tachycardia: Diagnosis and treatment. Cardiol Clin 15:599, 1997.
14. Morillo CA, Klein GJ, Thakur RK, et al: Mechanism of "inappropriate" sinus tachycardia: Role of sympathovagal balance. Circulation 90:873, 1994.
15. Liao D, Barnes RW, Chambless LE, et al: Age, race, and sex differences in autonomic cardiac function measured by spectral analysis of heart rate variability—the ARIC study. Atherosclerosis Risk in Communities. Am J Cardiol 76:906, 1995.
16. Stein PK, Kleiger RE, Rottman JN: Differing effects of age on heart rate variability in men and women. Am J Cardiol 80:302, 1997.
17. Huikuri HV, Pikkujamsa SM, Airaksinen KE, et al: Sex-related differences in autonomic modulation of heart rate in middle-aged subjects. Circulation 94:122, 1996.
18. Merri M, Benhorin J, Alberti M, et al: Electrocardiographic quantitation of ventricular repolarization. Circulation 80:1301, 1989.
19. Rautaharju PM, Manolio TA, Psaty BM, et al: Correlates of QT prolongation in older adults (the Cardiovascular Health Study). Cardiovascular Health Study Collaborative Research Group. Am J Cardiol 73:999, 1994.
20. Lehmann MH, Timothy KW, Frankovich D, et al: Age-gender influence on the rate-corrected QT interval and the QT-heart rate relation in families with genotypically characterized long QT syndrome. J Am Coll Cardiol 29:93, 1997.
21. Insulander P, Kenneback G, Straat E: Differences in dual AV nodal properties between men and women [abstract]. Eur Heart J 20:568, 1999.
22. Burke JH, Ehlert FA, Kruse JT, et al: Gender-specific differences in the QT interval and the effect of autonomic tone and menstrual cycle in healthy adults. Am J Cardiol 79:178, 1997.
23. Myerburg RJ, Cox MM, Interian A Jr, et al: Cycling of inducibility of paroxysmal supraventricular tachycardia in women and its implications for timing of electrophysiologic procedures. Am J Cardiol 83:1049, 1999.
24. Rosano GM, Leonardo F, Sarrel PM, et al: Cyclical variation in paroxysmal supraventricular tachycardia in women. Lancet 347:786, 1996.
25. Tawam M, Levine J, Mendelson M, et al: Effect of pregnancy on paroxysmal supraventricular tachycardia. Am J Cardiol 72:838, 1993.
26. Lee SH, Chen SA, Wu TJ, et al: Effects of pregnancy on first onset and symptoms of paroxysmal supraventricular tachycardia. Am J Cardiol 76:675, 1995.
27. Widerhorn J, Widerhorn AL, Rahimtoola SH, Elkayam U: WPW syndrome during pregnancy: Increased incidence of supraventricular arrhythmias. Am Heart J 123:796, 1992.
28. Stumpf WE, Sar M, Aumuller G: The heart: A target organ for estradiol. Science 196:319, 1977.
29. Johnson BD, Zheng W, Korach KS, et al: Increased expression of the cardiac L-type calcium channel in estrogen receptor-deficient mice. J Gen Physiol 110:135, 1997.
30. Drici MD, Burklow TR, Haridasse V, et al: Sex hormones prolong the QT interval and downregulate potassium channel expression in the rabbit heart. Circulation 94:1471, 1996.
31. Liu XK, Katchman A, Drici MD, et al: Gender difference in the cycle length–dependent QT and potassium currents in rabbits. J Pharmacol Exp Ther 285:672, 1998.
32. Hara M, Danilo P Jr, Rosen MR: Effects of gonadal steroids on ventricular repolarization and on the response to E4031. J Pharmacol Exp Ther 285:1068, 1998.
33. Larsen JA, Kadish AH: Effects of gender on cardiac arrhythmias. J Cardiovasc Electrophysiol 9:655, 1998.
34. Ng AV, Callister R, Johnson DG, Seals DR: Age and gender influence muscle sympathetic nerve activity at rest in healthy humans. Hypertension 21:498, 1993.
35. Shimizu W, Antzelevitch C: Cellular basis for the ECG features of the LQT1 form of the long-QT syndrome: Effects of beta-adrenergic ago-

nists and antagonists and sodium channel blockers on transmural dispersion of repolarization and torsade de pointes. Circulation 98:2314, 1998.
36. Shimizu W, Antzelevitch C: Cellular basis for long QT, transmural dispersion of repolarization, and torsade de pointes in the long QT syndrome. J Electrocardiol 32:177, 1999.
37. Shimizu W, Antzelevitch C: Effects of a K(+) channel opener to reduce transmural dispersion of repolarization and prevent torsade de pointes in LQT1, LQT2, and LQT3 models of the long-QT syndrome. Circulation 102:706, 2000.
38. Antzelevitch C, Shimizu W, Yan GX, et al: The M cell: Its contribution to the ECG and to normal and abnormal electrical function of the heart. J Cardiovasc Electrophysiol 10:1124, 1999.
39. Antzelevitch C: Ion channels and ventricular arrhythmias: Cellular and ionic mechanisms underlying the Brugada syndrome. Curr Opin Cardiol 14:274, 1999.
40. Rubart M, von der Lohe E: Sex steroids and cardiac arrhythmia: More questions than answers [editorial; comment]. J Cardiovasc Electrophysiol 9:665, 1998.
41. Wellman GC, Bonev AD, Nelson MT, Brayden JE: Gender differences in coronary artery diameter involve estrogen, nitric oxide, and Ca(2+)-dependent K+ channels. Circ Res 79:1024, 1996.
42. Elvan A, Rubart M, Zipes DP: NO modulates autonomic effects on sinus discharge rate and AV nodal conduction in open-chest dogs. Am J Physiol 272:H263, 1997.
43. Josephson ME, Kastor JA: Supraventricular tachycardia: Mechanisms and management. Ann Intern Med 87:346, 1977.
44. Josephson ME: Paroxysmal supraventricular tachycardia: An electrophysiologic approach. Am J Cardiol 41:1123, 1978.
45. Wu D, Denes P, Amat-y-Leon F, et al: Clinical, electrocardiographic and electrophysiologic observations in patients with paroxysmal supraventricular tachycardia. Am J Cardiol 41:1045, 1978.
46. Jackman WM, Beckman KJ, McClelland JH, et al: Treatment of supraventricular tachycardia due to atrioventricular nodal reentry, by radiofrequency catheter ablation of slow-pathway conduction. N Engl J Med 327:313, 1992.
47. Josephson ME, Miller JM: Atrioventricular nodal reentry: Evidence supporting an intranodal location. Pacing Clin Electrophysiol 16:599, 1993.
48. Guarnieri T, German LD, Gallagher JJ: The long R-P′ tachycardias. Pacing Clin Electrophysiol 10:103, 1987.
49. Kay GN, Epstein AE, Dailey SM, Plumb VI: Selective radiofrequency ablation of the slow pathway for the treatment of atrioventricular nodal reentrant tachycardia: Evidence for involvement of perinodal myocardium within the reentrant circuit. Circulation 85:1675, 1992.
50. Wellens HJ, Brugada P: Mechanisms of supraventricular tachycardia. Am J Cardiol 62:10D, 1988.
51. Wolbrette D, Patel H: Arrhythmias and women. Curr Opin Cardiol 14:36, 1999.
52. Calkins H, Langberg J, Sousa J, et al: Radiofrequency catheter ablation of accessory atrioventricular connections in 250 patients: Abbreviated therapeutic approach to Wolff-Parkinson-White syndrome. Circulation 85:1337, 1992.
53. Jackman WM, Wang XZ, Friday KJ, et al: Catheter ablation of accessory atrioventricular pathways (Wolff-Parkinson-White syndrome) by radiofrequency current. N Engl J Med 324:1605, 1991.
54. Swartz JF, Tracy CM, Fletcher RD: Radiofrequency endocardial catheter ablation of accessory atrioventricular pathway atrial insertion sites. Circulation 87:487, 1993.
55. Kannel WB, Wolf PA, Benjamin EJ, Levy D: Prevalence, incidence, prognosis, and predisposing conditions for atrial fibrillation: Population-based estimates. Am J Cardiol 82:2N, 1998.
56. Benjamin EJ, Wolf PA, D'Agostino RB, et al: Impact of atrial fibrillation on the risk of death. The Framingham Heart Study. Circulation 98:946, 1998.
57. Cameron A, Schwartz MJ, Kronmal RA, Kosinski AS: Prevalence and significance of atrial fibrillation in coronary artery disease (CASS Registry). Am J Cardiol 61:714, 1988.
58. Domanski MJ: The epidemiology of atrial fibrillation. Coron Artery Dis 6:95, 1995.
59. Feinberg WM, Blackshear JL, Laupacis A, et al: Prevalence, age distribution, and gender of patients with atrial fibrillation: Analysis and implications. Arch Intern Med 155:469, 1995.
60. Cooklin M, Gold MR: Implications and treatment of atrial fibrillation after cardiothoracic surgery. Curr Opin Cardiol 13:20, 1998.
61. Suttorp MJ, Kingma JH, Koomen EM, et al: Recurrence of paroxysmal atrial fibrillation or flutter after successful cardioversion in patients with normal left ventricular function. Am J Cardiol 71:710, 1993.
62. Cabin HS, Clubb KS, Hall C, Perlmutter RA, Feinstein AR: Risk for systemic embolization of atrial fibrillation without mitral stenosis. Am J Cardiol 65:1112, 1990.
63. Prystowsky EN, Benson DW Jr, Fuster V, et al: Management of patients with atrial fibrillation: A Statement for Healthcare Professionals. From the subcommittee on Electrocardiography and Electrophysiology, American Heart Association. Circulation 93:1262, 1996.
64. Wiener I: Clinical and echocardiographic correlates of systemic embolization in nonrheumatic atrial fibrillation. Am J Cardiol 59:177, 1987.
65. Petersen P, Kastrup J, Helweg-Larsen S, et al: Risk factors for thromboembolic complications in chronic atrial fibrillation. The Copenhagen AFASAK study. Arch Intern Med 150:819, 1990.
66. Aronow WS, Gutstein H, Hsieh FY: Risk factors for thromboembolic stroke in elderly patients with chronic atrial fibrillation. Am J Cardiol 63:366, 1989.
67. Anderson JL, Gilbert EM, Alpert BL, et al: Prevention of symptomatic recurrences of paroxysmal atrial fibrillation in patients initially tolerating antiarrhythmic therapy: A multicenter, double-blind, crossover study of flecainide and placebo with transtelephonic monitoring. Flecainide Supraventricular Tachycardia Study Group. Circulation 80:1557, 1989.
68. Pritchett EL, DaTorre SD, Platt ML, et al: Flecainide acetate treatment of paroxysmal supraventricular tachycardia and paroxysmal atrial fibrillation: Dose-response studies. The Flecainide Supraventricular Tachycardia Study Group. J Am Coll Cardiol 17:297, 1991.
69. Pritchett EL, McCarthy EA, Wilkinson WE: Propafenone treatment of symptomatic paroxysmal supraventricular arrhythmias: A randomized, placebo-controlled, crossover trial in patients tolerating oral therapy. Ann Intern Med 114:539, 1991.
70. Connolly SJ, Mulji AS, Hoffert DL, et al: Randomized placebo-controlled trial of propafenone for treatment of atrial tachyarrhythmias after cardiac surgery. J Am Coll Cardiol 10:1145, 1987.
71. Connolly SJ, Hoffert DL: Usefulness of propafenone for recurrent paroxysmal atrial fibrillation. Am J Cardiol 63:817, 1989.
72. Antman EM, Beamer AD, Cantillon C, et al: Long-term oral propafenone therapy for suppression of refractory symptomatic atrial fibrillation and atrial flutter [published erratum appears in J Am Coll Cardiol Jan; 13:264, 1989]. J Am Coll Cardiol 12:1005, 1988.
73. Brodsky MA, Allen BJ, Walker CJ 3rd, et al: Amiodarone for maintenance of sinus rhythm after conversion of atrial fibrillation in the setting of a dilated left atrium. Am J Cardiol 60:572, 1987.
74. Horowitz LN, Spielman SR, Greenspan AM, et al: Use of amiodarone in the treatment of persistent and paroxysmal atrial fibrillation resistant to quinidine therapy. J Am Coll Cardiol 6:1402, 1985.
75. Gold RL, Haffajee CI, Charos G, et al: Amiodarone for refractory atrial fibrillation. Am J Cardiol 57:124, 1986.
76. Gosselink AT, Crijns HJ, Van Gelder IC, et al: Low-dose amiodarone for maintenance of sinus rhythm after cardioversion of atrial fibrillation or flutter. JAMA 267:3289, 1992.
77. Gallagher JJ, Svenson RH, Kasell JH, et al: Catheter technique for closed-chest ablation of the atrioventricular conduction system. N Engl J Med 306:194, 1982.
78. Scheinman MM, Morady F, Hess DS, Gonzalez F: Catheter-induced ablation of the atrioventricular junction to control refractory supraventricular arrhythmias. JAMA 248:851, 1982.
79. Kay GN, Bubien RS, Epstein AE, Plumb VJ: Effect of catheter ablation of the atrioventricular junction on quality of life and exercise tolerance in paroxysmal atrial fibrillation. Am J Cardiol 62:741, 1988.
80. Bauernfeind RA, Amat YLF, Dhingra RC, et al: Chronic nonparoxysmal sinus tachycardia in otherwise healthy persons. Ann Intern Med 91:702, 1979.
81. Packer DL, Bardy GH, Worley SJ, et al: Tachycardia-induced cardiomyopathy: A reversible form of left ventricular dysfunction. Am J Cardiol 57:563, 1986.
82. Lee RJ, Kalman JM, Fitzpatrick AP, et al: Radiofrequency catheter modification of the sinus node for "inappropriate" sinus tachycardia. Circulation 92:2919, 1995.
83. Cossu SF, Steinberg JS: Supraventricular tachyarrhythmias involving the sinus node: Clinical and electrophysiologic characteristics. Prog Cardiovasc Dis 41:51, 1998.
84. Waspe LE, Chien WW, Merillat JC, Stark SI: Sinus node modification using radiofrequency current in a patient with persistent inappropriate sinus tachycardia. Pacing Clin Electrophysiol 17:1569, 1994.

85. Jayaprakash S, Sparks PB, Vohra J: Inappropriate sinus tachycardia (IST): Management by radiofrequency modification of sinus node. Aust N Z J Med 27:391, 1997.
86. Kalman JM, Olgin JE, Karch MR, et al: "Cristal tachycardias": Origin of right atrial tachycardias from the crista terminalis identified by intracardiac echocardiography. J Am Coll Cardiol 31:451, 1998.
87. Page RL: Treatment of arrhythmias during pregnancy. Am Heart J 130: 871, 1995.
88. Joglar JA, Page RL: Treatment of cardiac arrhythmias during pregnancy: Safety considerations. Drug Saf 20:85, 1999.
89. Chow T, Galvin J, McGovern B: Antiarrhythmic drug therapy in pregnancy and lactation. Am J Cardiol 82:581, 1998.
90. Mitani GM, Steinberg I, Lien EJ, et al: The pharmacokinetics of antiarrhythmic agents in pregnancy and lactation. Clin Pharmacokinet 12:253, 1987.

CHAPTER 36

Ventricular Tachycardia

Ali Massumi and Mohammad Hadi Kadivar

Certain ventricular arrhythmias are more common in women. Torsade de pointes, which is a distinctive form of polymorphic ventricular tachycardia with characteristic features including prolonged QT interval (especially in the acquired type), has been shown to occur more frequently in women.[1] Another form of ventricular tachycardia that occurs in the absence of structural heart disease is reported more frequently in the pregnant woman.[2] This idiopathic ventricular tachycardia, which originates in the right or left ventricle, is generally well tolerated but at times can cause fetal distress or demise. Most of these ventricular tachycardias in the normal heart are curable by newer catheter-based ablative procedures.

The true incidence, clinical course, and treatment responses of various arrhythmias in women have not been studied extensively.[3] Gender differences and response to antiarrhythmic drugs may also differ. Women have a longer QT and a higher resting heart rate, as well as smaller body and heart size.[4–7]

The incidence of coronary artery disease and related ventricular dysrhythmias, sustained ventricular tachycardia, and ventricular fibrillation, as well as sudden cardiac death, is significantly lower in women. The incidence of sudden cardiac death in women lags behind that in men by 20 years.[8] This is clearly related to the lower incidence of coronary artery disease in premenopausal women. Even after age 60, the incidence of sudden death in women for as yet unexplained reasons remains lower than in men.[9]

In this chapter, emphasis has been placed on aspects of ventricular tachycardias in women. The reader may refer to more detailed sources for a discussion of ventricular tachycardia in general.

ETIOLOGY OF VENTRICULAR TACHYCARDIA

Ventricular tachycardia is an abnormal rhythm consisting of three or more complexes originating distal to the bundle of His with a rate exceeding 100 beats per minute (bpm).[10] Chronic coronary artery disease with prior myocardial infarction is the most common cardiac disorder associated with ventricular tachycardia. A variety of other cardiac disorders are also associated with ventricular tachycardia (Table 36–1). A significant number of patients, 38% of those undergoing evaluation for ventricular tachycardia, have no evidence of heart disease.[11, 12]

Most patients with ventricular tachycardia of sufficient duration experience dizziness, syncope, distressing palpitations, or symptoms of congestive heart failure, as well as anginal chest discomfort.[13] Development of long-term electrocardiographic monitoring and electrophysiologic techniques has shown that many patients who die suddenly manifest ventricular tachycardia that deteriorates into ventricular fibrillation. Despite the expected symptoms, a significant group of patients with ventricular tachycardia either lack any symptoms or have limited and vague ones.[13] Absence of major symptoms should not mislead the observer into discarding the abnormal presenting rhythm as ventricular tachycardia and misdiagnosing it as supraventricular tachycardia.[13–16] Electrophysiologic studies have led to major advances in understanding the pathophysiologic mechanism of, as well as pharmacologic and nonpharmacologic (ablative or surgical) therapy for, ventricular tachycardia.

Ventricular Tachycardia—Definitions

Ventricular tachycardia is usually *paroxysmal*. However, occasionally an *incessant* form is encountered. An incessant ventricular tachycardia may be continuous or may be interspaced by occasional sinus beats or periods of sinus rhythm. A *repetitive* ventricular tachycardia, which is usually *monomorphic*, consists of a series of bursts of ventricular tachycardia ranging from 3 beats to less than 100 beats with intermittent sinus beats. The definition of *sustained ventricular tachycardia* is arbitrary; most often, sustained ventricular tachycardia is a ventricular tachycardia lasting more than 100 beats or longer than 15 to 30 seconds. Obviously, a ventricular tachycardia that requires medical intervention to terminate is regarded as sustained. *Nonsustained ventricular tachycardia* is defined as ventricular tachycardia consisting of 3 beats or more but less than 100 beats. Sustained ventricular tachycardia is a regular rhythm, whereas nonsustained ventricular tachycardia is often irregular. *Monomorphic ventricular tachycardia* has identical QRS complexes with a constant QRS width and cycle length. The

Table 36–1. ETIOLOGY OF VENTRICULAR TACHYCARDIA

Coronary artery disease
Acute ischemic event
Chronic ischemic state, post–myocardial infarction
Cardiomyopathy
Dilated cardiomyopathy
Hypertrophic cardiomyopathy
Restrictive cardiomyopathy
Valvular heart disease—presurgical and postsurgical intervention
Congenital heart disease—presurgical and postsurgical intervention
Metabolic disorders
Drug induction
Mitral valve prolapse
Acquired and congenital long QT syndrome
Right ventricular dysplasia
Left ventricular hypertrophy
Ventricular tachycardia in the absence of structural heart disease

axis remains constant. A *polymorphic ventricular tachycardia* has variable QRS morphology, width, axis, and cycle length. The *width* of QRS in ventricular tachycardia is in excess of 120 msec and usually in excess of 140 msec.

Fascicular types of ventricular tachycardia or ventricular tachycardias seen in the absence of structural heart disease have a shorter QRS width of 120 msec or even normal duration.[17]

Torsade de pointes is a unique type of ventricular tachycardia with twisting axis and polarity of the QRS, which can be distinguished by its features. This particular form of ventricular tachycardia, which was first described by Dessertenne in 1966,[18] is more common in women and is discussed later in this chapter.

The rate of ventricular tachycardia is usually in excess of 100 beats. The maximum rate of ventricular tachycardia is less than 250 bpm. Ventricular flutter is defined as a ventricular tachycardia whose rate is 250 bpm or more.

Ventricular Tachycardia—Electrocardiographic Features

Ventricular tachycardia has broad and bizarre complexes. The morphology of QRS complexes may be typical left (LBBB) or right bundle branch block (RBBB) but most frequently manifests intraventricular conduction defect (IVCD), which vaguely resembles LBBB or RBBB. This distinction is made on the basis of QRS voltage and polarity, and especially the polarity of the terminal portion of the QRS in lead VI.

The morphology and axis of QRS complexes depend on the site of origin and the course of the depolarization wavefront. The QRS axis is often abnormal, rightward or leftward, and indeterminate superior or inferior. A normal axis, however, does not exclude ventricular tachycardia.[17]

During ventricular tachycardia, the atria may be depolarized retrograde through the retrograde atrioventricular (AV) nodal conduction. Retrograde P waves can either be associated with the ventricular complexes in a 1:1 ratio[10] or demonstrate retrograde ventriculoatrial (VA) Wenckebach.[10] In the absence of VA conduction or when the rate of ventricular tachycardia is rapid, the atria are dissociated and exhibit their own independent rhythm, which could be sinus, atrial flutter or fibrillation, or a variety of other possibilities.

Capture beats and fusion beats are very helpful findings in favor of ventricular tachycardia; however, they are seen in a minority of ventricular tachycardia patients and usually are present when the ventricular tachycardia rate is relatively slow (i.e., less than 130 bpm). Capture beat is an occasional capture of the ventricle by the supraventricular rhythm. Fusion beat occurs when a dissociated atrial complex finds an opportunity to conduct to the ventricle but collides with the ventricular depolarization wave, which arrives at about the same time, resulting in a QRS complex showing activity from two sites.[19]

Features whose presence strongly favors ventricular tachycardia and that distinguishes ventricular tachycardia from supraventricular tachycardia with aberrancy include the following:

1. AV dissociation with capture and fusion beats
2. QRS width of 140 msec or greater[19]
3. Markedly abnormal QRS axis, especially superior axis
4. LBBB morphology or mono- or biphasic RBBB in V1
5. Negative QRS polarity in V1–V6 (negative concordance) (a positive concordance is less specific for ventricular tachycardia[10])
6. The presence of QS in V6
7. RS interval (from the onset of R to the nadir of S) of 100 msec or greater[20]
8. Absence of RS in all precordial leads[20]

Torsade de pointes is a particular form of ventricular tachycardia that occurs when the peaks of QRS complexes are twisted around the isoelectric line with changing amplitude, width, and cycle length.[18]

Bidirectional (fascicular) ventricular tachycardia characteristically has a narrow QRS, usually less than 140 msec with an RBBB pattern and shifting axis. There is a beat-to-beat shift in the frontal plane axis (alternating left and right axis).[21]

Ventricular Tachycardia—Electrophysiologic Observations

The underlying mechanisms of ventricular tachycardia are reentry, enhanced automaticity, and triggered activity.[22] The main mechanism for ventricular tachycardia is reentry. The anatomic substrate for reentry uses a circuit. Dispersion of refractoriness in one limb of the circuit permits slow conduction and produces unidirectional block in another limb. Slow conduction allows recovery of excitability within the circuit. Various patterns of reentrant excitation, including simple loop and figure-of-eight configurations, have been delineated. Damaged myocardium, anisotropy, and islands of fibrosis provide slow conduction and anatomic obstacles.[23] Several observations favor the reentrant process as the main mechanism for ventricular tachycardia in humans. These electrophysiologic observations include the following[24–27]:

- Initiation and termination of the arrhythmia during premature stimulation
- Transient entrainment of the tachycardia
- Resetting response to premature stimuli
- Response to antiarrhythmic drugs
- Direct myocardial mapping techniques

Initiation and termination of ventricular tachycardia in the electrophysiology laboratory is facilitated by programmed ventricular stimulation. Conventional[28, 29] and modified protocols[30–32] have been employed. A conventional protocol has four main components:

1. Site of stimulation
2. Stimulation current strength
3. Basic drive train cycle length
4. Number of extra stimuli

Most conventional induction protocols have used one, two, and three extra stimuli delivered at two ventricular sites (the right ventricular apex and the right ventricular outflow tract), often using basic drive train cycle lengths of 600, 500, and 400 msec. More recent protocols recommend using up to four extra stimuli and a basic drive cycle length of 400 msec.[30]

Programmed ventricular stimulation is used for a definitive diagnosis of ventricular tachycardia, as a guide to selection of antiarrhythmic agents, and for evaluation of patients before and after catheter ablation, device implantation, or surgical treatment.

Electrophysiologically, ventricular tachycardia is recognized by absence of a His potential before the onset of QRS. At times, because of retrograde activation of a His bundle during ventricular tachycardia, a very short or even negative H-V interval may be observed.[23] An exception is present in a rare form of ventricular tachycardia, called bundle branch reentry ventricular tachycardia, in which a His potential is present before each ventricular complex at the same or longer H-V time than the conducted sinus beat.[23] The presence of AV dissociation or retrograde partial VA conduction should be considered evidence for ventricular tachycardia.

Other mechanisms of ventricular tachycardia are triggered activity and enhanced automaticity. Triggered activity results from oscillations in membrane potentials that are divided into early and delayed after-depolarizations. Early after-depolarizations (EADs) have been observed in hypokalemia and are believed to be the mechanism responsible for torsade de pointes. Delayed after-depolarizations (DADs) are membrane oscillations that occur after repolarization has been achieved. An example is ventricular arrhythmias secondary to digitalis toxicity. DADs are believed to result from calcium loading. Unlike triggered activity, which requires a previous event (such as a pause) to trigger a response, enhanced automaticity and automatic rhythms occur spontaneously as a result of phase IV depolarization.

Ventricular Tachycardia—Clinical Features

Symptoms during ventricular tachycardia vary and depend on a variety of factors including left ventricular function, rate of ventricular tachycardia, the posture at the time of ventricular tachycardia onset, and the duration of ventricular tachycardia.[23] The patient may be asymptomatic or present with complaints of distressing palpitations, dizziness, or syncope, or symptoms of congestive heart failure. Sudden cardiac death may be the first presentation when unstable ventricular tachycardia degenerates rapidly into ventricular fibrillation.[23]

More than 95% of all regular wide QRS tachycardias seen in the emergency room of community hospitals are ventricular tachycardia.[24] A common mistake is to diagnose wide QRS tachycardia as a supraventricular tachycardia with aberrancy in patients who are either young, in a stable hemodynamic situation, or asymptomatic. The young age and the benign appearance of a patient should not rule out the diagnosis of ventricular tachycardia.[24]

Some of the physical findings depend on the P-to-QRS relationship. Examination of jugular venous pulsations may show evidence of AV dissociation. Absence of normal A and V waves with intermittent cannon A waves may be seen. If the atria are depolarized retrograde and regularly after each QRS complex, a regular cannon A wave is noted with each ventricular systole. A variable first heart sound may be rarely audible when the ventricular tachycardia rate is relatively slow and AV dissociation is present. Other findings include relative or severe hypotension, evidence of poor perfusion to the extremities, and congestive heart failure or murmur related to underlying heart disease, whether valvular, cardiomyopathic, or ischemic. In patients who present with recurrent sustained and monomorphic ventricular tachycardia due to left ventricular aneurysm, an abnormal segmental motion or bulging apex may be appreciated on physical examination, especially after restoration of normal sinus rhythm.

Idiopathic Ventricular Tachycardias

Ventricular tachycardias that occur in the absence of structural heart disease and are not associated with metabolic or electrolyte abnormalities or prolonged QT are considered idiopathic. In the strictest form, the absence of heart disease means normal cardiac function and structures as assessed by noninvasive and invasive studies, including right and left heart catheterization, coronary angiography, left ventriculography, and biopsy.[33] The presence of myocardial pathology, however, has not been excluded by myocardial biopsy in many patients reported to have this form of ventricular tachycardia. In clinical practice, however, invasive studies are rarely performed.[12]

Some common features of ventricular tachycardia in this population include the following[34]:

- No obvious structural heart disease
- Usually a single monomorphic configuration of QRS complex during ventricular tachycardia
- A less well-defined underlying electrophysiologic mechanism
- Generally a good prognosis in terms of arrhythmic mortality

Classification

Idiopathic ventricular tachycardias can be divided into those originating from the left or the right ventricle.

Idiopathic Left Ventricular Tachycardia

Idiopathic left ventricular tachycardia is characterized by QRS complexes that show an RBBB morphology and often left axis deviation complexes during ventricular tachycardia (Fig. 36–1). Most patients are 20 to 40 years old, and there is a similar frequency in men and women.[12] Tachycardia focus is located in the inferoapical portion of the left ventricle. This type of ventricular tachycardia is primarily seen in young people who have recurrent sustained, usually well-tolerated episodes of ventricular tachycardia and is often responsive to intravenous verapamil administration; thus this type is called verapamil-sensitive ventricular tachycardia.[12] Ventricular tachycardia can be induced by programmed stimulation. When the ventricular tachycardia rate is not fast, fusion and capture beats are noted.[35] During left ventricular mapping, a so-called "Purkinje spike" can be identified preceding the onset of the QRS complex.[35] Localized reentry or triggered activity is the most likely mechanism.[12, 35] Both

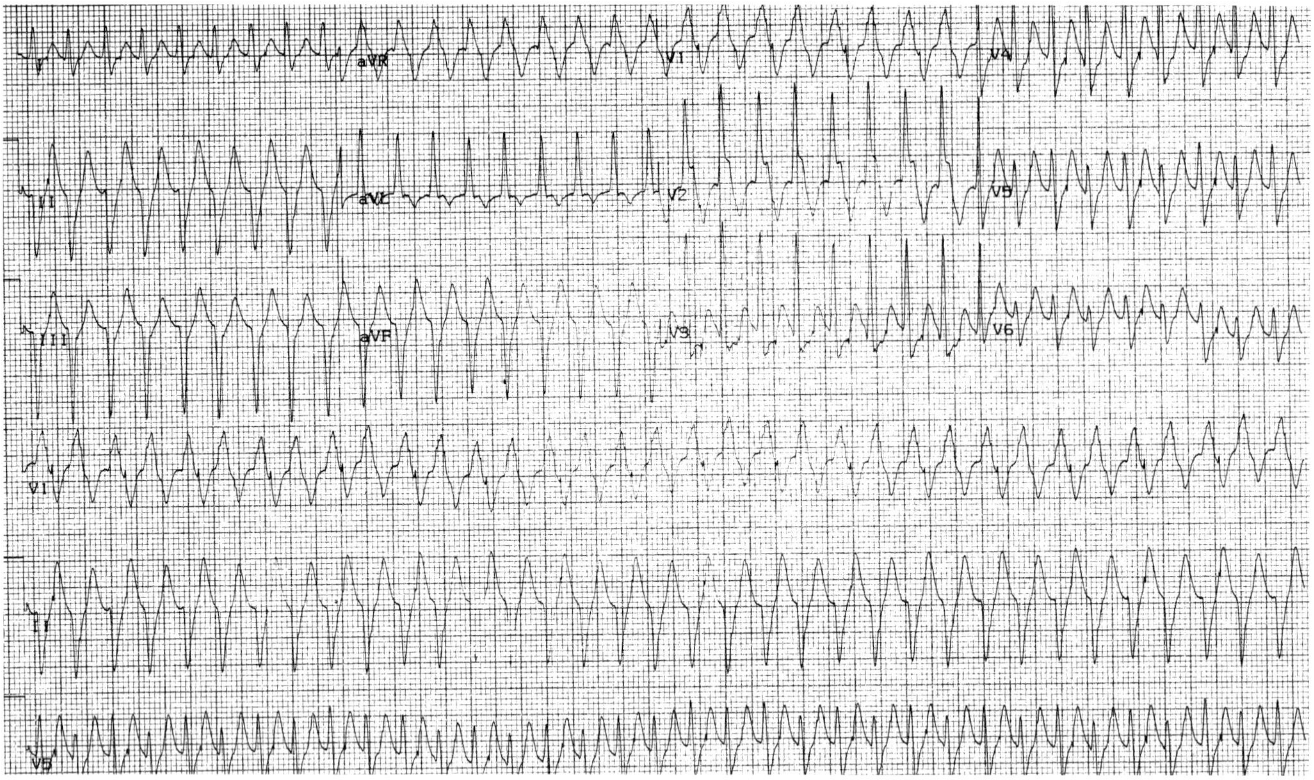

FIGURE 36–1. Idiopathic left ventricular tachycardia in a 26-year-old woman. Ventricular tachycardia rate is 210 beats per minute. There is right bundle branch block morphology with left axis deviation. The QRS width is 112 ms, which suggests that part of the conduction system is used in the tachycardia circuit; hence, the term "fascicular" tachycardia. This tachycardia is verapamil sensitive and should not be misinterpreted as supraventricular tachycardia. The patient was successfully treated with radiofrequency current delivered to the site of tachycardia origin in the posterior interventricular septum near the apex of the left ventricle.

mechanisms are slow channel activity dependent. Radiofrequency catheter ablation using radiofrequency current is an effective and curative treatment.[35, 36]

Idiopathic Right Ventricular Tachycardia

Idiopathic right ventricular tachycardia, which is seen in the absence of heart disease, is characterized by LBBB and usually inferior axis morphology of the QRS complex during ventricular tachycardia (Fig. 36–2).[37] The clinical presentation is often palpitation, but presyncope or syncope is not infrequent.[37] Idiopathic right ventricular tachycardia most often originates in the right ventricular outflow tract.[12] Because right ventricular tachycardia is frequently associated with exercise, it is described as exercise-induced, catecholamine-sensitive, or adenosine-responsive ventricular tachycardia.[12] It is thought that idiopathic right ventricular tachycardia is the result of cyclic adenosine monophosphate (AMP)–mediated triggered activity.[38] Some of these patients have inducible ventricular tachycardia with atrial and ventricular stimulation and, less commonly, premature ventricular stimulation.[37] Isoproterenol infusion may be necessary to produce sustained tachycardias.[37] Evidence for regional sympathetic denervation in patients with idiopathic right ventricular tachycardia using ^{123}I-meta-iodobenzyl guanidine (^{123}I-MIBG) scintigraphy has been described.[37]

Focal anatomic and functional wall motion abnormalities of right ventricular outflow in patients with idiopathic right ventricular tachycardia has been detected by cine magnetic resonance imaging (MRI).[39]

Radiofrequency catheter ablation has proved to be highly effective for treatment of idiopathic right ventricular tachycardia.[37, 39]

Repetitive Monomorphic Right Ventricular Tachycardia

The most prevalent form of idiopathic ventricular tachycardia is repetitive monomorphic right ventricular tachycardia, which is characterized by frequent ventricular extrasystoles, ventricular couplets, and salvos of nonsustained ventricular tachycardia lasting a few seconds to a few minutes with intervening sinus rhythm (Fig. 36–3). This arrhythmia was first described by Gallavardin in 1922.[40] In contrast to most other forms of idiopathic ventricular tachycardia, this tachycardia usually occurs at rest and is nonsustained. This tachycardia is seen more commonly in young and middle-aged patients.[41] Palpitations, dizziness, and rarely syncope are the presenting symptoms; however, in one third of patients, the arrhythmia is asymptomatic.[41] Repetitive monomorphic ventricular tachycardias are usually suppressed by exercise but may appear or become sustained in the recovery phase.[41] In the electrophysiology laboratory, repetitive monomorphic ventricular tachycardia may be induced by atrial or ventricular stimulation within a narrow pacing cycle window in only 22% of patients.[42] Infusion of isoproterenol may cause

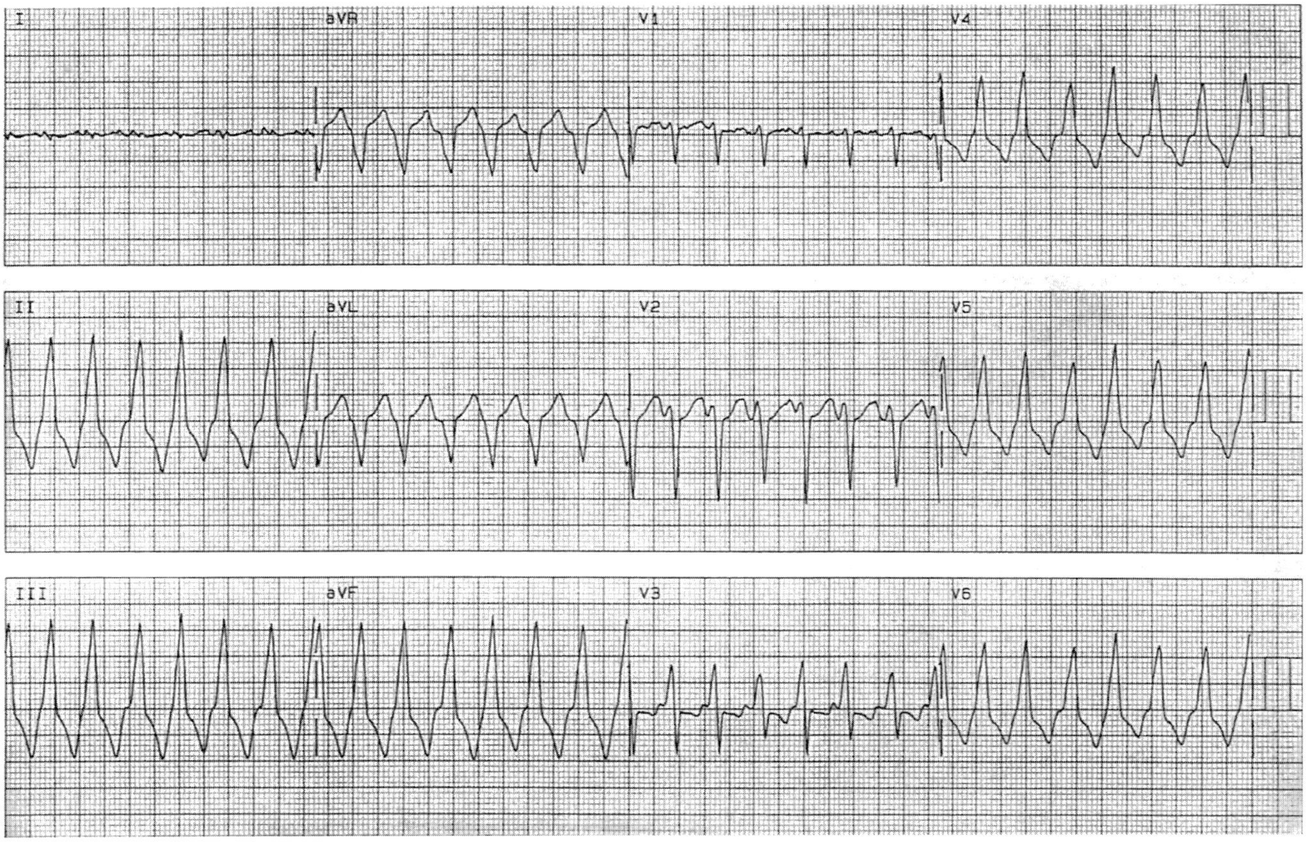

FIGURE 36–2. Sustained monomorphic ventricular tachycardia from the right ventricular outflow tract. Important features are the left bundle branch block morphology of the QRS with an inferior axis. Monophasic tall QRSs in inferior leads are typical. The patient was successfully treated with radiofrequency catheter ablation.

ventricular tachycardia in 40% or may abolish ventricular tachycardia.[42–44] The mechanism of ventricular tachycardia is cyclic AMP–mediated triggered activity.[12] Repetitive monomorphic ventricular tachycardia exhibits an LBBB pattern and an inferior or a normal QRS axis.[12] Patients may be asymptomatic, be mildly symptomatic, or rarely, have syncope. Medical therapy with oral beta-blocking drugs or verapamil yields inconsistent results. Class I-C agents have been shown to have good efficacy.[37] Radiofrequency catheter ablation has been used successfully for the treatment of this arrhythmia.

Arrhythmogenic Right Ventricular Dysplasia

Arrhythmogenic right ventricular dysplasia (ARVD) is a right ventricular cardiomyopathy that is manifested clinically by ventricular tachycardia usually of the LBBB morphology and is characterized by progressive replacement of myocardial cells with fibrous and adipose tissues.[45] The loss of myocardial cells in ARVD may result from cell death by apoptosis.[46] Apoptosis (or programmed cell death) in contrast to necrosis (or accidental cell death) is a series of tightly regulated events modulated by a genetic program. ARVD was first proposed by Fontaine and associates in 1977.[47] The clinical spectrum of this condition was described by Marcus.[45] ARVD is an uncommon but important source of ventricular tachycardia or sudden cardiac death.[48] ARVD must be considered in patients with frequent premature ventricular beats or transient or sustained ventricular tachycardia, particularly those with an LBBB configuration, who have no known cause for their arrhythmias.[45] ARVD primarily affects young adults, men more than women,[49] and is frequently diagnosed before age 40 years.[45] Patients may be very symptomatic with transient or sustained ventricular tachycardia with an LBBB configuration or may be asymptomatic. Ventricular tachycardia in ARVD is classically provoked by exertion.[50] Physical examination is typically normal. Surface electrocardiography can provide certain clues to the presence of arrhythmogenic right ventricular tachycardia such as an epsilon wave, which is visible as sharp discrete deflections at the terminal portion of the QRS complex or negative T waves, as well as an incomplete RBBB in right precordial leads. These waves are thought to arise from delayed activation of the diseased right ventricle.[51] Delayed activation is the electrocardiographic equivalent of late potentials seen on signal-averaged electrocardiogram (ECG).[51] Echocardiography,[52] MRI,[53] and contrast ventriculography[54] are very valuable tools in the diagnosis of arrhythmogenic right ventricular dysplasia.[54] A positive signal-averaged ECG in a patient with right ventricular arrhythmia and inducibility of ventricular tachycardia in the electrophysiology laboratory[46, 55] favor ARVD. The cause of ARVD is not known. There is occasional autosomal dominant inheritance.

Therapy

Medical treatment with beta blockers, amiodarone, or flecainide may be effective. Catheter ablation in patients who

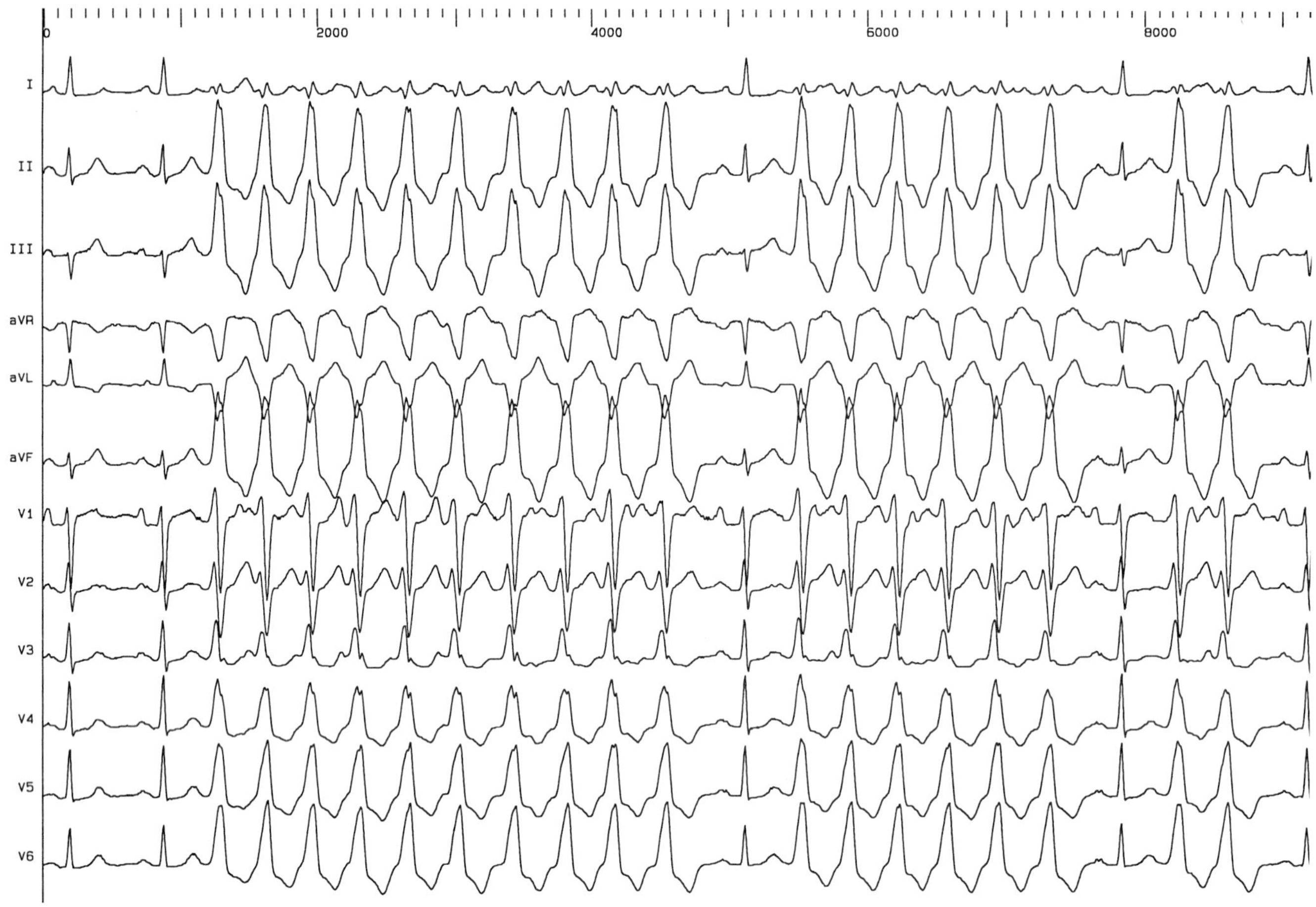

FIGURE 36–3. Repetitive monomorphic ventricular tachycardia in a young woman. Runs of monomorphic ventricular tachycardia with left bundle branch morphology and an inferior axis are interspaced with occasional sinus beats. Tall monophasic QRSs in inferior leads are typical of this type of ventricular tachycardia, which originates in the right ventricular outflow tract. The patient was successfully treated with radiofrequency catheter ablation.

are intolerant or refractory to antiarrhythmic therapy has limited success. Because disease is a progressive process, new ventricular tachycardia may develop later. Patients believed to be at high risk for sudden cardiac death are candidates for implantable cardioverter defibrillator (ICD) implantation.

Ventricular Tachycardia in Coronary Artery Disease

Coronary artery disease is the most common cause of sustained ventricular tachycardia. Ventricular tachycardia in these patients most commonly originates from the left ventricle. Ventricular tachycardia occurring after the acute stages of a myocardial infarction is thought to be caused by reentry within or adjacent to the infarct zone. Areas of fibrosis and streaks of fibrotic tissue adjacent to spared subendocardium or subepicardium and transmural extent of infarct region serve as anatomic ports of reentry.[23] Left ventricular aneurysm occurs in as many as 35% of patients after acute anterior wall myocardial infarction. Such left ventricular aneurysms are associated with a high incidence of serious ventricular arrhythmias.[56] Approximately 40% of patients with left ventricular aneurysms who do not manifest spontaneous ventricular tachycardia are inducible to ventricular tachycardia.[56] Patients who develop spontaneous, uniform sustained ventricular tachycardia have a larger aneurysm than do those without spontaneous ventricular activity.[56] It is also reported that aneurysms with fibroelastosis coating the endocardium are associated with ventricular tachycardia, whereas aneurysms with thrombus and fibrosis without elastic tissue coating the endocardium are not.[57]

Other factors determining the onset of ventricular tachycardia include changes in frequency of ventricular premature beats (VPBs), changes in autonomic tone,[58, 59] the presence of ischemia, or the use of antiarrhythmic agents.

Ventricular tachycardia is seen in patients with poor ventricular function.[57] Sustained ventricular tachycardia in patients with coronary artery disease has circadian variation in onset, occurring most frequently in the morning.[58] Prognosis of ventricular tachycardia in coronary artery disease depends on the following:

- Hemodynamic tolerance of ventricular tachycardia
- Overall left ventricular function
- Extent of coronary artery disease

In patients presenting with syncope, presyncope, or cardiac arrest, recurrence can be life threatening.

Ventricular Tachycardia in Dilated Cardiomyopathy

Sudden death is a major clinical problem in patients with idiopathic dilated cardiomyopathy. Severity of heart failure has been shown to be an important risk factor for sudden death in these patients.[60] The mechanism of ventricular tachycardia in dilated cardiomyopathy may be similar to that observed in coronary artery disease.[60] In most cases, the underlying mechanism is related to intramyocardial reentry circuits due to diseased myocardium or fibrosis.[61] A macro reentry circuit in the bundle branches produces a unique form of sustained monomorphic ventricular tachycardia in dilated cardiomyopathies, as well as ischemic cardiomyopathies, called bundle branch reentry.[35, 62–64] The right and left bundle branches, the His bundle, and transseptal ventricular muscle conduction are components of the reentrant circuit. Because ventricular activation occurs by way of bundle branches, the resultant QRS morphology has a typical LBBB or rarely an RBBB appearance.[23] Dilated heart and prolonged H-V interval at baseline sinus rhythm are usually required for this tachycardia. An electrocardiogram at baseline shows nonspecific intraventricular conduction defect or LBBB. During ventricular tachycardia, which is commonly manifesting an LBBB morphology, AV dissociation or VA block is present. On intracardiac electrogram, the His bundle potential precedes the ventricular activation with the H-V interval equal to or exceeding the H-V interval of sinus rhythm. A right bundle branch depolarization will also be recorded if a catheter is positioned next to the right bundle.[23] The clinical presentation in most patients is syncope and sudden death or palpitations in others.[63] The effective treatment of this particular form of ventricular tachycardia, which is seen in any dilated heart due to the ischemic or nonischemic type, is catheter ablation of the right bundle branch, which is easily performed and is curative.[60, 63–65] Drug therapy[66, 67] and ICD use are other modes of therapy.

TORSADE DE POINTES

Torsade de pointes, or twisting of the points, is a specific kind of ventricular tachycardia that occurs in patients with the long QT syndrome, regardless of whether it is congenital or acquired.[68] The term torsade de pointes was coined in 1966 by Dessertenne[18] to point out the distinctive undulating pattern of sequential QRS complexes and T waves during ventricular tachycardia.[68]

In torsade de pointes, the peaks of QRS complexes twist around an imaginary baseline on the ECG.[18] The phasic variation in the electrical polarity and amplitude of the QRS complexes should be looked for in preferably two or more simultaneously recorded leads.[23] By definition, a "torsade" covers several "pointes." The word is made plural only if the attacks of arrhythmia are recurrent.[69] The coupling interval of the first beat of the torsade is long. Marked prolongation of the QT interval, especially in bradycardia or after a pause, is part of the definition of torsade. Torsade de pointes may terminate spontaneously, or it may deteriorate into ventricular fibrillation.[70] In addition to having a prolonged QT interval, most of these patients also have abnormal T waves, which may be biphasic, bifid, or notched.[71]

The mechanism of initiation of torsade de pointes is triggered activity,[68] which is due to EAD. These EADs, which happen in situations in which repolarization is prolonged,[72] are calcium current dependent.[72] The mechanism responsible for the maintenance of torsade de pointes is not clear.[72] The association between torsade de pointes and marked QT prolongation may be congenital or acquired.

Gender Differences in QT Interval, Long QT Syndromes, and Torsade de Pointes

Gender differences in ECG parameters were noted as early as 1920.[4] Women are known to have longer QT intervals.[4–7] Global T-wave inversion on the ECG, which is believed to be a long QT pattern, is also much more common in women.[1, 3, 73] Symptomatic QT prolongation and especially torsade de pointes is more prevalent among women. Sex difference as a risk factor for torsade de pointes was reported by Makkar[1] in 1993, who found that in 332 reported cases, 70% of the cardiovascular drug-related torsade de pointes occurred in women. Women constituted the majority irrespective of the presence or absence of underlying heart disease, electrolyte abnormality, or level of corrected QT interval (QTC) at baseline. It was concluded that women are more prone than men to develop torsade de pointes during administration of drugs that prolong repolarization. Lehman[74] found that in 22 clinical trials involving 3135 adults who received d,l-sotalol, torsade de pointes developed in 4.1% of 799 women and 1.9% of 2336 men. Women had threefold greater odds of developing torsade de pointes than men.

There is evidence that inherited long QT disorders may be more common in women.[75] Moss and colleagues[7] found that 64% of patients enrolled in an international registry of subjects with long QT syndrome were female.

Sudden death in anorexia nervosa, which usually afflicts females, is associated with various QT interval prolongation resulting in syncope and ventricular tachyarrhythmias.[76] Women who use a liquid protein diet for weight reduction may develop hypokalemia and prominent U waves, as well as prolonged QU and ST- and T-wave abnormalities.[77] These patients may experience recurrent syncope or sudden death.

Congenital Long QT Syndromes

Various congenital long QT syndromes (LQT_1 through LQT_5) are inherited as autosomal dominant disorders,[68] which are characterized by syncope and sudden death from ventricular tachycardia.[75] Genetic markers have been identified on chromosomes 11, 7, 3, 4, and 21 corresponding to $LQT_{1–5}$.[68, 70]

Acquired Long QT Syndromes

In the acquired form, the QT prolongation seems to be mostly associated with the use of agents known to prolong myocardial repolarization.[23, 68, 69, 78] Secondary causes of acquired QT prolongation are many, including antiarrhythmic agents (Class IA, III), some antihistamines (terfenadine and astemizole), antibiotics (erythromycin, betoconazole, chloroquine, claritromycin, azithromycin), gastrointestinal factors (cisapride, liquid protein diets), psychotropic agents, diuretics, and electrolyte abnormalities (hypokalemia, hypomagnesemia, hypocalcemia).[68]

VENTRICULAR TACHYCARDIA IN PREGNANCY

There is an increased incidence of various arrhythmias during pregnancy.[79] Although supraventricular tachycardias are most common during pregnancy,[79, 80] ventricular tachycardias also occur in the pregnant woman with or without structural heart disease.

There is an increase in the incidence of ventricular tachycardias in the pregnant woman without heart disease.[2, 81] These ventricular tachycardias arise more commonly from the right side of the interventricular septum, namely the right ventricular outflow tract or the left side of the interventricular septum in the inferoposterior region of the septum. Those arising from the right ventricular outflow tract have an LBBB and inferior axis morphology, whereas those originating from the left side of the septum manifest RBBB and left axis deviation morphology (occasionally referred to as a fascicular ventricular tachycardia).

Brodsky and coworkers[2] reported seven cases and reviewed 23 other previously reported cases of new-onset ventricular tachycardia in pregnancy reported from 1931 to 1992; the great majority had no heart disease. Arrhythmia evaluation in the seven patients revealed an LBBB morphology in six of them, with the majority having a right (inferior) axis deviation consistent with a right ventricular outflow tract site of origin of ventricular tachycardia. There was evidence suggesting catecholamine-sensitive ventricular tachycardia, with the rate of tachycardia ranging from 110 to 250 bpm. Although ventricular tachycardia in the presence of a normal heart is usually well tolerated in pregnancy, maternal and fetal death have been reported.[2]

The mechanism of induction or exacerbation of ventricular tachycardia during pregnancy is not completely understood. Changes in autonomic tone, catecholamine sensitivity, and hormonal changes and the expected changes in cardiovascular function such as increase in cardiac output, basal heart rate, and intravascular volume play a role.

Antiarrhythmic Drug Therapy in Pregnancy

Indications for and choice of antiarrhythmic drug therapy in pregnancy depend on hemodynamic stability and symptoms of tachycardia, the safety of mother and fetus, and potential risks to the fetus, especially in the first 8 weeks. Although most antiarrhythmic medications appear to be safe,[82] a complete and absolute safety profile has not been established for any of Vaughan Williams' four classes of antiarrhythmic agents.[83] In general, it is best to avoid pharmacologic therapy during pregnancy; however, if drug therapy is necessary, Class II (beta-adrenergic blocking) agents may be the safest to try.[82] Propranolol has been used in pregnancy extensively, and its relative safety has been shown in the longest experience with Class II agents.[84, 85] Propranolol is reported to be rarely associated with intrauterine growth retardation. Cardioselective agents such as atenolol or metoprolol, which cause less interference with B_2-mediated peripheral vasodilation or uterine relaxation, are the preferred agents.[84–86] All commonly used antiarrhythmic drugs including Class I agents are capable of crossing the placental barrier.[82] Quinidine and procainamide have been used for the longest period,[87, 88] although uterine contraction,[89] premature labor,[90] neonatal thrombocytopenia,[91] and rarely, spontaneous abortions have been reported with quinidine.

Although intravenous lidocaine may be used for ventricular tachycardia,[84] phenytoin is contraindicated (Food and Drug Administration [FDA] Class X) owing to its teratogenic side effects, including mental and growth retardation.[84] Data on the Class IC agents flecainide and propafenone are limited, and they should be used with caution in pregnancy.[82]

Class III agents including sotalol and amiodarone have been used in pregnancy. Sotalol crosses the placenta, and transient neonatal bradycardia in response has been reported,[92] but it does not appear to cause significant adverse effects.[93] Amiodarone has been used during pregnancy[94–99] for resistant arrhythmias of the mother and rarely of the fetus.[95] Various reports have confirmed a limited transplacental passage of amiodarone and its active metabolite desethyl amiodarone (DEA).[96–98] Studies have shown a considerable amount of amiodarone in the breast milk.[96] Matsumura and associates[97] reported on nine pregnant women who received 200 mg of amiodarone a day. One neonate had abnormal thyroxine (T_4) and thyroid-stimulating hormone (TSH) levels, which normalized in 1 month. Plomp and colleagues reported on five pregnant women who were treated with amiodarone. One infant appeared hypothyroid, but after a few weeks of treatment, results of thyroid studies normalized.[96] Owing to limited data available, use of amiodarone in pregnancy should be limited to very resistant and symptomatic ventricular tachycardia. This drug should be used at the lowest effective dose, with careful attention to fetal thyroid function.

Clinical studies of verapamil in pregnant women have not demonstrated adverse effects on either the patient or fetus.[84] Intravenous verapamil may produce maternal hypotension and secondary fetal hypoperfusion.[100] Oral verapamil is capable of causing fetal bradycardia, heart block, or hypotension.[100] Diltiazem may cause skeletal abnormalities, decreased fetal weight, and even fetal death.[84, 101] Overall, adenosine[102] and β-blockers are the preferred treatment for supraventricular tachycardias in pregnancy.[82, 83] Intravenous procainamide and lidocaine, as well as DC shock, may be employed for treatment of ventricular tachycardia. Intravenous bretylium and amiodarone have not been studied extensively in pregnancy.

References

1. Makkar RR, Fromm BS, Skinman RT, et al: Female gender as a risk factor for torsades de pointes associated with cardiovascular drugs. JAMA 270:2590–2597, 1993.
2. Brodsky M, Doria R, Allen B: New-onset ventricular tachycardia during pregnancy. Am Heart J 123:933–941, 1992.

3. Albert CM, Ruskin JN: Arrhythmias and the use of implantable cardioverter-defibrillators. In Julian DG, Wenger NK (eds): Women and Heart Disease. St Louis, Mosby, 1997, pp 363–374.
4. Bazett M: An analysis of the time-relations of electrocardiograms. Heart 7:353–370, 1920.
5. Merri M, Benhorn J, Alberti M, et al: Electrocardiographic quantitations of ventricular repolarization. Circulation 80:1301–1308, 1989.
6. Ashman R: The normal duration of the QT interval. Am Heart J 23: 522–534, 1942.
7. Moss AJ, Schwartz PJ, Crampton RS, et al: The long QT syndrome: Prospective longitudinal study of 328 families. Circulation 84:1136–1144, 1991.
8. Kannel WB, Schatzkin A: Sudden death: Lessons from subsets in population studies. J Am Coll Cardiol 5:141B–149B, 1985.
9. Cupples LA, Gagnon DR, Kannel WB: Long and short term risk of sudden coronary death. Circulation 85:1-11–1-18, 1992.
10. Marriot HL: Ventricular tachycardia. In Wagner GS (ed): Practical Electrocardiography, 8th ed. Baltimore, Williams & Wilkins, 1988, p 311.
11. Slama R, Leclercq JF, Coumel PH: Paroxysmal ventricular tachycardia in patients with apparently normal hearts. In Zipes DP Jalife J (eds): Cardiac Electrophysiology and Arrhythmias. Orlando, Grune Stratton, 1985, pp 545–552.
12. Belhassen B, Viskin S: Idiopathic ventricular tachycardia and fibrillation. J Cardiovasc Electrophysiol 4:356–368, 1993.
13. Morady F, Shen EN, Bhandari A, et al: Clinical symptoms in patients with sustained ventricular tachycardia. West J Med 142:341–344, 1985.
14. Wellens HJJ, Bbar FW, Lie KL: The value of the electrocardiogram in the differential diagnosis of a tachycardia with a widened QRS complex. Am J Med 64:27–33, 1978.
15. Wellens HJJ, Bar FW, Vonagt EJ, et al: The differentiation between ventricular tachycardia and supraventricular tachycardia with aberrant conduction: The value of the 12-lead electrocardiogram. In Wellens HJJ, Kubertus HE (eds): What's New in Electrophysiology. The Hague, Martinus Nijhoff, 1987, pp 184–199.
16. Kindwall KE, Brown J, Josephson ME: Electrographic criteria for ventricular tachycardia in wide complex left bundle branch morphology tachycardias. Am J Cardiol 61:1279–1283, 1988.
17. Cohen HC, Gozo EG, Pick A: Ventricular tachycardia with narrow QRS complexes (left posterior fascicular tachycardia). Circulation 45: 1035–1043, 1972.
18. Dessertenne F: La tachycardie ventriculaire a deux foyers opposes variables. Arch Mal Coeur 59:263–272, 1966.
19. Wellens HJJ, Bar FW, Lie KL: The value of the electrocardiogram in the differential diagnosis of a tachycardia with a widened QRS complex. Am J Med 64:21–33, 1978.
20. Brugada P, Brugada J, Mont L, et al: A new approach to the differential diagnosis of a regular tachycardia with a wide QRS complex. Circulation 83:1649–1659, 1991.
21. Grimm W, Marchlinski FE: Accelerated idioventricular rhythm, bidirectional ventricular tachycardia. In Zipes DP, Jalife, J (eds): Cardiac Electrophysiology: From Cell to Bedside, 2nd ed. Philadelphia, W.B. Saunders, 1995, p 920.
22. Jazayeri MR, Sra JJ, Akhtar M: Wide QRS complexes: Electrophysiologic basis of a common electrocardiographic diagnosis. J Cardiovasc Electrophysiol 3:365–393, 1992.
23. Akhtar M: Clinical spectrum of ventricular tachycardia. Circulation 82:1561–1573, 1990.
24. Barold SS: Bedside diagnosis of wide QRS tachycardia. Pacing Clin Electrophysiol 18:2109–2115, 1995.
25. Fei LU, Statters DJ, Hratkova K, et al: Changes of autonomic influence on the heart immediately before the onset of spontaneous idiopathic ventricular tachycardia. J Am Coll Cardiol 24:1515–1522, 1994.
26. Zipes, DP: Ventricular tachycardia. In Braunwald E, ed: Heart Disease. Philadelphia, W.B. Saunders, 1997, p 677.
27. Jazayeri MR: Wide complex tachycardia. J Cardiovasc Electrophysiol 3:380–392, 1992.
28. Wellens HJJ, Schuilenburg RM, Durrer D: Electrical stimulation of the heart in patients with ventricular tachycardia. Circulation 46: 216, 1972.
29. Wellens HJJ, Lier KL, Durrer D: Further observations on ventricular tachycardia as studied by electrical stimulation of the heart: Chronic recurrent ventricular tachycardia during acute myocardial infarction. Circulation 49:647, 1974.
30. Hummel JD, Strickberger A, Daoud E, et al: Results and efficiency of programmed ventricular stimulation with four extrastimuli compared with one, two, and three extrastimuli. Circulation 90:2827–2832, 1994.
31. Ho DW, Cooper MJ, Richards DB, et al: Comparison of number of extra stimuli versus change in basic cycle length for induction of ventricular tachycardia by programmed ventricular stimulation. J Am Coll Cardiol 22:1711–1717, 1993.
32. Wellens HJJ, Duven DR, Lie KL: Observations on mechanism of ventricular tachycardia in man. Circulation 54:237–244, 1976.
33. Lerman BB, Stein KS, Engelstein ED, et al: Mechanism of repetitive monomorphic ventricular tachycardia. Circulation 92:421–429, 1995.
34. Brooks R, Burgess JH: Idiopathic ventricular tachycardia: A review. Medicine 67:271–294, 1988.
35. Zardini M, Thakur R, Klein GJ: Catheter ablation of idiopathic left ventricular tachycardia. Pacing Clin Electrophysiol 18:1255–1264, 1995.
36. Coggins DL, Lee RJ, Sweeney J, et al: Radiofrequency catheter ablation as a cure for idiopathic tachycardia of both left and right ventricular origin. J Am Coll Cardiol 23:1333–1341, 1994.
37. Nibley C. Wharton JM: Ventricular tachycardia with left bundle branch block morphology. Pacing Clin Electrophysiol 18:334–351, 1995.
38. Lerman BB, Belardinelli L, West GA, et al: Adenosine-sensitive ventricular tachycardia: Evidence suggesting cyclic AMP-mediated triggered activity. Circulation 74:279–280, 1986.
39. Carlson MD, White RD, Trohman RG, et al: Right ventricular outflow tract ventricular tachycardia: Detection of previously unrecognized anatomic abnormalities using cine magnetic resonance imaging. J Am Coll Cardiol 24:720–727, 1994.
40. Gallavardin L: Extra-systolic ventriculaire a paraoxysmes tachycardique prolonge. Arch Mal Coeur 15:298–306, 1922.
41. Ritchie AH, Kerr CR, Qi A, et al: Nonsustained ventricular tachycardia arising from the right ventricular outflow tract. Am J Cardiol 64: 594–598, 1989.
42. Buxton AE, Waxman HL, Marchlinski FE, et al: Right ventricular tachycardia: Clinical and electrophysiologic chracteristics. Circulation 68:917–927, 1983.
43. Rahilly GT, Prystowsky EN, Zipes DP, et al: Clinical and electrophysiological findings in patients with repetitive monomorphic ventricular tachycardia and otherwise normal electrocardiogram. Am J Cardiol 52:459–468, 1982.
44. Aliot E, Brembilla-Perrot B, Khalife K, et al: Ventricular tachycardias in individuals with apparently normal hearts. In Aliot E, Lazzara R, eds: Ventricular Tachycardias. From Mechanisms to Therapy. Dordrecht, The Netherlands, Martinus-Nighoff, 1987, pp 95–112.
45. Marcus FI, Fontaine GH, Guirandon G, et al: Right ventricular dysplasia: Report of 24 adult cases. Circulation 65:384–398, 1982.
46. Mallat Z, Tedgui A, Fontaliran F, et al: Evidence of apoptosis in arrhythmogenic right ventricular dysplasia. N Engl J Med 335:1190–1196, 1996.
47. Fontaine G, Guirandon G, Frank R, et al: Stimulation studies and epicardial mapping in ventricular tachycardia: Study of mechanisms and selection for surgery. In Rulbertus M (ed): Reentrant Arrhythmias. MTP, Lancaster, 1977, pp 334–350.
48. Thiene G, Nava A, Corrado D, et al: Right ventricular cardiomyopathy and sudden death in young people. N Engl J Med 318:129, 1988.
49. Manyari DE, Klein GJ, Gulamhusein S, et al: Arrhythmogenic right ventricular dysplasia: A generalized cardiomyopathy? Circulation 68: 251–257, 1983.
50. Leclercq J, Potenza F, Maison-Blance P, et al: Determinants of spontaneous occurrence of sustained monomorphic ventricular tachycardia in right ventricular dysplasia. J Am Coll Cardiol 28:720–724, 1996.
51. Leclercq JF, Coumel P: Late potentials in arrhythmogenic right ventricular dysplasia: Prevalence, diagnostic and prognostic values. Eur Heart J 14:80–83, 1993.
52. Rossi P, Massumi A, Gillette P, Hall RJ: Arrhythmogenic right ventricular dysplasia: Clinical features, diagnostic techniques, and current management. Am Heart J 102:414–420, 1982.
53. Ricci C, Longo R, Pagnan L, et al: Magnetic resonance imaging in right ventricular dysplasia. Am J Cardiol 70:1589–1595, 1992.
54 Marcus FI, Fontaine G: Arrhythmogenic right ventricular dysplasia/cardiomyopathy: A review. Pacing Clin Electrophysiol 18:1298, 1995.
55. Iesaka Y, Hiroe M, Aonuma K, et al: Usefulness of electrophysiologic study and endomyocardial biopsy in differentiating arrhythmogenic right ventricular dysplasia from idiopathic right ventricular tachycardia. Heart Vessels 5:65–69, 1990.

56. Miller JM, Vassalo JA, Kussmaul WG, et al: Anterior left ventricular aneurysm: Factors associated with the development of sustained ventricular tachycardia. J Am Coll Cardiol 12:375–382, 1988.
57. Bolic DR, Hackel DB, Reimer KA, et al: Quantitative analysis of myocardial infarct structure in patients with ventricular tachycardia. Circulation 6:1266–1279, 1986.
58. Lampert RL, Rosenfeld L, Batsford W, et al: Circadian variation of sustained ventricular tachycardia in patients with coronary artery disease and implantable cardioverter-defibrillators. Circulation 90:241–247, 1994.
59. Hohnloser SH, Klingenheben T, Loo A, et al: Reflex versus tonic vagal activity as a prognostic parameter in patients with sustained ventricular tachycardia or ventricular fibrillation. Circulation 89:1068–1073, 1994.
60. Turitto G, Ahuja RK, Caref EB, et al: Risk stratification for arrhythmic events in patients with non-ischemic dilated cardiomyopathy and nonsustained ventricular tachycardia: Role of programmed ventricular stimulation and the signal-averaged electrocardiogram. J Am Coll Cardiol 74:1523–1528, 1994.
61. Trappe HJ, Brugada P, Talajie M, et al: Prognosis of patients with ventricular tachycardia and ventricular fibrillation: Role of the underlying etiology. J Am Coll Cardiol 12:166–174, 1988.
62. Miles WM: Bundle branch reentry tachycardia: A chance to cure? J Cardiovasc Electrophysiol 4:263–265, 1993.
63. Black Z, Dhala A, Deshpande S, et al: Bundle branch reentrant ventricular tachycardia: Cumulative experience in 48 patients. J Cardiovasc Electrophysiol 4:253–262, 1993.
64. Caceres J, Jazayeri M, McKinnie J, et al: Sustained bundle branch reentry as a mechanism of clinical tachycardia. Circulation 79:256–270, 1989.
65. Black Z, Jazayeri M, Dhala A, et al: Bundle branch reentry: A mechanism of ventricular tachycardia in the absence of myocardial or valvular dysfunction. J Am Coll Cardiol 23:1718–1722, 1993.
66. Liem LB, Swerdlow CD: Value of electropharmacologic testing in idiopathic dilated cardiomyopathy and sustained ventricular tachyarrhythmias. Am J Cardiol 62:611–616, 1988.
67. Rae AP, Spielman SR, Kutalek SP, et al: Electrophysiologic assessment of antiarrhythmic drug efficacy for ventricular tachyarrhythmias associated with dilated cardiomyopathy. Am J Cardiol 59:291–295, 1987.
68. Zipes DP, Wellen HJJ: Sudden cardiac death. Circulation 98:2334–2351, 1998.
69. Leenhardt A, Coumel P, Slama R: Torsades de pointes. J Cardiovasc Electrophysiol 3:281–292, 1992.
70. Eggeling T, Oslerhues HH, Hochs M, et al: The arrhythmogenic substrate of the long QT syndrome: Genetic basis, pathology, and pathophysiologic mechanisms. Eur Heart J 14:73–79, 1993.
71. Emori T, Ohe T, Aihara N, et al: Dynamic relationship between the Q-aT interval and heart rate in patients with long QT syndrome during 24-hour Holter ECG monitoring. Pac Clin Electrophysiol 18: 1909–1918, 1995.
72. Lazzara R: Twisting of the points. J Am Coll Cardiol 29:843–844, 1997.
73. Walder LA, Spodnick DM: Global T wave inversion: Long term follow-up. J Am Coll Cardiol 21:1652–1656, 1993.
74. Lehmann MM, Hardy S, Archibald D, et al: Sex difference in risk of torsade de pointes with d,L-sotalol. Circulation 94:2535–2341, 1996.
75. Schwartz PJ, Periti M, Malliano A: The long QT syndrome. Am Heart J 89:399–411, 1975.
76. Isner JM, Roberts WC, Heymsfield SB: Anorexia nervosa and sudden death. Ann Intern Med 102:49–52, 1985.
77. Singh BN, Gaarder TD, Kanegae T, et al: Liquid protein diets and torsade de pointes. JAMA 240:115–119, 1978.
78. Kadish A, Morady F: Mechanism specific therapy of ventricular tachycardia. J Cardiovasc Electrophysiol 1:68–80, 1990.
79. Kadish AH: The effect of gender on cardiac electrophysiology and arrhythmias. In Zipes DP, Jalife J (eds): Cardiac Electrophysiology: From Cell to Bedside, 2nd ed. W.B. Saunders, Philadelphia, 1995, pp 1268–1275.
80. Mason BA, Ricci-Goodman J, Koos BJ: Adenosine in the treatment of maternal paroxysmal supraventricular tachycardia. Obstet Gyncol 80:478–480, 1992.
81. McMillan TM, Bellet S: Ventricular paroxysmal tachycardia: Report of a case in a pregnant girl of sixteen years with an apparently normal heart. Am Heart J 7:70–78, 1931.
82. Page RL: Treatment of arrhythmias during pregnancy. Am Heart J 130:871–876, 1995.
83. Chow T, Galvin J, McGovern B: Antiarrhythmic drug therapy in pregnancy and lactation. Am J Cardiol 82:581–621, 1998.
84. Cox JL, Gardner MJ: Treatment of cardiac arrhythmias during pregnancy. Prog Cardiovasc Dis 36:137–178, 1993.
85. Frishman WH, Chesner M: Beta-adrenergic blockers in pregnancy. Am Heart J 115:147–152, 1988.
86. Rubin PC, Butter SL, Clark D, et al: Obstetric aspects of the use in pregnancy-associated hypotension of the beta-adrenoceptor agonist atenolol. Am J Obstet Gynecol 150:389–392, 1984.
87. Elkayam V: Pregnancy and cardiovascular disease. In Braunwald E (ed): Heart Disease. W.B. Saunders, Philadelphia, 1992, pp 1790–1809.
88. Rotmensch HH, Elkayam V, Frishman W: Antiarrhythmic drug therapy during pregnancy. Ann Intern Med 98:487–497, 1983.
89. Meyer J, Lackner J, Schochet S: Paroxysmal tachycardia in pregnancy. JAMA 94:1901–1904, 1930.
90. Bellet S: Pregnancy. In Essentials of Cardiac Arrhythmias: Diagnosis and Management. W.B. Saunders, Philadelphia, 1972, pp 257–260.
91. Mauer A, Devaux L, Lakey M: Neonatal and maternal thrombocytopenic purpura due to quinidine. Pediatrics 19:84–87, 1957.
92. O'Hare MF, Murnaghan GA, Russel CJ, et al: Sotalol as a hypotensive agent in pregnancy. Br J Obstet Gynaecol 87:814–820, 1980.
93. Wagner X, Jouglard, Moulin M, et al: Coadministration of flecainide acetate and sotalol during pregnancy: Lack of teratogenic effects, passage across the placenta, and excretion in human breast milk. Am Heart J 119:700–702, 1990.
94. Widerhorn J, Bhandari AK, Bughi S, et al: Fetal and neonatal adverse effects profile of amiodarone treatment during pregnancy. Am Heart J 122:1162–1165, 1991.
95. De Catte L, De Wolf D, Smitz J, et al: Fetal hypothyroidism as a complication of amiodarone treatment for persistent fetal supraventricular tachycardia. Prenat Diagn 14:762–765, 1994.
96. Plomp TA, Valsma T, de Vijlder JJ: Use of amiodarone during pregnancy. Eur J Obstet Gynecol Reprod Biol 43:201–207, 1992.
97. Matsumura LK, Born D, Kunii IS, et al. Outcome of thyroid function in newborns from mothers treated with amiodarone. Thyroid 2:279–281, 1992.
98. Strange P, Frandsen J, Andreasen F: Amiodarone during pregnancy. Eur Heart J 9:108–109, 1988.
99. Robson DJ, Jeeva Raj MV, Storey GC: Use of amiodarone during pregnancy. Postgrad Med J 61:75–77, 1985.
100. Kleinman CS, Copel JH, Weinstein EM, et al: Treatment of fetal supraventricular tachyarrhythmias. J Clin Ultrasound 13:265–273, 1985.
101. Chaffman M, Brogden RN, Diltiazem: A review of its pharmacological properties and therapeutic efficacy. Drugs 29:387–454, 1985.
102. Elkayam V, Goodwin TM: Adenosine therapy for supraventricular tachycardia during pregnancy. Am J Cardiol 75:521–523, 1995.

CHAPTER

37 Heart Block

Carlos Rizo-Patron

The conduction system of the heart is responsible for the initiation and orderly transmission of an electrical impulse to the contracting myocardium and for synchronization of the atria and the ventricles. Conduction may be delayed or interrupted when any of the system's specialized structures is diseased or affected. This condition is referred to as *heart block*, a term initially coined by Gaskell[1] in 1882. All parts of the conduction system are potential sites of rhythm disturbances and heart block. Commonly seen blocks are sinoatrial (SA), atrioventricular (AV), and His-Purkinje blocks.

Heart block may be temporary or permanent and may involve one or more areas of the conduction system. Clinically, heart block is classified according to the severity of the conduction impairment. First-degree block, the mildest form of block, is manifested as a delay in conduction; however, impulses are always conducted, and this finding carries minimal clinical implications. Second-degree block is the intermittent interruption of conduction. Two forms have been described, one characterized by a progressive increase in the delay in conduction until block occurs (Mobitz type I) and another characterized by alternations between conduction and block (Mobitz type II). Third-degree block is the absence of conduction through a certain area of the conduction system.

Heart block should not be confused with functional "interference," in which the conduction delay or block occurs secondary to physiologic refractoriness created by a preceding impulse. Pauses resulting from interference of the conduction system are considered normal phenomena.

SINOATRIAL BLOCK

SA block occurs when the sinus impulse exits to the atria, and it is classified as first-, second-, or third-degree block. First-degree SA block theoretically occurs, although it cannot be recognized on a surface electrocardiogram (ECG) because the time of sinus impulse initiation cannot be seen.[2] Second-degree SA block is clinically demonstrable and is divided into Mobitz types I and II. Third-degree SA block results in the absence of atrial activation by the sinus node and is manifested as the lack of sinus P waves on a surface ECG.

Sinoatrial Block Mobitz Type I

SA block Mobitz type I is characterized by a cycle of progressive shortening of the PP interval followed by a pause (Fig. 37–1). The sinus pause is not a multiple of the PP intervals. When the block ratio is 3:2, it can simulate a sinus bigeminal pattern or "pseudobigeminy" (Fig. 37–2). This type of block can be a manifestation of high vagal tone, drug effect, or sick sinus syndrome. For clinical ECG recognition, at least a 4:3 ratio must be present. Diagnosis is difficult, especially when sinus arrhythmia is also present.

Sinoatrial Block Mobitz Type II

SA block Mobitz type II is the most common form of SA block.[2] It is characterized by an intermittent block in the SA area. Absence of one or more P waves results in a sinus pause that can be seen on a surface ECG (Fig. 37–3). The pauses are a multiple of the basic sinus rate or PP interval. When a 2:1 block occurs, patients may present with bradycardia, often with associated symptoms.[3, 4] Occasional high-degree SA block can occur, resulting in significant pauses leading to dizzy spells or episodes of syncope. Symptomatic block is an indication for implantation of a permanent pacemaker.

ATRIOVENTRICULAR BLOCK

AV block occurs when an atrial impulse is delayed or blocked at the level of the AV node or His bundle before it reaches the ventricles. Under normal circumstances, the AV node acts as a gatekeeper, protecting the ventricles from nonphysiologic high heart rates. In the case of atrial tachyarrhythmias, the AV node responds with physiologic delay and block as a result of its decremental conduction properties. Pathologic AV block can be considered only when the block occurs outside the physiologic block rates.

Differences in the conduction properties of the AV node and the His-Purkinje system and their responses to autonomic stimulation allow clinicians to infer the site of block from ECG characteristics, escape rates, and response to autonomic maneuvers.[5]

AV nodal blocks are commonly associated with a normal QRS complex, are worsened by vagal stimulation or sleep, and are improved by high sympathetic tone. His-Purkinje blocks are likely to be accompanied by a wide QRS complex and are not directly affected by vagal stimuli. Clinically, conduction might improve secondary to vagal slowing of the sinus rate. Acceleration of the sinus rate results in worsening of block.

Intracardiac His recordings may be useful in determining the site of block, particularly in the following situations: (1) second-degree AV block Mobitz type I with wide QRS complex,[6] (2) second-degree AV block Mobitz type II with normal QRS complex, and (3) second-degree AV block in which a concealed His extrasystole is suspected to be the cause of the block.[7]

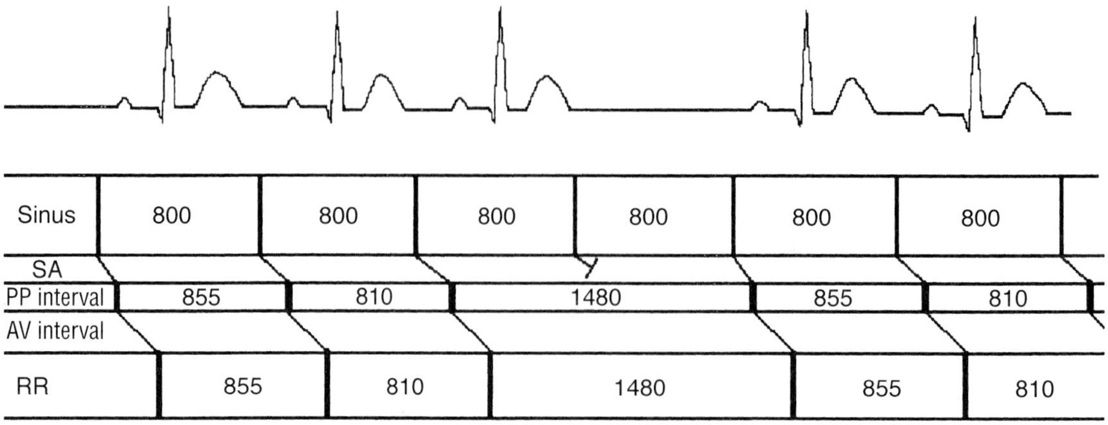

FIGURE 37–1. Sinoatrial block Mobitz type I.

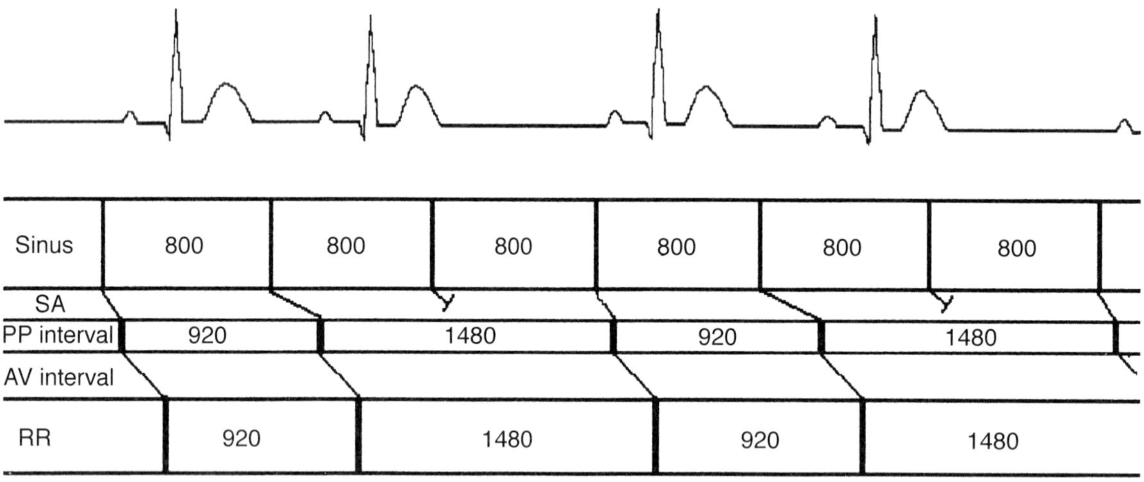

FIGURE 37–2. Sinoatrial block Mobitz type I with 3:2 ratio, simulating a sinus bigeminal pattern ("pseudobigeminy").

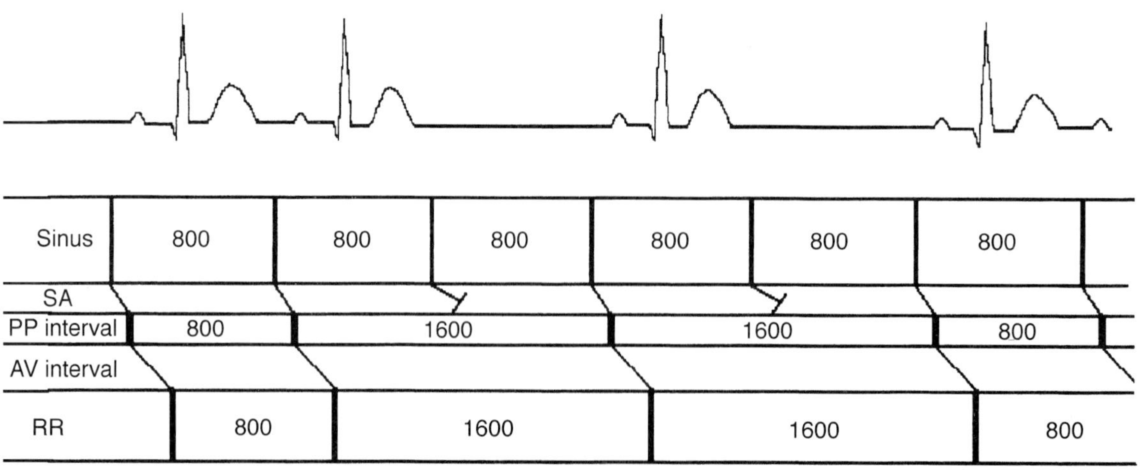

FIGURE 37–3. Sinoatrial block Mobitz type II.

Blocks in the AV node usually follow a predictable pattern, in contrast to His-Purkinje blocks, which are unpredictable and abrupt. Minor increases in atrial rates can produce profound changes in block. For this reason, an aggressive therapeutic strategy should be sought whenever intrahisian or infrahisian block is suspected. Profound bradycardia associated with heart block has been implicated as a cause of malignant ventricular arrhythmias.[8] Women seem to be at particular risk of developing torsades de pointes secondary to second- or third-degree heart block. Kawasaki and colleagues,[9] in a retrospective review of all reported cases of torsades de pointes related to acquired heart block, demonstrated that 72% of cases occurred in females, compared with an expected incidence of 52%.

First-Degree Atrioventricular Block

First-degree AV block is a delay in the conduction of a sinus or nonpremature atrial impulse to the ventricles. All atrial impulses are conducted, maintaining a 1:1 ratio between the atria and the ventricles. An atrial rhythm and a ventricular complex are seen on a surface ECG. The PR interval is longer than 0.20 sec (200 msec) and may vary with changes in the atrial rate. Slower atrial rates might result in normalization of the PR interval; faster rates, in longer PRs.

There are three possible mechanisms to explain first-degree AV block. Prolongation of the PR interval can result from slow AV nodal conduction (prolonged A-H interval), delayed conduction in the His-Purkinje system (prolonged H-V interval), or slow intra-atrial conduction (prolonged PA interval) (Fig. 37–4). The site of conduction delay can be determined only by using intracardiac His recordings.

A premature atrial impulse that does not originate in the sinus node and has a PR interval greater than 0.20 sec cannot be considered first-degree AV block. The conduction time between the site of atrial impulse origin and the AV node can be longer than that from the sinus node to the AV node. The conduction time is related to distance rather than delay, resulting in a prolonged PR interval.

Narula[10] found that the majority of clinical cases of prolonged PR intervals (79%) resulted from the presence of multiple sites of conduction delay. Puech and colleagues[11] found this to be true only 20% of the time. The significant site of delay in 83% of cases is the AV node.[10] The QRS duration may provide insight into the level of conduction delay. When the QRS is 0.11 sec or shorter, the delay is most likely to be in the AV node.[11] In rare instances, the delay occurs in the His bundle (as manifested by split His signals on intracardiac recordings) or by equal delays in both the right and left bundle branches. These also result in a narrow QRS on a surface ECG (Fig. 37–5).

When first-degree AV block and bundle branch block (QRS longer than 0.11 sec) occur together, the delay can be in the AV node or the His-Purkinje system and often in both.[11] Treatment with medications that can prolong infranodal conduction (e.g., class I antiarrhythmics) may precipitate Mobitz type II second-degree AV block and should be used cautiously. Intracardiac recordings to determine the site of block can be helpful in identifying patients at risk.

First-degree AV block occurs in a number of common clinical settings. High vagal tone in athletes and use of negative dromotropic drugs (e.g., beta blockers, calcium channel antagonists, digoxin, clonidine)[12] are common causes of AV conduction delay and first-degree AV block seen in clinical practice. These situations usually do not result in clinical symptoms; thus, therapy is not necessary.[6, 13] Disease states such as acute myocarditis, acute rheumatic fever, Lyme disease, and endocarditis can manifest with prolongation of the PR interval. Healthy individuals in whom the appearance of first-degree AV block is acute should be observed closely for the development of more advanced degrees of AV block that could require intervention. Frequently, patients with first-degree AV block experience

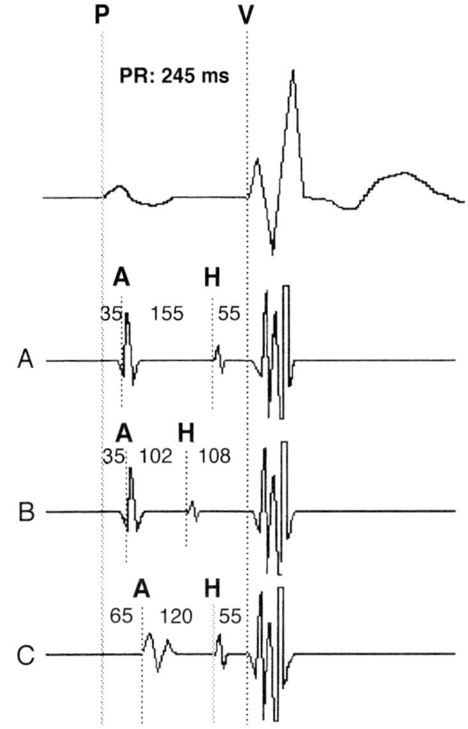

FIGURE 37–4. Mechanisms of first-degree atrioventricular (AV) block. *A*, Prolonged AV node conduction; *B*, prolonged infranodal conduction; *C*, prolonged atrial conduction times.

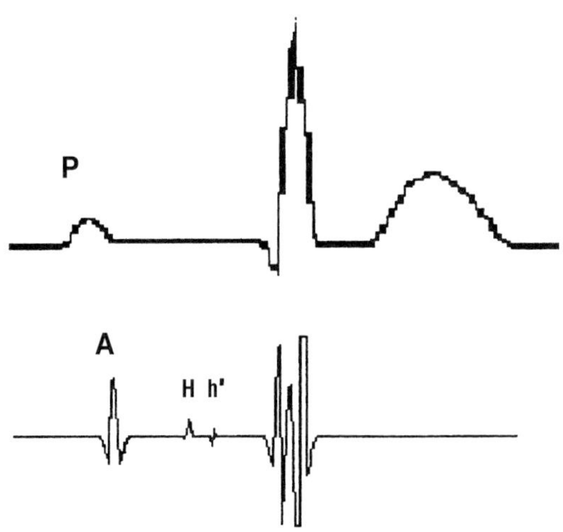

FIGURE 37–5. First-degree atrioventricular (AV) block due to intrahisian conduction delay.

transient Mobitz type I second-degree AV block when the sinus rate rises or during vagal maneuvers.

There are instances in which the PR interval can be as long as 0.6 to 0.8 sec. The atrial contraction occurs during ventricular systole, causing atrial stretching and the equivalent of pacemaker syndrome ("pacemaker syndrome without a pacemaker" or "pseudopacemaker syndrome").[14, 15] In these cases, patients may present with exercise intolerance, diastolic mitral regurgitation, and visible cannon waves in the jugular venous pulse. Barold[16] suggested that there could be a benefit from AV synchronization with the use of dual-chamber AV sequential pacing and that this syndrome should be considered a class II indication for dual-chamber pacing.

Patients with first-degree AV block, dilated cardiomyopathy, and congestive heart failure also seem to benefit from pacemaker implantation. This concept is currently considered investigational.[17, 18]

Second-Degree Atrioventricular Block

Second-degree AV block is the intermittent failure of conduction of certain atrial impulses to the ventricles secondary to conduction delays or to blocks in the AV junction or His-Purkinje system. Regular or irregular rhythms can result, depending on the frequency and periodicity of the intermittent conduction failure. Historically, this type of block was referred to as "incomplete block," a term that has been abandoned.

The first descriptions and classifications of second-degree AV block were made by Wenckebach[19] in 1899 and Hay[20] in 1906 and were based on clinical findings in the jugular venous pulses. In 1924, Mobitz[21] classified second-degree AV block into two types on the basis of electrocardiographic patterns. The advent of intracardiac His recordings allowed precise determination of the site of block.

Second-Degree Atrioventricular Block Mobitz Type I

Mobitz type I block (also known as the Wenckebach phenomenon) is the most common type of second-degree AV block.[11] The following four features characterize this type of block:

1. Progressive prolongation of the PR interval in consecutively conducted beats until one atrial impulse fails to be conducted (the increment by which the PR interval is prolonged decreases with each successive beat in the cycle).
2. Progressive shortening of the RR interval until a pause occurs.
3. A pause whose duration is shorter than twice the PP interval.
4. A sinus or atrial rate that is almost constant (equal PP intervals).

If all the criteria are met, the block is considered a typical Wenckebach phenomenon (Fig. 37–6), with varying conduction ratios (3:2, 4:3, 5:4, etc.) designating the relationship between atrial and ventricular depolarizations. In clinical practice, this typical block is seen with relatively low conduction ratios and accounts for less than 20% of spontaneous Mobitz type I blocks and approximately 35% of those induced by atrial pacing.[22]

In the more common atypical form, an initial progressive prolongation of the PR interval is followed by an almost

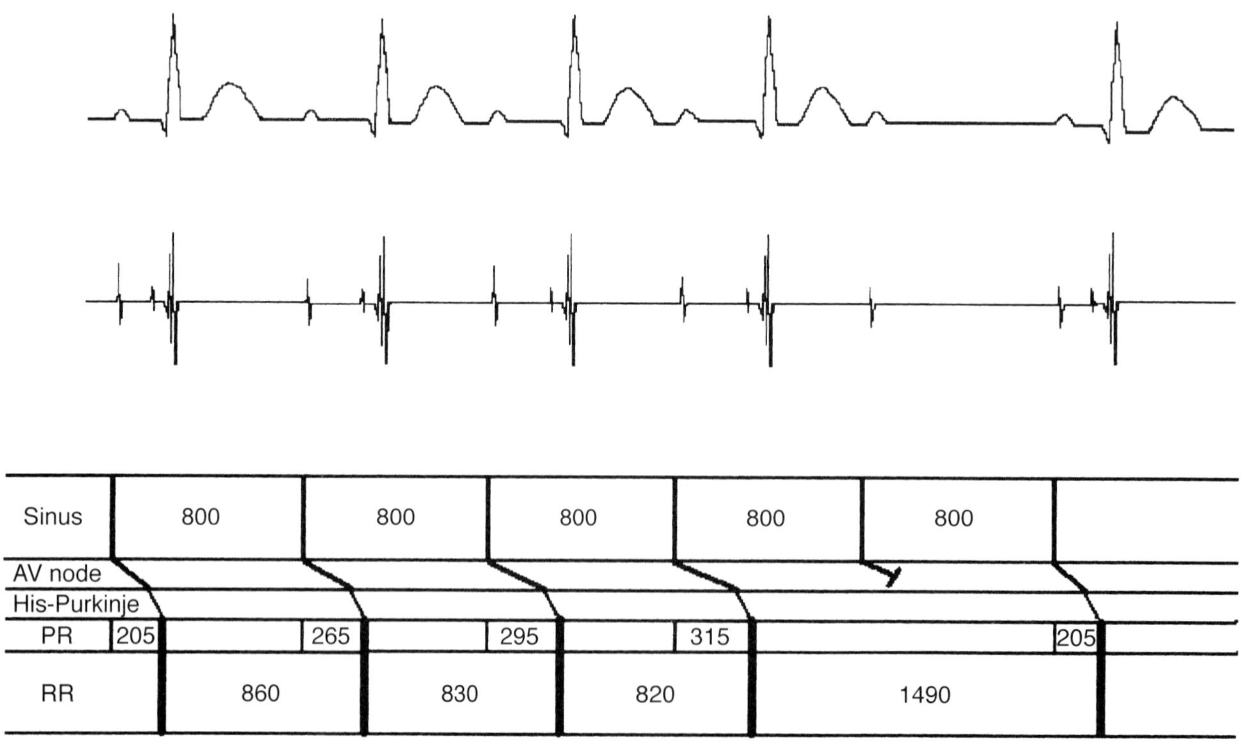

FIGURE 37–6. Second-degree atrioventricular (AV) block Mobitz type I (typical Wenckebach phenomenon).

constant long PR and a sudden nonconducted P wave. The pause following the nonconducted P is shorter than twice the PP interval. The first conducted beat following the dropped P has a shorter PR interval than that of the last conducted beat before the pause. The first PR interval is commonly prolonged; rarely does the last conducted beat have a PR interval shorter than 300 msec. In the atypical Wenckebach block, the PR interval of the last conducted beat may be prolonged significantly, suddenly lengthening the R-R interval and making the pause less apparent.

The presence of a Mobitz type I second-degree AV block and a normal QRS complex suggests the conduction delay or block is in the AV node.[11] In rare instances, 3:2 or 4:3 blocks can be seen in which the conducted beats have a normal QRS duration and a constant normal or mildly prolonged PR interval. This ECG finding is suggestive of intrahisian block (Fig. 37–7). When a Mobitz type I block is associated with a wide QRS complex, there could be multiple levels of block (i.e., in the AV node or the bundle branches or, in rare cases, a Wenckebach block at the level of the His-Purkinje system).[23]

Mobitz type I block occurs in some healthy people during periods of high vagal tone (e.g., in athletes,[24, 25] during sleep,[26] or as a consequence of using drugs that slow AV nodal conduction). In the elderly, Mobitz type I block occurs with mild dysfunction of AV nodal conduction. This type of second-degree AV block rarely results in clinical symptoms. Documented symptoms directly related to Mobitz type I block are the only indication for pacemaker therapy.

Second-Degree Atrioventricular Block Mobitz Type II

Second-degree AV block Mobitz type II is much less common than Mobitz type I but more clinically significant. The block almost always occurs at the level of the His-Purkinje system (35% within the His bundle and 65% distal to the His bundle).[11, 23, 27] This type of block is characterized by the following findings (Fig 37–8):

1. The periodic occurrence of nonconducted atrial impulses without a preceding Wenckebach phenomenon.
2. A constant PR interval (usually normal)[23] in all conducted beats and in the first beat after the pause.
3. R-R intervals that are multiples of PP intervals.
4. Common association with bundle branch blocks or fascicular blocks (although a narrow QRS complex is present in 35% of cases).[10]

In contrast to Mobitz type I, Mobitz type II block may be marked by sudden unexpected drops in conduction of an atrial beat or different ratios of AV conduction (1:1, 2:1, and 3:1) (see Fig. 37–8). These sudden changes can be seen with or without concomitant changes in the atrial rates. Mobitz type II is known to precede complete heart block and Stokes-Adams attacks. The presence of associated symptoms is a class I indication for pacemaker implantation.[28] Asymptomatic permanent and intermittent second-degree AV block Mobitz type II are considered class II indications for permanent pacing under current American College of Cardiology/American Heart Association (ACC/AHA) guidelines.[28] Pacemakers that maintain AV synchrony are preferred.

Second-Degree Atrioventricular Block with 2:1 Behavior

Second-degree AV block with a 2:1 AV conduction ratio is difficult to classify by Mobitz type, although the block is localized below the AV node in two thirds of cases.[10, 11]

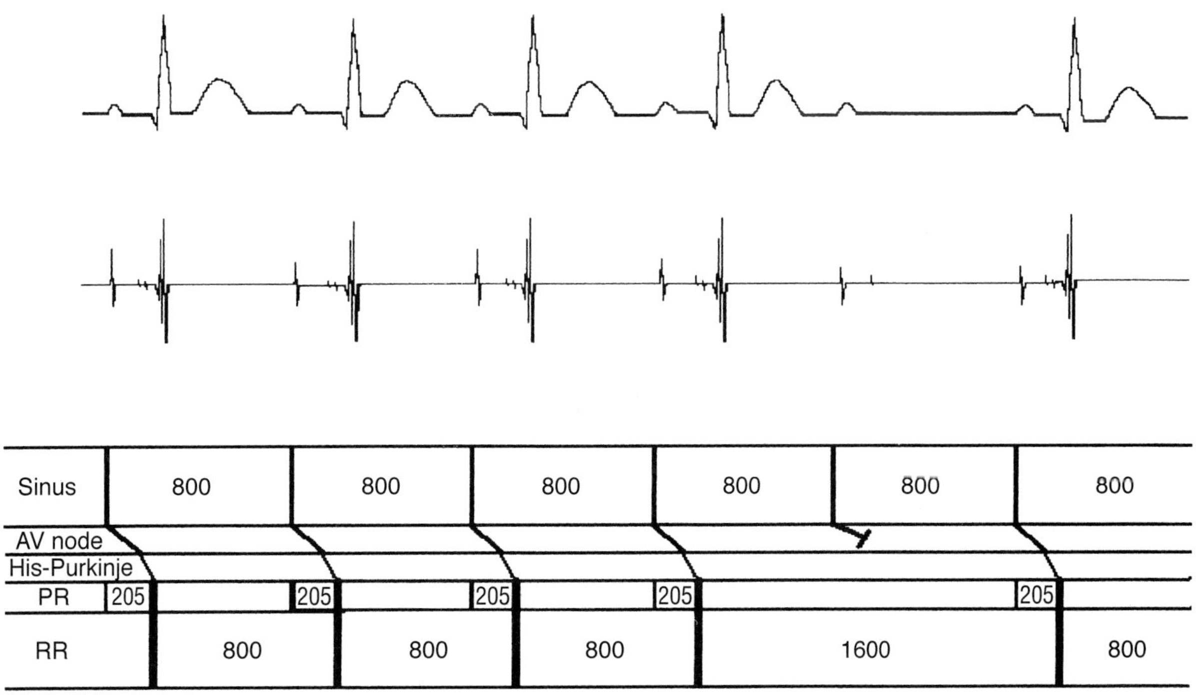

FIGURE 37–7. Intrahisian block.

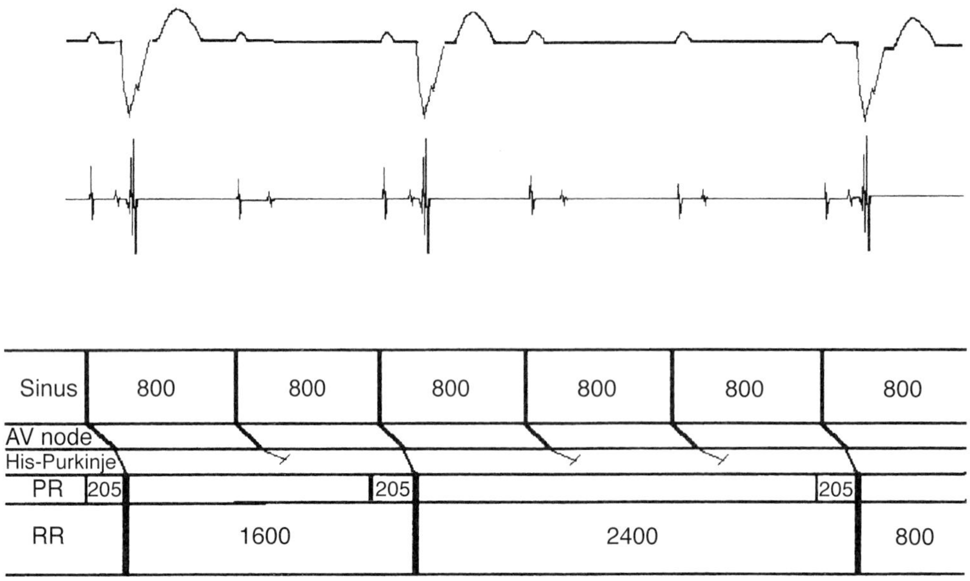

FIGURE 37–8. Second-degree atrioventricular (AV) block Mobitz type II.

The following clinical and ECG characteristics may aid in determining the type and level of block.

QRS Width. A 2:1 block with a narrow QRS interval is more commonly seen in cases of AV nodal involvement and is suggestive of Mobitz type I block. The presence of a bundle branch block does not help determine whether the level of block is AV nodal or infranodal tissue but makes Mobitz type II block the most likely diagnosis.

Wenckebach Periodicity on Electrocardiography. The presence of Wenckebach periodicity on ECG, before or after the appearance of the 2:1 block, suggests a Mobitz I type block. A 2:1 block is usually seen when the atrial rate accelerates or when a high vagal tone is present. When atropine is administered to patients with 2:1 Mobitz type I block, conduction improves, with recovery of 1:1 AV conduction or ratios of Wenckebach periodicity. In contrast, when atropine is given to patients with Mobitz type II block, block ratios can progress from 2:1 to 3:1 as a result of acceleration of the atrial rhythm with no improvement in infranodal conduction.

Vagal Maneuvers. When performed cautiously, vagal maneuvers can help differentiate the type of second-degree AV block. The decrease in atrial rate and worsening of AV node conduction create higher degrees of block in patients with Mobitz type I block. In patients with Mobitz type II block, slowing of the atrial rate can result in improvement of conduction to a 1:1 ratio without its passing through Wenckebach periodicity. Although these maneuvers are helpful, they do not always elicit the expected type of response.[29]

THIRD-DEGREE ATRIOVENTRICULAR BLOCK

Third-degree AV block is also referred to as *complete heart block*. It is characterized by the presence of independent atrial and ventricular rhythms and the inability of the atrial stimuli to be conducted to the ventricles (Fig. 37–9). In the majority of cases, the block is below the AV node, preferentially at the level of the bundle branches.[10, 11, 30] Block at the level of the AV node is seen in approximately 20% of cases. According to Puech and colleagues,[11] supra-His involvement when the escape rhythm QRS is narrow is seen in 53% of cases.

The escape rhythm in complete heart block comes from a subsidiary pacemaker at the level immediately below the site of block. In the case of AV nodal block or intrahisian block, the escape rhythm (40 to 60 bpm) comes from the AV junction or the His and demonstrates normal QRS morphologies in most cases[31] (Fig. 37–9*B*). If the block is in the distal His or the bundles, the escape rhythm (20 to 40 bpm) is fascicular or ventricular (Fig. 37–9*A*). Compared with men, elderly women have been shown to have a higher incidence of hisian block due to mitral ring calcification.[32]

In acquired third-degree AV block, symptoms depend on the rate of the escape rhythm. When the block is infranodal, Stokes-Adams syndrome, dizziness, and heart failure are common presenting symptoms and require immediate attention. Patients with symptomatic third-degree AV block and a temporary pacemaker catheter in place should be closely monitored, because overdrive suppression of the escape focus by pacing can result in prolonged periods of asystole. According to ACC/AHA guidelines, third-degree AV block is a class I indication for pacemaker implantation.[28]

ATRIOVENTRICULAR DISSOCIATION

AV dissociation is a generic term used in ECG to describe a phenomenon in which the atrial and ventricular rhythms are independent or dissociated. The term is not synonymous with AV block and is not mechanistically descriptive. Sometimes the AV dissociation is interrupted by conducted beats ("capture beats"), resulting in what has been referred to as "incomplete AV dissociation." This finding can be seen in AV dissociation due to default or usurpation (see later), but it is very uncommon in the presence of third-degree heart

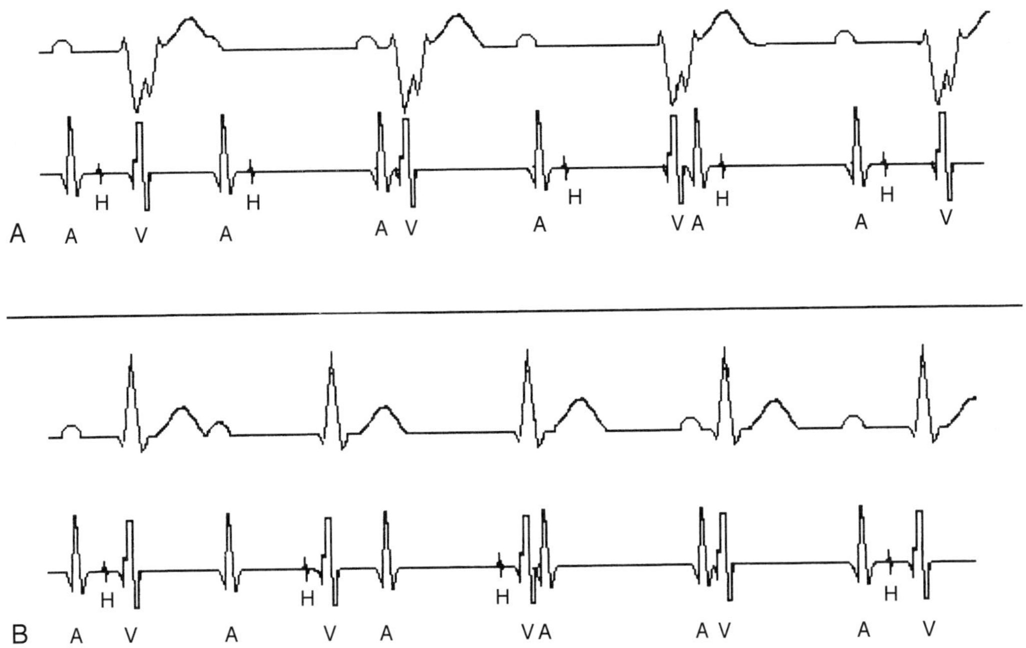

FIGURE 37–9. Third-degree atrioventricular (AV) block. *A,* Infranodal block, with wide complex idioventricular escape rhythm of 30-40 bpm. *B,* AV nodal block, with escape rhythm from low junction.

block. When the sinus and the subsidiary pacemaker have very similar rates (a phenomenon known as *isorhythmic dissociation*), it is difficult to establish a diagnosis of AV dissociation. AV dissociation is usually just a manifestation of a precipitating cause, and treatment is needed to correct the underlying disease.

Atrioventricular Dissociation by Default

AV dissociation by default occurs when the sinus node (the dominant pacemaker of the heart) slows its rate and a subsidiary pacemaker takes over. The escape rate of the subsidiary pacemaker is higher than the sinus bradycardia. As a consequence, the atria are activated through the sinus node, and the ventricles are activated at the rate of the next subsidiary dominant pacemaker, usually the AV junction. Considering that the escape rate of the junction is within normal limits, the patient will have bradycardia. No retrograde atrial activation is present.

Atrioventricular Dissociation by Usurpation

AV dissociation by usurpation occurs when the dominant pacemaker has a normal or slow rate of discharge but a subsidiary lower pacemaker has an accelerated discharge. The accelerated rhythm takes command of the ventricles, and the atria beat independently at the sinus rate. A condition for this occurrence is the absence of retrograde ventriculoatrial conduction.

Atrioventricular Dissociation Due to Third-Degree Atrioventricular Block

AV dissociation due to third-degree AV block is secondary to a conduction block at the level of the AV node or the His-Purkinje system. The atrial impulse is not transmitted down to the ventricles. Because the independent atrial and ventricular beatings usually occur at rates proper for their places in the pacemaker hierarchy, it is common to see normal sinus rates exceeding the ventricular rates (see Fig. 37–9).

Combined Atrioventricular Dissociation

When the above forms of AV dissociation are combined, slowing of the sinus node with junctional accelerated rhythms and AV block can occur. An example is AV dissociation caused by digitalis intoxication.

CONGENITAL HEART BLOCK

The structures of the cardiac conduction system arise from different embryologic sources.[33] The AV node and the His-Purkinje system develop as separate primordia that ultimately join.[34] Congenital complete heart block, first described by Morqui[35] in 1901, results from a discontinuity between the different parts of the conduction system. Congenital complete heart block is classified into (1) blocks associated with other congenital cardiac malformations and (2) blocks associated with otherwise normally structured hearts.[36] Pathologically it is also classified into (1) atrial-axis discontinuity, (2) nodoventricular discontinuity, and (3) intraventricular discontinuity.[36]

The association between maternal anti-Ro/SS-A and La/SS-B antibodies and congenital complete heart block has been well documented.[37–39] Li and colleagues[40] suggested that molecular similarities between laminin and La contribute to the pathogenesis of the disease. In cases of complete heart block related to the presence of maternal anti-Ro/SS-A and La/SS-B, the most common pathologic finding is discontinuity between the atria and the His conduction system, in which the AV node is replaced by fibrous tissue.[41] Heart block does not develop in all fetuses exposed to anti-Ro/SS-A.[42] There is a case report of twins—one born with complete heart block and the other with normal conduction—who both had anti-Ro/SS-A cord titers and similar HLA types.[43]

The mothers of patients with complete heart block are usually asymptomatic at the time of delivery[44] but have a high incidence of connective tissue disorders, such as undifferentiated autoimmune syndrome, systemic lupus erythematosus (SLE), and Sjögren's syndrome.[44, 45] Mothers of children with complete heart block also have a higher incidence of HLA-B8, HLA-DR3, and HLA-DQ than do healthy mothers and mothers with SLE who have normal children.[46]

Atrioventricular Block in the Fetus

Heart block in the fetus should be suspected in the presence of fetal bradycardia. The use of Doppler echocardiography helps confirm the diagnosis and identify any associated cardiac malformations.[47] Schmidt and colleagues[48] found that 29 of 55 fetuses (53%) with congenital complete heart block had associated cardiac malformations (e.g., left atrial isomerism, AV septal defects, aortopulmonary transposition, pulmonary stenosis, or atresia). The presence of heart failure or hydrops fetalis indicates a poor prognosis.[47, 49] The use of transplacental steroids to prevent progression and cause regression of AV block has reportedly been successful in some cases.[50, 51] Sympathomimetics administered by direct umbilical vein infusion can improve the ventricular rate and help control hydrops fetalis.[52] Groves and associates[47] successfully used salbutamol in treating three cases of complete heart block leading to fetal heart failure. Anandakumar and coworkers[49] used direct furosemide and digoxin in fetuses with some success, but at the risk of preterm labor and infection. Studies in fetal lambs have shown the feasibility of intrauterine transvenous[53, 54] and epicardial[55] pacing for this condition.

Not all echocardiographically detected heart blocks have a poor prognosis. Friedman and colleagues[56] reported cases in which fetal 2:1 AV block without hydrops spontaneously reverted to normal conduction before delivery.

Atrioventricular Block in Newborns and Children

Congenital complete heart block affects 1 in 20,000 to 25,000 live births.[57] In a study of 34 infants with congenital complete heart block and no other structural heart disease, 15% died in the first year.[58] In a study of 16 infants with congenital complete heart block, 3 (18.7%) died and 8 (50%) required permanent pacing for symptoms. Heart rates of less than 55 bpm associated with symptoms, congestive heart failure, ventricular ectopy, or prolonged QT interval indicate the need for permanent pacing in this population.[59]

Congenital Atrioventricular Block in Adults

In a long-term follow-up study by Michaelsson and associates,[60] a population of 102 patients (61 women and 41 men) with congenital heart block had a high incidence of Stokes-Adams attacks (27%); the attacks were fatal to 30% of the affected patients. More than 50% of patients required pacemaker implantation as treatment for symptoms of dizziness, fainting spells, effort dyspnea, ectopy, or low ventricular rate. Of note, the patients in this study showed a progressive decrease in subsidiary pacemaker rate.[60]

PATHOLOGIC CORRELATES OF ATRIOVENTRICULAR BLOCK

In the early 1900s, Tawara,[61] Humblet,[62] Hering,[63] and Mahaim[64] conducted the first pathologic studies to explain AV block. It is now known that conduction abnormalities can result from acute or chronic injuries to the conduction tissues caused by a wide range of disorders.

The disorder may involve the conduction tissue primarily or may arise from continuity with surrounding structures. Davies and colleagues[34] described their necropsy findings in 200 patients who had had AV block of at least 1 month's duration. Primary (idiopathic) degenerative disease of the conduction system accounted for 38% of cases, coronary disease for 17%, dilated cardiomyopathy for 13%, and calcific involvement by continuity for 11%. The remaining 20% of cases had miscellaneous causes, including infiltrative diseases, congenital disease, and acute myocarditis. In the same study, the most common site of involvement was the bundle branches, followed by the His bundle. The AV node or prenodal area was compromised in only 9%. In an earlier but conflicting study, Knieriem and Finkle[65] described the findings from 100 necropsies and concluded that fibrosis secondary to atherosclerotic coronary disease accounted for the great majority of cases of AV block.

Very few causes of AV block are reversible. Therefore, the only available therapy is the implantation of pacemakers.

Lev's Disease

In 1964, Lev[66] described an idiopathic entity in which loss of fibers at bifurcation and proximal portions of the left and right bundles leaves "ghost" structures. This degenerative process is usually associated with degeneration of the membranous septum, aortic-mitral annulus, and mitral annulus. Lev correlated the process with the presence of hypertensive heart disease and concluded that the progression from bundle branch disease to AV block can be a slow process that might take decades.[66]

Lenègre's Disease

In the same year that Lev's disease was first described, Lenègre first described a more diffuse disease affecting the distal portions of the bundle branches. In Lenègre's disease, the loss of fibers is replaced by fibrosis and does not leave "ghost" structures. This disease is less common than Lev's disease.[67] Intermediate forms between Lev's and Lenègre's diseases have also been described.[34]

ATRIOVENTRICULAR BLOCK ASSOCIATED WITH MYOCARDIAL INFARCTIONS

Atrioventricular block may develop in 5% to 13% of patients presenting with acute myocardial infarction (MI).[68–70] It occurs more frequently in inferoposterior infarcts than in anterior infarcts,[70] but anterior infarcts are associated with a higher incidence of permanent block.[71] In the presence of AV block, patients with MI have a higher in-hospital mortality[68, 70, 73–76] and worse ventricular dysfunction.[73, 74, 76, 77] The site of infarction, level of conduction involvement, escape rhythm, and hemodynamics determine the prognosis of patients with AV block.[68, 70]

Atrioventricular Block and Inferior Wall Myocardial Infarction

The incidence of AV block in inferoposterior MI is 10% to 20%.[68, 70, 73–75, 77, 78] There are two distinct clinical presentations of AV block in patients with inferoposterior MI. One is manifested as a sudden onset of high-degree AV block early in the course of the infarction (in the first 4 to 6 hours), is usually transient, and disappears in the first 24 hours. The second manifests later in the course of infarction (after 24 hours), is usually preceded by first-degree and second-degree AV block, and has a more prolonged course (average duration, 40 hours).[78, 79] Overlap between these two clinical presentations can be seen. There is controversy concerning the response of the early-onset type of AV block to atropine. Data from Feigl and colleagues[78] suggest that patients with early block show good response to atropine, whereas data from Sclarovsky and associates[79] and Onodera and coworkers[80] suggest that they do not.

Most of the information about AV block is from the prethrombolytic era. Data from two large-scale thrombolytic studies concerning the incidence of AV block in inferior MI—the Thrombolysis in Myocardial Infarction (TIMI) II trial[73] and the Thrombolysis and Angioplasty in Myocardial Infarction (TAMI) trial[77]—suggest that the condition and its negative prognostic risk remain unchanged. The presence of AV block continues to be associated with higher mortality (9.9% in the TIMI II trial[73] and 20% in the TAMI trial[77]), a rate 2.7 to 5 times higher than seen in patients with inferior MI who do not present with heart block. The infarct-related artery is more often the right coronary artery,[73] the artery is often occluded after administration of recombinant tissue plasminogen activator,[77] and there is a higher incidence of right ventricular infarction and right ventricular dysfunction.[73, 76, 81] The cause of death in this population is not heart block but is related to the extent of myocardial damage. Interestingly, in the TAMI trial, AV conduction block lasted less than 12 hours (median, 2.5 hours) in 75% of the cases in which plasminogen activator was administered[77]; nevertheless, block was still associated with higher mortality.

The current ACC/AHA guidelines for management of MI[82] recommend the immediate use of atropine in cases of symptomatic second- or third-degree AV block and narrow QRS complex accompanying inferior MI. If there is no response to atropine, temporary pacing is indicated. Transvenous temporary pacing is preferred to transcutaneous pacing in this setting because of the high probability that constant pacing will be required and the discomfort related to transcutaneous pacing. Permanent pacemaker implantation is indicated only if advanced AV block persists (class IIB ACC/AHA indication)[28] or if concomitant hisian or infrahisian disease is present (class I indication). There have been several reports of the successful use of theophylline to treat patients with atropine-resistant AV block.[83–86]

Atrioventricular Block and Anterior Myocardial Infarction

Although less common than heart block associated with inferoposterior infarcts, heart block associated with anterior MI is commonly associated with permanent damage to the conduction system (predominantly infranodal damage at the level of the bundle branches).[71, 87] Few studies have been reported in patients with this condition. Norris[70] reported a 75% mortality in patients with anterior MI associated with high-degree AV block. Another large-scale retrospective review found 70% mortality in patients who received pacing and 100% mortality in those who did not. Current guidelines suggest permanent pacing in patients with (1) persistent second-degree AV block with infranodal involvement and (2) third-degree AV block. When the block is located at the level of the AV node, permanent pacing is considered a class IIb indication.

Bundle Branch Block and Myocardial Infarction

New bundle branch block with MI occurs in approximately 8% to 13% of patients.[88–90] Patients who manifest bundle branch block are older, have larger infarcts, and have infarcts that are more often anterior (60%) than inferior (37%). The incidences of AV block, atrial fibrillation, and ventricular fibrillation as well as in-hospital mortality are higher than in patients without bundle branch block.[89, 90] Patients with anterior wall MI and bundle branch block have a high risk of progression to higher degrees of block and in-hospital mortality,[88, 89] particularly those with right bundle branch block.[91] Ricou and associates[91] found that patients with new right bundle branch block in association with anterior MI had poorer left ventricular function and higher rates of in-hospital and 1-year mortality.[91] Pathologically, there is a high incidence of necrosis at the right bundle. Thrombolytics have been shown to completely resolve right bundle branch block when used in association with reperfusion.[92]

References

1. Gaskell WH: On the rhythm of the heart of the frog and the nature of the action of the vagus nerve. Philos Trans R Soc Lond 17:993, 1882.
2. Narula OS: Disorders of sinus node: Electrophysiologic evaluation. In Narula OS (ed): Cardiac Arrhythmias: Electrophysiology, Diagnosis and Management. Williams & Wilkins, Baltimore, 1979, p 275.
3. Rosen KM, Loeb HS, Sinno MZ, et al: Cardiac conduction in patients with symptomatic sinus node disease. Circulation 43:836, 1971.
4. Rubenstein JJ, Schulman CL, Yurchak PM, et al: Clinical spectrum of the sick sinus syndrome. Circulation 46:5, 1972.
5. Mangiardi LM, Bonamini R, Conte M, et al: Bedside evaluation of atrioventricular block with narrow QRS complexes: Usefulness of carotid sinus massage and atropine administration. Am J Cardiol 49: 1136, 1982.
6. Gallastegui J, Hariman RJ: Indications for intracardiac electrophysiologic studies in patients with atrioventricular and intraventricular blocks not associated with acute myocardial infarction. Circulation 75:103, 1987.
7. Bhandari AK, Rahimtoola SH: Intracardiac electrophysiologic studies in patients with atrioventricular and intraventricular blocks not associated with acute myocardial infarction. Circulation 75:107, 1987.
8. Gladman G, Davis AM, Fogelman R, et al: Torsade de pointes, acquired complete heart block and inappropriately long QT in childhood. Can J Cardiol 12:683, 1996.
9. Kawasaki R, Machado C, Reinoehl J, et al: Increased propensity of women to develop torsades de pointes during complete heart block. J Cardiovasc Electrophysiol 6:1032, 1995.
10. Narula OS: Atrioventricular block. In Narula OS (ed): Cardiac Arrhythmias: Electrophysiology, Diagnosis and Management. Williams & Wilkins, Baltimore, 1979, p 85.
11. Puech P, Grolleau R, Guimond C: Incidence of different types of A-V block and their localization by His bundle recordings. In Wellens HJJ, Lie KI, Janse M (eds): The Conduction System of the Heart. HE Stenfert Kroese, Leiden, 1976, p 467.
12. Massumi RA: Atrioventricular block: A noninvasive approach to the problem. In Mandel W (ed): Cardiac Arrhythmias: Their Mechanisms, Diagnosis and Management. Philadelphia, JB Lippincott, 1987, p 343.
13. Mymin D, Mathewson FA, Tate RB, et al: The natural history of primary first-degree atrioventricular heart block. N Engl J Med 315: 1183, 1986.
14. Chirife R, Ortega DE, Salazar AL: "Pacemaker syndrome" without a pacemaker: Deleterious effects of first-degree AV block. RBM 12: 22, 1990.
15. Zornosa JP, Crossley GH, Haisty WK: Pseudopacemaker syndrome: A complication of radiofrequency ablation of the AV junction. Pacing Clin Electrophysiol 15:590, 1992.
16. Barold SS: Indications for permanent cardiac pacing in first-degree AV block: Class I, II, or III? Pacing Clin Electrophysiol 19:747, 1996.
17. Paul V, Cowell R, Morris-Thurgood J: First-degree heart block in heart failure: Is this a class one indication for dual-chamber pacing? Pacing Clin Electrophysiol 18:906, 1995.
18. Nishimura RA, Hayes DL, Holmes DR, et al: Mechanism of hemodynamic improvement by dual-chamber pacing for severe left ventricular dysfunction: An acute Doppler and catheterization hemodynamic study. J Am Coll Cardiol 25:281, 1995.
19. Wenckebach KF: Zur analyse des unregelmassigen pulses. Z Klin Med 37:475, 1899.
20. Hay J: Bradycardia and cardiac arrhythmia produced by depression of certain functions of the heart. Lancet 1:139, 1906.
21. Mobitz W: Uber die unvollstandige storung der erregungsuberleitung zwischen Vorhof und Kammer des menschilchen herzens. Z Gesamte Exp Med 41:180, 1924.
22. Denes P, Levy L, Pick A, et al: The incidence of typical and atypical A-V Wenckebach periodicity. Am Heart J 89:26, 1975.
23. Narula OS, Samet P: Wenckebach and Mobitz type II A-V block due to block within the His bundle and bundle branches. Circulation 41: 947, 1970.
24. Zepelli P, Fenici R, Sassara M, et al: Wenckebach second degree AV block in top ranking athletes: An old problem revisited. Am Heart J 100:281, 1980.
25. Meyles I, Kaplinsky E, Yahini J, et al: Wenckebach A-V block: A frequent feature following heavy physical training. Am Heart J 90: 426, 1974.
26. Brodsky M, Wu D, Denes P, et al: Arrhythmias documented by 24-hour continuous electrocardiographic monitoring in 50 male medical students without apparent heart disease. Am J Cardiol 39:390, 1977.
27. Narula OS: Clinical concepts of spontaneous and induced atrioventricular block. In Mandel W (ed): Cardiac Arrhythmias: Their Mechanism, Diagnosis and Management. JB Lippincott, Philadelphia, 1987, p 326.
28. Dreifus LS, Fisch C, Griffin JC, et al: Guidelines for implantation of cardiac pacemakers and antiarrhythmia devices. A report of the American College of Cardiology/American Heart Association Task Force on Assessment of Diagnostic and Therapeutic Cardiovascular Procedures (Committee on Pacemaker Implantation). J Am Coll Cardiol 18:1, 1991.
29. Jonas EA, Kosowsky BD, Ramaswamy K: Complete His-Purkinje block produced by carotid massage: Report of a case. Circulation 51:68, 1975.
30. Narula OS, Scherlag BJ, Samet P, et al: Atrioventricular block: Localization and classification by His bundle recordings. Am J Med 50:146, 1971.
31. Rosen KM, Dhingra RC, Loeb HS, et al: Chronic heart block in adults. Arch Intern Med 131:663, 1973.
32. Narula OS, Samet O: Predilection of elderly females for intra His bundle (BH) blocks. Circulation 50:195, 1974.
33. Anderson RH, Wenink ACG, Losekoot TG, Becker AE: Congenitally complete heart block: Developmental aspects. Circulation 56:90, 1977.
34. Davies MJ, Anderson RH, Becker AE: The Conduction System of the Heart. Butterworth, London, 1983.
35. Morquio L: Sur un maladie infantile et familiale caracteristique et la morte subite. Arch Med Enfantes 4:467, 1901.
36. Lev M: The pathology of complete atrioventricular block. Prog Cardiovasc Dis 6:317, 1964.
37. Scott JS, Maddison PJ, Taylor PV, et al: Connective tissue disease, antibodies to ribonucleoprotein, and congenital heart block. N Engl J Med 309:209, 1983.
38. Litsey SE, Noonan JA, O'Connor WN, et al: Maternal connective tissue disease and congenital heart block: Demonstration of immunoglobulin in cardiac tissue. N Engl J Med 312:98, 1985.
39. Behan WMH, Behan PO, Reid JM: Family studies of congenital heart block associated with Ro antibody. Br Heart J 62:320, 1989.
40. Li JM, Horsfall AC, Maini RN: Anti-La (SS-B) but not anti-Ro52 (SS-A) antibodies cross-react with laminin—a role in the pathogenesis of congenital heart block? Clin Exp Immunol 99:316, 1997.
41. Meilof JF, Frohn-Mulder IM, Stewart PA, et al: Maternal antibodies and congenital heart block: No evidence for the existence of a unique heart block–associated anti-Ro/SS-A autoantibody profile. Lupus 2: 239, 1993.
42. Watson RM, Scheel JN, Petri M, et al: Neonatal lupus erythematosus: Report of serological and immunogenetic studies in twins discordant for congenital heart block. Br J Dermatol 130:342, 1994.
43. Press J, Uziel Y, Laxer RM, et al: Long-term outcome of mothers of children with complete congenital heart block. Am J Med 100: 328, 1996.
44. Julkunen H, Kurki P, Kaaja R, et al: Isolated congenital heart block: Long-term outcome of mothers and characterization of the immune response to SS-A/Ro and to SS-B/La. Arthritis Rheum 36:1588, 1993.
45. Julkunen H, Siren MK, Kaaja R, et al: Maternal HLA antigens and antibodies to SS-A/Ro and SS-B/La: Comparison with systemic lupus erythematosus and primary Sjögren's syndrome. Br J Rheumatol 34: 901, 1995.
46. Olah KS, Gee H: Antibody mediated complete congenital heart block in the fetus. Pacing Clin Electrophysiol 16:1872, 1993.
47. Groves AMM, Allan LD, Rosenthal E: Therapeutic trial of sympathomimetics in three cases of complete heart block in the fetus. Circulation 92:3394, 1995.
48. Schmidt KG, Ulmer HE, Silverman NH, et al: Perinatal outcome of fetal complete atrioventricular block: A multicenter experience. J Am Coll Cardiol 17:1360, 1991.
49. Anandakumar C, Biswas A, Chew SS, et al: Direct fetal therapy for hydrops secondary to congenital atrioventricular heart block. Obstet Gynecol 87:835, 1996.
50. Buyon JP, Waltuck J, Kleinman C, Copel J: In utero identification and therapy of congenital heart block. Lupus 4:116, 1995.
51. Copel JA, Buyon JP, Kleinman CS: Successful in utero therapy of fetal heart block. Am J Obstet Gynecol 173:1384, 1995.
52. Lopes LM, Cha SC, Leone C, Zugaib M: Use of sympathomimetic agents in fetal atrioventricular heart block. Arq Bras Cardiol 63:297, 1994.
53. Murotsuki J, Okamura K, Watanabe T, et al: Production of complete heart block and utero cardiac pacing in fetal lambs. J Obstet Gynaecol 21:223, 1995.

54. Kikuchi Y, Shiraishi H, Igarashi H, et al: Cardiac pacing in fetal lambs: Intrauterine transvenous cardiac pacing for fetal complete heart block. Pacing Clin Electrophysiol 18:417, 1995.
55. Assad RS, Jatene MB, Moreira LF, Sales PC: Fetal heart block: A new experimental model to assess fetal pacing. Pacing Clin Electrophysiol 17:1256, 1994.
56. Friedman DM, Borg M, Rutkovsky L, Buyon JP: Benign fetal bradycardias diagnosed by echocardiography. Am J Perinatol 12:87, 1995.
57. Olah KS, Gee H: Antibody mediated complete congenital heart block in the fetus. Pacing Clin Electrophysiol 16:1872, 1993.
58. Brucato A, Gasparini M, Vignati G: Isolated congenital complete heart block: Long-term outcome of children and immunogenetic study. J Rheumatol 22:541, 1995.
59. O'Connor BK, Case CL, Gillette PC: Congenital heart block: Natural history and management. ACC Current Journal Review 4:63, 1995.
60. Michaelsson M, Jonzon A, Riesenfeld T: Isolated congenital complete atrioventricular block in adult life: A prospective study. Circulation 92: 442, 1995.
61. Tawara S: Das Reizleitungssystem des Saugetierkerzens. Gustav Fisher, Jena, 1906.
62. Humblet M: Allorythmic cardiaque par section du faisceau de His. Arch Int Physiol 3:330, 1905–1906.
63. Hering H: Die Durchschneidung des Uebergangsbundels beim. Saugetier herzen. 3 Mitt Pflugers Arch F Ges Physiol 3:298, 1906.
64. Mahaim I: Les Maladies Organiques du Faisceau de His-Tawara. Masson et Cie, Paris, 1931.
65. Knieriem HJ, Finkle E: Morphologie und Aetiologie des Totalen AV Blocks. Urban S Schuarzenberg, Munchen, 1974.
66. Lev M: The pathology of complete atrioventricular block. Prog Cardiovasc Dis 6:317, 1964.
67. Lenègre J: Etiology of bilateral bundle branch fibrosis in relation to complete heart block. Prog Cardiovasc Dis 6:317, 1964.
68. Kuo CT, Liu CY, Hsu TS, et al: Immediate prognostic significance of complete atrioventricular block in acute myocardial infarction. Taiwan Yi Xue Hui Za Zhi 88:712, 1989.
69. Kostuk WJ, Beanlands DS: Complete heart block associated with acute myocardial infarction. Am J Cardiol 26:380, 1970.
70. Norris RM: Heart block in posterior and anterior myocardial infarction. Br Heart J 31:352, 1969.
71. Hackel DB, Estes EH Jr: Pathologic features of atrioventricular and intraventricular conduction disturbances in acute myocardial infarction. Circulation 43:977, 1971.
72. Clemmensen P, Bates ER, Califf RM, et al: Complete atrioventricular block complicating inferior wall acute myocardial infarction treated with reperfusion therapy. TAMI Study Group. Am J Cardiol 67:225, 1991.
73. Berger PB, Ruocco NA, Ryan TJ, et al: Incidence and prognostic implications of heart block complicating inferior myocardial infarction treated with thrombolytic therapy: Results from TIMI II. J Am Coll Cardiol 20:533, 1992.
74. Dubois C, Pierard LA, Smeets JP, et al: Long-term prognostic significance of atrioventricular block in inferior acute myocardial infarction. Eur Heart J 10:816, 1989.
75. Behar S, Zissman E, Zion M, et al: Complete atrioventricular block complicating inferior acute wall myocardial infarction: Short- and long-term prognosis. Am Heart J 125:1622, 1993.
76. Kaul U, Hari Haran V, Malhotra A, Bhatia ML: Significance of advanced atrioventricular block in acute inferior myocardial infarction—a study based on ventricular function and Holter monitoring. Int J Cardiol 11:187, 1986.
77. Nicod P, Gilpin E, Dittrich H, et al: Long-term outcome in patients with inferior myocardial infarction and complete atrioventricular block. J Am Coll Cardiol 12:589, 1988.
78. Feigl D, Ashkenazy J, Kishon Y: Early and late atrioventricular block in acute inferior myocardial infarction. J Am Coll Cardiol 4:35, 1984.
79. Sclarovsky S, Strasberg B, Hirshberg A, et al: Advanced early and late atrioventricular block in acute inferior wall myocardial infarction. Am Heart J 108:19, 1984.
80. Onodera S, Ito M, Odakura H, et al: Atrioventricular block in acute inferior myocardial infarction [Japanese]. Kokyu To Junkan 40:255, 1992.
81. Strasberg B, Pinchas A, Arditti A: Left and right ventricular function in inferior acute myocardial infarction and significance of advanced atrioventricular block. Am J Cardiol 54:985, 1984.
82. Ryan TJ, Anderson JL, Antman EM, et al: ACC/AHA guidelines for the management of patients with acute myocardial infarction: A report of the American College of Cardiology/American Heart Association Task Force on Practice Guidelines (Committee on Management of Acute Myocardial Infarction). J Am Coll Cardiol 28:1328, 1996.
83. Goodfellow J, Walker PR: Reversal of atropine-resistant atrioventricular block with intravenous aminophylline in the early phase of inferior wall acute myocardial infarction following treatment with streptokinase. Eur Heart J 16:862, 1995.
84. Bertolet BD, McMurtrie EB, Hill JA, Belardinelli L: Theophylline for the treatment of atrioventricular block after myocardial infarction. Ann Intern Med 123:509, 1995.
85. Strasberg B, Bassevich R, Mager A, et al: Effects of aminophylline on atrioventricular conduction in patients with late atrioventricular block during inferior wall acute myocardial infarction. Am J Cardiol 67: 527, 1991.
86. Wesley RC Jr, Lerman BB, DiMarco JP, et al: Mechanism of atropine-resistant atrioventricular block during inferior myocardial infarction: Possible role of adenosine. J Am Coll Cardiol 8:1232, 1986.
87. Sutton R, Davies MJ: The conduction system in acute myocardial infarction complicated by heart block. Circulation 38:987, 1968.
88. Hollander G, Nadiminti V, Lichstein E, et al: Bundle branch block in acute myocardial infarction. Am Heart J 105:738, 1983.
89. Dubois C, Pierard LA, Smeets JP, et al: Short- and long-term prognostic importance of complete bundle-branch block complicating myocardial infarction. Clin Cardiol 11:292, 1988.
90. Gaspard P, Delahaye JP, Touboul P, et al: Long-term course of patients with myocardial infarction and bundle branch block. Arch Mal Coeur Vaiss 11:1287, 1980.
91. Ricou F, Nicod P, Gilpin E, et al: Influence of right bundle branch block on short- and long-term survival after acute anterior myocardial infarction. J Am Coll Cardiol 17:858, 1991.
92. Roth A, Miller HI, Glick A, et al: Rapid resolution of new right bundle branch block in acute anterior myocardial infarction patients after thrombolytic therapy. Pacing Clin Electrophysiol 16:13, 1993.

CHAPTER 38

Sudden Cardiac Death

Maureen Lowery, Agustin Castellanos, and Robert J. Myerburg

Sudden death, which accounts for approximately 50% of all cardiovascular-related deaths, is a formidable cause of premature death in the United States. The percentage of cardiovascular patients who die suddenly has remained constant despite the ongoing decline in total cardiovascular mortality.[1, 2] Each year in the United States, about 300,000 people of all ages, sexes, and socioeconomic groups experience sudden cardiac death (SCD).[3–5] Epidemiologic studies have clearly identified coronary heart disease (CHD) as the major cause of SCD in both men and women.[6, 7] From the Framingham data, SCD accounted for 40% of deaths resulting from coronary artery disease in men and 34% in women. However, significant gender differences were observed when the data were analyzed for predictive risk factors for SCD.[7, 8] Conventional risk factors independently predicted unexpected SCD in men but not in women.[9, 10] In addition, women are a more heterogeneous group at risk of SCD because of the variety of underlying structural heart disease in women.[11, 12] In this chapter, we review current information on SCD in women from four sources of data: epidemiologic studies, postmyocardial infarction outcome data, electrophysiologic characteristics of women, and studies of survivors of lethal or potentially lethal arrhythmias.

DEFINITIONS

SCD is defined as natural death from cardiac causes heralded by an abrupt loss of consciousness within 1 hour of the onset of acute symptoms in an individual with or without known pre-existing heart disease in whom the time and mode of death are unexpected.[2] Unexpected sudden death is defined as SCD in a person without prior overt or identified coronary heart disease.[9] The use of these definitions allows for better comparisons of epidemiologic and clinical data.

INCIDENCE AND ETIOLOGY

SCD is predominantly a syndrome of men; epidemiologic studies show a 3:1 male-to-female ratio.[8, 9] The high incidence of SCD in men is also observed in studies of prehospital cardiac arrest patients in which the percentage of men ranges from 75% to 89%.[13–15] SCD is rare in both sexes before the age of 45 years; however, SCD in women usually occurs 20 years later than in men. However, the incidence of SCD, which increases with age in both sexes, doubles with each decade of life.[10, 16]

Most SCDs are linked to the presence of CHD.[10, 17] In the Framingham study at the 30-year follow-up, 43% of all CHD deaths were sudden (46% in men versus 37% in women).[17] However, in persons without prior overt CHD, SCD occurred more often in women (67%) than in men (55%), especially in women younger than 65 years, in whom 90% of SCD occurred with no clinical evidence of pre-existing CHD.[10, 17]

Once overt CHD is established, the incidence of SCD increases in both sexes.[8, 10, 17] After a symptomatically recognized myocardial infarction (MI), the risk of SCD increases fourfold in men and threefold in women.[17] Over a 10-year period after a recognized MI, 5.3% of women and 11.9% of men died suddenly.[17] This gap in percentage between the sexes disappears after an unrecognized MI. In the 10 years after an unrecognized MI, 7.5% of women and 6.3% percent of men died of SCD.[17] Risk ratios comparing SCD in the general population after a recognized MI are 4.4 for men and 2.8 for women. Following an unrecognized MI, the risk ratio is 2.3 for men and 5.0 for women.[17] This finding is noteworthy because unrecognized MIs are more common in women (35%) than in men (28%).[17, 18]

The mechanisms responsible for SCD are complex and dynamic, and extend beyond the scope of this chapter.[19, 20] In SCD, the underlying form of structural heart disease, left ventricular (LV) function, and transient triggering events interact and lead to the ultimate cause of SCD, ventricular tachycardia (VT) or ventricular fibrillation (VF). Data from postmortem studies and studies from survivors of cardiac arrest show that the population of women who die suddenly is more heterogeneous than the population of men who die suddenly.[11, 12] In a retrospective study of 355 (271 men, 84 women) consecutive survivors of prehospital cardiac arrest referred for electrophysiologic testing, Albert and colleagues[11] found that coronary artery disease was the underlying form of structural heart disease in 80% of men but in only 45% of women. More women had both dilated cardiomyopathy and valvular heart disease. Several cardiac diseases were unique to women in the study by Albert and associates and have been recognized as being more common in women in other studies; these diseases include right ventricular dysplasia, congenital heart disease, coronary artery spasm, and long QT syndrome. Another noteworthy finding in the study by Albert and colleagues[11] was that more women (10%) than men (3%) had structurally normal hearts (Figs. 38–1 and 38–2). Together these results suggest women who die suddenly have less underlying CHD and are more likely to have structurally normal hearts. This gender difference in the type of underlying structural heart disease has been observed by others.[10, 12, 21, 22]

RISK FACTORS

Since the peak of the coronary artery disease epidemic in 1968, preventive efforts aimed at reducing risk factors of

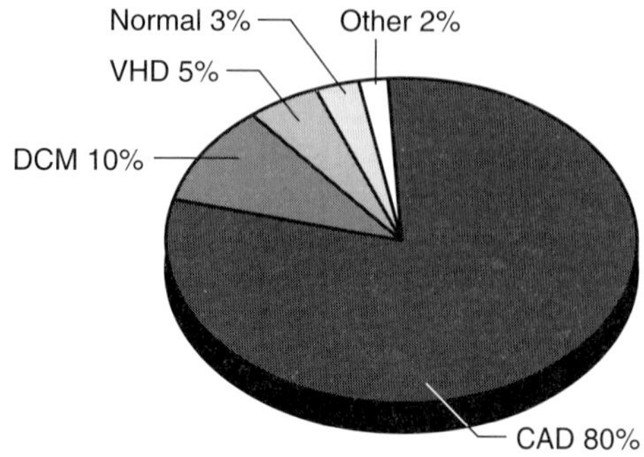

FIGURE 38–1. Pie chart indicating underlying structural heart disease in male survivors of cardiac arrest. (CAD, coronary artery disease; DCM, dilated cardiomyopathy; and VHD, valvular heart disease.) (From Albert CM, McGovern BA, Newel JB, Ruskin JN: Sex differences in cardiac arrest survivors. Circulation 93:1170, 1996.)

coronary artery disease have significantly decreased all causes of cardiovascular mortality, except SCD.[1, 2, 23] More than half of all coronary mortality is a result of SCD.[1, 24] Moreover, 50% of men and 64% of women who die suddenly have no history of recognized coronary artery disease.[6, 8, 10] If angina is excluded, 18% of men with coronary events and 24% of women present with sudden death as the first and only symptom.[10] Thus, identifying risk factors associated with SCD and any gender difference that may reflect the differences in the underlying cardiac pathology or pathophysiology is critical.

Epidemiologic studies attempt to clarify gender-specific risk profiles for SCD by regrouping the population studied into categories based on age, conventional risk factors, and presence of overt CHD and congestive heart failure (CHF).[6–10, 16] Both long- and short-term risk factors have been examined.[7]

SCD in women younger than 45 years is extremely uncommon. In the Framingham cohort, no woman younger than 45 years, with or without a history of CHD, died suddenly.[10] Krueger and coworkers[25] classified the causes of death among 338 women younger than 45 years whose deaths were attributed to acute MI on the death certificates and found that only 64 (19%) were caused by SCD (less than 1 hour). In addition, they noted that women who died suddenly were older (40 to 44 years), married, black, and had not been hospitalized.[25]

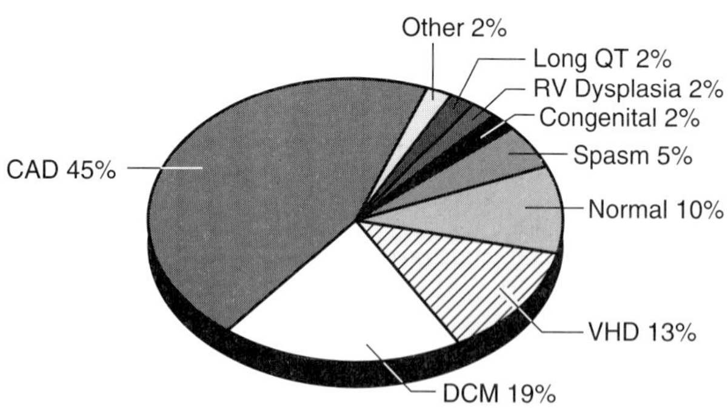

FIGURE 38–2. Pie chart indicating underlying structural heart disease in female survivors of cardiac arrest (CAD, coronary artery disease; DCM, dilated cardiomyopathy; RV, right ventricular; and VHD, valvular heart disease.) (From Albert CM, McGovern BA, Newel JB, Ruskin JN: Sex differences in cardiac arrest survivors. Circulation 93:1170, 1996.)

The conventional risk factors for CHD in men also predict SCD in men. This link between risk factors for CHD and SCD is not seen in women.[9] At the 26-year follow-up of the Framingham study, the risk factors for SCD in men were age, electrocardiographic left ventricular hypertrophy (ECG-LVH), systolic blood pressure, cigarette smoking, and total cholesterol, which are similar to the risk factors for atherosclerosis. In women, age, hematocrit, and vital capacity strongly predicted SCD, and glucose and cholesterol only marginally predicted SCD.[9, 16] In one study, cigarette smoking was not associated with SCD in women and could not be statistically associated with the increase in hematocrit or decrease in vital capacity.[9] The authors suggest that the inhalation patterns in women smokers differ from those in men.[16] However, this lack of an association between cigarette smoking and SCD in women has not been supported by other studies.[12, 25, 26] Krueger and associates[25] found an association between cigarette smoking and SCD in young women, and Talbott and associates[26] found a strong association with SCD in women who smoke more than a pack of cigarettes per day. In one retrospective study of autopsy results in women who died unexpectedly, 62% of women who died from CHD were heavy smokers, and the mean age at time of death was 19 years less in heavy smokers than in nonsmokers.[12]

The risk factors for SCD differ for men and women once overt coronary artery disease is manifest. In men with CHD, age, systolic blood pressure, cigarette smoking, and total cholesterol no longer predict an increased risk of SCD; ECG-LVH, glucose, and intraventricular block increase the risk of SCD.[16] In women with overt CHD, only hematocrit remained a significant predictor of SCD.[16]

Cupples and colleagues[7] assessed risk factors that were long-term predictors of SCD over 28 years and those that were short-term predictors over 2 years. Both long-term and short-term risk factors were analyzed in men and women with and without CHD and CHF. (The overall incidence of SCD in women in the long-term study was 32% of that in men; in the short-term study, 23%. The 10-year, age-adjusted incidence of SCD was 25.7/1000 in men and 6.7/1000 in women.) Using multivariate analysis, they reported that body mass index, cigarette smoking, glucose intolerance, ECG-LVH, serum cholesterol, and systolic blood pressure increased risk of SCD in men over the long term. In women, the predictors of long-term risk were systolic blood pressure, cigarette smoking, intraventricular block, and nonspecific ST- and T-wave changes.

The 2-year, short-term incidence of SCD in the study by Cupples and coworkers[7] was 5.9/1000 for men and 1.3/1000 for women, confirming the female advantage at any age of follow-up. The short-term predictors of SCD in men were serum cholesterol, heart rate, ECG-LVH, nonspecific ST- and T-wave changes, and intraventricular block. In women, only nonspecific ST- and T-wave changes and intraventricular block were significant predictors of short-term risk for SCD.

When the presence of CHD was added to the multivariate analysis, the long-term risk of SCD in men increased more than threefold and the short-term risk increased more than fivefold. In women, a similar trend of increased risk was seen in the presence of CHD but not to the same degree as that seen in men. The long-term risk of SCD in women with CHD increased about twofold and the short-term risk about threefold. When risk was analyzed according to CHF status, men with CHF had a greater long-term risk than short-term risk (4.8 versus 2.6, respectively). However, in women, only the increase in short-term risk was statistically significant (6.2 versus 1.5). Surprisingly, the data from electrophysiologic studies from survivors of cardiac arrest in other studies have not shown an association of a low ejection fraction (EF) (<40%) with inducibility of a lethal arrhythmia in women.[11, 27] Cupples and coworkers[7] determined the presence of CHF by symptoms and physical examination; left ventricular function was not directly measured. Thus, the absolute EF and the presence of systolic or diastolic failure may not be as important as the presence of pulmonary congestion in predicting short-term risk of SCD in women. In several studies of prognosis after acute MI, the incidence of CHF and in-hospital death was higher in women than in men, despite higher resting EFs in women.[28–31] In a study by Dittrich and associates,[29] the percentage of women who had an EF of less than 40% was similar in those who survived an acute MI (20%) and those who died (28%); however, pulmonary congestion was seen on chest radiograph in 48% of nonsurvivors and only 20% of survivors.

RISK OF LIFE-THREATENING ARRHYTHMIAS AFTER MYOCARDIAL INFARCTION

Most cases of SCD are caused by acute fatal arrhythmias: VT and VF.[2] Observations from coronary care units[32, 33] and from ambulatory Holter monitoring in survivors of acute MI have supported the hypothesis of the premature ventricular complex (PVC).[34–36] According to this hypothesis, the PVC triggers the initiation of VT/VF.[19] This electrogenic link between PVCs and fatal arrhythmias is not seen in women. In the Framingham study, patients who had PVCs on routine ECG were followed; the risk of SCD in men with PVCs increased three times, whereas no statistical increase in risk was seen in women.[37]

After a symptomatic MI, women have less than half the rate of SCD than men,[17] yet in studies of postinfarction risk that have assessed the relationship between PVCs and cardiac mortality, gender differences in arrhythmic risk have not been studied.[35, 36, 38] Most studies either excluded women or included too few for significant statistical analysis.[35, 36, 38]

The Myocardial Infarction Limitation Study (MILIS) examined 2-year mortality in 590 men and 226 women after MI.[28, 39] At 2 years, 36% of women and 21% of men had died. The higher cumulative mortality rate in women was independent of age.[28] The MILIS researchers found that frequent PVCs (>10/h) and LV dysfunction (EF <40%) independently increased the risk of SCD.[38] Unfortunately, no separate analysis assessing gender differences in PVC risk of SCD was conducted.

The Multicenter Postinfarction Research Group (MPRG) followed 673 men and 194 women for 2 years after MI for risk of death.[36, 40] These researchers, like the MILIS group, found that frequent PVCs (>10/h) and left ventricular dysfunction (EF <40%) increased the risk of SCD.[36] Again, risk was not studied by gender. Moss and colleagues[41] analyzed the data from the MPRG to evaluate gender differences in arrhythmic risk on 2-year mortality. Surprisingly, they found that ventricular ectopy did not significantly contribute to the 2-year mortality risk in women, despite similar distributions of frequent and repetitive PVCs.[41] However, left ventricular dysfunction significantly increased the 2-year risk of death in women and men.

More recently, Dittrich and associates[29] reported in-hospital and 1-year mortality data on 1551 men and 538 women after acute MI. Both in-hospital and 1-year mortality rates were similar for men and women when corrected for age. As in the MILIS and MPRG studies, complex PVCs and poor left ventricular function (EF<40%) were associated with death in men,[28, 29, 36, 39, 40] but neither complex PVCs nor a low EF separated women survivors from nonsurvivors.[29]

The data from the Framingham study that assessed PVCs and risk of death in a general population[37] and the data from Moss and coworkers[41] and Dittrich and colleagues[29] that assessed PVCs and risk of death in the higher risk postinfarction group imply that ventricular ectopy increases the risk of cardiac death in men but not in women. The reasons for this gender difference are not known. Further insight into arrhythmic risk of SCD in women is obtained from electrophysiologic studies in survivors of cardiac arrest.

FEMALE SURVIVORS OF CARDIAC ARREST

Freedman and colleagues[21] performed electrophysiologic studies in 150 consecutive survivors of cardiac arrest (111 men, 39 women). Patients with any inducible arrhythmia (sustained VT, nonsustained VT, or VF) were compared with those without an inducible arrhythmia. The strongest correlates for inducing a tachyarrhythmia were male sex and prior MI (Fig. 38–3). Arrhythmias were induced in 98 (88%) of 111 men versus 15 (39%) of 39 women. The probability of inducing an arrhythmia in men with a prior MI was 95% versus 72% in male cardiac arrest survivors without prior MI. The probability of inducing an arrhythmia in women with a prior MI was 77% versus only 19% in women with no prior MI. None of the 26 women with no prior MI had inducible sustained monomorphic VT.

Schoenfeld and associates[22] performed electrophysiologic studies in 261 consecutive patients (197 men, 64 women) with a history of spontaneous, ECG-documented ventricular tachyarrhythmias not associated with acute MI. Schoenfeld and coworkers,[22] like Freedman and associates,[21] showed that male sex and a prior MI were independent predictors of arrhythmia inducibility. Inducible arrhythmias were seen in 89% of patients presenting with sustained VT, in 61% of patients presenting with nonsustained VT, and in 66% of those presenting with VF. Atherosclerotic heart disease was present in 84% of patients presenting with sustained VT. In those presenting with nonsustained VT, 50% had nonatherosclerotic heart disease. Of the 64 women studied, 23 (36%) presented with nonsustained VT, 14 (15%) with sustained VT, and 27 (42%) with VF.

Three independent predictors of arrhythmia induction were identified by multivariate logistic regression analysis: the presenting arrhythmia, a history of one or more MIs, and male sex (Fig. 38–4). None of the women studied by Schoenfeld and associates had more than one prior MI, which may support the observation that women have less multivessel coronary artery disease.[42–44]

Albert and coworkers[11] retrospectively studied 355 (271 men, 84 women) consecutive survivors of out-of-hospital cardiac arrest. All patients underwent electrophysiologic testing. Gender differences in underlying pathology and predictors of both mortality and SCD were analyzed. Results of a baseline electrophysiologic study indicated that women were a more heterogeneous group with less coronary artery disease than men and that more women had structurally normal hearts. Inducible arrhythmias were seen in 46% of women but in only 27% of men. Of the women with an inducible arrhythmia, only 24% had inducible sustained monomorphic VT. When stratified by the presence of coronary artery disease, the data showed no significant gender difference in arrhythmia inducibility.

Important gender differences in predictors of mortality were seen (Table 38–1). A left ventricular ejection fraction of less than 40% predicted both total and cardiac mortality in men but not in women. These findings support those of Dittrich and colleagues,[29] who reported that a left ventricular ejection fraction (LVEF) less than 40% was found in similar numbers of women survivors and nonsurvivors. In the study by Albert and colleagues,[11] the presence of coronary artery disease was the most significant predictor of total and cardiac mortality in women. Women who survived cardiac arrest were less likely to have coronary artery disease; however, if coronary artery disease was present, women were 4.5 times more likely to die and 4.3 times more likely to die of a cardiac cause. Coronary artery disease alone, regardless of LVEF, predicts total mortality in women (Fig. 38–5).

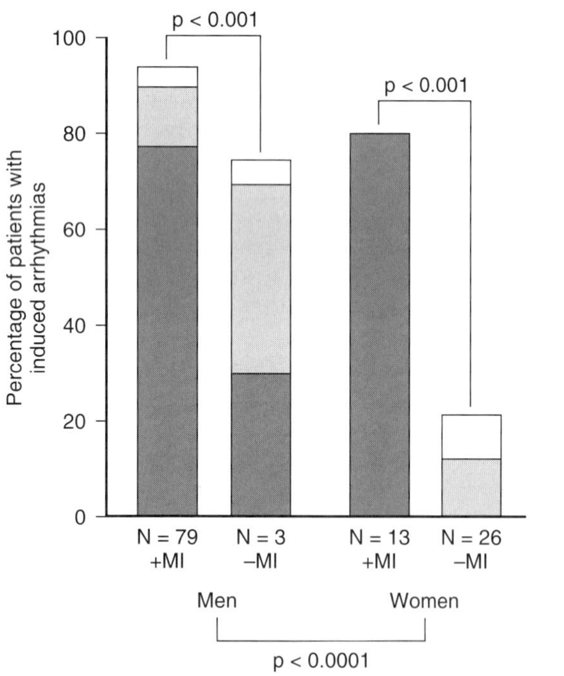

FIGURE 38–3. Probability of inducing sustained monomorphic ventricular tachycardia *(dark bars)*, ventricular fibrillation *(light bars)* and nonsustained ventricular tachycardia *(open bars)* by gender and history of myocardial infarction (MI) in four patient groups. The probability of inducing any arrhythmia was higher in men than in women. The number below each bar indicates the number of patients in the group. (From Freedman RA, Swerdlow CD, Soderholm-Diffatte V, et al: Clinical predictors of arrhythmia inducibility in survivors of cardiac arrest: Importance of gender and prior myocardial infarction. J Am Coll Cardiol 12:973, 1988, with permission.)

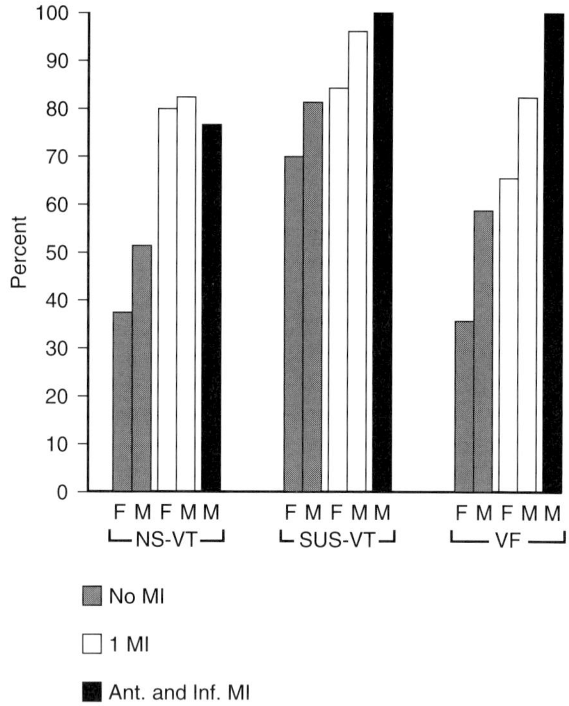

FIGURE 38–4. The probability of inducing ventricular arrhythmias in patients with a previously documented tachyarrhythmia is plotted as a function of the presenting clinical arrhythmia, sex of the patient, and presence of transmural myocardial infarction. (ANT, anterior; F, female, INF, inferior; M, male; MI, myocardial infarction; NO, none; NS, nonsustained; SUS, sustained; VF, ventricular fibrillation; VT, ventricular tachycardia.) (From Schoenfeld MH, McGovern B, Garan H, et al: Determinants of the outcome of electrophysiologic study in patients with ventricular tachyarrhythmias. J Am Coll Cardiol 6:298, 1985. Reprinted with permission from the American College of Cardiology.)

Gender differences were also seen in predictors of SCD. In men, sustained monomorphic VT and an LVEF of less than 40% increased the relative risk for SCD, whereas in women, the presence of a left ventricular aneurysm increased the risk more than fivefold. This finding is not surprising because a left ventricular aneurysm indicates residual myocardial damage from a previous large MI.

ARE WOMEN MORE SUSCEPTIBLE TO ARRHYTHMIAS RELATED TO PROLONGED REPOLARIZATION?

Makkar and coworkers[45] reported that more women than men are involved in cases of drug-related torsade de pointes, which suggests that women may be more likely than men to have an unexpected response to different medications. In a retrospective study, Kawasaki and colleagues[46] reanalyzed 72 previously reported cases of torsade de pointes in patients with complete heart block who were not taking drugs that could cause QT prolongation. The prevalence of women was greater than expected. They suggested that this finding may indicate gender variability in propensity to develop torsade de pointes in the wide spectrum of clinical entities associated with QT prolongation. The apparent increased propensity

Table 38–1. SEX-SPECIFIC MULTIVARIATE PREDICTORS OF MORTALITY

	RELATIVE RISK	95% Cs ON RELATIVE RISK	p*
Men (n = 271)			
Total mortality, 67 deaths			
LVEF <40%	2.82	1.61–4.95	.0001
Age	1.46	1.13–1.87	.002
Discharge on antiarrhythmics	1.82	1.00–3.35	<.05
Cardiac mortality, 48 deaths			
LVEF <40%	6.31	2.93–13.52	<.0001
ICD therapy	0.29	0.41–0.63	.006
SMVT on discharge EPS	4.29	1.71–10.82	.006
Sudden death, 21 deaths			
ICD therapy	0.05	0.01–0.39	.004
SMVT on discharge EPS	4.29	1.71–10.82	.006
LVEF <40%	2.58	0.93–7.16	.043
Women (n = 84)			
Total mortality, 19 deaths			
CAD	4.50	1.50–13.43	.003
Cardiac mortality, 14 deaths			
CAD	4.35	1.22–15.55	.012
Sudden death, 8 deaths			
LV aneurysm	5.15	1.20–21.99	.04

CAD, coronary artery disease; EPS, electrophysiologic studies; ICD, ischemic coronary disease; LV, left ventricle; LVEF, left ventricular ejection fraction; SMVT, sustained monomorphic ventricular tachycardia.

*p values are two-sided from Cox proportional-hazards model.

From Albert CM, McGovern BA, Newel JB, Ruskin JN: Sex differences in cardiac arrest survivors. Circulation 93:1170, 1996, with permission.

for women to develop this arrhythmia may result from a gender-dependent electrophysiologic mechanism rather than sex differences in metabolism of drugs known to cause QT prolongation. In fact, women normally have a slightly longer QTc interval than men,[46, 47] and long QT interval syndromes are more common in women.[48, 49] One study suggests that such differences appear during adolescence and disappear with aging. QTc intervals in women remain stable throughout a woman's lifetime, whereas intervals shorten in men during adolescence and return to levels similar to women in later life.[50]

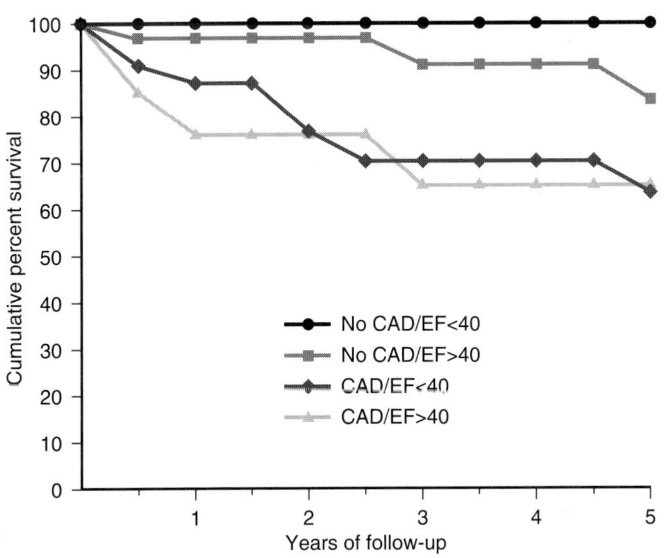

FIGURE 38–5. Plot of total mortality in women with and without coronary artery disease (CAD) stratified by left ventricular ejection fraction (EF). (From Albert CM, McGovern BA, Newel JB, Ruskin JN: Sex differences in cardiac arrest survivors. Circulation 93:1170, 1996.)

CONCLUSIONS AND CLINICAL IMPLICATIONS

Many of the studies on SCD have been conducted in men because the underlying disease, particularly coronary artery disease, is expressed earlier in men. However, the epidemiologic data available clearly demonstrate that sudden death is an important manifestation of heart disease among women. Although some epidemiologic patterns may differ between men and women, the frequency with which sudden death is the initial or terminal expression of underlying disease is comparable in men and women. Furthermore, some factors that may be important in the induction of potentially fatal arrhythmias, such as the duration of the QT interval, suggest the need for risk stratification in women. Life-threatening syndromes such as a long QT interval syndrome and proarrhythmic responses to various drugs are more common in women. Men and women have age-related differences in the risk of sudden death because of the delayed onset of CAD in women, but age-adjusted data show that the risk of sudden death in women is important.

References

1. Gillum RF: Sudden coronary death in the United States: 1980–1985. Circulation 79:756, 1989.
2. Myerburg RJ, Castellanos A: Cardiac arrest and sudden cardiac death. In Braunwald EB (ed): A Textbook of Cardiovascular Medicine, 4th ed. WB Saunders, Philadelphia, 1992, p 756.
3. Kuller L, Cooper M, Perper J: Epidemiology of sudden death. Arch Intern Med 129:714, 1972.
4. Myerburg RJ, Kessler KM, Castellanos A: Sudden cardiac death: Structure, function, and time-dependence of risk. Circulation 85(Suppl I):I-2, 1992.
5. Jiminez RA, Myerburg RJ: Sudden cardiac death: Magnitude of the problem, substrate/trigger interaction, and populations at high risk. Cardiol Clin 11:1, 1993.

6. Stokes J III, Kannel WB, Wolf PA et al: The relative importance of selected risk factors for various manifestations of cardiovascular disease among women and men from 35–64 years: 30 years of follow-up in the Framingham study. Circulation (Suppl V):V65, 1987.
7. Cupples AL, Gagnon DR, Kannel WB: Long- and short-term risk of sudden coronary death. Circulation 85(Suppl I):I11, 1992.
8. Lerner DJ, Kannel WB: Patterns of coronary heart disease morbidity and mortality in the sexes: A 26-year follow-up of the Framingham population. Am Heart J 111:383, 1986.
9. Schatzkin A, Cupples LA, Heeren T, et al: The epidemiology of sudden unexpected death: Risk factors for men and women in the Framingham Heart Study. Am Heart J 107:1300, 1984.
10. Kannel WB, Schatzkin A: Sudden death: Lessons from subsets in population studies. J Am Coll Cardiol 5:141B, 1985.
11. Albert CM, McGovern BA, Newel JB, Ruskin JN: Sex differences in cardiac arrest survivors. Circulation 93:1170, 1996.
12. Spain DM, Siegel H, Brudess VA: Women smokers and sudden death: The relationship of cigarette smoking to coronary disease. JAMA 224: 1005, 1973.
13. Liberthson RR, Nagel EL, Hirschman JC, et al: Prehospital ventricular fibrillation: Prognosis and follow-up course. N Engl J Med 291:317, 1974.
14. Baum RS, Alvarez H, Cobb LA: Survival after resuscitation from out-of-hospital ventricular fibrillation. Circulation 50:1231, 1974.
15. Myerburg RJ, Kessler KM, Estes D, et al: Long-term survival after prehospital cardiac arrest: Analysis of outcome during an 8-year study. Circulation 70:538, 1984.
16. Schatzhin A, Cupples LA, Heeren T, et al: Sudden death in the Framingham study: Differences in incidence and risk factors by sex and coronary artery disease status. Am J Epidemiol 120:888, 1984.
17. Kannel WB, Abbot RD: Incidence and prognosis of myocardial infarction in women: The Framingham study. In Eaker ED, Packard B, Wenger NK, et al (eds): Coronary Artery Disease in Women. National Heart, Lung, and Blood Institute, National Institutes of Health, Bethesda, MD, 1987, p 208.
18. Kannel WB, Abbott RD: Incidence and prognosis of unrecognized myocardial infarction: An update on the Framingham study. N Engl J Med 311:1144, 1984.
19. Myerburg RJ, Kessler KM, Kimura S, et al: Sudden cardiac death: Future approaches based on identification and control of transient risk factors. J Cardiovasc Electrophys 13:626, 1992.
20. Myerburg RJ, Kessler KM, Kimura S, et al: Life-threatening ventricular arrhythmias: The link between epidemiology and pathophysiology. In Zipes DP, Jalife J (eds): Cardiac Electrophysiology, 2nd ed. WB Saunders, Philadelphia, 1995, p 723.
21. Freedman RA, Swerdlow CD, Soderholm-Diffatte V, et al: Clinical predictors of arrhythmia inducibility in survivors of cardiac arrest: Importance of gender and prior myocardial infarction. J Am Coll Cardiol 12:973, 1988.
22. Schoenfeld MH, McGovern B, Garan H, et al: Determinants of the outcome of electrophysiologic study in patients with ventricular tachyarrhythmias. J Am Coll Cardiol 6:298, 1985.
23. Goldman L, Cook EF: The decline in ischemic heart disease mortality rates: An analysis of the comparative effects of medical intervention and changes in lifestyle. Ann Intern Med 101:825, 1984.
24. Lown B: Sudden cardiac death: The major challenge confronting contemporary cardiology. Am J Cardiol 43:313, 1979.
25. Krueger DE, Ellenberg SS, Bloom S, et al: Risk factors for fatal heart attacks in young women. Am J Epidemiol 113:357, 1981.
26. Talbott E, Kuller LH, Detri K, et al: Biologic and psychosocial risk factors of sudden death from coronary artery disease in white women. Am J Cardiol 39:858, 1977.
27. Vaitkus PT, Kindwall E, Miller JM, et al: Influence of gender on inducibility of ventricular arrhythmias in survivors of cardiac arrest with coronary artery disease. Am J Cardiol 67:537, 1991.
28. Tofler GH, Stone PH, Muller JE, et al: Effects of gender and race on prognosis after myocardial infarction: Adverse prognosis for women, particularly black women. J Am Coll Cardiol 9:473, 1987.
29. Dittrich H, Gilpin E, Nicod P, et al: Acute myocardial infarction in women: Influence of gender on mortality and prognostic variables. Am J Cardiol 62:1, 1988.
30. Tunstall-Pedoe H, Morrison C, Woodward M, et al: Sex differences in myocardial infarction and coronary deaths in the Scottish Monica population of Glascow 1985 to 1991. Circulation 93:1981, 1996.
31. Becker RC, Terrin M, Ross R, et al: Comparison of clinical outcomes for women and men after acute myocardial infarction. Ann Intern Med 120:638, 1994.
32. Lown B, Takhro AM, Hood WB, et al: The coronary care unit: New perspective and directions. JAMA 199:156, 1967.
33. Maynard C, Litwin PE, Martin JS, et al: Gender differences in the treatment and outcome of acute myocardial infarction. Results from the myocardial infarction triage and intervention registry. Arch Intern Med 152:972, 1992.
34. DeSoyza N, Meacham D, Murphy ML, et al: Evaluation of warning arrhythmia before paroxysmal ventricular tachycardia during acute myocardial infarction in men. Circulation 60:814, 1979.
35. Vismara LA, Amstudam BA, Mason DT: Relation of ventricular arrhythmia in the late hospital phase of acute myocardial infarction to sudden death after hospital discharge. Am J Med 59:6, 1975.
36. Ruberman W, Weinblatt M, Goldberg JD, et al: Ventricular premature complexes and sudden death after myocardial infarction. Circulation 64:297, 1981.
37. Bigger JT, Fleiss JL, Kleiger R, et al: The relationships among ventricular arrhythmias, left ventricular dysfunction, and mortality in the 2 years after myocardial infarction. Circulation 69:250, 1984.
38. Kannel WB, McGee DL: Epidemiology of sudden death: Insights from the Framingham Study. In Josephson ME (ed): Sudden Cardiac Death. FA Davis, Philadelphia, 1985, p 93.
39. The Coronary Drug Project Research Group: Prognostic importance of premature beats following myocardial infarction: Experience in the coronary drug project. JAMA 223:1116, 1973.
40. Mukharji J, Rude RE, Poole K et al: Risk factors for sudden death after acute myocardial infarction: Two-year follow-up. Am J Cardiol 54: 31, 1984.
41. The Multicenter Postinfarction Research Group: Risk stratification and survival after myocardial infarction. N Engl J Med 309:331, 1983.
42. Moss AJ, Carleen E, and the Multicenter Postinfarction Research Group: Gender differences in the mortality risk associated with ventricular arrhythmias after myocardial infarction. In Eaher ED, Packard B, Wenger NK, et al (eds): Coronary Heart Disease in Women. National Heart, Lung, and Blood Institute, National Institutes of Health, Bethesda, MD, 1987, p 204.
43. Chaitman BR, Bourassa MG, Lam J, et al: Noninvasive diagnosis of coronary artery disease in women. In Eaker ED, Packard B, Wenger NK, et al (eds): Coronary Heart Disease in Women. Haymarket Doyma, New York, 1987, p 222.
44. Chaitman BR, Bourassa MG, Davis K, et al: Angiographic prevalence of high risk coronary artery disease in patient subsets (CASS). Circulation 64:360, 1981.
45. Makkar RR, Fromm BS, Steinman RT, et al: Female gender as a risk factor for torsade de pointes associated with cardiovascular drugs. JAMA 270:2590, 1993.
46. Kawasaki R, Machado C, Reinoehl J, et al: Increased propensity of women to develop torsade de pointes during complete heart block. J Cardiovasc Electrophysiol 6:1032, 1995.
47. MacFarlane PW, Lawrie TDV: Comprehensive Electrocardiology: Theory and Practice in Health and Disease. Elmsford, NY, Pergamon Press, 1989, pp 407.
48. Merri M, Benhorin J, Alberti M, et al: Electrocardiographic quantitation of ventricular repolarization. Circulation 80:1301, 1989.
49. Moss AJ, Schwartz PJ, Crampton RS, et al: The long QT syndrome: Prospective longitudinal study of 328 families. Circulation 84:1136, 1991.
50. Rautaharju PM, Sophia HZ, Wong S, et al: Sex differences in the evolution of the electrocardiographic QT interval with age. Can J Cardiol 8:690, 1992.

Bibliography

Hashiba K: Hereditary QT prolongation syndrome in Japan: Genetic analysis and pathological findings of the conducting system. Jpn Circ J 42: 1133, 1978.

Jiang C, Atkinson D, Towbin J, et al: Two long QT syndrome loci map to chromosomes 3 and 7 with evidence for further heterogeneity. Nature Genet 8:141, 1994.

Keating M: Linkage analysis and long QT syndrome: Using genetics to study cardiovascular disease. Circulation 85:1973, 1992.

Lehmann MH, Hardy S, Archibald D, et al: Sex differences in risk of torsade de pointes with d,l-Sotalol. Circulation 94:2535, 1996.

CHAPTER 39

Neurally Mediated Syncopal Syndromes

Stephanie Grosz and Ali Massumi

Syncope is a sudden, transient loss of consciousness and postural tone that spontaneously resolves. Syncope signifies inadequate cerebral perfusion, which is most commonly secondary to a cardiovascular cause. The clinical syndrome of syncope is common and is estimated to account for 3% of all emergency department evaluations.[1] Contrary to popular belief, the incidence of syncope is similar in women and men, occurring in 3.5% and 3.0% respectively, according to data from the Framingham study.[2]

Evaluation of the patient with syncope is a challenging and sometimes frustrating task. A correct diagnosis is essential, because syncope is often recurrent and in certain cases may be the harbinger of a life-threatening disorder. A careful initial history and physical examination may provide clues to the etilogy of syncope in approximately 40% of cases[3]; however, initial impressions are sometimes misleading. For example, seizure-like jerking activity often accompanies a transient loss of cerebral blood flow and may be misinterpreted as an indication of a primary central nervous system disorder. Likewise, judicious interpretation of secondary diagnostic procedures is imperative, because they, too, may at times be misleading. For instance, it is essential to demonstrate correlation between abnormalities found at the time of electrocardiographic monitoring or electrophysiologic testing and the patient's symptoms.

CLASSIFICATION OF SYNCOPE

It is helpful to classify the etiology of syncope as cardiovascular or noncardiovascular, because this distinction significantly alters evaluation, prognosis, and treatment. The prognosis of syncope secondary to a cardiovascular cause is significantly worse than when symptoms are not attributable to structural heart disease.[5, 6] Cardiovascular causes include those that are secondary to structural cardiac, pulmonary, or vascular disease. A subgroup of patients with a cardiovascular cause of syncope are those with neurally mediated reflex syncope. Noncardiovascular causes include neurologic, metabolic, and psychiatric disorders (Table 39–1).[4]

The focus of this chapter is on neurally mediated reflex syncope and the syndromes that cause this disorder. Neurally mediated syncope is the most common cardiovascular cause of syncope.[7] The syncope in these cases is *independent* of any structural heart disease. These patients appear to be susceptible to unexpected, inappropriate, and paradoxical neurally mediated reflex activity, which results in excessive peripheral vascular capacity as well as paradoxic chronotropic and inotropic responses.[8]

DEFINITION AND CLASSIFICATION OF NEURALLY MEDIATED SYNDROMES

There are multiple types of neurally mediated reflex syncopal syndromes. These syndromes are caused by an inappropriate neurally mediated reflex arc. Each syndrome has a different trigger receptor with a final common efferent limb of the reflex arc.[8] The most common of these is the simple vasovagal faint, which usually has an easily identifiable, noxious stimulus (e.g., intravenous line insertion, sight of blood, pain). Carotid sinus hypersensitivity with syncope is the next most frequently encountered event. This occurs when mechanical pressure on the carotid sinus baroreceptors triggers and initiates the reflex arc. Neurally mediated syncope may also occur without any definite or readily identifiable trigger. There are other less common syndromes that result in neurally mediated syncope, such as those associated with increased intrathoracic pressure, gastrointestinal stimulation (e.g., swallowing, defecation), and genitourinary stimulation (e.g., postmicturition, pelvic examination, intrauterine device [IUD] insertion) (Table 39–2).[8, 9] A subgroup of patients with neurally mediated syncope manifests prolonged brady-

Table 39–1. CAUSES OF SYNCOPE

Cardiovascular
- Postural hypotension (dehydration, drug induced)
- Neurally mediated reflex syncope
  - Vasodepressor
  - Carotid sinus hypersensitivity
  - Other reflex-mediated syndromes
- Structural heart disease
  - Fixed cardiac output (left or right ventricular outflow tract obstruction–aortic stenosis, IHSS, etc.)
  - Severe coronary artery disease
  - Electrical disturbances
    - Bradyarrhythmias (sinus node dysfunction, AV block, pacemaker malfunction)
    - Tachyarrhythmias (supraventricular and ventricular)
- Vascular disease
  - Cerebrovascular (vertebral-basilar insufficiency, subclavian steal syndrome, severe carotid stenosis)
  - Aortic dissection

Noncardiovascular
- Metabolic
  - Hypoglycemia, profound hyperglycemia, hypercapnea
- Neurologic
  - Seizure
- Psychiatric
  - Conversion disorder
- Acute bleeding

AV, atrioventricular.

Table 39–2. NEURALLY MEDIATED REFLEX SYNCOPAL SYNDROMES

1. Vasovagal faint
2. Neurally mediated syncope without readily identifiable trigger
3. Carotid sinus syndrome
4. Exercise-related syncope
5. GI/GU stimulation syncope (swallow syncope, upper aerodigestive tract stimulation, post-micturition syncope)
6. Glossopharyngeal neuralgia syncope

GI/GU, gastrointestinal/genitourinary.

cardia and asystole, termed the malignant vasovagal syndrome.

PATHOPHYSIOLOGY

Various mechanoreceptors trigger the common reflex pathway that causes neurally mediated syncope. These are receptors throughout the cardiopulmonary circulation with sensory fibers that travel in the vagus nerves. These receptors are located primarily in the heart, at the venoatrial junction, and in the inferoposterior wall of the left ventricle.[10, 11] Activation of myelinated afferent receptors results in sympathoexcitation in some vascular beds and sympathoinhibition in others. Activation of the nonmyelinated component (C fibers) results in reflex vagal activation, with slowing of the heart rate and sympathoinhibition.[10, 11] Stimulation of these receptors trigger the reflex arc in patients with the simple vasovagal faint and likely is the responsible initiating factor in those with neurally mediated syncope without a readily identifiable cause.

These are arterial mechanoreceptors located in the carotid sinus and in the aortic arch have both baroreceptor and chemoreceptor function. The baroreceptors increase their discharge with increases in blood pressure, causing reflex cardiac slowing and peripheral vasodilation through parasympathetic activation and withdrawal of sympathetic activation. The opposite scenario occurs with hypotension. The afferent fibers travel through the glossopharyngeal nerve from the carotid sinus, and through the vagus nerve from the aortic arch to the medulla.[10] Activation of these receptors in the carotid sinus is responsible for the initiation of carotid sinus syncope.

Mechanoreceptors are also present in the pharynx, larynx, and esophagus. These receptors send afferent nerve fibers to the medulla through the vagus nerve. Normal and abnormal vagal reflexes may result from stimulation of the receptors and result in significant reflex changes in cardiac and vascular function, which may initiate syncope. It has been postulated that central crosstalk at the level of the medulla may facilitate abnormal vagally mediated events associated with pharyngeal and gastrointestinal stimulation,[12] which may cause syncope.

There are several factors involved in the pathophysiologic mechanism of neurally mediated syncope. It is hypothesized that augmented sympathetic tone is the critical event that initiates the complex reflex. As mentioned before, the triggering mechanisms vary with each syndrome. However, the efferent limb of the reflex arc is constant among the disorders.

The exact events that occur during each type of neurally mediated syncopal syndrome are not yet completely understood. The prototype description of the basic reflex arc applies to the series of events that occurs with a simple vasovagal faint and probably with neurally mediated syncope without a clear initiating event. The initial triggering event causes increased adrenergic stimulation.[8] This activates the cardiac mechanoreceptors found in the base of the right and left ventricle. The activation results in forceful cardiac contraction and sends signals through unmyelinated C fibers to the nucleus tractus solitarii in the medulla, which processes these afferent impulses. The intense mechanoreceptor stimulation is misinterpreted at the level of the medulla and mimics the conditions seen in hypertension. The paradoxic compensatory response results in peripheral vasodilation, hypotension, decreased heart rate,[5] and syncope.

At the beginning of this series of events, there are elevated levels of circulating epinephrine that confirm that an adrenergic discharge has occurred.[8] As events progress, there appears to be an imbalance between the levels of epinephrine and norepinephrine, with a blunted increase in norepinephrine levels in response to the profound hypotension seen during the syncopal event.[13] Simultaneously, there is an inadequate decrease in parasympathetic tone,[14] which further allows the profound hypotension and bradycardia to occur.

It is postulated that cerebral autoregulation is abnormal in patients predisposed to neurally mediated syncope. Recent studies using transcranial Doppler techniques have reported inappropriate cerebral vasoconstriction in the face of peripheral vasodilatation, which further decreases cerebral perfusion and facilitates syncope. This issue is particularly relevant in elderly patients, who may have underlying cerebrovascular disease and are more susceptible to changes in blood pressure.[15, 16]

Echocardiography has been helpful in studying the events that occur during neurally mediated syncope. During a tilt-provoked event, it has been shown that the rate of reduction of the end-diastolic volume index occurred more rapidly in patients with syncope than in controls.[17] Left ventricular (LV) cavity obliteration was seen more often in subjects with positive tilt responses.[18] This information further supports the theory that a sudden adrenergic surge has occurred, with intense inotropic stimulation. Paradoxically, a reduction in stroke volume index and in the ejection fraction, believed to be secondary to both increased peripheral translocation of blood and early vagal effects on ventricular contractility, was seen during the syncopal event.[17]

Recent work has explored the gender differences in the pathophysiologic response in tilt-induced neurocardiogenic syncope. Complete hemodynamic profiling was performed with radionuclide testing for evaluation of blood volume and its distribution, LV function, speed of circulation and vasoconstrictive responses to decreased preload. Autonomic testing was performed when indicated in this study. Several types of hemodynamic patterns were seen in patients, including a hyperdynamic circulatory response with increased cardiac output and decreased systemic vascular resistance (SVR). Other hemodynamic patterns identified in patients with tilt-induced syncope included increased venous pooling, autonomic insufficiency, and relative hypovolemia. Compared with male patients with a positive tilt test, this hyperkinetic pattern was more common in female patients and may predict favorable response to beta-blocker therapy.[19]

Having described the basic events, it should be noted that each neurally mediated syndrome is initiated by different mechanoreceptors. Stimulation of the carotid baroreceptors initiates the reflex arc responsible for the carotid sinus hypersensitivity syndrome. The final series of events is similar to the sequence seen in neurally mediated syncope described earlier.[8] In addition, mechanoreceptors in the upper digestive tract can stimulate spontaneous swallowing syncope.[20] Other receptors located in the gastrointestinal and genitourinary tracts are responsible for afferent limb activation in postmicturition syncope and syncope related to pelvic examination and instrumentation.[9, 21]

There are two manifestations of this reflex arc, the cardioinhibitory and vasodepressor components. The vagal stimulation causes bradycardia, with slowing of the sinus node discharge or atrioventricular (AV) block. This is the cardioinhibitory component of the response. The vasodepressor component causes hypotension and results from both sympathetic withdrawal and parasympathetic stimulation. The cardioinhibitory and vasodepressor responses may be seen separately, or patients may have a mixed response, with both slowing of the heart rate and hypotension.[8]

NATURAL HISTORY

The long-term prognosis for patients with neurally mediated syncope is generally excellent, with a low mortality rate. The condition may be associated with significant morbidity from injury, which may occur secondary to the syncopal event. In a natural history study, 56 patients with a diagnosis of neurally mediated syncope were followed for a mean of 16 months off therapy. There were no deaths, and the rate of recurrence was 7% at 1 year and 15% at 21 months.[22] Athletes with exercise-induced neurally mediated syncope were followed on therapy for a mean of 35 months. Again, no deaths occurred, and no patients had recurrent syncope. The majority of patients were able to return to athletics free of symptoms.[23] Therefore, the primary reason to diagnose and treat this condition is to prevent recurrence of syncope.

HEAD UPRIGHT TILT TABLE TESTING

Given the frequency of neurally mediated syncopal syndromes, much attention has focused on appropriate evaluation of these disorders. Head upright tilt table testing has received the most scrutiny in evaluating the neurally mediated syndromes, and some concerns remain regarding the specificity, reproducibility, and lack of standard methodology for this test.

The rationale for upright tilt testing lies in the observations that the bradycardia or hypotension produced during a positive upright tilt test mimics the spontaneous neurally mediated events. Patients experience a similar prodrome including nausea, diaphoresis, lightheadedness, pallor, and increased heart rate. It has been shown that the temporal sequences in spontaneous and induced events are similar. In addition, the plasma catecholamine levels during spontaneous and tilt-induced syncope have been shown to be similar, with a significant increase in circulating catecholamine levels before the fainting event.[24]

Indications for Head Upright Tilt Table Testing

The indications for head upright tilt table testing are still in evolution, but recent literature has identified general guidelines for when tilt table testing would be beneficial.[25–28] Patients who suffer from recurrent unexplained syncope without evidence of structural heart disease and with a history or prodrome suggestive of neurally mediated syncope are good candidates for testing. Patients who suffer even single syncopal episodes who have sustained injury or who have a high-risk profession (e.g., surgeon, pilot, driver) warrant tilt table testing. Patients with structural heart disease who have a history suggestive of neurally mediated syncope or in whom other causes of syncope have been excluded would likely benefit from tilt testing.[24–26]

There are other instances in which tilt testing may be useful, although not definitely indicated. Differentiating convulsive syncope from epilepsy with head upright tilt may be useful in patients with recurrent syncope associated with tonic-clonic activity, those who have normal electroencephalograms, and those who do not respond to antiseizure medication. In this instance, tilt table testing may correct a diagnostic error and facilitate appropriate treatment.[27] Tilt table testing may be helpful in the evaluation of elderly patients with recurrent unexplained falls. Follow-up testing of drug therapy for the treatment of neurocardiogenic syncope is controversial because the test has problems with reproducibility, which may limit accurate evaluation of treatment efficacy. Upright tilt table testing is potentially useful in evaluating recurrent vertigo associated with near-syncope or syncope. Tilt table testing has reproduced symptoms in a significant number of these patients and has been useful in identifying whether transient periods of autonomic dysfunction are the cause of the vertigo.[28] Finally, there have been reports that neurally mediated syncope may exacerbate chronic fatigue syndrome. Head upright tilt table testing may identify these patients, and therapy to control the neurally mediated syndrome may significantly improve their symptoms of chronic fatigue.[24, 29]

Tilt table testing is relatively contraindicated in patients with severe left ventricular outflow tract obstruction, severe mitral stenosis, severe proximal coronary artery disease, and critical cerebrovascular stenosis. These patients have fixed cardiac or vascular stenoses, and syncope that results during tilt table testing may not be related to a neurally mediated event. In addition, inducing hypotension in these patients with critical structural cardiac and vascular disease can potentially be dangerous as well as unhelpful.

Protocol

There have been multiple protocols for upright tilt table testing, with variable sensitivities and specificities reported throughout the literature. Tilt angles of 60, 70, 80, and 90 degrees with and without the use of pharmacologic agents have been used. We recommend a tilt angle of 70 degrees.

There is agreement in the literature that the use of saddle support tilt tables markedly reduces the specificity associated with tilt table testing, with positive tests occurring in as many as 67% of controls.[30] This is secondary to excessive compression of the leg and pelvic vessels. For this reason, it is recommended that footboard support tables be used for adequate testing. An appropriate tilt table should be designed to support the patient gently. It should permit accurate calibration of the tilt angle and should be able to move from supine to upright position relatively rapidly and smoothly.

The tilt table test should be supervised by a physician who is familiar with the procedure and with the interpretation of the various test results. A nurse or technician familiar with the technique and management of potential complications should be present.

The patient is brought to the room in the fasting state. It is recommended that the testing be performed in the morning, while the patient is well hydrated. If any delay in testing is encountered, intravenous fluids should be administered to prevent dehydration, because dehydration and orthostasis render the test invalid. Electrocardiographic and pulse oximetry monitoring is performed throughout the test. Blood pressure monitoring is performed every 2 minutes with the least intrusive method possible. A finger cuff is preferred. If monitoring with an arterial cannula is performed, then a 20- to 30-minute period of monitoring after placement of the arterial catheter is recommended to allow the patient to recover and reequilibrate. An intravenous line is placed for administration of medications either for the test procedure or for emergency resuscitation. The room should be comfortable and quiet for optimal testing.

The patient is usually monitored in the supine position for several minutes before tilting. The table is then raised to the desired angle (e.g., 70 degrees) for the duration of passive tilting, which ranges from 15 to 60 minutes. The most common duration is 45 minutes, based on data from Fitzpatrick,[30] who determined that the mean time to a positive test was 24 minutes, with 45 minutes representing an interval of 2 standard deviations. If the patient develops syncope or presyncope with hemodynamic compromise, the table is returned to the supine position. If the patient has a negative passive tilt table test, then carotid sinus massage should be performed while the patient is upright, unless bruits or known cerebrovascular disease is present. Firm circular pressure for 3 to 4 seconds should be applied to the left and then to the right carotid sinus with monitoring for decreases in heart rate and blood pressure. After carotid sinus massage is completed, the patient is returned to the supine position.

Pharmacologic provocation, usually with isoproterenol, may be performed to provoke the neurally mediated syncope. Isoproterenol acts directly to increase inotropism and circulating catecholamines, to stimulate cardiac C fibers, and to precipitate the reflex arc responsible for neurally mediated events. The addition of isoproterenol increases the sensitivity and overall positivity, although with a small but significant decrease in specificity. The most common starting dose for isoproterenol initiation is 1 μg per minute, with titration to achieve a 25% increase in heart rate, followed by a single 70-degree tilt for 10 to 15 minutes.[24] In other protocols, isoproterenol is administered at 1 μg per minute for 5 minutes followed by tilting for 10 to 15 minutes. If the test remains negative, the patient is returned to the supine position and the dosage is increased to a maximum of 4 μg per minute, or a heart rate of 150, followed by final tilting for 10 to 15 minutes.[24] Nitroglycerin may be used instead of isoproterenol to provoke neurally mediated syncope. Nitroglycerin acts indirectly by causing increased venous pooling and decreasing preload. This effect may precipitate syncope in susceptible individuals by amplifying the effect of upright posture and prompting the initial adrenergic surge as a compensatory response to peripheral venodilation. After the baseline tilt, nitroglycerin, 300 μg sublingually, may be administered, followed by repeat tilt table testing for 20 minutes.[31] There is no standard protocol for testing, and there are many variations in methodology. Comparable overall results have been achieved with provocative protocols using isoproterenol or nitroglycerin, although there is concern that different patients will become positive, depending on the provocative agent used. The variability of protocols has limited the interpretation of the literature with respect to sensitivity, specificity, and reproducibility of testing.

Classification of Responses During Tilt Table Testing

There are three classic responses seen during head upright tilt table testing—the cardioinhibitory, the vasodepressor, and the mixed type—although several other patterns can be seen. The most frequent type of response is a cardioinhibitory response[32] with an abrupt fall in heart rate to less than 40 bpm for greater than 10 seconds or asystole for greater than 3 seconds with or without preceding hypotension (Fig. 39–1).[33, 34] The bradyarrhythmia can be dramatic with prolonged asystole secondary to AV block or sinus node arrest. Figure 39–2 is an electrocardiogram of a patient who, 12 minutes into tilt table testing, developed first-degree AV block that rapidly progressed to high-grade AV block with ventricular asystole and syncope. In these instances, the cardioinhibitory response is present in its most exaggerated form, which is termed malignant vasovagal syndrome.[33, 34] The second type of result is a pure vasodepressor response, with an initial fall in diastolic blood pressure and then a fall in systolic blood pressure greater than 25 mm Hg or a fall in mean blood pressure greater than 15 mm Hg without a significant rise in heart rate and without associated bradycardia (Fig. 39–3). This is reported in one third of patients with a positive test.[32] Most often, patients manifest both of these patterns with a mixed response. Heart rate rises initially and then falls, but the ventricular rate does not fall to less than 40 bpm or falls to 40 bpm for less than 10 seconds with or without asystole of less than 3 seconds.[33] In each type of response, the initial adrenergic surge causes the heart rate to increase before the initiation of the reflex with hypotension or bradycardia. A less common orthostatic response, but one that is still neurally mediated, is present in some elderly patients. They may have a gradual parallel decline in systolic and diastolic blood pressure, followed by a sudden drop in heart rate and blood pressure, resulting in loss of consciousness (Fig. 39–4). The initial events can be ascribed to orthostasis, followed by subsequent activation of the reflex arc, with neurally mediated syncope. These patients often

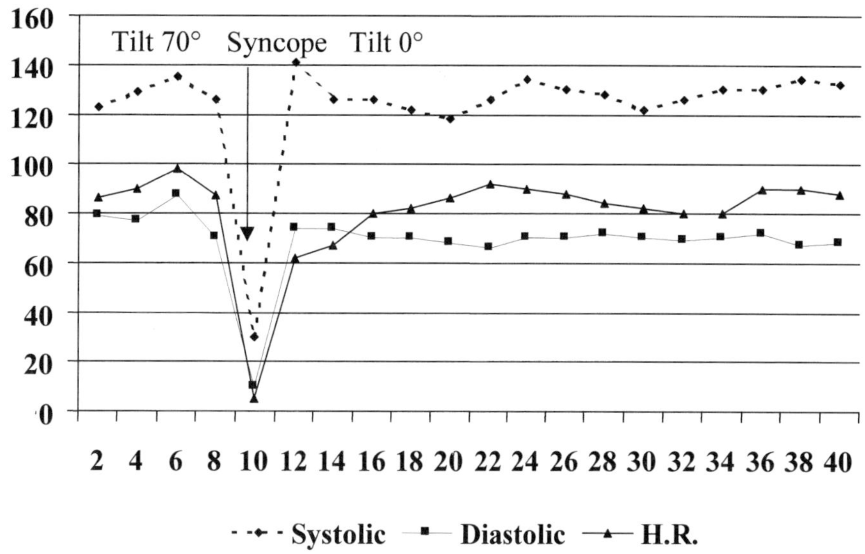

FIGURE 39–1. Cardioinhibitory response during tilt table testing. This is the most frequent type of response,[32] with an abrupt fall in heart rate to less than 40 bpm for more than 10 seconds, or asystole for more than 3 seconds with or without preceding hypotension.[33]

demonstrate other signs of autonomic dysfunction, such as orthostatic hypotension, in addition to this abnormal response to gravitational stress.[25] Other patients may have a psychogenic response during the tilt table test, with syncope and symptoms without any concomitant changes in blood pressure, electroencephalogram, or transcranial blood flow. This syncope is not neurally mediated but may signal a psychiatric illness that requires treatment.[25]

Sensitivity and Specificity of the Tilt Table Test

Determining the true sensitivity and specificity of upright tilt table testing is difficult because of the variety of protocols used and the lack of a true gold standard. Throughout the literature, there appear to be few false-positive tests, with a range of 0 to 11% positive tests in normal healthy volunteers during passive upright tilt testing.[30] The main difficulty with determining the specificity of this test is the potential for normal individuals without syncope to manifest this abnormal reflex during provocative conditions. Fitzpatrick and associates[30] provoked syncope in two of 27 normal controls and in five of 34 patients with known cardiac conduction system disease during tilting to 60 degrees for 60 minutes. Raviele and colleagues[35] reported no positive results in eight controls raised to 60 degrees for 60 minutes. Strasberg and associates[36] also reported no positive controls during 60-degree tilt for 60 minutes in 40 patients. In several studies, Grubb and coworkers had no positive controls during tilting to 80 degrees for 30 minutes; with isoproterenol (Isuprel) administration, no false-positive results occurred.[28, 37, 38] With brief passive tests, followed by Isuprel administration, more positive responses are seen in control patients. Almquist and coworkers reported that two of 18 control subjects developed syncope during the isoproterenol phase,[39] and Morillo and colleagues reported that 6.6% of control patients tested positive during the pharmacologic phase.[41] Although isoproterenol acts directly to increase inotropism and provokes a positive response, it may also cause abnormal activation of the reflex arc in patients who have not experienced syncope, which increases the false-positive rate.[39, 40]

Sensitivity is not as high as specificity during upright tilt table testing. Positive test percentages range from 26% to 90% during the passive phase of testing. Overall positive responses were reported in 49% of patients in a meta-analysis performed by Kapoor et al,[32] who reviewed 33 studies. Prolonged passive tilt at 60 degrees for 60 minutes resulted in positive tests in 53 of 71 patients (75%) in a study by Fitzpatrick and colleagues.[30] Strasberg and coworkers reported 37.5% positive results,[36] and Raviele and colleagues had a 50% positive rate[35] with a similar 60-degree protocol. Grubb and associates[38] reported a 64% overall positive rate, a 36% rate during baseline, and a 24% rate with Isuprel in 25 elderly patients, with 80-degree tilt. They also reported a 24% baseline positive rate and a 36% positive rate with Isuprel during a second study of nonelderly patients at 80-degree tilt.[37] Pongiglione and colleagues[41] reported an overall 80% positive rate in patients with 80-degree tilt with and without Isuprel. Morillo[40] reported a 61% positive rate with 60-tilt using Isuprel, and Almquist[39] had a 27% positive baseline and an 82% positive rate with Isuprel. The addition of isoproterenol increases the sensitivity and overall positivity of the tests, although with a small but significant decrease in specificity. As stated earlier, isoproterenol acts directly to increase inotropism and circulating catecholamines, stimulate cardiac C fibers, and precipitate the reflex arc responsible for neurally mediated events.

Several other drugs have been studied as adjuncts to increase further the sensitivity of tilt table testing, because of the concern of administering this drug to patients with angina or arrhythmias. Isoproterenol still remains the most commonly used and studied agent. Nitroglycerin has been used in several studies.[31, 42] Nitroglycerin acts indirectly by dilating the capacitance vessels, producing a significant pooling of blood within the vascular bed. This amplifies the effect of passive upright posture and increases the occurrence of neurally mediated syncope during testing. With the administration of intravenous nitroglycerin, a positive response occurred in 53% of patients, with 8% of controls having an abnormal test.[42] Sublingual nitroglycerin doubled the posi-

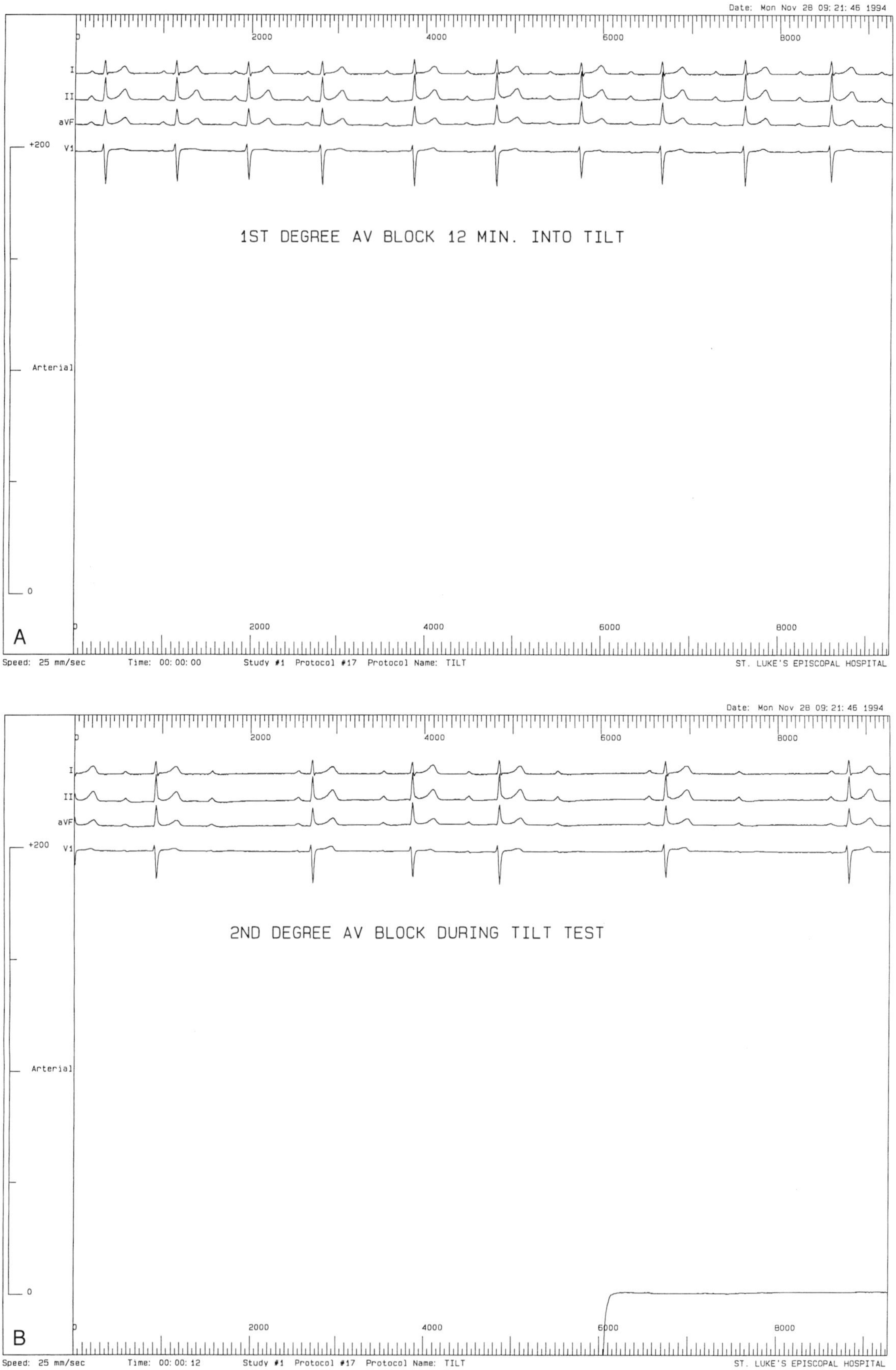

FIGURE 39–2. *A* and *B*, Twelve minutes into passive 70-degree tilt testing, the patient represented in Figure 39–1 began having first-degree AV block and then second-degree AV block.

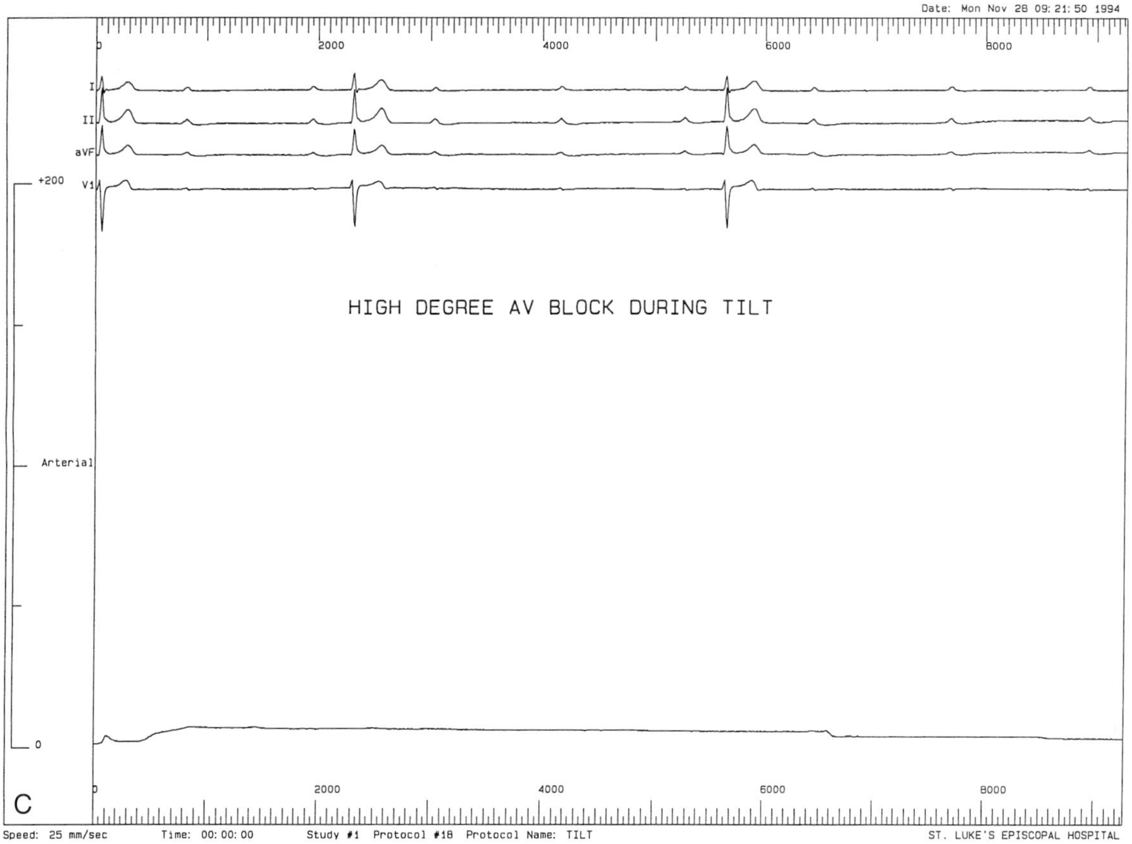

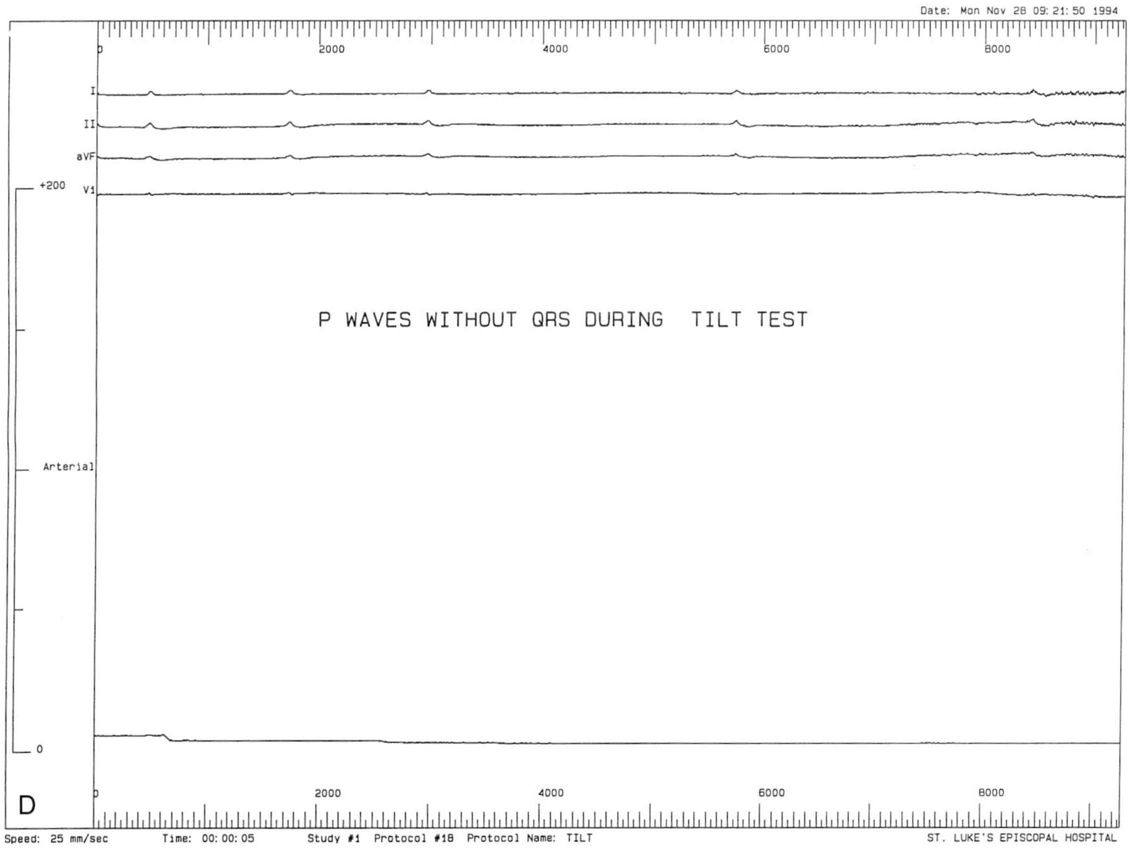

FIGURE 39–2 *Continued. C* to *E,* At the time of syncope, the patient experienced high-grade AV block with 18 seconds of ventricular asystole and seizure activity, before spontaneous return of rhythm. Blood pressure was not detectable at the time of syncope. Note the continuous P-wave activity during the period of ventricular asystole.

Illustration continued on following page

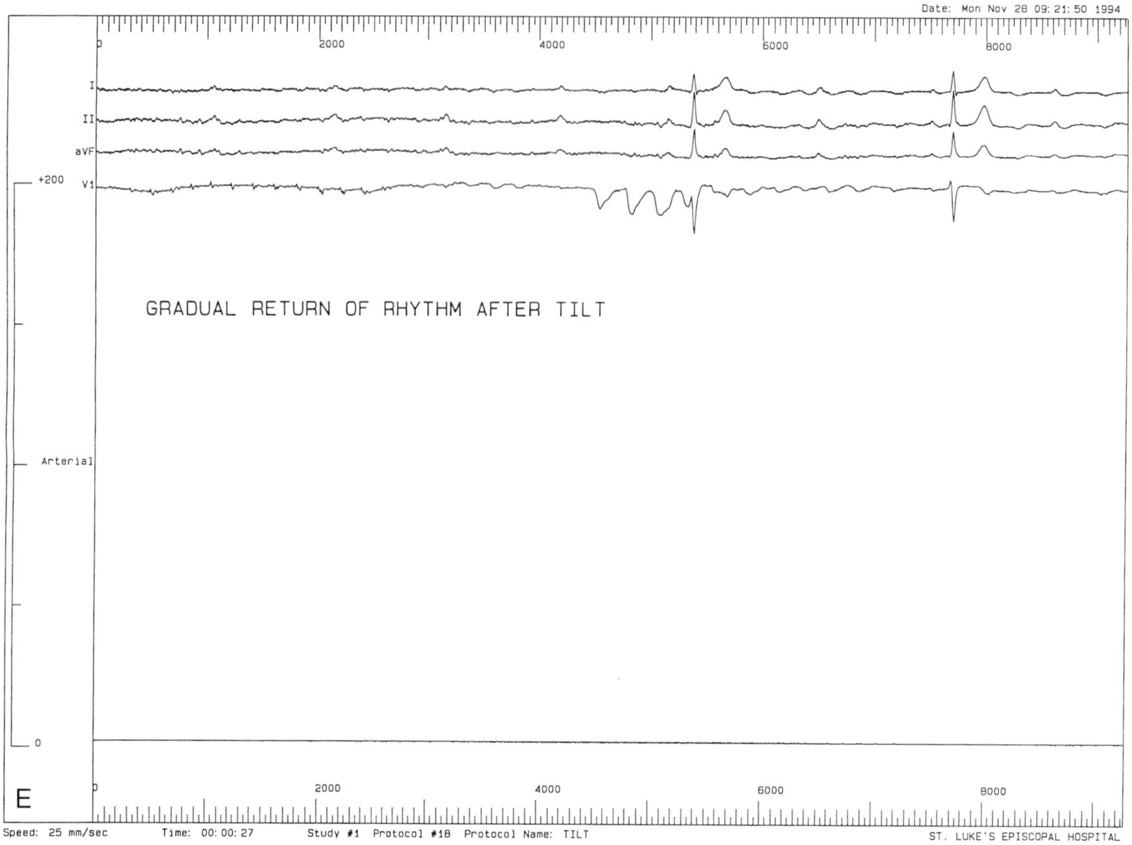

FIGURE 39–2. *Continued*

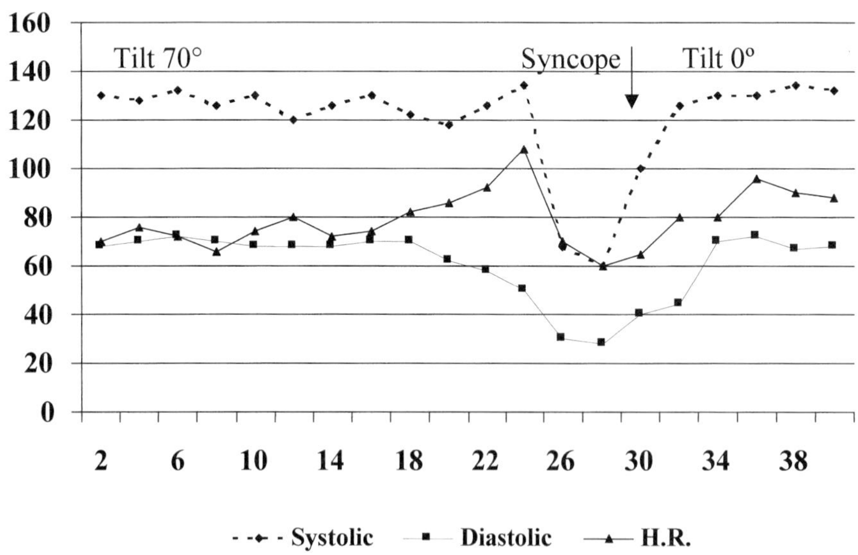

FIGURE 39–3. Vasodepressor response. A pure vasodepressor response is demonstrated, with an initial fall in diastolic blood pressure, and then a fall in systolic blood pressure greater than 25 mm Hg or a fall in mean blood pressure greater than 15 mm Hg without a significant rise in heart rate and without associated bradycardia.

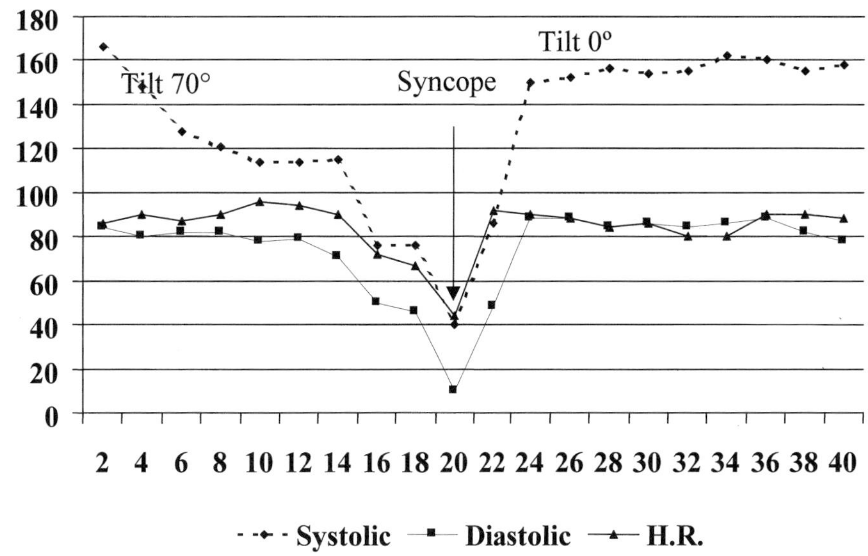

FIGURE 39–4. Orthostasic response. A less common, but still neurally mediated, response. Patients may have a gradual parallel decline in systolic and diastolic blood pressure, followed by a sudden drop in heart rate and blood pressure, resulting in loss of consciousness. The initial events can be ascribed to orthostasis, then subsequent activation of the reflex arc, with neurally mediated syncope.

tive response from 25% after the baseline tilt to 51% after nitroglycerin administration and repeat tilt.[31] Unfortunately, there was only a 33% correlation between tests performed using isoproterenol and nitroglycerin, and the utility of the nitroglycerin protocol is still not completely defined.

Edrophonium, which prevents acetylcholine degradation in the heart and peripheral vasculature, has been evaluated in tilt table testing, although its use is generally not common. Lurie and associates evaluated 45 patients with recurrent syncope. During the passive phase of the test, nine of 45 patients developed syncope with tilting to 60 degrees. After the administration of 10 mg of edrophonium, an additional 10 patients had classic neurocardiogenic events, with a pronounced bradycardic component. Of 20 controls, only one patient developed syncope with edrophonium.[43] This may be a useful drug to precipitate the bradycardia of the neurally mediated reflex.

Reproducibility of Syncope During Tilt Table Testing

The reproducibility of the head upright tilt table test is a critical issue, especially when considering testing the efficacy of various treatment regimens. To evaluate treatments, the means of diagnosis of a condition should be completely reliable. The reliability of head upright tilt table testing has been the focus of several recent studies. In general, the reproducibility of the test is reported to range from 60% to 100%. Concordance is the agreement between results in serial tests for the same patient. The concordance for patients with positive tests seems to be less than the concordance for those with negative tests.[44–47] Grubb and colleagues evaluated 21 patients with a history of syncope, with tilt table testing performed on different days. The overall concordance rate was quite acceptable, with 13 of 14 patients having a positive response on both tests and only one patient testing positive after an initial negative test.[44] A significant observation was that 36% of their patients required a different level of provocation to manifest an abnormal response. Patients with a longer clinical syndrome and with more frequent episodes of syncope were more often reproducibly abnormal during sequential tests. Brooks and coworkers[45] reported a very low rate of positive concordance of 37% between serial tests. Their protocol was a nonaggressive 15-minute, 70-degree tilt without pharmacologic provocation, and this may have significantly influenced their results. In this study, electrophysiologic testing on the same day of the tilt table test seemed to influence the test results, with more positive responses during tilt table tests performed on the same day as electrophysiologic testing than on separate days. Blanc and associates[47] evaluated 13 patients 7 days apart and found 62% of results correlated. Interestingly, patients with presyncopal syndromes more often had reproducible test results than patients with syncope.[47] An important finding reported by Fish and associates[48] was the frequent attenuated response during the second tilt table test. An overall reproducibility rate of 66% was reported among tests performed the same day, but the pattern of response was often different. The attenuated result obtained during repeat testing may limit the use of serial testing to assess treatment.[48] Chen and colleagues[46] reported a high rate of concordance (87%) and, significantly, there were no patients with initially negative test results who subsequently showed positive results. Overall, tilt table testing appears to have reasonable reproducibility, although the only truly reliable endpoint for assessing the efficacy of a treatment indicates the absence or presence of symptoms.

THERAPY OF NEURALLY MEDIATED SYNCOPE

Pharmacologic therapy has been the mainstay of treatment of most neurally mediated syndromes, with pacing therapy less commonly used. There are several approaches proposed to interrupt the reflex arc and prevent the vasovagal response. Drugs that decrease or block adrenergic stimulation (beta blockers) and inotropic response (beta blocker, disopyramide) may prevent stimulation of the cardiac C fibers and interrupt the afferent impulse responsible for the event.[25, 32, 49–51] Vagolytic drugs (atropine, scopolamine) may block the final efferent limb resulting in excessive vagal stimulation.[32, 49, 52] Theophylline may prevent neurally mediated syncope by blocking adenosine.[53] Volume-expanding agents (e.g., fludrocortisone) may increase intravascular reserve and decrease susceptibility to the initiating triggers.[32, 49] Drugs that oppose sympathetic withdrawal (etilefrine, methylphenidate, midodrine) may prevent the final vasodilation that characterizes the vasodepressor response.[49, 55–57] New reports show favorable responses to serotonin reuptake inhibitors, although these agents are not yet commonly used in these conditions.[49, 54]

Thus far, beta blockers are the most widely studied and safest medications for this disorder, and are thus considered first-line therapy for most recurrent neurally mediated syndromes. Reports show a positive response in 62% to 100% of affected patients, as evaluated by absence of syncope in follow-up, and by negative tilt table testing during therapy.[25, 32, 50, 51] A significant number of patients who report side effects with the medication are intolerant of beta blocker therapy. Disopyramide has been effective in some patients who fail or are intolerant of beta blocker therapy, although anticholinergic side effects relegate it to second-line therapy.[25, 52] Theophylline and scopolamine are less commonly used agents, with favorable results in small numbers of patients.[32, 53] The volume expander fludrocortisone is considered a useful drug, particularly in children, in adults with a dysautonomic component, and as an adjuvant treatment in refractory cases. Side effects, such as fluid retention and hypertension, may necessitate discontinuation of therapy. Support stockings can be helpful in patients with an orthostatic component to decrease peripheral venous pooling and decrease susceptibility to syncope.

Recent literature has shown that serotonin reuptake inhibitors may be effective, especially in cases of refractory neurocardiogenic syncope.[54] The exact mechanism by which these drugs work is still unknown. It is postulated that sympathoinhibitory serotonergic mechanisms may be activated during acute hemorrhage—a model that mimic the situation during vasovagal syncope—and this causes vasodilitation and bradycardia. Both fluoxetine and sertraline have been evaluated, with as many as 50% of refractory patients responding favorably to these agents.[54]

The final class of agents to consider are those that block sympathetic withdrawal. Methylphenidate was evaluated in seven women who were refractory to traditional therapies, and rendered six of the seven asymptomatic.[55] This drug acts by releasing stored catecholamines from the presynaptic pool and preventing their reuptake. Peripheral vascular effects are primarily those of vasoconstriction. Because of a significant side effect profile, including anorexia, nausea, anxiety, worsening of angina pectoris, and the potential for addiction, this drug is considered only in refractory patients. New data on midodrine, an alpha agonist, have shown that this agent can prevent the neurocardiogenic response in patients unresponsive to beta blocker therapy, and it may be indicated as a second tier of treatment for this subgroup of patients.[56, 57]

Implantation of permanent pacing devices for the treatment of neurocardiogenic syncope has been a controversial topic. Many of the affected patients are young, and the natural history of the disorder is benign with frequent spontaneous remissions. Permanent pacing can have psychological sequelae for these patients. In addition, pacing does not always prevent syncope in these patients. In a recent study[58] comparing the effectiveness of cardiac pacing with drug therapy, temporary pacing during tilt testing did not alleviate the hypotension caused by the vasodepressor component of the response.[58] Temporary pacing did not alleviate symptoms of syncope and presyncope in these patients. Ninety-four percent of the patients in this study were treated with drug therapy alone, with no recurrence in symptoms. A patient treated with dual-chamber pacing had recurrent syncope and required drug treatment for control of symptoms. Others have found that pacing may treat the cardioinhibitory component of the event but often does not prevent syncope.[59] Pacing may attenuate the hemodynamic response, and there may be a role for pacing as adjuvant therapy in refractory or elderly patients. Pacing is generally not indicated in the treatment of neurocardiogenic syncope except in certain select cases.

There are several subgroups of patients in whom pacemaker therapy may be considered. Elderly patients with or without carotid sinus hypersensitivity and with an asystolic response to carotid sinus massage may benefit from pacing therapy, although a significant vasodepressor component may still be present in these patients, that pacing does not alleviate.[60] Pacing in the malignant vasovagal syndrome is controversial. Most patients can be managed with pharmacologic therapy alone, but occasionally, pacing therapy may be used in conjunction with medication to control symptoms in these patients. Careful evaluation of patients with neurocardiogenic syncope allows identification of this subgroup of patients with prolonged asystole during tilt table testing of greater than 4 seconds' duration. These patients have a more severe clinical syndrome with more frequent and severe episodes without a prodrome. Although the majority of these patients, as many as 60%, can be managed with pharmacologic therapy alone, because of the severity of symptoms, pacing therapy can be helpful in conjunction with medication. Dual-chamber pacing is superior to single-chamber pacing, with less fall in systemic blood pressure, often converting sudden dramatic episodes to less severe events with a warning prodrome. Pacing therapy has a role in the subgroup of patients with asystolic neurocardiogenic syncope unresponsive to medical therapy as well as in the elderly.[60]

CONCLUSIONS

Neurocardiogenic syncope is a common disorder that has been more frequently diagnosed since the advent of head upright tilt table testing. The natural history is generally benign, with the primary goals of treatment being prevention of the morbidity associated with this condition and improving the quality of life in these generally healthy patients. The pathophysiology involves a complex reflex arc with multiple triggers. The end results of this series of events are vagally mediated bradycardia and systemic hypotension with syncope. Future areas of research should involve further evaluation and standardization of the many tilt table protocols, their reproducibility, and the applicability in assessing the effectiveness of therapy. Several new therapies are available, and testing is under way to find the best tolerated therapies to control this disorder and prevent this type of syncopal syndrome from negatively impacting on patients' lives.

References

1. Day SC, Cook EF, Funkenstein H, Goldman L: Evaluation and outcome of emergency room patients with transient loss of consciousness. Am J Med 73:15–23, 1982.
2. Savage DD, Corwin L, McGee D, et al: Epidemiologic features of isolated syncope: The Framingham Study. Stroke 16:626–669, 1985.
3. Kapoor W, Snustall O, Peterson I, et al: Syncope in the elderly. Am J Med 80:419, 1986.
4. Benditt D, Remole S, Milstein S, Bailin S: Syncope: Causes, clinical evaluation, and current therapy. Ann Rev Med 43:283–300, 1992.
5. Kapoor WN, Karpf M, Wieand S, et al: A prospective evaluation and follow-up of patients with syncope. N Engl J Med 309:197–204, 1983.
6. Benditt D: Syncope. In Willerson JT, Cohn J (eds): Cardiovascular Medicine. Churchill Livingstone, New York, 1995, p 1411.
7. Kapoor WN: Evaluation and outcome of patients with syncope. Medicine 69:160, 1990.
8. Benditt D, Goldstein M, Adler S, et al: Neurally mediated syncopal syndromes—pathophysiology and clinical evaluation. In Mandel W (ed): Cardiac Arrththmias, 3rd ed. J.B. Lippincott, Philadelphia, 1995, pp 879–906.
9. Chi, I-C, Wildens L, Siemens A, Lippes J: Syncope and other vasovagal reactions at interval insertion of Lieppes Loop D. Contraception 33: 179–187, 1986.
10. Smith M, Carlson, M, Thames M: Reflex control of the heart and circulation: Implications for cardiovascular electrophysiology. J Cardiovasc Electrophysiol 2:441–449, 1991.
11. Pelletier C, Shepherd J: Circulatory reflexes from mechanoreceptors in the cardio-aortic area. Circ Res 33:131–138, 1973.
12. Cunningham E, Ravich W, Jones B, Donner M: Vagal reflexes referred from the upper aerodigestive tract: An infrequently recognized cause of common cardiorespiratory responses. Ann Intern Med 116:575–582, 1992.
13. Sra J, Murthy V, Natale A, et al: Circulatory and catecholamine changes during head-up tilt testing in neurocardiogenic (vasovagal) syncope. Am J Cardiol 73:33–37, 1994.
14. Lippman N, Stein K, Lerman B: Failure to decrease parasympathetic tone during upright tilt predicts a positive tilt-table test. Am J Cardiol 75:591–595, 1995.
15. Grubb B, Gerard G, Roush K, et al: Cerebral vasoconstriction during head-upright tilt induced syncope: A paradoxic and unexpected response. Circulation 84:1157–1164, 1991.
16. Janosik D, Gomez C, Njemaze P, et al: Abnormalities in cerebral blood flow autoregulation during tilt induced neurocardiogenic syncope (abstract). Pacing Clin Electrophysiol 15:592, 1992.
17. Yamanouchi Y, Jaalouk S, Shehadeh A, et al: Changes in left ventricular volume during head-up tilt in patients with vasovagal syncope: An echocardiographic study. Am Heart J 131 1:73–80, 1996.
18. Nwosu E, Rahko P, Hanson P, Grogan E: Hemodynamic and volumetric response of the normal left ventricle to upright tilt testing. Am Heart J 128:106–113, 1994.
19. Wattar AR, Patel C, Jaeger F, Fouad Torazi F: Gender differences in tilt-induced neurocardiogenic syncope (abstract). Pacing Clin Electophysiol 20(Part II):1161, 1997.
20. Palmer E: The abnormal upper gastrointestinal vagovagal reflexes that affect the heart. Am J Gastroenterol 66:513–522, 1976.
21. Chi I-c, Wilkens R, Siemens AJ, Potts M: Rare events occurring at insertion of an intrauterine device—a review of an international experience. Adv Contracept 3:49–71, 1987.
22. Ruiz G, Peralta A, Gonzalez-Zuelgaray J, Duce E: Evolution of patients with clinical neurocardiogenic (vasovagal) syncope not subjected to specific treatment. Am Heart J 130:345–350, 1995.
23. Calkins H, Seifert M, Morady F: Clinical presentation and long-term follow-up of athletes with exercise-induced vasodepressor syncope. Am Heart J 129:1159–1164, 1995.
24. Benditt D, Ferguson DW, Grubb BP, et al: Tilt table testing for assessing syncope. ACC expert consensus document. J Am Col Cardiol 28:263–275, 1996.
25. Grubb B, Kosinski D, Samoil D: Recurrent unexplained syncope: The role of head upright tilt table testing. Heart Lung 22:502–508, 1993.
26. Samoil D, Grubb B: Head upright tilt table testing for recurrent unexplained syncope. Clin Cardiol 16:763–766, 1993.
27. Grubb B, Gerard G, Rousch K, et al: Differentiation of convulsive syncope and epilepsy with head upright tilt. Ann Intern Med 115: 871–876, 1991.
28. Grubb B, Rubin A, Wolfe D, et al: Head upright tilt table testing: A useful tool in the evaluation and management of recurrent vertigo of unknown origin associated with near-syncope or syncope. Otolaryngol Head Neck Surg 107:570–576, 1992.
29. Rowe P, Bou-Holaigah I, Kan J, Calkins H: Is neurally mediated hypotension an unrecognized cause of chronic fatigue? Lancet 345: 623–624, 1995.
30. Fitzpatrick A, Theodorakis G, Vardas P, Sutton R: Methodology of head upright tilt testing in patients with unexplained syncope. J Am Coll Cardiol 17:125–130, 1991.
31. Raviele A, Menozzi C, Brignole M, et al: Value of head-up tilt testing potentiated with sublingual nitroglycerin to assess the origin of unexplained syncope. Am J Cardiol 76:267–272, 1995.
32. Kapoor W, Smith M, Miller N: Upright tilt testing in evaluating syncope: A comprehensive literature review. Am J Med 97:78–88, 1994.
33. Benditt D, Lurie K, Adler S, Sakaguchi S: Rationale and methodology of head-up tilt table testing for evaluation of neurally mediated (cardioneurogenic) syncope. In Zipes D, Jalife J (eds): Cardiac Electrophysiology–From Cell to Bedside. WB Saunders, Philadelphia, 1995, pp 1115–1128.
34. Fitzpatrick A, Theodorakis G, Vardas P, et al: The incidence of malignant vasovagal syndrome in patients with recurrent syncope. Eur Heart J 12:389–394, 1991.
35. Raviele A, Gasparini G, Di Pede F, et al: Usefulness of head upright tilt testing in evaluating patients with syncope of unknown origin and negative electrophysiologic study. Am J Cardiol 65:1322–1327, 1990.
36. Strasberg B, Rechavia E, Sagie A, et al: The head-up tilt table test in patients with syncope of unknown origin. Am Heart J 118(Pt. 9): 923–927, 1989.
37. Grubb B, Temesy-Armos P, Hahn H, Elliot L: Utility of upright tilt table testing in the evaluation and management of syncope of unknown origin. Am J Med 90:6–10, 1991.
38. Grubb B, Wolfe D, Samoil D, et al: Recurrent unexplained syncope in the elderly: The use of head-upright tilt table testing in evaluation and management. J Am Geriatr Soc 40:1123–1128, 1992.
39. Almquist A, Goldenberg I, Milstein S, et al: Provocation of bradycardia and hypotension by isoproterenol and upright posture in patients with unexplained syncope. N Engl J Med 320: 346–351, 1989.
40. Morillo C, Klein G, Zandri S, Yee R: Diagnostic accuracy of a low-dose isoproterenol head-up tilt protocol. Am Heart J 129:901–906, 1995.
41. Pongiglione G, Fish F, Strasburger J, Benson W: Heart rate and blood pressure response to upright tilt in young patients with unexplained syncope. J Am Coll Cardiol 16:165–170, 1990.
42. Raviele A, Gasparini G, DiPede F, et al: Nitroglycerin infusion during upright tilt: A new test for the diagnosis of vasovagal syncope. Am Heart J 127:103–111, 1994.
43. Lurie K, Dutton J, Mangat R, et al: Evaluation of edrophonium as a provocative agent for vasovagal syncope during head-up tilt table testing. Am J Cardiol 72:1286–1290, 1993.
44. Grubb B, Wolfe D, Temesy-Armos P, et al: Reproducibility of head upright tilt table test results in patients with syncope. Pacing Clin Electrophysiol 15(Part I):1477–1481, 1992.
45. Brooks R, Ruskin J, Powell A, et al: Prospective evaluation of day-to-day reproducibility of upright tilt-table testing in unexplained syncope. Am J Cardiol 71:1289–1292, 1993.
46. Chen X, Chen M, Remole S, et al. Reproducibility of head-up tilt-table testing for eliciting susceptibility to neurally mediated syncope in patients without structural heart disease. Am J Cardiol 69:755–760, 1992.
47. Blanc J, Mansourati J, Maheu B, et al: Reproducibility of a positive passive upright tilt test at a seven-day interval in patients with syncope. Am J Cardiol 72:469–471, 1993.
48. Fish F, Strasburger J, Benson D: Reproducibiity of a symptomatic response to upright tilt in young patients with unexplained syncope. Am J Cardiol 70:605–609, 1992.
49. Elder CA, Spinler SA: Upright tilt-table testing and drug therapy for recurrent vasovagal syncope. Ann Pharmacother 26:786–788, 1992.
50. Cohen M, Snow J, Grasso V, et al: Efficacy of pindolol for treatment of vasovagal syncope. Am Heart J 130:787–790, 1995.
51. Mahanonda N, Bhuripanyo K, Kangkagate C, et al: Randomized double-blind, placebo-controlled trial of oral atenelol in patients with unexplained syncope and positive upright tilt table test results. Am Heart J 130:1250–1253, 1995.
52. Morillo C, Leitch J, Yee R, Klein G: A placebo-controlled trial of intravenous and oral disopyramide for prevention of neurally mediated

syncope induced by head-up tilt. J Am Coll Cardiol 22:1843–1888, 1993.
53. Nelson SD, Stanley M, Love CJ, Schaal SF: Chronic oral theophylline for the management of vasodepressor syncope (abstract). Circulation 82 (Suppl III):III-707, 1990.
54. Grubb B, Samoil D, Kosinski D, et al: Use of sertraline hydrochloride in the treatment of refractory neurocardiogenic syncope in children and adolescents. J Am Coll Cardiol 24:490–494, 1994.
55. Grubb B, Kosinski D, Mouhaffel A, Pothoulakis A: The use of methylphenidate in the treatment of refractory neurocardiogenic syncope. Pacing Clin Electrophysiol 19:836–840, 1996.
56. Ghaly N, Gessman L, White M, et al: Efficacy of midodrine hydrochloride in the treatment of refractory neurocardiogenic syncope (abstract). Pacing Clin Electrophysiol 20(Part II): 1159, 1997.
57. Klingenheben T, Sticherling C, Li Y, et al: A two-step treatment strategy in neurocardiogenic syncope: Midodrine as second-line treatment in patients refractory to beta-receptor-blockers (abstract). Pacing Clin Electrophysiol 20(Part II):1159, 1997.
58. Sra J, Jazayeri M, Avitall B, et al: Comparison of cardiac pacing with drug therapy in the treatment of neurocardiogenic (vasovagal) syncope with bradycardia or asystole. N Engl J Med 328:1085–1090, 1993.
59. Ko C, Hou Z, Chiou C, Chen C: Pacing may not prevent neurocardiogenic syncope: The importance of correct diagnosis. Int J Cardiol 43: 207–209, 1994.
60. Menozzi C, Brignole M, Lolli G, et al: Follow-up of asystolic episodes in patients with cardioinhibitory, neurally mediated syncope and VVI pacemaker. Am J Cardiol 72:1152–1155, 1993.
61. Grubb B, Temesy-Armos P, Moore J, et al: Head-upright tilt-table testing in the evaluation and management of the malignant vasovagal syndrome. Am J Cardiol 69:904–908, 1992.

SECTION

XII

PULMONARY HYPERTENSION

CHAPTER

40

Pathophysiology, Clinical Recognition, Diagnosis, and Management

Adaani E. Frost

Pulmonary hypertension is a disorder of the pulmonary vascular bed. Morbidity and mortality associated with pulmonary hypertension usually result from the secondary cardiac failure it produces. The finite capacity of the right side of the heart to generate cardiac output in the face of high pulmonary vascular resistance is responsible for most of the signs and symptoms of pulmonary hypertension and often for the mortality associated with this disease. Recent advances in our understanding of primary pulmonary hypertension, which is a rare disorder, have led to a greater understanding of the pathophysiology of all forms of pulmonary hypertension. The following review of the pathophysiology, diagnosis, and management of pulmonary hypertensive disorders excludes neonatal and pediatric issues outside of those relating to the development of the pulmonary vascular bed.

PATHOPHYSIOLOGY OF THE NORMAL PULMONARY CIRCULATION

The pulmonary circulation is a low-pressure, high-flow, high-capacity system[1] with a large surface area designed to provide an interface with the alveoli and to facilitate effective gas exchange. The smallest unit of the pulmonary vascular bed is the septal capillary, which is composed of alveolar epithelial lining cells supported by minimal stroma closely approximated to the vascular endothelium of the pulmonary capillary. Oxygen and carbon dioxide diffuse across the endothelial and epithelial layers because of the pressure differential between dissolved gas and alveolar gas, which is enhanced by the reversible binding of hemoglobin to both oxygen and carbon dioxide.

Flow across the large surface area of the pulmonary vascular bed is determined by the viscosity of the fluid flowing through the system and the length and radius of the vessels. This relationship is expressed in Poiseuille's law, which describes flow through rigid cylindrical tubes as $R = 8nL/r^4$, where R = resistance, n = viscosity of fluid, L = length of the cylinder, and r = radius. The principles of this equation can be used to understand pressure and flow across the pulmonary vascular bed; however, the vessels within the circulation are not rigid cylinders, and the pathology of the pulmonary circulation often reflects this fact. If flow and blood viscosity are constant, then changes in resistance across the pulmonary vascular bed should reflect changes in vessel radius. In the clinical setting, resistance to flow across the pulmonary vascular bed is expressed as a function of the pressure gradient across the vascular bed, the mean pulmonary artery pressure [PA_{mean}] minus pulmonary capillary wedge pressure [LA_{mean}], and is inversely proportional to the cardiac output. Thus, an increase in resistance can be reflected by an increase in the mean pulmonary artery pressure, or by a decrease in the cardiac output. Similarly, if pulmonary vascular resistance remains constant, an increase in cardiac output results in an increase in mean pulmonary artery pressure, whereas a decrease in cardiac output is associated with a decrease in pulmonary artery pressure. Recognition of these simple concepts is crucial to understanding and evaluating the pulmonary vascular bed in the clinical setting. Pulmonary artery pressure can increase with a change in pulmonary vascular resistance (produced by a decrease in the vessel radius or an increase in fluid viscosity), an increase in cardiac output, or an increase in the mean left atrial pressure (as seen in pulmonary hypertension caused by left-sided heart failure or valve disease).

The normal adult at sea level has a systolic pulmonary artery pressure of approximately 22 mm Hg, a diastolic pressure of approximately 8 mm Hg, and a mean pulmonary arterial pressure of 13 mm Hg.[2] These measurements reflect the larger capacity and lower resistance of the pulmonary vascular bed relative to the systemic vascular bed. The pulmonary vascular resistance in normal individuals decreases with increased flow, and the pulmonary artery pressure remains relatively stable with significant increases in blood flow.[3–5] Possible reasons include an increase in the radius of these highly compliant vessels resulting from vessel distention and vessel recruitment. This low resistance circuit is characterized histologically by thinner, less muscular pulmonary arteries that have fewer adrenergic nerve endings than systemic vessels of similar size. Pulmonary hypertension has been defined clinically[6, 7] as a mean pulmonary artery pressure greater than 25 mm Hg at rest or greater than 30 mm Hg during exercise.

Understanding the development of the pulmonary circulation and the normal responses of the pulmonary vascular bed to various stimuli is important to understanding the pathophysiology of pulmonary hypertension. In utero, the unventilated fetal lung has no role in gas exchange. Fetal pulmonary vascular resistance approximates systemic vascular resistance after birth. Blood flows primarily from the systemic venous return to the right atrium, through the foramen ovale, into the left atrium, and out into the systemic arterial circulation through the left ventricle.[8, 9] During fetal life, approximately one fourth of the systemic venous return reaches the right ventricle, whereas the remainder enters the left ventricle through the foramen ovale. Approximately two thirds of the right ventricular output bypasses the pulmonary vascular bed and enters the descending aorta through the ductus arteriosus. Thus, only a small fraction of the venous return enters the pulmonary vascular bed and perfuses the lung. Fetal (and to a lesser extent, adult) pulmonary vascular resistance is labile and is affected by autonomic nerve stimulation, pharmacologic agents, and arterial pO_2, pCO_2, and pH. In the systemic circulation, elevations in pCO_2 and decreases in pO_2 produce vasodilation.[10] In contrast, hypoxia[11, 12] and hypercapnia in the pulmonary vascular bed produces vasoconstriction. Acidemia, together with pCO_2 and pO_2 levels, produces further vasoconstriction. The resulting hypoxic vasoconstriction may contribute to intrauterine elevation of pulmonary vascular resistance.

Following birth, hypoxic vasconstriction is an important homeostatic mechanism for optimizing blood oxygenation in the face of acute or chronic pulmonary parenchymal abnormalities like pneumonia and emphysema. Although the alveoli were initially thought to be the major sites of hypoxic vasoconstriction, oxygen sensing does not occur exclusively in the alveolar capillaries.[13] In fact, Kato and Staub[14] provided histologic confirmation that the small muscular pulmonary arteries at the level of the terminal respiratory bronchioles are the major site of hypoxic vasoconstriction. Their work was confirmed by Nagasaka and associates,[15] who determined that the main site of hypoxic vasoconstriction lies within the small pulmonary arteries (30 to 50 μm) and that the remaining vascular resistance arises from the capillaries and the venous system.

Although alveolar or airway hypoxia alone is sufficient to stimulate hypoxic vasoconstriction, a reduction in the oxygenation of the mixed venous blood returning to the right ventricle has an additional effect on pulmonary vasoconstriction.[16, 17] When the lungs expand after birth, the pulmonary vascular resistance falls dramatically and pulmonary blood flow increases. By the end of the first week of life, the ductus arteriosus is functionally closed, and pulmonary vascular remodeling has decreased smooth muscle within the intra-acinar pulmonary arteries. An increase in the compliance of the pulmonary vascular bed accompanies this remodeling and by the age of 6 months, pulmonary vascular resistance achieves adult levels. Vasoconstrictive stimuli (such as hypoxia, hypercapnia, and acidemia) that persist are thought to inhibit the normal regression of pulmonary smooth muscle within the neonatal lung, to induce the proliferation of smooth muscle, and to extend fibroblasts and smooth muscle into the intra-acinar arteries. Adult development of persistent pulmonary hypertension in response to various chronic vasoconstrictive stimuli results from similar mechanisms.

ETIOLOGIES OF PULMONARY HYPERTENSION

Primary and secondary pulmonary hypertension result from disorders of the pulmonary arteries, capillaries, venules, or left heart (Table 40–1).

Elevations of Left Atrial Pressure

The most common cause of pulmonary hypertension is cardiac disease that produces an increase in left atrial pressures. This increase can result from elevated left ventricular end-diastolic pressure associated with almost any form of left ventricular failure or valvular disease (such as mitral stenosis, aortic stenosis, or aortic insufficiency). Furthermore, space-occupying lesions of the left atrial or ventricular cavities such as myxomas, thrombus, or rarely, tumor can increase left atrial pressure. The presentation of left ventricular dysfunction and valvular disease and their diagnosis and management are discussed in Sections III and IV of this text.

Table 40–1. SECONDARY CAUSES OF PULMONARY HYPERTENSION

LUNG DISEASE
Parenchymal disease: interstitial lung disease evidenced by reduction in TLC of > 2 SD from predicted norm and associated pulmonary infiltrates on chest x-ray study or high-resolution CT; obstructive lung disease evidenced by hypoxemia and reduced flow rates (FEV_1/FVC ratio > 2 SD from predicted norm)[56]
Ventilation disorders
Congenital anomalies of lungs, thorax, or diaphragm
Hypoxia-induced disease
HEART DISEASE
Elevated left heart filling pressures
Congenital systemic to pulmonary shunts
ANATOMIC OBSTRUCTION OF THE PULMONARY VASCULAR BED
Pulmonary thromboembolism
Mediastinal fibrosis
Congenital stenosis of pulmonary artery or vein
Foreign bodies (talc)
TUMOR
HEMOGLOBINOPATHIES (SICKLE CELL)
SCHISTOSOMIASIS
COLLAGEN VASCULAR DISEASES
TOXINS OR DRUGS
Anorexic agents
Toxic rapeseed oil
L-Tryptophan
Crack cocaine
PULMONARY HYPERTENSION–ASSOCIATED DISEASES
HIV infection
Portal hypertension
Gaucher's disease

FEV_1, forced expiratory volume (in 1 second); FVC, forced vital capacity; HIV, human immunodeficiency virus; SD, standard deviation; TLC, total lung capacity.

Disorders of the Pulmonary Veins

Congenital or acquired obstruction of pulmonary venous drainage is a rare cause of pulmonary venous hypertension. Acquired obstruction is associated both with mediastinal irradiation and with idiopathic mediastinal fibrosis. Pulmonary veno-occlusive disease is discussed under the heading of primary pulmonary hypertension because it is a primary disorder of the pulmonary vascular bed that results in pulmonary hypertension.

Pulmonary Parenchymal Disease

Pulmonary vascular disease is a common and serious complication both of chronic obstructive and of restrictive pulmonary parenchymal disease. About 50% of patients with chronic obstructive pulmonary disease (COPD) older than 50 years of age develop pulmonary hypertension, which significantly reduces survival[18] and impairs quality of life.

The development of pulmonary hypertension in pulmonary parenchymal disease is associated with a variety of factors. An absolute reduction in the cross-sectional area of the pulmonary vascular bed occurs in many of the pulmonary parenchymal diseases, most notably emphysema. The destruction of alveoli and of the alveolar septa containing the capillaries defines the parenchymal disease. However, even in very severe emphysema, pulmonary artery pressures rarely increase to the levels seen in other pulmonary disorders associated with similar reductions in FEV_1. Mean pulmonary artery pressures rarely exceed 40 mm Hg in COPD.[19] The loss of vascular surface area caused by destruction of lung parenchyma or compression of the vasculature by hyperinflation may play an important role in the development of pulmonary hypertension in some patients with severe emphysema.[20] However, in several studies both the level and the rate of progression of arterial hypoxemia correlate with the severity and the rate of progression of pulmonary hypertension[21, 22] rather than with the degree of derangement in pulmonary function studies. The incomplete hemodynamic response to long-term oxygen therapy in hypoxemic patient with COPD suggests that other factors contribute to pulmonary vascular disease in this setting.[23]

Although supplemental oxygen therapy is the only form of treatment that improves survival in hypoxemic patients with COPD, no clear relationship exists between improved survival and reduction in pulmonary vascular resistance with oxygen therapy. Some evidence suggests that patients in whom oxygen therapy reverses pulmonary hypertension to some degree (defined as a drop in mean pulmonary artery [PA] pressure of 5 mm Hg or more) survive longer than those who do not respond.[24]

In contrast to COPD, the fibrosing and inflammatory pulmonary disorders, such as idiopathic pulmonary fibrosis and sarcoidosis, are frequently associated with major increases in pulmonary artery pressure. This secondary pulmonary hypertension is caused, in part, by inflammatory or fibrosing changes that occur within the pulmonary arteries (both small and medium arteries and capillaries). Secondary pulmonary hypertension contributes significantly to morbidity and mortality in patients with these diseases.

In addition to affecting the pulmonary vascular bed directly, pulmonary parenchymal disease produces pulmonary hypertension by the vasoconstricting effects of alveolar and airway hypoxemia, hypercapnia, and mixed venous hypoxemia. The normal physiologic response to hypoxemia is the induction of erythropoietin production. Erythropoietin, which is produced by the kidney, acts on the bone marrow to increase hemoglobin production by decreasing the programmed cell death that normally regulates the release of circulating erythrocytes from the marrow. The resulting abnormal elevations in hemoglobin increase blood viscosity according to Poiseuille's law and contribute to the elevation in pulmonary artery pressures.

Similarly, the normal cardiovascular response to hypoxemia is to increase cardiac output—initially with effort and ultimately even at rest. This increase in cardiac output, which has no effect on pulmonary vascular resistance, further increases pulmonary artery pressures, thereby creating an additional load on the right ventricle.

Pulmonary Arterial Disease

The development of pulmonary hypertension by directly involving the precapillary pulmonary arterial bed occurs as a consequence of anatomic, reactive (vasoconstrictive), or inflammatory obstruction.

Pulmonary Thromboembolic Disease

Anatomic obstruction occurs in pulmonary thromboembolic disease, which is a common and frequently fatal disease. Of 5 million episodes of deep venous thrombosis detected from clinical and autopsy data, approximately 10% (representing 600,000 patients) result in pulmonary emboli.[25] Only 0.4% of pulmonary emboli result in the development of pulmonary hypertension associated with chronic pulmonary thromboembolic disease.[26] These cases represent approximately 2000 new cases of chronic pulmonary hypertension each year in the United States that can be attributed to pulmonary embolic disease. Demographic data on the frequency of this disease in men and women are conflicting. Most clinical series contain more men than women, with an overall ratio as high as 5:1 suggested by surgical data from San Diego.

Pulmonary hypertension following thromboembolism may be attributed to the following mechanisms: major proximal occlusion of the vascular bed by a single large clot; reactive vasoconstriction in the remaining vascular bed; proximal propagation of clot; or in situ thrombosis within smaller arterioles that occurs as a consequence of intimal damage produced by cytokine mediators, vasoconstriction, hypoxia, coagulation disturbances, or turbulent flow resulting from large vessel obstruction. Interestingly, the distal vasculature in proximal large vessel thromboembolic disease is usually patent but not normal. Distal histopathologic changes in the proximally obstructed vascular bed identical to the features of pulmonary hypertension have been reported in both an early case report[27] from 1946 and in more recent data.[28, 29] In addition, similar changes have been produced in dogs by proximal ligation of the pulmonary artery—even in the absence of pulmonary hypertension.[30, 31] These data suggest that these histopathologic changes are not mediated by flow or pressure. Despite the histologic changes (e.g., intimal proliferation, medial hypertrophy, and plexiform lesions) characteristic of pulmonary hypertension, removing the proximal obstruction alleviates the pulmonary hypertension. Studies have suggested that endothelial injury in the distal vasculature results from proximal large vessel obstruction.[32–34] This putative endothelial injury may contribute to the development of the pulmonary edema that characterizes reperfusion of the lung after successful surgical extraction of an organized thrombus.

Schistosomiasis

Although conventional thromboembolic disease is the most common pulmonary arterial vascular obstruction seen in the

United States, the parasitic disease schistosomiasis is common worldwide[35] and is associated with pulmonary vascular obstruction. In schistosomiasis, obstruction is caused both by the anatomic presence of the parasite and by the intense inflammatory vasculitic response that occurs when the parasite breaks down. In endemic areas such as Egypt, schistosomiasis is the most common cause of cor pulmonale. Significant liver disease is always present when such pulmonary changes occur.

Pulmonary Hypertension Associated with Liver Disease

Pulmonary hypertension was first associated with chronic liver disease and portal hypertension in 1951.[36] Since then, numerous case reports and series have confirmed this association.[37] Pulmonary hypertension associated with liver disease, although rare,[38] has major implications for patients who are being considered for liver transplant or who are being evaluated for the diagnosis and management of pulmonary hypertension. The survival rate of patients with pulmonary hypertension associated with portal hypertension is lower than that in patients with isolated primary pulmonary hypertension.[32] Hypoxemia is found frequently in patients with cirrhosis because of the presence of intrapulmonary shunts[39] (the hepatopulmonary syndrome). In patients with hypoxemia without pulmonary hypertension, liver transplantation is usually successful. The effect of pulmonary hypertension on patient survival after liver transplantation is unclear. In some studies, pulmonary hypertension has increased the mortality rate[40] and complicated postoperative care in liver transplant patients[41]; however, in multivariate analyses, pulmonary hypertension had no effect on graft or patient survival.[42]

Pulmonary Hypertension Associated with Human Immunodeficiency Virus Infection

Human immunodeficiency virus (HIV) infection is emerging as one of the more common causes of new-onset primary pulmonary hypertension.[43–45] This association has triggered interest in potential viral mechanisms for the onset of pulmonary hypertension.[46] The overall survival rate of HIV-infected patients with pulmonary hypertension is poor. In fact, the survival rate is equal to or worse than that for non–HIV-infected patients with primary pulmonary hypertension. The effect of the newer antiretroviral drugs on patients with pulmonary hypertension is unknown. Antiretroviral drugs have not been shown to affect the hemodynamic or clinical markers of pulmonary hypertension. Experience with continuous intravenous prostacyclin, however, while anecdotal, is very promising. The pathology of pulmonary hypertension in HIV-infected patients can include classic plexogenic arteriopathy. Intravenous drug use can be associated with pulmonary veno-occlusive disease,[47] and unexplained thrombotic primary pulmonary hypertension has been reported in an HIV-infected patient.[48]

Miscellaneous Causes of Pulmonary Hypertension

Pulmonary hypertension has been associated with Gaucher's disease, a rare storage disease characterized by hepatosplenomegaly and portal cirrhosis. Pulmonary hypertension has been described in association with the presence of Gaucher's cells within the pulmonary parenchyma. The effect of treatment of Gaucher's disease with the synthetic glucocerebrosidase (alglucerase [Ceredase]) on pulmonary hypertension is unknown; however, pulmonary hypertension has been diagnosed after treatment.[49]

The use of appetite suppressants has been associated with the development of primary pulmonary hypertension and has primarily affected women. An epidemic of primary pulmonary hypertension in the mid to late 1960s was associated with the use of aminorex fumarate.[50] More recent, carefully documented reports on the association between derivatives of fenfluramine and new-onset pulmonary hypertension[51, 52] suggest that the use of these anorexiants for longer than 3 months significantly increases the risk of developing pulmonary hypertension (a 23-fold increase in the odds ratio). In addition, this pulmonary hypertension does not respond to discontinuing the anorexiants. The pathologic appearance of anorexiant-associated pulmonary hypertension is indistinguishable from that of primary pulmonary hypertension. Whether affected patients have an inherent predisposition to developing pulmonary hypertension is unknown.

L-Tryptophan was first associated with pulmonary hypertension in 1989 when an epidemic characterized by diffuse myalgia and eosinophilia occurred. The eosinophilia-myalgia syndrome was attributed to the use of over-the-counter L-tryptophan. The pathology of this particular type of pulmonary hypertension is characterized by widespread non-necrotizing vasculitis, which involves veins and arteries with perivascular and interstitial infiltration by lymphocytes and eosinophils.[53]

Primary Pulmonary Hypertension

In 1891, Romberg[54] described the case of a woman with pulmonary hypertension that could not be explained by the usual mechanisms. In 1959, Dresdale and coworkers[55] reported a series of 39 cases of this unexplainable pulmonary hypertension and coined the term primary pulmonary hypertension. By 1971, more than 600 cases of primary pulmonary hypertension had been reported, making this entity a rare though increasingly recognized diagnosis. Primary pulmonary hypertension is defined clinically[56] as the presence of pulmonary hypertension (mean pulmonary artery pressure greater than 25 mm Hg at rest or greater than 30 mm Hg during exercise), normal pulmonary artery wedge pressure, and the absence of secondary causes. The term primary pulmonary hypertension includes a spectrum of pathologic pictures and acknowledges associations with other diseases: HIV-associated pulmonary hypertension, toxin-induced pulmonary hypertension, and pulmonary hypertension associated with portal hypertension.

The recognition that a disorder of vascular homeostasis within the pulmonary circulation can result in pulmonary hypertension and its attendant morbidity and mortality has increased scientific focus on this entity. Although primary pulmonary hypertension was originally thought to be limited to relatively young women, data from the Patient Registry for the Characterization of Primary Pulmonary Hypertension[57] indicate otherwise. The sex distribution of the initial 187 registrants showed that the female-to-male ratio was 1.7:1. The age distribution differed between the sexes; the highest frequency was in the third decade of life for women and the fourth decade for men. The disease is not confined to younger age groups; 10% of the patients were 60 years or older.

The primary pulmonary vasculopathies have been divided into three subsets: pulmonary arteriopathy, pulmonary veno-occlusive disease, and pulmonary capillary hemangiomatosis.

Pulmonary Arteriopathy

Historically, plexogenic pulmonary arteriopathy was thought to be pathognomonic of primary pulmonary hypertension and was thought to have prognostic and therapeutic ramifications. In fact, studies on patients with primary pulmonary hypertension, thromboembolic pulmonary hypertension,[58] and pulmonary hypertension secondary to congenital cardiac disease have shown similar pathologic pictures with varying degrees of thrombosis and classic plexogenic pulmonary arteriopathy. Plexogenic pulmonary arteriopathy should be considered a histologic description of a nonspecific response to hemodynamic injury that does not correlate with the etiology, hemodynamic features, or prognosis of the disease.[59]

The pathogenesis of pulmonary arteriopathy is not fully understood although vasoconstriction and thrombosis appear to be significant factors in the development and perpetuation of the disease. Several clinical studies suggest that a coagulation disorder contributes to the progression and mortality of this disease, but other data are conflicting. The histopathology includes features of in situ thrombosis. Studies of anticoagulation with warfarin have indicated that anticoagulation increases survival, especially in patients who are unresponsive to vasodilator therapy.[60, 61] In a study by Eisenberg and colleagues,[62] patients with primary pulmonary hypertension had increased thrombin activity, as shown by plasma concentrations of fibrinopeptide A, which is a marker of the action of thrombin on fibrinogen. This finding suggests a procoagulant tendency in patients with primary pulmonary hypertension. In the same study, the normal fibrinolytic response to clot formation was limited as shown by increased activity of plasminogen activator inhibitor-1. A similar study by Huber and associates[63] demonstrated a prothrombotic tendency both in primary pulmonary hypertension patients and in patients with pulmonary hypertension secondary to thromboembolic disease compared with patients with Eisenmenger's physiology and controls. These authors based their conclusions on evidence of coagulation activation (indicated by fibrinogen levels) and impaired fibrinolysis (indicated by t-PA and plasminogen activator-1 inhibitor).

The putative vasoconstrictive mechanism that results in primary pulmonary hypertension is also not fully understood. Clinical studies indicate that vasodilators increase functional capacity and possibly improve survival.[51] These studies imply that vasoconstriction is a factor in the onset and progression of this disease. Further clinical studies have suggested that vasoconstriction may be mediated either by excessive production of vasoconstrictors such as thromboxane,[64] endothelin,[65, 66] and serotonin,[67] or by inadequate production of endogenous vasodilators such as prostacyclin.[55] The plexiform lesions of pulmonary hypertension, although no longer considered pathognomonic of primary pulmonary hypertension, are still considered histologic markers of pulmonary hypertension. The presence of these lesions has been associated with evidence of increased endothelial cell growth and with features of inflammation (specifically increased numbers of T and B lymphocytes and macrophages). These findings suggest an increased production of cytokines and growth factors, which might contribute both to the development of the plexiform lesions and to the progression of pulmonary hypertension.[68] Transforming growth factor-β has been one of the cytokines implicated in this response.[69]

Pulmonary Veno-occlusive Disease

Pulmonary veno-occlusive disease, an uncommon cause of pulmonary hypertension, is thought to be caused by a primary obstructive thrombotic disorder of the pulmonary venules and veins. The veins show medial hypertrophy and arterialization; the alveolar capillaries are extremely congested, and the alveoli contain numerous hemosiderin-laden macrophages. These characteristics contrast sharply with pulmonary arteriopathy, which almost completely spares the alveoli and alveolar capillaries. Changes in the pulmonary arteries in pulmonary veno-occlusive disease are thought to be secondary to the venous obstructions.[70] Like classic primary pulmonary hypertension caused by pulmonary arteriopathy, the cause of pulmonary veno-occlusive disease is unknown. Pulmonary veno-occlusive disease has been observed after chemotherapy,[71, 72] and familial cases have been reported.[73, 74]

Pulmonary Capillary Hemangiomatosis

Pulmonary capillary hemangiomatosis is a rare condition characterized by proliferating thin-walled microvessels that infiltrate the lung parenchyma, pleura, and peribronchial and perivascular interstitium.[75] These infiltrating microvessels cause fibrous obstruction of the lumen of affected vessels. Medial hypertrophy of the muscular arteries and muscularization of the arterioles also occurs. Because of their thin walls, these vessels are predisposed to bleeding with hemoptysis and its pathologic corollary, hemosiderin-laden macrophages in the alveolar spaces and interstitium.

DIAGNOSTIC EVALUATION OF PULMONARY HYPERTENSION

General Clinical Features

The common signs and symptoms of pulmonary hypertension (Table 40–2) are often subtle and can be confounded by the presence of associated or underlying diseases that

Table 40–2. SIGNS AND SYMPTOMS OF PULMONARY HYPERTENSION

SIGNS
Right ventricular heave
Palpable prominent P2
Jugular venous distention
Hepatojugular reflux
Right-sided S3 or S4
Hepatomegaly (often pulsatile)
Ascites
Splenomegaly
Peripheral edema
Anasarca
Supraventricular arrhythmia
Peripheral or central cyanosis
SYMPTOMS
Fatigue
Dyspnea
Syncope
Near-syncope
Cough
Hoarseness
Edema
Increasing abdominal girth
Palpitations
Raynaud's phenomenon

contribute to the development of the pulmonary hypertension. The most common symptoms include exertional dyspnea, fatigue, chest pain (which often mimics angina in character, location, radiation, and aggravating and alleviating factors), syncope, and near-syncope.

In patients with intrinsic pulmonary parenchymal disease, a decrease in exercise tolerance without commensurate decreases in airway obstruction or restriction suggests the development or progression of pulmonary vascular disease. Assessing a decrease in exercise tolerance in this patient population, however, is often confounded by steroid-associated myopathy and deconditioning.

Syncope is a particularly ominous symptom because it indicates significant compromise of cardiac output. The presence of edema or anasarca usually correlates with severe right-sided heart failure, and the severity of right-sided heart failure, as reflected in right atrial pressure elevation, correlates with mortality, as seen in patients with primary pulmonary hypertension and in patients with isolated cardiac disease awaiting heart transplantation. In both groups, right atrial pressures less than or equal to 10 mm Hg are associated with survival, whereas those with right atrial pressures greater than or equal to 20 mm Hg have a predicted 6-month mortality rate of 100%. Hoarseness is found frequently and relates to compression of the left recurrent laryngeal nerve by the hugely dilated pulmonary artery and the adjacent aorta.

Raynaud's phenomenon is frequently present in patients with primary pulmonary hypertension (reportedly between 6% and 20%) and is seen in 25% to 30% of patients with pulmonary hypertension associated with collagen vascular disease.

Abdominal distention and, occasionally, disturbances in bowel function can indicate passive congestion of the liver and portal hypertension. Liver capsular distention with associated right upper quadrant pain can occur in the presence of acute or rapidly progressive right-sided heart failure. If right-sided heart failure and liver congestion are severe or persistent, then jaundice can be present.

Clinical Features of Primary Pulmonary Hypertension

The Primary Pulmonary Hypertension Registry documented many of the initial presenting features of primary pulmonary hypertension. Dyspnea, which was the most common initial symptom, was reported in 60% of patients but was present in 98% of patients by the time they had been diagnosed and enrolled in the registry. The mean time from onset of symptoms to diagnosis was 2.03 $\pm$ 4.9 years.[57] The initial symptoms in descending order of frequency were fatigue (19%), syncope (8%), chest pain (7%), near-syncope (5%), palpitations (5%), and leg edema (3%). However, at the time of enrollment, fatigue was present in 73% of patients, chest pain in 47%, near-syncope in 41%, syncope in 36%, edema in 37%, and palpitations in 33%. Only 10% of the patients in the initial review of registrants reported symptoms of Raynaud's phenomenon. Of that 10%, almost all (95%) were women. The incidence of Raynaud's phenomenon in this group does not differ significantly from that in the general population (6%).[76] The registry data also showed that the rates of smoking (45%), oral contraceptive use (54% of the females), and parity (2.3 live births per female patient) were similar to those in the general population.

General Physical Examination Findings in Pulmonary Hypertension

Findings on physical examination can reflect the features of pulmonary hypertension and the underlying disease. Patients may be cyanotic in the presence of a severe V/Q mismatch, underlying lung disease, or a right-to-left shunt (either congenital or acquired). Chest examination may show features of intrinsic parenchymal lung disease, for example, hyperinflation with reduced breath sounds in the case of emphysema, or diffuse fine dry crackles in the presence of pulmonary fibrosis. However, the chest examination may be normal in keeping with pure pulmonary vascular disease. Prominent bibasilar "moist" inspiratory crackles, or pleural fluid along with appropriate cardiovascular findings would suggest that the source of the pulmonary hypertension is left ventricular dysfunction. However, the interdependence of right and left ventricular function, confined as the ventricles are within the pericardial sac, can confound the physical examination. Bibasilar crackles compatible with interalveolar pulmonary edema and classic left-sided heart failure can occur when deteriorating cardiac output and massive dilation of the right ventricle are present. Although the left ventricular ejection fraction is preserved in patients with right ventricular pressure overload, the left ventricular cavity is underfilled.[77–79] This situation may occur because of elevated left ventricular end-diastolic pressure arising from compromise of the left ventricular cavity by paradoxical septal shift. In addition, pleural effusions can occur with pulmonary hypertension associated with collagen vascular disease, primary pulmonary hypertension, and of course, pulmonary hypertension associated with pulmonary embolic disease. Therefore, their presence does not necessarily imply a predominantly left-sided etiology for pulmonary hypertension.

Cardiovascular findings can be striking; however, in early pulmonary hypertension, abnormal findings may be absent. In fact, cardiac function may be normal at rest. Jugular venous distention may be present, which indicates increased right ventricular filling pressures. However, jugular venous distention may indicate increased intrathoracic pressure, which is attributable to significant intrinsic pulmonary disease in the absence of elevated pulmonary arterial pressures. Jugular venous distention with associated paradoxical pulse marks severe airway obstruction. In these patients, syncope and near-syncope usually reflect limited venous return caused by elevated intrathoracic pressures, rather than limited cardiac output resulting from pulmonary arterial hypertension. Under these circumstances, the pulmonary examination indicates either a pulmonary vascular or a pulmonary parenchymal etiology for syncope.

The presence of A waves indicates elevated right ventricular filling pressure, and v waves indicate tricuspid regurgitation. A precordial heave or lift can be palpated over the sternum and is related both to the proximity of the distended right ventricle to the sternum (with obliteration of the retrosternal air space) and to the increased contractile force of the hypertrophied and dilated right ventricle. Occasionally, a pulmonary arterial pulse can be palpated at the left sternal border second interspace in cases of massive distention of the pulmonary arteries. Auscultation may reveal an accentuated P2 component of the second heart sound, which may also be palpable. A right-sided S4 is not uncommon in moderately severe pulmonary hypertension, but the presence of a right-sided S3 gallop indicates a more severe right ventricular failure. A holosystolic murmur compatible with tricuspid insufficiency is another common finding. With severe right ventricular dilation, a pulmonary insufficiency murmur (diastolic, low pitched, blowing) may be heard at the left sternal border, second or third interspace. Fixed splitting of the second heart sound suggests an unrecognized congenital cardiac defect (atrial septal defect). The presence of a pulmonary flow murmur heard over the major pulmonary artery branches during a breath hold has been associated with pulmonary artery branch interruption caused by stenosis or by chronic large vessel proximal thromboembolic disease.[80]

Hepatomegaly, ascites, or edema indicate right-sided heart failure. However, portal hypertension resulting from intrinsic liver disease is associated with the development of pulmonary hypertension caused by unknown mechanisms. The presence of these physical findings, particularly in the absence of marked jugular venous distention, would suggest that portal hypertension is the cause rather than the effect of pulmonary hypertension.

Peripheral cyanosis is an ominous sign that indicates a significant reduction in cardiac output. Central cyanosis can reflect intrinsic pulmonary parenchymal disease, significant ventilation-perfusion mismatching from pulmonary parenchymal or vascular disease, or the presence of a right-to-left shunt (either congenital or acquired). Recent onset suggests the opening of a foramen ovale (a common occurrence in patients with chronically elevated right-sided pressures) or the development of Eisenmenger's physiology in patients with congenital cardiac disease.

The pathophysiology of digital clubbing remains unclear, although the presence of precapillary shunts (at the level of the liver or the lung) with release of megakaryocytes into the systemic circulation has been proposed as a potential mechanism. The megakaryocytes occlude capillaries and are thought to release platelet-derived growth factors (and other factors) that increase endothelial permeability and stimulate the activity and proliferation of fibroblasts and other connective tissue cells.[81] Digital clubbing rarely occurs in primary pulmonary hypertension and only if a right-to-left shunt is present. However, it is a common feature of congenital cardiac disease, septic and fibrosing pulmonary disease, and liver disease.

Laboratory Evaluation for Pulmonary Hypertension

An extensive laboratory evaluation is required to establish a diagnosis of pulmonary hypertension and to discover its underlying cause (Table 40–3). Baseline tests should initially be conducted when pulmonary hypertension is suspected. Secondary studies are initiated based on the results of a physical examination, history, or preliminary results of the initial baseline evaluations.

Chest radiographs may show significant pulmonary parenchymal disease, features such as Kerley B lines that suggest left ventricular dysfunction, or radiologic features of pulmonary hypertension (Table 40–4). Enlargement of the major hilar pulmonary arteries indicates pulmonary hypertension.

Table 40–3. LABORATORY EVALUATION OF PULMONARY HYPERTENSION

BASELINE
Chest x-ray
Electrocardiogram
Pulmonary function tests
Echocardiogram
Ventilation-perfusion lung scan
Hemoglobin and hematocrit
Liver function tests
SECONDARY
Heart catheterization
Pulmonary angiogram
Sleep study
Venous Doppler scan
Collagen vascular evaluation
ESR, ANA, RF, anti-DNA
Scleroderma antibodies
Anticardiolipin antibodies
Lupus anticoagulant
Coagulation screen
Protein C, protein S, antithrombin III
Factor V resistance to activated protein C (Leiden mutation)
Homocysteine
Prothrombin 20210A
Ferritin (hemochromatosis)
Hemoglobin electrophoresis
Liver biopsy
Abdominal ultrasound

ANA, antinuclear antibodies; ESR, erythrocyte sedimentation rate; RF, rheumatoid factor.

Table 40–4. RADIOLOGIC FEATURES OF PULMONARY HYPERTENSION

GENERAL	
	Right ventricular enlargement
	Loss of retrosternal air space (on lateral film) resulting from right ventricular distention
	Pulmonary arterial dilation (upper limit of normal = 16 mm right interlobar artery)
SPECIFIC	
	Pulmonary plethora—as in congenital or left ventricular cardiac disease
	Asymmetric oligemia—due to pulmonary arterial occlusions
	Diffuse oligemia—Eisenmenger's physiology, primary pulmonary hypertension
	Proximal pulmonary arterial calcification—longstanding increases in PVR, for example, Eisenmenger's physiology

PVR, pulmonary vascular resistance.

The normal maximum diameter of this artery on inspiration is 16 mm in adult men and 15 mm in adult women.[82] Further enlargement may be considered indicative of the presence of pulmonary hypertension.

Electrocardiography may show the characteristic signs of right ventricular hypertrophy: QRS axis less than 110 degrees (right axis deviation), RSR′ in V_1 and V_2, incomplete right bundle branch block, and P pulmonale (peaked P waves in inferior and right precordial leads indicative of right atrial enlargement). Acute severe CO_2 retention or severe hypoxemia can produce acute pulmonary hypertension with all the associated electrocardiographic, echocardiographic, and radiologic manifestations of pulmonary hypertension. Although they are markers of the severity of the underlying parenchymal lung disease, acute severe CO_2 retention and severe hypoxemia are dramatically and rapidly reversed by initiating appropriate bronchodilator and anti-inflammatory therapy, by administering oxygen, and by providing mechanical ventilatory support (either invasive or noninvasive—e.g., continuous positive airway pressure).

Echocardiography may show right ventricular hypertrophy and dilation, and associated hypokinesis. Flattening of the interventricular septum during systole and diastole or frank paradoxical displacement of the interventricular septum into the left ventricular cavity can occur with increasing right ventricular distention and pressure overload. Echocardiograms (aided, if necessary, by contrast with agitated saline) can estimate pulmonary artery pressures, left atrial pressure, and cardiac output. In addition, echocardiograms can indicate the location and size of right-to-left shunts (intrapulmonary shunts as described in the hepatopulmonary syndrome, atrial septal defects, ventricular septal defects, patent foramen ovale) and provide data on valve areas, transvalvular gradients, and left ventricular function.

Pulmonary function tests show significant pulmonary parenchymal disease as the cause of pulmonary hypertension. As discussed earlier, significant abnormalities of pulmonary function or diffusion capacity have to be present (usually with reductions in diffusing capacity of the lung for carbon monoxide [DLCO] below 50%) before the pulmonary hypertension can be attributed to parenchymal disease. The inflammatory pulmonary parenchymal diseases (pulmonary fibrosis, sarcoidosis, bronchiectasis) are more commonly associated with significant pulmonary hypertension than are the purely obstructive diseases.

Ventilation-perfusion lung scanning is a critical adjunct to the assessment of pulmonary hypertension, even though fatalities have been associated with the injection.[83, 84] Lung scans are not indicated when clinical or radiologic evidence of pulmonary parenchymal disease is available; however, in the presence of a normal parenchyma on chest radiograph, multiple segmental unmatched defects reflect a high probability of pulmonary hypertension associated with thromboembolic disease. The lung scan is usually normal in primary pulmonary hypertension and in those forms of pulmonary hypertension associated with collagen vascular disease when the pulmonary parenchyma is preserved. However, by their nature, the abnormalities, when present, are not segmental defects but patchy, irregular, and usually peripheral perfusion defects. The presence of macroaggregates of ^{131}I-labeled albumin on a postinfusion scan of the head and kidneys can provide additional information about the presence of significant right-to-left shunts.

TREATMENT OF PULMONARY HYPERTENSION

The treatment of pulmonary hypertension should, to a certain extent, be tailored to the specific underlying cause of the pulmonary hypertension. However, many of the predisposing causes, such as intravenous drug abuse, the use of anorexiants, pulmonary parenchymal disease, and Gaucher's disease, may no longer be amenable to treatment likely to reverse the process.

The first-line approach to managing pulmonary hypertension is to remove potential aggravating factors like vasoconstrictors (such as over-the-counter pseudoephedrine, neosynephrine compounds, inhaled adrenalin), hypoxemia, cigarette smoke (which has a vasoconstricting effect[85]), and residence at high altitude.

The other aspects of treating pulmonary hypertension relate to therapy designed to decrease pulmonary vascular resistance and increase right ventricular contractility. Therapy should include judicious management of blood viscosity by phlebotomy because an increase in red cell mass is an appropriate and necessary physiologic response to tissue demands for oxygen delivery in patients who are hypoxic or who have low cardiac output. The use of phlebotomy to improve exercise tolerance, myocardial function, and tissue oxygen delivery in hypoxemic polycythemic patients has been studied in patients with COPD. In these patients, reducing the hematocrit from 62% to 56% by phlebotomy improved exercise performance[86] and left ventricular function.[87] Extrapolating from COPD patients to pulmonary hypertensive patients with limited cardiac output is not unreasonable. However, no data are available on the effect of phlebotomy in pulmonary hypertensive patients.

Lung or heart-lung transplantation is the final therapeutic option for patients with severe, progressive pulmonary hypertension unresponsive to therapy and who are classified as New York Heart Association (NYHA) class III or worse.

Treatment of Pulmonary Hypertension Secondary to Pulmonary Parenchymal Disease

Clearly, the underlying disease should be treated. As previously discussed, oxygen administration has some capacity to reverse hypoxic vasoconstriction. In one report, the use of steroids was effective in treating the inflammatory pulmonary disorder sarcoidosis.[88] Vasodilator therapy improved pulmonary vascular resistance and cardiac output in COPD-associated pulmonary hypertension,[89] but clinical benefits were not shown in studies of exercise tolerance.[90] The use of digoxin in the absence of associated left ventricular dysfunction to improve right ventricular function has not been clinically useful.[91] This finding is not surprising because patients with COPD usually die of hypoxia or hypercapnia rather than from low cardiac output. The benefits of vasodilators in patients with severe pulmonary parenchymal disease and associated severe cor pulmonale must be weighed against the risks of increasing arterial hypoxemia by disturbing hypoxic pulmonary vasoconstriction.

Treatment of Pulmonary Thromboembolic Disease

The treatment of pulmonary hypertension associated with pulmonary thromboembolism is predicated on preventing subsequent thromboembolism. Anticoagulation has not been shown to affect disease progression. Histologic studies and studies of the activation of the coagulation system suggest the presence of ongoing thrombosis or thromboembolism. The mortality rate with medical management of pulmonary hypertension is 39% at a mean follow-up of 4 to 5 years, and in 30% to 40% of cases,[92] progression of pulmonary hypertension is caused by recurrent pulmonary embolism.[92] Placing an inferior vena caval filter (a bird's nest or a Greenfield filter) is considered mandatory, but whether caval filters affect long-term disease progression is unknown.

Pulmonary thromboendarterectomy, a revascularization procedure, has been extremely successful. Mortality is remarkably low (recently reported as 8.7%[93]) considering the severity of illness, the complexity of the surgery, and the mortality associated with severe pulmonary hypertension alone. A risk analysis of a large surgical series[94] failed to identify preoperative predictors of mortality, which would permit optimal candidate selection. In that analysis, the variables assessed had been identified as potential risk factors in earlier studies and included age, NYHA class, and pulmonary vascular resistance. Pulmonary vascular resistance approached but did not achieve statistical significance. Postoperative predictors of mortality in the same study included failure to lower the pulmonary vascular resistance by more than 50% and prolonged time on bypass. The causes of postoperative mortality include intraoperative myocardial infarction, recurrent thrombosis, technical surgical problems (perforation of the pulmonary artery), and multiorgan failure, which is usually a consequence of hypotension caused by right ventricular failure or failure to adequately reduce the pulmonary vascular resistance.

Treatment of Primary Pulmonary Hypertension

At present, anticoagulation and high-dose calcium channel blockers are used in conventional therapy for primary pulmonary hypertension. Patients who respond to calcium channel blockers have a better prognosis than patients who do not respond. Initiating calcium channel blockers (in patients who respond) significantly improves pulmonary artery pressures and pulmonary vascular resistance, which is maintained over time and may improve survival.[95]

Prostacyclin,[96, 97] adenosine,[98] and nitric oxide[99] have been used for rapid screening for acute vasoreactivity (which selects those patients most likely to respond to calcium channel blockers). The rapid reversibility of these agents makes them a good choice for screening because the negative effect of the conventional calcium channel blockers is sustained for the half-life of the drug. Nifedipine and diltiazem have been the two calcium channel blockers most frequently used. However, newer shorter acting calcium channel blockers with less negative inotropic effect (nicardipine) are being used with increasing frequency to establish optimum treatment doses in pulmonary hypertension; longer acting calcium channel blockers with little or no negative inotropic effect (amlodipine) are used in stable patients who have demonstrated vasoreactivity.[100]

For patients in whom conventional therapy fails and clinical or hemodynamic parameters worsen, continuous intravenous prostacyclin is the treatment of choice before considering lung transplantation. The benefits of prostacyclin were established in a 12-week study that compared survival, hemodynamic, and functional parameters in patients with primary pulmonary hypertension who were randomized to receive either conventional therapy (calcium channel blockers and anticoagulation) or conventional therapy and a continuous intravenous infusion of synthetic prostacyclin (epoprostenol). In this study, prostacyclin improved survival, hemodynamic measurements (which was not predicted by the initial response to the drug), and functional capacity.[101] Prostacyclin may achieve its benefits through several mechanisms: by directly affecting vasodilation, by acting on endothelial cells,[102] or by decreasing platelet-associated production of thromboxane A_2. Case reports have suggested that prostacyclin may be useful in the long-term management of other causes of pulmonary hypertension.[103, 104] The role of digoxin in these patients is uncertain, but clinical experience suggests that the positive inotropic effect of digoxin is useful in these patients because morbidity and mortality are usually related to failure of right ventricular output. The maximum pressure of the untrained right ventricle is limited; however, chronic increases in afterload induce both dilation and hypertrophy. Theoretically, the hypertrophied right ventricle should respond to digoxin in a manner similar to the left ventricle. Although digoxin has a vasoconstrictive effect on both pulmonary and systemic vasculature, this effect appears to be outweighed by the benefit produced by increased contractility; therefore, the current practice is to treat patients who have primary pulmonary hypertension with digoxin.[105]

The presence or development of a patent foramen ovale is associated with improved survival.[106] Patients with primary pulmonary hypertension usually die because of progressive right-sided failure with a reduced cardiac output. The presence of a patent foramen ovale reduces the right ventricular afterload, and the cardiac output improves at the expense of oxygenation. For both adults[107, 108] and children[109] in whom medical management has failed to relieve primary pulmonary hypertension (or in some cases, secondary hypertension related to congenital cardiac disease—mitral atresia or stenosis[110]), balloon and blade septostomy have been used. This procedure creates physiology similar to that achieved with the natural reopening of the vestigial foramen ovale in the atrial septum. Although it is not widely used, this procedure has resolved symptoms and improved survival. The patient is usually transfused to a hemoglobin level of 15 to 16 g to improve oxygen-carrying capacity. An ambulatory protocol of continuous inhaled nitric oxide has been successful in treating a few cases of primary pulmonary hypertension.[111] However, technical refinements in the ambulatory nitric oxide protocol are required before it can be widely used to treat primary pulmonary hypertension.

Treatment for Pulmonary Hypertension Secondary to Collagen Vascular Disease

The treatment of pulmonary hypertension secondary to collagen vascular disease is based on the same principles as those described earlier; however, few data are available. Calcium channel blockers[112] improve hemodynamic variables in many patients. Comparative studies of vasodilator therapies have not been conducted. In patients with connective tissue diseases in the scleroderma spectrum, angiotensin-converting enzyme inhibitors have been effective in some studies[113] but not in others.[114] A large randomized study comparing continuous epoprostenol with conventional therapy has established the efficacy of this drug in patients with pulmonary hypertension secondary to the scleroderma spectrum of disease.[115]

Treatment for Eisenmenger's Complex

Management of patients with Eisenmenger's complex has changed little over the years. Conventional wisdom has been to avoid oxygen therapy because it does not improve oxygen delivery to the tissues owing to the presence of shunt physiology. Oxygen therapy is associated with nasal dryness, inconvenience, and expense. Although the vascular bed should have the capacity to vasodilate (because it can vasoconstrict) and, therefore, increasing alveolar oxygen should have a vasodilator effect, the benefits of oxygen therapy in patients with Eisenmenger's complex are unproved. Although reduced oxygen saturation requires a higher hematocrit to increase the oxygen-carrying capacity of the blood and to maintain tissue oxygen delivery, once viscosity increases to a hematocrit greater than 60%, tissue oxygen delivery decreases. However, oxygen delivery improves when the hematocrit is approximately 56%. Thus, phlebotomy should be used judiciously in these patients. The effectiveness of vasodilators in congenital heart diseases that result in Eisenmenger's complex is largely unknown. In anecdotal reports, the use of alpha-adrenergic receptor blockade,[116] calcium channel blockers,[117] and prostacyclin[118] has improved hemodynamic measurements and function. Vasodilator therapy runs the risk of increasing right-to-left shunting and aggravating hypoxemia. These drugs should be used in a closely controlled setting with careful hemodynamic monitoring.

Future Directions in Therapy for Pulmonary Hypertension

Ongoing research is aimed at identifying the genetic locus associated with familial primary pulmonary hypertension.[119] Identifying the gene and its product should provide information on the mechanism of pulmonary hypertension and provide insight into new treatment regimens. Primary pulmonary hypertension is a unique model for studying the mechanisms involved in the evolution of pulmonary hypertension in other diseases. Oral synthetic prostacyclin analogues,[120] inhaled and dermal prostacyclin,[121] endothelin receptor antagonists, and ambulatory inhaled nitric oxide are other therapies currently being investigated, while the underlying abnormality producing pulmonary hypertension remains to be discovered.

References

1. Perloff JK, Szidon JP: Pulmonary hypertension: Etiologies, recognition, consequences. In Willerson JT, Sanders CA (eds): Clinical Cardiology. Grune & Stratton, New York, 1977, p 419.
2. Guyton AC: The pulmonary circulation. In Textbook of Medical Physiology, 6th ed. WB Saunders, Philadelphia, 1981, p 289.
3. Banchero N, Sime F, Penaloza D, et al: Pulmonary pressure, cardiac output and arterial oxygen saturation during exercise at high altitude, and at sea level. Circulation 33:249, 1966.
4. Holmgren A, Jonsson B, Sjostrant T: Circulatory data in normal subjects at rest and during exercise in recumbent position, with special reference to the stroke volume at different work intensities. Acta Physiol Scand 49:343, 1960.
5. Donald KW, Bishop JM, Cumming G, et al: Effect of exercise on the cardiac output and circulatory dynamics of normal subjects. Clin Sci 14:37, 1955.
6. Rich S, Dantzker DR, Ayres SM, et al: Primary pulmonary hypertension: A national prospective study. Ann Intern Med 107:216, 1987.
7. Rubin LJ: ACCP Consensus Statement: Primary Pulmonary Hypertension. Chest 104:236, 1993.
8. Dawes GS: Changes in the circulation at birth. Br Med Bull 17: 148, 1961.
9. Wagenwoort CA, Neufeld NN, Edward JE: The structure of the pulmonary arterial tree in fetal life and early postnatal life. Lab Invest 10:751, 1961.
10. Staub NC: Site of hypoxic vasoconstriction. Chest 88(Suppl):240S, 1955.
11. Von Euler US, Liljestrand G: Observation on the pulmonary arterial blood pressure in the cat. Acta Physiol Scand 12:301, 1946.
12. Cutaia M, Rounds S: Hypoxic pulmonary vasoconstriction. Physiologic significance, mechanism, and clinical relevance. Chest 97:706, 1990.
13. Doyle JT, Wilson JS, Warren JV: The pulmonary vascular response to short-term hypoxia in human subjects. Circulation 5:263, 1952.
14. Kato M, Staub NC: Response of small pulmonary arteries to unilobar hypoxia and hypercapnia. Circ Res 19:426, 1966.
15. Nagasaka Y, Bhattacharya F, Nanjo S, et al: Micro puncture measurement of lung microvascular pressure profile during hypoxia in cats. Circ Res 54:90, 1984.
16. Marshall BE, Marshall C, Benumoff J, et al: Hypoxic pulmonary vasoconstriction in dogs: Effects of lung segment size and oxygen tension. J Appl Physiol 51:153, 1981.
17. Marshall C, Marshall BE: Influence of perfusate PO_2 on hypoxic pulmonary vasoconstriction in rats. Circ Res 52:691, 1983.
18. Burrows B, Kettel LJ, Niden AH, et al: Patterns of cardiovascular dysfunction in chronic obstructive pulmonary disease. N Engl J Med 286:912, 1972.
19. Salvaterra CG, Rubin LJ: Clinical Commentary: Investigation and management of pulmonary hypertension in chronic obstructive pulmonary disease. Am Rev Respir Dis 148:1414, 1993.
20. Rubin LJ, Tod ML, Yoshimura K: Effects of nitrendipine and hypoxia on pulmonary vascular resistance in experimental emphysema. Am Rev Respir Dis 142:625, 1990.

21. Bishop JM, Cross KW: Use of other physiological variables to predict pulmonary arterial pressure in patients with chronic obstructive pulmonary disease: Multicentre Study. Eur Heart J 2:509, 1981.
22. Weitzenblum E, Sautegeau A, Ehrhart M, et al: Long-term course of pulmonary arterial pressure in chronic obstructive pulmonary disease. Am Rev Respir Dis 130:993, 1984.
23. Timms RM, Khaja FU, William GW, et al: Hemodynamic response to oxygen therapy in chronic obstructive pulmonary disease. Ann Intern Med 102:29, 1985.
24. Ashutosh K, Mead J, Dunsky M: Early effect of oxygen administration and prognosis in chronic obstructive pulmonary disease and cor pulmonale. Am Rev Respir Dis 127:399, 1983.
25. Dalen JE, Alpert JS: Natural history of pulmonary embolism. In Sasahara AA, Sonnenblick EH, Lesch M (eds): Pulmonary Embolism. Grune & Stratton, New York, 1975, p 77.
26. Paraskos JA, Adelstein SJ, Smith RE, et al: Late prognosis of acute pulmonary embolism. N Engl J Med 289:55, 1973.
27. Castleman B, Bland EF: Organized emboli of the tertiary pulmonary arteries. An unusual cause of cor pulmonale. Arch Pathol 42:581, 1946.
28. Moser KM, Bloor CM: Pulmonary vascular lesions occurring in patients with chronic major vessel thromboembolic hypertension. Chest 103:685, 1993.
29. Moser KM, Daily PO, Peterson KL, et al: Thromboendarterectomy for chronic major-vessel thromboembolic pulmonary hypertension. Immediate and long term results in 42 patients. Ann Intern Med 107: 560, 1987.
30. Shure D, Bloor CM: Heparin prevents pulmonary artery remodeling in post-obstructive pulmonary arteriopathy in dogs. Chest 93:154S, 1988.
31. Shure D, Swain JA, Abraham JL, et al: Pulmonary arterial hypertensive changes distal to a central vascular obstruction in the dog. Am Rev Respir Dis 129:A331, 1984.
32. Huber GL, Edmunds LH Jr: Pulmonary artery occlusion. II. Morphologic studies. J Appl Physiol 22:1002, 1967.
33. Shure D, Jacobs K: Endothelial injury consequent to prolonged pulmonary artery obstruction. Am Rev Respir Dis 139:A174, 1989.
34. Barie PS, Malik AB: Effect of pulmonary arterial occlusion on lung fluid and protein exchange. J Appl Physiol 53:543, 1982.
35. Jawalurz KI, Karpas CM: Pulmonary schistosomiasis: A detailed clinicopathological study. Am Rev Respir Dis 88:517, 1965.
36. Mantz FA, Craige E: Portal axis thrombosis with spontaneous portocaval shunt and resultant cor pulmonale. AMA Arch Pathol 52:91, 1951.
37. Robalino BD, Moodie DS: Association between primary pulmonary hypertension and portal hypertension: Analysis of its pathophysiology and clinical, laboratory and hemodynamic manifestations. J Am Coll Cardiol 17:492, 1991.
38. Edwards BS, Weir EK, Edwards WD, et al: Coexistent pulmonary and portal hypertension: Morphologic and clinical features. J Am Coll Cardiol 10:1233, 1987.
39. Krowka MJ, Dickson R, Cortese D: Hepatopulmonary syndrome: Clinical observation and lack of therapeutic response to somatostatin analogue. Chest 104:515, 1993.
40. Hobeika J, Houssin D, Bernard O, et al: Orthotopic liver transplantation in children with chronic liver disease and severe hypoxemia. Transplantation 57:224, 1994.
41. Taura P, Garcia-Valdecasas JC, Beltran J, et al: Moderate primary pulmonary hypertension in patients undergoing liver transplantation. Anesth Analg 83:675, 1996.
42. Castro M, Krowka MJ, Schroeder DR, et al: The frequency and clinical implications of increased pulmonary artery pressures in liver transplant patients. Mayo Clin Proc 71:543, 1996.
43. Petitpretz P, Brenot F, Azarian R, et al: Pulmonary hypertension in patients with human immunodeficiency virus infection. Comparison with primary pulmonary hypertension. Circulation 89:2722, 1994
44. Bray GL, Martin GR, Chandra R: Idiopathic pulmonary hypertension, hemophilia A, and infection with human immunodeficiency virus. Ann Intern Med 111:689, 1989.
45. Himmelman RB, Dohrmann M, Goodman P, et al: Severe pulmonary hypertension and cor pulmonale in the acquired immunodeficiency syndrome. Am J Cardiol 64:1396, 1989.
46. Mette SA, Palevsky HI, Pietra GG, et al: Primary pulmonary hypertension in association with human immunodeficiency virus infection: A possible viral etiology for some forms of hypertensive pulmonary arteriopathy. Am Rev Respir Dis 145:1196, 1992.
47. Escamilla R, Hermant C, Berjaud J, et al: Pulmonary veno-occlusive disease in a HIV-infected intravenous drug abuser. Eur Respir J 8: 1982, 1995.
48. Heron E, Laaban J-P, Capron F, et al: Thrombotic primary pulmonary hypertension in an HIV + patient. Eur Heart J 15:394, 1994.
49. Dawson A, Elias DJ, Rubenson D, et al: Pulmonary hypertension developing after alglucerase therapy in two patients with type 1 Gaucher disease complicated by the hepatopulmonary syndrome. Ann Intern Med 125:901, 1996.
50. Gurtner HP: Aminorex and pulmonary hypertension. A review. Cor Vasa 27:160, 1985.
51. Abenhaim L, Moride Y, Rich S, et al: The International Primary Pulmonary Hypertension Study (IPPHS). Chest 105:37S, 1994.
52. Abenhaim L, Moride Y, Brenot F, et al: Appetite-suppressant drugs and the risk of primary pulmonary hypertension. N Engl J Med 335: 609, 1996.
53. Tazelaar HD, Myers JL, Drage CW, et al: Pulmonary disease associated with L-tryptophan–induced eosinophilic myalgia syndrome: Clinical and pathology features. Chest 97:1032, 1990.
54. Romberg E: Veber Sklerose der Lungenartera. Deutsch Arch Klin Med 48:197, 1891.
55. Dresdale DT, Schultz M, Michtom RJ: Primary pulmonary hypertension: I. Clinical and hemodynamic study. Am J Med 11:686, 1951.
56. Lewis RJ: ACCP Consensus Statement: Primary pulmonary hypertension. Chest 104:236, 1993.
57. Rich S, Dantzker DR, Ayres SM, et al: Primary pulmonary hypertension. A National Prospective Study. Ann Intern Med 107:216, 1987.
58. Moser KM, Bloor CM: Pulmonary vascular lesions occurring in patients with chronic major vessel thromboembolic pulmonary hypertension. Chest 103:685, 1993.
59. Palevsky HI, Schloo BL, Pietra GG, et al: Primary pulmonary hypertension: Vascular structure, morphometry and responsiveness to vasodilator agents. Circulation 80:1207, 1989.
60. Fuster V, Steele PM, Edwards WD, et al: Primary pulmonary hypertension: Natural history and the importance of thrombosis. Circulation 70:580, 1984.
61. Rich S, Kaufmann E, Levy PS: The effect of high doses of calcium-channel blockers on survival in primary pulmonary hypertension. N Engl J Med 327:76, 1992.
62. Eisenberg PR, Lucore C, Kaufman L, et al: Fibrinopeptide A levels indicative of pulmonary vascular thrombosis in patients with primary pulmonary hypertension. Circulation 82:841, 1990.
63. Huber K, Beckmann R, Frank H, et al: Fibrinogen, t-PA, and PAI-1 plasma levels in patients with pulmonary hypertension. Am J Respir Crit Care 150:929, 1994.
64. Christman BW, McPherson CD, Newman JH, et al: An imbalance between the excretion of thromboxane and prostacyclin metabolites in pulmonary hypertension. N Engl J Med 327:70, 1992.
65. Giaid A, Yanagisawa M, Langleben D, et al: Expression of endothelin-1 activity in the lungs or patients with pulmonary hypertension. N Engl J Med 328:1732, 1993.
66. Giaid A, Polak JM, Gaitonde V, et al: Distribution of endothelin-like immunoreactivity and mRNA in the developing and adult human lung. Am J Respir Cell Mol Biol 4:50, 1991.
67. Herve P, Launay J-M, Scrobohaci M-L, et al: Increased plasma serotonin in primary pulmonary hypertension. Am J Med 99:249, 1995.
68. Tuder RM, Groves B, Badesch DB, et al: Exuberant endothelial cell growth and elements of inflammation are present in plexiform lesions of pulmonary hypertension. Am J Pathol 144:275, 1994.
69. Botney MD, Bahadori L, Gold LI: Vascular remodeling in primary pulmonary hypertension. Am J Pathol 144:286, 1994.
70. Wagenvoort CA, Wagenvoort N: The pathology of pulmonary veno-occlusive disease. Virch Arch (A) 364:69, 1974.
71. Ellis DA, Capewell SJ: Pulmonary veno-occlusive disease after chemotherapy. Thorax 41:415, 1986.
72. Lombard CM, Churg A, Winokur S: Pulmonary veno-occlusive disease following therapy for malignant neoplasms. Chest 92:871, 1987.
73. Davies P, Reid L: Pulmonary veno-occlusive disease in siblings: Case report and morphometric study. Hum Pathol 13:911, 1982.
74. Voordes CG, Kuipers JRG, Elema JD: Familial pulmonary veno-occlusive disease: A case report. Thorax 32:763, 1977.
75. Wagenvoort CA, Beetstra A, Spijker J: Capillary hemangiomatosis of the lung. Histopathology 2:401, 1978.
76. Zahavi I, Chagnac A, Hering R, et al: Prevalence of Raynaud's phenomenon in patients with migraine. Arch Intern Med 144:742, 1984.
77. Louie EK, Lin SS, Reynertson SI, et al: Pressure and volume loading

of the right ventricle have opposite effects on the left ventricular ejection fraction. Circulation 92:819, 1995.
78. Jessup M, Sutton M St. J, Wever KT, et al: The effect of chronic pulmonary hypertension on left ventricular size, function, and interventricular septal motion. Am Heart J 113:114, 1987.
79. Nootens M, Kaufmann E, Wolfkiel C, et al: Right and left ventricular systolic interaction at rest and exercise in pulmonary hypertension. J Am Coll Cardiol 23(special issue):418A, 1994.
80. Moser KM, Auger WR, Fedullo PF, et al: Chronic thromboembolic pulmonary hypertension: Clinical picture and surgical treatment. Eur Respir J 5:334, 1992.
81. Dickinson CJ, Martin JF: Megakaryocytes and platelet clumps as the cause of finger clubbing. Lancet 2:1434, 1987.
82. Chang CH: The normal roentgenographic measurement of the right descending pulmonary artery in 1,085 cases. Am J Roentgenol 87: 929, 1962.
83. Williams JO: Death following injection of lung scanning agent in a case of pulmonary hypertension. Br J Radiol 47:61, 1974.
84. Child JS, Wolfe JD, Tashkin D, et al: Fatal lung scan in a case of pulmonary hypertension due to chronic obliterative pulmonary hypertension. Chest 67:308, 1975.
85. Liu SQ, Fung YC: Material coefficients of the strain energy function of pulmonary arteries in normal and cigarette smoke-exposed rats. J Biomech 26:1261, 1993.
86. Chetty KG, Light RW, Stansbury DW, et al: Exercise performance of polycythemic chronic obstructive pulmonary disease patients. Effect of phlebotomies. Chest 98:1073, 1990.
87. Milne N, Light RW, Chetty KG: Exercise-induced changes in left ventricular function after phlebotomy in patients with polycythemic COPD. J Thorac Imaging 5:68, 1990.
88. Rodman DM, Lindenfeld JA: Successful treatment of sarcoidosis-associated pulmonary hypertension with corticosteroids. Chest 97: 500, 1990.
89. Rubin LK, Tod ML, Yoshimura K: Effects of nitrendipine and hypoxia on pulmonary vascular resistance in experimental emphysema. Am Rev Respir Dis 142:625, 1990.
90. Dal Nogare AR, Rubin LJ: The effects of hydralazine on exercise capacity in pulmonary hypertension secondary to chronic obstructive pulmonary disease. Am Rev Respir Dis 133:385, 1986.
91. Mathur PN, Powles ACP, Pugsley SO, et al: Effect of digoxin on right ventricular function in severe chronic airflow obstruction: A controlled clinical trial. Ann Intern Med 95:283, 1981.
92. Presbitero P, Aiello E, Aruta E, et al: Thromboembolic pulmonary hypertension. Cardiologia 36(Suppl 1):203, 1991.
93. Jamieson SW, Auger WR, Fedullo PF, et al: Experience and results with 150 pulmonary thromboendarterectomy operations over a 29-month period. J Thorac Cardiovas Surg 106:116, 1993.
94. Daily PO, Dembitsky WP, Iversen S, et al: Risk factors for pulmonary thromboendarterectomy. J Thorac Cardiovasc Surg 99:670, 1990.
95. Rich S, Kaufmann E, Levy PS: The effect of high doses of calcium-channel blockers on survival in primary pulmonary hypertension. N Engl J Med 327:76, 1992.
96. Palevsky HI, Long W, Crow J, et al: Prostacyclin and acetylcholine as screening agents for acute pulmonary vasodilator responsiveness in primary pulmonary hypertension. Circulation 82:2018, 1990.
97. Raffy O, Azarian R, Brenot F, et al: Clinical significance of the pulmonary vasodilator response during short-term infusion of prostacyclin in primary pulmonary hypertension. Circulation 93:484, 1996.
98. Nootens M, Schrader B, Kaufmann E, et al: Comparative acute effects of adenosine and prostacyclin in primary pulmonary hypertension. Chest 107:54, 1995.
99. Pepke-Zaba J, Higenbottam TW, Tuan D-X, et al: Inhaled nitric oxide as a cause of selective pulmonary vasodilatation in pulmonary hypertension. Lancet 338:1173, 1991.
100. Woodmansey PA, O'Toole L, Channer KS, et al: Acute pulmonary vasodilatory properties of amlodipine in humans with pulmonary hypertension. Heart 75:171, 1996.
101. Barst R, Rubin L, Long WA, et al: A comparison of continuous intravenous epoprostenol (prostacyclin) with conventional therapy for primary pulmonary hypertension. The Primary Pulmonary Hypertension Study Group. N Engl J Med 30:334, 1996.
102. Boyer-Neumann C, Brenot F, Wolf M, et al: Continuous infusion of prostacyclin decreases plasma levels of t-PA and PAI-1 in primary pulmonary hypertension. Thromb Haemost 73:735, 1995.
103. Jones K, Higenbottam T, Wallwork J: Pulmonary vasodilation with prostacyclin in primary and secondary pulmonary hypertension. Chest 96:784, 1989.
104. Long WA, Rubin LJ: Prostacyclin and PGE_1 treatment of pulmonary hypertension. Am Rev Respir Dis 136:773, 1987.
105. Palevsky HI, Fishman AP: The management of primary pulmonary hypertension. JAMA 265:1014, 1991.
106. Rozkovec A, Montanes P, Oakley CM: Factors that influence the outcome of primary pulmonary hypertension. Br Heart J 55:449, 1986.
107. Nihill MR, O'Laughlin MP, Mullins CE: Effects of atrial septostomy in patients with terminal cor pulmonale due to pulmonary vascular disease. Cathet Cardiovasc Diagn 24:166, 1991.
108. Hausknecht MJ, Sims RE, Nihill MR, et al: Successful palliation of primary pulmonary hypertension by atrial septostomy. Am J Cardiol 65:1045, 1990.
109. Kerstein D, Levy PS, Hsu DT, et al: Blade balloon atrial septostomy in patients with severe primary pulmonary hypertension. Circulation 91:2028, 1995.
110. Thanopoulos BC, Georgakopoulos D, Tsaousis GS, et al: Percutaneous balloon dilatation of the atrial septum: Immediate and midterm results. Heart 76:502, 1996.
111. Snell GI, Salamonsen RF, Bergin P, et al: Inhaled nitric oxide used as a bridge to heart-lung transplantation in a patient with end-stage pulmonary hypertension. Am J Respir Crit Care Med 151:1263, 1995.
112. Alpert MA, Pressly TA, Mukerji V, et al: Acute and long-term effects of nifedipine on pulmonary and systemic hemodynamics in patients with pulmonary hypertension associated with diffuse systemic sclerosis, the CREST syndrome and mixed connective tissue disease. Am J Cardiol 68:1687, 1991.
113. Albert MA, Pressly TA, Mukerji V, et al: Short- and long-term hemodynamic effects of captopril in patients with pulmonary hypertension and selected connective tissue disease. Chest 102:1407, 1992.
114. Niarchos AP, Whitman HH, Goldstein DE, et al: Hemodynamic effects of captopril in pulmonary hypertension of collagen vascular disease. Am Heart J 104:834, 1982.
115. Badesch DB, Tapson VF, McGoon MD, et al: Continuous intravenous epoprostenol for pulmonary hypertension due to the scleroderma spectrum of disease: A randomized, controlled trial. Ann Intern Med 132:425, 2000.
116. Watanabe K, Mori C, Haneda N, et al: Chronic alpha 1 blockade in a patient with Eisenmenger syndrome. Pediat Cardiol 12:52, 1991.
117. Wong CK, Yeung DW, Lau CP, et al: Improvement of exercise capacity after nifedipine in patients with Eisenmenger's syndrome complicating ventricular septal defect. Clin Cardiol 14:957, 1991.
118. Gildein HP, Wildberg A, Mocellin R: Comparative studies of hemodynamics under prostacyclin and nifedipine in patients with Eisenmenger syndrome. Z Kardiol 84:55, 1995.
119. Loyd JE, Butler MG, Foroud TM, et al: Genetic anticipation and abnormal gender ratio at birth in familial primary pulmonary hypertension. Am J Respir Crit Care Med 152:93, 1995.
120. Tetsuro A, Miyazaki M, Toda N: Vasodilator actions of tRK-100 a new prostaglandin I_2 analogue. Br J Pharmacol 89:703, 1986.
121. Zwissler B, Welte M, Messmer K: Effects of inhaled prostacyclin as compared with inhaled nitric oxide on right ventricular performance in hypoxic pulmonary vasoconstriction. J Cardiothorac Vasc Anesth 9: 283, 1995.

SECTION

XIII

CONNECTIVE TISSUE DISEASE

CHAPTER 41

Pathophysiology, Clinical Recognition, Diagnosis, and Management

Frank C. Arnett and James T. Willerson

The multisystem connective tissue diseases include diseases in which immunologic mechanisms play central roles in pathogenesis. Each disease is characterized by distinctive clinical patterns, host susceptibility factors, and in many, serologic markers useful in diagnosis. For each disorder, however, different cardiac and vascular structures may be affected, resulting in a variety of clinical cardiovascular abnormalities.

SYSTEMIC LUPUS ERYTHEMATOSUS

Systemic lupus erythematosus (SLE) is a multisystem autoimmune disease characterized by the potential for inflammatory lesions in many organs.[1] SLE occurs in people of any age or race, but young women in the childbearing years are most susceptible, especially blacks and Asians. The etiology of SLE is unknown; however, genetic factors are known to be important, especially hereditary deficiencies of the complement system and certain class II HLA genes (HLA-DR2 and DR3 haplotypes).[1,2]

Autoantibodies to intracellular nuclear constituents, such as DNA, ribonucleoproteins (e.g., Sm, RNP, Ro, La), and histones, occur characteristically and account for positive antinuclear antibody (ANA) tests in more than 95% of patients.[1] Autoantibodies to double-stranded DNA and Sm are most disease specific but occur in the minority of patients. Additional autoantibodies are also common, including those to cellular elements (e.g., red blood cells, lymphocytes, platelets, neurons) and plasma components (e.g., IgG, phospholipids). Individual patients with SLE demonstrate their own distinctive profiles of autoantibodies.[1] Many of these autoantibodies are associated with and are probably causal for specific clinical manifestations, either through the deposition of antigen-antibody immune complexes or through antibody-mediated tissue damage. Recent studies suggest that individual autoantibodies are mediated by different genetically determined HLA class II (HLA-DQ) molecules.[2]

The spectrum of SLE, including its cardiac manifestations and its prognosis, has changed considerably over the last 40 years.[3] With the advent of more sophisticated serologic tests, milder and earlier cases are now recognized. Treatment with corticosteroids and other immunosuppressive agents, as well as appropriate antibiotics, antihypertensives, and other drugs, has improved survival from less than 50% at 5 years in the 1950s[4] to more than 90% at 10 years (Fig. 41–1).[5,6] Concomitantly, the prevalence of lupus carditis has decreased considerably, from being nearly universally present, especially at autopsy, in the precorticosteroid era to 55% in 1954, 38% in 1971, and 18% in 1978.[3] At the same time, there has been an increasing appreciation of premature atherosclerosis as a complication of the vascular injury and possibly of corticosteroid therapy, nephrotic syndrome, and other factors.[3,7] It is extremely important that hyperlipidemia, that is, hypercholesterolemia, and increases in low-density lipoprotein (LDL) be aggressively corrected by diet and statin therapy in these patients. In addition, associations or causal relationships have been established between specific autoantibodies and certain cardiac manifestations. Examples include congenital heart block with anti-Ro (SS-A) and La (SS-B) antibodies,[8,9] valvular disease (Libman-Sacks endocarditis), other cardiac lesions, and intravascular thromboses with antiphospholipid antibodies.[10–12]

Any cardiac structure may be involved in SLE.[3,13–15] The presence and extent of pathologic cardiac lesions, however, correlate poorly with clinical manifestations. Acute or healed inflammatory lesions scattered focally or diffusely throughout the pericardium, myocardium, valves, and coronary vasculature have been well described, especially in necropsy series. Immunofluorescence studies have demonstrated extensive granular deposits of immunoglobulins and C3, which correlate with the histopathologic changes in these tissues.[16] Therefore, immune complex–mediated injury is believed to be the major cause of lupus cardiac lesions.[17] In situ thrombotic events on cardiac valves, other endocardial surfaces, and extracardiac vascular surfaces due to antiphospholipid antibodies also represent a potential major pathogenic mechanism.[10–12,18,19]

Pericardial Disease

Pericarditis is the most common cardiac complication, occurring in 19% to 48% of SLE patients and as the presenting feature in 1% to 2% of patients.[3,13,14] Clinical features include the typical substernal, position-related, pleuritic chest pain, sometimes, but not usually, confirmed by an auscultatory pericardial rub and typical electrocardiographic (ECG) changes. Atrial arrhythmias, including flutter and fibrillation, may occur in this setting owing to the close proximity of the SA node to the pericardium. Echocardiography usually reveals a small pericardial effusion; however, large fluid accumulations with tamponade have been rarely reported. Constrictive pericarditis is rare.[20]

Pericardial fluid associated with SLE shows a mild to moderate inflammatory exudate, occasionally bloody, with

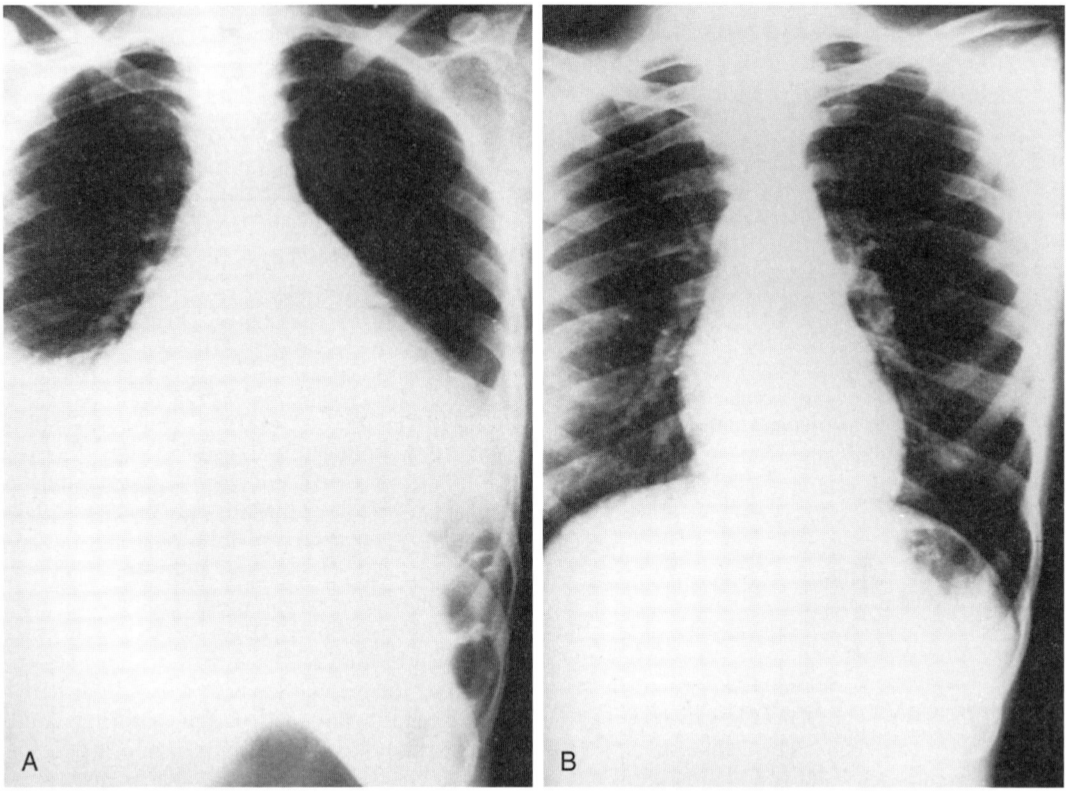

FIGURE 41–1. Chest radiographs of a patient with SLE. *A*, Massive pericardial effusion and bilateral pleural effusions. *B*, Complete resolution of effusions 4 weeks after treatment with corticosteroids. (From Willerson J, Cohn J [eds]: Cardiovascular Medicine. Churchill Livingstone, New York, 1995, p 1669.)

white blood cell counts usually in the 2000 to 5000/mm^3 range, a mildly elevated protein level, and normal glucose values. Lupus erythematosus (LE) cells or ANAs may be found in the pericardial fluid of seropositive patients, but they do not discriminate lupus effusions from those with other causes. Complement levels are typically low, and immune complexes have been demonstrated.[3, 21] Pericardiocentesis is rarely necessary for diagnostic purposes, because concomitant pleural effusions exhibiting similar characteristics are usually present and can be aspirated more safely. Prompt removal of pericardial fluid is lifesaving when pericardial tamponade is present. It may be diagnostically necessary when infectious pericarditis is suspected.

The therapy for lupus pericarditis should be dictated by its severity. For mild symptomatic pericarditis, especially without significant pericardial effusion or other serious disease manifestations, indomethacin, 75 to 150 mg/day in three divided doses, may be effective. Sometimes larger doses are required. This medication should be given after meals and with milk, if possible, to avoid gastrointestinal injury. Other nonsteroidal anti-inflammatory agents, including salicylates, in doses recommended for arthritis may be used alternatively. Many patients, however, require low- to moderate-dose corticosteroids (10 to 40 mg of prednisone equivalent/day) to relieve symptoms or resolve effusions. When a single daily dose of prednisone is effective, it should be given at 7 to 8 AM each day to mimic the typical diurnal variations in systemic steroid levels. Large effusions or pericardial tamponade dictate prompt initiation of high doses of intravenous corticosteroids (60 to 100 mg of prednisone equivalent/day in divided doses).

Myocarditis

Myocardial involvement is clinically evident in 8% to 25% of reported cases.[3] Several pathologic forms have been recognized, including diffuse small vessel obliteration and myocyte destruction, probably as the result of immune complex deposition,[3, 22] myocardial cell degeneration and lymphocyte infiltration associated with skeletal myositis, elevated CK levels, anti-nRNP antibodies,[23] and global myocardial ischemia and dysfunction due to multiple thrombi in small vessels associated with antiphospholipid antibodies.[18, 19]

The earliest clinical manifestations of myocarditis include resting tachycardia, atypical chest discomfort, third heart sounds, and nonspecific ST-T wave changes on ECG. More overt signs include cardiomegaly in the absence of pericardial fluid or other causes of cardiac enlargement, congestive heart failure (CHF), and arrhythmias. Echocardiography usually reveals multichamber enlargement, global myocardial hypokinesia, and a reduced ejection fraction. Myocardial biopsy may be necessary for diagnosis and for determining the type and activity of the disease process.[22] Differential diagnosis should include other causes of myocardial dysfunction, such as hypertension, diabetes mellitus, premature atherosclerotic heart disease, viral myocarditis, and a rare form of vacuolar myocardiopathy associated with chloroquine and other antimalarials sometimes used in the treatment of SLE.[24]

Active myocarditis requires aggressive corticosteroid therapy, along with appropriate measures to control arrhythmias and congestive failure. Prednisone, 60 to 100 mg/day in divided doses, should be given immediately and the patient's cardiac status monitored closely clinically and by ECG, echocardiography, and levels of creatinine kinase (and isoenzyme of creatine kinase with muscle and brain subunits [CK-MB isoenzyme]). CHF should be treated as necessary with diuretics, digoxin, nitrates, or unloading intervention in the form of angiotensin-converting enzyme (ACE) inhibitors or angiotensin II receptor inhibitors. Serious ventricular arrhythmias should be suppressed with appropriate drugs (i.e., lidocaine, procainamide, or possibly, amiodarone). Although procainamide may induce a lupus-like syndrome, it does not usually exacerbate idiopathic SLE and can be used safely in such patients. Anticoagulation should also be used to prevent the formation of mural thrombi, especially when antiphospholipid antibodies, which promote intravascular thrombosis, are present. Once signs of active myocarditis have resolved, prednisone should be tapered slowly over weeks to months, with close monitoring for recurrences of symptoms and signs indicative of renewal of SLE activity.

Coronary Heart Disease

Occlusive disease of major coronary arteries with myocardial infarction (MI) has been reported in approximately 4% of patients with SLE.[3, 25] Several studies have confirmed a higher than expected rate of MI in women with SLE. Compared with SLE patients without infarctions, these patients tend to be older and to have a longer duration of disease. There are well-documented cases of MIs occurring in patients in their 20s, often after having had the onset of lupus in childhood.[26, 27] The basis for coronary artery disease in most patients with SLE is due to premature atherosclerosis, possibly as a consequence of acute and chronic vasculitis with or without an influence of corticosteroid therapy. In some patients, the additional effects of the nephrotic syndrome or hypertension may be factors. Previous endothelial cell damage from immune complex disease may be contributory to atheroma formation. Diagnosis and treatment are the same as for usual acute coronary syndromes, and all patients receiving corticosteroids should be monitored and treated appropriately for hypercholesterolemia and hypertension.

Coronary artery occlusion resulting from an active vasculitis is rare, but it has been documented.[28] The condition should be suspected when the patient has active signs of lupus, especially vasculitis, affecting other organs. Coronary angiography also may prove helpful diagnostically when a beaded pattern or small aneurysms are seen in the coronary artery system. Treatment requires high-dose corticosteroids.

More recently, spontaneous coronary artery (and other arterial) thrombosis secondary to the presence of antiphospholipid antibodies has been recognized.[29, 30] It is usually suggested by the presence of a prolonged partial thromboplastin time (PTT) that does not correct with the addition of normal plasma. Sometimes, the serum prothrombin time (PT) is also prolonged. The patient may have no other symptoms of active SLE. The presence of a positive lupus anticoagulant with a prolonged PTT, a positive test for anticardiolipin antibodies, or a biologic false-positive test for syphilis should raise clinical suspicion of this syndrome. Therapy with antiplatelet agents, such as aspirin and sometimes Plavix (clopidogrel bisulfate) should be initiated. In complicated cases, long-term anticoagulation with Coumadin (warfarin sodium) may be needed.

Valvular Lesions

Valvular involvement in SLE is often recognized, especially at autopsy. Libman and Sacks in 1924[31] first described a sterile verrucous endocarditis affecting the underside of the mitral leaflets. Necropsy studies have found Libman-Sacks endocarditis in approximately 43% of lupus patients, with the mitral valve involved in 24%, the aortic valve in 5%, the tricuspid valve in 5%, and the pulmonic valve in 3%.[7, 32] The vegetations appear as small, flat, or slightly raised projections adherent to the valve margins, commissures of the leaflets, chordae tendineae, and papillary muscles (Fig. 41–2). Histologically, the vegetations are composed of lymphocytes, plasma cells, fibrous tissue, fibrin, and platelet thrombi, with hematoxylin bodies occasionally observed.[7, 33] Their pathogenesis is believed to arise from fibrin platelet thrombi that subsequently organize on the valve. Ultimately, valvular thickening and fusion of commissures may lead to either valvular regurgitation or stenosis. Although clinical reports most often describe mitral or aortic regurgitation, obstruction of both valves has been well documented but is very rarely a clinical problem.[34, 35] Occasionally, emboli to the coronary or cerebral circulations occur.[34]

Transthoracic echocardiographic studies have documented clinically important valvular lesions in approximately 18% of patients with SLE.[12] Approximately half of these patients had verrucous endocarditis and the remainder had rigid and thickened valves with stenosis, regurgitation, or both. Over 5 years of follow-up, almost one half of these patients, especially those with valvular thickening, required surgical treatment. In one study, 54 patients with SLE were evaluated by transesophageal echocardiography.[36] Approximately 50% were found to have leaflet thickening, of whom 73% had valve regurgitation and 50% had valve masses.

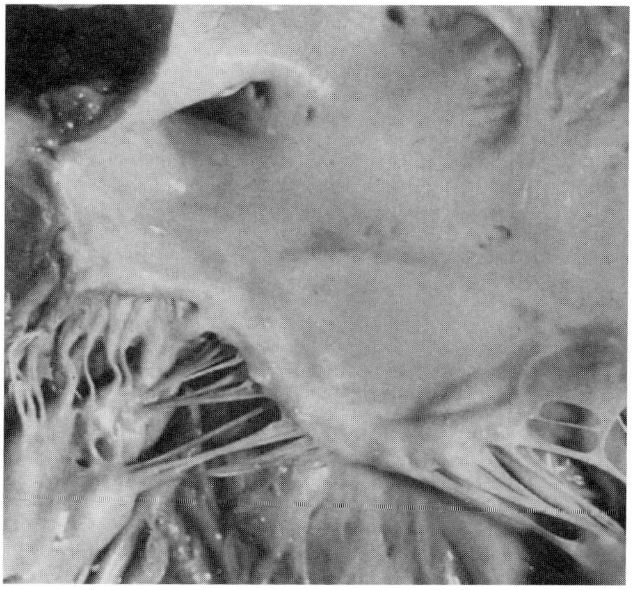

FIGURE 41–2. Necropsy specimen of left atrium and mitral valve of a patient with SLE. Note focal thickening of mitral leaflet and chordae tendineae. (Courtesy of William C. Roberts, M.D., National Institutes of Health, Bethesda, Maryland. Adapted from Bulkley BH, Roberts WC: The heart in systemic lupus erythematosus and the changes induced in it by corticosteroid therapy. Am J Med 58:243, 1975, with permission from Excerpta Medica Inc.)

Overall, valve regurgitation was noted in 59% to 64% of patients, and it was moderate to severe in one quarter.[36] A strong association of valvular lesions with circulating antiphospholipid antibodies has been noted in some[10, 11] but not all studies.[36] Antiphospholipid antibodies are present in approximately 30% of SLE patients when they are directly measured by anticardiolipin immunoassays and in approximately 7% to 15% when detected as a lupus anticoagulant by various coagulation assays.[37, 38] A biologic false-positive test for syphilis is another indirect indicator of these autoantibodies. Paradoxically, these antibodies may prolong clotting indices, especially the PTT in vitro (thus the name lupus anticoagulant). However, in vivo they promote intravascular clotting. Therefore, patients who have antiphospholipid antibodies may develop spontaneous venous or arterial thromboses, including superficial or deep venous clots with pulmonary embolization, cerebrovascular clots with cerebrovascular accidents or other neurologic syndromes, digital or extremity ischemia, and a variety of other thrombotic phenomena, including involvement of the cardiac valves. In addition, antiphospholipid antibodies have been associated with recurrent spontaneous abortions, the skin abnormality livedo reticularis, and thrombocytopenia.

Other than surgical repair of severely damaged cardiac valves, a therapeutic strategy to prevent valvular damage has not yet been developed.[37] Minimally, low-dose aspirin (80 mg/day) probably has merit. Antimalarials, such as hydroxychloroquine (200 mg/day), may be useful in lowering antiphospholipid antibody levels. Corticosteroids for isolated valvular disease are probably not useful. A primary antiphospholipid antibody syndrome has been described in patients who have clinical thrombotic events associated with positive anticardiolipin antibodies or lupus anticoagulants but who do not have any other features of SLE.[39, 40] These patients typically have prolonged PTTs that are not corrected by the addition of normal plasma. An echocardiographic study demonstrated cardiac valvular lesions similar to those of SLE in 36% of these patients.[41]

SLE patients, as well as those with primary antiphospholipid antibody syndrome, may also present with acute coronary artery thromboses or global myocardial dysfunction due to diffuse small vessel thrombosis.[18, 19] Mural thrombi mimicking atrial myxoma have also been described, as well as the aortic arch syndrome.[42, 43] Therapy should definitely include attempts at thrombolysis, especially early in the course of the disease, and anticoagulation, including aspirin and warfarin. Whether corticosteroids are effective is unknown, but in acute situations these agents are probably worthy of a trial (60 to 100 mg of prednisone/day); however, their administration should be delayed until after infarct healing has occurred, that is, perhaps 6 to 8 weeks after MI has occurred.

Pulmonary Hypertension

Pulmonary hypertension is a rare complication of SLE.[44–46] The majority of patients reported also have had Raynaud's phenomenon or other features that suggest overlapping with scleroderma. Similarly, the pathologic findings in small pulmonary arteries are similar to those seen in scleroderma[47, 48] and primary pulmonary hypertension[49] (i.e., that of an obliterative arteriopathy characterized by prominent proliferation of the intima). Many of these patients have positive rheumatoid factor (RF) tests. Prostacyclin analogues and/or nitric oxide given as an inhalant have recently been shown to lower pulmonary artery pressures and improve symptoms and function in some patients.

Congenital Heart Block

The neonatal lupus syndrome (NLE), which includes complete heart block as its most serious manifestation, is a rare disorder that is strongly associated with and probably caused by transplacental passage of maternal autoantibodies to the ribonucleoproteins Ro (SS-A) and La (SS-B).[9, 50] NLE is most commonly manifested as a transient lupus rash in the infant, which disappears 4 to 6 months postpartum, commensurate with the dissipation of maternal antibodies. The majority of anti-Ro/La–positive mothers who bear infants with NLE or congenital complete heart block (CCHB) are usually asymptomatic at the time but subsequently develop symptoms of Sjögren's syndrome or SLE.[51] Only a fraction of anti-Ro–positive women produce an abnormal infant, and they almost invariably possess the genetically determined HLA-DR3, DQw2 haplotype. The infants' human leukocyte antigen (HLA) genes do not appear to be relevant to disease predisposition.[50] Moreover, maternal autoantibodies to certain subspecies of the Ro (52 kD) and La (48 kD) particles increase the likelihood that infants will have the cardiac abnormality.[8] Women who have one child with NLE or CCHB are at high risk (25%) for having another affected infant.

Pathologic studies of fetal hearts have shown cellular infiltrates of lymphocytes and plasma cells spread throughout the atrium and ventricle in fetuses that die during the second trimester, whereas calcification and fibrosis have been found in those that die later.[21] In some cases, atrial axis discontinuity was present, along with replacement of the atrioventricular (AV) node by fibrosis or fatty tissue but a normal distal conducting system. Immunofluorescence studies have revealed widespread deposition of immunoglobulins, C3, and fibrin. However, it remains unclear whether the immune reactants contain the anti-Ro or anti-La antibodies.[52–54] Experimental evidence suggests that Ro or La antigens may be externally expressed on developing fetal cardiac cells, unlike adult heart tissue, and may serve as targets for direct injury by the autoantibodies.[8]

CCHB appears in the fetus between 18 and 30 weeks of gestation, at a time when maternal IgG antibody transfer across the placenta is reaching its peak.[8] Unexpected fetal bradycardia, detected during routine monitoring or at the time of premature labor, is the first sign. The diagnosis is confirmed by fetal ECG, the absence of congenital structural cardiac abnormalities on ultrasonography, and the presence of maternal anti-Ro/La antibodies. When fetal heart block occurs early, death in utero is common; when fetal heart block occurs late, a viable infant is usually delivered, who may at the time or later require a cardiac pacemaker. In many cases, a pacemaker may not be needed until teenage years, when the young adult becomes symptomatic as a result of the relatively slow heart rate. In addition, the extent of myocardial damage, usually assessed by ultrasonography, provides another element critical to survival. Early detection in utero of an affected but viable fetus provides several potential therapeutic options, including dexamethasone, which crosses the placenta and may suppress cardiac inflammation, and plasmapheresis of the mother to lower anti-Ro/La antibody levels.[55]

Drug-Induced Lupus

Several drugs have been reported to cause a lupus-like syndrome, and a definite association has been established for a few.[56, 57] High-dose, long-term procainamide induces a positive ANA in 50% to 75% of treated patients, and a lupus-like syndrome occurs in up to 30% of patients. Men and women are affected equally in drug-induced lupus. Arthralgias and arthritis are the most common clinical manifestations, followed by pleuropulmonary disease in 33% to 52%. Pericarditis occurs in 14% to 18% and rarely has been reported to cause tamponade or constriction. Other cardiac complications have been reported; however, procainamide, like chlorpromazine, may also induce formation of antiphospholipid antibodies.[58] Quinidine less commonly may induce lupus or an arthritis syndrome resembling rheumatoid arthritis (RA) or polymyalgia rheumatica.[59, 60] Renal disease and antibodies to double-stranded DNA are uncommon in drug-induced lupus, and the prognosis in these patients is generally excellent, with the SLE-like illness usually disappearing when the drug is discontinued.

RHEUMATOID ARTHRITIS

RA is primarily a chronic progressive polysynovitis of unknown etiology. It leads to progressive joint destruction and disability, as well as to a variety of extra-articular inflammatory lesions (rheumatoid nodules, interstitial lung disease, scleritis, vasculitis, and cardiac lesions) (Fig. 41–3). RA is more common in women than in men. Autoantibodies to immunoglobulin G (IgG) (RFs) are present in the sera and synovia of 80% of patients, and immune complexes of anti-IgG/IgG are believed to participate in the articular and extra-articular inflammatory lesions. Genetic predisposition is strongly associated with certain class II major histocompatibility complex (MHC) alleles, especially HLA-DR4 and DR1, which share a specific amino acid sequence in their third hypervariable regions. The severity of joint disease and the occurrence of extra-articular manifestations correlate strongly with high-titer serum RF and homozygosity for the HLA class II susceptibility sequence.[61–64]

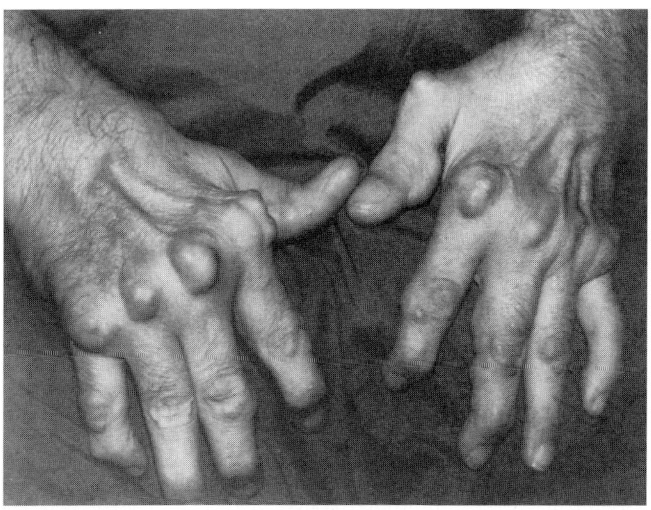

FIGURE 41–3. Rheumatoid arthritis of hands and wrists with symmetric joint swelling, swan-neck deformities, and ulnar deviation of the fingers. Multiple subcutaneous (rheumatoid) nodules are also present. (From Willerson J, Cohn J [eds]: Cardiovascular Medicine. Churchill Livingstone, New York, 1995, p 1666.)

Cardiac structures that may be involved in RA include the pericardium, myocardium, endocardial valves, and coronary arteries.[65, 66]

Pericardial Disease

Pericardial disease is most common, with inflammation, granuloma formation, fibrous thickening, or usually small effusions detected in approximately 30% of patients by echocardiography.[65, 66] However, clinically evident pericarditis with chest pain, fever, and an auscultatory rub is infrequent, occurring in only 2% to 4% of patients.[65–67]

Constrictive pericarditis due to pericardial thickening and contracture or enlarging effusion is infrequent, but when it occurs, it is a serious problem.[65, 67, 68] The earliest symptoms are usually those of right-sided heart failure with progressive pedal edema and ascites. Later, or when pericardial fluid accumulates rapidly (tamponade), symptoms of left-sided cardiac failure predominate and include dyspnea, orthopnea, and paroxysmal nocturnal dyspnea. Findings on examination include a rapid, weak pulse, distended jugular veins accentuated during inspiration (Kussmaul's sign), distant heart sounds, hepatomegaly, and less frequently, a pericardial rub or knock. The knock has mid-diastolic timing and is a higher frequency sound than the typical S3. Paradoxical blood pressures (i.e., pulsus paradoxus) occur uniformly with larger pericardial effusions that limit cardiac filling and emptying (i.e., pericardial tamponade) but relatively infrequently with constrictive pericarditis. Clinical suspicion is most important in diagnosis and should lead to a prompt echocardiographic study, which, if not definitive, should be followed by cardiac catheterization with pressure studies. With pericardial tamponade and constrictive pericarditis, one expects to find an equalization of pressures in the right side of the heart, including elevation of mean right atrial and right ventricular end-diastolic and pulmonary artery diastolic pressures, which are also equal or within 1 to 2 mm Hg of one another. The mean pulmonary capillary wedge pressure may also be the same as the right atrial pressure (RAP), right ventricular end-diastolic pressure (RVEDP), and pulmonary artery diastolic pressure (PADP).

When constrictive pericarditis is a consideration, a magnetic resonance imaging study or rapid-speed CT is capable of allowing one to estimate pericardial thickness; one of 4 mm or greater is abnormal. In urgent situations in which tamponade is suspected, emergency pericardiocentesis may provide a diagnosis and may be lifesaving. Rheumatoid pericardial effusions are typically bloody, with elevated white blood cell counts (2000–10,000/mm^3), very low or absent glucose levels, and low complement levels.[69] Bacterial, mycobacterial, or fungal infections and malignancy should always be excluded by appropriate stains and cultures of the pericardial fluid, because patients with RA are often taking corticosteroids or other immunosuppressive drugs.

Relief of cardiac compression and prevention of recurrence are the primary therapeutic goals. Surgical stripping of the pericardium is usually necessary for constrictive pericarditis or compressive pericardial effusions.[67, 70] Pericardiocentesis is used to remove fluid to relieve cardiac compression on an emergency basis to treat pericardial tamponade or to provide a diagnosis of connective tissue disease, infection, or neoplastic process. In the patient with a large pericardial effusion, high doses of oral or intravenous corticosteroids (60 to 100 mg of prednisone equivalent/day), and sometimes cyclophosphamide (2 mg/kg/day orally or intravenously), should be given to prevent reaccumulation of the pericardial fluid often associated with pericardiocentesis when the fluid accumulation causes hemodynamic problems.[65, 67]

Myocardial Involvement

This finding is common at autopsy but is rarely clinically important.[5, 6] Rheumatoid granulomas have been reported in 3% to 5% of cases, and focal nonspecific changes are even more common. Clinical sequelae and treatment depend on the location and extent of myocardial nodules. Conduction disturbances may require electrical pacing and arrhythmias appropriate pharmacologic suppression. Heart failure is rare, and if the condition is unresponsive to high doses of corticosteroids and cyclophosphamide (see earlier), it is usually not amenable to other therapies.

Valvular Dysfunction

Valvular dysfunction may also result rarely from rheumatoid nodule deposition with attendant narrowing or regurgitant valvular lesions, but it is rarely of clinical significance.[65]

Coronary Vasculitis

Vasculitis of the medium and small coronary arteries is rare but may occur with generalized systemic vasculitis.[71] It may lead to MI or CHF resulting from diffuse myocardial ischemia or necrosis. Other signs of systemic vasculitis are usually present. These signs include fever; mononeuritis multiplex; ischemic skin, nail, and digital lesions; leukocytosis (often with eosinophilia); and thrombocytosis. Aggressive therapy with high-dose corticosteroids is recommended, usually 80 to 100 mg of prednisone equivalent/day (orally or intravenously and in divided doses), and may be preceded by 3 days each of 1000 mg of prednisone equivalent IV (pulse therapy). Consideration should also be given to early initiation of cyclophosphamide (2 mg/kg/day orally or intravenously) because of the life-threatening nature of this complication. Once cardiac and systemic signs of active vasculitis resolve, prednisone (and later cyclophosphamide) should be tapered slowly over weeks to months with close follow-up of the patient for signs of recurrence of vasculitis.

Still's Disease

This systemic disorder was originally described in children and was subsequently classified, probably erroneously, within the heterogeneous spectrum of juvenile RA.[72, 73] Adult-onset Still's disease is now well recognized. Typical clinical features include high-spiking fever; an evanescent salmon-colored rash occurring during times of fever; arthritis; pleurisy or pericarditis; lymphadenopathy; splenomegaly; and leukocytosis. Serologic testing for RF and ANAs is typically negative. The disease usually runs a relapsing course over several months and then enters remission without permanent sequelae. However, serious pericardial effusion or myocarditis occurs rarely. Serious complications such as cardiac disease require treatment with corticosteroids. Prednisone, 60 to 80 mg/day orally or intravenously and in divided doses, should be initiated and continued until cardiac abnormalities resolve or stabilize. Then, the daily dose should be tapered over weeks (or months), with frequent monitoring of cardiac signs and symptoms, echocardiograms, and erythrocyte sedimentation rates (ESRs).

SCLERODERMA

Scleroderma or systemic sclerosis (SSc) is a chronic multisystem disease characterized by widespread fibrosis and obliterative vascular lesions of the skin and lungs, heart, kidneys, and gastrointestinal tract.[74] Raynaud's phenomenon occurs in more than 90% of cases and is the first symptom in many patients. Typically, skin thickening begins in the distal extremities and progresses centrally, resulting in progressive joint contractures, muscle atrophy, and restricted movement. A limited form of the disease is the CREST (calcinosis, Raynaud's phenomena, esophageal dysmotility, sclerodactyly, and telangiectasia) syndrome, in which skin and major organ involvement is limited and the prognosis is a better one than in the absence of these findings (Fig. 41–4). Even more localized cutaneous forms of scleroderma include morphea and linear scleroderma, which are not associated with Raynaud's phenomenon or visceral involvement.

Clinical features of SSc often overlap with those of SLE, myositis, and RA, especially in the entity known as mixed connective tissue disease (MCTD).[75] Moreover, in many ways SSc resembles chronic graft-versus-host disease.[76] ANAs are present in 90% of patients with SSc, and include some targets that are highly disease specific, such as anticentromere, antitopoisomerase I (Scl-70), and a variety of antinucleolar antibodies.[77–79] Different autoantibodies tend to be markers of certain clinical manifestations of SSc. For example, anticentromere antibodies are found in the majority of patients with the CREST syndrome or mild scleroderma and indicate a generally good prognosis. Conversely, antitopoisomerase I antibodies correlate with diffuse skin and visceral involvement, and anti-nRNP and anti-PM-Scl antibodies are associated with complicating myositis. Because of these observations, an immunologic basis for SSc is strongly suspected but poorly understood.

Cardiac involvement in SSc may be caused primarily by the disease itself (myocardial or pericardial scleroderma) or secondarily by pulmonary or systemic hypertension.

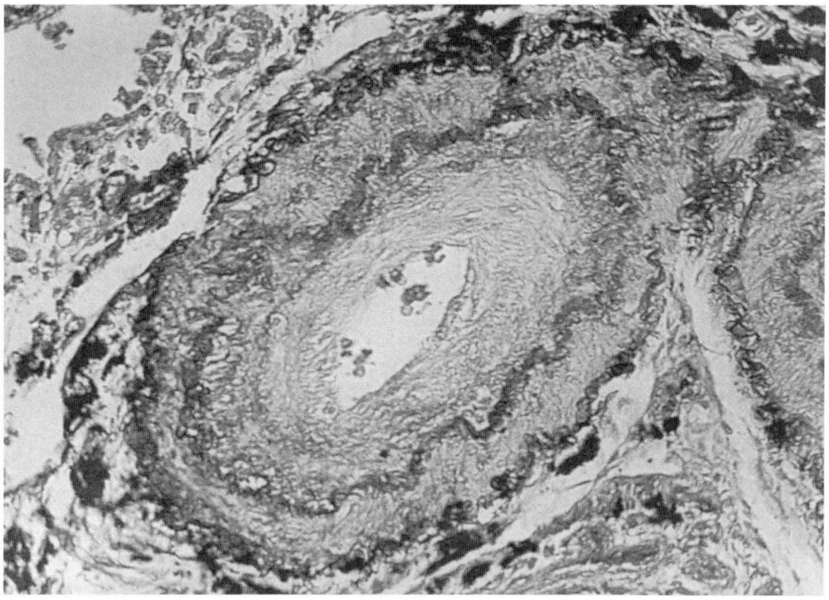

FIGURE 41–4. Photomicrograph of a small pulmonary artery in a patient with scleroderma and rapidly progressive pulmonary hypertension. Note extensive obliterative proliferation of the intima and the lack of inflammatory cells. Similar vascular lesions characterize the digital, cardiac, renal, and other organs involved. (Courtesy of William C. Roberts, M.D., National Institutes of Health, Bethesda, Maryland.)

Myocardial Involvement

The characteristic myocardial lesion of SSc is a patchy fibrosis distributed randomly throughout the right and left ventricles.[47, 74, 80–85] Myocardial fibrosis is frequently found at autopsy, but its actual prevalence in SSc remains unknown. Unlike the fibrosis of coronary atherosclerosis, it does not spare the subendocardial layer and it is not associated with hemosiderin deposition. Ventricular size and weight are usually normal unless pulmonary or systemic hypertension is also present. Myocardial tissue appears to be replaced rather than infiltrated by fibrosis. The cause of the fibrosis is unknown, but there is considerable evidence suggesting ischemic injury from diseased intramyocardial small arteries and arterioles.[47, 74] The epicardial coronary artery system is usually normal. An obliterative vasculopathy of intramyocardial arteries and arterioles, similar to that found in lungs, kidneys, and digital arteries, has been reported in several necropsy studies (see Fig. 41–4).[47, 48] Contraction band necrosis has been described in postmortem hearts, suggesting that reperfusion injury may be a factor in the fibrosis.[80, 85] This observation first led to the concept of myocardial Raynaud's phenomenon,[80] which has subsequently been supported further by the findings of reversible cold-induced abnormalities of myocardial perfusion observed by thallium-201 scintigraphy.[86, 87] Transient segmental areas of hypokinesis demonstrated by two-dimensional echocardiography appear to correlate with these lesions. In some studies, these abnormalities appeared to be prevented by the use of nifedipine.[87] The concept of recurrent vasospasm of intramural coronary arteries leading to transient ischemia, reperfusion injury, and subsequent fibrosis is compelling but controversial.[88] More recently, mast cells that may induce fibrosis after degranulation have been demonstrated in the skin and myocardium of scleroderma patients, and may serve as an additional or alternative mechanism through which extensive fibrosis develops.[89]

The clinical consequences of myocardial fibrosis may be conduction disturbances or biventricular CHF. Approximately 50% of SSc patients have a normal ECG and no significant myocardial dysfunction, as assessed by radionuclide ventriculography. On the other hand, 58% of SSc patients with normal ECGs have been found to have fixed thallium perfusion abnormalities suggesting myocardial fibrosis. Infarction patterns on ECG, especially septal, have been well documented in asymptomatic SSc patients with no evidence of extramural coronary artery disease.

The prevalences of various conduction disturbances in SSc patients have been estimated widely.[90–94] Representative frequencies from ECG studies are shown in Table 41–1.[74] The most serious are progressive heart block, asystole, and ventricular ectopy, which may lead to syncope or sudden death. Clements and colleagues[91] demonstrated a correlation of resting ECG abnormalities and clinical symptoms of palpitations and syncope with significant atrial and ventricular arrhythmias found on 24-hour monitoring. Compared with normal subjects, there is a significant increase in exercise-induced arrhythmias, possibly due to myocardial fibrosis, because arrhythmias correlate with fixed abnormalities of

Table 41–1. ESTIMATED PREVALENCES OF ELECTROCARDIOGRAPHIC FINDINGS IN SYSTEMIC SCLEROSIS BASED ON 436 CASES

FINDING	INCIDENCE
Normal ECG	56%
PR prolongation	5%
Right bundle branch block	2%
Left bundle branch block	1%
Left anterior fascicular block	5%
Nonspecific conduction abnormality	4%
Second- or third-degree block	1%
Left ventricular hypertrophy	7%
Right ventricular hypertrophy	7%
Low voltage QRS	5%
Nonspecific T-wave abnormality	7%
Atrial ectopy	7%
Ventricular ectopy	5%

Adapted from Follansbee WP, Curtiss EI, Rahko PS, et al: The electrocardiogram in systemic sclerosis (scleroderma). Am J Med 79:183, 1985.

thallium perfusion and rarely occur in SSc patients with normal thallium scans. Patients with the CREST syndrome are less likely to have serious myocardial disease than those with diffuse scleroderma; however, serious ventricular arrhythmias have been documented in CREST patients, as well as myocardial defects of thallium perfusion.[94] Clinically evident myocardial disease in scleroderma is a poor prognostic sign. Heart disease is second only to pulmonary failure as a cause of death.[95]

There is no known specific therapy for scleroderma heart disease. Corticosteroids are ineffectual. Whether D-penicillamine, an agent that appears beneficial in scleroderma itself, is effective for the myocardial fibrosis is unknown, but it is worthy of consideration.[96] Because of the possibility of a vasospastic component to the myocardial disease, nifedipine or other calcium channel blockers both for therapy and as prophylaxis should be considered, because they have proved beneficial in peripheral Raynaud's phenomenon.[97] Because of their efficacy in scleroderma renal disease, ACE inhibitors may be useful for cardiac scleroderma, especially when the patient has hypertension.[98, 99]

In addition to chronic, fibrotic myocardial disease, an acute inflammatory myocarditis has been reported to occur rarely.[100] These patients with SSc typically have accompanying peripheral myositis and elevated CK-MB fractions. CHF or conduction disturbances are the primary clinical manifestations. High-dose corticosteroids (60 to 100 mg of prednisone equivalent/day in divided doses) appear to be effective in this subset of patients (see recommendations for lupus myocarditis).

Pericardial Involvement

Clinically evident pericarditis in the absence of renal disease occurs in 10% to 15% of patients with SSc, and asymptomatic pericardial involvement, including pericardial fibrosis or small to moderate effusions, has been found by echocardiography or autopsy in 40% to 60%.[74, 101, 102] Acute pericarditis with fever, chest pain, an auscultatory rub, and leukocytosis is unusual. Sudden death, probably from tachyarrhythmias, has been reported in such patients. Chronic pericardial effusions are more common, and tamponade has been reported. Constrictive pericarditis is rare. The characteristics of the pericardial fluid have been described in only a few cases. In general, the fluid is an exudate with only mild inflammatory changes, including low white blood cell counts (4 to 400/mm^3), normal glucose levels, slightly elevated proteins, and no evidence of immune complexes or complement consumption.[103]

Small to moderate pericardial effusions do not require specific therapy. Large effusions usually do not respond to corticosteroids, but acute pericarditis may be responsive. Pericardiocentesis or a pericardial window, or both, are required for effusions that compromise cardiac function.

Secondary Cardiac Complications

Pulmonary hypertension with right-sided heart failure may develop slowly in patients with progressive pulmonary fibrosis or, more rapidly, in those with a predominantly obliterative vasculopathy of small pulmonary arteries. Indeed, cor pulmonale (right-sided heart failure secondary to lung disease) is the most common cardiac complication of SSc. The latter form of pulmonary hypertension, without interstitial fibrosis, also tends to occur as a late manifestation of the CREST syndrome (Fig. 41–5).[104] The pulmonary arterial lesions are similar to those in primary pulmonary hypertension (PPH), demonstrating prominent intimal proliferation and, at times, a plexiform lesion (Fig. 41–6).[62] The prognosis for such patients is poor. Prostacyclin analogues and/or inhaled nitric oxide have recently been shown to be effective, at least temporarily. Lung transplantation is a consideration, but it is unknown whether similar lesions might develop in the allograft.

Systemic arterial hypertension, typically severe, accompanied by a microangiopathic hemolytic anemia, usually precedes scleroderma renal crisis. Increased systemic renin levels with rapid deterioration of renal function and oliguria occur over days to weeks. Left-sided heart failure is a common consequence. Obliterative arteriolar lesions, similar to those seen elsewhere in SSc (see Fig. 41–4), are found in renal arcuate arteries. Aggressive, prompt lowering of blood pressure, especially with ACE inhibitors, may reverse or stabilize renal failure.[98, 99] Hemodialysis is indicated for those with severe or irreversible azotemia. Renal transplantation has been successful in many cases. If chronic rejection of the grafted kidney occurs, it cannot be distinguished histopathologically from recurrent renal scleroderma.

POLYMYOSITIS AND DERMATOMYOSITIS

The idiopathic inflammatory myopathies polymyositis and dermatomyositis are characterized by lymphocytic cellular infiltrates and by degeneration and necrosis of proximal skeletal muscles (see Fig. 41–6).[105, 106] There is evidence that cell-mediated autoimmunity to skeletal muscle may play an

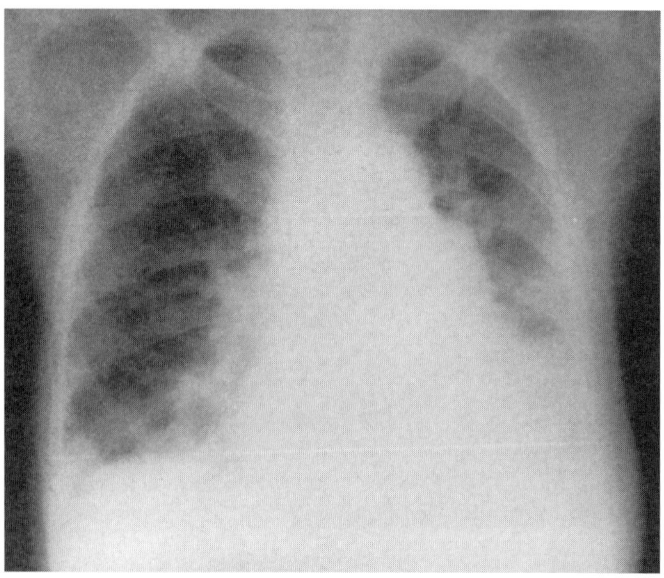

FIGURE 41–5. Chest radiograph of a patient with long-standing CREST variant of scleroderma who has developed pulmonary hypertension. Note cardiomegaly with prominence of pulmonary artery and lack of pulmonary fibrosis. Histopathology of pulmonary vessels of such a patient would appear as in Figure 42–4. (From Willerson J, Cohn J [eds]: Cardiovascular Medicine. Churchill Livingstone, New York, 1995, p 1675.)

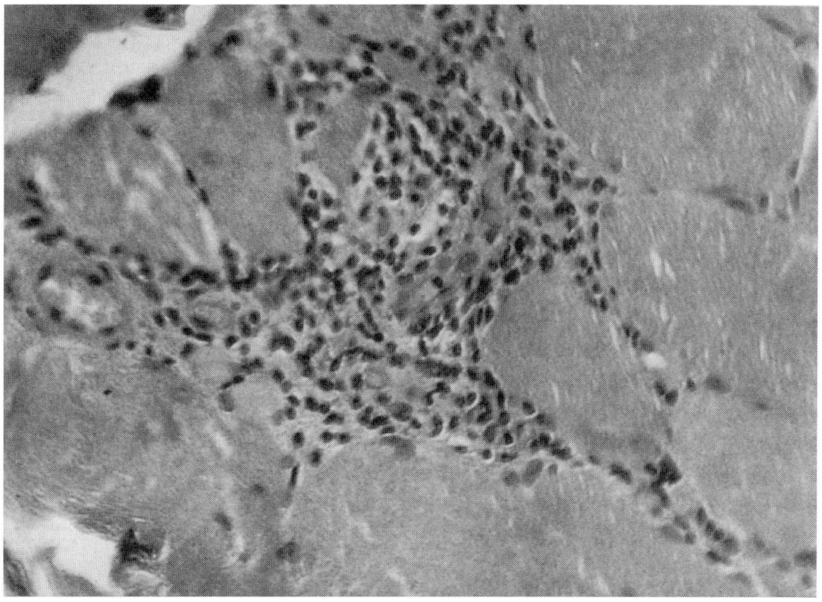

FIGURE 41–6. Photomicrograph of a proximal skeletal muscle of a patient with poly- or dermatomyositis. Note round cell infiltration between muscle bundles. Similar inflammatory lesions may involve the myocardium. (From Willerson J, Cohn J [eds]: Cardiovascular Medicine. Churchill Livingstone, New York, 1995, p 1676.)

important pathogenic role; however, the etiology of these disorders is unknown. In approximately 10% of patients, especially those older than 50 years, an underlying malignancy is present, usually a carcinoma. In addition, a similar myositis may accompany the other connective tissue diseases, scleroderma, and SLE.

The dominant clinical features are progressive proximal muscle weakness involving the shoulder and pelvic girdles, neck flexors, and the pharyngeal musculature.[105, 106] Distal and respiratory muscle weakness is uncommon except in longstanding or untreated disease. CK levels are typically elevated. Electromyography shows a typical myopathic pattern, and biopsy of an affected muscle shows typical histopathologic changes.[105] ANAs are present in 80% to 90% of patients, and several specificities (anti-Jo-1, anti-Mi-2) are highly correlated with subsets of these diseases.[107] For example, autoantibodies to tRNA synthetases, such as anti-Jo-1 (his tRNA synthetase) and to other intracellular translation factors, correlate strongly with an inflammatory interstitial lung disease,[108] which over time may lead to cor pulmonale.

Myocardial inflammation, histologically similar to skeletal myositis, may occur. The frequency of cardiac involvement is unknown; however, evidence of myocardial muscle inflammation, as well as small vessel disease, was reported in 30% of 20 patients examined at autopsy.[109] The most common clinical manifestations of myocarditis are subtle and nonspecific and include resting tachycardia, atypical chest pain, and nonspecific ST–T-wave changes on ECG. Overt CHF, heart block, and arrhythmias have all been reported.[110–112] Myocarditis appears to parallel active skeletal myositis. Serum CK and myoglobin levels are typically elevated. An elevated CK-MB fraction and/or troponin level should raise suspicion of myocardial involvement, although an elevated CK-MB fraction may also be the result of regenerating skeletal muscle.[113] Clinical suspicion of myocarditis raised by examination and ECG should be pursued by studies of myocardial function, including ejection fraction. At times, endomyocardial biopsy may be necessary to establish the diagnosis.[114]

Therapy for active myocarditis should be aimed at prompt suppression of the inflammatory response. Corticosteroids in high doses should be given intravenously and the patient monitored closely. Divided doses of 60 to 100 mg of prednisone equivalent/day represent a reasonable starting point, and frequent monitoring of CK levels provides the most sensitive measure of response. In patients who are not improving clinically and with falling CK levels, intravenous pulses of up to 1000 mg of prednisone equivalent may be necessary. Steroid tapering should begin only after CK levels have normalized and should proceed slowly over weeks to months, using the CK as a guide. If the CK levels again begin to rise while the patient remains at a high corticosteroid dose, or if serious steroid side effects are occurring, an immunosuppressive drug, such as methotrexate (15 to 25 mg/week) or azathioprine (2 mg/kg/day) should be added as a steroid-sparing agent. Arrhythmias, heart failure, and AV block should be managed in the usual manner.

PRIMARY VASCULITIDES

The primary vasculitides include a group of disorders, each of unknown etiology, characterized primarily by a necrotizing vasculitis.[115] These entities are clinically and serologically distinct from the previously described connective tissue diseases, in which vasculitis also may be a prominent complication. Moreover, each of the primary vasculitides demonstrates its own distinctive clinical picture of organ involvement, size of vessel affected,[116] host predisposition, and serologic markers. Classification criteria for most have been established recently.[117–122] However, considerable overlap may occur and may make specific diagnosis impossible. Immune complexes are believed to cause the vascular disease in most cases.[115]

Polyarteritis Nodosa

Polyarteritis nodosa (PAN) is the classic prototype of a widespread, necrotizing vasculitis.[115–120] Medium-sized muscular arteries are most prominently involved, usually in a patchy, segmental pattern and often at arterial bifurcations. Small aneurysms may develop and may either rupture or become thrombosed (Fig. 41–7). Less commonly, small arteries, arterioles, or veins also may be involved. Necropsy studies in the precorticosteroid era demonstrated myocardial arteritis and infarction in 62% of patients, myocardial hypertrophy in 64%, and pericarditis in 33%.[123]

The typical patient is a middle-aged man or, less commonly, woman. A frank MI, CHF, or pericarditis may be the presenting manifestation of PAN, although other features are usually present, most commonly myalgias, arthralgias, weight loss, peripheral neuropathy, hypertension, or renal insufficiency. Common laboratory abnormalities include low-grade anemia, leukocytosis, thrombocytosis, an elevated ESR, liver function abnormalities, and, in approximately 20% to 30% of patients, a positive test for hepatitis B surface antigen.[124] The diagnosis of PAN is based on histopathologic demonstration of necrotizing vasculitis, usually in muscle, sural nerve, or testicular biopsy specimens, or angiographic demonstration of small arterial aneurysms in the celiac or mesenteric arteries (see Fig. 41–7).[125] ANAs and antineutrophil cytoplasmic antibodies (ANCA) are typically negative, but RF tests are frequently positive. Treatment with high doses of corticosteroids is mandatory. Prednisone equivalent of 60 to 100 mg/day is usually initially effective, but most patients require the addition of cyclophosphamide (2 mg/kg/day) or azathioprine (2 mg/kg/day).[126, 127] Tapering of prednisone must be accomplished slowly and should be guided by a lack of clinically apparent active vasculitis and laboratory variables (e.g., ESR, platelet counts, urinary sediment abnormalities). The prognosis for PAN is generally poor; however, if the disease can be controlled early with vigorous therapy, many patients appear to have a self-limited course.[124]

Wegener's Granulomatosis

This condition is characterized by a necrotizing granulomatous vasculitis of the upper respiratory tract, lungs, and kidneys.[115, 119, 128] Small and medium-sized arteries and veins are typically involved. Recently, anti-neutrophil cytoplasmic antibodies (ANCAs) have been reported in approximately 90% of such patients, and frequently also in microscopic polyarteritis, a recently recognized similar disease affecting small vessels.[129, 130] Clinical cardiac abnormalities in Wegener's granulomatosis are infrequent. Pericarditis has been reported in 6% of patients and myocardial involvement in less than 2%.[128] Corticosteroids alone are not effective therapy for Wegener's granulomatosis but should be used initially in doses of 40 to 60 mg of prednisone equivalent/day to suppress systemic symptoms. Instead, immunosuppressive agents, especially cyclophosphamide (2 mg/kg/day), should be started promptly, and after several weeks or months, prednisone may be tapered and discontinued. Useful variables to follow include sinus and chest x-rays, renal function, and serum ANCA levels. The prognosis has improved considerably with this approach, and some patients can be tapered from all drugs after 1 to 2 years.[119, 128]

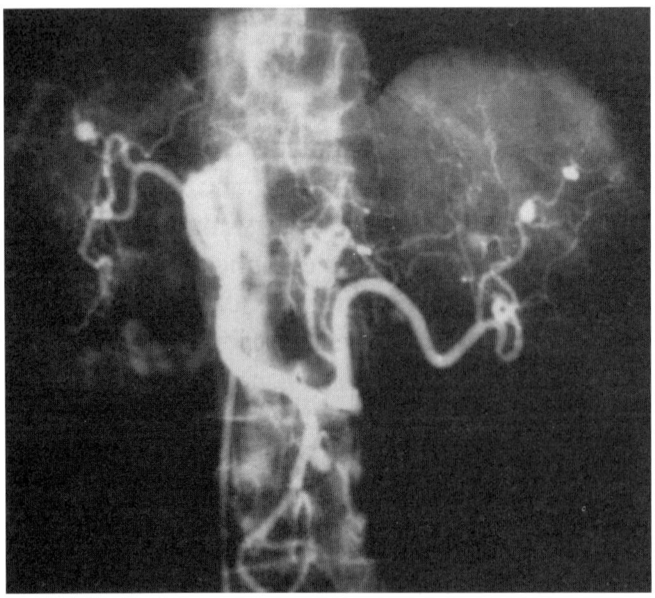

FIGURE 41–7. Celiac arteriogram of a patient with polyarteritis nodosa, showing multiple aneurysms. (From Willerson J, Cohn J [eds]: Cardiovascular Medicine. Churchill Livingstone, New York, 1995, p 1677.)

Churg-Strauss Angiitis

This condition represents another form of granulomatous vasculitis, primarily affecting the lungs, which occurs in patients with longstanding asthma.[115, 118, 131] Eosinophilia is typically present. Cardiac involvement is similar to that seen in PAN.

Hypersensitivity Angiitis

Hypersensitivity angiitis is a common disease of small arteries and veins and is usually heralded by a rash. It is classically associated with allergic reactions to drugs, such as sulfonamides, penicillins, and allopurinol.[115, 117] The coronary vasculature may be involved as well as the pericardium. Treatment includes discontinuation of the offending drug and administration of high-dose corticosteroids (60 to 100 mg of prednisone equivalent/day) when there is serious organ involvement.

Giant Cell Arteritis

This condition, also termed temporal, cranial, or granulomatous arteritis, typically affects older persons (older than 50 years), most often whites.[121, 132] Medium-sized cranial arteries are affected by a granulomatous inflammation that leads to symptoms of headache, scalp tenderness, jaw claudication, and sudden loss of vision. Some patients also have muscle pain and stiffness around the shoulder and pelvic girdles (polymyalgia rheumatica). Large vessel involvement of the aorta or its major branches occurs in 9% to 14% of cases, leading to aortic arch syndrome, intermittent claudication, cerebral ischemic attacks, abdominal angina, aortic aneurysm and rupture, and aortic valvular insufficiency.[133, 134] Coronary insufficiency with angina or MI, or both, has been reported infrequently.[132, 135] The diagnosis should be suspected in any older patient complaining of pain about the head, neck, or shoulders. An elevated ESR is typically found but may occasionally be normal. Diagnosis is usually made by biopsy of a temporal artery or clinical response to a trial of moderate- to high-dose corticosteroids. Coronary or large vessel involvement should be confirmed by appropriate angiographic studies.[133] Corticosteroids in doses adequate to suppress the inflammatory process, usually 50 to 80 mg of prednisone equivalent/day, is the initial treatment of choice. Most patients respond to corticosteroids alone, and additional immunosuppressive agents (e.g., azathioprine, cyclophosphamide) are rarely needed. Useful parameters to follow and guide steroid tapering include the patient's symptoms and the ESR. If vascular insufficiency of large vessels fails to respond, indicating irreversible arterial obstruction, or if aneurysms continue to enlarge, vascular surgical approaches are indicated.[133]

Takayasu's Arteritis

Also known as pulseless disease, Takayasu's arteritis is another form of granulomatous arteritis affecting the aorta and its major branches.[122, 136–138] The disease occurs most commonly in young Asian women but has been reported in all races. HLA-B52 is increased in persons of Japanese descent.[139] CHF due to systemic hypertension is the most common cardiac manifestation. Hypertension occurs in 37% to 50% of patients and is caused by renal artery or proximal aortic involvement.[138] Coronary insufficiency or MI may result from aortic involvement at the origin of the coronary system. Coronary arteritis per se is rare. Aortic root dilatation may result in aortic valvular insufficiency. Diagnosis is based on symptoms of aortic arch syndrome, intermittent claudication, or cerebral ischemia associated with pulse deficits and/or bruits over large arteries on examination, as well as typical findings on aortic angiography (Fig. 41–8).[138] Treatment should include moderate to high doses of corticosteroids (40 to 60 mg of prednisone equivalent/day), occasionally with immunosuppressives[140] and, when necessary, vascular surgical bypass or grafting procedures.

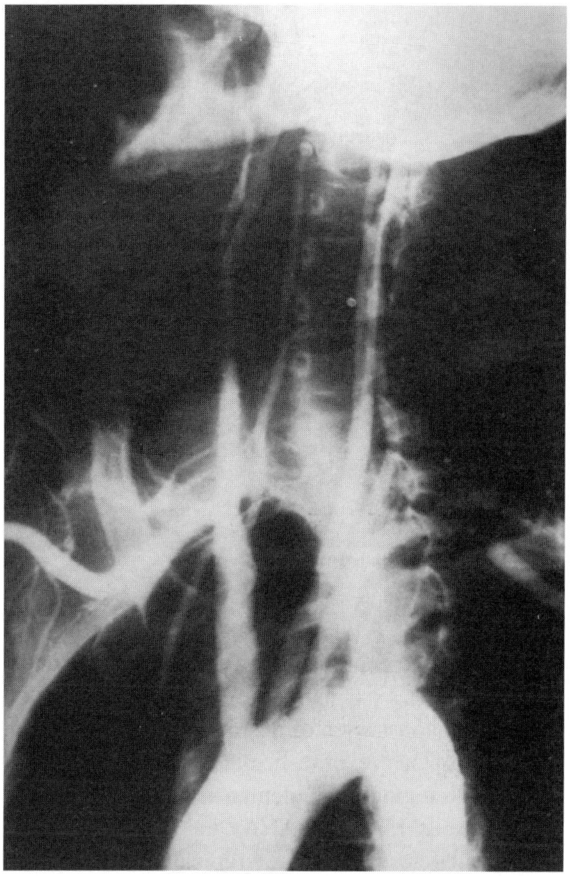

FIGURE 41–8. Arch arteriogram of a patient with Takayasu's arteritis. Note irregularity or narrowing of innominate, right carotid, and left subclavian arteries. (From Willerson J, Cohn J [eds]: Cardiovascular Medicine. Churchill Livingstone, New York, 1995, p 1678.)

Kawasaki's Disease

This condition, also known as mucocutaneous lymph node syndrome, is primarily an acute disease of infants or small children[141] and rarely affects adults.[142] It is characterized by fever, lymphadenopathy, a desquamative skin rash, and mucous membrane lesions (strawberry tongue, urethritis, conjunctivitis). Cardiac involvement occurs in approximately 5% of cases and most commonly manifests as coronary artery aneurysms or coronary thromboses.[141] Other reported complications include ventricular aneurysms, myocarditis, pericarditis, cardiac tamponade, and CHF. Sudden death attributable to cardiac arrhythmias or MI has been reported in 1.7% of cases.[141] Coronary thromboarteritis with aneurysmal dilatation found at autopsy of children who died of Kawasaki's disease is similar to that previously described in infantile polyarteritis.[143] Diagnosis is based on the clinical features of the disease. When clinical examination or ECG suggests cardiac involvement, coronary angiography is indicated. Therapy should include high-dose aspirin to prevent coronary thromboses (80 to 100 mg/day in four divided doses or maintenance of a serum salicylate level of 20 to 25 mg/dl), which should be continued for at least 2 months when coronary aneurysms are present. Corticosteroids appear to promote coronary aneurysm formation and are contraindicated. Recently, intravenous gamma globulin has been reported to be the most effective therapy for Kawasaki's disease, and it may prevent the coronary lesions.[144] The optimal dosing schedule remains controversial. Variously, 400 mg/kg/day for 4 days, 1 g/kg once, and 2 g/kg once have all been reported to abbreviate the acute symptoms and prevent coronary artery aneurysms.

Behçet's Disease

This entity is characterized by recurrent episodes of oral and genital ulcers and uveitis.[145, 146] Other manifestations include recurrent meningoencephalitis, pustulonecrotic skin lesions after trauma (pathergy), arthritis, bowel ulceration, pulmonary artery aneurysms (Hughes-Stovin syndrome),[147] and systemic vasculitis.[145, 146] The disease is most common in young adults of Japanese, Middle Eastern, and Southern European extraction. In these ethnic groups, the histocompatibility antigen HLA-B51 is strikingly increased in patients with Behçet's disease but not in similarly affected Americans or Northern Europeans.[148] The cardiovascular manifestations of Behçet's disease relate to vasculo-occlusive disease, often with aneurysm formation, of small, medium, and large vessels, more often veins than arteries.[149] Superficial thrombophlebitis, usually recurrent, is most common, but deep venous occlusion of the superior and inferior vena cavae and of the subclavian, common iliac, femoral, and hepatic veins has been reported. Arterial occlusions of aneurysms of subclavian, renal, carotid, pulmonary, and femoral arteries may also occur. Although coronary vessel involvement should be possible in theory, there is only rare documentation of heart disease per se in this disorder.

Treatment of Behçet's disease begins with corticosteroid therapy, with doses commensurate with the severity of disease.[146] Colchicine[146] and thalidomide[150] also have been reported to be useful. Chlorambucil[151] or azathioprine[152] may be effective in more severe disease, especially ocular disease.

References

1. Hahn BH, Wallace DJ (eds): Dubois Lupus Erythematosus. Lea & Febiger, Philadelphia, 1993.
2. Arnett FC, Reveille JD: The genetics of lupus erythematosus. Rheum Dis Clin North Am 18:865, 1992.
3. Stevens MB: Systemic lupus erythematosus and the cardiovascular system. In Lahita RG (ed): Systemic Lupus Erythematosus. John Wiley & Sons, New York, 1987, pp 673.
4. Harvey AM, Shulman LE, Tumulty PA, et al: Review of the literature and clinical analysis of 138 cases. Medicine 33:219, 1954.
5. Hochberg MC, Dorsch CA, Feinglass EJ, Stevens MB: Survivorship in systemic lupus erythematosus. Arthritis Rheum 24:54, 1981.
6. Reveille JD, Bartolucci A, Alarcon GS: Prognosis in systemic lupus erythematosus. Arthritis Rheum 33:37, 1990.
7. Bulkley BH, Roberts WC: The heart in systemic lupus erythematosus and the changes induced in it by corticosteroid therapy. Am J Med 58:243, 1975.
8. Buyon JP: Complete heart block and antibodies to the SSA/Ro-SSB/La antigen systems. Clin Asp Autoimmun 4:8, 1990.
9. Scott JS, Maddison PJ, Taylor PV, et al: Connective-tissue disease, antibodies to ribonucleoprotein, and congenital heart block. N Engl J Med 309:209, 1983.
10. Straaton KV, Chatham WW, Reveille JD, et al: Clinically significant valvular heart disease in systemic lupus erythematosus. Am J Med 85: 645, 1988.
11. Leung WH, Wong KL, Lau CP, et al: Association between antiphospholipid antibodies and cardiac abnormalities in patients with systemic lupus erythematosus. Am J Med 89:411, 1990.
12. Galve E, Candell-Riera J, Pigrau C, et al: Prevalence, morphologic types, and evolution of cardiac valvular disease in systemic lupus erythematosus. N Engl J Med 319:817, 1988.
13. Shearn MA: The heart in systemic lupus erythematosus. Am Heart J 58:452, 1959.
14. Hejtmancik MR, Wright JC, Quint R, Jennings FL: The cardiovascular manifestations of systemic lupus erythematosus. Am Heart J 68:119, 1964.
15. James TN, Rupe CE, Monto RW: Pathology of the cardiac conduction system in systemic lupus erythematosus. Ann Intern Med 63:402, 1965.
16. Bidani AK, Roberts JL, Schwartz MM, Lewis EJ: Immunopathology of cardiac lesions in fatal systemic lupus erythematosus. Am J Med 69:849, 1980.
17. Das SK, Cassidy JT: Antiheart antibodies in patients with systemic lupus erythematosus. Am J Med Sci 265:275, 1973.
18. Gur H, Keren G, Averbuch M, Levo Y: Severe congestive lupus cardiomyopathy complicated by an intracavitary thrombus: A clinical and echocardiographic follow-up. J Rheumatol 15:1278, 1988.
19. Kattwinkel N, Villanueva AG, Labib SB, et al: Myocardial infarction caused by cardiac microvasculopathy in a patient with the primary antiphospholipid syndrome. Ann Intern Med 116:974, 1992.
20. Jacobson EJ, Reza MJ: Constrictive pericarditis in systemic lupus erythematosus. Arthritis Rheum 21:972, 1978.
21. Hunder GG, Mullen BJ, McDuffie FC: Complement in pericardial fluid of lupus erythematosus. Ann Intern Med 80:453, 1974.
22. Berg G, Bodet J, Webb K, et al: Systemic lupus erythematosus presenting as isolated congestive heart failure. J Rheumatol 12:1182, 1985.
23. Borenstein DG, Frye WB, Arnett FC, Stevens MB: The myocarditis of systemic lupus erythematosus. Ann Intern Med 89:619, 1978.
24. Ratliff NB, Estes ME, Myles JL, et al: Diagnosis of chloroquine cardiomyopathy by endomyocardial biopsy. N Engl J Med 316:191, 1987.
25. Hosenpud JD, Montanaro A, Hart MV, et al: Myocardial perfusion abnormalities in asymptomatic patients with systemic lupus erythematosus. Am J Med 77:286, 1984.
26. Homcy CJ, Liberthson RR, Fallon IT, et al: Ischemic heart disease in systemic lupus erythematosus in the young patient: Report of 6 cases. Am J Cardiol 49:478, 1982.
27. Spiera H, Rothenberg RR: Myocardial infarction in four young people with SLE. J Rheumatol 10:464, 1983.
28. Korbet SM, Schwartz MM, Lewis EJ: Immune complex deposition and coronary vasculitis in systemic lupus erythematosus. Am J Med 77:141, 1984.
29. Asherson RA, Mackay IR, Harris EN: Myocardial infarction in a young man with systemic lupus erythematosus, deep vein thrombosis, and antibodies to phospholipid. Br Heart J 56:190, 1986.
30. Maaravi Y, Raz E, Gilon D, Rubinow A: Cerebrovascular accident and myocardial infarction associated with anticardiolipin antibodies in a young woman with systemic lupus erythematosus. Ann Rheum Dis 48:853, 1989.
31. Libman E, Sacks B: A hitherto undescribed form of valvular and mural endocarditis. Arch Intern Med 33:701, 1924.
32. Ropes MW: Systemic Lupus Erythematosus. Cambridge University Press, Cambridge, UK, 1976.
33. Shapiro RF, Gample CN, Wiesner KB, et al: Immunopathogenesis of Libman-Sacks endocarditis. Ann Rheum Dis 36:508, 1977.
34. Pritzker MR, Ernst JD, Caudill C, et al: Acquired aortic stenosis in systemic lupus erythematosus. Ann Intern Med 93:434, 1980.
35. Lerman BB, Thomas LC, Abrams GD, Pitt B: Aortic stenosis associated with systemic lupus erythematosus. Am J Med 72:707, 1982.
36. Roldan CA, Shively BK, Lau CC, et al: Systemic lupus erythematosus valve disease by transesophageal echocardiography and the role of antiphospholipid antibodies. J Am Coll Cardiol 20:1127, 1992.
37. Petri M: The clinical syndrome associated with antiphospholipid antibodies. J Rheumatol 19:505, 1992.
38. Love PE, Santoro SA: Antiphospholipid antibodies: Anticardiolipin and the lupus anticoagulant in systemic lupus erythematosus (SLE) and in non-SLE disorders. Ann Intern Med 112:682, 1990.
39. Asherson RA, Khamashta MA, Ordi-Ros J, et al: The primary antiphospholipid syndrome: Major clinical and serological features. Medicine 68:366, 1989.
40. Asherson RA: The catastrophic antiphospholipid syndrome. J Rheumatol 19:508, 1992.
41. Galve E, Ordi J, Barquinero J, Evangelista A, et al: Valvular heart disease in the primary antiphospholipid syndrome. Ann Intern Med 116:293, 1992.
42. Leventhal LJ, Borofsky MA, Bergey PD, Schumacher HR Jr: Antiphospholipid antibody syndrome with right atrial thrombosis mimicking an atrial myxoma. Am J Med 87:111, 1989.
43. Fereante FM, Myerson GE, Goldman JA: Subclavian artery thrombosis mimicking the aortic arch syndrome in systemic lupus erythematosus. Arthritis Rheum 25:1501, 1982.
44. Nair SS, Askari AD, Popelka CG, Kleinerman JF: Pulmonary hypertension and systemic lupus erythematosus. Arch Intern Med 140: 109, 1980.
45. Hodson P, Klemp P, Meyers OL: Pulmonary hypertension in systemic lupus erythematosus: A report of four cases. Clin Exp Rheumatol 1: 241, 1983.
46. Gladman DD, Sternberg L: Pulmonary hypertension in systemic lupus erythematosus. J Rheumatol 12:365, 1985.
47. D'Angelo WA, Fries JF, Masi AT, Shulman LE: Pathologic observations in systemic sclerosis (scleroderma). Am J Med 46:428, 1969.
48. Norton WL, Nardo JM: Vascular disease in progressive systemic sclerosis (scleroderma). Ann Intern Med 73:317, 1970.
49. Rich S, Dantzker DR, Ayres SM, et al: Primary pulmonary hypertension. Ann Intern Med 107:216, 1987.
50. Watson RM, Lane AT, Barnett NK, et al: Neonatal lupus erythematosus. Medicine 63:362, 1984.
51. McCune AB, Weston WL, Lee LA: Maternal and fetal outcome in neonatal lupus erythematosus. Ann Intern Med 106:518, 1987.

52. Lee LA, Coulter S, Erner S, Chu H: Cardiac immunoglobulin deposition in congenital heart block associated with maternal anti-Ro autoantibodies. Am J Med 83:793, 1987.
53. Litsey SE, Noonan JA, O'Connor WN, et al: Maternal connective tissue disease and congenital heart block. N Engl J Med 312:98, 1985.
54. Taylor PV, Scott JS, Gerlis LM, et al: Maternal antibodies against fetal cardiac antigens in congenital complete heart block. N Engl J Med 315:667, 1986.
55. Buyon JP, Swersky SH, Fox HE, et al: Intrauterine therapy for presumptive fetal myocarditis with acquired heart block due to systemic lupus erythematosus. Arthritis Rheum 30:44, 1987.
56. Harmon CE, Portanova JP: Drug-induced lupus: Clinical and serological studies. Clin Rheum Dis 8:121, 1982.
57. Hess EV, Mongey AB: Drug-related lupus. Bull Rheum Dis 40:1, 1991.
58. Edwards RL, Rick ME, Wakem CJ: Studies on a circulating anticoagulant in procainamide-induced lupus erythematosus. Arch Intern Med 141:1688, 1981.
59. Cohen MG, Kevat S, Prowse MV, Ahern MJ: Two distinct quinidine-induced rheumatic syndromes. Ann Intern Med 108:369, 1988.
60. West SG, McMahon M, Portanova JP: Quinidine-induced lupus erythematosus. Ann Intern Med 100:840, 1984.
61. Arnett FC, Edworthy SM, Bloch DA, et al: The American Rheumatism Association 1987 revised criteria for the classification of rheumatoid artheritis. Arthritis Rheum 31:315, 1988.
62. Harris ED Jr: Rheumatoid arthritis. Pathophysiology and implications for therapy. N Engl J Med 322:1277, 1990.
63. Gregersen PK, Silver J, Winchester RJ: The shared epitope hypothesis. An approach to understanding the molecular genetics of susceptibility to rheumatoid arthritis. Arthritis Rheum 30:1205, 1987.
64. Weyand CM, Hicok KC, Conn DL, Goronzy JJ: The influence of HLA-DRB1 genes on disease severity in rheumatoid arthritis. Ann Intern Med 117:801, 1992.
65. Pizzarello RA, Goldberg J: The heart in rheumatoid arthritis. In Utsinger PD, Zuaifler NJ, Ehrlich GE (eds): Rheumatoid Arthritis. Etiology, Diagnosis, Management. JB Lippincott, Philadelphia, 1985, pp 431–440.
66. Sigal LH, Friedman HD: Rheumatoid pancarditis in a patient with well controlled rheumatoid arthritis. J Rheumatol 16:368, 1989.
67. Hara KS, Ballard DJ, Ilstrup DM, et al: Rheumatoid pericarditis: Clinical features and survival. Medicine 69:81, 1990.
68. Escalante A, Kaufman RL, Quismorio P Jr, Beardmore TD: Cardiac compression in rheumatoid pericarditis. Semin Arthritis Rheum 20: 148, 1990.
69. Franco AE, Levine HD, Hall AP: Rheumatoid pericarditis: Report of 17 cases diagnosed clinically. Ann Intern Med 77:837, 1972.
70. John JT Jr, Hough A, Sergent JS: Pericardial disease in rheumatoid arthritis. Am J Med 66:385, 1979.
71. Voyles WF, Searles RP, Bankhurst AD: Myocardial infarction caused by rheumatoid vasculitis. Arthritis Rheum 23:860, 1980.
72. Pouchot J, Sampalis JS, Beaudet F, et al: Adult Still's disease: Manifestations, disease course, and outcome in 62 patients. Medicine 70: 118, 1991.
73. Bank I, Marboe CC, Redberg RF, Jacobs J: Myocarditis in adult Still's disease. Arthritis Rheum 28:452, 1985.
74. Follansbee WP: The cardiovascular manifestations of systemic sclerosis (scleroderma). Curr Probl Cardiol 11:245, 1986.
75. Sharp GC, Singsen BH: Mixed connective tissue disease. In McCarty DJ (ed): Arthritis and Allied Conditions. Lea & Febiger, Philadelphia, 1989, pp 1080–1091.
76. Furst DE, Clements PJ, Graze P, et al: A syndrome resembling progressive systemic sclerosis after bone marrow transplantation. Arthritis Rheum 22:904, 1979.
77. Weiner ES, Earnshaw WC, Senecal JL, et al: Clinical associations of anticentromere antibodies and antibodies to topoisomerase I. Arthritis Rheum 31:378, 1988.
78. Chevalier J, Kazatchkine MD: Distribution in cluster of complement receptor type 1 (CR1) on human erythrocytes. J Immunol 142:2031, 1989.
79. Okano Y, Steen VD, Medsger TA Jr: Autoantibody to U3 nucleolar ribonucleoprotein (fibrillarin) in patients with systemic sclerosis. Arthritis Rheum 35:95, 1992.
80. Ridolfi RL, Bulkley BH, Hutchins GM: The cardiac conduction system in progressive systemic sclerosis. Am J Med 61:361, 1976.
81. Leinwand I, Duryee AW, Richter MN: Scleroderma (based on a study of over 150 cases). Ann Intern Med 41:1003, 1954.
82. Bulkley BH, Ridolfi RL, Salyer WR, Hutchins GM: Myocardial lesions of progressive systemic sclerosis. Circulation 53:483, 1976.
83. Sackner MA, Heinz ER, Steinberg AJ: The heart in scleroderma. Am J Cardiol 17:542, 1966.
84. Oram S, Stokes W: The heart in scleroderma. Br Heart J 23:243, 1961.
85. Follansbee WP, Miller TR, Curtiss EI, et al: A controlled clinicopathologic study of myocardial fibrosis in systemic sclerosis (scleroderma). J Rheumatol 17:656, 1990.
86. Alexander EL, Firestein GS, Weiss JL, et al: Reversible cold-induced abnormalities in myocardial perfusion and function in systemic sclerosis. Ann Intern Med 105:661, 1986.
87. Ellis WW, Baer AN, Robertson RM, et al: Left ventricular dysfunction induced by cold exposure in patients with systemic sclerosis. Am J Med 80:385, 1986.
88. Follansbee WP, Curtiss EI, Medsger TA, et al: Physiologic abnormalities of cardiac function in progressive systemic sclerosis with diffuse scleroderma. N Engl J Med 310:142, 1984.
89. Lichtbroun AS, Sandhaus LM, Giorno RC, et al: Myocardial mast cells in systemic sclerosis: A report of three fatal cases. Am J Med 89: 372, 1990.
90. Gottdiner JS, Moutsopoulos HM, Decker JL: Echocardiographic identification of cardiac abnormality in scleroderma and related disorders. Am J Med 66:391, 1979.
91. Clements PJ, Furst DE, Cabeen W, et al: The relationship of arrhythmias and conduction disturbances to other manifestations of cardiopulmonary disease in progressive systemic sclerosis (PSS). Am J Med 71: 38, 1981.
92. Roberts NK, Cabeen WR, Moss J, et al: The prevalence of conduction defects and cardiac arrhythmias in progressive systemic sclerosis. Ann Intern Med 94:38, 1981.
93. Kostis JB, Seibold JR, Turkevich D, et al: Prognostic importance of cardiac arrhythmias in systemic sclerosis. Am J Med 84:1007, 1988.
94. Follansbee WP, Curtiss EI, Rahko PS, et al: The electrocardiogram in systemic sclerosis (scleroderma). Am J Med 79:183, 1985.
95. Altman RD, Medsger TA Jr, Bloch DA, Michel BA: Predictors of survival in systemic sclerosis (scleroderma). Arthritis Rheum 34:403, 1991.
96. Jiminez SA, Sigal SH: A 15-year prospective study of treatment of rapidly progressive systemic sclerosis with D-penicillamine. J Rheumatol 18:1496, 1991.
97. Coffman JD, Clement DL, Creager MA, et al: International study of ketanserin in Raynaud's phenomenon. Am J Med 87:264, 1989.
98. Lopez-Ovejero JA, Saal SD, D'Angelo WA, et al: Reversal of vascular and renal crisis of scleroderma by oral angiotensin-converting-enzyme blockade. N Engl J Med 300:1417, 1979.
99. Whitman III HH, Case DB, Laragh JH, et al: Variable response to oral angiotensin-converting-enzyme blockade in hypertensive scleroderma patients. Arthritis Rheum 25:241, 1982.
100. West SG, Killian PJ, Lawless OJ: Association of myositis and myocarditis in progressive systemic sclerosis. Arthritis Rheum 24:662, 1981.
101. McWhorter JE, Leroy EC: Pericardial disease in scleroderma (systemic sclerosis). Am J Med 57:566, 1974.
102. Smith JW, Clements PJ, Levisman J, et al: Echocardiographic features of progressive systemic sclerosis (PSS). Correlation with hemodynamic and postmortem studies. Am J Med 66:28, 1979.
103. Gladman DD, Gordon DA, Urowitz MB, Levy HL: Pericardial fluid analysis in scleroderma (systemic sclerosis). Am J Med 60:1064, 1976.
104. Stupi AM, Steen VD, Owens GR, et al: Pulmonary hypertension in the CREST syndrome variant of systemic sclerosis. Arthritis Rheum 29:515, 1986.
105. Dalakas MC: Polymyositis, dermatomyositis, and inclusion-body myositis. N Engl J Med 325:1487, 1991.
106. Strongwater SL: Overview and clinical manifestations of inflammatory myositis: Polymyositis and dermatomyositis. Mount Sinai J Med 55: 435, 1988.
107. Reichlin M, Arnett FC: Multiplicity of antibodies in myositis sera. Arthritis Rheum 27:1150, 1984.
108. Targoff IN, Arnett FC: Clinical manifestations in patients with antibody to PL-12 antigen (alanyl-tRNA synthetase). Am J Med 88:241, 1990.
109. Denbow CE, Lie JT, Tancredi RG, Bunch TW: Cardiac involvement in polymyositis. A clinicopathologic study of 20 autopsied patients. Arthritis Rheum 22:1088, 1979.
110. Askari AD: Cardiac abnormalities. Clin Rheum Dis 10:31, 1984.
111. Tymms KE, Webb J: Dermatopolymyositis and other connective tissue diseases: A review of 105 cases. J Rheumatol 12:1140, 1985.

112. Hochberg MC, Feldman D, Stevens MB: Adult onset polymyositis/dermatomyositis: An analysis of clinical and laboratory features and survival in 76 patients with a review of the literature. Semin Arthritis Rheum 15:168, 1986.
113. Larca LJ, Coppola JT, Honig S: Creatine kinase MB isoenzyme in dermatomyositis: A noncardiac source. Ann Intern Med 94:341, 1981.
114. Weiss J, Shark W, Fishbein M, et al: The use of endomyocardial biopsy in a serious cardiac abnormality associated with polymyositis: A case report. J Rheumatol 9:299, 1982.
115. Fauci AS, Haynes BF, Katz P: The spectrum of vasculitis. Ann Intern Med 89:660, 1978.
116. Lie JT, Members and consultants of the American College of Rheumatology, Subcommittee on Classification of Vasculitis: Illustrated histopathologic classification criteria for selected vasculitis syndromes. Arthritis Rheum 33:1074, 1990.
117. Calabrese LH, Michel BA, Bloch DA, et al: The American College of Rheumatology 1990 criteria for the classification of hypersensitivity vasculitis. Arthritis Rheum 33:1108, 1990.
118. Masi AT, Hunder GG, Lie JT, et al: The American College of Rheumatology 1990 criteria for the classification of Churg-Strauss syndrome (allergic granulomatosis and angiitis). Arthritis Rheum 33:1094, 1990.
119. Leavitt RY, Fauci AS, Bloch DA, et al: The American College of Rheumatology 1990 criteria for the classification of Wegener's granulomatosis. Arthritis Rheum 33:1101, 1990.
120. Lightfoot RW Jr, Michel BA, Bloch DA, et al: The American College of Rheumatology 1990 criteria for the classification of polyarteritis nodosa. Arthritis Rheum 33:1088, 1990.
121. Hunder GG, Bloch DA, Michel BA, et al: The American College of Rheumatology 1990 criteria for the classification of giant cell arthritis. Arthritis Rheum 33:1122, 1990.
122. Arend WP, Michel BA, Bloch DA, et al: The American College of Rheumatology 1990 criteria for the classification of Takayasu arteritis. Arthritis Rheum 33:1129, 1990.
123. Holsinger DR, Osmundson PJ, Edwards JE: The heart in periarteritis nodosa. Circulation 25:610, 1962.
124. Sergent JS, Lockshin MD, Christian CL, Gocke DJ: Vasculitis with hepatitis B antigenemia: Long-term observations in nine patients. Medicine 55:1, 1976.
125. Dahlbert PJ, Lockhart JM, Overholt EL: Diagnostic studies for systemic necrotizing vasculitis. Arch Intern Med 149:161, 1989.
126. Fauci AS, Katz P, Haynes BF, Wolff SM: Cyclophosphamide therapy of severe systemic necrotizing vasculitis. N Engl J Med 301:235, 1979.
127. Leib ES, Restivo C, Paulus HE: Immunosuppressive and corticosteroid therapy of polyarteritis nodosa. Am J Med 67:941, 1979.
128. Hoffman GS, Kerr GS, Leavitt RY, et al: Wegener granulomatosis: An analysis of 158 patients. Ann Intern Med 116:488, 1992.
129. Specks U, Wheatley CL, McDonald TJ, et al: Anticycloplasmic antibodies in the diagnosis and followup of Wegener's granulomatosis. Mayo Clin Proc 64:28, 1989.
130. Flak RJ, Hogan S, Carey TS, Jennette C, and the Glomerular Disease Collaborative Network: Clinical course of antineutrophil cytoplasmic autoantibody-associated glomerulonephritis and systemic vasculitis. Ann Intern Med 113:656, 1990.
131. Lanham JG, Elkon KB, Pusey CD, Hughes GR: Systemic vasculitis with asthma and eosinophilia: A clinical approach to the Churg-Strauss syndrome. Medicine 63:65, 1984.
132. Hamilton CR Jr, Shelley WM, Tumulty PA: Giant cell arteritis: Including temporal arteritis and polymyalgia rheumatica. Medicine 50:1, 1971.
133. Klein RG, Hunder GG, Stanson AW, Sheps SG: Large artery involvement in giant cell (temporal) arteritis. Ann Intern Med 83:806, 1975.
134. Klinkhoff AV, Reid GD, Moscovich M: Aortic regurgitation in giant cell arteritis. Arthritis Rheum 28:582, 1985.
135. Kay RH, Pooley R, Herman MV: Unsuspected giant cell arteritis diagnosed at open heart surgery. Arch Intern Med 142:1378, 1982.
136. McKusick VA: A form of vascular disease relatively frequent in the Orient. Am Heart J 63:57, 1962.
137. Judge RD, Currier RD, Gracie WA, Figley MM: Takayasu's arteritis and the aortic arch syndrome. Am J Med 32:379, 1962.
138. Ishikawa K: Natural history and classification of occlusive thromboaortopathy (Takayasu's disease). Circulation 57:27, 1978.
139. Isohisa I, Numano F, Maezawa H, Sasazuki T: HLA-Bw52 in Takayasu disease. Tissue Antigens 12:246, 1978.
140. Shelhamer JH, Bolkman DJ, Parrillo JE, et al: Takayasu's arteritis and its therapy. Ann Intern Med 103:121, 1985.
141. Kawasaki T, Kosaki F, Okawa S, et al: A new infantile acute febrile mucocutaneous lymph node syndrome (MLNS) prevailing in Japan. Pediatrics 54:271, 1974.
142. Milgrom H, Palmer EL, Slovin SF, et al: Kawasaki disease in a healthy young adult. Ann Intern Med 92:467, 1980.
143. Glanz S, Bittner SJ, Berman MA, et al: Regression of coronary-artery aneurysms in infantile polyarteritis nodosa. N Engl J Med 294:939, 1976.
144. Barron KS, Sher MR, Silverman ED: Intravenous immunoglobulin therapy: Magic or black magic. J Rheumatol 19:94, 1992.
145. Shimizu T, Ehrlich GE, Inaba G, Hayashi K: Behçet disease. Arthritis Rheum 8:223, 1979.
146. James DG: Behçet's disease. Br J Clin Pract 44:364, 1990.
147. Durieux P, Bletry O, Huchon G, et al: Multiple pulmonary arterial aneurysms in Behcet's disease and Hughes-Stoven syndrome. Am J Med 71:736, 1981.
148. Ohno S, Ohguchi M, Hirose S, et al: Close association of HLA-Bw51 with Behcet's disease. Arch Ophthalmol 100:1455, 1982.
149. James DG: Recognition of the diverse cardiovascular manifestations in Behçet's disease. Am Heart J 103:457, 1982.
150. Hamza MH: Treatment of Behçet's disease with thalidomide. Clin Rheumatol 5:365, 1986.
151. O'Duffy JD, Robertson DM, Goldstein NP: Chlorambucil in the treatment of uveitis and meningoencephalitis of Behçet's disease. Am J Med 76:75, 1984.
152. Yazici H, Halit P, Barnes CG, et al: A controlled trial of azathioprine in Behçet's syndrome. N Engl J Med 322:281, 1990.

INDEX

Note: Page numbers followed by the letter f refer to illustrations; page numbers followed by the letter t refer to tables.

B

C

D

E

Q

R

S

ISBN 0-443-07900-5

90038

9 780443 079009